HYPERTROPHIC CARDIOMYOPATHY

Collected Reprints (1968-2016)

By

William C. Roberts, MD

and

Colleagues

ISBN: 979-8-88680-089-0
Printed in the United States of America on acid-free paper.

Preface

It is a bit unfair to list this large collection of articles on hypertrophic cardiomyopathy (HC) as originating from the brain or pen of William C. Roberts. Numerous ones came from the mind and pen of my dear friend Dr. Barry Maron, who generously included me as an author in many manuscripts created by him. HC was put on the map originally by Dr. Eugene Braunwald, and its definitive therapy (surgical ventricular septectomy for the obstructive variety) by Dr. Andrew G. Morrow, both of whom worked together at the National Institutes of Health in Bethesda, Maryland. Ironically, Dr. Morrow, who did his operation in >300 patients with obstructive HC, had the disease himself, as did two of his three offspring. Thus, the 1960s provided the opportunity to study numerous patients with HC. In the 1970s and afterwards, Dr. Barry Maron became the top guru in HC, and he and his colleagues continue to add information on this fascinating condition.

—William C. Roberts, MD

Table of Contents

*Articles are numbered based on WCR's CV.

Muscular Subaortic Stenosis

Clinical and Pathologic Observations in an Elderly Patient*

GORDON A. EWY, M.D., FRANK I. MARCUS, M.D., OSHIN BOHAJALIAN, M.D., HENRY L. BURKE, M.D. *and* WILLIAM C. ROBERTS, M.D., F.A.C.C.

Washington, D. C. and Bethesda, Maryland

SINCE Brock's description in 1957,[1] muscular obstruction to left ventricular outflow, variously called idiopathic hypertrophic subaortic stenosis,[2,3] hypertrophic obstructive cardiomyopathy,[4] and muscular subaortic stenosis,[5–7] has become a well recognized entity. In the majority of patients the cause of the outflow obstruction is unknown (idiopathic).[2–5] The congenital and familial varieties strongly suggest a genetic basis for the disorder.[2–4,8–11] In some subjects, however, the subaortic muscular obstruction appears to be secondary to valvular aortic stenosis or systemic hypertension.[1,12–15] The present report describes the oldest known patient with clinically diagnosed and pathologically demonstrated muscular subaortic stenosis. She had systemic hypertension for several years and shortly before death demonstrated the clinical findings of muscular subaortic stenosis. At necropsy, the anatomic features of muscular subaortic stenosis were present.

CASE REPORT

A 74 year old Negro woman was admitted to the District of Columbia General Hospital in October 1966 with hemiplegia, pneumococcal pneumonia and bacteremia. She had been under medical care elsewhere since 1961 for systemic hypertension; her blood pressure before treatment in 1962 was 230/115 mm. Hg. There was no record of a precordial murmur at that time. During the last four years she had received reserpine and thiazides. She had been relatively asymptomatic until 1963 when she complained of dizziness, palpitations and exertional dyspnea. During the next two years the blood pressure varied from 120/65 to 205/105 mm. Hg. A precordial murmur that varied markedly in intensity was heard throughout the three years before death.

On examination, the blood pressure was 150/70 mm. Hg, temperature 102° F., pulse 100 beats/min. and respirations 28/min. There was a prominent *a* wave in the jugular venous pulse. The carotid impulse was brisk-rising. The left ventricular apical impulse was diffuse and displaced laterally. This impulse was sustained throughout systole and bifid (Fig. 1D). A grade 3/6 long, rough, pansystolic murmur was heard loudest at the apex and radiated to the mid-axillary line (Fig. 1B). The murmur also was heard at the lower left sternal border, but was not well transmitted to the base of the heart or to the neck. No diastolic murmur was audible. A marked increase in the intensity of the murmur was noted with the postpremature beat. The first heart sound was of normal intensity. At the upper left sternal edge the second heart sound was narrowly split with very little respiratory movement. At the apex a loud atrial diastolic gallop sound preceded the first heart sound (Fig. 1A); the second heart sound was followed by a soft ventricular diastolic gallop.

The electrocardiogram (Fig. 2) was consistent with loss of inferiorly and anteriorly directed QRS electrical forces manifested by prominent Q waves in leads II, III, aVF, and V_2 through V_6. Chest roentgenogram (Fig. 3) three and one-half months before death showed mild cardiomegaly. A roentgenogram 25 days before death revealed an infiltrate in the left lower lobe and calcium in the mitral annular region. Calcium was not present in the aortic valve region.

Laboratory studies showed evidence of pneumonia and bacteremia due to Diplococcus pneumoniae which cleared promptly with penicillin. Nevertheless, the patient became increasingly obtunded and was comatose during the latter half of her hospitalization. Three episodes of tachycardia and tachypnea associated with diffuse bilateral basilar rales occurred while she was in the hospital.

At necropsy, she weighed 107 pounds and measured 62 inches in length. Death appeared to be the result

* From the Georgetown University Medical Division, the Department of Pathology, District of Columbia General Hospital, Washington, D. C., and the Laboratory of Pathology, Clinic of Surgery, National Heart Institute, National Institutes of Health, Bethesda, Md. This study was supported in part by grants from the National Heart Institute, National Institutes of Health and Special Cardiac Research Fund.

Address for reprints: Gordon A. Ewy, M.D., Georgetown University Medical Division, District of Columbia General Hospital. 19th and Mass. Ave., S. E. Washington, D. C. 20003.

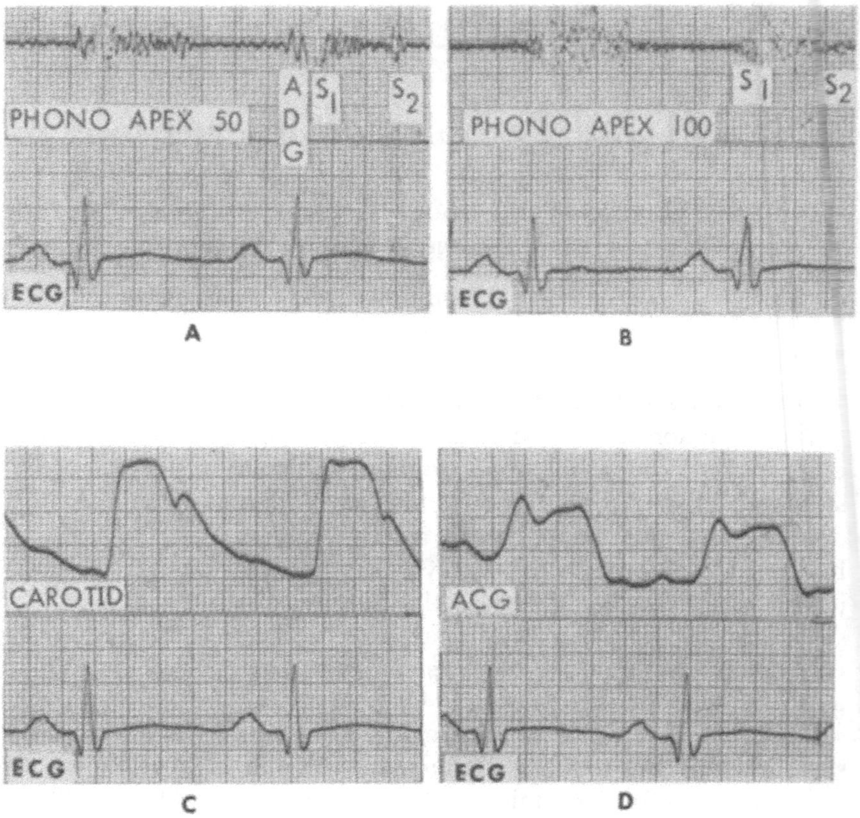

Figure 1. *Phonocardiograms, carotid pulse recording and apex cardiogram.* **A,** low frequency phonocardiogram illustrating the atrial diastolic gallop (ADG). **B,** medium frequency phonocardiogram demonstrating the pansystolic murmur. **C,** external carotid pulse recording. **D,** apex cardiogram.

Phonocardiograms were recorded utilizing a Sanborn heart sound pickup (Model 350-1700-C10) and a Sanborn heart sound amplifier (Model 350-1700 B). The carotid impulse and apex cardiogram were recorded utilizing a Statham physiologic pressure transducer (Model No. PR 23-2G-300) and a Sanborn carrier preamplifier (Model 350-1100-AS). A funnel type contact device (diameter 2.5 cm.) was used for the carotid pulse recording and a cup-shaped chest wall contact device (diameter 5 cm.) for that of the apex impulse. The recordings were made with a Sanborn 2-channel direct writing (Model 296) recorder.

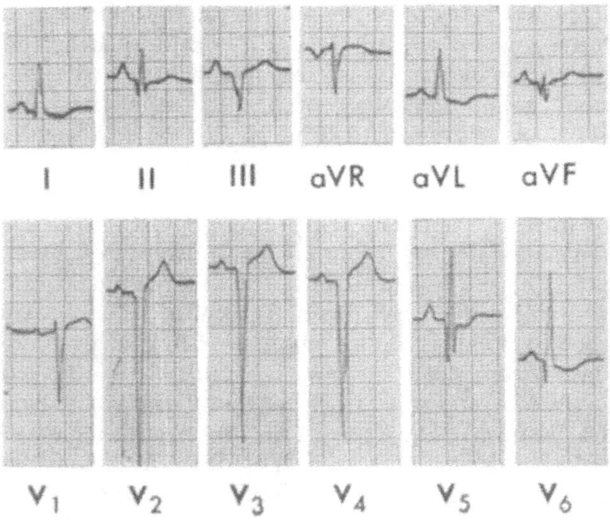

Figure 2. *Twelve lead scalar electrocardiogram* with standardization of 1 mv. equal to 10 mm. Tracing is consistent with myocardial infarction.

of aspiration of gastric contents into the tracheobronchial tree. A branch of the left pulmonary artery was obstructed by a recent embolus, but there was no pulmonary infarct.

The heart (Fig. 4 to 6) weighed 650 gm. There was left ventricular hypertrophy (free wall up to 2.5 cm. thick), particularly the cephalad portion of the muscular ventricular septum (3.7 cm. thick). The left ventricular outflow tract was clearly narrowed by the extremely hypertrophied ventricular septal myocardium. There was mild endocardial thickening in

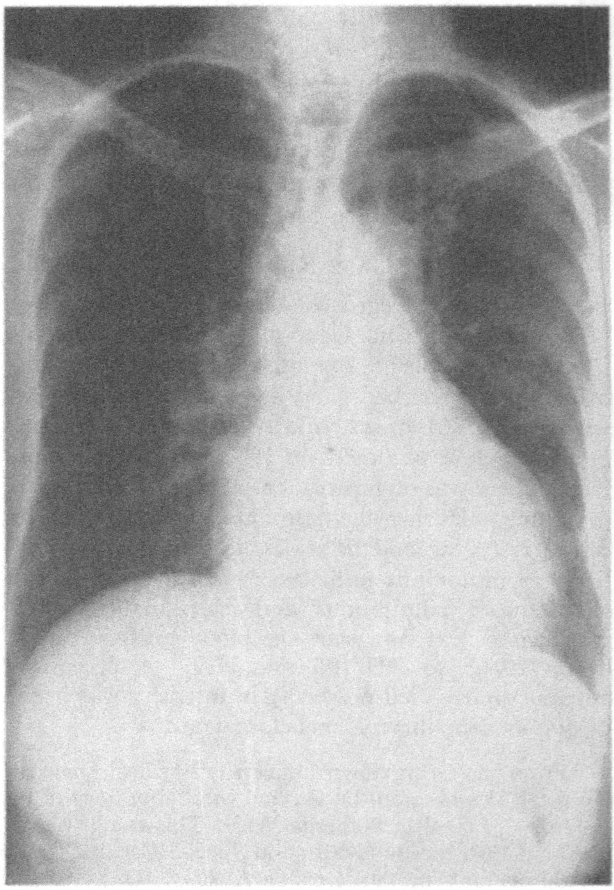

Figure 3. *Chest roentgenogram* taken three months before death showing cardiomegaly.

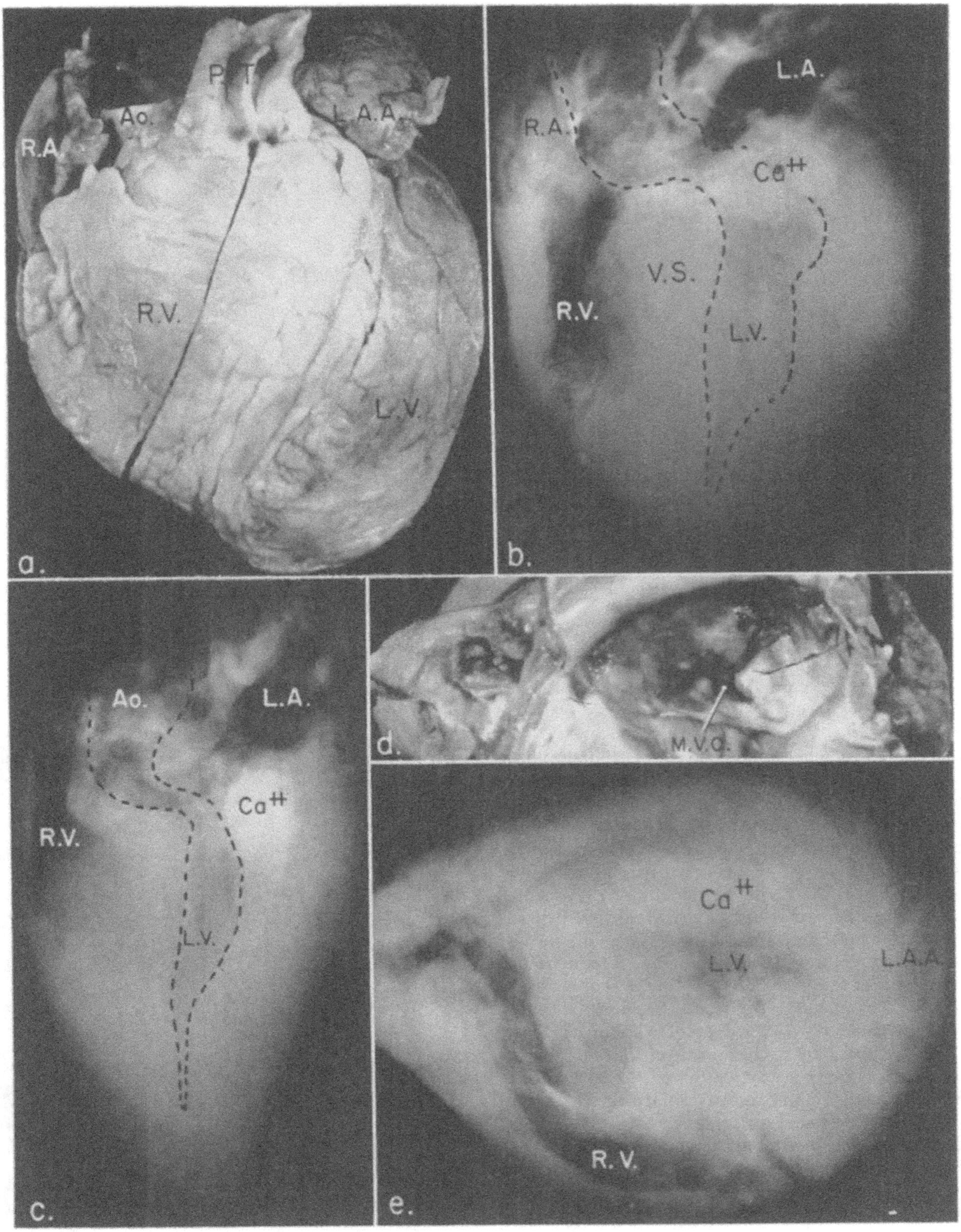

Figure 4. *Heart.* **a,** *exterior* disclosing marked left ventricular (L.V.) hypertrophy. R.V. = right ventricle; R.A. = right atrium; L.A.A. = left atrial appendage; Ao. = aorta; P.T. = pulmonary trunk. **b,** *anteroposterior radiograph of the heart specimen.* The left ventricular (L.V.) cavity is small (enclosed by dashes), and the ventricular septum (V.S.) is severely hypertrophied. Ca^{++} = calcium deposit in mitral annulus and behind the posterior mitral leaflet; L.A. = left atrium. **c,** *lateral radiograph of the specimen.* The interior lining of the small left ventricular cavity is outlined by the dashed lines. **d,** *view of the small mitral valve orifice* (M.V.O.) as seen from the opened left atrium. **e,** *radiograph of specimen taken from above.* This view again illustrates the small size of the left ventricular cavity, and the marked hypertrophy of the left ventricular free walls and ventricular septum.

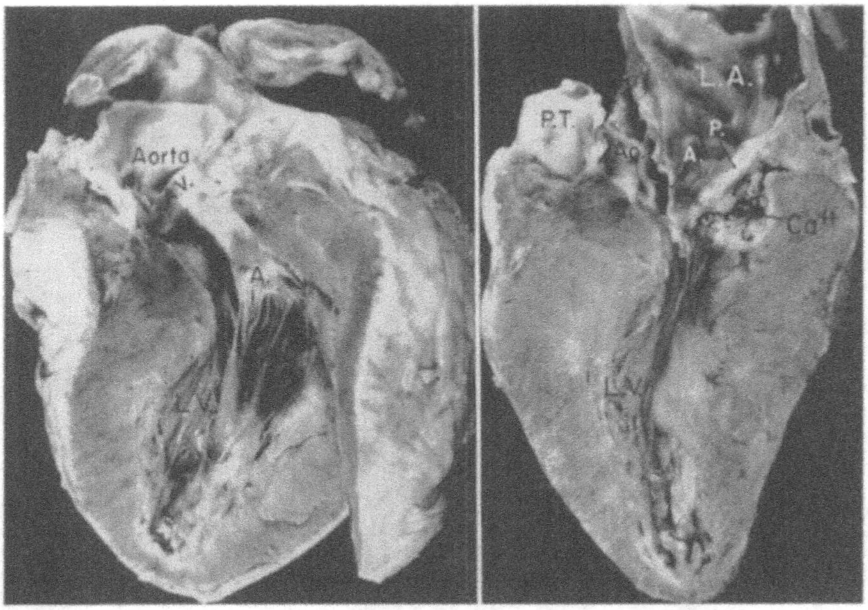

Figure 5. *Opened left side of heart.* **Left,** the left ventricle (L.V.), aortic valve (A.V.) and aorta are opened. The cephalad portion of the muscular ventricular septum is severely hypertrophied, and the endocardium covering it is thickened. **Right,** the lateral portions of the anterior and posterior walls of the left ventricle and mitral leaflets have been removed. The degree of hypertrophy of the cephalad portion of the muscular ventricular septum is even better appreciated in this view. The anterior mitral leaflet (A.) contacts the endocardium of the muscular ventricular septum. An inverted S would be produced if an imaginary line were drawn from the apex of the left ventricle to the aortic root. The posterior mitral leaflet (P.) is plastered down to the free wall myocardium by the large calcium (Ca^{++}) deposit. L.A. = left atrium; P.T. = pulmonary trunk.

the left ventricular outflow tract. The three aortic valve cusps were normal. The anterior mitral leaflet was focally thickened as were its attached chordae tendineae. Huge deposits of calcium adhered the posterior mitral leaflet to the underlying myocardium. The mitral valve orifice was narrowed and permitted passage of only the tip of the index finger. This narrowing was the result of the heavy calcium deposits behind the posterior mitral leaflet protruding into the orifice and the limited motion of the anterior mitral leaflet due to severe hypertrophy of the cephalad portion of the muscular ventricular septum. The left ventricular cavity was small, and the left atrial cavity, moderately dilated. The lumen of the anterior descending coronary artery was narrowed up to 50 per cent, and that of the right coronary artery and left circumflex coronary artery, up to 25 per cent. A fibrous scar was present at the apex of the left ventricle. The right ventricular wall was hypertrophied (0.7 cm. thick), but there was no evidence of right ventricular outflow obstruction.

Comments

The clinical diagnosis in this elderly patient was suggested by the brisk-rising carotid pulse, the bifid apical impulse, the loud atrial diastolic gallop and the long apical systolic murmur with postpremature beat accentuation. Because of

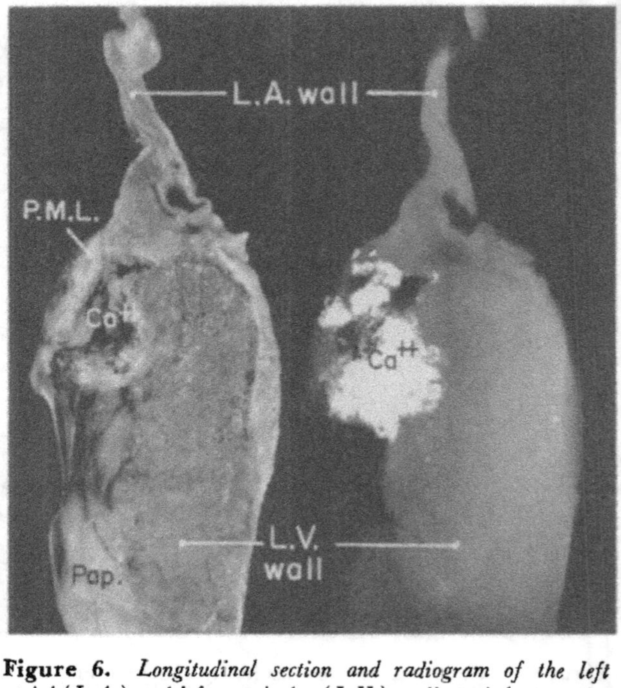

Figure 6. *Longitudinal section and radiogram of the left atrial (L.A.) and left ventricular (L.V.) walls and the posterior mitral leaflet (P.M.L.).* The mass of calcium (Ca^{++}) adheres this leaflet to the myocardial wall behind it. Thus, this leaflet is immobile. Although the deposit of calcium did not appear to be a factor in causing the subaortic stenosis, it probably did act as an impediment to left atrial emptying. Pap. = papillary muscle.

the paucity of reported clinical and pathologic correlations in muscular subaortic stenosis, we comment on each of these diagnostic features as they applied to this patient.

The carotid pulse was brisk-rising to palpation, even when the patient was afebrile. The indirect recording of the carotid pulse (Fig. 1) did not have the spike-dome configuration that has been described[16,17] and recorded in many younger patients with muscular subaortic stenosis but not mentioned in reports of elderly patients.[11,18] The absence of the typical spike dome in our patient may have been due to alterations of the central arterial distensibility that accompanies the aging process. Freis and associates[19] have demonstrated, utilizing an instrument with good response characteristics, that the externally recorded carotid impulse consists of two systolic maximums and that aging or hypertension or both result in an increase in the height of the second systolic maximum in relation to the height of the first. They suggest that these changes reflect changes in central arterial distensibility. Thus, aging and possibly other factors may alter the configuration of the externally recorded impulse of muscular subaortic stenosis. It should be stressed that a normal carotid impulse by palpation does not exclude this diagnosis.

The bifid left ventricular apical impulse in our patient was consistent but not diagnostic of muscular subaortic stenosis. Careful recordings of the left ventricular precordial impulse in muscular subaortic stenosis have shown that the bifid nature of this impulse may be due to either a forceful presystolic impulse followed by a systolic impulse[20] or a twin systolic impulse. On rare occasions all three impulses (presystolic impulse followed by the twin systolic impulse) can be palpated and recorded. The same combination of impulses can be recorded in patients with left ventricular hypertrophy of other causes and therefore is not pathognomonic of muscular subaortic stenosis (unpublished data).

An atrial diastolic gallop is frequent in muscular subaortic stenosis.[3–5] It may also occur in patients with mitral regurgitation of recent onset, such as rupture of chordae tendineae,[21] but is distinctly unusual in chronic rheumatic mitral regurgitation.[22,23]

The apical pansystolic murmur had several possible causes. Calcification of the mitral annulus may rarely produce mitral regurgitation.[24] The electrocardiographic findings consistent with myocardial infarction suggested that papillary muscle dysfunction may have been the cause of the mitral regurgitation.[25,26] The positive blood cultures made us consider that the murmur was secondary to active bacterial endocarditis of the mitral valve. Rheumatic heart disease with mitral insufficiency could not be excluded. However, the definite ***postpremature beat accentuation of the systolic murmur*** suggested that the murmur was not entirely due to mitral insufficiency. Murmurs secondary to ventricular outflow obstruction increase in intensity with the postpremature beat, but murmurs of mitral insufficiency react with little change or may even decrease in intensity.[23,27,28] Our experience (unpublished data) is that the murmur in muscular subaortic stenosis likewise augments with the postpremature beat. Figure 7 illustrates the phenomenon of postpremature beat accentuation of the systolic apical murmur

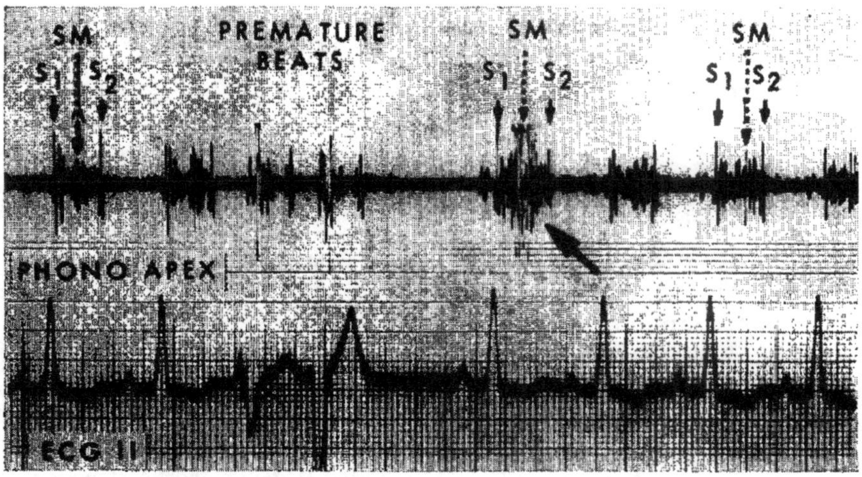

Figure 7. *Phonocardiogram* **demonstrating postpremature beat accentuation of the systolic apical murmur in another patient (not included in this report) with muscular subaortic stenosis.**

in another patient with muscular subaortic stenosis. Even though pansystolic, the murmur responded in the manner of an outflow obstructive murmur. The lack of radiation of the murmur into the neck and the brisk-rising carotid pulse was not consistent with aortic obstruction of the more common fixed valvular variety, and was in accord with that found in patients with muscular subaortic stenosis.

There are three anatomic features which characterize muscular subaortic stenosis: (1) severe hypertrophy of the cephalad portion of the ventricular septum; (2) thickening of the endocardium in the outflow portion of the left ventricle; and (3) abnormal mitral valve, usually with focal fibrous thickening of the leaflets, particularly the anterior one, and abnormalities in length of the chordae tendineae. In addition, the left atrial cavity is almost always dilated. In contrast to the almost constant changes of the aortic valve in the discrete form of subaortic stenosis, the cusps are usually not deformed in muscular subaortic stenosis.

Our patient fulfilled each of these criteria. It is not possible anatomically to separate the idiopathic form of muscular subaortic stenosis from that secondary to fixed valvular aortic stenosis or systemic hypertension. The role played by the elevated blood pressure in our patient is uncertain. The extensive deposition of calcium in the mitral annulus area is viewed as an incidental associated lesion which is unrelated to the muscular subaortic stenosis. There is some evidence that the thick-walled, but small-chambered left ventricle in patients with muscular subaortic stenosis may act as an impediment to left atrial emptying. Almost certainly the protrusion of the posterior mitral leaflet into the mitral orifice by the underlying calcium deposits further retarded left atrial emptying (or left ventricular filling) in our patient.

Summary

The clinical and pathologic findings in a 74 year old Negro woman with muscular subaortic stenosis are reported. The clinical diagnosis was suggested by the combination of a brisk-rising carotid pulse, a bifid left ventricular precordial impulse, a prominent atrial diastolic gallop and an apical pansystolic murmur with post-premature beat accentuation. At necropsy there was severe hypertrophy of the cephalad portion of the ventricular septum, thickening of the endocardium of the outflow portion of the left ventricle and focal fibrous thickening of the mitral valve leaflets.

Acknowledgment

We acknowledge the cooperation of Dr. A. V. Jones, who followed the patient during the four years before her death.

References

1. Brock, R. C. Functional obstruction of the left ventricle: Acquired aortic subvalvular stenosis. *Guy's Hosp. Rep.*, 106: 211, 1957.
2. Braunwald, E., Morrow, A. F., Cornell, W. P., Aygen, M. M. and Hilbish, R. F. Idiopathic hypertrophic subaortic stenosis: Clinical, hemodynamic and angiographic manifestations. *Am. J. Med.*, 29: 924, 1960.
3. Braunwald, E., Lambrew, C. T., Rockoff, S. D., Ross, J., Jr. and Morrow, A. G. Idiopathic hypertrophic subaortic stenosis. *Circulation*, 29: (Suppl. 4): 1, 1964.
4. Cohen, J., Effat, H., Goodwin, J. F., Oakley, C. M. and Steiner, C. M. Hypertrophic obstructive cardiomyopathy. *Brit. Heart J.*, 26: 16, 1964.
5. Wigle, E. D., Heimbecker, R. O. and Gunton, R. W. Idiopathic ventricular septal hypertrophy causing muscular subaortic stenosis. *Circulation*, 26: 325, 1962.
6. Manchester, G. Muscular subaortic stenosis. *New England J. Med.*, 269: 300, 1963.
7. Gorlin, R., Cohen, L. S., Elliott, W. C., Klein, M. D. and Lane, F. J. Hemodynamics of muscular subaortic stenosis. In: Cardiomyopathies, Ciba Symposium, p. 76. London, 1964. Churchill, Ltd.
8. Davies, L. G. A familial heart disease. *Brit. Heart J.*, 14: 206, 1952.
9. Wood, R. S., Taylor, W. J., Wheat, M. W., Jr. and Schiebler, G. L. Muscular subaortic stenosis in childhood: Report of occurrence in three siblings. *Pediatrics*, 30: 749, 1962.
10. Brent, L. B., Aburano, A., Fisher, D. L., Moran, T. J., Myers, J. D. and Taylor, W. J. Familial muscular subaortic stenosis: An unrecognized form of "idiopathic" heart disease: With clinical and autopsy observations. *Circulation*, 21: 167, 1960.
11. Sanders, C. A., Austin, W. G., Jordan, J. C. and Scannell, J. G. Idiopathic hypertrophic subaortic stenosis in two elderly siblings. *New England J. Med.*, 274: 1254, 1966.
12. Brock, R. Functional obstruction of the left ventricle. *Guy's Hosp. Rep.*, 108: 126, 1959.
13. Brachfeld, N. and Gorlin, R. Subaortic stenosis: A revised concept of the disease. *Medicine*, 38: 415, 1959.
14. Beard, E. F., Cooley, D. A. and Latson, J. R. Combined subaortic stenosis and infundibular subpulmonic stenosis. *Arch. Int. Med.*, 100: 647, 1957.
15. Morrow, A. G., Sharp, E. H. an Braunwald, E. Congenital aortic stenosis. *Circulation*, 18: 1090, 1958.
16. Benchimol, A., Dimond, E. G. and Shen, Y. Ejection time in aortic stenosis and mitral stenosis.

Comparison between the direct and indirect arterial tracings with special references to pre and postoperative findings. *Am. J. Cardiol.*, 6: 728, 1960.

17. Benchimol, A., Legler, J. F. and Dimond, E. G. The carotid tracing and apex cardiogram in subaortic stenosis and idiopathic myocardial hypertrophy. *Am. J. Cardiol.*, 11: 427, 1963.
18. Warkentin, D. L. and Korns, M. E. Hypertrophic subaortic stenosis in the aged. *Am. Heart J.*, 73: 106, 1967.
19. Freis, E. D., Heath, W. C., Luchsinger, P. C. and Snell, R. E. Changes in the carotid pulse which occur with age and hypertension. *Am. Heart J.*, 71: 757, 1966.
20. Nagle, R. E., Boicourt, O. W., Gillam, P. M. S. and Mounsey, J. P. D. Cardiac impulse in hypertrophic obstructive cardiomyopathy. *Brit. Heart J.*, 28: 419, 1966.
21. Cohen, L. B., Mason, D. T. and Braunwald, E. Significance of an atrial gallop sound in mitral regurgitation: A clue to the diagnosis of ruptured chordae tendineae. *Circulation*, 35: 112, 1967.
22. Perloff, J. K. and Harvey, W. P. Auscultatory and phonocardiographic manifestations of pure mitral regurgitation. *Progr. Cardiovas. Dis.*, 5: 172, 1962.
23. Brigden, W. and Leatham, A. Mitral incompetence. *Brit. Heart J.*, 15: 55, 1953.
24. Korn, D., DeSanctis, R. W. and Sell, S. Massive calcification of the mitral annulus. *New England J. Med.*, 267: 900, 1962.
25. Burch, G. and DePasquale, N. The syndrome of papillary muscle dysfunction. *Ann. Int. Med.*, 59: 508, 1963.
26. Bashour, F. A. Mitral regurgitation following myocardial infarction: The syndrome of papillary mitral regurgitation. *Dis. Chest*, 48: 113, 1965.
27. Alhomme, P., Welti, J. J. and Facquet, J. Postextrasystolic accentuation of the murmur of aortic stenosis: Its importance in the clinical diagnosis of systolic murmurs. *Arch. mal coeur.*, 51: 493, 1958.
28. Hultgren, H. and Leo, T. Phonocardiographic features of combined mitral stenosis and insufficiency. *Medicine*, 38: 103, 1959.

DRUGS IN USE

080 Anticoagulants	66-01-00 Hematologic Anticoagulant	U 0323/79 Heparin (Sodium)	4/68 - 1527

Experimental Design	Diagnosis	Results	Adverse Reactions
Females 26 Males 15 No. Patients 41 Age: 20-81 yrs. Dosage & Duration: 10,000 I.U. followed by 5,000 I.U. on preop. evening & morning resp.; maint. 5,000 I.U., b.i.d. as required Route: s.c.	Operations: Struma resection 12 Cholecystectomy 11 Stomach resection 8 Misc. 10 Reason for Use Prophylaxis of postop. pulmonary embolism	Pulmonary embolism: Yes: Fatal 2 Recovery 1 No 38	No.Pts. Hemorrhage, massive 6* Hematoma, at inj. site 6 Necorsis, s.c., at inj. site 1 *Discont. therapy & treated with protamine sulfate; reoperation required in 2 pts.

Author's Comment

Incidence of pulmonary embolism was not reduced by heparin. Because of this failure & of adverse reactions, heparin is not recommended as a prophylactic therapy of this postop. complication.

Giehl, H.-J. (Bezirkskrankenhaus Altstadt, Magdeburg, Ger.)
Zur Lungenembolie - mit einem Bericht uber erste Erfahrungen mit der subkutanen Heparinprophylaxe.
Deutsch. Gesundh. 22: 1829-1832 (Sept. 28) 1967.

Prepared by Paul de Haen Inc. for the drug index card system, "de Haen Drugs in Use."

Pulmonary Parenchymal Ossific Nodules in Idiopathic Hypertrophic Subaortic Stenosis

L. MAXIMILIAN BUJA, MD
and WILLIAM C. ROBERTS, MD, FACC
Bethesda, Maryland

Attention is called to the occurrence of pulmonary parenchymal ossific nodules in 2 siblings, both young adults, with idiopathic hypertrophic subaortic stenosis. This association has not been described previously.

Ossific nodules in the pulmonary parenchyma frequently are observed radiographically and morphologically in patients with rheumatic mitral valvular disease, especially stenosis.[1–3] Similar nodules have been observed rarely in patients with interstitial pulmonary fibrosis (Hamman-Rich syndrome)[4] and in at least 1 patient with each of the following conditions: left atrial myxoma, constrictive pericarditis, systemic hypertension, coronary arterial disease and aortic regurgitation.[5,6] This report describes pulmonary ossific nodules in 2 siblings with idiopathic hypertrophic subaortic stenosis. The association of such nodules with this entity has not been recorded previously, and we did not observe them at autopsy examination of the lungs of 7 other patients with idiopathic hypertrophic subaortic stenosis.

Case Reports

Case 1. At age 26, this man was asymptomatic when examined at the National Heart Institute, Bethesda, Md. A grade 2–3/6 systolic murmur was heard over the left sternal border and apex. Electrocardiogram showed sinus rhythm, biatrial enlargement and T wave abnormalities. Chest roentgenograms (Fig. 1) showed cardiomegaly and multiple densities throughout both lung fields. (These lesions were reported to have been observed on a chest roentgenogram taken 5 years earlier.) Repeated radiograms during the subsequent 7 years showed no increase in the number or size of the pulmonary parenchymal nodules. Results of the histoplasmin skin test were positive; those of skin tests for blastomycosis, coccidiomycosis and tuberculosis were negative. On cardiac catheterization the intravascular pressures (mm Hg) were right atrial mean 3; right ventricular 35/3; pulmonary arterial 35/24; left atrial mean 16, with *a* waves 26 and *v* waves 20; simultaneous left ventricular and brachial arterial 150/26 and 120/70, respectively, yielding a 30 mm Hg peak systolic gradient at rest which increased to 85 mm Hg with provocation (ouabain). The cardiac index was 2.1 liters/min per m^2.

At age 33 (6 months before death) exertional and nocturnal dyspnea and atrial fibrillation developed. Three weeks before death the patient was again hospitalized. The precordial systolic murmur was now only intermittently audible. Electrocardiogram showed atrial fibrillation and intraventricular conduction defect. The rhythm reverted to normal after transthoracic electrical countershock.

From the Section of Pathology, National Heart and Lung Institute, National Institutes of Health, Bethesda, Md. 20014. Manuscript received December 30, 1968, accepted February 25, 1969.

Address for reprints: Dr. William C. Roberts, Section of Pathology, National Heart and Lung Institute, National Institutes of Health, Bethesda, Md. 20014.

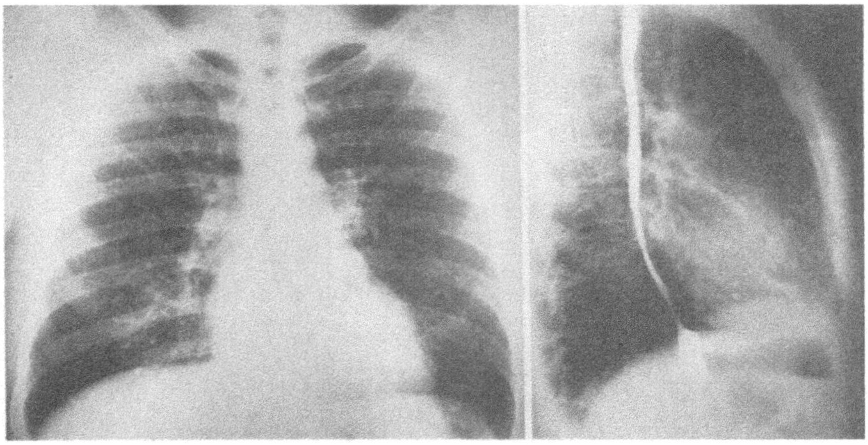

Figure 1. Case 1. Chest roentgenograms taken at age 26. Anteroposterior **(left)** and lateral **(right)** views.

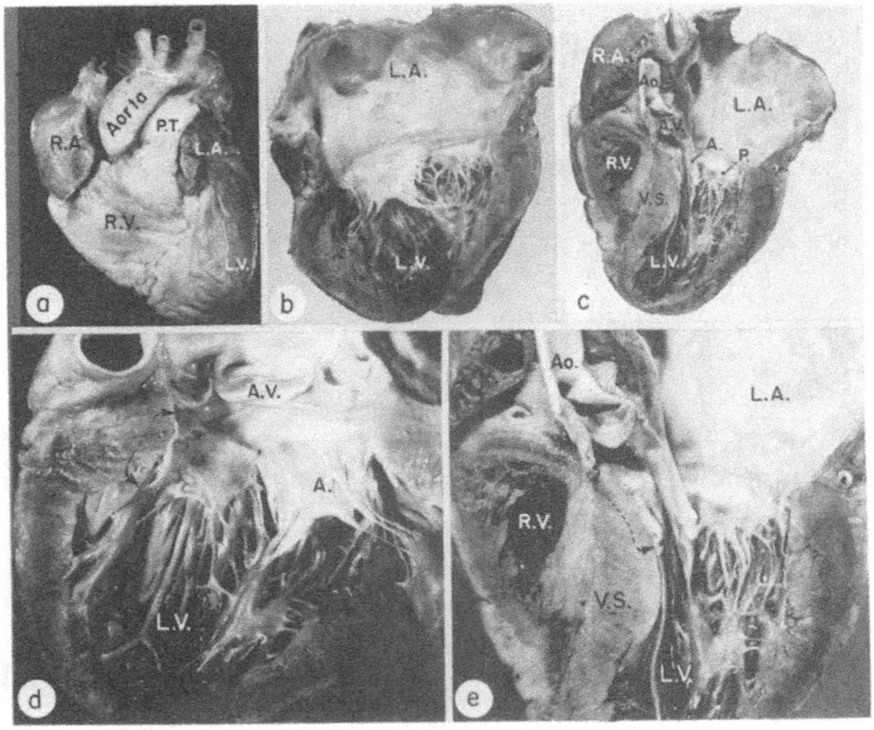

Figure 2. Case 1. Heart at autopsy. **a,** exterior view. All chambers are enlarged L.A. = left atrium; L.V. = left ventricle; P.T. = pulmonary trunk; R.A. = right atrium; R.V. = right ventricle. **b,** open left side showing dilated left atrium, focally thickened mitral leaflets and chordae and hypertrophied left ventricle. A thrombus is present at the apex of the left ventricle. **c,** coronal section. The ventricular septum (V.S.) is thicker than the free wall of the left ventricle. A close-up view of the outflow tract is shown in **e.** A. and P. = anterior and posterior mitral leaflets, respectively; Ao. = aorta. **d,** opened aorta, aortic valve (A.V.) and left ventricle. The endocardium in the outflow tract is thickened, and this thickening corresponds to similar thickening on the ventricular aspect of the anterior mitral leaflet (A.). The aortic valve is normal.

Repeat catheterization showed the pulmonary arterial pressure to be 52/25; mean pulmonary arterial wedge 22, with *a* waves 24 and *v* waves 26; and simultaneous left ventricular and brachial arterial pressures 120/26 and 120/80 mm Hg, respectively. A 33 mm Hg gradient was provoked by isoproterenol. The cardiac index was 2.0 liters/min per m^2. Six days after catheterization atrial fibrillation recurred, and 4 days later sudden unilateral hemiparesis appeared. The next day the left femoral arterial pulse was absent, and the patient died.

At necropsy the left external iliac, right internal iliac and left internal carotid arteries were completely occluded by thromboembolic material, as were several small mesenteric arteries. A thrombus (1.5 by 1.5 by 1.5 cm) was present in the apex of the left ventricle. Several renal and splenic infarcts were present.

The heart (Fig. 2) weighed 450 g. The ventricular septum was 2.7 cm thick, and the left ventricular free wall was 1.3 cm thick. An endocardial plaque was present in the left ventricular outflow tract. The mitral valve leaflets and several chordae tendineae were thickened. The left atrium was dilated, and the endocardium of its posterosuperior wall was thickened. There was narrowing of the lumens of the anterior descending (25 to 50 percent), left circumflex (50 to 75 percent) and left marginal (90 percent) coronary arteries.

The lungs together weighed 1,050 g. On postmortem radiograms and plastic (vinyl) cast preparations (Fig. 3) circumscribed nodules measuring between 0.1 to 0.6 cm were observed in all lobes. The ossific nodules (Fig. 3) consisted of mature lamellar bone with osteocytes and bone marrow but no iron or sim-

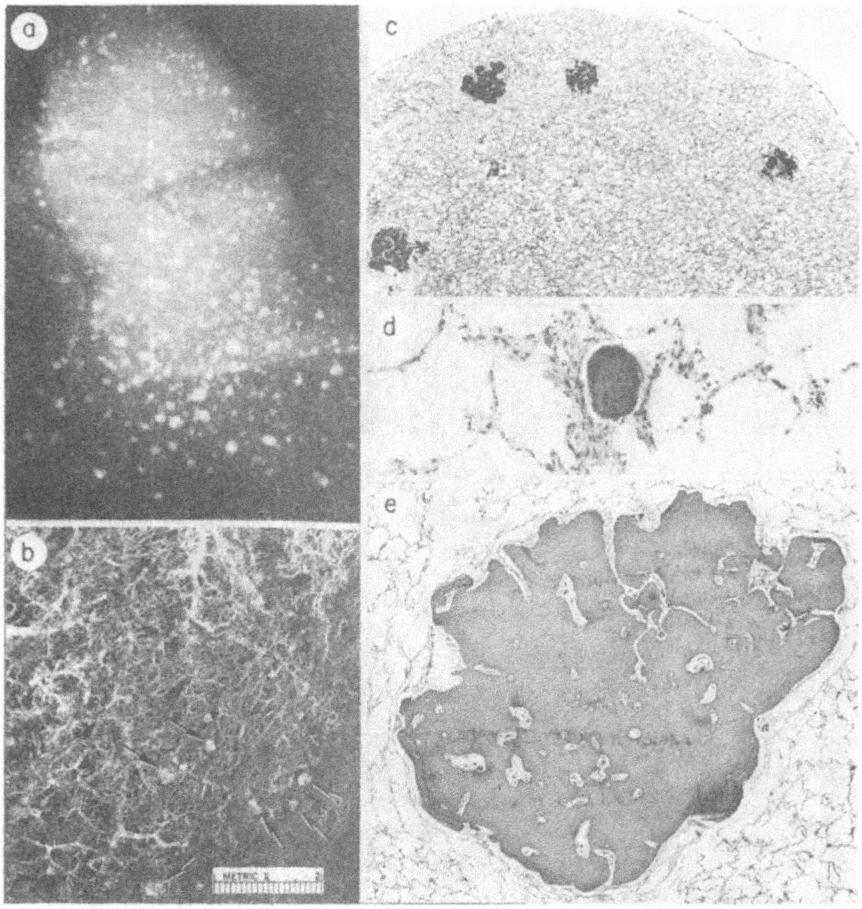

Figure 3. Case 1. Lung at autopsy. **a,** postmortem radiograph of left lung showing numerous pulmonary parenchymal ossific nodules. **b,** a plastic (vinyl) cast preparation of right lung demonstrating normal pulmonary arteries. Pulmonary ossific nodules are indicated by arrows. **c,** photomicrograph of lung showing four ossific nodules. Elastic van Gieson, × 6, reduced by 39 percent. **d,** minute ossific nodule located entirely within an alveolus. Hematoxylin and eosin stain, × 160, reduced by 39 percent. **e,** more usual-sized ossific nodule consisting of mature, lamellar bone with osteocytes in lacunae and spaces containing bone marrow. Hematoxylin and eosin, × 20, reduced by 39 percent.

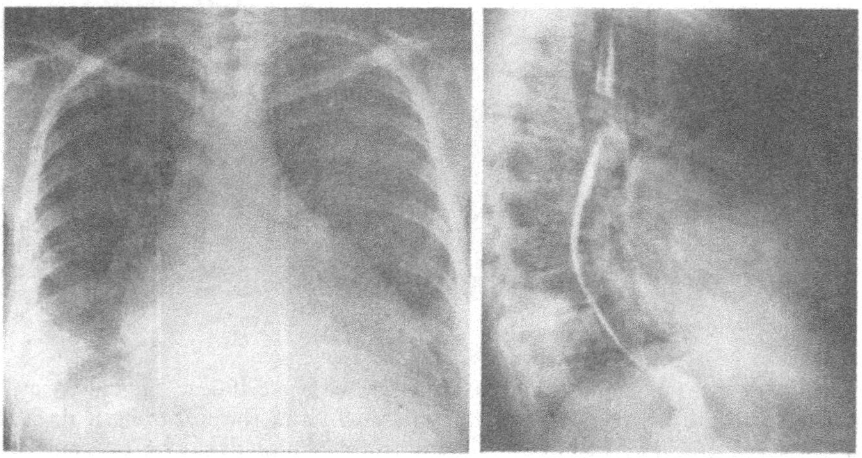

Figure 4. Case 2. Chest roentgenograms taken at age 25. Anteroposterior (left) and lateral (right) views.

ple calcium salts (Prussian blue and Von Kossa stains).* Hemosiderin-laden macrophages were present in a few alveoli. No microorganisms were seen. The capillaries were congested, and the interlobular septa were edematous. The pulmonary blood vessels were normal histologically.

* The Von Kossa method stains the phosphate and carbonate ions of calcium phosphate and carbonate molecules that remain in tissue after the calcium has been removed to facilitate histologic sectioning. The method is positive only for simple molecules and is negative once the calcium phosphate and carbonate are formed into the complex crystals of mature bone. Thus, the stain is positive only in areas of recent calcific deposition or areas of bone destruction.

Case 2. This 26 year old woman was the sister of the patient in Case 1. She had had exertional and nocturnal dyspnea and persistent dependent subcutaneous edema for 3 years before she was examined at the National Heart Institute at age 25. A grade 3/6 blowing systolic murmur was heard over the apex, left axilla and left sternal border. The feet were edematous. Electrocardiogram showed atrial fibrillation, left ventricular hypertrophy with strain, left ventricular conduction delay and an occasional premature contraction. Chest roentgenograms (Fig. 4) showed left atrial enlargement and right pleural effusion. On cardiac catheterization the intravascular pressures (mm Hg) were right atrial mean 10; right ventricular

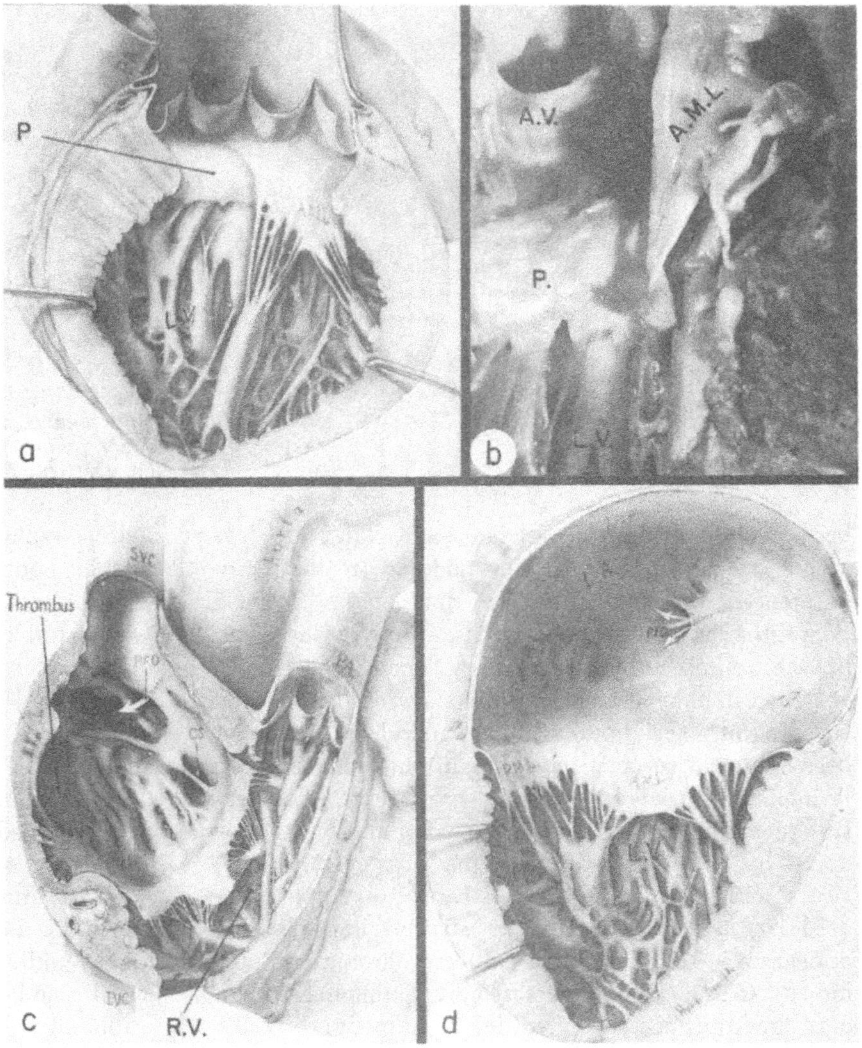

Figure 5. Case 2. Heart at autopsy. **a,** drawing of opened aorta and hypertrophied left ventricle (L.V.). A thick endocardial plaque (P) covers the left ventricular aspect of the cephalad portion of the ventricular septum which is severely hypertrophied. The anterior leaflet of the mitral valve (A.M.L.) and some of the chordae tendineae are thickened. P.A. = pulmonary trunk; L.A. = left atrium. **b,** a close-up of an actual photograph of the left ventricular outflow tract. A.V. = aortic valve. **c,** drawing of the opened right side of the heart. The right atrium is dilated and contains a thrombus. The fossa ovale region is probe-patent but valvular-competent (P.F.O.). The tricuspid valve is normal, and the right ventricular (R.V.) cavity is very small. S.V.C. = superior vena cava; C.S. = ostium of coronary sinus; I.V.C. = inferior vena cava. **d,** drawing of opened left atrium (L.A.), thickened mitral valve and left ventricle. The left atrium is dilated. P.M.L. = posterior mitral leaflet.

50/8; pulmonary arterial 40/25; left atrial mean 19—with *v* waves 23; left ventricular 103/2; and aortic 95/55. The cardiac index was 1.8 liters/min per m^2. Symptoms of cardiac dysfunction progressed, and she died with severe congestive heart failure 1 year later at another hospital.

At autopsy the heart weighed 350 g and was very similar to the heart of the patient's brother (Case 1). The cephalad portion of the ventricular septum was disproportionally thickened, and an endocardial plaque present in the left ventricular outflow tract corresponded to fibrous thickening of the ventricular aspect of the anterior mitral leaflet (Fig. 5). The left atrium was dilated, and the aortic valvular cusps were normal. An antemortem thrombus was present in the right atrium. The coronary arteries appeared normal.

The lungs showed changes of severe chronic pulmonary congestion and pulmonary hypertension. The alveolar septa were focally but extensively thickened; many alveoli contained hemosiderin-laden macrophages; parenchymal cholesterol granulomas were frequent;[7] acute pneumonia was present in the right lower lobe; large areas of atelectasis were present bilaterally; the visceral pleura over the lower lobes was thick; and many ossific nodules, similar to those seen in the lungs in Case 1, were found throughout the pulmonary parenchyma (Fig. 6).

The muscular pulmonary arteries and arterioles showed medial hypertrophy and intimal proliferation. A few smaller pulmonary arteries contained organized thromboemboli. The lumens of the pulmonary veins also were severely narrowed by fibrous intimal tissue.

Discussion

Differential diagnosis: The pulmonary parenchymal nodules observed in these 2 cases were similar radiographically and morphologically to those seen in patients with rheumatic mitral valvular disease.[1–3] Such nodules consist of mature lamellar bone. They measure 0.1 to 1.0 cm in diameter and are located within the pulmonary parenchyma, often purely intra-alveolar. They may be present in any lobe, most frequently the lower lobes, and they may contain

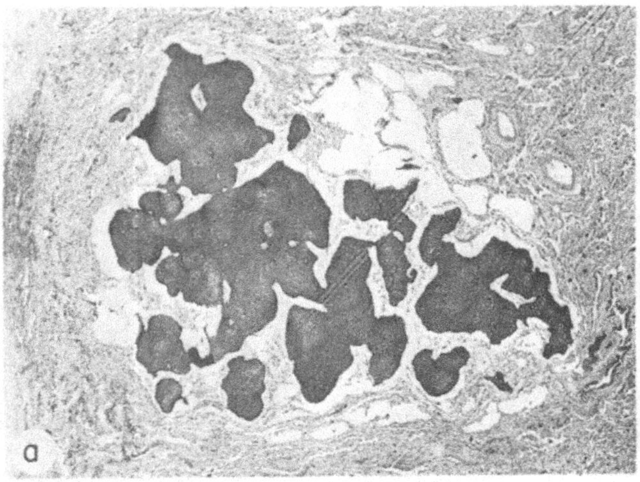

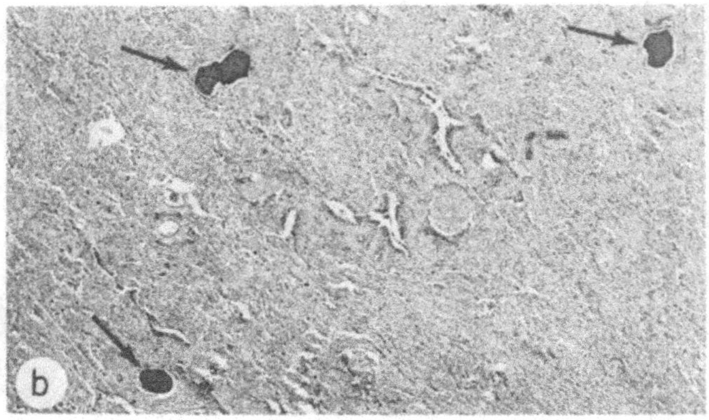

Figure 6. Case 2. pulmonary ossific nodules. **a,** large ossific nodule. **b,** three small nodules (arrows). The pulmonary parenchyma is atelectatic. Hematoxylin and eosin, each × 25, reduced by 23 percent.

bone marrow or iron or calcium salts. They are free of microorganisms. The ossific nodules are distinctly different morphologically from pulmonary alveolar microliths,[8] pulmonary corpora amylacea[9] and branching interstitial pulmonary bone occasionally observed in older patients.[1] Pulmonary ossific nodules, corpora amylacea and alveolar microliths have not been reported to occur together in the same patient. Pulmonary alveolar microlithiasis presents a distinctive roentgenographic appearance similar to that produced by acute pulmonary edema. However, the patients with pulmonary microliths are asymptomatic at least initially despite the striking radiographic appearance. Later in these subjects chronic cor pulmonale may develop. Interestingly, pulmonary alveolar microlithiasis is familial.[8] Pulmonary ossific nodules as occurred in each of our 2 cases have not been reported previously in more than 1 member of a single family. Pulmonary corpora amylacea are not visible radiographically, and there is no evidence that they produce pulmonary dysfunction.

The nodules observed on chest roentgenograms of patients with healed histoplasmosis, miliary tuberculosis, chickenpox or some pneumoconioses may simulate the radiographic appearance of pulmonary parenchymal ossific nodules. The nodules in the lungs of Patient 1 were diagnosed radiographically during life as healed histoplasmosis.

Mechanism of formation of pulmonary parenchymal ossific nodules: The mechanism of formation is speculative. The only finding that appears to be common to patients with these nodules is pulmonary venous hypertension, but the exact relation of the increased pressure to the ossific nodules is unknown.[2,3,5] Pulmonary nodules have been observed in patients with[3,5] and without[2] overt congestive cardiac failure. Organization of pulmonary edema fluid to form osteoid and finally bone has been suggested as a possible mechanism of formation of the pulmonary parenchymal ossific nodules.[2,3,5] Development of the ossific nodules by transformation of intraalveolar hemosiderin deposits also has been suggested[10] but seems unlikely. Ossific nodules may be observed in portions of lung entirely free from hemosiderin deposits, and ossific nodules have not been described in subjects with idiopathic pulmonary hemosiderosis, a condition that produces the largest deposition of iron in the alveolar spaces.[11] The ossific nodules were not observed at various stages of formation in either of our 2 patients. Indeed, whether the nodules were large or small, their morphologic features were similar. This fact suggests that all of the ossific nodules in an individual patient formed at the same time. Ossific nodules have been observed experimentally in rabbits given irradiation to the lungs 1 to 2 months before sacrifice.[12]

Relation of ossific nodules to degree of cardiac dysfunction: Although pulmonary venous hypertension occurred in our 2 cases, neither the number nor the size of the pulmonary ossific nodules was proportional to the degree of rise in pulmonary venous pressure. Patient 2 had severe cardiac failure for several years with extensive pulmonary parenchymal and vascular changes of chronic congestion. In contrast, Patient 1 was asymptomatic until 6 months before death, and his lungs were virtually normal except for the presence of numerous ossific nodules. Although Patient 2 had far more evidence of chronic pulmonary congestion than did Patient 1, she had far fewer ossific nodules. However, at autopsy the hearts of both patients were strikingly similar although the degree of cardiac dysfunction was quite different.

Acknowledgment

We thank Doctors Eugene Braunwald and Stephen E. Epstein for use of the clinical information in the 2 cases described.

References

1. **Wells HG, Dunlap CE:** Disseminated ossification of the lungs. Arch Path (Chicago) 35:420–426, 1943
2. **Fleming HA, Robinson CLN:** Pulmonary ossification with cardiac calcification in mitral valve disease. Brit Heart J 19:532–538, 1957
3. **Galloway RW, Epstein EJ, Coulshed N:** Pulmonary ossific nodules in mitral valve disease. Brit Heart J 23:297–307, 1961
4. **Ventura JC:** Disseminated nodular pulmonary ossification with Hamman-Rich syndrome. J Lancet 86:60–63, 1966
5. **Epstein EJ, Chapman R, Coulshed N, et al:** Pulmonary ossific nodule formation in the absence of mitral valve disease. A report of four cases. Amer Heart J 65:816–825, 1963
6. **Hudson REB:** Cardiovascular Pathology, Vol. I. Baltimore, Williams & Wilkins, 1961, p 1015
7. **Glancy DL, Frazier PD, Roberts WC:** Pulmonary parenchymal cholesterol-ester granulomas in patients with pulmonary hypertension. Amer J Med 45:198–210, 1968
8. **Sosman MC, Dodd GD, Jones WD, et al:** The familial occurrence of pulmonary alveolar microlithiasis. Amer J Roentgen 77:947–1012, 1957
9. **Michaels L, Levine C:** Pulmonary corpora amylacea. J Path Bact 74:49–56, 1957
10. **Ellman P, Gee A:** Pulmonary hemosiderosis. Brit Med J 2:384–390, 1951
11. **Soergel KH, Sommers SC:** Idiopathic pulmonary hemosiderosis and related syndromes Amer J Med 32:499–511, 1962
12. **Engelstad RB:** Über die Wirkungen der Röntgenstrahlen auf die Lungen. Acta Radiol (Stockholm) 15: Suppl 19:1–93, 1934

Operative Treatment of Hypertrophic Obstructive Cardiomyopathy

The Case Against Mitral Valve Replacement

WILLIAM C. ROBERTS, MD, FACC
Bethesda, Maryland

In the January 1973 issue of this Journal, Cooley et al.[1] proposed that "mitral valve replacement should be considered the surgical procedure of choice in patients with advanced hypertrophic stenosis." This conclusion was based on "excellent" operative results from mitral valve replacement in nine patients, two of whom died, with hypertrophic obstructive cardiomyopathy. Cooley and associates switched from partial resection of the ventricular septum in this condition to mitral valve replacement because (1) valve replacement relieved both the left ventricular outflow systolic pressure gradient and the mitral regurgitation; (2) postoperative conduction disturbances were reduced; (3) the septectomy procedure failed "to obtain complete or even acceptable relief of the stenotic gradient;" and (4) "many of the patients who initially obtained an adequate result [from septectomy] later experienced gradual recurrence of the obstructive hypertrophy." Because Cooley et al. did not discuss or reference results of others using the partial septectomy technique, it seemed appropriate to summarize reported results from the septectomy procedure and to discuss the advantages and disadvantages of partial septectomy versus mitral valve replacement for hypertrophic obstructive cardiomyopathy in light of these results.

Results of septectomy performed by five different surgeons are summarized in Table I.[2-6] Results in 26 patients operated on by Cooley using the septectomy technique also are included. The mortality rate for the 167 patients was 19 percent. Ninety-five of the 126 survivors (75 percent) of the operative procedure were in functional class III or IV (New York Heart Association classification) preoperatively and only 6 (5 percent) were in class III or IV postoperatively. Thus, *clinical improvement by septectomy is usually excellent.*

Septectomy usually completely alleviates the left ventricular outflow tract gradient. In 68 of the tabulated 167 patients, left ventricular and systemic arterial pressures were measured both pre- and postoperatively (Table II). In 80 percent (54 patients) no left ventricular outflow tract pressure gradient at rest was present postoperatively; in another 16 percent the pressure gradient was ≤20 mm Hg, and only 4 percent had a gradient >20 mm Hg postoperatively. Small (<25 mm Hg) gradients could be provoked postoperatively in most patients.[2,4,5] Resting gradients have been observed at catheterization during the first year postoperatively when no gradients were evident at later studies.[2,4] In no reported cases has there been any recurrence or exacerbation of outflow obstruction at any time after operation.

The left ventricular end-diastolic pressure usually decreases after septectomy. Left ventricular end-diastolic pressure decreased in 55 of 76 patients (72 percent) in whom it was measured both before and after septectomy (Table III). Preoperatively, it was increased (>12 mm Hg) in 54 patients (71 percent), and postoperatively in 36 patients (47 percent). The left ventricular end-diastolic pressure in the 76 patients averaged 19 mm Hg preoperatively and 13 mm Hg postoperatively.

Mitral regurgitation, a well recognized accompaniment of hypertrophic obstructive cardiomyopathy, usually disappears after septectomy. In 14 patients operated on by Morrow et al.[2] in whom adequate left ventricular contrast studies were obtained both pre- and postoperatively, mitral regurgitation was evident before operation in 13, and postoperatively in 2 (mild in each). Of 21 patients operated on by Barratt-Boyes[4] in whom postoperative angiographic studies were performed, 18 had no mitral regurgitation, 2 had mild and 1 had moderate regurgitation.

Cooley et al. also were among those (Table I) describing favorable results with partial ventricular septectomy: "with two exceptions, striking clinical inprovement followed septal myocardiectomy in nearly every surviving patient who was symptomatic before operation."[6] Septectomy was carried out from a right ventricular approach in 10 of their 26 patients, in part because this approach prevented "damage to the mitral valve suspension."[6] Cooley et al. subsequently abandoned septectomy, however,

Address for reprints: William C. Roberts, MD, Section of Pathology, National Heart and Lung Institute, National Institutes of Health, Bethesda, Md. 20014.

TABLE I

Results of Septectomy

Authors	Patients (total no.)	Preoperative Functional Class of Survivors I	II	III	IV	Postoperative Functional Class of Survivors I	II	III	IV	Deaths
Morrow et al.[2]	43	0*	1*	17*	13*	22*	9*	0*	0*	6
Tajik et al.[3]	43	2*	3*	23*	0*	12*	13*	2*	1*	11
Barratt-Boyes and O'Brien[4]	30	1	12	7	7	24	2	1	0	3
Adelman et al.[5]	25	2	3	14		8	11	0	0	6
Cooley et al.[6]	26	2	5	14	0	19		2	0	5
Totals	167	31 (25%)		95 (75%)		120 (95%)		6 (5%)		31
		126				126				(19%)

* Includes only those patients followed up more than 12 months after septectomy.

and now consider mitral valve replacement the operative procedure of choice for hypertrophic obstructive cardiomyopathy. This conclusion is based on early (up to 18 month follow-up) results in only nine patients, two of whom died; results in the other seven are described as "excellent." A "low profile disc valve with full orifice design" was employed (Biork-Shiley tilting disc valve or the Cooley-Cutter disc valve). Cardiac catheterization (performed 2 weeks to 8 months postoperatively) in eight of the nine patients disclosed small (5 to 15 mm Hg) left ventricular to systemic arterial peak systolic pressure gradients in eight and no gradient in one. Left ventricular end-diastolic pressure averaged 21 mm Hg preoperatively, and 12 mm Hg postoperatively.

A major reason given by Cooley et al. for advocating mitral valve replacement rather than septectomy was that valve replacement alleviated both the left ventricular outflow obstruction and, at the same time, the accompanying mitral regurgitation. But septectomy also relieves both disorders and it relieves the outflow gradient more completely. In only 1 of the 7 surviving patients of Cooley et al. was the left ventricular outflow gradient in fact totally relieved by mitral valve replacement, whereas in 80 percent of 68 patients treated by septectomy (Table II), the left ventricular outflow gradient was totally obliterated. Moreover, mitral regurgitation (as proved by left ventricular angiography) is infrequent after septectomy.[2,4] It is assumed that mitral regurgitation was also obliterated in the patients of Cooley et al., but left ventricular angiography was not performed postoperatively in any of them, and the clinical diagnosis of mitral regurgitation after mitral valve replacement may be difficult without left ventricular angiography.[7]

Cooley et al. also stressed that the mitral valve leaflets are anatomically abnormal and that their chordal attachments are bizarre in hypertrophic cardiomyopathy. Fibrous thickening of these leaflets and chordae, well recognized in this condition,[8-13] is not the cause of the regurgitation because the latter

TABLE II

Effect of Septectomy on Left Ventricular Outflow Tract Obstruction

Author	Patients Undergoing Septectomy (no.)	Patients with Both Pre- and Postop Catheterization Data (no.)	Postoperative: Patients with No PSG (no.)	Patients with PSG ≤20 mm Hg (no.)	Patients with PSG >20 mm Hg (no.)
Morrow et al.[2]	43	29	27	2	0
Tajik et al.[3]	43	0	...	...	...
Barratt-Boyes and O'Brien[4]	30	22	18	2	2
Adelman et al.[5]	25	11	8	3	0
Cooley et al.[6]	26	6	1	4	1
Totals	167	68	54 (80%)	11 (16%)	3 (4%)

Postop = postoperative; PSG = peak systolic pressure gradient at rest between left ventricle and systemic artery.

TABLE III

Effect of Septectomy on Left-Ventricular End-Diastolic Pressure (LVEDP)

		Preoperative				Postoperative			
Author	Patients (total (no.)	Patients with Pre- and Postop LVEDP Recorded (no.)	Patients with LVEDP $>$12 mm Hg (no.)	Patients with LVEDP $\leq$12 mm Hg (no.)	Average LVEDP (mm Hg)	Patients with LVEDP $>$12 mm Hg (no.)	Patients with LVEDP $\leq$12 mm Hg (no.)	Patients with Reduced LVEDP ↓ (no.)	Average LVEDP (mm Hg)
Morrow et al.[2]	43	29	21	8	20	17	12	24	12
Tajik et al.[3]	43	...	...	...	...	...	...	...	...
Barratt-Boyes and O'Brien[4]	30	22	12	10	13	4	18	13	8
Adelman et al.[5]	25	19	16	3	21	12	7	14	16
Cooley et al.[6]	26	6	5	1	21	3	3	4	17
Totals	167	76	54 (71%)	22 (29%)	19	36 (47%)	40 (53%)	55 (72%)	13

disappears after septectomy.[2,4] Rather, the regurgitation appears to result from malalignment of the left ventricular papillary muscles,[14] particularly the anterolateral one. The bending of these structures by the disproportionally thickened ventricular septum is relieved by septectomy, but it is uncertain whether it is relieved by mitral valve replacement.

Another advantage of mitral valve replacement over septectomy according to Cooley et al. is that there are fewer postoperative conduction disturbances. In nearly all patients undergoing septectomy from the left ventricular side left bundle branch block or hemiblock develops, and in nearly all undergoing septectomy from the right side right bundle branch block develops. Complete heart block is infrequent. It appears unlikely, however, that left bundle branch block produced by septectomy has the same prognostic significance as that produced by its more common cause, coronary atherosclerosis. But if the patient has right bundle branch block preoperatively—and this occurs in about 3 percent of patients with hypertrophic obstructive cardiomyopathy[15]—septectomy, at least from the left side, should not be performed. Thus, conduction disturbances are consequences of septectomy, but they infrequently cause major complications, and these complications do not compare to those associated with prosthetic cardiac valves.

Cooley's major criticism of the septectomy procedure was that it failed "to obtain complete or even acceptable relief of the stenotic gradient," and that "many of the patients who initially obtained an adequate result [from septectomy] later experienced gradual recurrence of the obstructive hypertrophy." Both claims are incorrect. Hemodynamic data (Table II) show that the outflow gradient is usually completely abolished by septectomy. Furthermore, left ventricular outflow obstruction has never been reported to develop after septectomy in any patient during long postoperative follow-up periods. Symptomatic improvement also has been long-lasting.[2-4]

Thus, mitral valve replacement has few advantages and several disadvantages compared to septectomy as the operative procedure of choice for patients with hypertrophic obstructive cardiomyopathy. Because complications inherent to prosthetic valves are so common, results of valve replacement for this condition must be unequivocally better than those from the other procedure (septectomy) to justify this radical approach. To conclude, as did Cooley et al., that "mitral valve replacement should be considered the surgical procedure of choice in patients with advanced hypertrophic stenosis"[1] on the basis of their preliminary and incomplete data in nine patients is unjustified and dangerous. No information, for example, regarding the hemodynamic status of the mitral valve prostheses was presented. That mitral regurgitation was eliminated has not been documented and, of more concern, there is no evidence that mitral stenosis has not been added. Some degree of prosthetic obstruction occurs after every mitral valve replacement utilizing a low-profile prosthesis.[16] When replacement is carried out in patients with a small left ventricular cavity, as is the case with hypertrophic obstructive cardiomyopathy, the likelihood of considerable prosthetic obstruction is much greater. The left ventricle in hypertrophic obstructive cardiomyopathy is too small to accommodate a caged-ball type mitral prosthesis—indeed, its insertion in this condition has proved disastrous—and low-profile valves even of "smaller than usual diameter"[1] and of the central flow type do not assure against prosthetic dysfunction. Impairment to left ventricular filling occurs naturally in hypertrophic obstructive cardiomyopathy,[17] and this impairment may well be increased after mitral valve replacement. The need for anticoagulant agents in patients with a prosthetic mitral valve adds another serious long-term disadvantage to this procedure.

The most dangerous aspect of valve replacement for hypertrophic obstructive cardiomyopathy, however, is that a new disease—namely, "prosthetic cardiac valve"—is introduced and *it has a higher 5 year mortality rate than does symptomatic hypertrophic obstructive cardiomyopathy,* whether or not septectomy is performed. Of 100 patients who underwent mitral valve replacement for stenosis or regurgitation, or both, by Morrow,[18] only 63 percent are alive 5 years after operation and only 51 percent after 8 years, and these long-term results are as good as any reported. There have been several changes in prostheses subsequently but there is no proof that the presently employed prostheses, including the Cooley-Cutter disc valve, will provide better long-term results than those obtained by Levine et al.[18] The survival rate for symptomatic hypertrophic obstructive cardiomyopathy even without septectomy is better.[19] Of 56 patients followed up at the National Heart and Lung Institute for up to 12 years (average 32 months) with hypertrophic obstructive cardiomyopathy, 47 (84 percent) are alive and all were in functional class II, III or IV (New York Heart Association) when initially examined.

Mitral valve replacement cannot be justified by the facts presented here or by any theoretical considerations. Mitral replacement for hypertrophic obstructive cardiomyopathy is not directed at the primary fault, namely, disproportional hypertrophy of the ventricular septum; that is, the septum is considerably thicker than the left ventricular free wall.[8,10-13,20,21] Ultrastructural[22] and histologic studies[21] have shown that the myocardial fibers in the ventricular septum are bizarre in appearance and have abnormal orientations one to another. In contrast, the orientations of the myocardial fibers in the free walls are normal. The left ventricular outflow obstruction is produced by contact of the anterior mitral leaflet and the thickened ventricular septum during systole. Fibrous thickening of the mitral valve leaflets and chordae results from this contact, which is alleviated by septectomy. Mitral valve replacement also nearly obliterates the left ventricular outflow gradient, as Cooley et al. have nicely shown, but the vigorous contractions of the ventricular septum may remain. After septectomy, the left ventricular cavity dilates to near normal proportions,[21] that is, similar to those of the left ventricular free wall. In contrast, there is no indication that the septum gets thinner or that the left ventricular cavity increases to normal size after valve replacement. Because the cavity is still small and the septum still disproportionally hypertrophied, the septum may contact the inserted prosthetic mitral valve during ventricular systole as it does the anterior mitral leaflet before replacement. This contact could produce prosthetic dysfunction.

In an occasional patient with hypertrophic obstructive cardiomyopathy the ascending aorta is too small to allow septectomy by way of the aorta alone. An alternate surgical procedure, therefore, is necessary in these patients. Septectomy by way of the right ventricle rather than mitral valve replacement may still be the more reasonable procedure because of complications inherent to valvular prostheses, and because left ventricular incisions may lead to incisional aneurysms.

In summary, the conclusion of Cooley et al. that mitral valve replacement is "the surgical procedure of choice" for patients with hypertrophic obstructive cardiomypathy is at best premature and potentially dangerous. The mortality rate from the prosthesis alone is greater than that for the underlying disease, hypertrophic obstructive cardiomyopathy. Furthermore, everything that can be accomplished by mitral valve replacement can be better accomplished by septectomy. Septectomy more completely abolishes the left ventricular outflow tract pressure gradient and at the same time alleviates the associated mitral regurgitation. Moreover, septectomy, by attacking the primary fault, abolishes the disproportional hypertrophy of the ventricular septum, and in so doing allows the left ventricular cavity to dilate to normal dimensions. There is no evidence at this time that the disproportional ventricular septal hypertrophy is relieved or that the left ventricle dilates after mitral valve replacement. And, finally, there is no evidence that the mitral prosthesis, inserted in the small left ventricle, functions normally.

References

1. **Cooley DA, Leachman RD, Wukasch DC:** Diffuse muscular subaortic stenosis: surgical treatment. Amer J Cardiol 31:1–6, 1973.
2. **Morrow AG, Epstein SE, Rodgers BM, et al:** Idiopathic hypertrophic subaortic stenosis: a current assessment of the results of operative treatment. In, Hypertrophic Obstructive Cardiomyopathy (Wolstenholme GEW, O'Connor M, ed). London, J & A Churchill, 1971, p 140–149
3. **Tajik AJ, Giuliani ER, Frye RL, et al:** Idiopathic hypertrophic subaortic stenosis (IHSS); results of long-term surgical follow-up (abstr). Amer J Cardiol 31:161, 1973
4. **Barratt-Boyes BG, O'Brien KP:** Surgical treatment of idiopathic hypertrophic subaortic stenosis using a combined left ventricular-aortic approach. In Ref 2, p 150–159
5. **Adelman AG, Wigle ED, Ranganathan N, et al:** The clinical course in muscular subaortic stenosis. A retrospective and prospective study of 60 hemodynamically proved cases. Ann Intern Med 77:515–525, 1972
6. **Cooley DA, Bloodwell RD, Hallman GL, et al:** Surgical treatment of muscular subaortic stenosis. Results from septectomy in twenty-six patients. Circulation 35 & 36: suppl I: I-124–I-132, 1967
7. **Rockoff SD, Ross J Jr, Oldham NN Jr, et al:** Ventriculo-atrial regurgitation following prosthetic replacement of the mitral valve. Angiocardiographic and hemodynamic findings. Amer J Cardiol 17:817–824, 1966
8. **Morrow AG, Roberts WC, Ross J Jr, et al:** Obstruction to left ventricular outflow. Current concepts of management and operative treatment. Ann Intern Med 69:1255–1286, 1968
9. **Ewy GA, Marcus FI, Bohajalian O, et al:** Muscular subaortic stenosis. Clinical and pathologic observations in an elderly patient. Amer J Cardiol 22:126–132, 1968
10. **Roberts WC:** Pathologic aspects of valvular and subvalvular (discrete and diffuse) aortic stenosis. In, The Natural History and Progress in Treatment of Congenital Heart Defects. An International Symposium Sponsored by the Ontario Heart Foundation in Cooperation with the Hospital for Sick Children and the University of Toronto (Kidd BSL, Keith JD, ed). Springfield, Ill, Charles C Thomas, 1971, p 221
11. **Roberts WC, Perloff JK:** Mitral valvular disease. A clini-

copathologic survey of the conditions causing the mitral valve to function abnormally. Ann Intern Med 77:939–975, 1972
12. **Roberts WC:** Valvular, subvalvular, and supravalvular aortic stenosis: morphologic features. Cardiovasc Clin 7:140–121, 1973
13. **Roberts WC, Dangel JC, Bulkley BH:** Non-rheumatic valvular cardiac disease. A clinico-pathologic survey of 27 different conditions causing valvular dysfunction. Cardiovasc Clin 5:332–446, 1973
14. **Adelman, AG, McLoughlin MJ, Marquis Y, et al:** Left ventricular cineangiographic observations in muscular subaortic stenosis. Amer J Cardiol 24:689–697, 1969
15. **Braunwald E, Lambrew CT, Rockoff SD, et al:** Idiopathic hypertrophic subaortic stenosis: I. A description of the disease based upon an analysis of 64 patients. Suppl. to Circulation 29 & 30: suppl IV: IV-3–IV-119, 1964
16. **Hawe A, Frye RL, Ellis FH Jr:** Late hemodynamic studies after mitral valve surgery. J Thorac Cardiovasc Surg 65:351–358, 1973
17. **Stewart S, Mason DT, Braunwald E:** Impaired rate of left ventricular filling in idiopathic hypertrophic subaortic stenosis and valvular aortic stenosis. Circulation 37:8–14, 1968
18. **Levine FH, Copeland JG, Morrow AG:** Prosthetic replacement of the mitral valve: continuing assessments of the 100 patients operated upon during 1961–1965. Circulation 47:518–526, 1973
19. **Frank S, Braunwald E:** Idiopathic hypertrophic subaortic stenosis. Clinical analysis of 126 patients with emphasis on the natural history. Circulation 37:759–788, 1968
20. **Henry WL, Clark CE, Epstein SE:** Asymmetric septal hypertrophy. Echocardiographic identification of the pathognomonic anatomic abnormality of IHSS. Circulation 47:225–233, 1973
21. **Roberts WC, Ferrans VJ:** The pathologic anatomy of the cardiomyopathies (idiopathic dilated and hypertrophic types, infiltrative types and endomyocardial disease with and without eosinophilia). Circ Res: suppl: in press
22. **Ferrans VJ, Morrow AG, Roberts WC:** Myocardial ultrastructure in idiopathic hypertrophic subaortic stenosis. A study of operatively excised left ventricular tract muscle in 14 patients. Circulation 45:769–792, 1972

Differences in Distribution of Myocardial Abnormalities in Patients with Obstructive and Nonobstructive Asymmetric Septal Hypertrophy (ASH)

Light and Electron Microscopic Findings

By Barry J. Maron, M.D., Victor J. Ferrans, M.D., Ph.D., Walter L. Henry, M.D., Chester E. Clark, M.D., David R. Redwood, M.D., William C. Roberts, M.D., Andrew G. Morrow, M.D., and Stephen E. Epstein, M.D.

SUMMARY

Previous studies have shown that abnormal cellular morphology is present in the ventricular septum of patients with asymmetric septal hypertrophy (ASH). The present study was undertaken to determine whether these morphologic abnormalities are limited to the ventricular septum of patients with ASH or are more diffusely distributed throughout the heart, and whether different patterns of distribution of the cellular abnormalities exist in patients with and patients without left ventricular outflow obstruction. Myocardium was obtained at operation or necropsy from 22 patients, including 14 with obstructive and eight with non-obstructive ASH, and studied by both light and electron microscopy. Many hypertrophied, bizarrely shaped, and abnormally arranged cardiac muscle cells, presumably a morphologic manifestation of the genetically transmitted myocardial defect in ASH, were present in the ventricular septum of all patients. In patients with obstructive ASH, these abnormalities were either absent or rarely found in muscle from the left and right ventricular free walls. This observation suggests that functional limitation in these patients is due largely to left ventricular outflow obstruction. In contrast, numerous disorganized cells were extensively distributed in the left and right ventricular feee walls from seven of eight symptomatic patients with non-obstructive ASH, suggesting that these abnormalities probably contribute importantly to functional impairment in such patients.

Additional Indexing Words:

Ultrastructure | Idiopathic hypertrophic subaortic stenosis | Myocardium | Hypertrophic cardiomyopathy | Ventricular hypertrophy

ASYMMETRIC septal hypertrophy (ASH) comprises a disease spectrum in which only some patients have obstruction to left ventricular outflow under basal conditions; in most patients, however, obstruction is absent.[1, 2] Despite this hemodynamic difference, virtually all patients with this disease have disproportionate hypertrophy of the ventricular septum with respect to the posterobasal left ventricular wall.[1-4]

Light and electron microscopic studies have demonstrated that the ventricular septum in patients with ASH and left ventricular outflow obstruction contains many hypertrophied, bizarrely shaped, and abnormally arranged cardiac muscle cells.[5-7] Because these histologic abnormalities are present only rarely in other forms of heart disease,[5, 8] we believe that this bizarre cardiac architecture may be a manifestation of the genetically transmitted[9] myocardial defect in ASH. Furthermore, it has been suggested that the left ventricular free wall thickening present in some patients indicates that the myocardial disorder is diffusely distributed in the heart.[10] This concept has led some investigators to view the role of operative intervention, even in patients who have obstruction, with extreme skepticism.[11] On the other hand, it has been shown that operation is of benefit to virtually all patients with ASH and obstruction,[12] suggesting that the myocardial defect in these patients is not diffuse.

In order to resolve this controversy, and to define further the extent and severity of myocardial abnormalities in the hearts of patients with obstructive and

From the Cardiology Branch, Section of Pathology and Clinic of Surgery, National Heart and Lung Institute, Bethesda, Maryland.

Address for reprints: Dr. Barry J. Maron, Cardiology Branch, National Heart and Lung Institute, Bldg. 10, Room 7B-15, Bethesda, Maryland 20014.

Received November 1, 1973; revision accepted for publication April 3, 1974.

nonobstructive ASH, two studies were undertaken. The first study, which forms the basis of this communication, describes the distribution of morphologic abnormalities in the heart by light and electron microscopy. The second study[13] describes the distribution of wall thickening as determined by echocardiography and by examination of necropsy specimens.

Methods

Patient Selection

The morphologic studies reported in this communication were made on myocardium obtained from 22 patients with ASH. The diagnosis of ASH (i.e., the ratio of the thickness of the ventricular septum to that of the posterobasal left ventricular wall is greater than 1.3) was established in all 22 patients by echocardiography,[1] necropsy examination, or both. Patients were selected for operation (left ventricular myotomy-myectomy) if they had cardiac symptoms sufficient to produce significant functional limitation (New York Heart Association functional classes 3 or 4) and did not respond adequately to propranolol.

Clinical and hemodynamic data from the patients (12 men and ten women; aged 8 to 67 years) are summarized in table 1. Measurements of the peak systolic pressure gradient between left ventricle and a systemic artery were obtained in all patients under basal conditions and during provocative interventions (Valsalva maneuver or administration of isoproterenol). Patients were divided into three groups on the basis of the magnitude of the gradient: 1) *Obstructed group:* any gradient present under basal conditions. This group includes 12 patients with gradients of 65 to 162 mm Hg under basal conditions; 2) *Provocable obstruction group:* no basal gradient but provocable gradients greater than 30 mm Hg. This group includes two patients who had no gradients under basal conditions but developed gradients greater than 30 mm Hg after provocative maneuvers; 3) *Nonobstructed group:* no pressure gradient under basal conditions and a provocable peak gradient of less than 30 mm Hg. This group includes eight patients.

None of the patients without obstruction had had clinical evidence of obstruction prior to the time of cardiac catheterization (i.e., murmurs louder than grade II were not described and carotid tracings did not demonstrate the typical bisferious contour characteristic of most patients with obstruction). Mitral regurgitation was demonstrated by angiocardiogram in seven patients (severe in patient #18,

Table 1

Clinical and Hemodynamic Data in 22 Patients with ASH

				Pressures (mm Hg)						
				PA	RV	LV	Aorta	PSG		CI
Pt. no.	Age	Sex	FC	(S/D)	(S/D)	(S/D)	(S/D)	Basal	Provoked	(L/min/m²)
1	47	M	3	32/15	32/5	190/12	125/75	65	150	—
2	44	M	3	22/10	22/6	180/11	110/75	70	90	1.8
3	61	M	3	36/14	38/8	190/24	115/70*	75	95	2.2
4	39	F	3	32/16	32/9	180/12	100/68	90	—	5.0
5	61	F	3	24/11	24/7	200/12	110/65	90	100	1.8
6	24	F	3	22/11	25/4	210/16	115/70	95	—	3.4
7	49	F	3	24/12	24/6	180/20	80/45	100	90	3.1
8	67	F	3	40/15	40/5	205/11	105/65	100	130	2.2
9	22	M	3	42/18	42/10	220/32	118/60	102	140	3.1
10	57	M	4	24/8	30/6	220/20	105/80	115	—	2.1
11†	34	F	3	23/12	20/3	160/18	85/50*	75	125	2.0
12†	19	F	3	62/12	28/20	260/20	98/75	162	—	—
13	18	M	3	—	—	130/12	130/92	0	70	3.8
14	59	M	3	22/12	24/6	135/12	135/75	0	70	1.7
	62§		3	55/10	70/11	140/24	140/55	0	10	—
15†	28	F	3	48/26	48/10	108/34	114/64*	0	6	—
	32		4	—	—	95/20	97/52*	0	0–34	2.3
16†	33	M	3	52/25	52/15	120/26	120/80*	0	29	2.0
17†	30	M	3	29/14	29/7	115/28	117/70*	0	17	2.4
18†	40	F	4	34/17	34/5	112/11	122/65*	0	0	1.6
19†	29	F	3	70/30	70/17	130/38	130/80	0	0	1.2
20‡	59	M	3	30/14	30/7	115/22	115/65	0	0	2.4
21¶	24	M	2	22/12	22/7	110/10	110/70	0	0	3.2
22†	8	M	3	90/55	90/27	90/34	105/60	0	—	1.6

*Brachial artery pressure.

†Died.

‡Associated coronary arterial disease.

§Ventricular septal defect (Pulmonary-to-systemic flow ratio = 2.4), which had been produced during the course of left ventricular myotomy-myectomy three years previously.

¶Pulmonary sarcoidosis demonstrated on open lung biopsy; myocardial biopsy showed no evidence of sarcoidosis.

Abbreviations: FC = functional class (New York Heart Association); PA = pulmonary artery; RV = right ventricle; S/D = systolic/diastolic; LV = left ventricle; PSG = peak systolic gradient; CI = cardiac index.

moderate in patients #2 and #20, and mild in patients #10, #14, #15, and #16). The period of time between cardiac catheterization and operative biopsy ranged from one week to 11 months (median, two months), and between cardiac catheterization and death (for the patients studied at necropsy) from one day to three years (median, four months).

Eight patients in this study had died; two of these had obstructive ASH (#11, #12) and the remaining six patients had nonobstructive ASH (#15–19, #22). Four patients (#11, #15, #17 and #22) died suddenly (presumably of their cardiac disease); three (#12, #18 and #19) died at operation, and one (#16) died of severe congestive heart failure and thromboemboli to the brain. In addition to ASH, one patient (#16) was found at necropsy to have severe coronary arterial luminal narrowing by atherosclerotic plaques.

Selection and Preparation of Tissue

In 14 patients myocardial biopsies were taken only at operation. In seven other patients myocardium was obtained only at necropsy and in one other patient (#19) myocardium was taken at both operation and necropsy.

Operative biopsies

In 12 patients myocardium was taken during the course of left ventricular myotomy-myectomy. Eleven of these patients had obstructive ASH. The other patient (#19) was severely symptomatic with nonobstructive ASH and continued to deteriorate rapidly in spite of intensive medical therapy; myotomy-myectomy was attempted to increase left ventricular compliance. Myocardium was obtained in the other three patients at the time of thoracotomy for other conditions: patient #21 had a diagnostic lung biopsy for suspected sarcoidosis; patient #20 had an aorto-coronary artery saphenous vein bypass operation for coexistent coronary arterial disease, and patient #14 underwent closure of a ventricular septal defect which had been produced during the course of left ventricular myotomy-myectomy three years previously.

The sites from which myocardial tissues were obtained included: the cephalad portion of the left side of the ventricular septum (12 patients); the cephalad portion of the right side of the ventricular septum (two patients); the left ventricular apex (13 patients); the left ventricular posterior wall, about halfway between the left ventricular apex and the atrioventricular groove (12 patients), and the right ventricular anterior wall, in the area of the outflow tract (seven patients).

In patients undergoing left ventricular myotomy-myectomy, tissue (about 10 x 10 x 15 mm) was resected from the ventricular septum after 20 to 40 min of cardiopulmonary bypass and after a period of 10 to 12 min of cardiac arrest. During the latter period the aorta was clamped, the heart was cooled to approximately 30°C, and the coronary arteries were not perfused.

Biopsies from the left and right ventricular free walls were obtained after 2 to 5 min of cardiopulmonary bypass but before institution of cardiac arrest. Cylindrical biopsies (about 2 x 10 mm), representing either approximately three-fourths of the thickness or the full thickness of the ventricular wall, were obtained by epicardial puncture of the left ventricular posterior wall and right ventricular anterior wall with a 14 gauge Vim-Silverman biopsy needle (modified Franklin type) having a 16 gauge split inner cannula. Biopsies of the left ventricular apex (about 3 x 4 x 5 mm) were taken with a scalpel.

The myocardial specimens were immediately fixed with cold 3% glutaraldehyde in 0.1 M phosphate buffer, pH 7.2. After washing with several changes of cold 5% sucrose in 0.1 M phosphate buffer, pH 7.2, the tissues were post-fixed with 1% osmium tetroxide in Millonig's phosphate buffer, pH 7.2, dehydrated with a graded series of ethanols and propylene oxide and embedded in Maraglas.[14] Semithin (0.5 μ thick) sections were cut from all tissue blocks from each biopsy, stained with alkaline toluidine blue, and examined by light microscopy. Five to 40 semithin sections, each measuring 1-4 mm^2 in area, were available from each biopsy for analysis. Final choice of tissue areas for electron microscopic study was limited to those areas that contained artifact-free, longitudinally oriented muscle cells. Ultrathin sections were stained with uranyl acetate and lead citrate and examined with an RCA EMU-3G electron microscope.

Necropsy Specimens

Myocardium was obtained at necropsy from eight patients, including six with nonobstructive ASH and two with obstructive ASH. In each patient, multiple blocks of myocardium were taken from the full thickness of the ventricular septum, the left ventricular anterior and posterior walls, and the right ventricular anterior wall. Tissue was sectioned at 6 μ thickness and stained with hematoxylin and eosin.

Microscopic Analysis

The pattern of arrangement of cardiac muscle cells was analyzed by light and electron microscopy (electron microscopic analysis was not performed on the necropsy specimens) and rated independently by two investigators (B. J. M. and V. J. F.) according to the grading system presented in table 2. The purposes of this assessment were to determine whether or not cardiac muscle cells in a given area of tissue were normal in shape and normally aligned with respect to each other; i.e., arranged in parallel and connected at their ends by intercellular junctions (intercalated discs). For this reason, evaluation of cellular arrangement was limited to cardiac muscle cells in longitudinal or slightly oblique sections. Transverse diameters of muscle cells were measured from sections of biopsy tissue with a calibrated micrometer eyepiece. Measurements were made on 35 to 50 longitudinally oriented muscle cells and the average of these measurements was used to define the cell diameters characteristic of each biopsy.

Results

Arrangement, Size, and Shape of Cardiac Muscle Cells in the Ventricular Septum

The morphology of cardiac muscle cells from the ventricular septum was indistinguishable in patients with or without left ventricular outflow tract obstruction and corresponded to that previously described[5] in patients with obstructive ASH (typical IHSS). Many of the cells in the ventricular septum demonstrated great variation in size and were irregularly shaped (figs. 1–4); many were markedly enlarged, with transverse diameters ranging from 10 to 70 μ (average 28 μ; normal 10–15 μ). Multiple intercalated discs, presumably representing lateral cytoplasmic processes

Table 2

*Morphologic Assessment of Cellular Arrangement in 22 Patients with ASH**

Patient #	VS	LV PW	LV APEX	RV ANT
		ASH with Obstruction		
1	1+	0	0	0
2	1+	0	0	0†
3	1+	0	0	0§
4	2+	—	0	—
5	1+	0†	0†	0†
6	2+	—	0	—
7	2+	0	0†	—
8	2+	0	0†	—
9	2+	—	0	—
10	1+	0	0	0
11‡	2+	0†	—	0
12‡	2+	0§	—	0
		ASH with Provocable Obstruction		
13	1+	0	0	—
14	1+	1+	0	0†
		ASH Without Obstruction		
15‡	2+	2+	—	2+
16‡	2+	2+	—	2+
17‡	2+	2+	—	2+
18‡	2+	2+	—	2+
19¶	2+	2+	2+	2+
20	1+	0	—	—
21	—	1+	—	—
22‡	2+	2+	—	2+

*Grading system: 0 = normal cellular arrangement; 1+ = mild to moderate disorganization of cells; 2+ = severe disorganization of cells; — = not examined.

†Myofibrillar and/or myofilament disarray present which involved only a few cells of a tissue block area. Muscle cells were hypertrophied but normally arranged.

‡Necropsy data.

§Small, rare foci of hypertrophied, bizarrely shaped, and disoriented cardiac muscle cells; all other cells were hypertrophied but normally arranged.

¶Necropsy and biopsy data.

Abbreviations: VS = ventricular septum; PW = posterior wall; LV = left ventricle; RV = right ventricle; ANT = anterior.

of muscle cells,[15] were common. Adjacent muscle cells often demonstrated loss of their normal parallel relation and were arranged obliquely or perpendicularly to each other. In some areas, however, the muscle cells were hypertrophied and rectangularly shaped in longitudinal section, were arranged in parallel and were connected predominantly by end-to-end intercellular junctions. The observations on arrangement of muscle cells are summarized in table 2.

In addition, in five patients small bundles of hypertrophied but otherwise normally appearing cardiac muscle cells coursed in a disorderly fashion through larger normally arranged bundles (fig. 5). These abnormally arranged muscle bundles were, however,

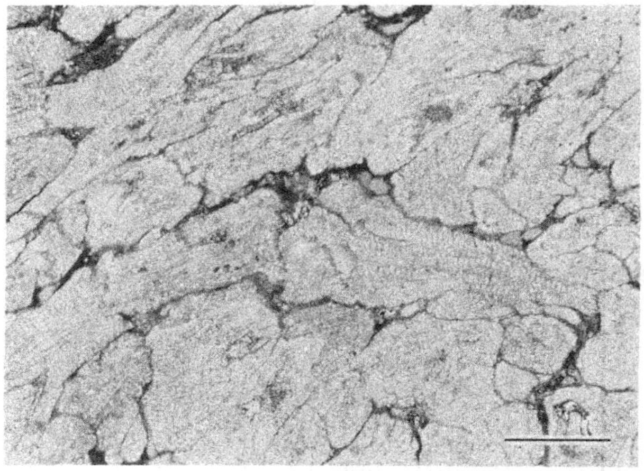

Figure 1

Light micrograph of semithin section of myocardium from the ventricular septum of patient #19 with nonobstructive ASH. Muscle cells are hypertrophied, irregularly shaped, and oriented in different directions. Alkaline toluidine blue stain. X 335. Scale bar = 40 μ.

rare features of the hearts of patients with ASH, when compared with the commonly observed bizarrely shaped and disorganized cardiac muscle cells.

Arrangement, Size, and Shape of Cardiac Muscle Cells in the Left and Right Ventricular Free Walls

The morphology of cardiac muscle cells in the ventricular free walls differed distinctly in patients with obstruction compared to those without obstruction (table 2).

ASH with obstruction

In the 12 patients having ASH and left ventricular outflow obstruction, the vast majority of muscle cells

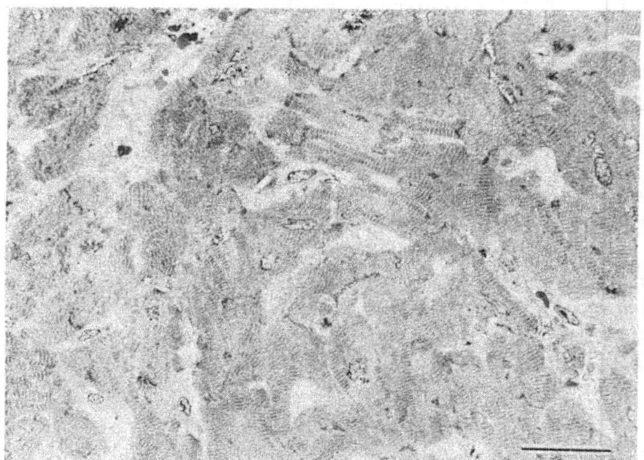

Figure 2

Light micrograph of semithin section from the ventricular septum of patient #19. Muscle cells and myofibrils are arranged obliquely and perpendicularly to each other. Alkaline toluidine blue stain. X 400. Scale bar = 50 μ.

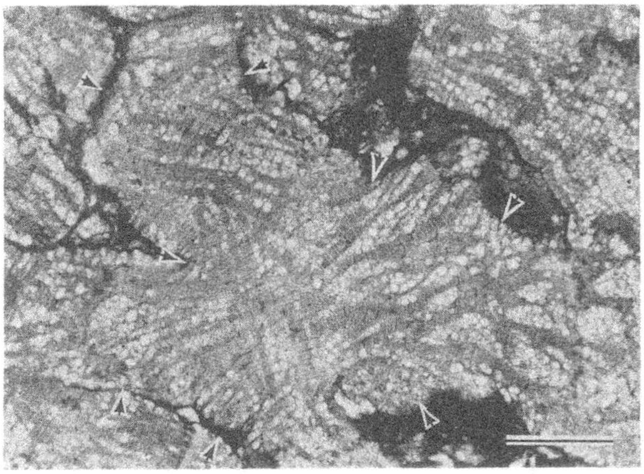

Figure 3

Light micrograph of semithin section from ventricular septum of patient #4 with obstructive ASH. A hypertrophied, stellate-shaped muscle cell with obliquely and transversely oriented myofibrils is shown in the center. The outline of this cell is indicated by arrowheads. Compare with figure 11 which shows an electron micrograph of a similar area. Alkaline toluidine blue stain. X 675. Scale bar = 20 μ.

from the left and right ventricular free walls did not show the bizarre shapes or severe malalignment characteristic of cells in the ventricular septum. Cells from the ventricular free walls usually appeared rectangular in longitudinal section and were relatively uniform in size and shape (figs. 6–8). These cells, however, were hypertrophied with transverse cell diameters ranging from 10 to 66 μ (average 28 μ). The degree of cellular enlargement did not differ in the left ventricular apex, left ventricular posterior wall, or ventricular septum. Muscle cells from the right ventricular free wall ranged from 10 to 45 μ (average 23 μ) in diameter. Cardiac muscle cells from the left ventricular free wall of five patients with moderate to severe aortic valvular stenosis (gradients of 40 to 90 mm Hg) were studied for comparison and showed transverse cell diameters of 13 to 70 μ (average 28 μ). Of the 12 patients with ASH and left ventricular outflow obstruction, only two (#3 and #12) demonstrated rare, small foci of hypertrophied, abnormally arranged cardiac muscle cells in the left or right ventricular free walls.

ASH Without Obstruction

In seven of the eight patients having ASH without outflow obstruction, the majority of cardiac muscle cells from the left and right ventricular free walls were hypertrophied, bizarrely shaped, and abnormally arranged (figs. 9, 10). Some cardiac muscle cells from these seven hearts were hypertrophied but regularly shaped and normally arranged. The remaining patient (#20) was severely symptomatic but had coexisting coronary arterial disease; this patient had large, abnormally arranged cardiac muscle cells in a biopsy specimen from the ventricular septum but normally arranged cells in a biopsy from the left ventricular posterior wall.

The transverse diameters of cells from the left ventricular posterior wall in patients with nonobstructive ASH were increased, ranging from 10 to 63 μ (average 33 μ). The right ventricular muscle cells also were greatly enlarged (average transverse diameter 37 μ) in patient #19 with nonobstructive ASH and severe pulmonary arterial hypertension.

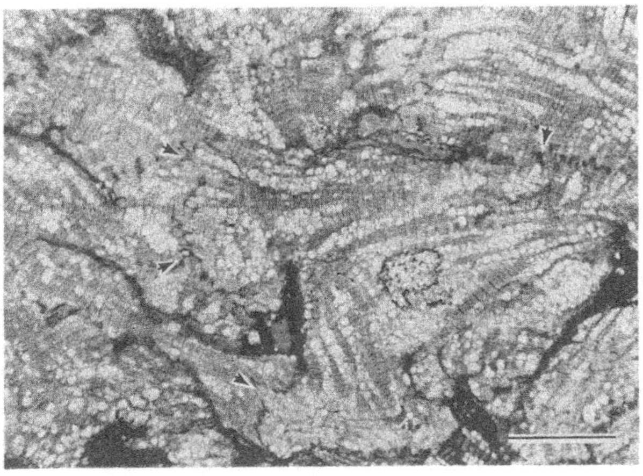

Figure 4

Light micrograph of semithin section from ventricular septum of patient #4 with obstructive ASH. The hypertrophied, bizarrely shaped cardiac muscle cell in the center has disorganized myofibrils and forms intercellular connections (arrowheads) with several adjacent cells. Alkaline toluidine blue stain. X 675. Scale bar = 20 μ.

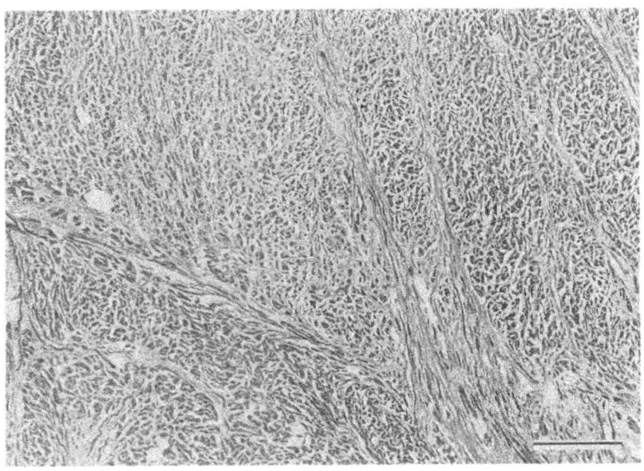

Figure 5

Light micrograph of ventricular septum from patient #17 with nonobstructive ASH. Several small bundles of cardiac muscle cells associated with connective tissue elements course in a disorderly fashion through larger, normally arranged bundles of cells. Hematoxylin and eosin stain. X 20. Scale bar = 500 μ.

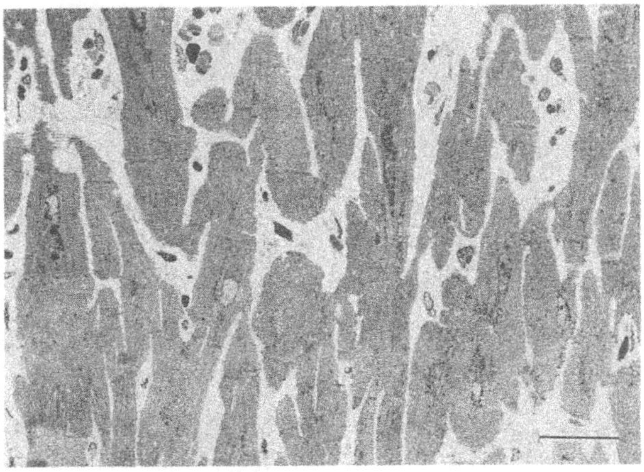

Figure 6

Light micrograph of semithin section from right ventricular free wall of patient #1 with obstructive ASH. The mildly hypertrophied muscle cells have a parallel arrangement and are joined by end-to-end intercellular junctions. Compare with figure 7 which shows an electron micrograph of a similar area. Alkaline toluidine blue stain. X 200. Scale bar = 50 μ.

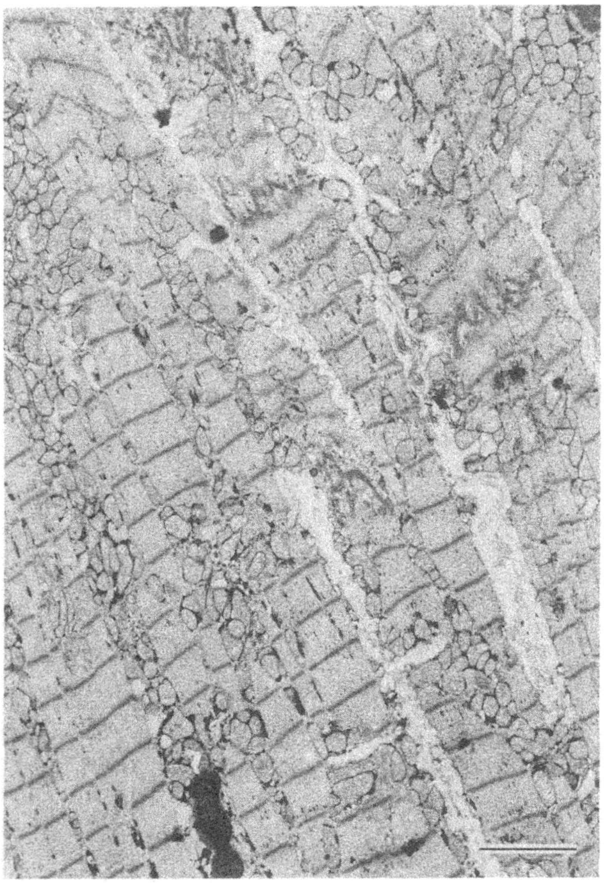

Figure 7

Low power electron micrograph of parts of two muscle cells in the left ventricular posterior wall from patient #8 with obstructive ASH. There are minimal irregularities in cell shapes but the myofibrils are normally arranged. Compare with figure 6 which shows a light micrograph of a similar area. X 4200. Scale bar = 3 μ.

ASH with Provocable Obstruction

In one of the two patients (#13) in this intermediate category, abnormally arranged muscle cells were found in the ventricular septum but not in a left ventricular free wall biopsy. In the other patient (#14), however, large, bizarrely shaped, and disorganized cardiac muscle cells were present in biopsy specimens from both the ventricular septum and left ventricular posterior wall.

Arrangement of Myofibrils and Myofilaments in the Ventricular Septum and Ventricular Free Walls

In six of the 12 patients with obstructive ASH and six of the eight patients with nonobstructive ASH,

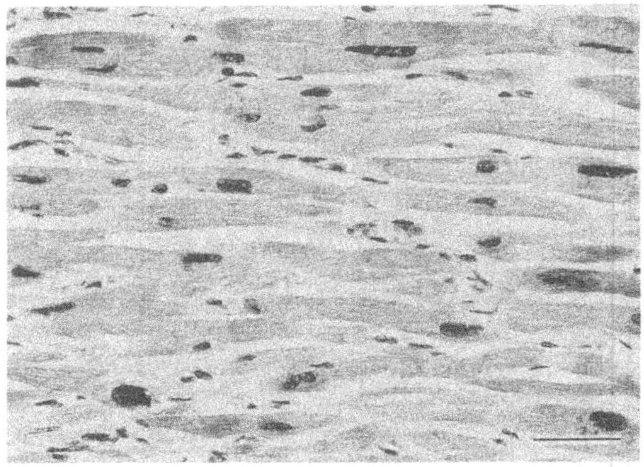

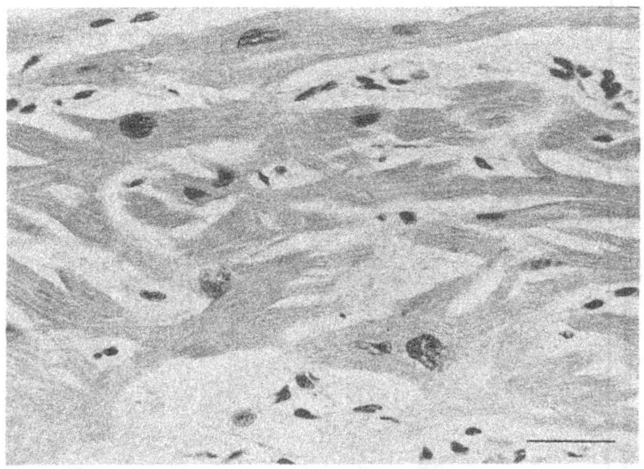

Figure 8 (top)

Light micrograph of the left ventricular free wall of patient #12 with obstructive ASH. The muscle cells are hypertrophied, regularly shaped, and normally arranged. Hematoxylin and eosin stain. X 225. Scale bar = 50 μ.

Figure 9 (bottom)

Light micrograph of left ventricular free wall of patient #16 with nonobstructive ASH. Muscle cells are irregularly shaped and arranged obliquely and perpendicularly to each other. Hematoxylin and eosin stain. X 225. Scale bar = 50 μ.

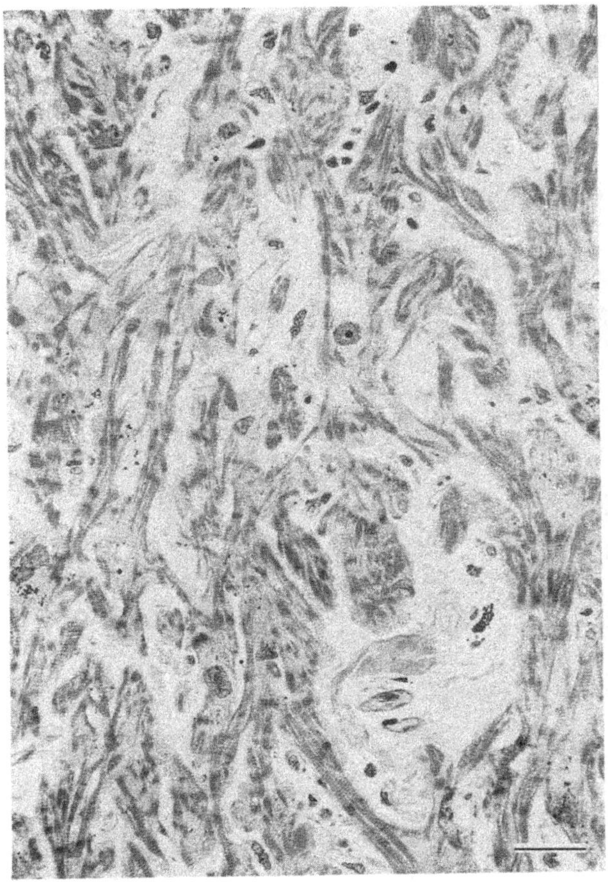

Figure 10

Light micrograph of semithin section from left ventricular posterior wall of patient #19 with nonobstructive ASH. The muscle cells have bizarre shapes and are markedly disorganized. Alkaline toluidine blue stain. X 200. Scale bar = 50 μ.

many of the bizarrely shaped muscle cells from the ventricular septum contained myofibrils that showed marked disarray. Adjacent myofibrils were oriented obliquely or perpendicularly to each other (figs. 2–4, 9, 11, 12). In the left and right ventricular free walls, disorganized myofibrils were often found in hypertrophied, abnormally arranged cardiac muscle cells of three patients with nonobstructive ASH and occasionally in hypertrophied, normally arranged muscle cells of four patients with obstructive ASH and one patient with provocable obstruction (table 2). In addition, myofilaments commonly originated from the Z band of one myofibril and inserted into the Z bands of other myofibrils (fig. 12).

Alterations in Other Cellular Components

Several other ultrastructural abnormalities were identified in myocardium from the ventricular septum and ventricular free walls in the 15 patients with operative biopsies. The extent and severity of these additional abnormalities did not differ in patients with obstructive ASH, ASH with provocable obstruction, or nonobstructive ASH.

Abnormalities in Z *band* structure were present in muscle from 12 patients and were generally most prominent in the ventricular septum. These abnormalities consisted of widening and spreading of Z bands (fig. 12) and increased amounts of Z band-like material at points of attachment of myofibrils to intercellular junctions (intercalated discs). These alterations in Z band structure were of the type considered suggestive of the formation of new sarcomeres.[16]

Mitochondrial damage was present in 14 patients and consisted of swelling of mitochondria and disruption of cristae. These abnormalities were more marked in the ventricular septum than in the left ventricular free walls in 11 of the 14 patients, and may have been due to the cardiac arrest under hypothermic and hypoxic conditions.[17]

Markedly convoluted *intercellular junctions* (intercalated discs) were a consistent finding in biopsies from all 15 patients. Side-to-side intercellular junctions were present instead of, or in addition to, the more usual end-to-end junctions of muscle cells in seven patients. These side-to-side junctions were usually seen in muscle cells from the ventricular septum in areas of myofibrillar disarray. Areas of separation of the plasma membranes of the undifferentiated segments of intercellular junctions were present in 12 patients (fig. 13). These abnormalities, which resemble those described in other forms of cardiac hypertrophy,[18] were more marked in the left and right ventricular walls than in the ventricular septum in 11 of the 12 patients.

In 11 of the 15 patients, all *glycogen* granules in cardiac muscle cells were in the usual monoparticulate β-form (diameter 225 to 375 Å); in the other four patients, some glycogen particles were in the form of large rosettes (α-glycogen) with diameters of 1300 to 2400 Å.[19]

Dilatation of the *transverse tubular system* was present in 11 of the 15 patients and was most prominent in the left ventricular wall in seven patients (fig. 14). The *sarcoplasmic reticulum* was normal in hypertrophied cardiac muscle cells from all patients. A few markedly enlarged *nuclei* with bizarre convolutions of the nuclear membrane were found in biopsies from all patients and were most common in the ventricular septum. *Ribosomes* were present in increased numbers in most cells from both the ventricular septum and ventricular free walls, and were usually free in perinuclear areas, between myofibrils and near intercellular junctions as well as attached to the membranes of the sarcoplasmic reticulum. *Lipofuscin*

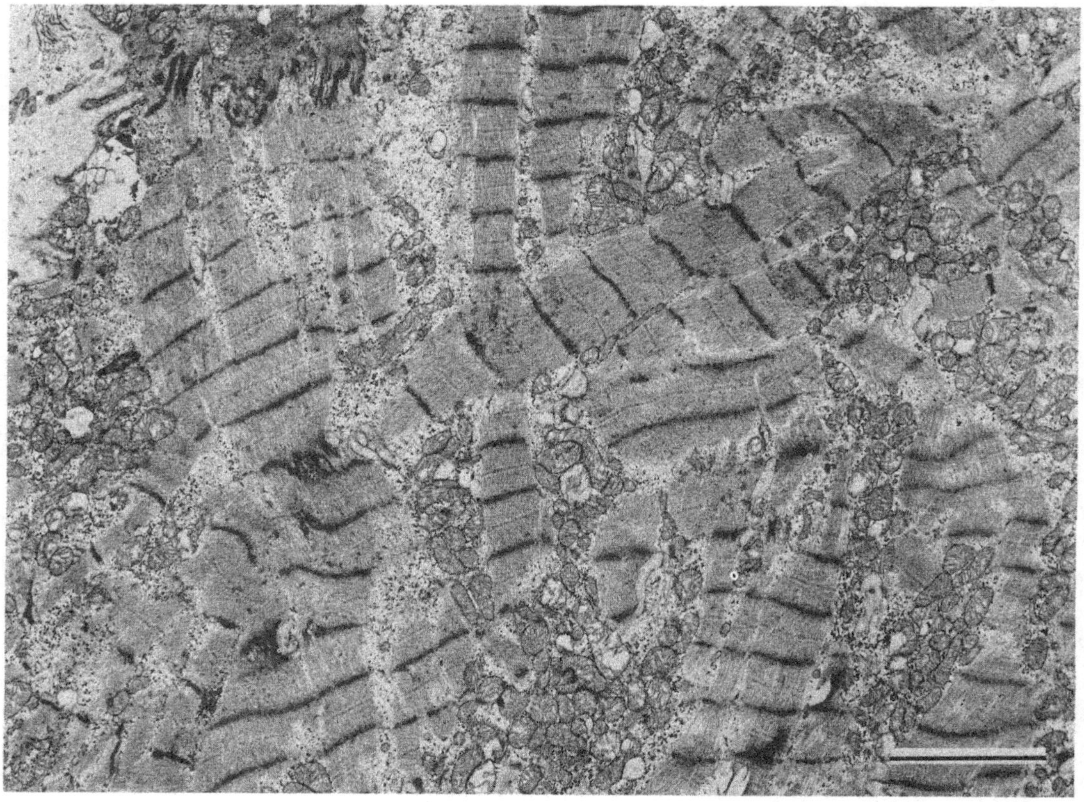

Figure 11

Electron micrograph of part of a cardiac muscle cell showing an area of myofibrillar disarray. Compare with figure 3 which shows a light micrograph of a similar area. Ventricular septum from patient #8 with obstructive ASH. X 5,900. Scale bar = 4 μ.

granules were increased in number in all hearts. Variable amounts of *interstitial fibrosis*, characterized by increased numbers of mature and developing collagen fibrils, were present in myocardium from the ventricular septum and ventricular free walls of all patients.

Degenerated cardiac muscle cells were present in the ventricular septum or left ventricular free wall in six patients. These cells were usually present in areas of fibrosis and often appeared isolated, having no contact with other muscle cells. These degenerated cells demonstrated the following features: preferential loss of thick myofilaments; accumulations of abnormal Z band-like material attached to thin myofilaments; decreased numbers of myofibrils and T tubules; many small mitochondria; proliferation and dilatation of sarcoplasmic reticulum; and thickening of the basement membranes.[20] Cardiac muscle cells of this type are not unique to ASH but are also seen in left ventricular myocardium from patients with aortic valvular stenosis and/or regurgitation.[20]

Discussion

This investigation confirms the data of previous studies[5-7] showing that cardiac muscle cells which are hypertrophied, bizarrely shaped, and abnormally arranged are invariably present in the ventricular septum of patients with ASH and left ventricular outflow tract obstruction. The observations in this communication further demonstrate that these cells also are found in the ventricular septum of patients without obstruction. The occurrence of these cells in patients with ASH and no present or previous evidence of outflow obstruction suggests that high ventricular pressure is not the primary mechanism responsible for their unusual morphologic features or their increased size. Moreover, cells with these characteristics are rarely found in patients with cardiac hypertrophy from causes other than ASH. For example, we have observed foci of bizarrely shaped and abnormally arranged cardiac muscle cells in some patients with congenital heart diseases associated with right ventricular outflow tract obstruction[8] (and unpublished observations), but have not observed these cells in patients with congestive cardiomyopathies or in patients with left ventricular hypertrophy due to aortic valvular disease. Thus, it appears reasonable to assume that these hypertrophied, bizarrely shaped,

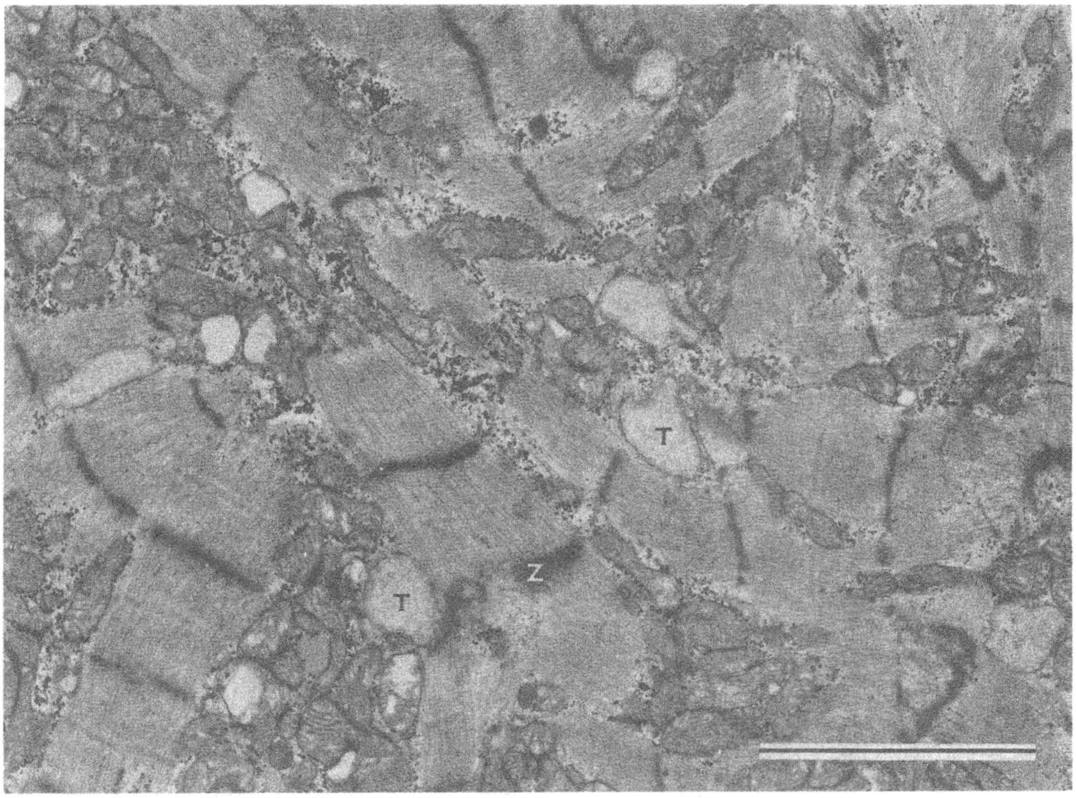

Figure 12

Electron micrograph of part of a cardiac muscle cell showing marked disorganization of myofibrils and myofilaments, thickening of some of the Z bands (Z) and mild dilatation of T tubules (T). Ventricular septal muscle from patient #8 with obstructive ASH. X 13,400. Scale bar = 2 μ.

and disorganized cardiac muscle cells, while not an absolutely specific finding in patients with

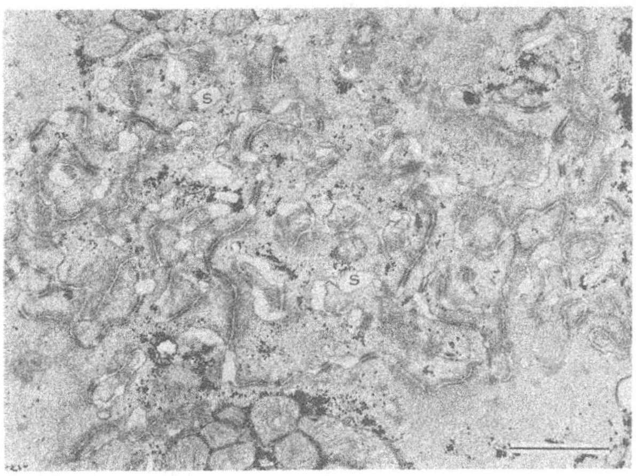

Figure 13

Electron micrograph showing a markedly convoluted intercellular junction (intercalated disc) between two hypertrophied cardiac muscle cells. There are prominent areas of separations (S) of the plasma membranes of the undifferentiated areas of the intercellular junction. Left ventricular posterior wall from patient #5 with obstructive ASH. X 12,300. Scale bar = 1 μ.

ASH,[5, 8] are morphologic manifestations of a genetically transmitted myocardial defect.

Although all patients with either obstructive or non-obstructive ASH have this cellular abnormality in the

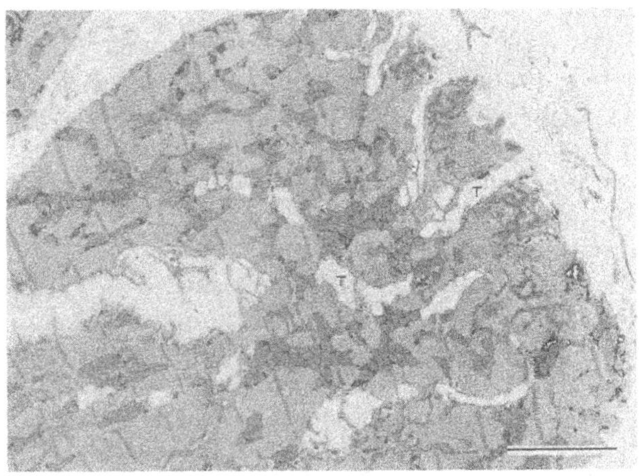

Figure 14

Electron micrograph showing parts of several cardiac muscle cells with dilated T tubules (T) and thickened basement membranes. Left ventricular posterior wall from patient #5 with obstructive ASH. X 4,600. Scale bar = 3 μ.

ventricular septum, the distribution of these bizarre cells in other areas of myocardium is markedly different in these two groups of patients. The abnormal cardiac muscle cells were distributed widely in the left and right ventricular free walls of symptomatic patients with nonobstructive ASH. In contrast, these bizarre cells were absent or rarely found in the left and right ventricular free walls of symptomatic patients with ASH who had outflow obstruction. In fact, the majority of cardiac muscle cells found in tissue sections from the left ventricular free wall of patients with obstructive ASH were indistinguishable from those hypertrophied and normally arranged cardiac muscle cells present in the left ventricular free wall of patients with fixed left ventricular outflow obstruction. This observation suggests that the hypertrophy present in the left ventricular free wall of patients with obstructive ASH is due to high ventricular pressures. It should be emphasized that these morphologic observations were made primarily in severely symptomatic patients; therefore, it is possible that the bizarrely shaped and maloriented cardiac muscle cells are not as widely distributed in the hearts of asymptomatic patients with nonobstructive ASH. Indeed, the one patient with nonobstructive ASH and mild symptoms (patient #21) had only mild disorganization of muscle cells in the left ventricular posterior wall.

Two patients (#13 and #14) in this study had no outflow obstruction under basal conditions, but had large gradients after provocative interventions. Hypertrophied, bizarrely shaped, and abnormally arranged muscle cells were present in a biopsy from the left ventricular posterior wall of one of these two patients, while no abnormal cells were present in the left ventricular free wall biopsies from the other patient. Definitive conclusions cannot be drawn from the data of this small subgroup of patients. It is interesting to speculate, however, that the left ventricular free wall in patients with provocable gradients may be involved by cellular abnormalities that are intermediate in extent between those found in patients with outflow obstruction under basal conditions and in patients without outflow obstruction.

Some normally or abnormally oriented cardiac muscle cells from patients with ASH showed intracellular abnormalities such as disarray of myofibrils and myofilaments. Such morphologic abnormalities are relatively nonspecific findings, since they occur in patients with other forms of ventricular hypertrophy in which bizarrely shaped and disorganized cells are not present.[5, 21] Thus, the precise significance of myofibrillar and myofilament disarray in cardiac muscle cells of patients with ASH is presently unclear. In addition, we observed small muscle bundles (composed of hypertrophied, but otherwise normal cells) coursing in a disorderly fashion through larger, normally arranged bundles. These bundles, although distinctive in appearance, were an inconsistent and uncommon feature of the hearts studied; the relation of these muscle bundles to the genetically transmitted myocardial defect in ASH is uncertain.

The bizarrely shaped and abnormally arranged cardiac muscle cells present in patients with ASH were greatly hypertrophied, having transverse diameters ranging from 10–70 μ (average of 28 μ). Cells present in the left ventricular free wall of patients with obstructive ASH or severe aortic valvular stenosis, however, also had transverse diameters within the same range. Although these data suggest that the degree of hypertrophy of the muscle cells is the same in ASH and in fixed left ventricular outflow obstruction, we do not believe that this is actually the case. We consider that the measurement of transverse diameter is a poor index of cell size when cells are stellate shaped rather than cylindrical. Indeed, we had the distinct impression that the area (in contrast to the transverse diameter) of the bizarrely shaped cells characteristic of ASH was considerably greater than that of the hypertrophied cells present in patients with fixed left ventricular outflow obstruction.

The biopsy technique employed in this study yielded a relatively small amount of tissue and thus the possibility of a sampling error must be considered. Indeed, other investigators have shown that the abnormal muscle cells in patients with ASH are irregularly distributed within the heart[5, 22] and may be found predominantly in the middle layer of the ventricular septum and ventricular free walls.[23] The morphologic characteristics of the cardiac muscle cells from tissue removed at operation in this study were, however, remarkably consistent within each of the two groups of patients (obstructive and nonobstructive ASH). More importantly, the morphologic findings in the necropsy specimens, in which multiple full thickness blocks from different areas of the ventricular walls were examined, were similar to those in the operative biopsies. Thus, it appears unlikely that the biopsy data were significantly influenced by sampling error.

In conclusion, our observations indicate that hypertrophied, bizarrely shaped, and disorganized cardiac muscle cells, presumably a morphologic manifestation of the myocardial defect in ASH, are invariably present in the ventricular septum of patients with nonobstructive and with obstructive ASH. These abnormal cells involve the ventricular free walls extensively in symptomatic patients with nonobstructive ASH and probably are responsible for functional impairment. In symptomatic patients with obstructive ASH, however, the abnormal cells are localized principally to the ventricular septum, an observation suggesting that the functional limitation in this group is due largely to left ventricular outflow tract obstruction.

References

1. Henry WL, Clark CE, Epstein SE: Asymmetric septal hypertrophy (ASH): Echocardiographic identification of the pathognomonic anatomic abnormality of IHSS. Circulation **47:** 225, 1973
2. Henry WL, Clark CE, Epstein SE: Asymmetric septal hypertrophy (ASH): The unifying link in the IHSS disease spectrum. Observations regarding its pathogenesis, pathophysiology and course. Circulation **47:** 827, 1973
3. Menges H, Brandenburg RO, Brown AL: The clinical, hemodynamic, and pathologic diagnosis of muscular subvalvular aortic stenosis. Circulation **24:** 1126, 1961
4. Roberts WC: Valvular, subvalvular, and supravalvular aortic stenosis: morphologic features. Cardiovasc Clin **5:** 104, 1973
5. Ferrans VJ, Morrow AG, Roberts WC: Myocardial ultrastructure in idiopathic hypertrophic subaortic stenosis. A study of operatively excised left ventricular outflow tract muscle in 14 patients. Circulation **45:** 769, 1972
6. Teare D: Asymmetrical hypertrophy of the heart in young adults. Br Heart J **20:** 1, 1958
7. Meesen H, Poche R: Beiträge zur pathologischen Anatomie der Fallotschen Fehler und zur idiopathischen Herzhypertrophie. Anglo-German Med Rev **4:** 73, 1967
8. Maron BJ, Ferrans VJ, White RI: Unusual evolution of infundibular stenosis in patients with ventricular septal defect: Clinical and morphologic observations. Circulation **48:** 1092, 1973
9. Clark CE, Henry WL, Epstein SE: Familial prevalence and genetic transmission of idiopathic hypertrophic subaortic stenosis. New Engl J Med **289:** 709, 1973
10. Goodwin JF, Oakley CM: The cardiomyopathies (Editorial). Br Heart J **34:** 545, 1972
11. Oakley CM: Hypertrophic obstructive cardiomyopathy: Patterns of progression. *In* Hypertrophic Obstructive Cardiomyopathy, CIBA Foundation Symposium, edited by Wolstenholme GEW, O'Connor M. London, J & A Churchill, 1971, p 9
12. Morrow AG, Epstein SE, Rodgers BM, Braunwald E: Idiopathic hypertrophic subaortic stenosis: A current assessment of the results of operative treatment. *In* Hypertrophic Obstructive Cardiomyopathy, CIBA Foundation Symposium, edited by Wolstenholme GEW, O'Connor M. London, J & A Churchill, 1971, p 140
13. Henry WL, Clark CE, Roberts WC, Morrow AG, Epstein SE: Differences in distribution of myocardial abnormalities in patients with obstructive and nonobstructive asymmetric septal hypertrophy (ASH): Echocardiographic and gross anatomic findings. Circulation, in press
14. Freeman J, Spurlock B: A new epoxy embedment for electron microscopy. J Cell Biol **13:** 437, 1962
15. Maron BJ, Ferrans VJ: Significance of multiple intercalated discs in hypertrophied human myocardium. Am J Pathol **73:** 81, 1973
16. Legato MJ: Sarcomerogenesis in human myocardium. J Molec Cell Cardiol **1:** 425, 1970
17. De Gasperis C, Miani A, Donatelli R: Ultrastructural changes in human myocardium associated with ischemic arrest. J Molec Cell Cardiol **1:** 169, 1970
18. Kawamura K, James TN: Comparative ultrastructure of cellular junctions in working myocardium and the conduction system under normal and pathologic conditions. J Molec Cell Cardiol **3:** 31, 1971
19. Maron BJ, Ferrans VJ: Occurrence of α-glycogen in cardiac muscle cells. J Molec Cell Cardiol **6:** 85, 1974
20. Maron BJ, Ferrans VJ, Roberts WC: Myocardial ultrastructure in patients with chronic aortic valvular disease. Am J Cardiol, in press
21. Ferrans VJ, Massumi RA, Shugoll GI, Ali N, Roberts WC: Ultrastructural studies of myocardial biopsies in 45 patients with obstructive or congestive cardiomyopathy. *In* Recent Advances in Studies on Cardiac Structure and Metabolism, Vol. 2, The Cardiomyopathies, edited by Bajusz E, Rona G, Brink AJ, Lochner A. Baltimore, University Park Press, 1973, p 231
22. Olsen EGJ: Morbid anatomy and histology in hypertrophic obstructive cardiomyopathy. *In* Hypertrophic Obstructive Cardiomyopathy, CIBA Foundation Symposium, edited by Wolstenholme GEW, O'Connor M. London, J & A Churchill, 1971, p 183
23. Wigle ED, Adelman AG, Silver MD: Pathophysiological consideration in muscular subaortic stenosis. *In* Hypertrophic Obstructive Cardiomyopathy, CIBA Foundation Symposium, edited by Wolstenholme GEW, O'Connor M. London, J & A Churchill, 1971, p 63

Differences in Distribution of Myocardial Abnormalities in Patients with Obstructive and Nonobstructive Asymmetric Septal Hypertrophy (ASH)

Echocardiographic and Gross Anatomic Findings

By WALTER L. HENRY, M.D., CHESTER E. CLARK, M.D., WILLIAM C. ROBERTS, M.D., ANDREW G. MORROW, M.D., AND STEPHEN E. EPSTEIN, M.D.

SUMMARY

Patients with typical idiopathic hypertrophic subaortic stenosis (IHSS) represent only one subgroup of a cardiac disease in which the characteristic anatomic abnormality is asymmetric septal hypertrophy (ASH). In most patients with ASH, left ventricular outflow obstruction is absent and cardiac dysfunction presumably is due to widespread involvement of the left ventricle by an underlying myocardial abnormality. In other patients with ASH, left ventricular outflow obstruction is present (typical IHSS) and constitutes a major feature of the hemodynamic and physical findings. To determine whether patients with outflow obstruction also have the underlying myocardial abnormality diffusely involving the left ventricle, the gross morphology of hearts from patients with and without outflow obstruction were studied both by necropsy and by echocardiography. Echocardiographic studies revealed that the ventricular septum was thicker in obstructive ASH, a finding confirmed by the postmortem studies. The necropsy studies also indicated that although the left ventricular free wall was thickened in both obstructive and nonobstructive ASH, the configuration of the left ventricular free wall was distinctly different in the two groups. In obstructive ASH, the free wall was hypertrophied and identical in appearance to that seen in valvular aortic stenosis. Moreover, echocardiographic studies indicated that the thickening of the free wall behind posterior mitral leaflet appeared to regress after operative relief of the outflow obstruction. In contrast, the left ventricular free wall of severely symptomatic patients without outflow obstruction had a markedly different and unique appearance; the free wall of left ventricle directly behind the posterior mitral leaflet was of normal or less than normal thickness, whereas the remaining free wall was nonuniformly thickened. On the basis of these findings and the microscopic data presented in the companion paper, we conclude that the myocardial abnormality in obstructive ASH (typical IHSS) is localized largely to the ventricular septum, with left ventricular free wall thickening occurring as a consequence of outflow obstruction. In symptomatic patients with nonobstructive ASH, however, the data suggest that the left ventricle, including free wall, is extensively involved with a primary myocardial abnormality.

Additional Indexing Words:

Hypertrophic cardiomyopathy
Left ventricular outflow obstruction
Idiopathic hypertrophic subaortic stenosis
Septal myotomy-myectomy

RECENT ECHOCARDIOGRAPHIC and pathologic studies have revealed that patients with typical idiopathic hypertrophic subaortic stenosis (IHSS) represent only one subgroup of a cardiac disease in which the characteristic anatomic abnormality is asymmetric septal hypertrophy (ASH).[1-3] In most patients with ASH, left ventricular outflow obstruction is absent; cardiac dysfunction, when present, presumably is due to widespread involvement of the left ventricle with an underlying myocardial abnormality.[4-8] In other patients with ASH, outflow obstruction is present (typical IHSS) and constitutes a major feature of the hemodynamic and physical findings.[5, 9-11] Since outflow obstruction can be abolished by septal myotomy-myectomy, operation has been proposed as a useful therapeutic procedure in selected patients.[12-14] The benefit provided by this operation however, ultimately depends on whether or not symptoms are due mainly to outflow obstruction or are a

From the Cardiology Branch and Clinic of Surgery, National Heart and Lung Institute, Bethesda, Maryland.

Address for reprints: Dr. Walter L. Henry, Cardiology Branch, National Heart and Lung Institute, Bldg. 10, Room 7B-15, Bethesda, Maryland 20014.

Received November 1, 1973; revision accepted for publication May 22, 1974.

consequence of the underlying myocardial abnormality. Some investigators hold the latter view[15, 16] and state that operation is not beneficial.[16] Our operative experience is at variance with this position.[12-14]

As a result, two studies, described in this and in the companion paper, were undertaken. Preliminary results of these studies were summarized previously.[3] In the companion paper, the distribution within the myocardium of cellular abnormalities was analyzed by light and electron microscopy.[17] In the present study, the distribution of wall thickening was studied by echocardiography which measured 1) septal and left ventricular postero-basal free wall thickness in patients with ASH who had varying degrees of left ventricular outflow obstruction and 2) postero-basal free wall thickness in patients with ASH in whom severe obstruction had been abolished several years earlier by septal myotomy-myectomy. In addition, the configuration and thickness of the ventricular septum and left ventricular free wall was evaluated in necropsy specimens from patients with obstructive and nonobstructive ASH.

Methods

Echocardiographic Assessment of Wall Thickness

One hundred adult patients with echocardiographic evidence of asymmetric septal hypertrophy (ASH) were studied. No patient had been operated upon before the echocardiographic study. Patients with disproportionate septal thickening due to right ventricular hypertension were excluded. ASH was considered to be present if the ventricular septum was at least 1.3 times as thick as the postero-basal free wall (fig. 1).[1] Septal thickness was measured below (caudal to) the level of the distal margins of the mitral valve. Postero-basal left ventricular free wall thickness was measured with the transducer oriented so that part of the echocardiographic signal was reflected from the posterior mitral leaflet. Both septal and postero-basal free wall thickness measurements were made during the phase of the cardiac cycle that occurs after rapid ventricular filling but before atrial systole. By restricting measurements to this portion of the cardiac cycle, the thinning of the walls caused by atrial systole was avoided. Of particular importance was the use of the T scan technique to reduce the error that occurs when the ultrasound beam passes obliquely through the left ventricular cavity.[1] In brief, this technique involves identification of the long axis of the left ventricle (by defining the angle of motion of the transducer that incorporates first the anterior and posterior mitral leaflets and then the aortic valve). Once this is known, the left ventricle is scanned perpendicular to the long axis at a point just below the tip of the mitral leaflets. Measurements of wall thickness are made in that portion of the record in which transverse ventricular dimension is maximal. The left ventricular outflow gradient also was estimated from the echocardiogram for each patient while in the supine position and in a basal state.[18]

Subdivision of Patients

Cardiac catheterization was carried out in 67 of the 100 patients. In all 67 patients the left ventricular outflow gradient was first recorded when the patient was supine and in a basal condition, and then during or following several provocative maneuvers (i.e., a premature ventricular contraction, a Valsalva maneuver, or an isoproterenol infusion). The 67 catheterized patients were initially subdivided into three groups on the basis of the magnitude of the left ventricular outflow pressure gradient: 1) *nonobstructed* group: no pressure gradient under basal conditions and a peak provocable gradient less than 30 mm Hg; 2) *provocable* obstruction group: no basal gradient but provocable gradients greater than 30 mm Hg (in most instances exceeding 50 mm Hg); 3) *obstructed* group: gradients present under basal conditions. In 63 of the 67 patients the cardiac catheterization, echocardiographic, and physical examination data all were consistent. The four exceptions were patients catheterized before 1964 in whom the physical findings had changed between the time of catheterization and recent echocardiographic study. Since in all four cases the physical findings and the echocardiograms were compatible, the patients were reassigned to a subgroup based on the echocardiographic data.

Subdivision of the remaining 33 noncatheterized patients was based on an estimation of the gradient by echocardiography. Two of the 33 patients had an obstruction index[18] indicating an outflow pressure gradient under basal conditions. Because provocative maneuvers were not employed in the echocardiographic studies, patients were placed in the nonobstructed group when no systolic forward movement of the anterior mitral leaflet was observed. Patients with anterior movement of the mitral leaflet during systole but an

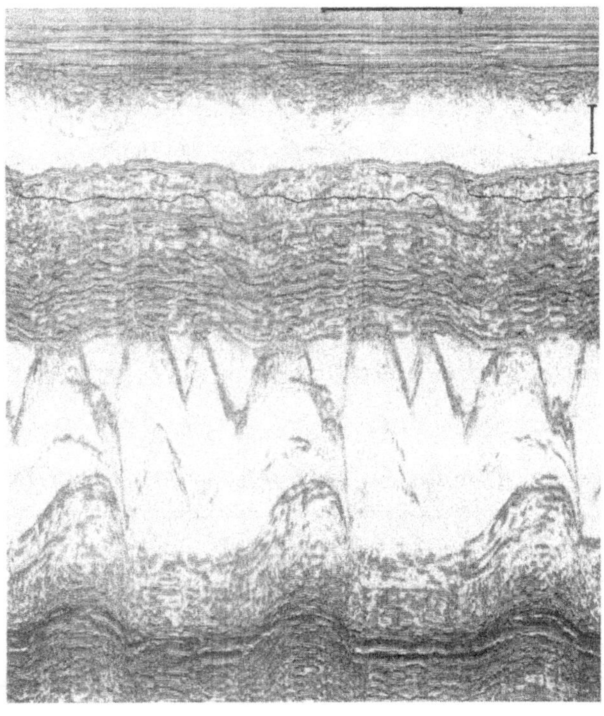

Figure 1

Unretouched echocardiogram from a patient with asymmetric septal hypertrophy (ASH). In this example, the thickness of the ventricular septum is 2.2 times that of the postero-basal left ventricular free wall.

obstruction index that did not indicate an outflow pressure gradient were placed in the group with provocable obstruction. (A gradient usually can be elicited upon provocation in patients without resting obstruction when the mitral leaflet moves forward even slightly during systole. Unpublished observations). Of the 33 noncatheterized patients, 27 were classified as nonobstructive, four as obstructive only by provocation, and two as obstructive. When both catheterized and noncatheterized patient groups were combined (total, 100 patients), 51 were classified as nonobstructive, 14 as provocable obstruction only, and 35 as obstructive.

Effects of Operation on Wall Thickness in Obstructive ASH

Echocardiograms were obtained from three groups of patients: a) 16 adult patients in whom septal myotomy-myectomy for obstructive ASH (typical IHSS) had been performed at least two years previously (range 2.5 to 12.3 years, mean 6.5 years); b) 13 adult patients in whom septal myotomy-myectomy had been performed within the past year; and c) 22 normal subjects (mean age 22 years, range 18–41 years). The 16 obstructive ASH patients operated upon at least two years previously did not have preoperative echocardiograms because the technique was not available. Both preoperative and postoperative (6–12 months after operation) catheterization was performed in all 16, however, and in each, operation totally abolished the basal gradient demonstrated preoperatively. The 13 adult patients more recently operated upon for obstructive ASH had preoperative echocardiograms but serial assessment of changes in wall thickness was not possible because operation had been performed within the past 12 months. Comparison of the preoperative hemodynamic data in the 16 long-term postmyectomy patients with the 13 recent postmyectomy patients revealed no significant differences in cardiac indices, left ventricular end-diastolic pressures, left ventricular outflow pressure gradients (table 1), or cardiac symptoms.

Necropsy Assessment of Wall Configuration and Thickness

The hearts of 23 patients with a premortem diagnosis of either IHSS or hypertrophic nonobstructive cardiomyopathy were reviewed. Ten were male and 13 female. Because many deaths occurred before the availability of echocardiography, ASH had not been demonstrated prior to death. In each patient, however, premortem catheterization data, including left ventricular angiography, were available. Outflow obstruction under basal conditions was present in 13 (the diagnosis of IHSS was made by previously described criteria[19]). In the remaining ten patients no resting gradients were recorded and maximum provocable gradients were less than 30 mm Hg. In the latter ten patients the diagnosis of hypertrophic nonobstructive cardiomyopathy was made when angiography demonstrated a hypertrophied ventricle with a small cavity in a patient who did not have systemic hypertension or fixed left ventricular outflow obstruction. The age at time of death averaged 43 ± 6 years (range 18 to 62 years) for the patients with outflow obstruction, and 31 ± 4 years (range 12 to 52 years) for those without outflow obstruction. Two obstructed and three nonobstructed patients died of noncardiac causes. All 18 remaining patients had been in functional class III or IV (New York Heart Association classification) before death. Of these 18, six died during or shortly after septal myotomy-myectomy.

Results

Echocardiography

Nonoperated Patients

Septal thickness of 22 normal subjects and the 100 patients with ASH is plotted in figure 2. Mean septal thickness was 9.9 ± 0.1 mm (range 8–12) in normals, 18.5 ± 0.4 mm (range 13–30) in nonobstructed patients, 23.2 ± 0.9 mm (range 17–32) in patients with only provocable obstruction, and 24.1 ± 0.6 mm (range 17–33) in obstructed patients. By definition, mean thickness of the ventricular septum for each of the three groups of patients with ASH was significantly different from that of the normal subjects. Mean septal thickness of obstructed patients and those with provocable obstruction was significantly greater in both than that of nonobstructed patients ($P < 0.01$). Whether this increased septal thickness is partly responsible for the outflow obstruction or merely a consequence of the elevated intraventricular pressure is unclear.

Postero-basal left ventricular free wall thickness for the same three groups of patients is shown in figure 3. Mean wall thickness was 9.5 ± 0.1 mm (range 8–11) in normals, 10.3 ± 0.1 mm (range 8–14) in nonobstructed patients, 12.0 ± 0.3 mm (range 10–17) in

Table 1

Hemodynamic Parameters in Recent and Long-Term Postmyectomy Patients

Preoperative hemodynamic parameters	Obstructive patients — premyectomy (Recent)	Obstructive patients — postmyectomy (Long-term)	Statistical significance (P = 0.05) of difference
Resting LV outflow gradient mm Hg	74 ± 10	80 ± 12	NS
Provocable LV outflow gradient mm Hg	144 ± 10	138 ± 10	NS
Cardiac index liters/min/m^2	2.85 ± 0.32	2.79 ± 0.17	NS
LV end-diastolic pressure mm Hg	19.3 ± 2.4	18.6 ± 1.7	NS

patients with provocable obstruction and 13.3 ± 0.4 mm (range 10–19) in obstructed patients. Mean postero-basal free wall thickness of obstructed patients was significantly greater ($P < 0.01$) than that of both normals and nonobstructed patients. In non-obstructed patients, mean postero-basal free wall thickness was less than 1 mm greater than that of the normal subjects, but the difference was significant ($P < 0.01$). As shown in figure 3, free wall thickness was 12 mm or greater in three of 51 (6%) non-obstructed patients. In contrast, 28 of 35 (80%) obstructed patients had free wall thicknesses of 12 mm or greater.

Post Myotomy-myectomy Patients

Postero-basal left ventricular free wall thickness of 16 long-term postmyectomy patients (third column, fig. 4) was 11.4 ± 0.4 mm (range 10 to 16). This was significantly ($P < 0.01$) less than the postero-basal free wall thickness (mean 13.2 ± 0.5 mm, range 10–16) measured preoperatively in the 13 patients who had septal myotomy-myectomy within the past year (last column, fig. 4).

Necropsy

General Description

Photographs of two hearts from patients with ASH are shown in figure 5. On the left is the heart from a patient with outflow obstruction, while the heart on the right is from a patient without outflow obstruction. A diagrammatic summary of the findings in 23 necropsy specimens of patients with ASH is shown in

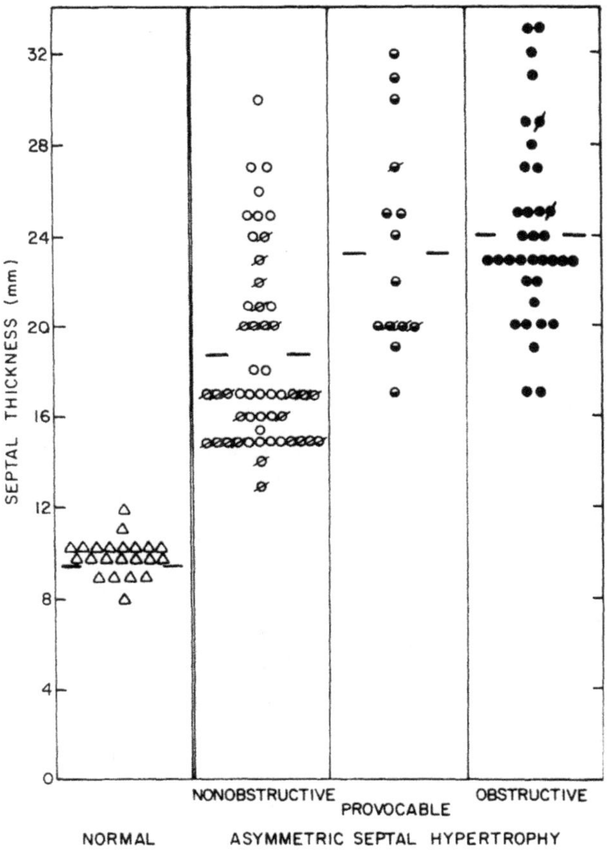

Figure 2

Thickness of the ventricular septum in millimeters (measured echocardiographically) is shown for 22 normal subjects, and 100 patients with asymmetric septal hypertrophy (ASH). The patients with ASH were subdivided into three groups (nonobstructive, provocable, obstructive) on the basis of the left ventricular outflow pressure gradient. Patients who were not catheterized are identified by a diagonal line through the data point. Mean values are indicated by the horizontal lines. Mean septal thickness of obstructive patients and those with provocable obstruction were both significantly greater than nonobstructive patients (P < 0.01).

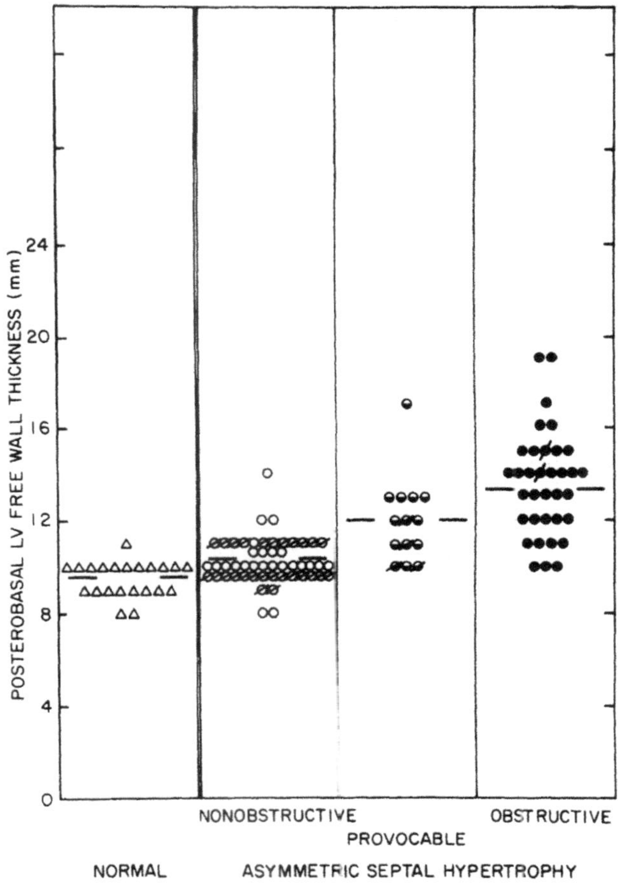

Figure 3

Thickness of the postero-basal left ventricular free wall in millimeters (measured echocardiographically) is shown for 22 normal subjects, and 100 patients with asymmetric septal hypertrophy (ASH). The patients with ASH were subdivided into three groups (nonobstructive, provocable, obstructive) on the basis of the left ventricular outflow pressure gradient. Patients who were not catheterized are identified by a diagonal line through the data point. Mean values are indicated by the horizontal lines. The thickness of the postero-basal free wall of the obstructive and provocable patients was significantly greater than that of the non-obstructive patients (P < 0.01).

figure 6. All hearts had marked thickening of the ventricular septum. While the left ventricular free wall also was thickened in most patients, its configuration was distinctly different in patients with outflow obstruction compared to those without obstruction. In each of the 13 hearts with outflow obstruction, the left ventricular free wall was identical to that seen in patients with valvular aortic stenosis or systemic hypertension: the free wall directly behind the posterior mitral leaflet was thickened and rounded; the free wall immediately caudal to and to either side of the posterior mitral leaflet was similarly thickened; and the free wall progressively decreased in thickness from base to apex (as seen also in the normal heart).

In the hearts from the ten patients without outflow obstruction, the left ventricular free wall had a distinctly different configuration: the free wall directly *behind* posterior mitral leaflet, especially in the longitudinal axis that included the postero-medial papillary muscle, tapered as it approached the atrioventricular ring, and was normal or less than normal in thickness (fig. 6); the free wall caudal to and just lateral or medial to the posterior leaflet, however, was thickened; and the normal decrease in wall thickness from base to apex was absent.

Thickness Measurements in Obstructive ASH

Maximum thickness of the ventricular septum in the 13 hearts with obstructive ASH ranged from 20 to 45 mm (mean 29.8 ± 1.9), and maximum left ventricular free wall thickness ranged from 17 to 32 mm (mean 20.5 ± 1.3). In all but one of the hearts studied, maximum septal thickness was at least 1.3 times the maximum thickness of the left ventricular free wall. In every heart, no significant difference was noted between free wall thickness directly behind the posterior mitral leaflet and maximum left ventricular free wall thickness.

Thickness Measurements in Nonobstructive ASH

Maximum thickness of the ventricular septum in the ten hearts with nonobstructive ASH ranged from

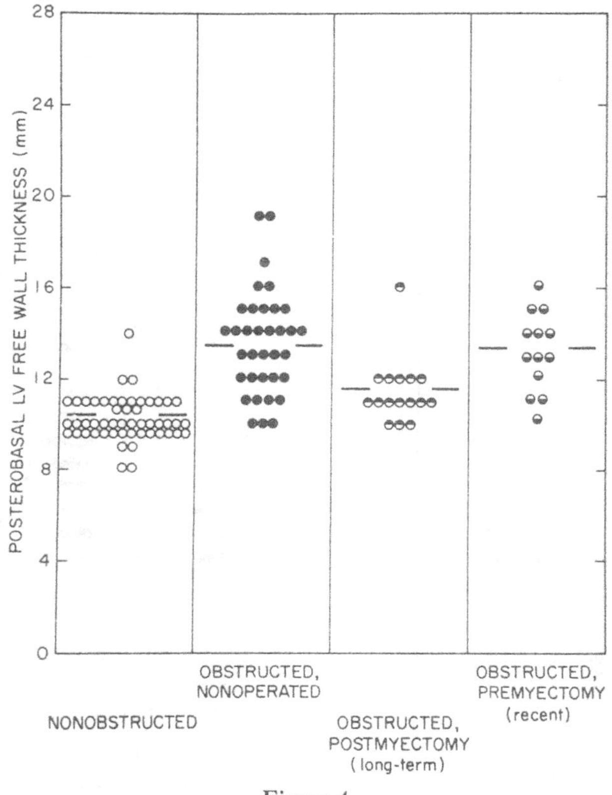

Figure 4

Thickness of the postero-basal left ventricular free wall in millimeters (measured echocardiographically) is shown for 51 nonobstructed patients (first column), and for 35 obstructed patients (second column) who had not been operated upon prior to echocardiographic study. Postero-basal left ventricular free wall thickness of 16 patients (third column), all of whom had been operated upon at least 2½ years earlier (mean 6.5 years, range 2.5 to 13.3) also are shown along with the wall thickness measured preoperatively in 13 patients (last column) who had undergone septal myotomy-myectomy within the past year. Preoperative wall thickness of the patients recently operated upon was similar to the nonoperated obstructed patients. The wall thickness of the patients operated upon several years earlier, however, was significantly less (P < 0.01) than either of these two groups, suggesting that regression of postero-basal wall thickness had occurred.

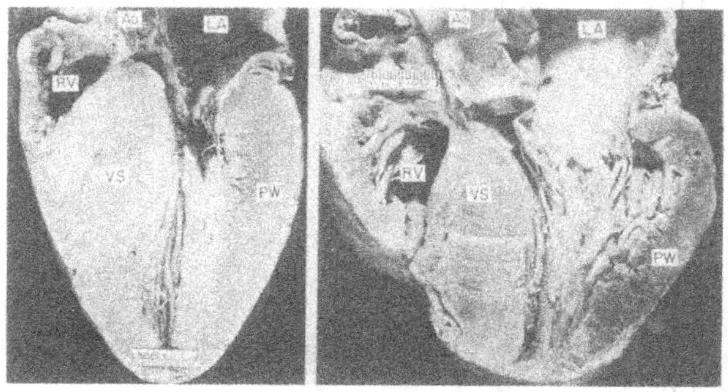

Figure 5

Two hearts with asymmetric septal hypertrophy (ASH), one with obstruction (left) and one without obstruction (right). The left ventricular free wall behind the posterior mitral leaflet is thickened in the patient with obstruction, but in the patient without obstruction the wall behind the posterior mitral leaflet is of normal thickness. In each, the ventricular septum is much thicker than the left ventricular free wall (asymmetric septal hypertrophy). Ao = aorta; LA = left atrium; RV = right ventricle; VS = ventricular septum; PW = posterior left ventricular free wall.

The patient whose heart is shown on the left was a 36-year-old woman. The peak systolic pressure gradient between left ventricle and systemic artery was 75 mm Hg at rest, and 125 mm Hg with provocation (Valsalva maneuver).

The patient whose heart is shown on the right was a 33-year-old woman. The peak systolic pressure gradient between left ventricle and systemic artery was zero at rest and 10 mm Hg with provocation (isoproterenol infusion).

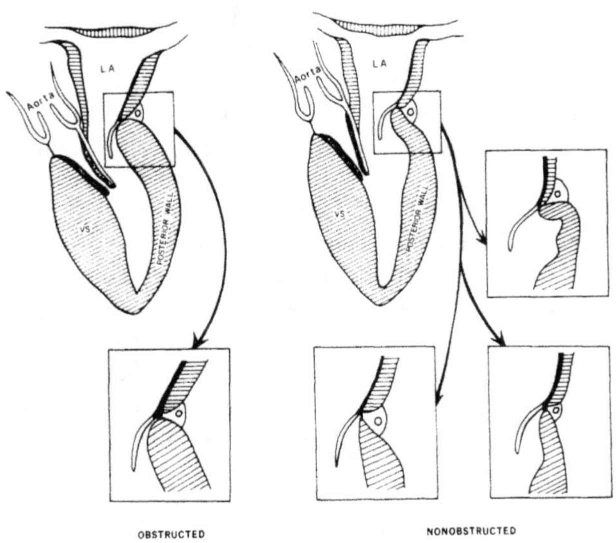

Figure 6

Diagram depicting representative configurations and thicknesses of the postero-basal left ventricular free wall just behind the posterior mitral leaflet in obstructive and nonobstructive asymmetric septal hypertrophy (ASH). In obstructive ASH, the most basal portion of free wall is rounded and thick and similar in appearance to that seen in patients with valvular aortic stenosis. This same region is distinctly different, however, in nonobstructive ASH. In both obstructive and nonobstructive ASH, the ventricular septum is much thicker than the left ventricular free wall. Also the mural endocardium of the left ventricular outflow tract and the anterior mitral leaflet in apposition to it are thickened in both groups.

17 to 40 mm (mean 25.4 ± 2.5), and maximum thickness of the left ventricular free wall ranged from 13 to 26 mm (mean 17.7 ± 1.2). In these hearts without obstruction, thickness of the posterobasal left ventricular free wall, measured directly behind the posterior leaflet at approximately its midportion (in the plane of the postero-medial papillary muscle), ranged from 6 to 14 mm (mean 9.3 ± 0.9). This value was significantly less ($P < 0.01$) than the maximum free wall thickness. In each of these ten hearts, maximum septal thickness was at least 1.3 times the thickness of the left ventricular free wall that was directly behind the posterior mitral leaflet. When maximum free wall thickness was used instead of the postero-basal wall thickness, two of the ten patients had septal-free wall ratios less than 1.3.

Discussion

The results of the present study and that of the companion paper[17] are compatible with the hypothesis that left ventricular free wall thickening in patients with obstructive ASH is a consequence of left ventricular outflow obstruction, while thickening in patients with nonobstructive ASH is due to the underlying myocardial abnormality. In obstructive ASH, several lines of evidence lead to this hypothesis. First, the portion of the left ventricular free wall directly behind the posterior mitral leaflet (as measured echocardiographically) was thickened in patients with resting obstruction, tended to be less so in patients with only provocable gradients, and differed only slightly from normal in patients without obstruction (fig. 3). Second, postero-basal free wall thickness in patients whose left ventricular outflow obstruction was abolished several years previously by operation was significantly less than that measured preoperatively in a similar group of patients with obstruction operated upon within the past year, suggesting that the thickening present in patients with obstructive ASH can be at least partially reversed by operative abolition of the obstruction. (This latter conclusion can be regarded as only tentative, however, because regression of free wall thickening has not yet been measured serially in the same patients pre- and postoperatively. Of note, those studies obtained six months postoperatively thus far have not revealed a significant decrease in postero-basal free wall thickness suggesting that regression may occur over a long time period). Third, the configuration of the left ventricular free wall in hearts with obstructive ASH examined at necropsy was indistinguishable from that seen in valvular aortic stenosis. And last, the microscopic data presented in the companion paper revealed that hypertrophied, bizarrely shaped, and abnormally arranged cells, believed to be a manifestation of the genetic abnormality in ASH, were abundantly present in the ventricular septum but not the left ventricular free wall. The myocardial cells in the left ventricular free wall were hypertrophied and morphologically identical to those found in patients with valvular aortic stenosis. Thus, anatomic, echocardiographic, and microscopic data are all consistent with the concept that left ventricular free wall thickening in obstructive ASH is a consequence of left ventricular outflow obstruction.

Examination of the left ventricular free wall of patients with nonobstructive ASH, however, suggested that a different mechanism leading to wall thickening is operative in these patients. If high intraventricular pressure were the only factor responsible for free wall thickening in all patients with ASH, the left ventricular free wall of patients without outflow obstruction should have been normal in thickness and similar in configuration to that of normal subjects. Our echocardiographic studies and those of others[20] suggested that this was the case. Necropsy examination of hearts from patients with nonobstructive ASH, however, revealed that the portion of left ventricular free wall directly behind posterior mitral leaflet was normal in thickness (confirming the echocardiographic findings), but that major portions of the remainder of the left ventricular free wall were thickened. Moreover, the microscopic morphology of the left ventricular free wall in nonobstructive ASH was distinctly different from that present in obstructive ASH,[17] in that the hypertrophied, bizarrely shaped, and abnormally arranged cells were present not only in the septum, but were also extensively distributed in the free wall. Finally, other secondary causes of hypertrophy such as left ventricular outflow obstruction or systemic hypertension could not be demonstrated in these patients. Thus, the gross anatomic and microscopic data are compatible with the concept that left ventricular free wall thickening in nonobstructive ASH is due to the underlying myocardial abnormality.

That patients with and without outflow obstruction have the same disease is indicated by studies demonstrating both forms of the disease in members of the same family.[21] Also, both groups of patients have disproportionate septal thickening that appears to be transmitted as an autosomal dominant trait.[21] Finally, the ventricular septum of both groups contains the same bizarrely-shaped and abnormally-arranged cells, which are found only rarely in other forms of heart disease.[17] It should be noted that some patients with right ventricular hypertension have disproportionate septal thickening.[3, 22] Such patients usually are easily identified on clinical grounds and should not be included in the ASH disease spectrum. In the present study, 23 of the 24 catheterized patients with nonobstructive ASH had right ventricular systolic pressures less than 35 mm Hg. ASH in these patients, therefore, cannot be ascribed to right ventricular hypertension.

One important point regarding echocardiographic, angiographic, or anatomic examination of hearts of patients with nonobstructive ASH deserves emphasis. In most patients without obstruction, the postero-basal wall that is not thickened is sharply limited to the region directly behind the posterior mitral leaflet. This fortuitously is the region of the posterior wall that is measured echocardiographically when the ultrasound beam passes through the posterior mitral leaflet. When studying the heart at necropsy, it is important that this same region be examined because sections cut lateral or medial to the longitudinal plane, which includes postero-medial papillary muscle, may be significantly thickened. In these instances the diagnosis of concentric hypertrophy, rather than ASH, might erroneously be made. In addition, the basal portion of the *anterior* free wall in one of the ten hearts from patients with nonobstructive ASH was thicker than the ventricular septum, a finding demonstrating that in rare cases portions of the left ventricular free wall may be thicker than the ventricular septum. Despite the unusual distribution of thickening observed in the hearts with nonobstructive ASH, in every instance, the septum was at least 1.3 times the thickness of that portion of the left ventricular free wall directly behind the posterior mitral leaflet.

When the echocardiographic, gross anatomic, and microscopic data are considered, it would appear that a cardiac disease spectrum exists in which asymmetric septal hypertrophy (ASH) is the characteristic anatomic abnormality (fig. 7). A recent study of the familial incidence of ASH indicates that ASH is transmitted genetically as an autosomal dominant trait.[21] We suggest that the hypertrophied, bizarrely-shaped, and abnormally-oriented muscle cells are a manifestation of this genetic abnormality. The data from this and the companion study[17] indicate that in all patients with ASH these cellular abnormalities are present in the ventricular septum and the septum is thickened. In some patients with ASH, outflow obstruction is present (i.e., typical IHSS), and in these patients, the cellular abnormalities are localized largely to the ventricular septum; they are absent, or only rarely seen, in the left ventricular free wall. As a result of the elevated intraventricular pressure, cellular hypertrophy and gross anatomic thickening occurs secondarily throughout the left ventricle including the already thickened septum. Despite the secondary free wall thickening, however, the ventricular septum with rare exception is thicker than the free wall. In the necropsy specimens, the one exception to this observation was a patient with severe, long-standing left ventricular outflow obstruction. We also have studied two patients echocardiographically (one with left ventricular outflow obstruction and one with previously documented severe obstruction that subsequently disappeared), who have the same degree of thickening in the septal and postero-basal free wall. These cases suggest that, in rare instances, secondary hypertrophy of the postero-basal left ventricular free wall may result in the septal-free wall ratio being less than 1.3. In our experience, however, such cases are unusual.

In patients with ASH and no outflow obstruction, the cellular abnormalities are widely distributed throughout the left ventricle (in addition to the septum). Because such patients do not have outflow obstruction, it seems reasonable to assume that the gross anatomic thickening of the free wall is due to their genetic defect, one manifestation of which is the hypertrophied, bizarrely-shaped, and abnormally-oriented myocardial cells. Finally, in some patients with ASH, outflow obstruction occurs only after provocative maneuvers. We suggest that such patients represent an intermediate group in the spectrum of

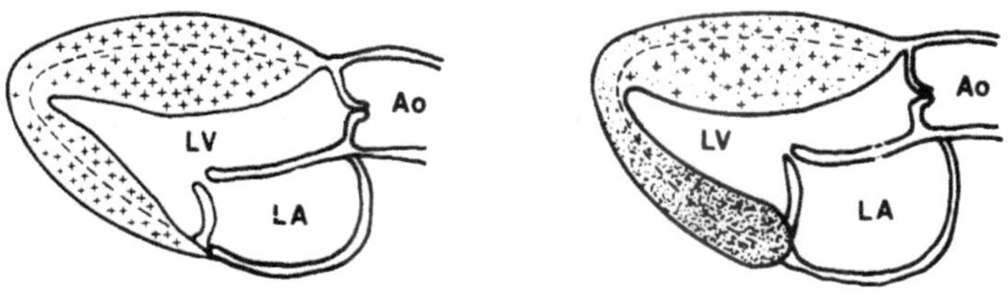

OUTFLOW OBSTRUCTION	ABSENT	PRESENT
SEPTUM		
Myocardial cells	Hypertrophied; abnl shape, arrangement	Hypertrophied; abnl shape, arrangement
Gross pathology	Thickened	Thickened
FREE WALL		
Mycardial cells	Hypertrophied; abnl shape, arrangement	Hypertrophied; normal shape, arrangement
Gross pathology	Thickened (nonuniform)	Thickened secondarily (uniform)

+++ Myocardial cellular abnormalities
Hypertrophy secondary to increased LV pressure

Figure 7

Diagram of a proposed pathophysiologic spectrum of asymmetric septal hypertrophy (ASH). In nonobstructive ASH (left), abnormal myocardial cells are widespread and present in both the ventricular septum and free wall. Wall thickening in these patients presumably is a result of the cellular abnormalities. In obstructive ASH (right), however, the abnormal myocardial cells are localized largely in the ventricular septum and the free wall appears to be thickened as a consequence of the left ventricular outflow obstruction.

ASH. Wall thickening in these patients may be due to cellular hypertrophy resulting from the intermittently elevated ventricular pressures, but it also may in part be caused by the presence of hypertrophied, bizarrely-shaped, and abnormally-arranged myocardial cells. If this concept of the pathophysiology of ASH is correct, it suggests that in patients with obstructive ASH (i.e., typical IHSS), the relief of symptoms that occurs immediately following abolition of the outflow obstruction by septal myotomy-myectomy need not be followed inevitably by clinical deterioration due to primary myocardial dysfunction.

Acknowledgment

The authors would like to thank Mrs. Joyce McKay, Ms. Cora Burn, and Mrs. Estelle Cohen for their assistance in this study.

References

1. Henry WL, Clark CE, Epstein SE: Asymmetric septal hypertrophy (ASH): Echocardiographic identification of the pathognomonic anatomic abnormality of IHSS. Circulation **47:** 225, 1973
2. Roberts WC: Valvular, subvalvular, and supravalvular aortic stenosis: Morphologic features. Cardiovasc Clin **5:** 104, 1973
3. Henry WL, Clark CE, Epstein SE: Asymmetric septal hypertrophy (ASH): The unifying link in the IHSS disease spectrum: Observations regarding its pathogenesis, pathophysiology, and course. Circulation **47:** 827, 1973
4. Braunwald E, Aygen MM: Idiopathic myocardial hypertrophy without congestive heart failure or obstruction to blood flow. Am J Med **35:** 7, 1963
5. Braunwald E, Lambrew CT, Rockoff SD, Ross J Jr, Morrow AG: Idiopathic hypertrophic subaortic stenosis: I. A description of the disease based upon an analysis of 64 patients. Circulation **30:** 3, 1964
6. Goodwin JF: Cardiac function in primary myocardial disorders. Br Med J **1:** 1527, 1964
7. Goodwin JF: Congestive and hypertrophic cardiomyopathies: A decade of study. Lancet **1:** 731, 1970
8. Goodwin JF, Oakley CM: The cardiomyopathies. Br Heart J **34:** 545, 1972
9. Goodwin JF, Hollman A, Cleland WP, Teare RD: Obstructive cardiomyopathy simulating aortic stenosis. Br Heart J **22:** 403, 1960
10. Braunwald E, Morrow AG, Cornell WP, Aygen MM, Hillbish TF: Idiopathic hypertrophic subaortic stenosis: Clinical, hemodynamic and angiographic manifestations. Am J Med **29:** 924, 1960
11. Wigle ED, Heimbecker RO, Gunton RW: Idiopathic ventricular septal hypertrophy causing muscular subaortic stenosis. Circulation **26:** 325, 1962
12. Morrow AG, Epstein SE, Rodgers BM, Braunwald E: Idiopathic hypertrophic subaortic stenosis: A current assessment of the results of operative treatment. *In* Hypertrophic Obstructive Cardiomyopathy, edited by Wolstenholme GEW, O'Connor M. London, J & A Churchill, 1971, p 140
13. Henry WL, Stinson EB, Clark CE, Morrow AG, Epstein SE: Long-term effects of operation on obstruction and LV hypertrophy in IHSS. (abstr) Clin Res **21:** 425, 1973
14. Epstein SE, Morrow AG, Henry WL, Clark CE: The role of operative treatment in patients with idiopathic hypertrophic subaortic stenosis. Circulation **48:** 677, 1973
15. Goodwin JF: Changing concepts of hypertrophic obstructive cardiomyopathy in the last decade. *In* Hypertrophic

Obstructive Cardiomyopathy, edited by WOLSTENHOLME GEW, O'CONNOR M. London, J & A Churchill, 1971, p 4

16. OAKLEY CM: Hypertrophic obstructive cardiomyopathy: Patterns of progression. *In* Hypertrophic Obstructive Cardiomyopathy, edited by WOLSTENHOLME GEW, O'CONNOR M. London, J & A Churchill, 1971, p 9
17. MARON BJ, FERRANS VJ, HENRY WL, CLARK CE, REDWOOD DR, ROBERTS WC, MORROW AG, EPSTEIN SE: Differences in distribution of myocardial abnormalities in patients with obstructive and nonobstructive asymmetric septal hypertrophy (ASH): Light and electron microscopic findings. Circulation **50:** , 1974
18. HENRY WL, CLARK CE, GLANCY DL, EPSTEIN SE: Echocardiographic measurement of the left ventricular outflow gradient in idiopathic hypertrophic subaortic stenosis. N Engl J Med **288:** 989, 1973
19. GLANCY DL, EPSTEIN SE: Differential diagnosis of type and severity of obstruction to left ventricular outflow. Progr Cardiovasc Dis **14:** 153, 1971
20. ABBASI AS, MACALPIN RN, EBER LM, PEARCE ML: Left ventricular hypertrophy diagnosed by echocardiography. N Engl J Med **289:** 118, 1973
21. CLARK CE, HENRY WL, EPSTEIN SE: Familial prevalence and genetic transmission of idiopathic hypertrophic subaortic stenosis. N Engl J Med **289:** 709, 1973
22. GOODMAN DJ, HARRISON DC, POPP RL: Echocardiographic features of primary pulmonary hypertension. Am J Cardiol **33:** 438, 1974

Original Contributions

PATHOLOGIC ANATOMY OF THE CARDIOMYOPATHIES

Idiopathic Dilated and Hypertrophic Types, Infiltrative Types, and Endomyocardial Disease with and without Eosinophilia

*William C. Roberts, M.D.,**
and Victor J. Ferrans, Ph.D., M.D.†

Abstract

This presentation summarizes necropsy observations in patients with three types of cardiomyopathy: idiopathic, infiltrative, and endomyocardial disease. The idiopathic variety is subdivided into two types depending on the size of the ventricular cavity. In the dilated ventricular type the left ventricular wall is frequently less than 1.5 cm. thick, intracardiac thrombi are common, the atrioventricular valve rings usually are mildly dilated, and focal myocardial and endocardial scars are common. In the nondilated type (hypertrophic cardiomyopathy), the ventricular septum is usually thicker than the left ventricular free wall, which also is thick (> 1.5 cm.). When the septum is similar in thickness to the left ventricular free wall (symmetric), left ventricular outflow obstruction does not occur. When the septum is thicker than the left ventricular free wall (asymmetric), left or right ventricular outflow obstruction may or may not be present. The orientation of myocardial fibers one to another in the ventricular septum in the nondilated (hypertrophic) type is abnormal, whereas it is normal in the dilated ventricular type. Intracardiac thrombi are rare and atrioventricular valve rings are never dilated in the nondilated type of idiopathic cardiomegaly.

The infiltrative types of cardiomyopathies include iron, calcium, lipids, mucopolysaccharides, granulomas, amyloid, and neoplasms. The first four usually are located within myocardial cells and the latter three, between myocardial cells. It is probable that all these myocardial infiltrates are capable of producing cardiac dysfunction, primarily on a restrictive basis.

Endomyocardial disease may or may not be associated with eosinophilia. When the latter occurs, the eosinophils are structurally normal. Death is related to congestive cardiac failure. This category in actuality also is idiopathic.

*Clinical Professor of Pathology and Medicine (Cardiology), Georgetown University, Washington, D.C. Chief, Section of Pathology, National Heart and Lung Institute, National Institutes of Health, Bethesda, Maryland.

†Senior Investigator, Section of Pathology, National Heart and Lung Institute, National Institutes of Health, Bethesda, Maryland.

TABLE 1. Hypertrophic Cardiomyopathy: Clinical and Necropsy Observations in 40 Patients

Groups	No. pts.	FH of HD	Ages (yr.) Range (avg.)	Sex F	Sex M	Systemic hyper-tension[a]	LV-SA PSG (mm. Hg) (rest)	LV-SA PSG (mm. Hg) (provo-cation)	Heart weight (gm.) Range (avg.)	VS > LVFW[h]	"Small" or normal sized RV and LV cavities	Endo. plaque LVO	Thick mitral valve	LVFW behind PML normal thick-ness	Di-lated left atrium	Normal aortic valve	No. pts. with CA >50% narrowed
I. With sub-aortic stenosis	20	6	18–70 (43)	12	8	7	8–170 (85)	56–140[b] (100)	390–1250 (654)	17	20	19	19	0	20	18	7[c]
II. Without subaortic stenosis	13	9[d]	9–55 (28)	6[e]	7	1	0	0–150[f]	350–1020 (683)[g]	10	13	6	6	11	13	13	0
III. No catheteri-zation	7	0	49–78 (67)	5	2	5	-	-	430–710 (518)	6	7	4	4	0	7	7	0
TOTALS	40	15	9–78 (42)	23	17	13	0–170	0–150	350–1250 (634)[g]	33[h]	40	29	29	11	40	38	7[c]

[a]Systemic blood pressure by cuff > 140 systolic or >90 mm. Hg diastolic or both.
[b]The PSG increased in each of the 11 patients provoked (by isoprotorenol or Valsalva maneuver).
[c]Transmural left ventricular fibrosis in only one patient.
[d]No information available in two patients.
[e]Two patients were asymptomatic. One died suddenly; the second committed suicide.
[f]Of 10 patients provoked, PSG remained zero in four and increased to 10–150 mm. Hg in seven. In only one of the latter was the PSG with provocation >32 mm. Hg.
[g]Heart weights of four children are excluded. The hearts of the 22 women averaged 551 gm.; those of the 14 men, 759 gm.
[h]Defined as thickest portion of ventricular septum > thickest portion of left ventricular free wall.
Abbreviations: CA = coronary artery; Endo = endocardial; FH = family history; HD = heart disease; LV = left ventricle; LVFW = left ventricular free wall; LV = left ventricular outflow tract; PML = posterior mitral leaflet; PSG = peak systolic gradient; SA = systemic artery; VS = ventricular septum; RV = right ventricle.

Although much has been written about the various cardiomyopathies, surprisingly few reports have focused on the pathologic anatomy of these conditions. This communication focuses on the structural alterations in the heart in the dilated and nondilated (hypertrophic) types of idiopathic cardiomyopathy, in the infiltrative types of cardiomyopathy, and in endomyocardial disease with and without eosinophilia (Table 1). The secondary cardiomyopathies, those associated with known conditions (collagen diseases, endocrine disorders, generalized infections, metabolic and neurologic disorders, physical forces, drugs, and metals), are not included. Concrete data from patients studied at necropsy by the authors are presented in addition to information derived from reports of others.

IDIOPATHIC CARDIOMYOPATHY

Dilated Ventricular Type (Congestive Type, Primary Myocardial Disease)

We have studied at necropsy 64 patients with idiopathic cardiomegaly of the dilated type (Figs. 1 to 11). In each, the ventricles were dilated, the coronary arteries were free of significant luminal narrow-

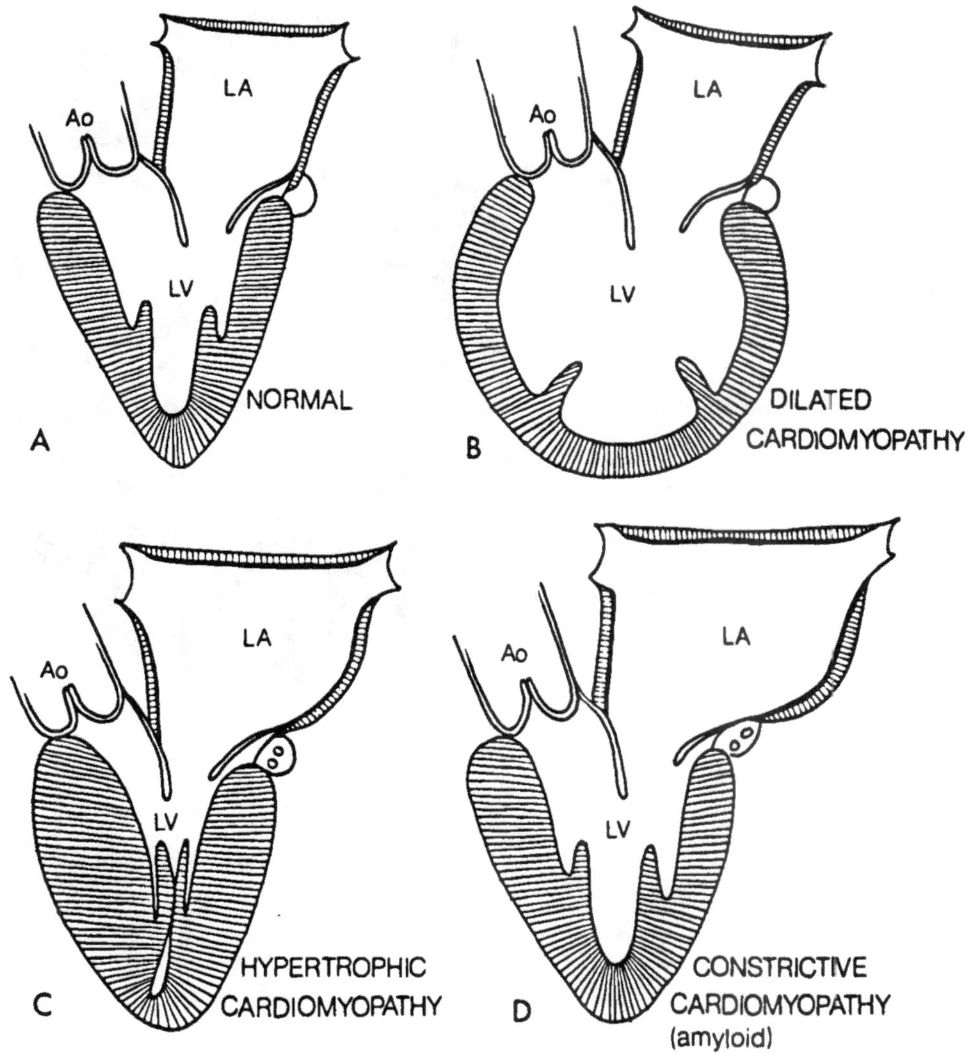

Figure 1. Diagram illustrating the various types of cardiomyopathies, compared to the normal, discussed herein. In the hypertrophic type of cardiomyopathy the left ventricular cavity is small, and in the constrictive variety, as illustrated by amyloidosis, the left ventricular cavity is of normal size. In the dilated type the largest circumference of the left ventricle is not at its base but midway between the apex and base.

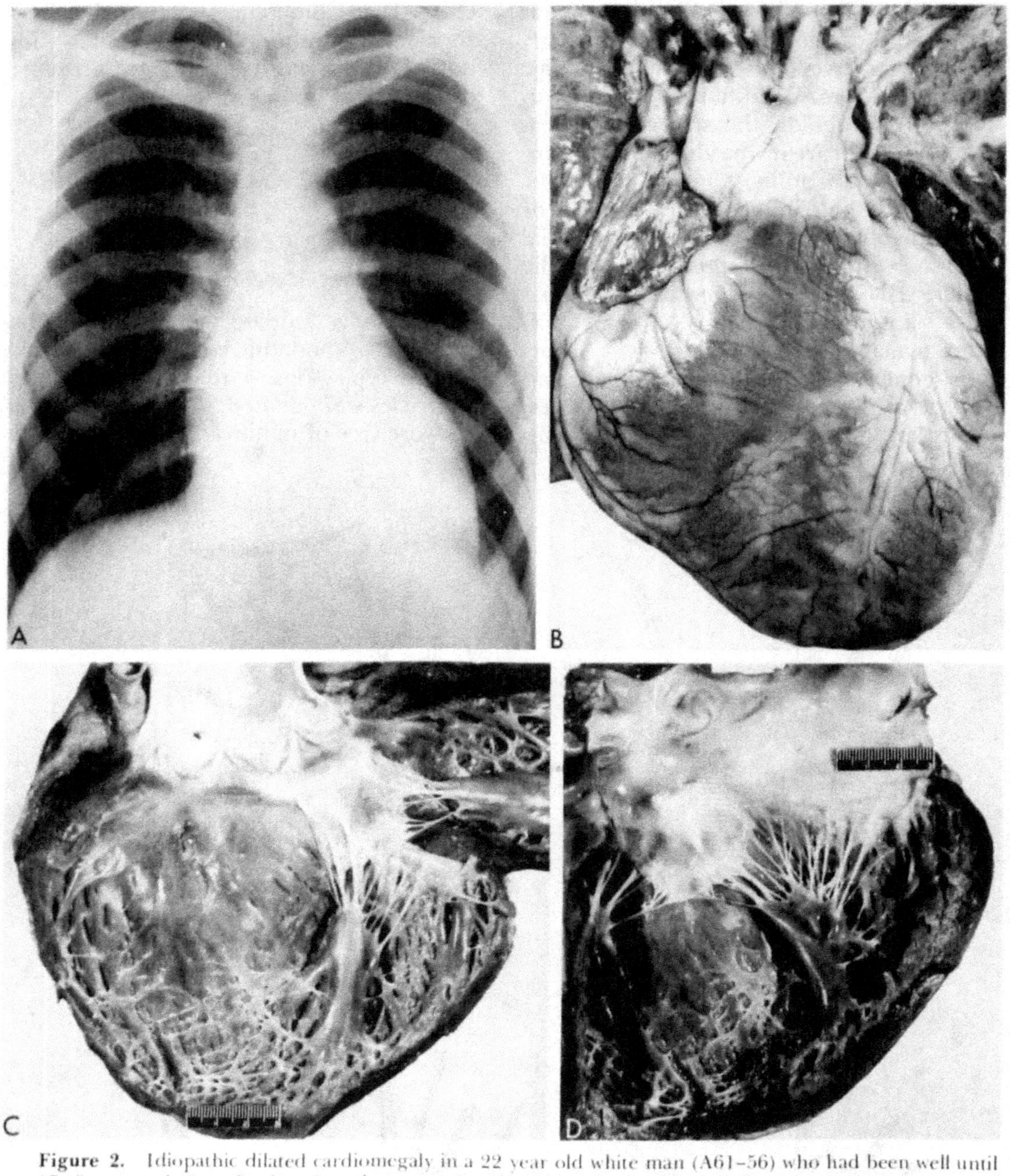

Figure 2. Idiopathic dilated cardiomegaly in a 22 year old white man (A61–56) who had been well until age 17 (five years before death), when the onset of a pleuritic type of pain was followed by congestive cardiac failure. The electrocardiogram showed nonspecific T wave changes. After a four month hospitalization, he was entirely well until two months before death when an upper respiratory infection resulted in overt congestive heart failure. Thereafter the heart failure progressively worsened and the heart enlarged. A grade 2/6 apical systolic murmur appeared. At necropsy the heart weighed 570 gm. and both ventricles were very dilated. The valves and coronary arteries were normal. Histologic sections of left ventricular wall showed only mild interstitial fibrosis. *A*, Chest roentgenogram during last week of life. *B*, Anterior aspect of heart. The pericardial sac contained 50 ml. of serous fluid. *C*, Opened left ventricle, aortic valve, and aorta. Small focal endocardial thickenings are present. *D*, Opened left atrium, mitral valve, and left ventricle. The mitral anulus is not dilated.

ing, the valves were normal except for occasional focal thickening of the atrioventricular valve leaflets, and there was not significant or prolonged systemic hypertension. The ages of the 64 patients ranged from 13 to 96 years (average, 46): the 43 males averaged 44 years and the 21 females, 49 years. Forty patients were black.

Twenty-three of the 64 patients were known to be chronic alcoholics. Twelve patients (seven women) had had documented systemic hypertension at some time (systolic pressure > 140 mm. Hg or diastolic pressure > 90 mm. Hg, or both). In most the blood pressure elevation was associated with congestive cardiac failure, but in at least one patient hypertension, which had been present for many years, disappeared when congestive failure appeared. In five patients other family members also had a cardiomyopathy: in two of the five the cardiomyopathy in other family members

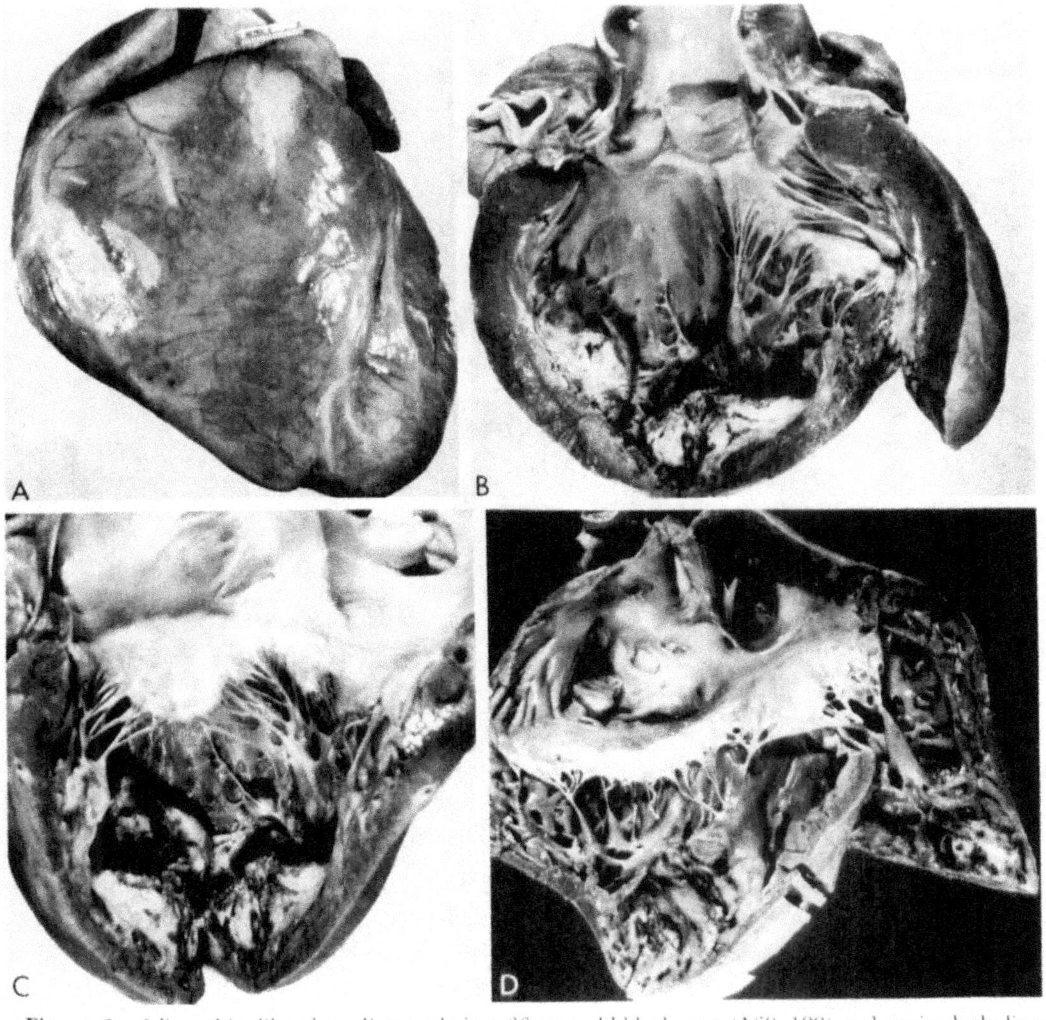

Figure 3. Idiopathic dilated cardiomegaly in a 36 year old black man (A69–199), a chronic alcoholic who had been well until two years before death, when evidence of congestive cardiac failure appeared. The latter gradually worsened and various arrhythmias also appeared. Finally pulmonary infiltrates, proved to be secondary to pulmonary emboli, precipitated death. By radiography the heart was markedly enlarged. An electrocardiogram showed low voltage, Q and T wave changes suggesting old infarction, and an intraventricular conduction defect. He never had chest pain, hypertension, or a precordial murmur. At necropsy the heart with the intracardiac thrombi weighed 750 gm. "Milk spots" were present over the anterior surface of the right ventricle and at the left ventricular apex *(A)*. Thrombi were present in the apex of both ventricles *(B, C, D)* and in the right atrial appendage *(D)*. Histologically, large foci of replacement and interstitial fibrosis were seen in the left ventricular wall. Both left ventricular papillary muscles were atrophied and severely scarred. *A*, Heart as viewed anteriorly. This is better seen in Figure 4. The notch present at the junction of the left ventricular apices was considered at one time to be diagnostic of the African condition, endomyocardial fibrosis, but this is not the case as shown by this patient. *B*, Opened left ventricle, aortic valve, and aorta showing the large apical thrombus. *C*, Opened left atrium, mitral valve, and left ventricle. The mitral anulus is not dilated. *D*, Open right atrium, tricuspid valve, and right ventricle showing a thrombus at the apex of the ventricle.

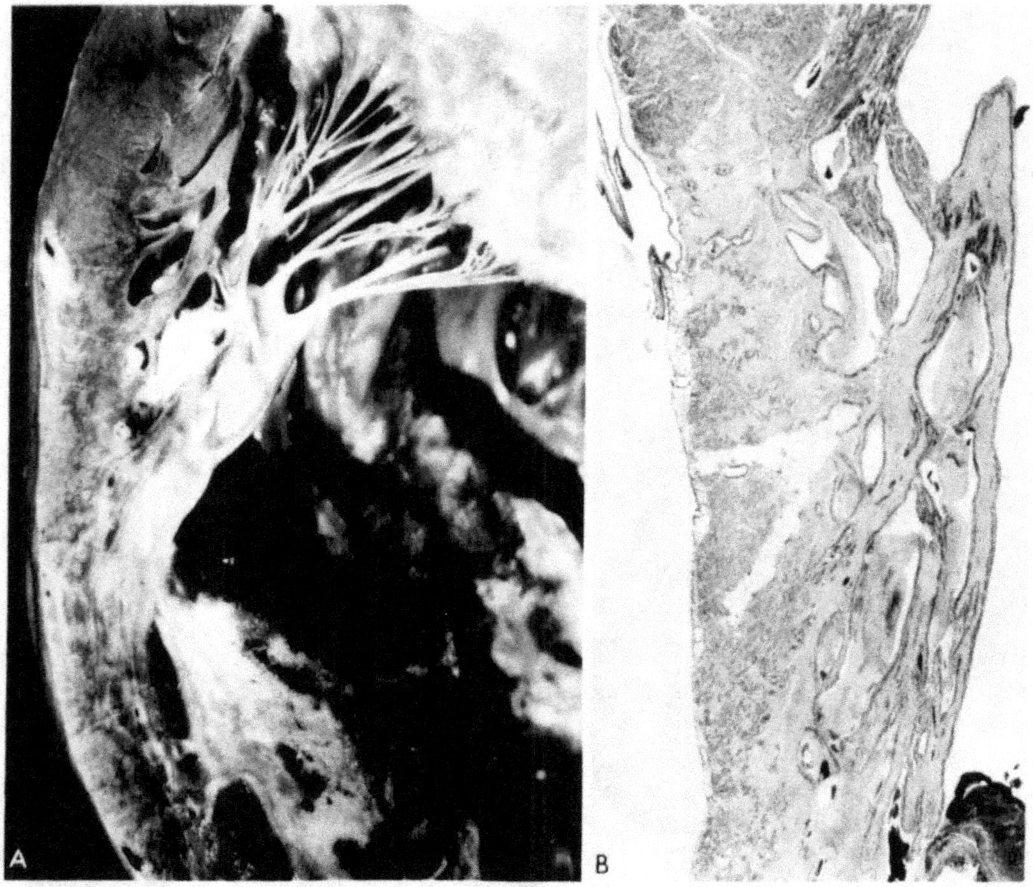

Figure 4. Papillary muscle fibrosis in idiopathic dilated cardiomyopathy. Anterolateral left ventricular papillary muscle in patient (A69–199) described in Figure 3. The papillary muscle is diffusely fibrotic, and much of the free wall beneath the papillary muscle also is scarred. This case shows that replacement myocardial fibrosis may be extensive at times in patients with primary myocardial disease. (*B*, Phosphotungstic acid–hematoxylin stain, ×3.)

was of the hypertrophic (asymmetric) type and not of the dilated type. Two patients had "peripartum cardiomyopathy" with the onset of congestive cardiac failure one and three months, respectively, after delivery. Eight patients had diabetes mellitus (adult onset type). Eleven patients had episodic chest pains, four of whom clinically were believed to have had acute myocardial infarcts in the past. At necropsy six of the 11 had left ventricular scars, but each was small. One patient, a 30 year old man, died suddenly and unexpectedly without previous symptomatic evidence of cardiac dysfunction. His heart weighed 780 gm. and was known to have been enlarged for 16 years. All remaining 63 patients had evidence of cardiac dysfunction (congestive cardiac failure) ranging from one to 240 months (average, 47); 12 patients had had evidence of congestive cardiac failure for more than 60 months and 21 patients, for less than 24 months. Sixteen patients had atrial fibrillation and 19 patients had complete bundle branch block (left in 13, right in two, and indeterminate in four). Death in most patients was the result of progressive congestive cardiac failure, but at least 15 patients died suddenly without apparent worsening of the congestive cardiac failure.

At necropsy the hearts ranged in weight from 350 to 860 gm. (average, 597): the hearts of the 21 females ranged from 350 to 860 gm. (average, 576) and those of the 43 males from 400 to 830 gm. (average, 610). All four cardiac chambers were dilated in all 64 patients. In some patients the left ventricular walls were more than 1.5 cm. thick, and in others the walls were of normal thickness. The greater the dilatation of the left ventricle, the less the likelihood that the walls were thickened. By histiologic examination, however, most myocardial cells in the walls of all four cardiac chambers appeared hypertrophied; a few fibers in the walls of all four chambers appeared atrophied.

Intracardiac fibrin-platelet thrombi were found in 36 patients (56 per cent). The most common location was the left ventricle (30 patients). The right ventricle contained thrombi in 16 patients, the right atrial appendage in 14, and the left atrial appendage in eight. In 22 patients more than one cardiac chamber contained thrombi. The apices of the ventricles were the locations of most ventricular thrombi, which usually were multiple. Huge thrombi were present in the left ventricle in two patients, and in one left ventricular outflow obstruction (24 mm. Hg peak systolic pressure gradient) appeared to result from extension of the thrombus into the outflow tract. In only one patient was a thrombus present in the body of an atrium (right). The myoendocardium beneath some ventricular thrombi was scarred but this was not always the case. In 12 patients focal endocardial fibrous thickening, without superimposed thrombus, was observed, particularly in the apices of the ventricles or in the atrial appendages. These lesions may have resulted from organization of thrombi. If these lesions are interpreted as evidence of "healed" or organized endocardial thrombi, then 48 (75 per cent) of the 64 patients had intracardiac thrombi at some time. Many patients had diffuse, uniform, endocardial thickening of the left ventricle, usually of a minimal degree, and occasionally also of the right ventricle.

Foci of intramural fibrosis were observed grossly in the left ventricular walls in 23 patients. The scarring was most frequent in one or both left ventricular papillary muscles and, next, in the subendocardial portions of the free wall. In seven patients the scarring was transmural. By histologic examination, however, foci of fibrosis, mainly interstitial (intermyocardial and perivascular) rather then replacement, were observed in the walls of all four cardiac chambers of virtually every heart. Foci of myocardial necrosis and inflammatory cell infiltrates were absent in the cardiac walls of all 64 patients. In most patients the extramural coronary arteries grossly were free of atherosclerotic plaques or other lesions. In the patients in whom some atherosclerotic plaques were observed, the lumens in none were narrowed more than 50 per cent. No significant abnormality of intramural coronary arteries was observed by histologic examination in any patient.

Except for focal fibrous thickening of one or more leaflets of the tricuspid or mitral valves or both, the valves were normal. The minimal focal scarring was of no functional significance. In most patients the circumferences of the tricuspid and mitral valve anuli were mildly dilated. The tricuspid anuli ranged from 10.5 to 16.5 cm. (average, 13.0) and the mitral anuli from 9.0 to 12.5 cm. (average, 11). Normally the tricuspid anulus in adults averages 11.0 cm. (range, 8.5 to 13.5) and the mitral anulus, 9.0 cm. (range, 7.0 to 10.5). The circumferences of the pulmonary trunk and ascending aorta usually were normal (< 8 cm.). The circumference of the base of the left ventricle (this excludes the distance of the basal attachment of the anterior mitral leaflet) and the longitudinal distances between the bases of the aortic valve (or the base of the posterior mitral leaflet) and the left ventricular apex were increased in all patients.

In addition to studying 64 necropsy patients with idiopathic cardiomegaly of the dilated type, we examined by electron microscopy biopsy specimens of ventricular myocardium (obtained either with a Konno catheter or with a Menghini needle[1]) from 31 living patients with the same condition.[2] Three main findings were observed (Figs. 8 to 11):

1. Interstitial fibrosis, i.e., increased numbers of mature and developing collagen fibrils in interstitial spaces.

2. Cellular hypertrophy, consisting of increased transverse diameters of the muscle cells; increased size of nuclei and Golgi complexes; and increased numbers of mitochondria, myofibrils, glycogen granules, and free and membrane bound ribosomes.

3. Changes considered as probably degenerative, such as cellular edema; increased numbers of lipid droplets, lysosomes, and lipofuscin granules; dilatation of tubules of the sarcoplasmic reticulum and the T system; myofibrillar damage; and various mitochondrial alterations, in-

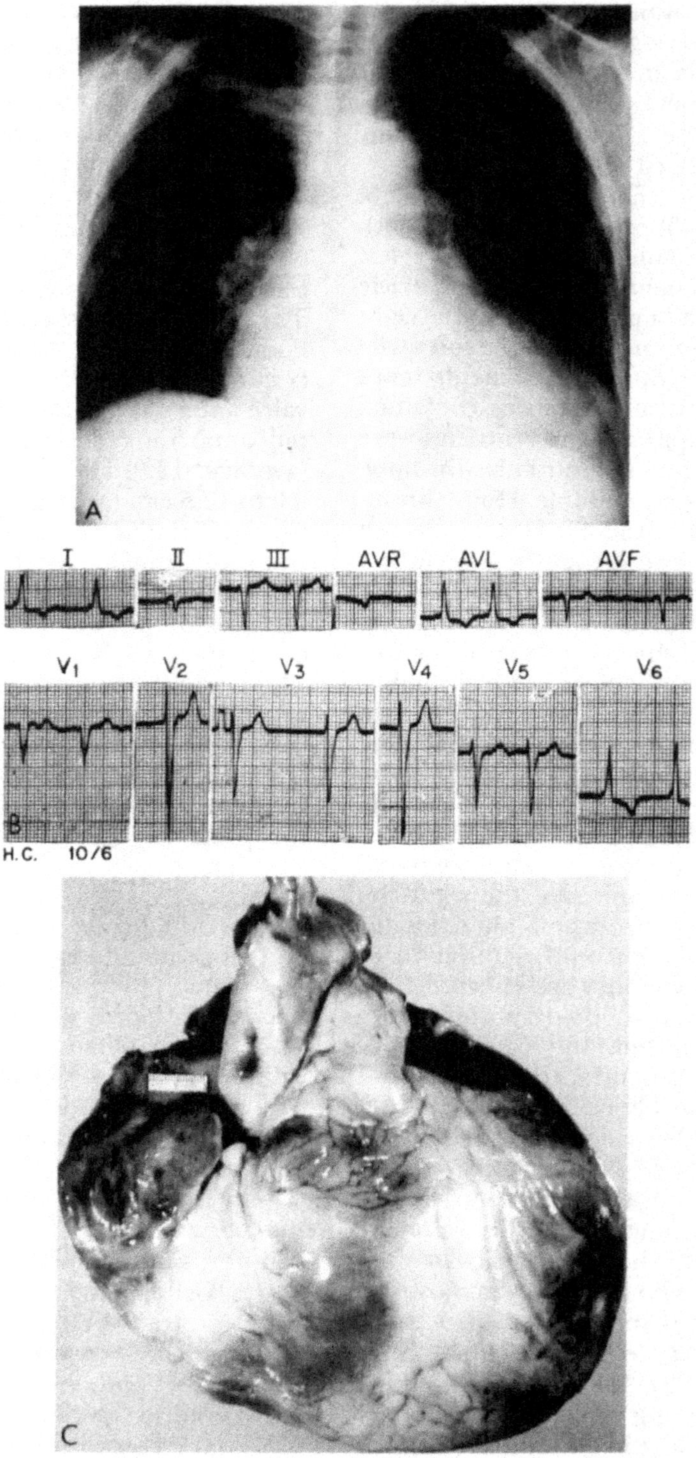

Figure 5. Idiopathic dilated cardiomyopathy in a 50 year old black woman (A72–216) who had been well until five years before death, when congestive cardiac failure appeared. During the next five years the heart progressively enlarged. Left bundle branch block and atrial fibrillation appeared about two years before death. It was stated that she had had systemic hypertension for several years, but during each hospitalization most blood pressure recordings were normal. On admission to the National Heart and Lung Institute she was in severe congestive cardiac failure (functionally class IV [New York Heart Association]). Grade 3/6 pansystolic blowing murmurs were present: one over the apex and another along the lower left sternal border. The latter murmur increased with inspiration. At catheterization the pressures in mm. Hg were: pulmonary artery 70/40, right ventricle 70/24, right atrium m26 v30, left ventricle 100/30, and brachial artery 110/75. Left ventricular cineangiogram showed a severely dilated, poorly contracting ventricle, 3+ to 4+ mitral regurgitation, and a large

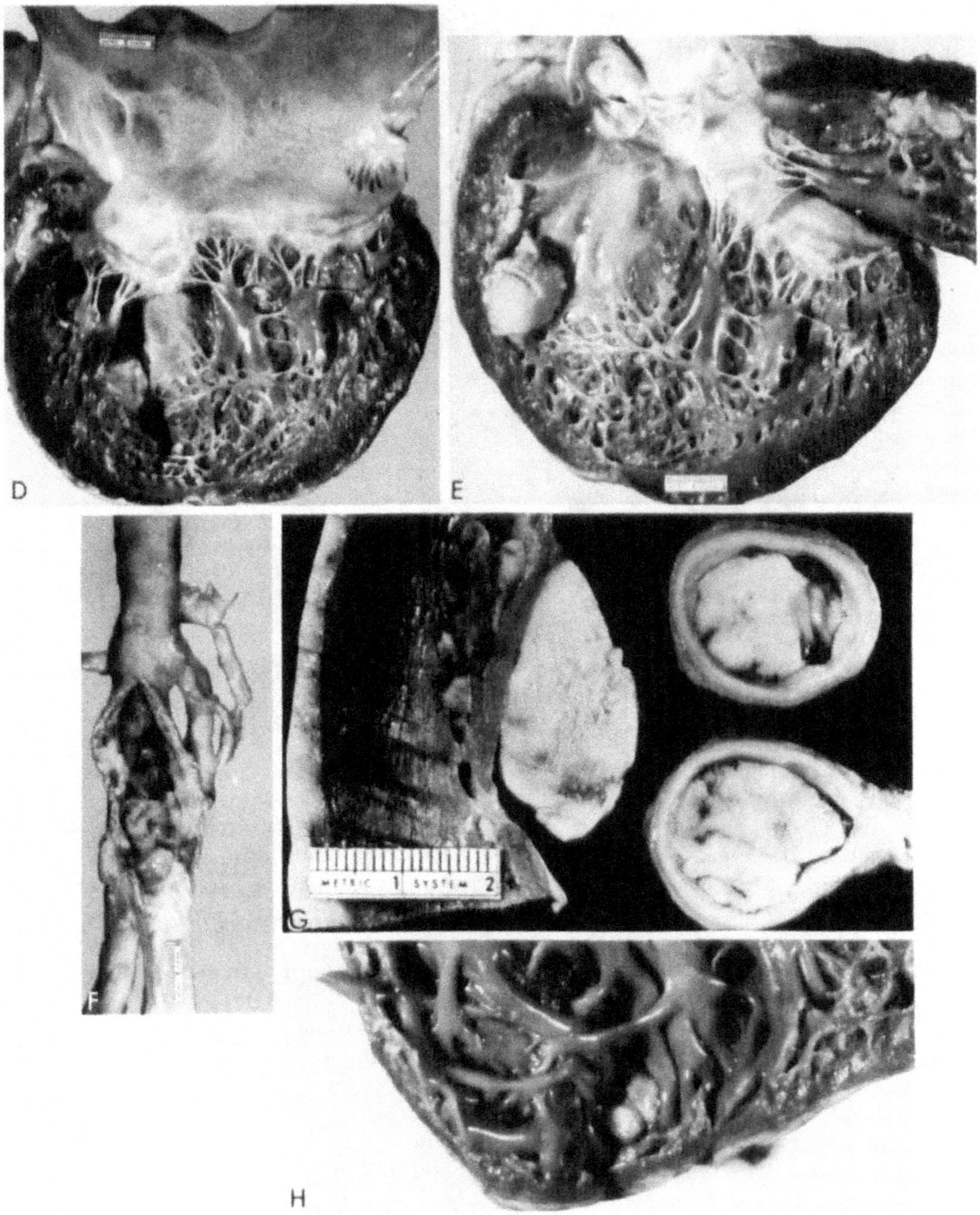

Figure 5. *Continued.* left atrium. This patient was considered clinically to have severe mitral and tricuspid regurgitation, probably due to rheumatic disease, and valve replacement was recommended. However, she had a stroke and died shortly before scheduled operation. *A*, Chest roentgenogram showing a large cardiac silhouette. *B*, Electrocardiogram 24 days before death. *C*, Dilated heart weighing 700 gm., exterior view. *D*, Opened left atrium, mitral valve, and left ventricle and *(E)* opened left ventricle and aortic valve. Mural thrombi are present in the ventricle. The mitral and aortic valves are normal. *F*, Opened abdominal aorta showing occluding embolus. A cross section of the occluded aorta is shown in *G* along with a longitudinal view of the thrombus attached to the wall of the left ventricle. The material in the aorta is identical to that in the left ventricle. A small mural thrombus also is present in the apex of the right ventricle *(H)*.

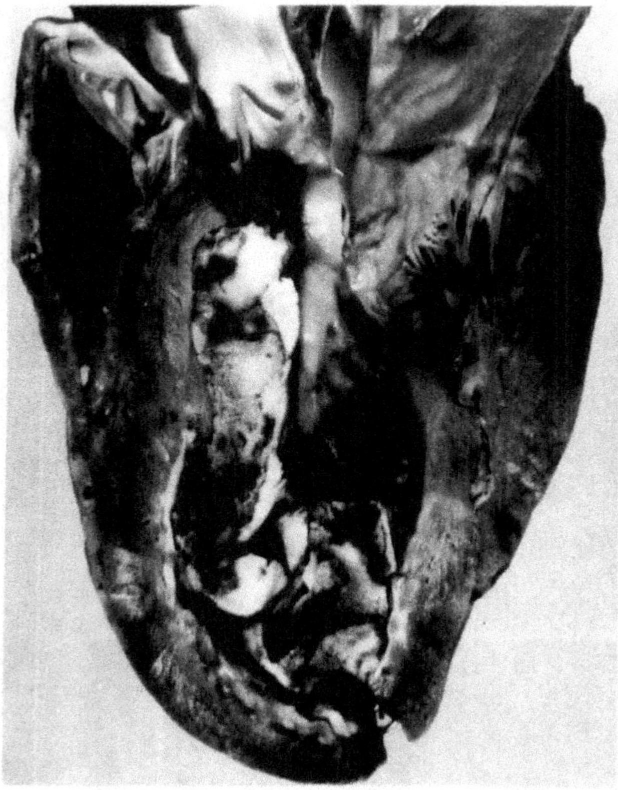

Figure 6. Idiopathic dilated cardiomyopathy. Posterior half of both ventricles exposed to show a huge left ventricular thrombus extending from the apex to just below the aortic valve in a 31 year old black man (DCGH 71A–273) who had had evidence of congestive cardiac failure with cardiomegaly for eight years. A grade 2/6 pansystolic apical murmur was present. Electrocardiogram disclosed left ventricular hypertrophy with ischemia. At catheterization, pullback pressures from the left ventricle to the ascending aorta were 126/26 and 102/67 mm. Hg, respectively. The 24 mm. Hg peak systolic pressure gradient probably resulted from the large thrombus that extended into the left ventricular outflow tract. Pulsus alternans was noted in the left ventricular and aortic pressure tracings. The patient died of pulmonary infarction from emboli. At necropsy the heart weighed 550 gm. and the left ventricular thrombus weighed 50 gm. The coronary arteries and valves were normal.

cluding mitochondrial swelling, intramitochondrial concentric lamellae, and loss of mitochondria cristae.

In addition, the mitochondria in most patients showed wide ranges in size, frequently with a predominance of mitochondria that were smaller than normal. No viral particles were observed. Abnormalities of myofibrillar orientation were observed in biopsy specimens from three of the 31 patients and were minimal. Edematous and damaged myocardial capillaries were observed in nine patients. Morphologic findings in patients with histories of chronic alcoholism were indistinguishable from those in patients without chronic alcoholism. The degree to which degenerative changes occurred in individual biopsy specimens generally correlated with the duration and severity of symptoms of cardiac dysfunction.

Comments on Idiopathic Cardiomegaly of the Dilated Type. By definition, the cause of the dilated type of cardiomyopathy is uncertain. If a viral etiology or other etiology is established as the cause, the cardiomyopathy is no longer "idiopathic" and with time it is hoped that the number of cases in the idiopathic category will decrease. This diagnosis is made by exclusion both clinically and at necropsy. Although valvular regurgitation (tricuspid or mitral or both) may occur, the valvular leaflets and chordae are normal except for occasional minimal focal thickening. Furthermore, although chest pain and electrocardiographic changes consistent with healed myocardial infarction may occur in this cardiomyopathy, the extramural coronary arteries are free of "significant" luminal narrowing. But how much coronary arterial luminal narrowing is permissible before a diagnosis of idiopathic cardiomegaly is permitted? We have chosen 50 per cent luminal narrowing as the upper limit. The presence of chronic pulmonary parenchymal disease, other than pulmonary infarction from emboli or of congenital cardiac malformations, even one such as atresia of the ostium of the coronary sinus,[3] also disallows a diagnosis of primary myocardial disease.

The level of the systemic blood pressure obviously is an essential piece of in-

(Text continued on page 302.)

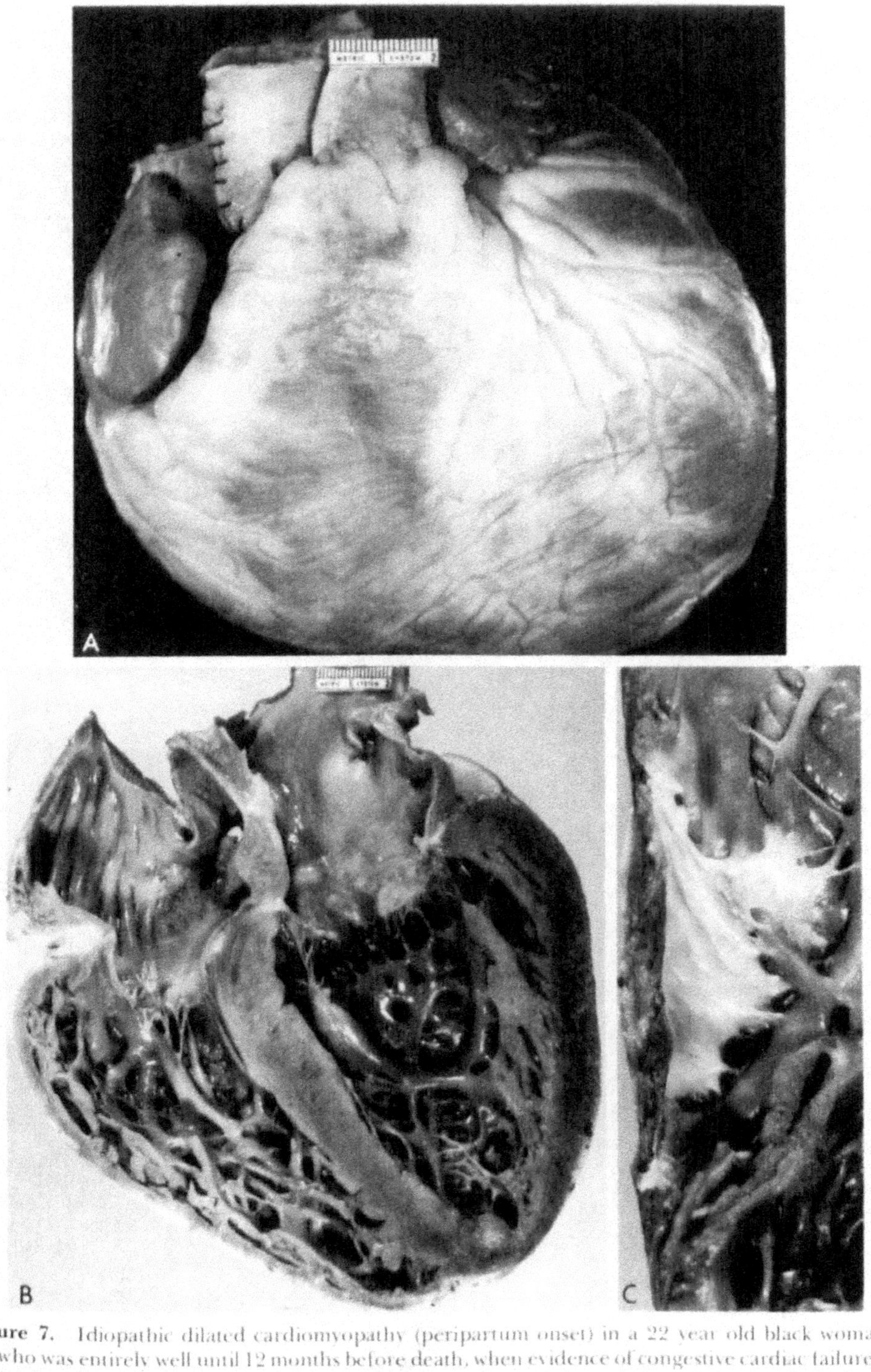

Figure 7. Idiopathic dilated cardiomyopathy (peripartum onset) in a 22 year old black woman (DCGH 73A–2) who was entirely well until 12 months before death, when evidence of congestive cardiac failure appeared six weeks after delivery of her first child. The failure progressed thereafter until death. She had evidence of multiple pulmonary emboli during the illness. There was no precordial murmur. An electrocardiogram showed ST-T wave changes and right atrial abnormality. *A*, The heart weighed 440 gm. All four chambers are dilated. The mitral anular circumference is considerably less than the circumference of the midportion of the left ventricle (*B*). The mural endocardium in the right ventricle is focally thickened (*C*). This lesion probably results from the organization of thrombus.

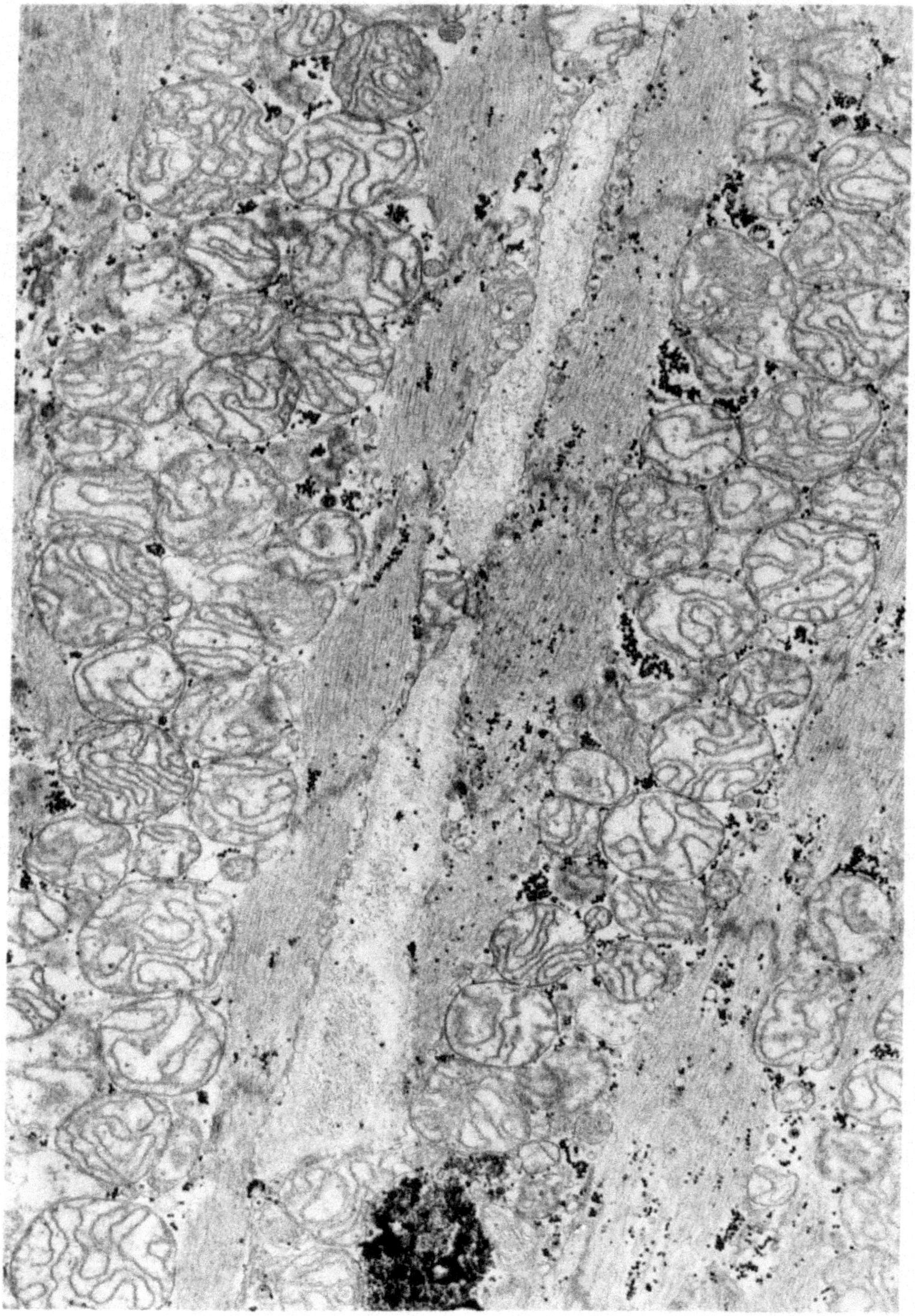

Figure 8. Dilated cardiomyopathy in a 25 year old man. Mitochondria in two adjacent cardiac muscle cells show swelling, clearing of matrix, and reduction in the numbers of cristae. (× 20,000.)

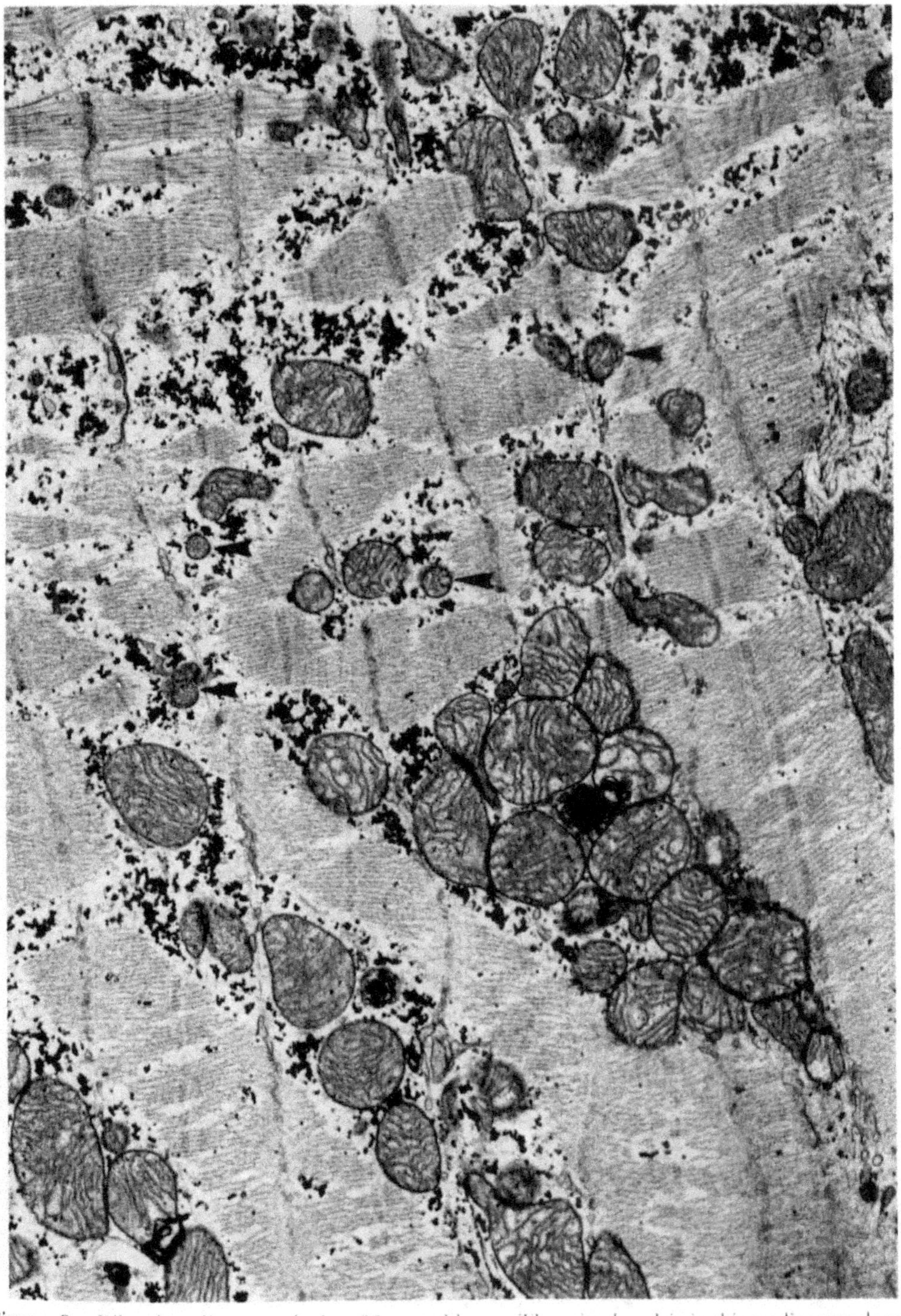

Figure 9. Dilated cardiomyopathy in a 28 year old man. The mitochondria in this cardiac muscle cell vary in size from very small (arrowheads) to normal. (× 17,000.)

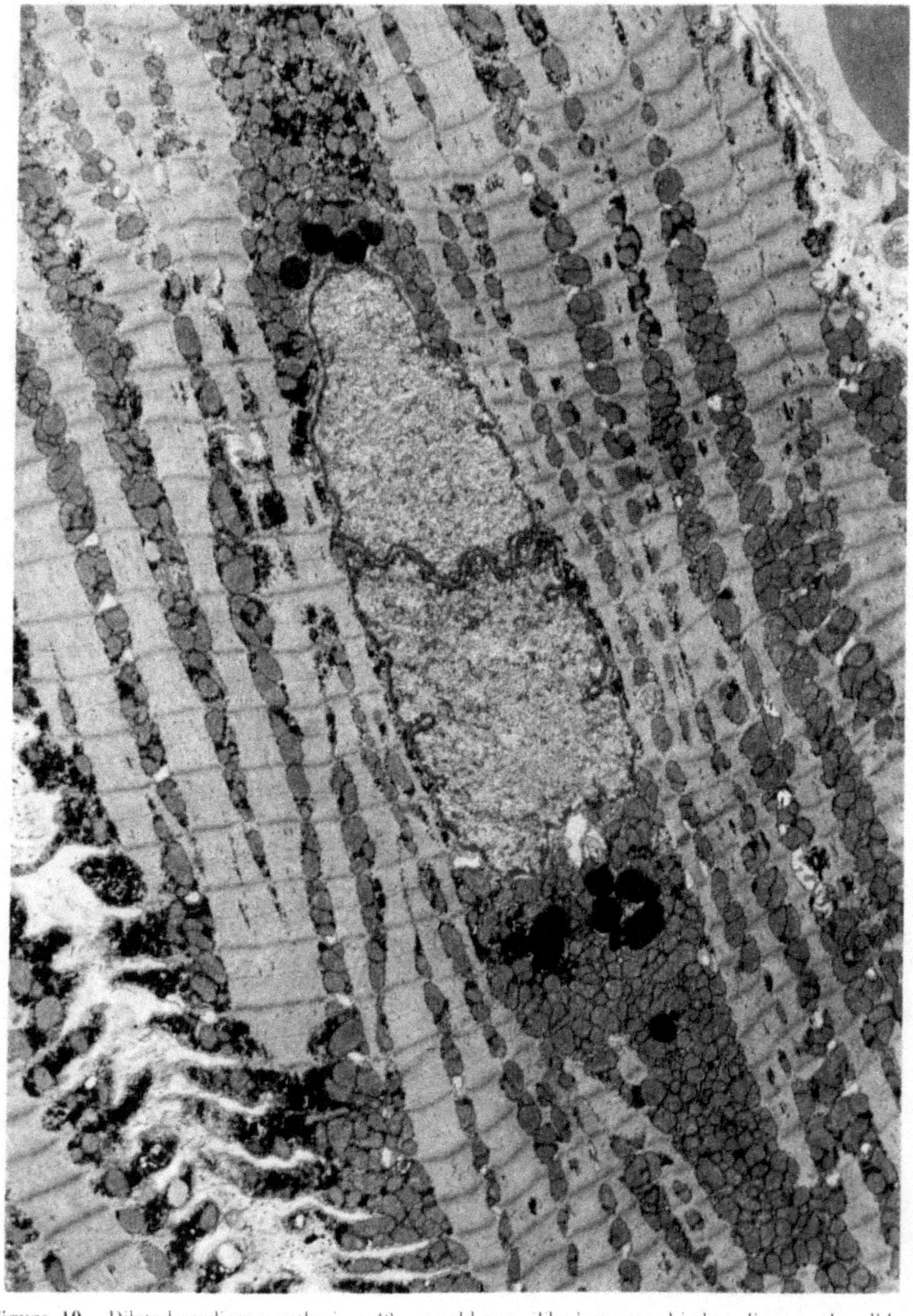

Figure 10. Dilated cardiomyopathy in a 43 year old man. The hypertrophied cardiac muscle cell has two nuclei, large perinuclear zones filled with mitochondria and a few lipofuscin granules, and normally arranged myofibrils. (× 6200.)

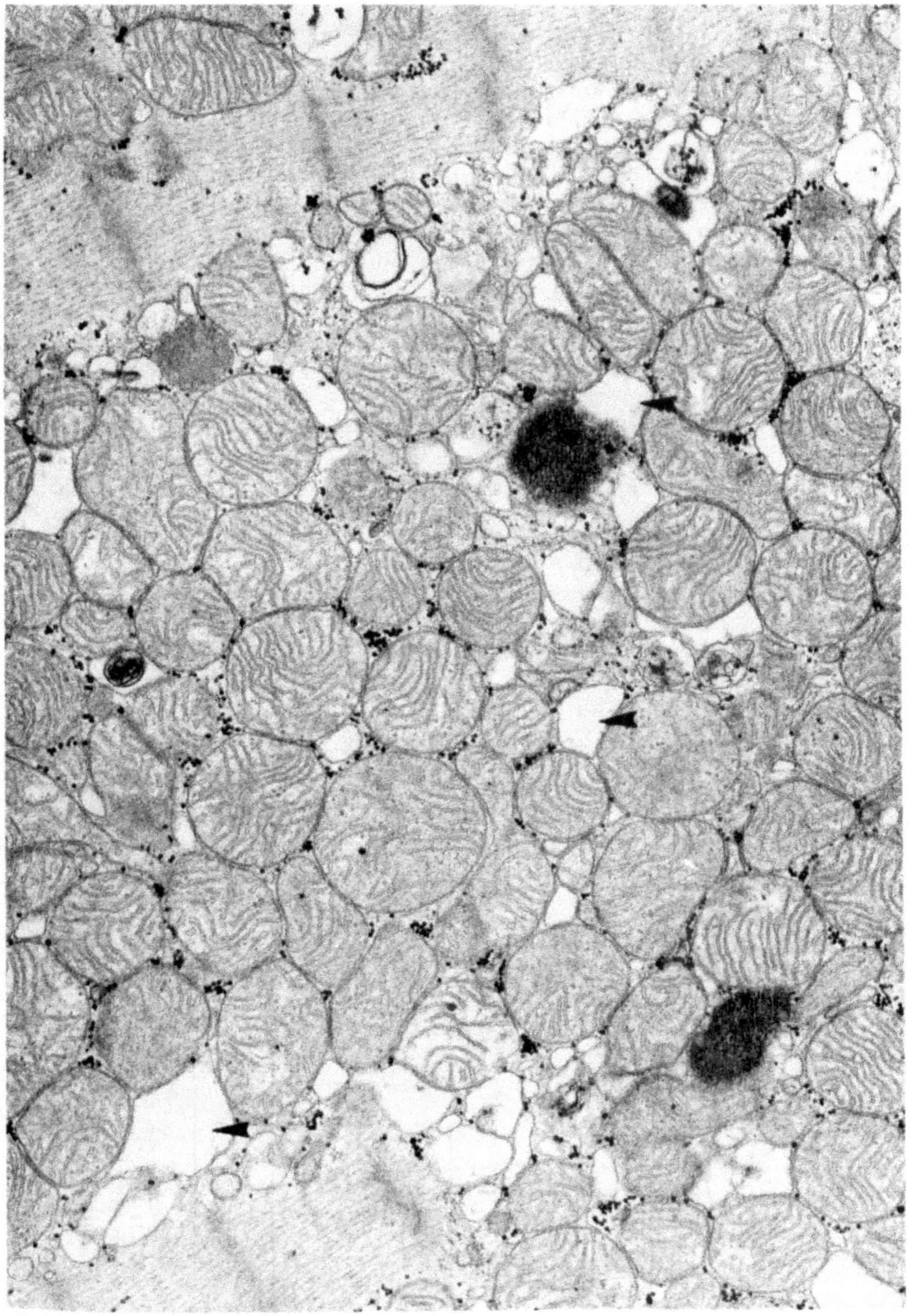

Figure 11. Dilated cardiomyopathy in a 31 year old man with chronic alcoholism. The sarcoplasmic reticulum (arrowheads) is dilated in this muscle cell. (× 24,500.)

formation. At necropsy, the heart of a hypertensive patient with fatal chronic congestive cardiac failure may simulate the heart of a patient with idiopathic cardiomegaly of the dilated type. It is probable that a number of patients considered to have idiopathic cardiomegaly, particularly those in older age groups may have had normal blood pressures during their symptomatic illness but elevated pressures years earlier. Eight of our 64 patients were known to have had systemic hypertension several years before presenting with normal blood pressure and severe congestive cardiac failure; four others had mild systolic systemic hypertension during their terminal illnesses. Although elevations of blood pressure may occur in idiopathic cardiomegaly, and may be of importance in its pathogenesis, it is unlikely that hypertension plays a major role in causing fatal congestive cardiac failure in primary myocardial disease, and consequently these 12 patients were included in our study. None had morphologic evidence of chronic hypertension in the kidney or spleen.

The inclusion in this study of a 96 year old patient might raise questions as to proper diagnosis. This patient had had evidence of congestive cardiac failure for about six months without chest pain or previously known systemic hypertension. Although the clinical diagnosis was coronary heart disease, at necropsy the coronary arteries were wide open, actually dilated; the four valves were normal, the myocardial walls were free of fibrosis or necrosis except for scarring of the papillary muscles, and the heart weighed 630 gm. Thus, by exclusion, this patient is included. Of the 64 patients, only three were more than 65 years of age and two were less than 21 years of age.

Study of the myocardium in these

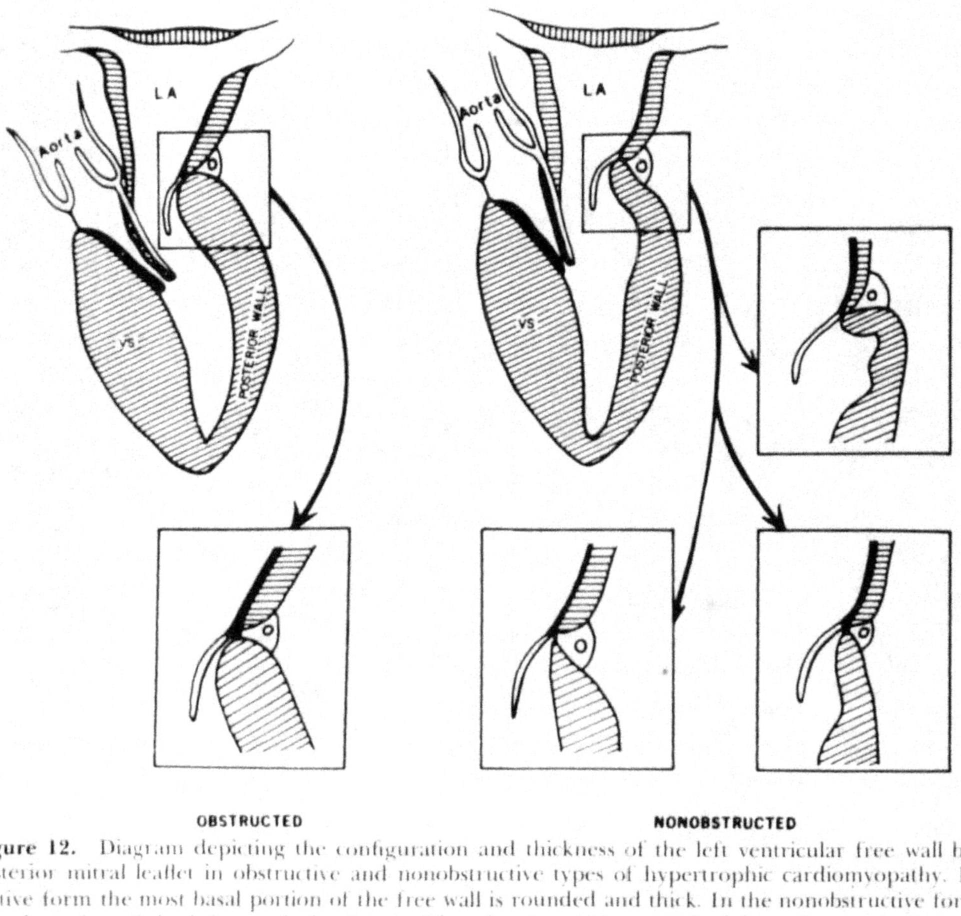

Figure 12. Diagram depicting the configuration and thickness of the left ventricular free wall behind the posterior mitral leaflet in obstructive and nonobstructive types of hypertrophic cardiomyopathy. In the obstructive form the most basal portion of the free wall is rounded and thick. In the nonobstructive form the most basal portion of the left ventricular free wall is pointed, or thin, or arched. In each type the ventricular septum is much thicker than the left ventricular free wall; the mural endocardium in the left ventricular outflow tract and the anterior mitral leaflet in apposition to it are thickened.

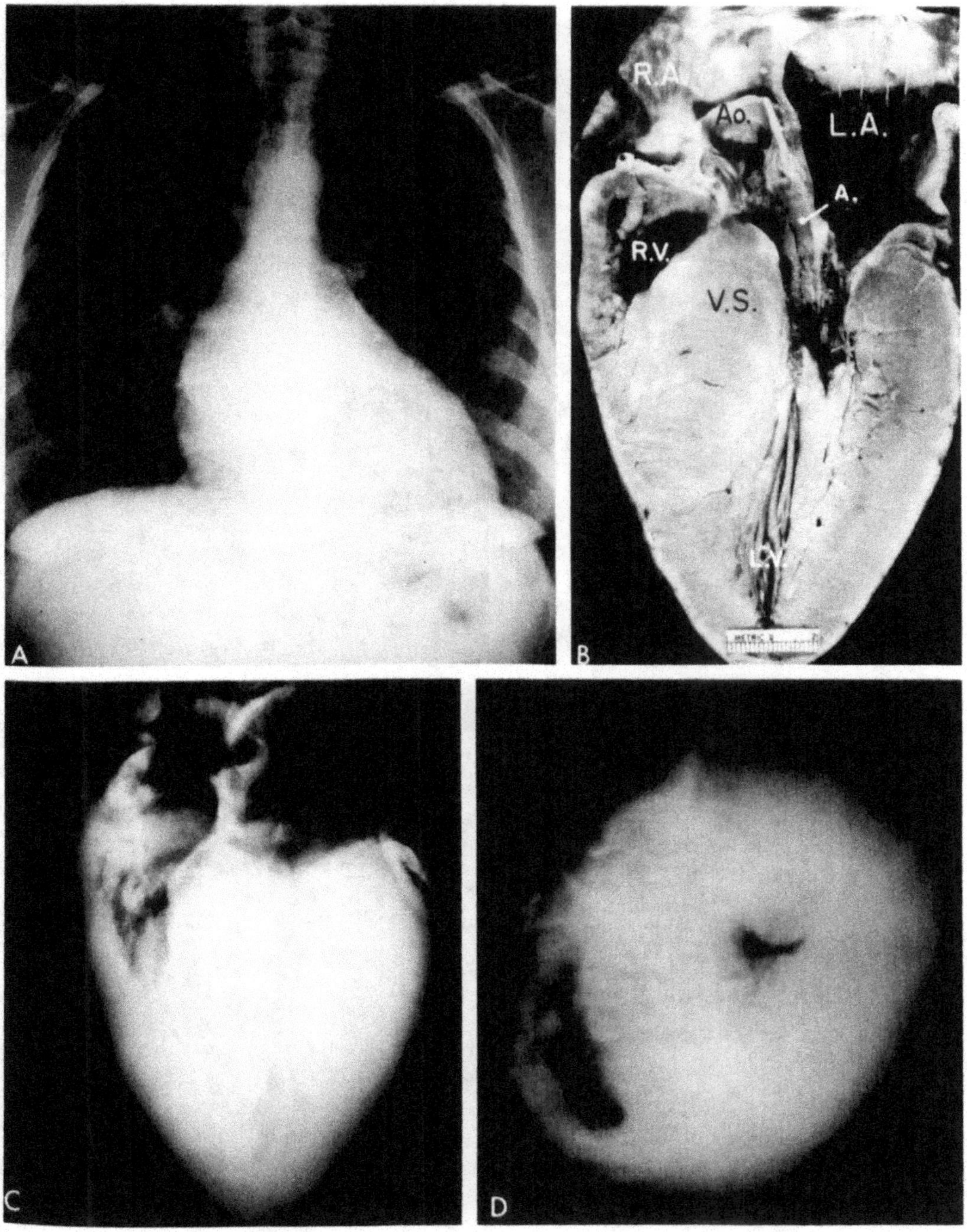

Figure 13. Hypertrophic asymmetric obstructive cardiomyopathy. This 36 year old woman (A67-121) developed congestive cardiac failure during her second pregnancy at age 32. When studied at age 34, she had a grade 3/6 precordial systolic murmur, loudest over the apex, and audible third and fourth heart sounds. An electrocardiogram showed bilateral bundle branch block with left axis deviation and prolongation (0.23 sec.) of the P-R interval. Catheterization disclosed a 75 mm. Hg peak systolic pressure gradient at rest between the left ventricle (160/18) and femoral artery (85/50) and a 125 mm. Hg gradient with provocation (Valsalva). The premature ventricular response was positive for idiopathic hypertrophic subaortic stenosis. She died during an episode of rapid heart action. She was known to have had multiple premature ventricular contractions on occasion. At necropsy the heart was enlarged (*A*), weighing 450 gm., the left ventricular cavity was small (*B, C, D*), and the ventricular septum was much thicker than the left ventricular free wall. There was little room in the left ventricular cavity for the mitral leaflets, and contact lesions (fibromas) were present on the ventricular aspect of the anterior mitral leaflet and on the adjacent left ventricular mural endocardium (*B*). This is the typical "muscle bound" heart in which the ventricular cavities are minute in comparison to the mass of ventricular muscle. Both atria are dilated.

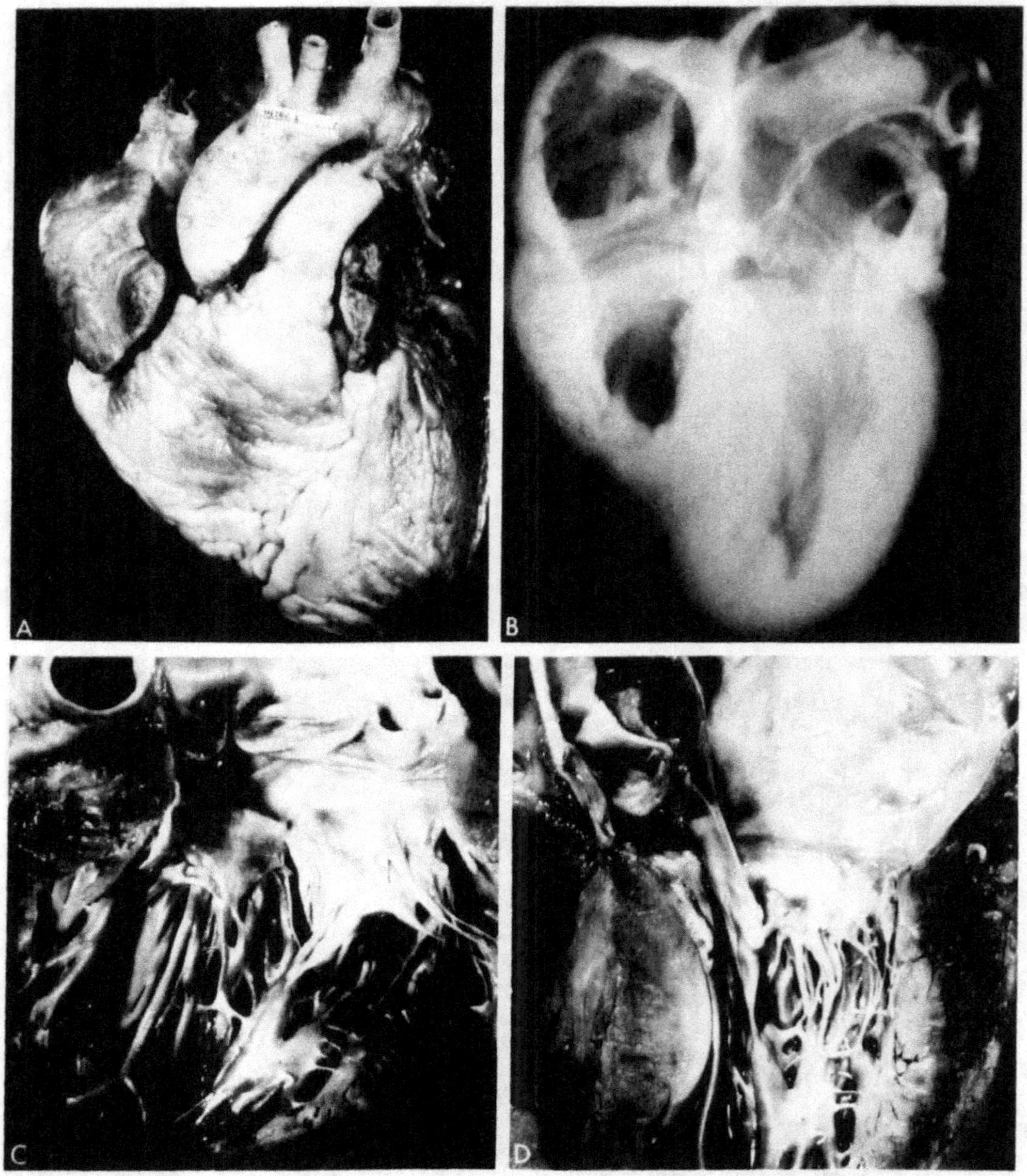

Figure 14. Hypertrophic asymmetric nonobstructive cardiomyopathy. This 33 year old man (A68–185) had no systolic pressure gradient at rest between the left ventricle and brachial artery, but a 33 mm. Hg gradient was provoked by isoproterenol. He died of sudden unilateral hemiparesis, which appeared six days after the catheterization. He had been asymptomatic when examined at age 26, when a grade 2 to 3/6 precordial systolic murmur, loudest at the apex, was heard. Catheterization at that time showed a 30 mm. Hg peak systolic gradient at rest between the left ventricle and brachial artery, and it rose to 85 mm. Hg with ouabain provocation. He became symptomatic (exertional and nocturnal dyspnea) six months before death, when atrial fibrillation appeared. The precordial murmur then was only intermittently audible. At necropsy the heart weighed 450 gm.; both atria were dilated but neither ventricle was dilated *(A)*. The ventricular septum was thicker than the left ventricular free wall *(B)*. A mural endocardial plaque was present in the left ventricular outflow tract, and the corresponding anterior mitral leaflet was thickened (*C*, *D*). The longitudinal cut of the heart in *D* clearly shows that the ventricular septum is thicker than the left ventricular free wall.

patients either by light or by electron microscope discloses only nonspecific findings. It is disappointing that the electron microscope has not been more useful from a diagnostic standpoint in this condition. Electron microscopic observations in the dilated type of idiopathic cardiomegaly, however, have been limited, and therefore it is possible that more specific findings will be appreciated with further study. Our knowledge of myocardial changes in the early stages of primary myocardial disease is limited. It is apparent, however, that once myocardial degeneration occurs, it can lead to a vicious cycle of further cardiac failure and further degeneration. Progression of degenerative changes in cardiac muscles may be responsible for the clinical deterioration and therapeutic unresponsiveness of patients with advanced stages of idiopathic cardiomegaly of the dilated type. There is not enough scarring in the walls of these hearts to account for the poor cardiac function.

Intracardiac mural thrombi in the idiopathic dilated type of cardiomyopathy probably represent anatomic manifestations of relative stasis of blood within the heart as a result of an extremely depressed cardiac output. The areas of greatest stasis appear to be the apices of the ventricles and the atrial appendages. On rare occasion left ventricular thrombi may be large enough to obstruct the blood flow within this chamber.

Although the typical heart in idiopathic cardiomyopathy of the dilated type has greatly dilated ventricles and ventricular walls of normal thickness, some patients with this condition have relatively thick ventricular walls and only mildly dilated cavities. The size of the left ventricular cavity appears to be roughly proportional to the severity and duration of symptomatic congestive heart failure; the larger the cavity, the longer the duration of symptoms and vice versa.

The myocardium in patients with the dilated type of cardiomyopathy occurring in the puerperium appears to be similar to that in patients with idiopathic dilated cardiomyopathies occurring in nonpuerperal states.[4,5] Fatty change in cardiac muscle cells, however, a common finding in pa-

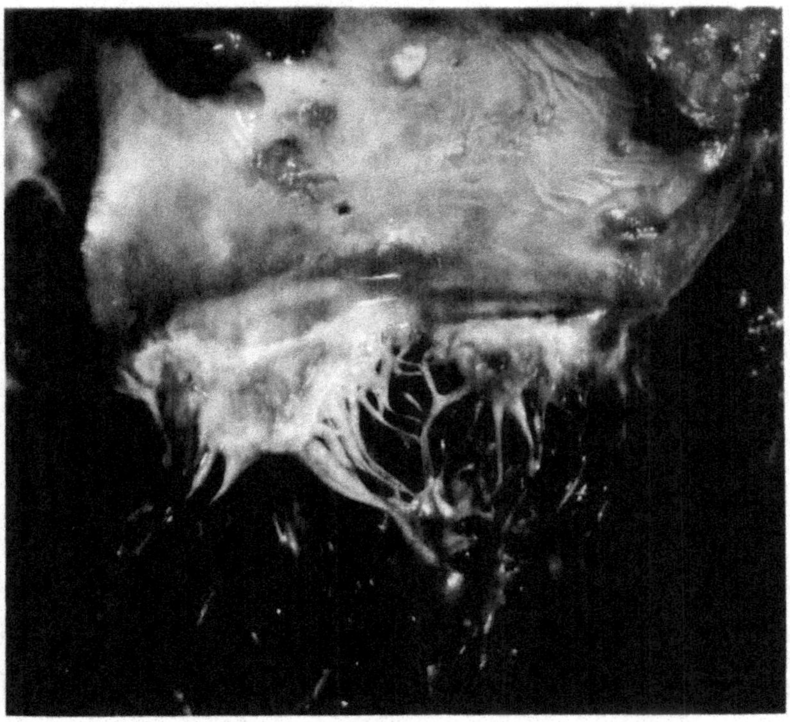

Figure 15. Hypertrophic asymmetric obstructive cardiomyopathy. Opened mitral valve showing that both posterior and anterior leaflets are thickened in the patient described in Figure 14 (A68–185). This type of leaflet thickening is typical of hypertrophic cardiomyopathy.

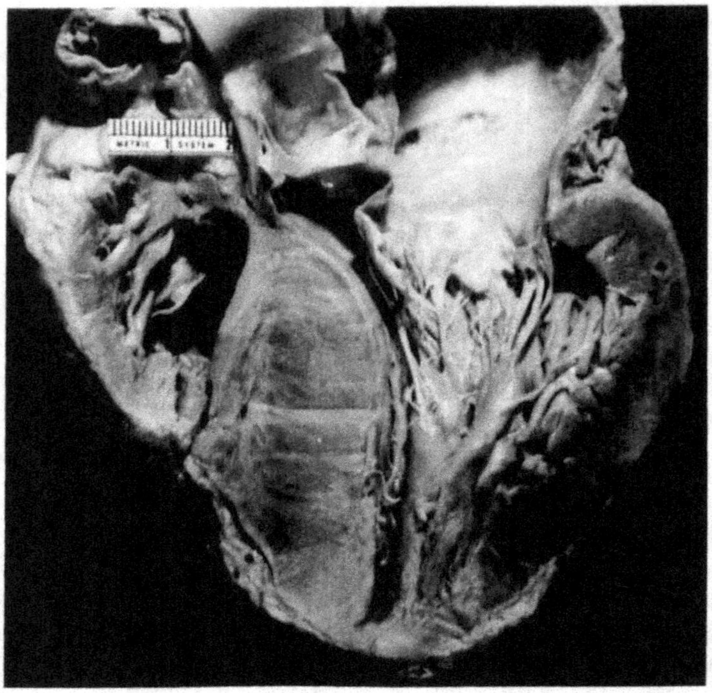

Figure 16. Hypertrophic asymmetric nonobstructive cardiomyopathy. This 33 year old woman (A67-70) became mildly symptomatic when she was 15 years of age. She had three pregnancies without difficulty, but during the fourth she had overt congestive cardiac failure. When admitted to the National Heart and Lung Institute at age 28, she had exertional dyspnea, chest pain, and occasional episodes of dizziness. Several other family members had idiopathic hypertrophic subaortic stenosis. A grade 2/6 precordial systolic murmur, loudest at the apex, and a fourth heart sound were audible. An electrocardiogram showed left bundle branch block and premature ventricular contractions. The cardiac silhouette was enlarged by radiography. No systolic gradient was present between the left ventricle (108/34 mm. Hg) and the brachial artery (114/64 mm. Hg) at rest. By age 30, the angina, dyspnea, and dizziness were more frequent and worse; the syncope had occurred once. On repeat catheterization there was still no systolic gradient present between the left ventricle (97/30 mm. Hg) and the femoral artery (102/58) at rest, but a 9 mm. Hg gradient was provoked by isoproterenol. The premature ventricular contraction response was normal. Repeat catheterization two years later yielded virtually identical findings. The left ventricular angiocardiogram was interpreted as showing "cavity obliteration." She was found dead in bed at home four months later. At necropsy the heart weighed 430 gm. The ventricular septum was much thicker than the left ventricular free wall, which was of normal thickness. The mitral leaflets were only slightly thickened and no endocardial mural plaque was present in the left ventricular outflow tract. Both atria were dilated. This case is typical of the nonobstructive variety of hypertrophic asymmetric cardiomyopathy and is characterized by normal thickness of at least the basal portion of the left ventricular free wall.

tients with nonpuerperal dilated cardiomyopathy and chronic alcoholism,[6,7] may be less frequent in puerperal cardiomyopathy.

Nondilated (Hypertrophic) Cardiomyopathy

This section summarizes observations in 40 patients with hypertrophic cardiomyopathy studied at necropsy by the authors (Figs. 12 to 28). The findings in some of these patients have been described previously.[8-11] The 40 patients ranged in age from nine to 78 years (average, 42): 23 were women and 17 were males. Other family members of 15 patients had similar cardiac conditions. Thirteen patients had systemic hypertension; five, anemia (blood hematocrit < 35 per cent); nine, atrial fibrillation; nine, bundle branch block (left in three, indeterminate in five, and bilateral in one); and one, complete heart block (the latter was preceded by left bundle branch block). Eighteen patients died naturally of the cardiac condition (13 suddenly, five in progressive congestive cardiac failure), nine after cardiac operations, three of complications of cardiac catheterization, one of acute myocardial infarction, and nine of noncardiac causes.

The 40 patients were divided into three groups on the basis of documentation by cardiac catheterization of the presence or absence of peak systolic pressure gradients

(Text continued on page 313.)

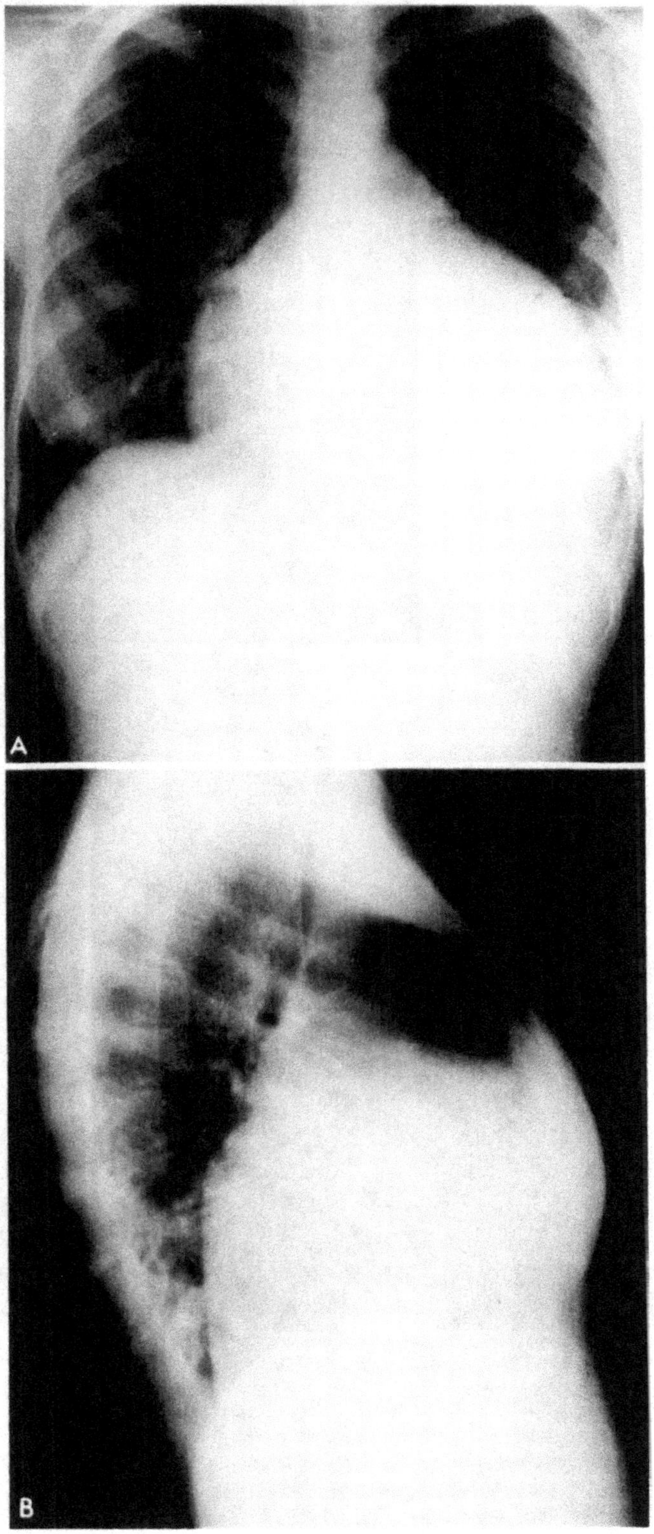

Figure 17. Hypertrophic asymmetric obstructive cardiomyopathy in a 20 year old woman (A72–197). A precordial murmur had been heard at age 11, and symptoms (exertional dyspnea and palpitations) appeared at age 12 years. Catheterization at age 14 disclosed a 50 mm. Hg peak systolic pressure gradient between the left ventricle (158/10) and the brachial artery (108/57) and an abnormal premature ventricular response. A left ventricular cineangiocardiogram was consistent with idiopathic hypertrophic subaortic stenosis and showed considerable mitral regurgitation. The left ventricular cavity was small. From age 14 to 20 she had no overt congestive cardiac failure, but there were episodic palpitations and rarely chest pain relieved by rest. During this time she was functionally class II (New York Heart Association). Three months before death she had clinical, electrocardiographic, and enzymatic changes typical of acute transmural (anterolateral wall) myocardial infarction. During the period of infarction there was evidence of congestive cardiac failure. After discharge she continued to have mild dyspnea and episodic chest pain. She died shortly after the sudden appearance of features of acute pulmonary edema. The radiographs shown here were taken four years before death (age 16 years). The cardiac silhouette is massively enlarged. At necropsy the heart weighed 1250 gm. and she weighed only 47 kg. This may be one of the largest hearts ever recorded in a woman.

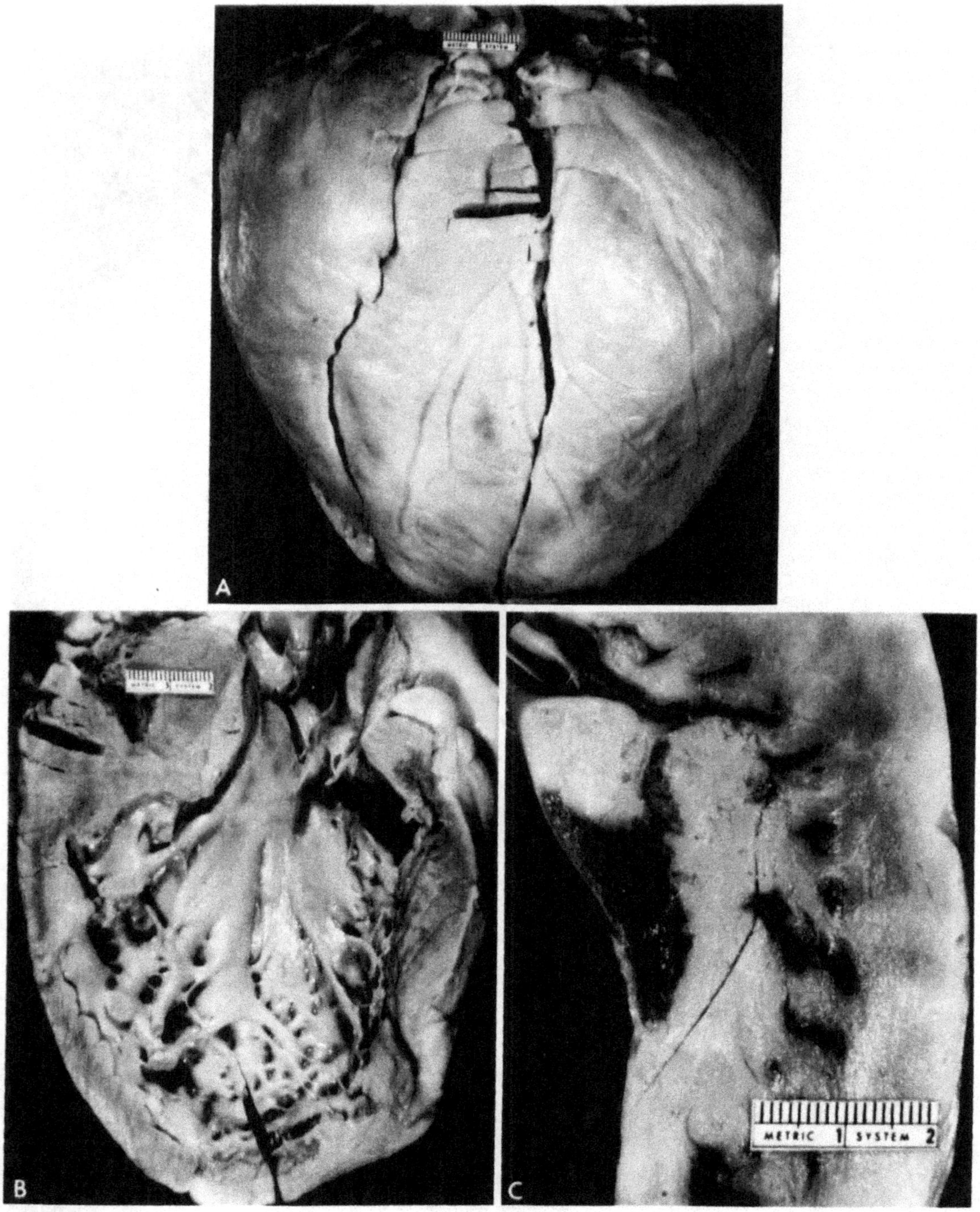

Figure 18. Hypertrophic asymmetric obstructive cardiomyopathy in the patient described in Figure 17 (A72–197). The unusual feature here is the massive degree of the cardiac hypertrophy (1250 gm.; *A*), the absence of an endocardial fibrous plaque in the left ventricular outflow tract, the absence of thickening of the mitral leaflets (*B*), and the occurrence of myocardial necrosis (acute myocardial infarction) without coronary arterial luminal narrowing. The ventricular septum is enormously thickened. Both the anterior and the posterior left ventricular free walls are thinned, presumably a result of the acute myocardial infarction three months before death. A longitudinal section showing necrosis in one left ventricular papillary muscle is shown in *C*. The left ventricular cavity in this patient is dilated (*B*), but the dilatation is probably the result of the myocardial infarction rather than idiopathic hypertrophic subaortic stenosis, because a left ventricular angiogram several years before the infarction had shown a "small" left ventricular cavity.

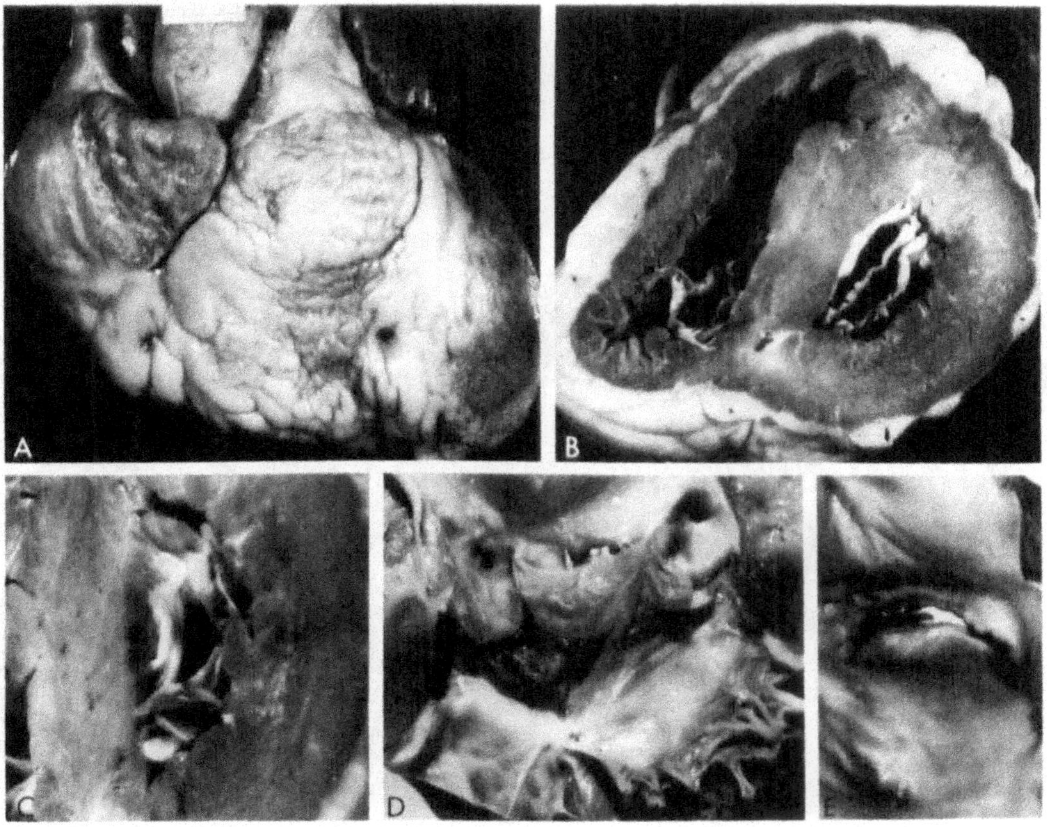

Figure 19. Hypertrophic symmetric (nonobstructive) cardiomyopathy. This 46 year old woman (A72-15), who was noted to have a precordial murmur at age 16, was asymptomatic until age 29, when features of congestive cardiac failure appeared. At age 36 she was studied at the National Heart and Lung Institute. Her father had died of heart disease at age 42, and two siblings in their 30's had had heart disease of an unknown type. A grade 4/6 precordial systolic murmur, loudest at the apex, and a fourth heart sound were audible. An electrocardiogram showed left axis deviation, atrial abnormality, and left ventricular hypertrophy. At catheterization the pressures (in mm. Hg) were: pulmonary artery 36/16; right ventricle 42/4; left atrium m14, a24, v15, and simultaneous left ventricle and brachial artery 162/16 and 96/60, respectively, giving a 66 mm. Hg peak systolic gradient. This gradient increased with isoproterenol infusion. The typical premature ventricular beat response of idiopathic hypertrophic subaortic stenosis was present. A left ventricular cineangiocardiogram was diagnostic of idiopathic hypertrophic subaortic stenosis. From age 36 to 44 she did well and at age 43 could swim, hike two miles, and climb one flight of stairs with difficulty. At age 44 exertional dyspnea became bothersome again, and intermittent claudication of the right leg appeared. At age 45 episodic tachycardia and angina pectoris appeared, and six months before death she had two episodes of syncope, one followed by transient hemiplegia. She was readmitted to the National Heart and Lung Institute one month before death and was functionally class III (New York Heart Association). Examination showed that now no precordial murmur was present, but loud third and fourth heart sounds were audible. The liver was enlarged and all pulses in both legs were absent. Electrocardiogram showed sinus rhythm, a prolonged P-R interval (>0.20 sec.), left axis deviation, low voltage, and Q waves in II, III, and AVF. Radiography showed enlargement of both the left atrium and the left ventricle. The serum cholesterol and triglyceride levels were normal. During the first several days in the hospital she lost 5 kg. and felt better. Shortly thereafter, however, she became febrile and had a grand mal seizure. Her course thereafter was progressively downhill, characterized by complete heart block, atrial fibrillation, low urine output, and hypotension. It is likely that no outflow gradient was present during her last year of life because during this period no precordial murmur was heard. At necropsy the atria were dilated, the ventricular cavities were not dilated, and the ventricular septum was identical in thickness to the left ventricular free wall (*A, B*). An endocardial mural plaque was present in the left ventricular outflow tract (*C, D*) and the ventricular aspect of the anterior mitral leaflet was thickened. *A*, View of heart from anterior aspect. The atria are prominent. *B*, Transverse section of ventricles. The mural endocardial plaque in the left ventricular outflow tract is apparent. *C*, Close-up view of endocardial plaque. *D*, Opened left ventricular outflow tract. *E*, Mitral orifice viewed from left atrium. This orifice is always "small" in hypertrophic cardiomyopathy because the left ventricular cavity is not dilated.

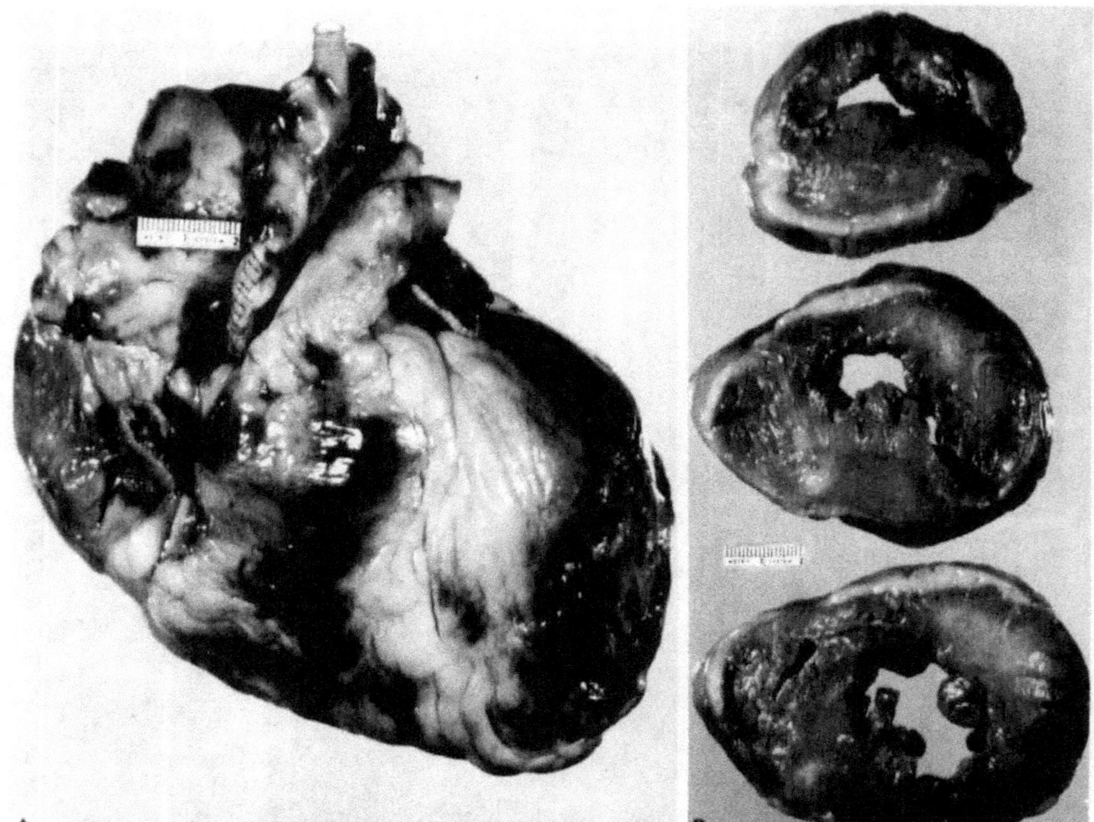

A B

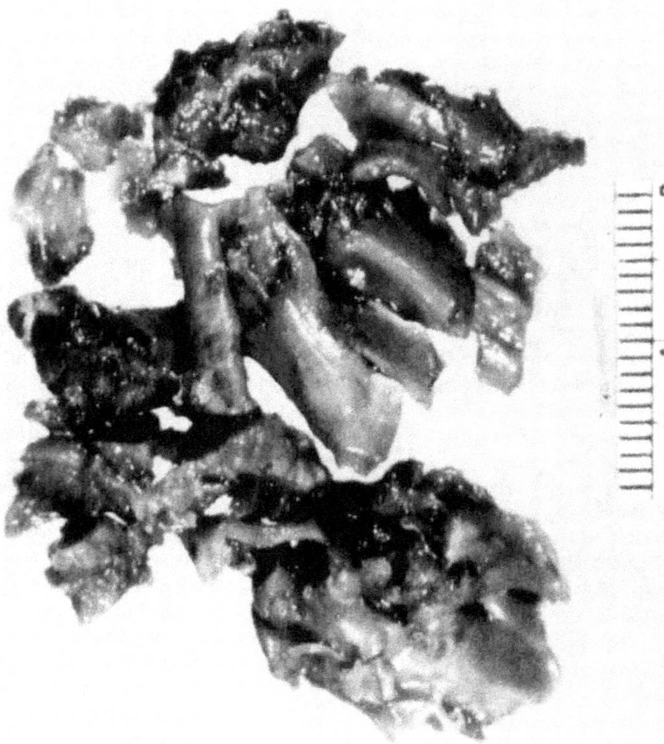

C

Figure 20. Hypertrophic symmetric (nonobstructive) cardiomyopathy. This 25 year old woman (A72–200) developed exertional dyspnea at age 21. During the next four years congestive heart failure progressed and angina pectoris appeared. She had a grade 2 to 3/6 precordial systolic murmur, loudest at the apex, and the murmur was increased in intensity by the Valsalva maneuver. Catheterization at age 23 disclosed no systolic pressure gradient between the left ventricle (124/25 mm. Hg) and the femoral artery (125/83). A repeat study at age 25 (10 months before death) was similar: left ventricle 130/38 and femoral artery 130/80 mm. Hg. On cineangiocardiography the left ventricular cavity was minute and there was mild mitral regurgitation. Because of a lack of improvement with propanolol therapy, a left ventricular myotomy and myectomy was performed. Because the aorta was so small, the resection had to be carried out via a left ventriculotomy incision. Approximately 8 gm. of myocardium was excised *(C)*. *A*, Anterior view of heart. *B*, Transverse sections of ventricles. The top one is near the apex and the bottom one near the base. The anterior free wall near the apex and the posterior free wall near the base are of normal thickness.

Figure 21. Hypertrophic asymmetric obstructive cardiomyopathy. This 19 year old girl (A70–278), who was found to have a precordial murmur at age six, was asymptomatic until age 19 (22 months before death), when she developed fever, supraventricular arrhythmias, and alpha streptococcal septicemia two months after some dental work. Because of a marked deterioration in effort tolerance, cardiac catheterization was performed (16 months before death). A peak systolic pressure gradient of 162 mm. Hg was recorded between the left ventricle (260/20) and the ascending aorta (98/75), and a 38 mm. Hg gradient between the right ventricle (62/12) and the pulmonary trunk (28/20). A left ventricular cineangiocardiogram was typical of idiopathic hypertrophic subaortic stenosis. Mitral regurgitation was trivial. The apical portion of the left ventricle was not visualized on angiography. The coronary arteries appeared normal following aortic root injection. An electrocardiogram showed biventricular hypertrophy. At an operation (left ventricular outflow myotomy and myectomy) performed nine days before death a left ventricular apical aneurysm, noted here, was observed. A left ventricular aneurysm is indeed rare in idiopathic hypertrophic subaortic stenosis except after left ventricular incision during operative therapy. This aneurysm is unique in that its wall consists of myocardium similar to that in other portions of the left ventricular free wall. (Most aneurysms at this site obviously consist entirely of fibrous tissue, the result of healing of an acute myocardial infarction, and myocardial fibers are infrequently observed in the aneurysmal wall.) The mechanism of formation of this "myocardial aneurysm" is uncertain. It might be reasoned that the extremely high left ventricular systolic pressure (260 mm. Hg) simply caused bulging of the thinnest portion of the left ventricular free wall, i.e., the apex. Because left ventricular outflow was obstructed, this high pressure was exerted onto the apex with resulting aneurysmal formation. This high a systolic left ventricular pressure in idiopathic hypertrophic subaortic stenosis is unusual at any age but particularly so in childhood, and the latter in some way also may have been a factor. At autopsy the heart weighed 730 gm. and the ventricular septum was disproportionally hypertrophied. The left ventricular cavity was minute. The apical aneurysm was free of thrombus; its wall consisted of myocardial fibers, many of which had been made necrotic by the ligature that had been placed about the base of the aneurysm at operation nine days earlier.

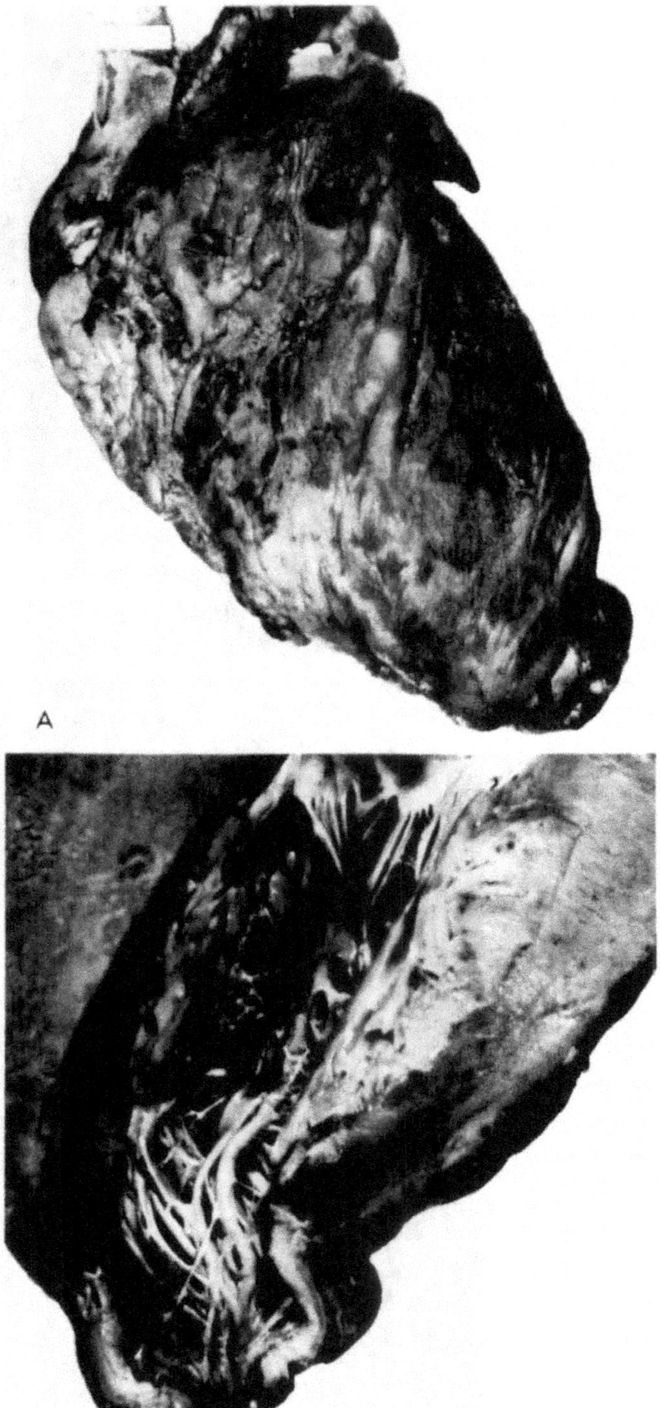

A

B

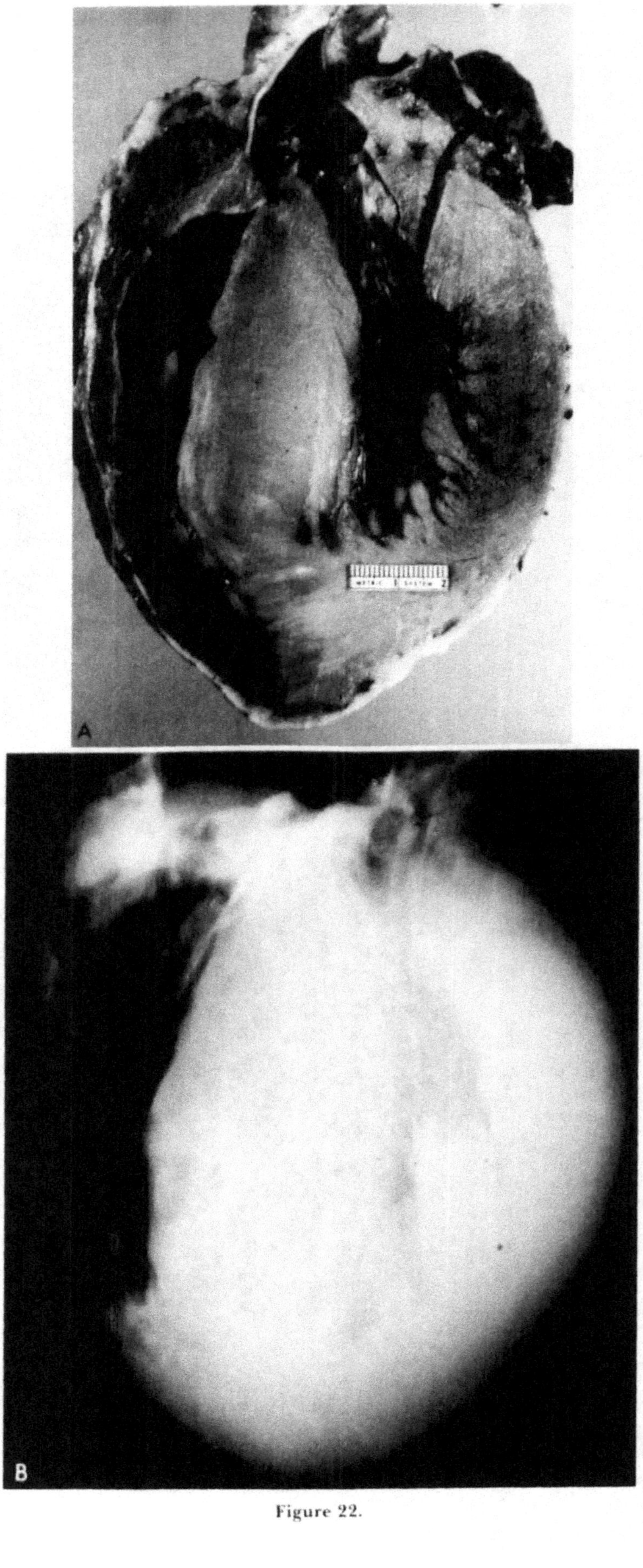

Figure 22.

at rest between the left ventricle and a systemic artery (Table 1). Twenty patients had subaortic stenosis with a peak systolic pressure gradient at rest of 20 to 170 mm. Hg (average, 93; group I). Thirteen patients with zero pressure gradients at rest comprise group II; provocation in 11 patients produced gradients (range, 10 to 150 mm. Hg) in seven. In only one patient was the provoked peak systolic pressure gradient greater than 32 mm. Hg. The seven patients in whom cardiac catheterization was not performed comprise group III. The diagnosis of idiopathic hypertrophic subaortic stenosis was established preoperatively in 19 of 20 patients in group I, in 11 of 13 patients in group II, and in only two of seven patients in group III. The only undiagnosed patient in group I was studied in 1956 before this disorder was recognized as a distinct entity. The two undiagnosed patients in group II clinically had pure mitral regurgitation, believed to be on a rheumatic basis, but again each was studied before the clinical and hemodynamic features of idiopathic hypertrophic subaortic stenosis were well recognized; one died in 1961 and the second in 1963.

At planned mitral valve replacement in one, the left ventricular wall was found to be thick and the cavity, small; idiopathic hypertrophic subaortic stenosis therefore was suspected and later confirmed at postoperative catheterization. The clue to the proper diagnosis in each of the two patients in group II was the rapidly rising systemic arterial pulses. An additional clue in one patient was the increased intensity of the precordial systolic murmur during beats following premature ventricular contractions.[9] The diagnosis of idiopathic hypertrophic subaortic stenosis in each of the eight patients in whom this diagnosis was not established clinically was made at necropsy by observing anatomic cardiac findings identical to those in patients in whom the diagnosis was established by clinical means.

The 20 patients in group I averaged 43 years of age; the 13 in group II, 28 years; and the seven in group III, 67 years. All patients in group I had symptoms of cardiac dysfunction; two patients in group II and four in group III were asymptomatic. Whereas only six patients in group I had histories of similar heart disease in other family members, nine patients in group II had positive histories. Precordial systolic murmurs ranging in intensity from grades 3/6 to 5/6 were present at some time in all 20 patients in group I. In one patient, however, a grade 3/6 systolic precordial murmur was audible eight years before death when the peak systolic pressure gradient was 70 mm. Hg, but when she was examined during the last year of life, no precordial murmur was audible. Similar murmurs occurred in 11 of 13 patients in group II, but the intensity was less (grade

Figure 22. Hypertrophic asymmetric obstructive (right sided) cardiomyopathy. This 18 year old boy (A72-78), described in detail elsewhere,[12] was studied initially when he was asymptomatic at age eight years because his brother had just died suddenly at age nine from idiopathic hypertrophic subaortic stenosis (left sided obstruction). At catheterization, no systolic pressure gradient was observed between the left ventricle and the systemic artery, but a 35 mm. Hg systolic pressure gradient was recorded between the right ventricle (56/5) and the pulmonary artery (21/9). An electrocardiogram showed right axis deviation, right ventricular hypertrophy, and a right ventricular conduction delay. The child remained asymptomatic until age 12, when he developed chest pain while playing football. Precordial pain recurred frequently thereafter and was precipitated by exertion of decreasing intensity so that he was forced to limit his activities to a sedentary level. When he was restudied at age 13, a grade 4/6 systolic ejection type of precordial murmur was heard, loudest along the left sternal border. Electrocardiography now showed more severe right ventricular hypertrophy. Catheterization showed a 118 mm. Hg peak systolic pressure gradient between the right ventricle (135/7) and pulmonary artery (17/7) and there was no systolic gradient between the left ventricle (108/4) and the brachial artery (108/63 mm. Hg). Resection of the right ventricular outflow myocardium with insertion of a patch at the right ventriculotomy was performed, and catheterization seven months postoperatively showed virtually no systolic pressure gradient between the right ventricle (30/4 mm. Hg) and the pulmonary artery (28/12). He was asymptomatic. Electrocardiography now showed a right bundle branch block. This boy apparently remained asymptomatic until the day of death, when he felt faint while driving a car. He pulled over to the side of the road and collapsed. No anatomic explanation for death was provided by necropsy. His heart weighed 660 gm. The right ventricular outflow tract was wide open. The ventricular septum was much thicker than the left ventricular free wall (4.0 compared to 1.9 cm.), and the right ventricular wall was of normal thickness. The endocardium of the left ventricular outflow tract was not thickened and the mitral valve was normal. Mild interstitial fibrosis involved the ventricular septum. *A*, A longitudinal section of the ventricles shows the disproportional ventricular septal hypertrophy. The right ventricular cavity is larger than the left. *B*, The radiograph of the heart was taken before it was opened.

3/6 in three patients, grade 2/6 in five, grade 1/6 in three). Systolic murmurs were audible in six (grade 4/6 in one, grade 3/6 in four) of seven patients in group III. Four of 20 patients in group I, two of 12 in group II, and one of seven in group III had atrial fibrillation. Of 15 patients in group I in whom left ventricular angiographic studies were performed, seven had mitral regurgitation; of nine patients in

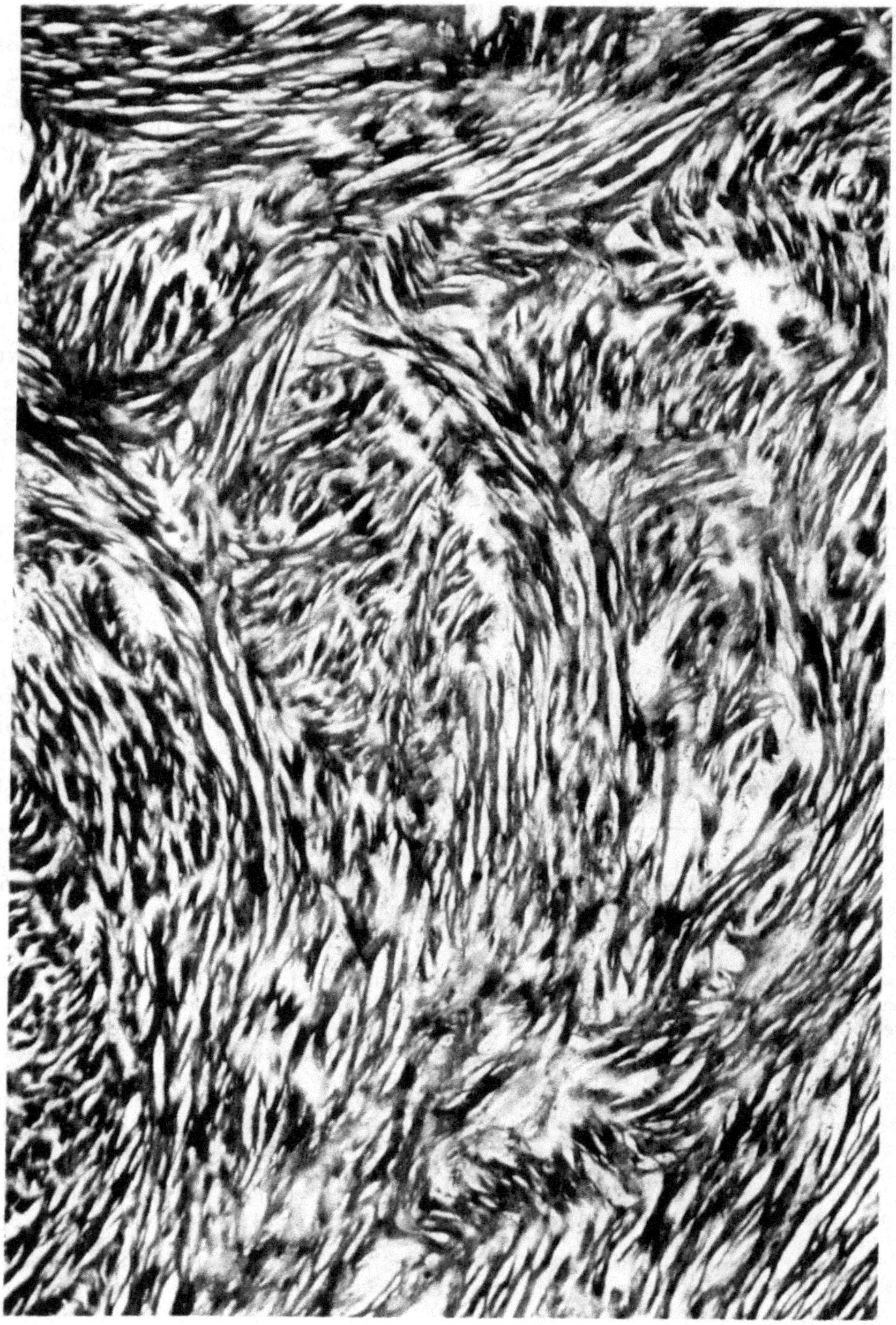

Figure 23. Histologic section of ventricular septal myocardium from 19 year old man with hypertrophic obstructive cardiomyopathy. The bundles of muscle cells are irregularly arranged and course in various directions. (Masson stain, × 60.)

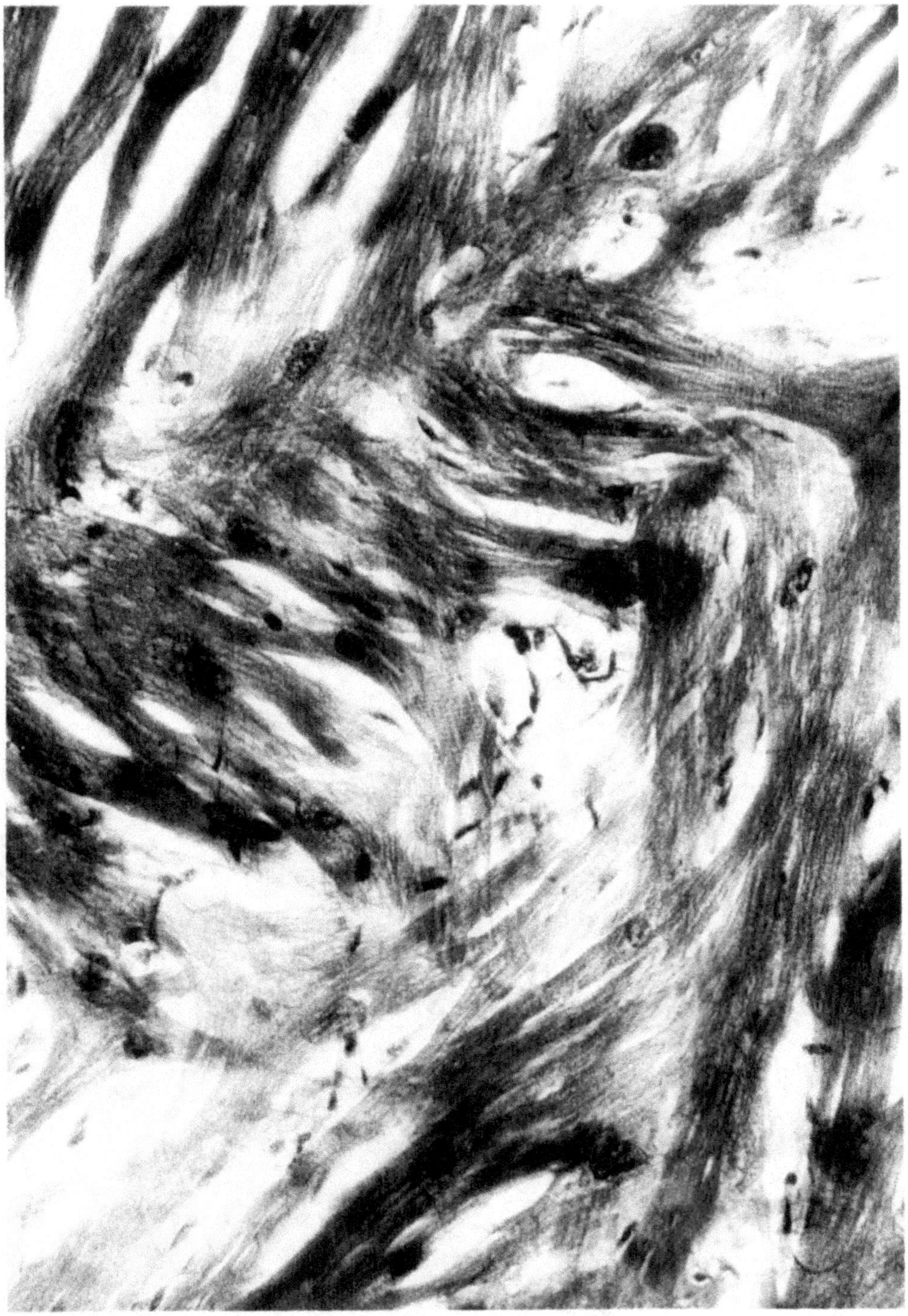

Figure 24. High power view of same tissue as in Figure 23, showing marked divergence in the orientation of adjacent muscle cells. (Masson stain. × 300.)

group II with left ventricular angiograms, five had mitral regurgitation. Seven patients in group I and four in group II had systolic pressure gradients between the right ventricle and pulmonary trunk. One of the latter patients had a 128 mm. Hg peak systolic pressure gradient between the right ventricular body and pulmonary trunk and none between the left ventricle and systemic artery.[12] His brother, how-

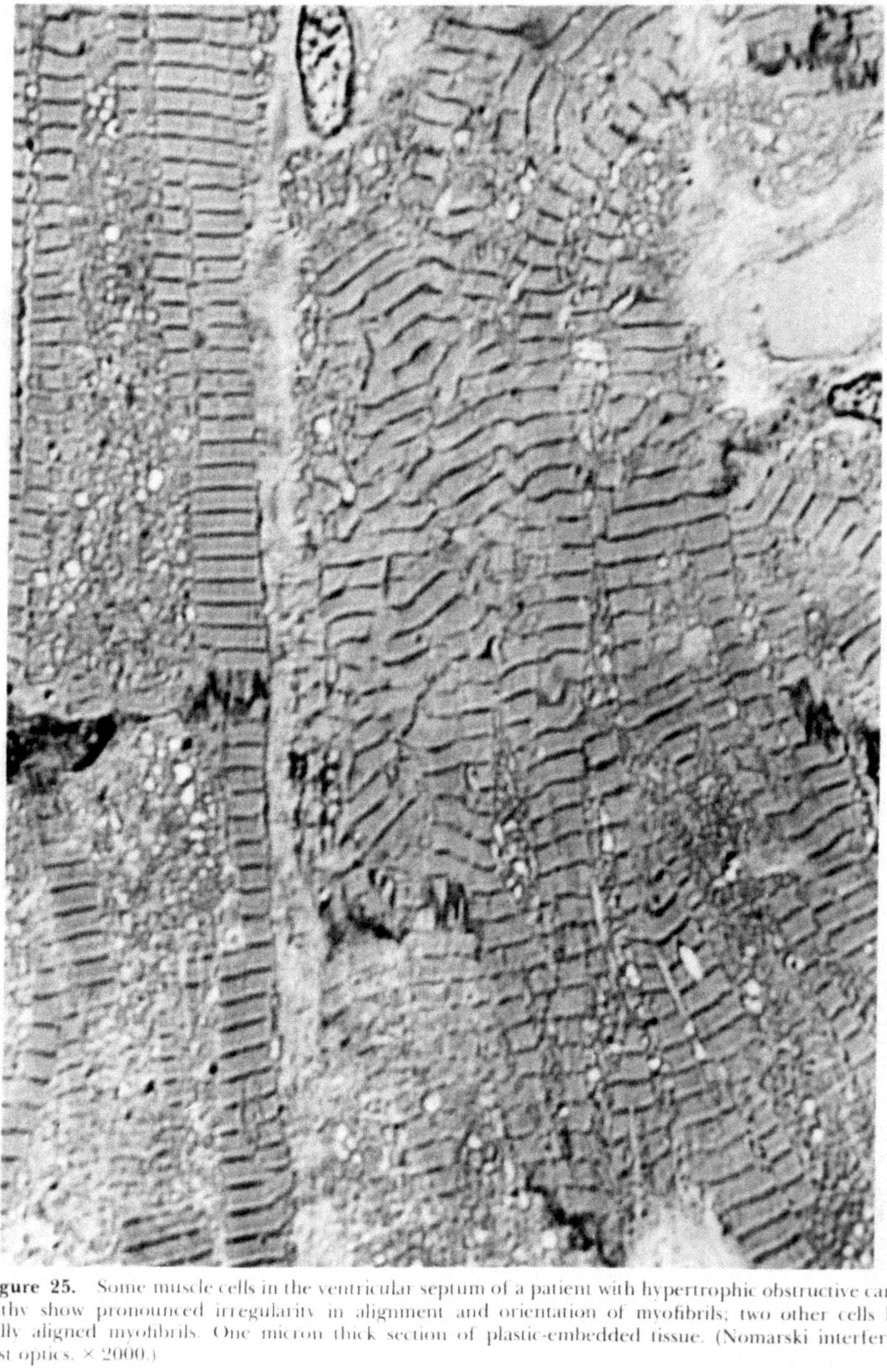

Figure 25. Some muscle cells in the ventricular septum of a patient with hypertrophic obstructive cardiomyopathy show pronounced irregularity in alignment and orientation of myofibrils; two other cells have normally aligned myofibrils. One micron thick section of plastic-embedded tissue. (Nomarski interference contrast optics. × 2000.)

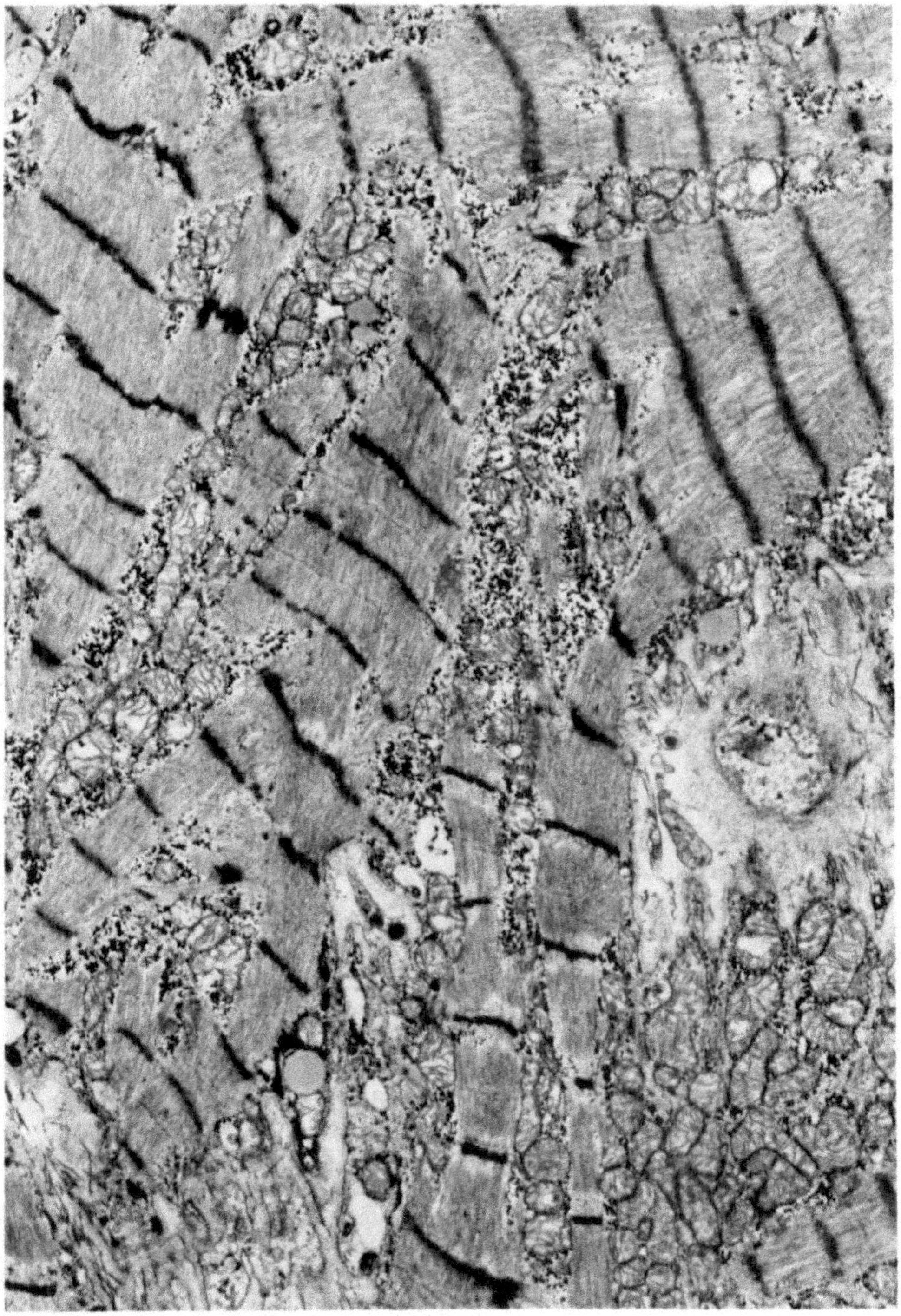

Figure 26. Part of muscle cell in ventricular septum of 29 year old woman with hypertrophic nonobstructive cardiomyopathy showing abnormal myofibrillar orientation and focal thickening of Z bands. (× 8000.)

ever, had typical left sided idiopathic hypertrophic subaortic stenosis. Four patients in group I and five in group II had pulmonary hypertension; in two patients the pulmonary systolic pressure was greater than 50 mm. Hg. Six of 11 patients in group I and seven of nine patients in group II had elevated left atrial pressures; all 12 patients with elevated left atrial pressures had either mitral regurgitation or elevated left ventricular end diastolic pressures. Twelve patients in group I and nine in group II had elevated (≥ 12 mm. Hg) left ventricular end diastolic pressures.

The necropsy cardiac observations in 40 patients are summarized in Table 1. The hearts of the 40 patients ranged from 350 to 1250 gm. (average, 634). In 33 patients the ventricular septa were unequivocally thicker than the thickest portion of left ventricular free wall. In all 20 patients with documented left ventricular outflow obstruction at rest, the left ventricular free walls (anterior, lateral, and posterior) were hypertrophied and to similar degrees at all corresponding levels (Fig. 15). In contrast, the left ventricular free walls behind the posterior mitral leaflets were not thickened in 11 of 13 patients without obstruction at rest, and in two of them the entire free wall was of normal thickness. In 40 patients both ventricular cavities appeared smaller than normal or normal in size. The mural endocardium of the left ventricular outflow tract in apposition to the anterior mitral leaflet was thickened in 29 patients. The mitral valve leaflets, particularly the anterior ones, were thickened by fibrous tissue in 29 patients. Both left and right atria were dilated in 40 patients. Except for fibromas in two patients, the aortic valve cusps were normal. Foci of fibrosis were observed grossly in the left ventricular papillary muscles in 38 patients, and these structures appeared smaller than normal in all of them. Other subendocardial scars were present grossly in most patients. Only one had a transmural scar and it was small. Excluding the nine patients who died during or soon after cardiac operations, foci of myocardial necrosis were present in only one patient. She was a 21 year old woman who had an acute myocardial infarct beginning three months before death. The coronary arteries were normal, but her heart weighed 1250 gm. (body weight, 47 kg.). Histologic examination of sections of the left ventricular free wall and of the ventricular septum disclosed interstitial fibrosis of varying degrees in all patients and, usually, small foci of replacement fibrosis as well. Varying degrees of disorientation of myocardial fibers were observed in histologic sections of ventricular septa in all 40 patients. The intramural coronary arteries in the ventricular septae appeared increased in number and their walls were thick in one patient.

The myocardium in the left ventricular outflow tract of patients with idiopathic hypertrophic subaortic stenosis is distinctive by light and electron microscopy. Ferrans et al.[13] studied by electron microscope the operatively excised left ventricular outflow tract muscle in 14 patients with this disorder. Distinctive abnormalities were found in each patient. Bundles of muscle cells were severely disorganized with cells running in different directions instead of in parallel. Muscle cells were wider and shorter than in hypertrophy due to other causes and showed increased cellular branching, extensive side-to-side intercellular junctions, widened Z bands, and evidence of formation of new sarcomeres. Some myofibrils were oriented obliquely or perpendicular to the longitudinal axes of the cells, and some myofilaments that originated from a single Z band inserted into the Z bands of other myofibrils. Examination of the left ventricular apical myocardium in two of the 14 patients disclosed hypertrophied but normally arranged muscle cells. The abnormal architecture of the muscle cells appears to be a unique feature of hypertrophic cardiomyopathy.

Comments on Idiopathic Cardiomyopathy of the Hypertrophic Type. Study of our patients with hypertrophic cardiomyopathy disclosed several characteristic anatomic features of this entity: disproportional hypertrophy of the ventricular septum, small or normal sized left and right ventricular cavities, endocardial mural plaque of the left ventricular outflow tract, thickened mitral valve, dilated atria, hypertrophied (focal or diffuse) free walls of all four cardiac chambers, normal or nearly normal aortic valve cusps, normal sized ascending aorta, and severe abnormalities involving the organization of mus-

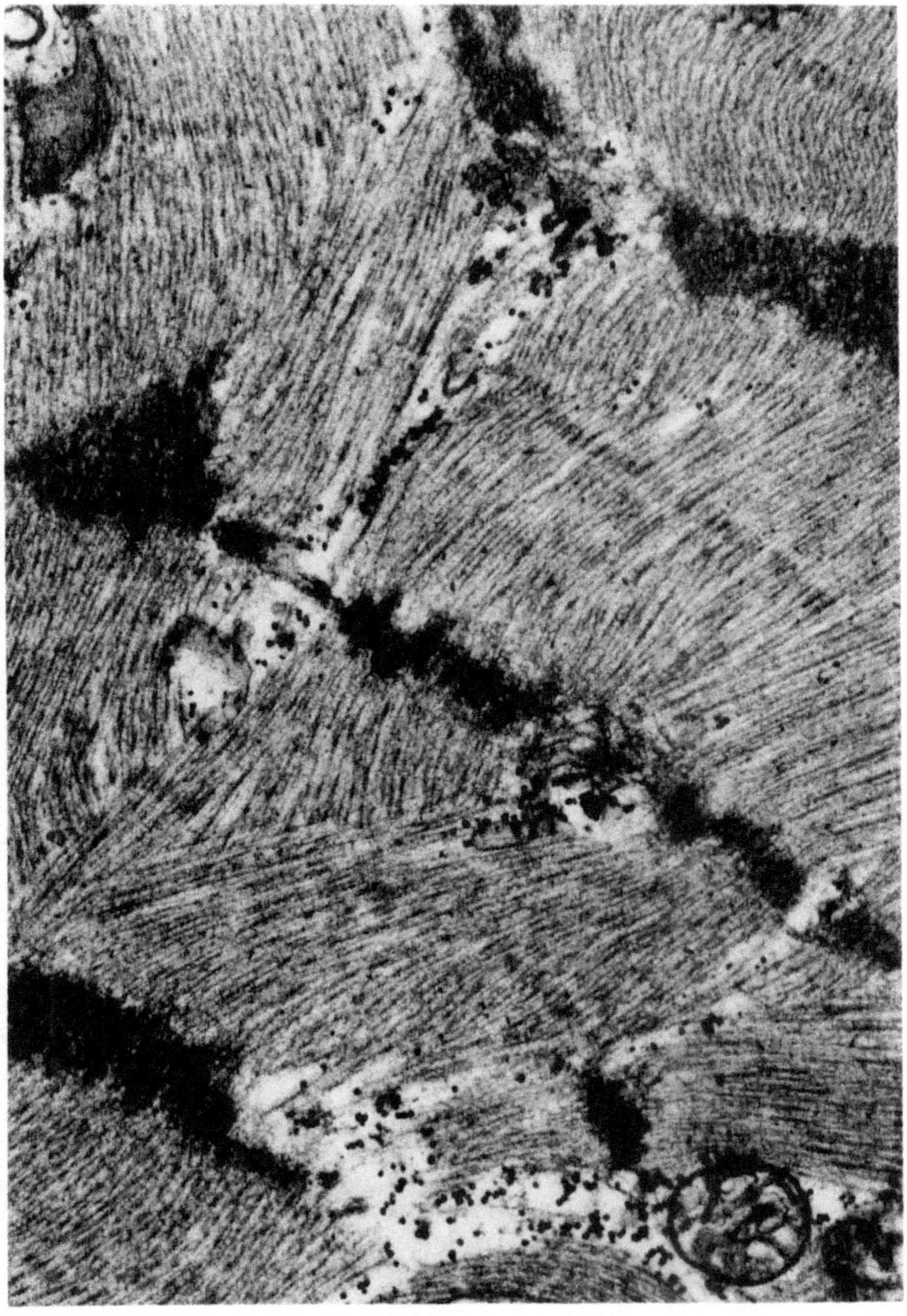

Figure 27. Marked thickening of Z bands and interweaving of myofilaments coursing in several different directions are shown in part of muscle cell from ventricular septum of 39 year old woman with hypertrophic obstructive cardiomyopathy. (× 47,000.)

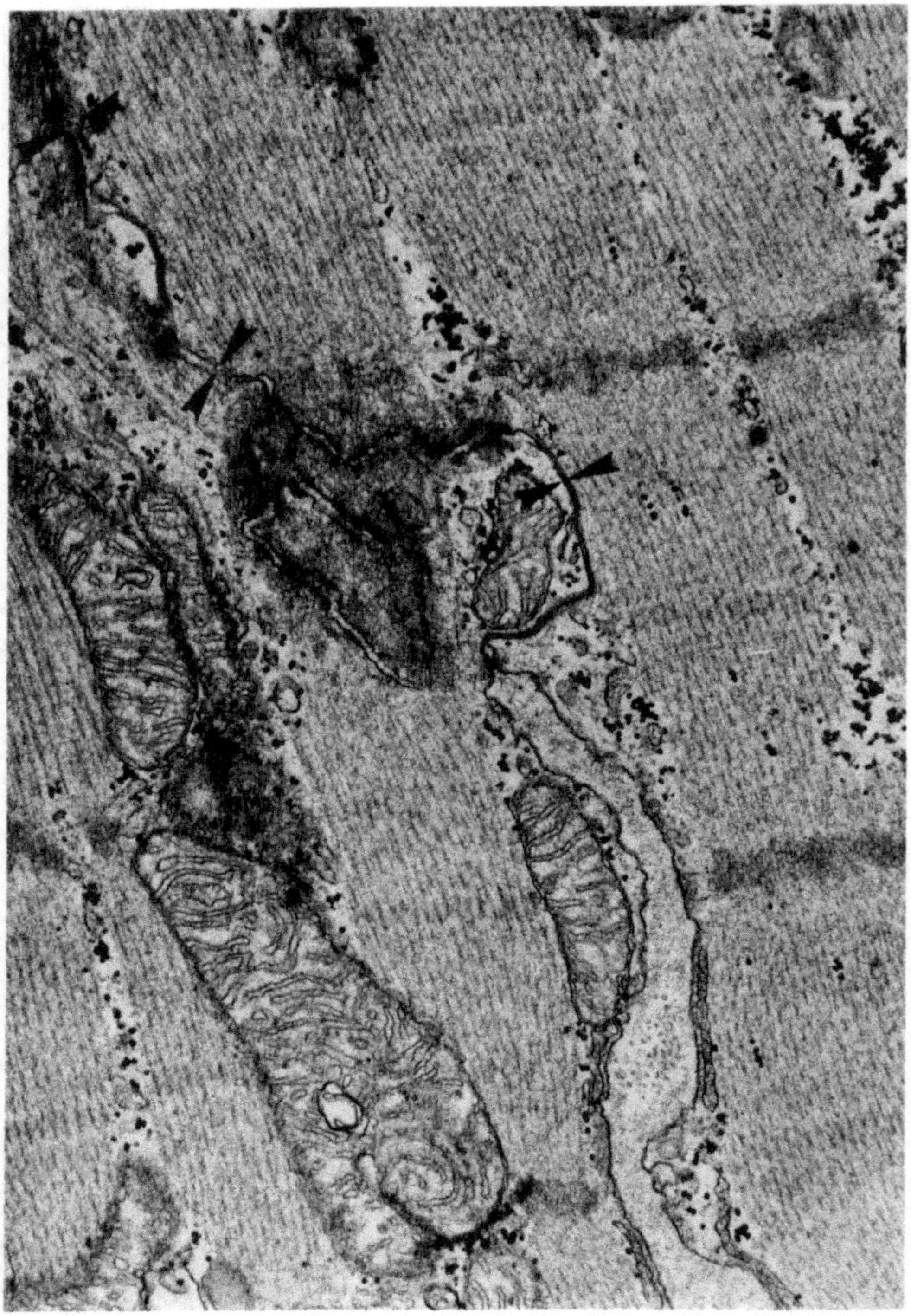

Figure 28. Area of side-to-side junction (arrowheads) between two adjacent muscle cells in ventricular septum of 30 year old man with hypertrophic obstructive cardiomyopathy. (× 40,000.)

cle cell bundles and the arrangement and orientation of myofibrils and myofilaments of individual muscle cells in the ventricular septum.

The major gross anatomic feature of hypertrophic cardiomyopathy is disproportional hypertrophy of the ventricular septum; i.e., the ventricular septum is thicker than the left ventricular free wall. Normally, at all ages, the ventricular septum and left ventricular free wall are equal in thickness. Disproportional or asymmetric septal hypertrophy is the characteristic anatomic feature of hypertrophic cardiomyopathy. Disproportional septal hypertrophy and disorganization of the septal muscle fibers are probably the only anatomic features of hypertrophic cardiomyopathy present from birth. The other features appear to be secondary to these basic defects and are acquired later. Originally it was believed that the thickest portion of the ventricular septum in this condition was that portion just below the aortic valve. Study of our 40 necropsy patients, however, clearly demonstrates that the thickest portion of the septum is about midway between the base of the aortic valve cusps and the apex of the left ventricle. The thickest portion of the septum also is usually just opposite the apex of the right ventricle. Thus, an adequate myotomy or myectomy in idiopathic hypertrophic subaortic stenosis must include interruption or excision of the myocardium located in the middle third of the septum and not just that portion close to the aortic valve.

Six of the 40 patients had symmetric rather than asymmetric hypertrophic cardiomyopathy. By definition, the thickest portion of the ventricular septum was equal in thickness to the thickest portion of the left ventricular free wall. In all six patients, however, that free wall immediately behind the posterior mitral leaflet was thinner than the thickest portion of the ventricular septum. It is probable that typical asymmetric septal hypertrophy had been present at one time in four of them, because each had mural endocardial fibrous plaques in the left ventricular outflow tract and correspondingly thickened anterior mitral leaflets. One (a 46 year old woman) of these three had had a 70 mm. Hg peak systolic pressure gradient between the left ventricle and a systemic artery and a loud systolic murmur eight years before death, but no murmur was audible during her last several months of life. It is possible that the ventricular septum thinned and outflow obstruction (and the murmur) disappeared as a consequence.

Another (a 62 year old woman) of these three patients had systemic hypertension, and a huge (170 mm. Hg) peak systolic pressure gradient was measured shortly before operation. Also preoperatively, an echocardiogram showed no disproportional septal hypertrophy. At operation disproportional septal hypertrophy was not observed, and pressure recordings in the operating room showed no systolic gradient between the left ventricle and the systemic artery. The third patient (a 53 year old man) had had systemic hypertension for years, and at catheterization at age 46 the peak systolic pressure gradient between the left ventricle and the systemic artery at rest was 8 mm. Hg and with provocation, 56 mm. Hg. The last of these four patients (a 65 year old woman) also had systemic hypertension but never underwent catheterization. The fifth patient (a 25 year old woman) with symmetric hypertrophy had no mural or valvular endocardial thickening and no peak systolic pressure gradient between the left ventricle and the systemic artery at rest or after provocation. The sixth patient (a nine year old boy) had massive cardiomegaly (670 gm. heart) and he weighed less than 50 kg. Injection of contrast material into the right and left ventricles at the same time showed that the ventricular septum was not disproportionally hypertrophied. This child died suddenly.

In addition to the six patients with symmetric hypertrophic cardiomyopathy already discussed, three others at necropsy also had ventricular septa identical in thickness to the left ventricular free walls. Each of them, however, had undergone left ventricular myotomy and myectomy (septectomy) for idiopathic hypertrophic subaortic stenosis 31 to 57 months earlier. One of them died of suicide, another of acute myocardial infection from severe coronary disease, and the third of progressive congestive cardiac failure. With the exception of the latter patient, not only had the ventricular septa returned to normal thickness but the ventricular cavities had dilated to normal dimensions. The heart of the patient dying of congestive failure looked like the heart in the dilated type of cardiomyopathy—the ventricular cavities were quite dilated and the ventricular septum was of the same thickness as the left ventricular free wall.

The presence or absence of hypertrophy of the left ventricular free wall is helpful in separating patients with the obstructive type from those with the nonobstructive type of hypertrophic cardiomyopathy.[14, 15] The left ventricular free wall was uniformly hypertrophied in all 20 patients with hypertrophic cardiomyopathy and subaortic stenosis at rest (true idiopathic hypertrophic subaortic stenosis). In contrast, the most basal portion of the left ventricular free wall (i.e., that portion immediately behind the posterior mitral leaflet) was of normal thickness in 11 of the 13 patients with hypertrophic cardiomyopathy and no subaortic stenosis. In two of the latter patients the entire left ventricular free wall was of normal thickness. The absence of hypertrophy in the left ventricular free wall behind the posterior mitral leaflet is detectable by echocardiogram, and thus has made possible the clinical separation of nonobstructive from obstructive patients with hypertrophic cardiomyopathy by this noninvasive technique.[14, 15]

The small systolic pressure gradients between the right ventricular body and the pulmonary trunk in some patients with hypertrophic cardiomyopathy almost certainly result from severe hypertrophy of the ventricular septum, because these gradients often disappear after left ventricular myotomy with or without myectomy. The cause of the hypertrophy of the right ventricular free wall in patients with idiopathic hypertrophic subaortic stenosis without right ventricular systolic hypertension or outflow obstruction is uncertain.

Both ventricular cavities in hypertrophic cardiomyopathy are smaller than normal or are normal in size. Most commonly the left ventricular cavity is slitlike with an S-shaped configuration. The papillary muscles probably contact one another during ventricular systole as do the anterior mitral leaflet and the mural endocardium in the outflow tract. Fibromas, which appear to result from abnormal contact of surfaces during ventricular contraction, were present in two of our patients. A saccular aneurysm was present at the apex of the left ventricle in one patient, a 19 year old girl with a 162 mm. Hg outflow tract gradient (Fig. 21). It consisted entirely of myocardium, but its thickness was considerably less than that of the wall in other areas.

The small left ventricular cavity appears to be responsible for the thickening of the mural endocardium in the left ventricular outflow tract and also for the fibrous thickening of the mitral leaflets. It is important to recall that the mitral valve resides in the left ventricle, which being relatively small in hypertrophic cardiomyopathy, causes abnormal contact of the mitral leaflets with each other and causes the anterior leaflet to contact the mural endocardium in the left ventricular outflow tract. The caudal margin of the mural endocardial plaque corresponds precisely to the distal margin of the anterior mitral leaflet. The focal fibrous thickening of the posterior leaflet probably results from contact of the mitral leaflets during ventricular systole, because there is not enough room in the left ventricular cavity to accommodate the leaflets and chordae easily. The ventricle and mitral leaflets in this respect may be regarded as being similar to an accordion. The mitral leaflet thickening in hypertrophic cardiomyopathy is somewhat analogous to that which occurs normally as a consequence of aging. With aging the left ventricular cavity becomes smaller, presumably in response to the lowered cardiac output; the mitral leaflets, thicker; and the left ventricular muscle, less compliant. The left atrium dilates in response to the increased work required to fill the small left ventricle. Similar mechanisms appear to be accelerated in idiopathic hypertrophic subaortic stenosis.

Most patients with hypertrophic cardiomyopathy have some degree of mitral regurgitation. It is not related to anular dilatation because the mitral anulus in this condition is not dilated. Furthermore, the leaflet thickening is not extensive enough to cause valvular regurgitation. The most likely explanation appears to be abnormal bending of the papillary muscles, particularly the anterolateral one.[16, 17] These structures may be bent abnormally by the bulging ventricular septum with resulting excessive tension on the chordae tendineae, preventing closure of the mitral orifice. Although usually present in hypertrophic cardiomyopathy, focal papillary muscle scarring cannot account for the regurgitation. Mitral regurgitation, usually mild, may be the predominant clinical feature of this condition. Mitral valve replacement in idiopathic hypertrophic subaortic stenosis, despite contrary views,[18] is hazardous because the small left ventricular cavity is rarely capable of freely accommodating a prosthesis.[19]

The aortic valve cusps are usually normal in patients with hypertrophic cardiomyopathy. By contrast, in discrete subaortic stenosis they are the sites of jet lesions produced by blood being ejected under high force and velocity through the area of narrowing, which is only about 1 cm. below the base of the aortic cusps. In hypertrophic obstructive cardiomyopathy (idiopathic hypertrophic subaortic stenosis) the area of obstruction is farther down in the left ventricular cavity, almost certainly at the caudal margin of the left ventricular outflow endocardial plaque, which corresponds to the distal margin of the anterior mitral leaflet. This site is considerably below the aortic valve cusps, so that if a jet is produced it is diffused before reaching the valve cusps.

The recent electron microscope studies of Ferrans et al.[13] clearly demonstrate distinctive morphologic abnormalities in hypertrophic cardiomyopathy. They consist of severe disorganization of the bundles of muscle cells and of the architecture of individual muscle cells in the ventricular septum. Similar findings are rare in the left ventricular free wall in patients with idiopathic hypertrophic subaortic stenosis or in the crista supraventricularis muscle of patients with the tetralogy of Fallot. Abnormalities of the organization of muscle bundles and muscle cells were observed in only 10 per cent of the patients with idiopathic cardiomegaly of the dilated type and were minimal in degree and uncommon.[2] The biopsy specimens in the latter patients, however, were from the caudal portion of the right ventricle or from the left or right ventricular free walls, and not from the cephalad portion of the ventricular septum as in the patients with idiopathic hypertrophic subaortic stenosis. The disorganization of the muscle fibers in the latter disorder also can be appreciated by light microscopic examination, by which method disorganization is infrequent in subjects with idiopathic cardiomegaly of the dilated type and is virtually always present in patients with idiopathic hypertrophic subaortic stenosis.

INFILTRATIVE CARDIOMYOPATHIES

The infiltrative cardiomyopathies include various infiltrates into the walls of the cardiac chambers. The infiltrates may be localized to the myocardial interstitium (amyloid, granulomas, neoplasms, acid mucopolysaccharides), or they may be within myocardial cells (calcium, iron, glycogen, and lipids). Some infiltrates, such as calcium, may involve both interstitium and myocardial fibers.

Amyloid

We have studied at necropsy 18 patients with cardiac amyloidosis extensive enough to cause cardiac dysfunction during life (Fig. 29). Fifteen were described elsewhere.[20] The 18 patients ranged in age from 21 to 89 years (average, 59): 12 were men and six were women. Fifteen patients had congestive cardiac failure; in none was the failure lessened by the administration of digitalis. Conduction disturbances or arrhythmias developed in 11 patients—in 10 of them while they were receiving digitalis. All three patients without congestive cardiac failure had gastrointestinal disturbances and peripheral neuropathy. Congestive cardiac failure was the cause of death in 15 of the 18 patients. Although three had had a history of elevated blood pressure in the past, no patient had systemic hypertension during the last three months of life. Electrocardiograms disclosed low voltage (sum of the total R and S wave voltage in leads I, II, and III $\leq$ 1.5 millivolts) in 15 patients and patterns simulating old anterior (poor R wave progression in leads V_1-V_3) or posterior (Q wave in leads II, III, and aVF) myocardial infarction in 12 patients. Chest roentgenograms showed cardiomegaly in 15 patients. None, how-

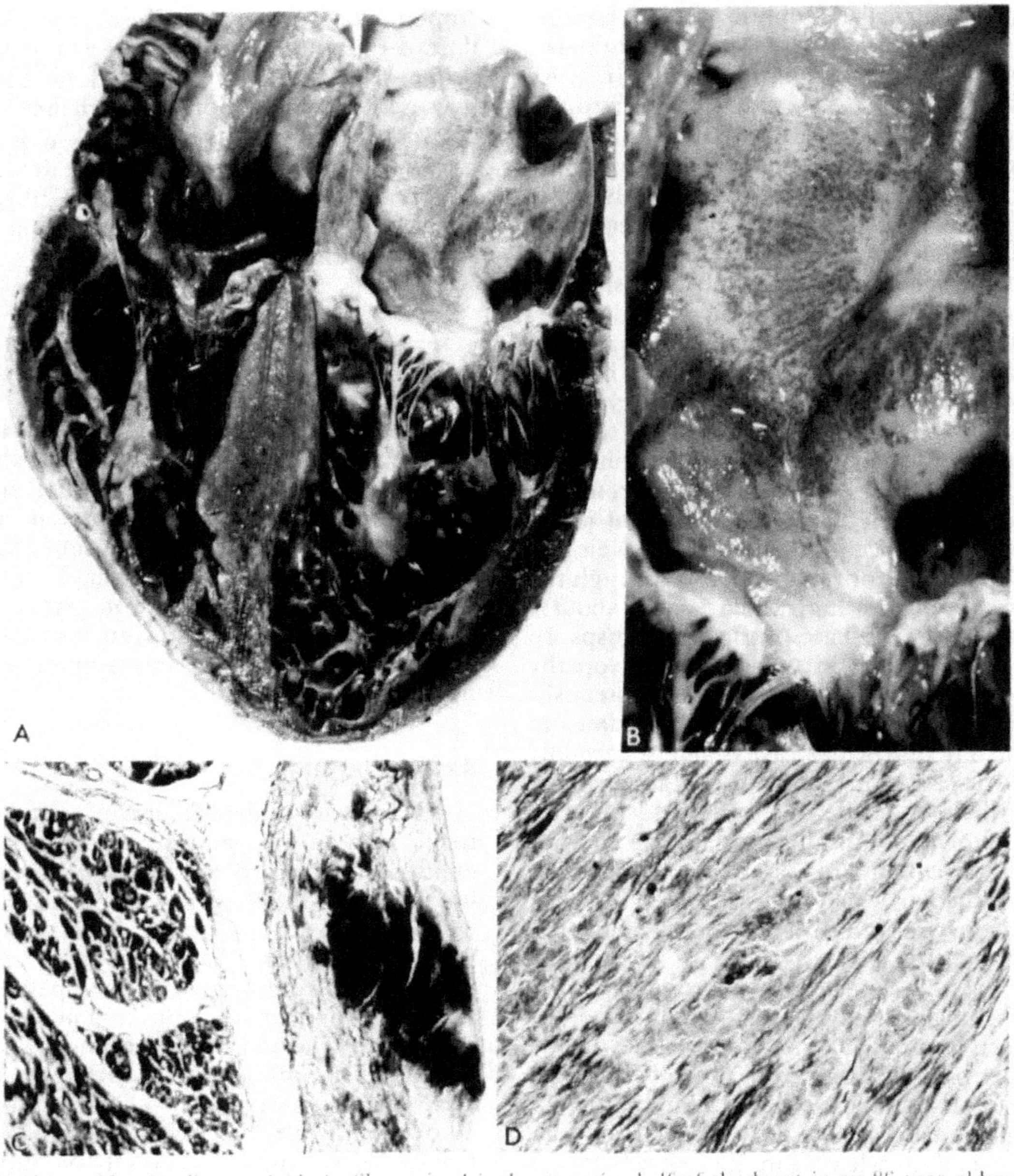

Figure 29. Cardiac amyloidosis. Shown in *A* is the posterior half of the heart in an 86 year old man (A68–18) who had angina pectoris and a healed myocardial infarction as well as large amyloid deposits. A close-up view of left atrial endocardium is shown in *B*. The wavy lesion on this endocardium represents amyloid deposits, which were extensive in the ventricules. *C*. Photomicrograph of left atrial endocardial amyloid deposit. *D*. Amyloid has extensively infiltrated a left ventricular papillary muscle. (Crystal violet stain. *C*. × 107. *D*. × 32.)

ever, had massive enlargement. Two patients had clinical and hemodynamic findings suggesting constrictive pericarditis and one underwent thoracotomy for planned pericardiectomy.

In 14 patients amyloidosis was not associated with another systemic disease (primary amyloidosis), and in four patients another systemic disease (multiple myeloma) was present (secondary amyloidosis). In 16 patients amyloid was present in many body orgáns (systemic amyloidosis) and in two patients amyloid was present only in the heart (isolated amyloidosis). In four patients more than one family member had amyloidosis (familial amyloidosis); each had peripheral neuropathy and three had vitreous opacities. The diagnosis of amyloidosis was established during life by biopsy in 13 of the 16 patients with systemic amyloidosis.

At necropsy the hearts weighed 370 to

700 gm. (average, 498). The ventricular myocardium in each patient was firm, rubbery, and noncompliant. Histologically, amyloid was present between many myocardial cells in each heart. Focal small deposits of amyloid, replacing areas of myocardium, also were found in most hearts. Both left ventricular papillary muscles in all 18 patients contained amyloid. The sinus node or atrioventricular bundle or both showed amyloid in five of eight patients in whom these tissues were examined. Tan, waxy appearing, focal deposits of amyloid were visible grossly in the endocardium of both the right and left atria of every patient and also in the ventricular endocardium in 12 patients. One or more cardiac valves in each patient contained amyloid, but in no patient did the deposits appear to impair valvular function. Amyloid occurred in the adventitia and media of intramural coronary arteries and veins in every patient, and in half of them the lumens of the intramural coronary vessels were narrowed by intimal amyloid deposits. Four patients had severe (> 75 per cent) narrowing of the extramural coronary arteries by old atherosclerotic plaques, but in none were intimal amyloid deposits found in these arteries. In two patients, however, small amyloid deposits were observed in the media of extramural coronary arteries. In Congo red preparations the amyloid deposits stained orange and showed green birefringence. The deposits were metachromatic when stained by crystal violet. By electron microscopy (one patient) the cardiac amyloid deposits consisted of nonbranching fibrils 80 to 130Å in diameter (average, 100).

The foregoing data and those of others indicate that amyloid in the heart must be extensive in order to produce cardiac dysfunction. The hearts that function improperly because of amyloid infiltration have firm, rubbery, noncompliant ventricular walls. Although the ventricular walls are firm, the ventricular cavities are usually not dilated.* The atria, however, usually are dilated, and the enlargement of the cardiac silhouette in this condition may well be related to the atrial dilatation rather than to the ventricular wall thickening. Most patients with symptomatic cardiac amyloidosis have congestive cardiac failure unresponsive to digitalis therapy, electrocardiographic low voltage, and conduction or rhythm disturbances. The latter are particularly common after digitalis administration, which may be contraindicated in this condition. A diagnosis of clinically significant cardiac amyloidosis should be questioned in the absence of congestive cardiac failure and electrocardiographic low voltage.

*Cardiac amyloidosis thus joins hypertrophic cardiomyopathy and constrictive pericarditis as a cause of congestive cardiac failure not associated with ventricular dilatation.

Granuloma (Giant Cell Myocarditis)

Granulomas with giant cells have been observed in the myocardium in a number of conditions (Table 2). We found giant cells in the myocardium at necropsy in 16 patients, excluding those with acute rheumatic fever (Table 3; Figs. 30 to 32). Four patients had sarcoidosis. Each of them had granulomas in other body organs as well as in the myocardium. Two other patients with numerous myocardial granulomas also probably had sarcoidosis, but other organs and tissues were not available for examination. In each of these six patients the granulomatous inflammation in the myocardium was widespread, always involving the entire thickness of the right and left ventricular walls at some sites (transmural; Figs. 30, 31). In one of the six patients the granulomas completely replaced both left ventricular papillary muscles and much of the free wall beneath them (Fig. 30). This patient presented shortly before death with mitral regurgitation from papillary muscle dysfunction.[16] Each of these six patients died as a result of myocardial involvement:

TABLE 2. Conditions Associated with Giant Cells in Myocardium

1. Infection
   A. Tuberculosis
   B. Parasites
   C. Fungi
   D. Spirochetes (syphilis)
2. Systemic noninfectious diseases
   A. Sarcoidosis
   B. Wegener's granulomatosis
   C. Panarteritis (pulseless disease)
3. Rheumatic heart disease or acute rheumatic fever
4. Rheumatoid arthritis
5. Coronary heart disease
6. Hypertensive heart disease
7. Thymoma or myasthenia gravis or myositis
8. Idiopathic

TABLE 3. GIANT CELL MYOCARDITIS: DATA IN 16 NECROPSY PATIENTS

Patient	*Age (years)*	*Race*	*Sex*	*Associated disease*	*CHF*	*ECG*	*Mode of death*	*Myocardial giant cells* $(1^+–4^+)$	*Extracardiac giant cells*
1	48	W	F	–	+	–	CHF Arrhythmia	++++	–
2				–	+	CHB	CHF	+++	–
3	40	W	F	Sarcoid	+	LVH	RF CHF	+++	+ (liver)
4	26	B	F	Sarcoid	+	CHB	Arrhythmia CHF	++++	+ (liver, L, LN)
5	44		F	Sarcoid	+	SB $\uparrow$ G-T	Arrhythmia****	++++	+ (liver, L, LN, spleen)
6	30	B	M	Sarcoid	0	RBBB	Arrhythmia****	+++	+ (liver, L, LN)
7	26	B	M	IE (active)	+	AMI	AMI 2° embolus	+***	0
8	17	W	F	IE (active)	+	RVH, RAD	CHF	+	0
9	42	W	M	IE (healed)	+	AF, LVH	CHF	+	0
10	10	W	F	IE (healed)*	+	–	CHF	++	+ (L)
11	65	W	F	RA	+	LBBB $\uparrow$ P-R	CHF	++	+ (L, SC)
12	73	B	M	RA	+	LAD	Sudden	++	+ (SC)
13	15	B	M	Panarteritis	0	PVC	Operation	+**	+ (arteries)
14	38	B	M	CAD	+	IVCD	CHF	+	+ (liver, L)
15	50	W	M	CAD	+	OMI	Operation	+	0
16	61	W	F	HCVD Cancer, uterus	0	LVH	Shock	+	0

Abbreviations:
+ = positive; 0 = negative; – = information not available; $\uparrow$ = increased; AF = atrial fibrillation; AMI = acute myocardial infarction; CAD = coronary heart disease; CHB = complete heart block; CHF = congestive heart failure; ECG = electrocardiogram; HCVD = hypertensive cardiovascular disease; IE = infective endocarditis; IVCD = intraventricular conduction defect; LAD = left axis deviation; LBBB = left bundle branch block; L = lung; LN = lymph nodes; OMI = old myocardial infarction; P-R = P-R interval; PVC = premature ventricular contractions; RA = rheumatoid arthritis; RAD = right axis deviation; RBBB = right bundle branch block; RF = renal failure; RVH = right ventricular hypertrophy; SB = sinus bradycardia; SC = subcutaneous tissue.

* = complex congenital malformation of heart and great vessels also.
** = giant cell arteritis also involved the coronary arteries but produced no significant obstruction.
*** = septic coronary embolus occluding left anterior descending artery.
**** = paroxysmal ventricular tachycardia several times in past.

all had either episodic arrhythmias, usually ventricular in origin, or severe congestive cardiac failure or both.

The numbers of multinucleated and mononucleated inflammatory cells in the myocardium in the other 10 patients was minimal compared to that observed in the six with definite or probable sardoidosis (Table 3). Four had infective endocarditis.[21–23] In these patients the granulomas may represent organization of septic coronary emboli. Two patients had rheumatoid arthritis with rheumatoid nodules (which contain giant cells) in the myocardium and endocardium.[24, 25] Another had giant cell arteritis of the aorta and its major branches, leading to absent pulses (pulseless disease).[26] Foci of granulomatous inflammation containing giant cells were present in the left ventricular wall. Their etiology is uncertain, but presumably the aortitis and the myocarditis have the same cause. The origin of the myocardial giant cells in the two patients with fatal coronary atherosclerosis and in the one patient with fatal hypertension also is uncertain. The giant cells in these three patients were located in areas of myocardial fibrosis.

It is evident from this and other reports that there are many causes of giant cell formation in the myocardium. Idiopathic giant cell myocarditis affects all ages without predilection for sex or race. Congestive cardiac failure, arrhythmias, and sudden death are common, and often the conducting as well as the working myocardium is extensively damaged. At the other end of the spectrum are patients who die from other conditions and at necropsy are found to have giant cells in the myocardium. The number of myocardial giant cells in the latter group of patients is usually small and of no functional significance. Patients with giant cells in the myocardium often also have giant cells in other organs or tissues.

It is difficult to distinguish idiopathic giant cell myocarditis with extracardiac involvement from sarcoidosis involving the heart and other organs. Although it rarely causes death, cardiac involvement occurs in about 20 per cent of the patients with sarcoidosis.[27] The noncaseating granulomas are usually located in the ventricular septa and free walls and occasionally in the pericardium. The myocardial granulomas may progress to fibrous scar formation without residual granulomatous inflammation, as in two other patients studied by us (Fig. 32). Degeneration of myocardial cells may occur also.[28] Arrhythmias, conduction disturbances, and sudden death occur. Probably some patients previously reported as having idiopathic giant cell myocarditis actually had sarcoidosis.

Giant cell myocarditis has a varied etiology and probably represents an unusual reaction of the myocardium to antigens or stimuli of varying types. Clinically the diagnosis of giant cell myocarditis cannot be established without myocardial biopsy and a negative biopsy report does not rule out this entity.

Neoplasm

Neoplastic disease of the heart has received through publications (many of which

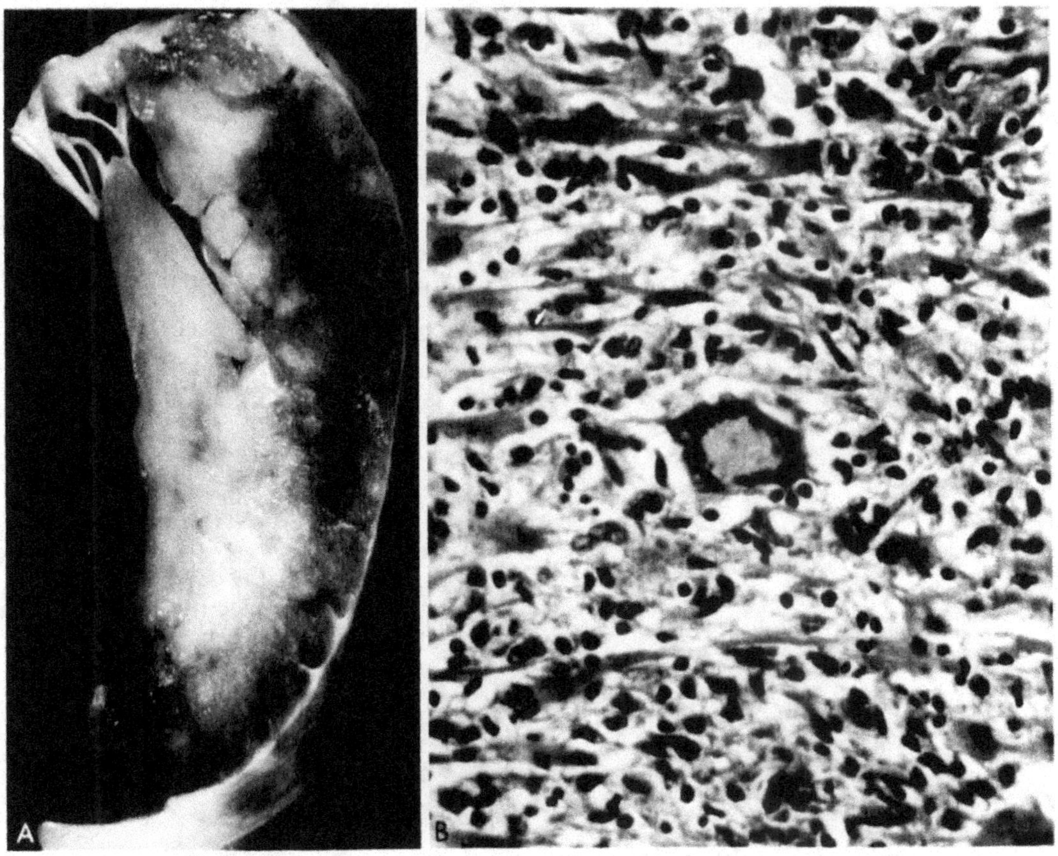

Figure 30. Giant cell myocarditis secondary to sarcoidosis. Shown in *A* is a longitudinal section through an anterolateral papillary muscle in a 26 year old woman (PGGH A-70-541) who had been asymptomatic until 10 days before death, when dyspnea appeared. The dyspnea rapidly worsened, and when hospitalized on the day of death she was in acute pulmonary edema. The blood pressure was 80/70 mm. Hg, the heart rate 160 beats per minute; a grade 3-4/6 pansystolic blowing murmur radiated to the axilla. Chest roentgenography showed congested lungs, cardiomegaly, and prominent hilar adenopathy. An electrocardiogram showed nonspecific ST-T wave changes and atrial hypertrophy. She developed complete heart block and died shortly thereafter. At necropsy large firm white deposits were present in the walls of all four cardiac chambers and completely replaced both left ventricular papillary muscles (*A*). On histologic section the firm white areas represented hard granulomas typical of sarcoidosis (*B*). Similar hard granulomas were present in lymph nodes, liver, spleen, and lung. Stains for acid-fast organisms; other bacteria, and fungi were negative. (*B*, Hematoxylin and eosin stain. × 400.)

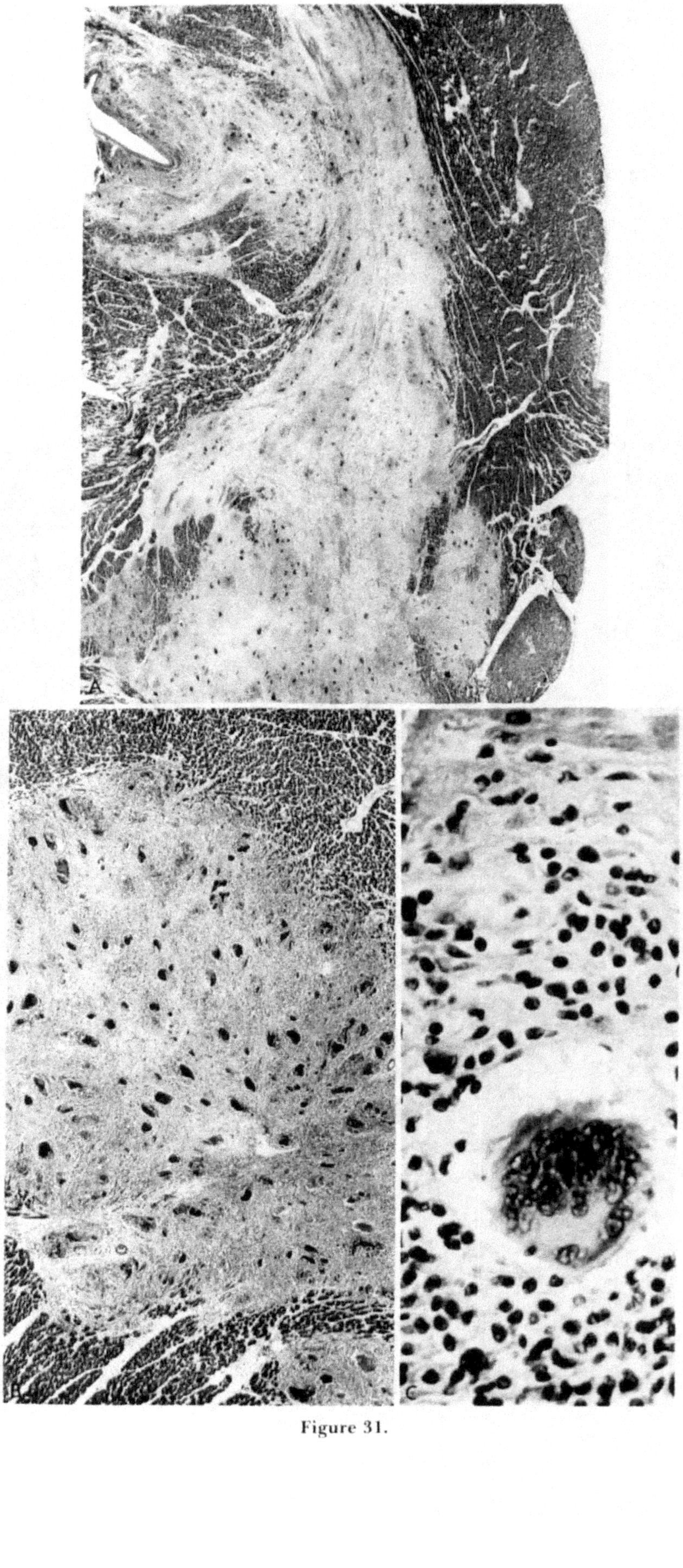

Figure 31.

are case reports) far more attention than it deserves. Most tumors in the heart represent metastases from primaries elsewhere, the most common being the lung and breast. The majority of secondary tumors invade only the epicardium (tumors limited to parietal pericardium should not be considered as involving the heart) and relatively few of them penetrate into the myocardium. Secondary tumors, which initially attach to the endocardium and then invade the myocardium, are far less frequent, although this pathway is the usual one for tumors originating in the kidney or adrenal gland. Primary tumors of the heart more often originate from the endocardium, the most frequent one being myxoma, which is benign. Primary malignant tumors of the heart are rare indeed and usually are sarcomas (Fig. 33).

One of us (WCR) has examined at necropsy the hearts of 686 patients who died of acute leukemia (420 patients),[29] or lymphoma (196 patients),[30] or malignant melanoma (70 patients).[31] Several observations that resulted from these studies may be summarized as follows. Although metastases to the heart in these three malignant disorders were relatively frequent (64 per cent in melanoma; 37 per cent in acute leukemia; 24 per cent in lymphoma), symptoms of cardiac dysfunction were infrequent. Indeed, in the case of leukemia and lymphoma, the frequency of dyspnea, chest pain, effusions into body cavities, precordial murmurs, ventricular gallops, edema, and electrocardiographic disturbances was similar in patients with and in those without cardiac leukemia or lymphoma, and these clinical findings most often were the result of mediastinal, pleural, or pulmonary leukemia or lymphoma, anemia, hypoalbuminemia, or an underlying cardiac condition. Electrocardiograms were abnormal in 61 per cent of 33 patients with cardiac lymphoma and in 62 per cent of 104 patients with lymphoma but without tumor nodules in the heart.

Controls of this type for patients with secondary cardiac neoplasms were not found in previous reports of cardiac metastases. Signs or symptoms of cardiac dysfunction could be attributed to lymphomatous involvement of the heart in only five of the 48 patients with cardiac lymphoma and in less than 20 of the 156 patients with cardiac leukemia cell infiltrates. Most patients with cardiac symptoms had extensive neoplastic involvement with hemorrhage in the pericardium or huge tumor deposits within a chamber or a cardiac wall. Most often, however, even huge tumor nodules in a cardiac chamber or wall were clinically silent. It is possible, however, that cardiac symptoms were masked or overshadowed by clinical manifestations of tumor deposits in other body organs or tissues.

The foregoing three reports are discussed because they were the first to our knowledge in which necropsy data were obtained by re-examination of the hearts, both grossly and histologically, by only one or two observers, rather than by accepting the information listed in the autopsy protocols. Moreover, the clinical data were obtained in patients with the same neoplasm but no cardiac metastases as well as in patients with cardiac metastases. These studies also demonstrated that many previously proposed criteria for clinically determining the presence of cardiac metastases were unreliable. In a patient with a malignant neoplasm and without previous cardiac disease, the following clinical findings strongly suggest the presence of cardiac metastases: acute pericarditis, cardiac tampon-

Figure 31. Giant cell myocarditis, idiopathic type, in a 49 year old obese Indian woman who had been well until two months before death, when syncope appeared. When she was hospitalized, an electrocardiogram disclosed complete heart block with a ventricular rate of 32 beats per minute. The blood pressure was 140/70 mm. Hg. No murmurs were audible. A chest radiograph showed moderate cardiomegaly. One month after the episode of syncope, acute pneumonia developed, followed shortly by evidence of congestive cardiac failure. Three days before death, substernal chest pain occurred and the electrocardiogram then showed changes consistent with acute myocardial infarction. Congestive heart failure persisted. Cardiac arrest followed a seizure. At necropsy the heart weighed 430 gm. Large white firm infiltrates were present in the cephalad portion of the muscular ventricular septum and in the anterolateral papillary muscle of the left ventricle. Histologic examination of the infiltrates disclosed them to be composed of fibrous tissue containing numerous giant cells and some mononuclear cells (*A* to *C*). Special strains for acid fast organisms, other bacteria, and fungi were negative. The heart was the only organ containing granulomas. *A*, Full thickness of ventricular septum showing the extensiveness of the infiltrates. *B* and *C*, Progressive higher power photomicrographs of the giant cell infiltrates. Some of the giant cells contained over 50 nuclei. (Hematoxylin and eosin stain. *A*, × 11. *B*, × 35. *C*, × 85.)

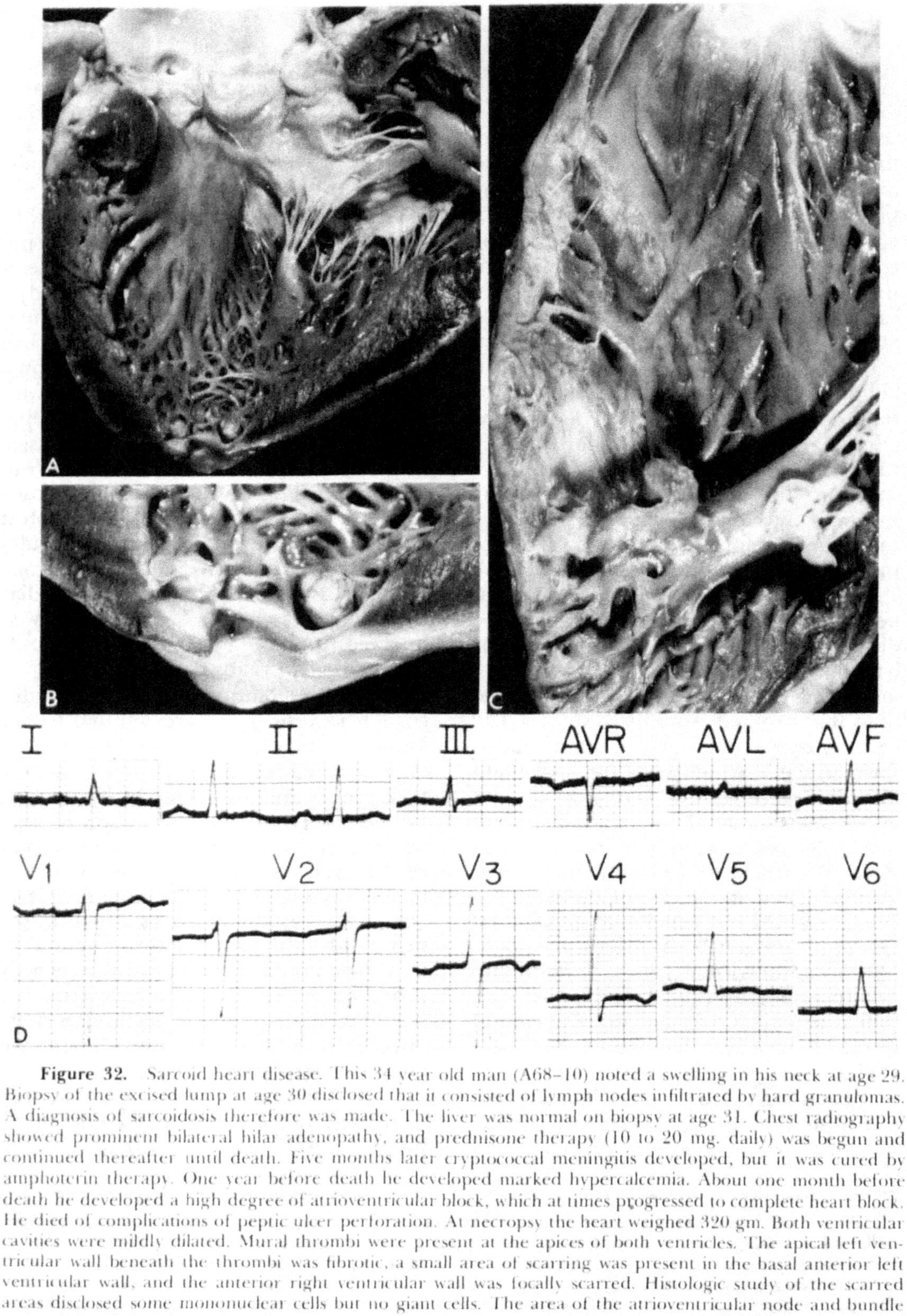

Figure 32. Sarcoid heart disease. This 34 year old man (A68–10) noted a swelling in his neck at age 29. Biopsy of the excised lump at age 30 disclosed that it consisted of lymph nodes infiltrated by hard granulomas. A diagnosis of sarcoidosis therefore was made. The liver was normal on biopsy at age 31. Chest radiography showed prominent bilateral hilar adenopathy, and prednisone therapy (10 to 20 mg. daily) was begun and continued thereafter until death. Five months later cryptococcal meningitis developed, but it was cured by amphoterin therapy. One year before death he developed marked hypercalcemia. About one month before death he developed a high degree of atrioventricular block, which at times progressed to complete heart block. He died of complications of peptic ulcer perforation. At necropsy the heart weighed 320 gm. Both ventricular cavities were mildly dilated. Mural thrombi were present at the apices of both ventricles. The apical left ventricular wall beneath the thrombi was fibrotic, a small area of scarring was present in the basal anterior left ventricular wall, and the anterior right ventricular wall was focally scarred. Histologic study of the scarred areas disclosed some mononuclear cells but no giant cells. The area of the atrioventricular node and bundle was serially sectioned: considerable scarring with some mononuclear cells was present in the conduction tissue, but the node and bundle and proximal bundle branches were not interrupted at any point. Although no granulomas were observed in this patient's heart, it is nevertheless highly likely that the myocardial scars were the result of "healed" sarcoid granulomas. The myocardial scarring, for example, was similar to that observed in the lymph nodes, and the coronary arteries were normal. The healing appears to have been the result of steroid therapy given for three years. *A*, Opened left ventricle. At the apex is a thrombus, better seen in *B*. The myocardium beneath the thrombus is scarred. *C*, Right ventricular wall showing severe focal scarring. The electrocardiogram was recorded three days before death.

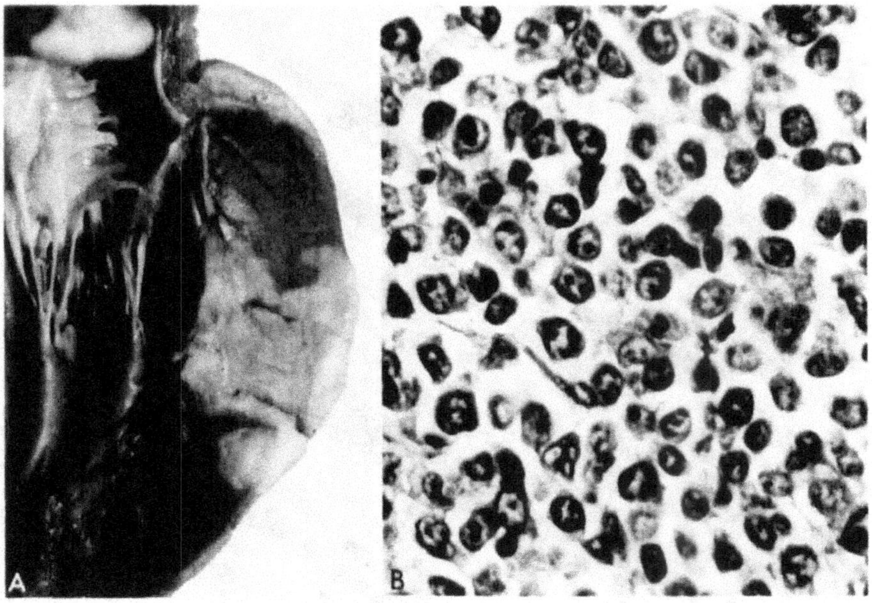

Figure 33. Secondary tumor (undifferentiated lymphoma) to heart in a 59 year old woman (A63–119) who had extensive deposits of tumor in the right atrium, left ventricle, and pericardium but no signs or symptoms of cardiac dysfunction. Tumor was present at necropsy in 16 organs and tissues. *A*, Longitudinal section of portions of left ventricular wall showing a through-and-through tumor deposit. *B*, Photomicrograph of an area of tumor nodule. (Hematoxylin and eosin stain. × 628.)

ade or constriction, rapid increase in the size of the cardiac silhouette by roentgenogram, onset of ectopic tachycardia, development of second or third degree atrioventricular block, and onset of unequivocal cardiac failure. Cytologic examination of the pericardial fluid and angiography obviously increase the ability to diagnose cardiac metastases.

Calcium

Calcium is most commonly observed in the heart in the coronary arteries, mitral anulus, aortic and scarred mitral valve cusps, large myocardial scars, and pericardium. In these circumstances the calcific deposits are extracellular. This discussion, however, concerns calcific deposits within individual myocardial fibers, also a frequent occurrence. Focal calcific deposits in myocardial cells are frequently observed in patients dying after periods of prolonged shock or in renal failure.[32] We have observed this lesion most frequently in patients dying soon after cardiac operations (Fig. 34).[33] Its cause is uncertain, although severe hypoxia is the most likely explanation and the lesion may be produced experimentally by this means.[34] High serum levels of calcium also may be a factor. The fibers infiltrated by calcium are always necrotic. Probably normal myocardial cells will not calcify. Thus, so-called metastatic calcification of the heart does not occur. Deposition of calcium salts into individual myocardial cells represents dystrophic calcification. When the lesions are extensive, it is probable that cardiac dysfunction may result. We have observed the heart of a patient who died with severe uremia in whom nearly every myocardial fiber was calcified. The myocardium felt like shark's skin. We also have observed huge deposits of calcium throughout the left ventricular wall in a 19 year old man from Uganda; the cause was unknown. Massive myocardial calcification has been reported by others.[35]

Iron

It is now clear that extensive iron deposits in myocardial cells cause cardiac dysfunction (Fig. 35). Buja and Roberts[36] studied 19 patients with cardiac iron deposits: the ventricular iron deposits were visible grossly in nine patients and by light

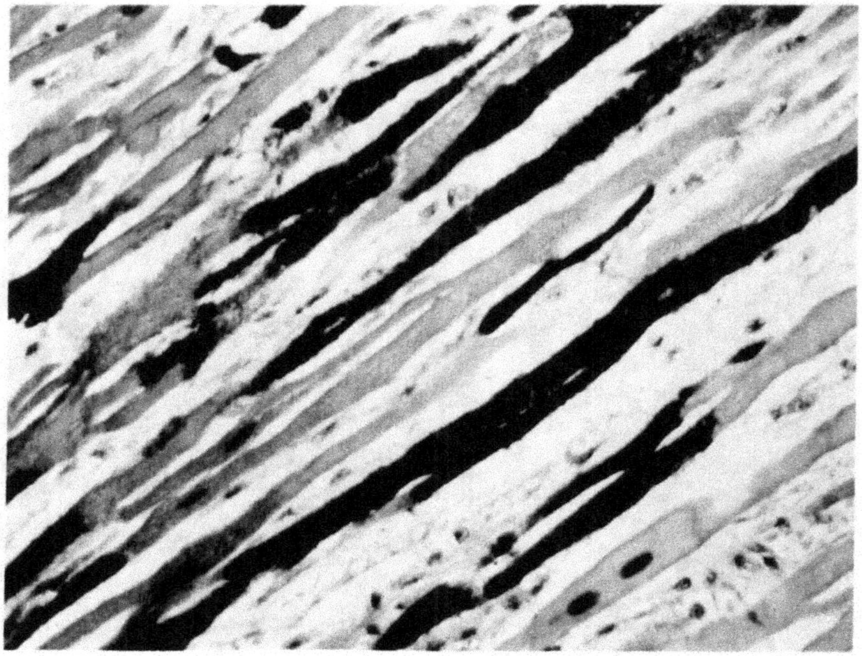

Figure 34. Myocardial fiber calcification in a 46 year old woman (A66–146) who died 20 days after replacement of stenotic mitral and incompetent tricuspid valves with prostheses. Postoperatively she had evidence of severely low cardiac output. Calcification of individual myocardial fibers was widespread at necropsy. The cause of this lesion is uncertain, but hypoxia probably plays a role in its formation. (Hematoxylin and eosin stain. ×200.)

microscopy only in the other 10. Each of the nine patients with grossly visible iron had clinical evidence of cardiac dysfunction (congestive cardiac failure in seven), whereas none of the 10 with only microscopically visible iron had cardiac dysfunction. All nine patients with grossly visible iron had abnormal electrocardiograms, mainly arrhythmias and conduction disturbances. Cardiac iron deposits were not distributed uniformly. The deposits were always most extensive in ventricular myocardium, less in atrial myocardium, the least in conducting as contrasted to working myocardium. The patients with supraventricular arrhythmias, however, had the largest atrial deposits of iron. Extensive cardiac iron deposits occurred not only in patients with idiopathic hemochromatosis but also in patients who received more than 100 units of whole blood (500 ml. per unit), unless bleeding diatheses coexisted, and in patients with chronic anemia and hepatic cirrhosis receiving less than 100 units of blood. The iron heart is not a strong heart but a weak one.

Glycogen

A deficiency of one or more of the enzymes involved in the biosynthesis and degradation of glycogen produces glycogen storage disease, of which at least eight types have been described.[37] Cardiac involvement occurs in types II, III, and IV. Most cases of glycogen storage disease causing cardiomegally belong to type II (Pompe's disease), caused by a deficiency of α-1,4-glucosidase, a lysosomal enzyme that hydrolyzes glycogen to glucose. The glycogen within the cardiac muscle cells is biochemically and morphologically normal (β particles, 250 to 400 Å in diameter), but is present in excessive amounts both within lysosomes and free in the cytoplasm.[38,39] As a result the heart enlarges, sometimes to a marked degree, and congestive cardiac failure supervenes. Survival rarely extends beyond infancy or early childhood.

Microscopically the muscle cells show a characteristic lacework pattern, with large clear central spaces (which represent the sites of glycogen deposition) and a peripheral rim of compressed cytoplasm. Endocardial fibroelastosis of at least the left ventricle usually is present also.[40] Although the deposits of glycogen usually involve all myocardial cells relatively uniformly, on occasion the fibers in the ventricular septum may contain disproportionately excessive quantities of glycogen and lead to subaortic stenosis.[41]

Myocardial involvement occurs to a variable extent in type II glycogenosis (glycogen debranching enzyme deficiency).[37] In type IV glycogenosis (branching enzyme deficiency) deposits of abnormal glycogen are found free in the cytoplasm of cardiac muscle cells, hepatocytes, and a variety of other types of cells.[42] These glycogen deposits are basophilic (in contrast to those in other glycogenoses, which are unstained in hematoxylin-eosin preparations) and are composed of nonbranching fibrils that measure 40 to 80 Å in diameter. These fibrils resemble those of the basophilic carbohydrate deposits in basophilic degeneration of the heart.[43, 44] It has been suggested that congenital rhabdomyoma of the heart, in which the tumor cells contain large amounts of glycogen, may be a localized form of glycogen storage disease.[45] Small foci of basophilic degeneration of the heart are common findings at necropsy, particularly in the older age group. Extensive basophilic degeneration is found frequently in myxedema and occasionally in congestive and hypertrophic cardiomyopathy. Its functional significance is unknown.

In addition to the observations mentioned, glycogen deposits have been reported in cardiac muscle cells in idiopathic cardiomyopathy in infants[46] and in adults with beer drinker's cardiomyopathy[47] or in familial cardiomyopathy.[48] Except in the latter patients, the glycogen deposits were localized within myocardial cell mitochondria. Recently Buja et al.[49] showed that intramitochondrial glycogen deposits develop in canine myocardium as a delayed response to prolonged periods (30 to 45 minutes) of anoxic cardiac arrest. Furthermore, we have observed intramitochondrial glycogen in the myocardium of patients with Fallot's tetralogy. It would appear, therefore, that such deposits in cardiac muscle cells represent a type of response to injury rather than a specific type of cardiomyopathy.

Lipids and Mucopolysaccharides

Infiltration of the cytoplasm of cardiac muscle cells by lipid droplets (fatty degeneration) occurs as a nonspecific finding in a great variety of disorders, including hypoxia.

Fabry's disease (angiokeratoma corporis diffusum universale) may be singled out among the lipid storage diseases as the one in which extensive and clinically significant (cardiomegaly and congestive cardiac failure) accumulation of glycolipid occurs in cardiac muscle cells.[50] In this condition glycolipid deposits also are present in the endothelium and vascular smooth muscle as well as in most other tissues of the body. The disease results from a deficiency of ceramide trihexosidase, an enzyme that hydrolyzes ceramide trihexoside. This glycolipid accumulates in the form of birefringent granules composed of concentric or parallel lamellae spaced 40 to 65 Å apart. In ordinary histologic preparations the deposits are dissolved and the cardiac muscle cells resemble those in type II glycogenosis. In cardiac muscle cells of a patient with Hurler's disease we also observed small lipid deposits composed of parallel or concentric lamellae. The deposits, the composition of which is unknown, were extensive in the smooth muscle cells of coronary arteries also.

ENDOMYOCARDIAL DISEASE

A cardiomyopathy of unknown etiology characterized by severe focal endocardial fibrosis of one or both ventricles, with underlying subendocardial fibrosis and with or without associated eosinophilia is discussed under this heading. We have studied at necropsy eight patients with extensive ventricular endomyocardial fibrosis associated with severe blood eosinophilia (Figs. 36 to 39). Two of the eight patients were described earlier.[51, 52] Five patients were diagnosed as having eosinophilic leukemia. One patient had a positive Philadelphia chromosome. We prefer to call this condition endomyocardial disease with eosinophilia. All eight patients were males, aged 13 to 52 years. Each had symptoms for 11 to 44 months (average, 29). The highest leukocyte counts ranged from 79,000 to 150,000 per cu. mm. and the highest percentage of eosinophils on differential smears of the peripheral blood ranged from 19 to 90 per cent. Although greatly increased in number, the eosinophils appeared structurally normal in each patient. Each patient had overt right and left sided congestive cardiac failure, which was the dominant clinical feature and usually the cause of death.

At necropsy the hearts weighed 420 to 530 gm. (average, 472). All four cardiac chambers were mildly dilated and the walls of all four chambers were mildly thickened. The endocardium in the left ventricular inflow tract and apex was markedly thickened by dense fibrous tissue in each patient, and this fibrosis, devoid of elastic fibrils, was overlain by fibrin-platelet-leukocyte-erythrocyte thrombi in all but one pa-

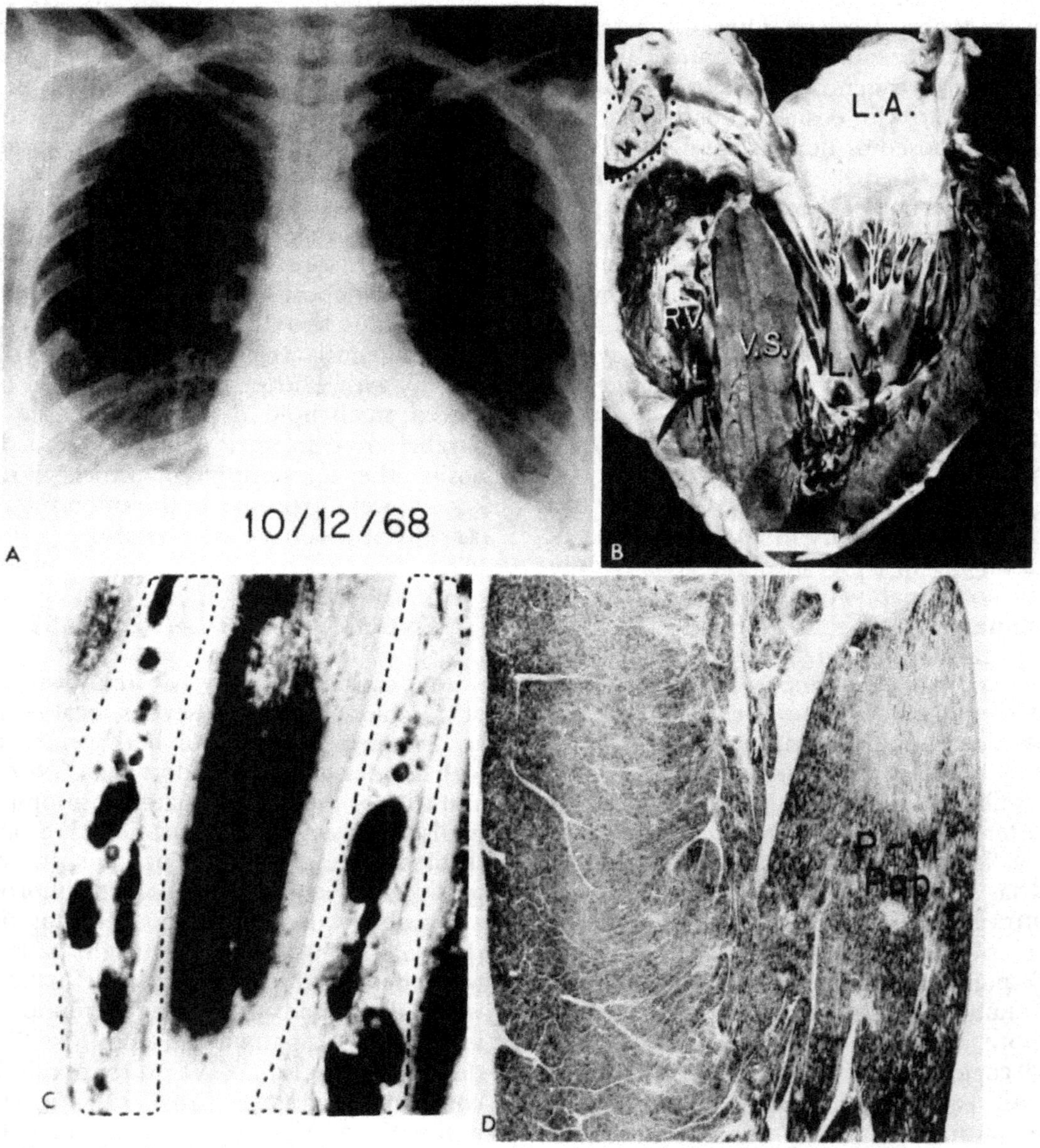

Figure 35. Cardiac hemosiderosis in a 42 year old woman (A68–327) with sickle cell anemia. She had received 260 units of blood when congestive cardiac failure developed six years before death. *A*, A chest roentgenogram showed cardiomegaly. By the time of death she had received 359 units of blood (90 gm. of iron). *B*, At necropsy the walls of the right and left ventricles and left atrium were rusty brown owing to extensive iron deposits. The right atrial wall in contrast was tan, and only minute particles of iron were present in it by histologic examination. *C*, Photomicrograph of several myocardial cells containing huge deposits of iron. Despite large deposits of iron in the working myocardium, no iron deposits were observed in the conducting myocardium. Longitudinal sections of left ventricular walls, including posteromedial (P-M) and anterolateral (A-L) papillary muscles, are shown in *D* and *E*, respectively. Foci of necrosis and fibrosis are present in each papillary muscle. These necrotic and fibrotic areas probably are anatomic indicators of chronic myocardial hypoxia, a result of the chronic anemia. (Prussian blue iron stains. *C*, × 628. *D*, × 3. *E*, × 2.)

tient. Right ventricular apical endocardial scars were present in all but one patient, and in two they extended cephalad toward the tricuspid valve in the inflow portion of this chamber. Mural thrombi overlay these right ventricular fibrous plaques in two patients. The left ventricular myocardium immediately beneath the fibrous plaques showed some degree of replacement and interstitial fibrosis in each patient, but in all the myocardial scarring was limited to the inner half of the wall (subendocardium). No right ventricular myocardial scarring was observed. Eosinophilic leukocytes, usually few in number, were found in sections of heart. In two patients several intramural coronary arteries were plugged by fibrin-platelet thrombi with resulting foci

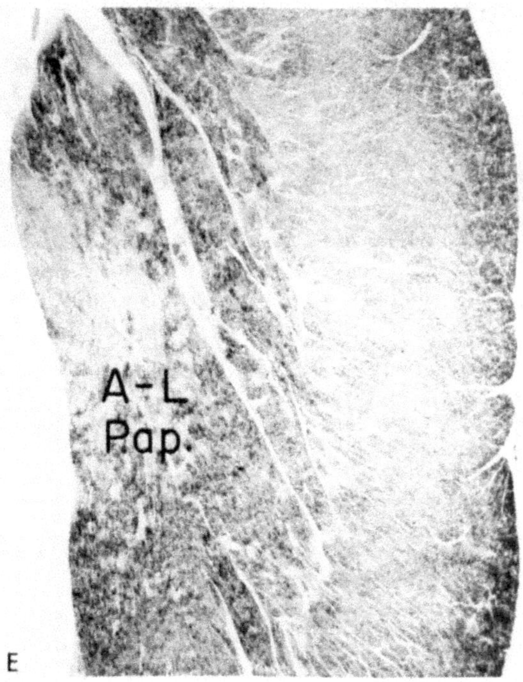

E

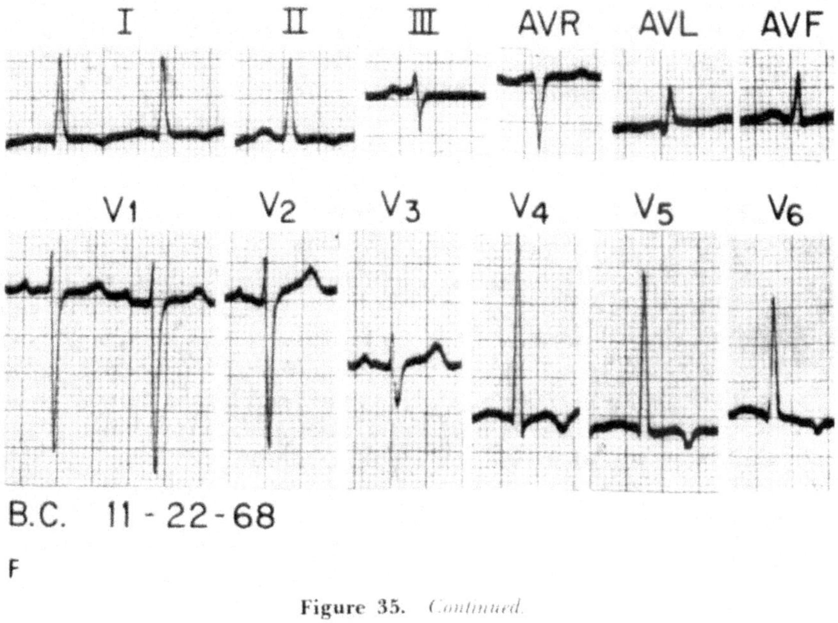

F

Figure 35. *Continued.*

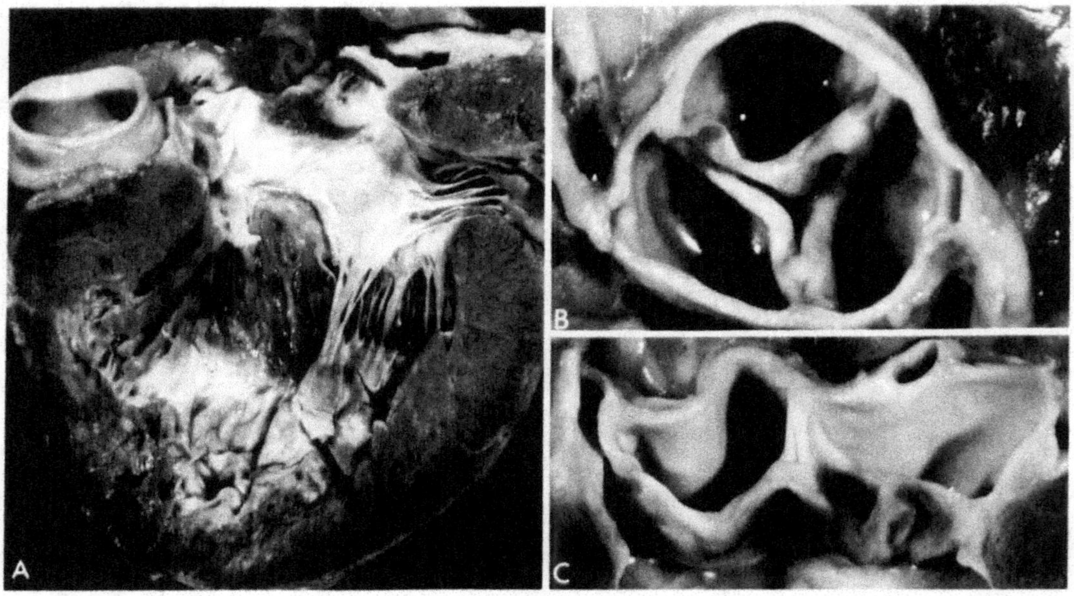

Figure 36. Endomyocardial disease and eosinophilia. Opened left ventricle in a 46 year old man (A71-250) who died after a complicated illness of 42 months. He had progressive congestive cardiac failure, leukocytosis (96,000 white blood cells per cu. mm.) with 90 per cent eosinophils on peripheral blood smear. He also had murmurs typical of aortic stenosis and regurgitation. At necropsy the heart weighed 520 gm., and large endocardial plaques were present in the apex of left ventricle (*A*) and small ones in apex of right ventricle. No intracardiac thrombi were present. *B*, Aortic valve from above, showing thickened cusps and fusion of two of the three commissures. *C*, Opened aortic valve showing fibrin material at the site of the fused commissure. The cause of the aortic valve disease is uncertain, but presumably it was caused by the same process affecting the mural endocardium in the apex of the left ventricle.

of myocardial necrosis. Except for one patient with extensive coronary arterial atherosclerosis, the extramural coronary vessels were normal. No patient had had clinical evidence of acute myocardial infarction, but one patient had had systemic hypertension at one time. The liver (1800 to 2800 gm. [average, 2200]) was enlarged in all eight patients but the lymph nodes were not prominent. Splenic weights, available in three patients (splenectomies elsewhere in two), were 480, 560, and 1500 gm. The weights were definitely larger than those in patients with idiopathic cardiomegaly of either the dilated or hypertrophic type. Several body organs, including lung, contained emboli with infarcts.

In addition to the eight American patients with endomyocardial disease and eosinophilia just described, one of us (WCR) has examined* the hearts of 24 patients who died in Kampala, Uganda, with endomyocardial fibrosis without significant eosinophilia. To our knowledge, none had peripheral blood eosinophilia (> 15 per cent). Their ages (known in 17 of the 24) ranged from three to 50 years (average, 27); three patients were over age 40 and six, under age 21 years. Of 16 patients in whom the sex was known, 11 were males and five were females. The duration of symptoms of cardiac dysfunction (known in 16 patients) ranged from two weeks to 24 months (average, seven months).

At necropsy the hearts were usually only mildly increased in weight, ranging from 370 to 500 gm. Endocardial plaquing (fibrous tissue devoid of elastic fibers) was present in the left ventricle in all 24 patients: in 14 it was severe, in five moderate, and in five minimal. Right ventricular endocardial plaquing was present in 18 and absent in six patients: in nine it was severe, in two moderate, and in seven minimal. Thus, endocardial fibrosis involved both ventricles in 18 (75 per cent) of the 24 patients. The endocardial fibrosis was located almost exclusively in the inflow tracts of the ventricles, and when the plaquing was severe it extended from the ventricular apices to beneath the posterior mitral or

*Through the courtesy of Doctors J. N. P. Davies and Monica Bishop at Albany, New York. Professor Davies, whose name should be attached to this entity,[53] brought these specimens to Albany when he moved there from Kampala, Uganda.

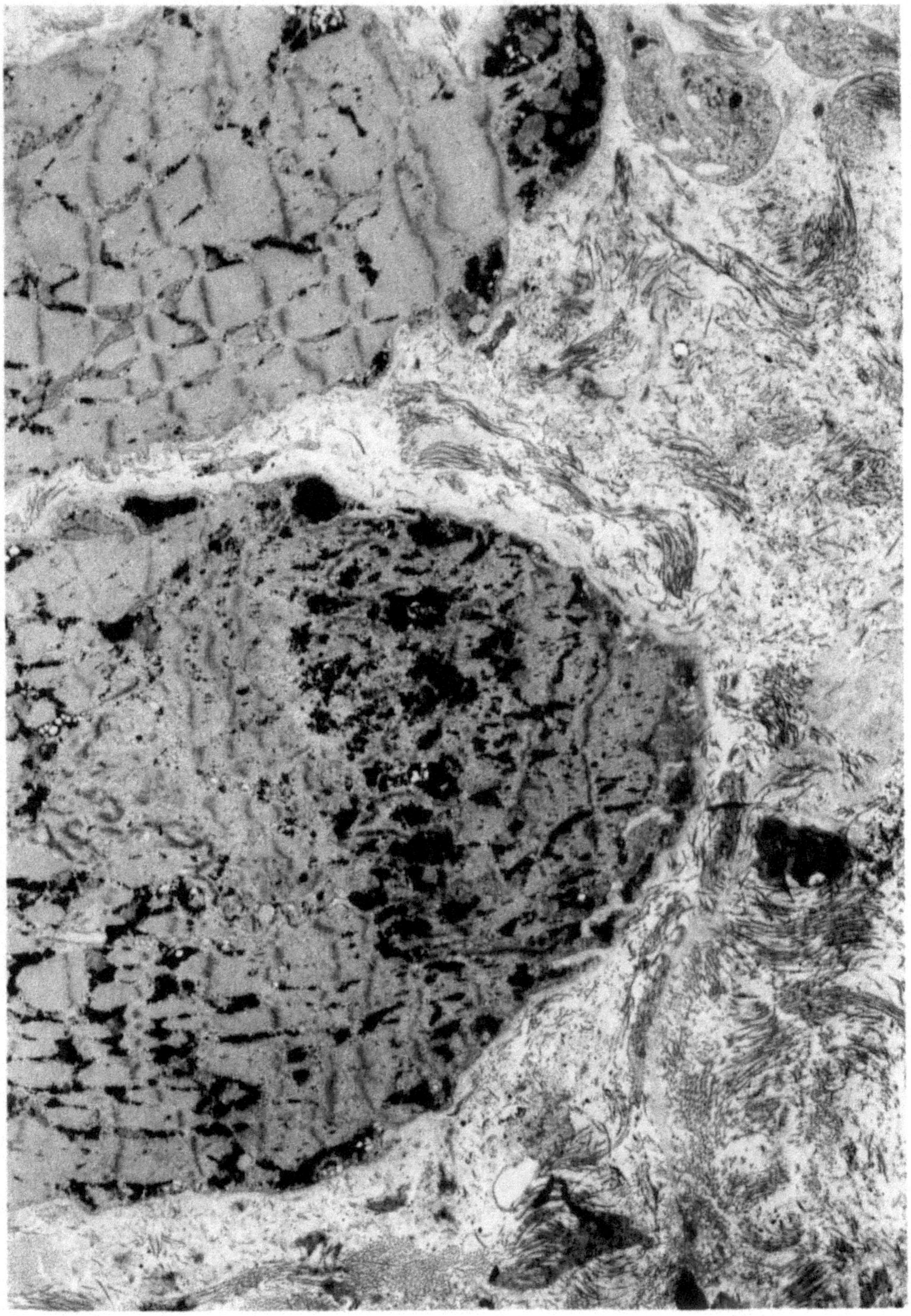

Figure 37. Muscle cells are surrounded by dense collagenous bundles in the right ventricular subendocardium of a man with eosinophilia and endomyocardial fibrosis. (× 5000.)

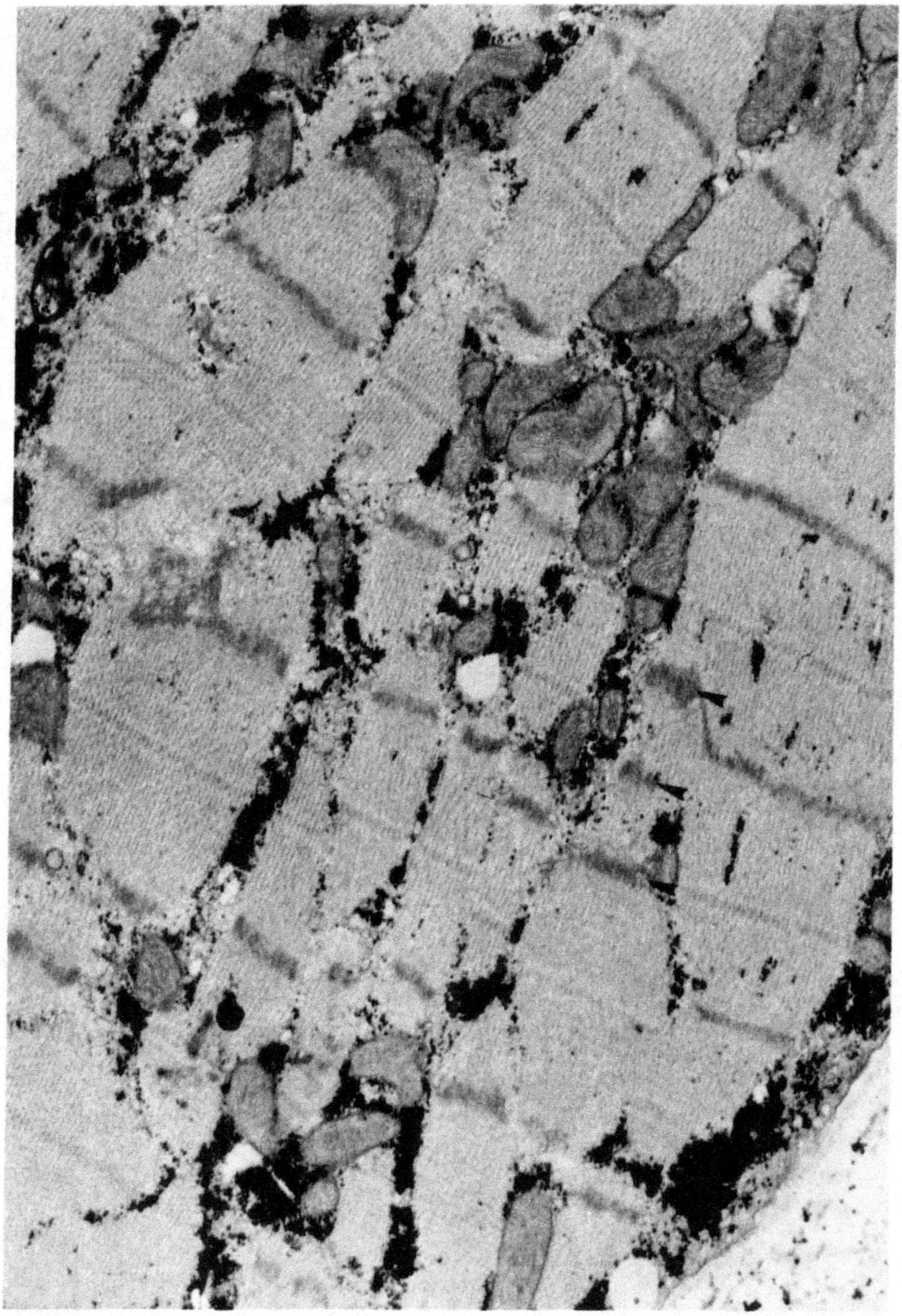

Figure 38. Myofibrils in cardiac muscle cell in a man with eosinophilia and endomyocardial fibrosis, showing loss of registration and focal widening of Z bands. Small sarcomeres (arrowheads) are considered to be in process of formation. (×21,000.)

posterior and septal tricuspid valve leaflets. When the endocardial scars were mild, they were usually limited to the ventricular apices. The configuration of the heart (i.e., the size of the various cardiac chambers and of the pulmonary trunk) depended primarily on which ventricle contained the largest deposits of endocardial scar tissue or superimposed thrombi. When the amount of endocardial plaquing was severe in the left ventricle and absent, mild, or moderate in the right ventricle, the heart

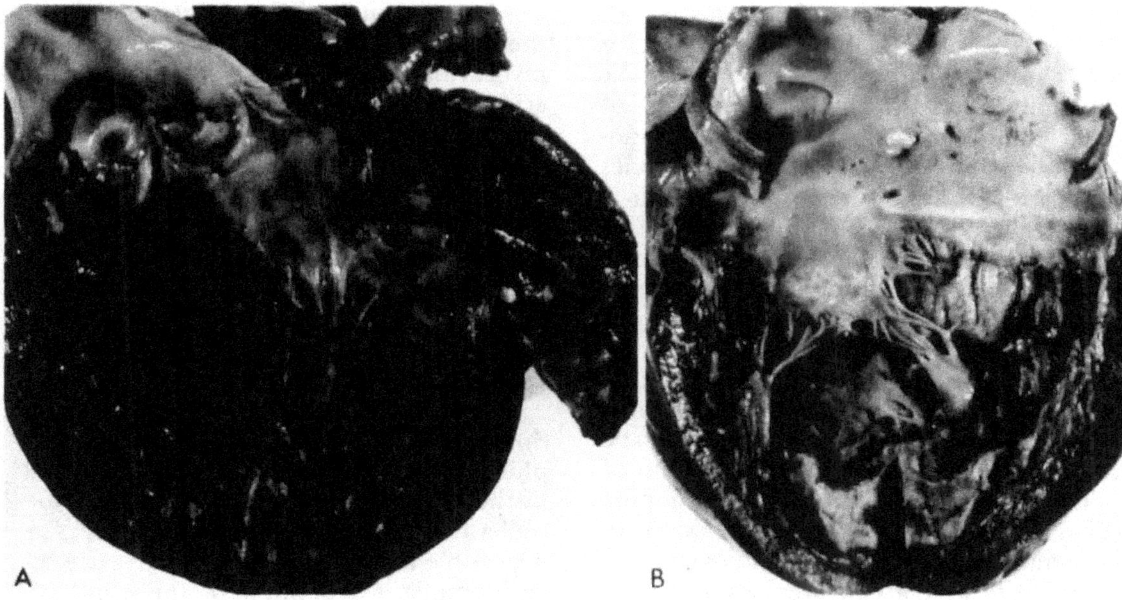

Figure 39. Davies' endomyocardial fibrosis in a Uganda native. *A*, Opened left ventricle, aortic valve, and aorta. *B*, Opened left atrium, mitral valve, and left ventricle. A large thrombus is present over the left ventricular apex, and the posterior mitral leaflet is adherent to the underlying mural endocardium. The process involves the endocardium of the entire inflow portion of the left ventricle. The presence of the large thrombus and the absence of dense endocardial fibrous tissue probably indicate that the process in this patient was of relatively recent onset. (The photographs were given to WCR by Dr. Gregory T. O'Connor, who spent two years in Kampala, Uganda.)

usually had the appearance of a mitral stenotic heart; i.e., the left atrium, pulmonary trunk, right ventricle and right atrium were dilated and the left ventricular cavity was small, being constricted by the extensive endocardial scarring. The left ventricle in this situation appears to be noncompliant and acts to some extent as an impediment to flow. The mitral lesion in this circumstance, however, is not stenotic unless another disease (e.g., rheumatic) coexists, but the mitral orifice in endomyocardial fibrosis is frequently made incompetent by the mural endocardial fibrosis, which adheres to the undersurface of the posterior mitral leaflet, causing the latter to be immobile. When the right ventricular endocardial scarring is more severe than that in the left ventricle, the right ventricle acts as an impediment to flow. The right atrium dilates, at times even to giant proportions as it did in one of the 24 patients; the right ventricle is usually constricted, and the left atrium and left ventricle remain more or less normal in size. This type of heart may be viewed as the tricuspid incompetent one. When the amount of endocardial plaquing is similar in both ventricles, each atrium becomes quite dilated and the ventricular cavities usually remain small or at least not dilated.

Although it is usually confined to the inflow tract, the ventricular endocardial plaquing in endomyocardial fibrosis on rare occasion may extend into the left ventricular outflow tract as it did in one of the 24 patients, and it also may be present in the atria. Also in one of the 24 patients both atria contained large endocardial plaques. Infective endocarditis appears to be a frequent complication in endomyocardial fibrosis. Three of the 24 patients had superimposed bacterial endocarditis of the mitral valve causing rupture of several chordae tendineae in each patient.

Comments on Endomyocardial Fibrosis with and without Eosinophilia. Löffler[54] in 1936 described two patients with "fibroplastic parietal endocarditis with blood eosinophilia." During his lifetime Löffler saw two patients with this condition, which bears his name. From 1936 to 1957, 24 other patients with this condition were reported,[51] and in the same year Bousser[55] summarized the clinical and pathologic findings in 13 patients with "eosinophilic leukemia" reported between 1944 and

1956. Since then many other patients with Löffler's "fibroplastic parietal endocarditis with blood eosinophilia" and "eosinophilic leukemia" have been described.[56] Each of these conditions is characterized by endocardial fibrosis of one or both ventricles and severe blood eosinophilia. Death is usually the result of congestive cardiac failure. From examination of previous reports and of our eight necropsy cases, it appears that the clinical and pathologic findings in patients with eosinophilic leukemia and Löffler's endocarditis are similar and that these two conditions are indeed the same disease. Whether this entity deserves to be called leukemia remains unclear. One of our eight patients had the Philadelphia (Ph 1) chromosome, a finding believed to be diagnostic of chronic granulocytic leukemia. Although greatly increased in number, the eosinophils in all eight patients appeared normal morphologically, an observation quite at variance with the usual concept of leukemia. The enlargement of the liver and spleen in these cases, however, is out of proportion to that found in most patients with congestive cardiac failure and tends to support the concept that this entity is in the leukemic category.

Certain similarities also exist between endomyocardial fibrosis of the African variety and endomyocardial fibrosis with eosinophilia, described by others as Löffler's endocarditis or eosinophilic leukemia. The mural endocardial thickening in the ventricles is seen in both conditions. Blood eosinophilia recently has been emphasized as a feature of endomyocardial fibrosis. Davies[57] in his initial report of 36 patients mentioned that "they sometimes show an eosinophilia for which none of the causes of eosinophilia account." Of 40 necropsy patients with endomyocardial fibrosis studied by Ive and associates,[58] 17 (43 per cent) had eosinophilia (absolute count > 1000 per cu. mm. or a differential count > 20 per cent of the total leukocyte count). Davies speculated that the earliest lesion in endomyocardial fibrosis is infiltration of the myocardium by round cells and eosinophils leading to necrosis of the endocardium and subendocardial myocardium. Thrombi form over the necrotic areas. As the mural thrombi and necrotic cardiac tissue become organized, the inflammatory cells disappear and only dense fibrous tissue remains.

In a recent study by Conner et al.[53] of the hearts of 16 patients dead from endomyocardial fibrosis, excessive amounts of acid mucopolysaccharide were found in the endocardium and inner myocardium, and these authors suggested that this was "a fundamental and possibly unique change" in endomyocardial fibrosis. These authors did not mention eosinophilic cell infiltration in endomyocardial fibrosis, but indeed these cells may be absent or rare in cases of Löffler's endocarditis or eosinophilic leukemia.[51, 52, 54]

It appears that some patients with endomyocardial fibrosis may have eosinophilia and that others may not. Löffler, in his initial report, emphasized that eosinophilia is inconstant and may disappear. It is possible that the presence or absence of eosinophilia is dependent on the length of the illness.

The possibility that Löffler's fibroplastic parietal endocarditis, eosinophilic leukemia (without abnormal myelopoiesis), and endomyocardial fibrosis of Davies are the same disease at different states of development is an attractive hypothesis. Patients with eosinophilia associated with a transient benign febrile illness, such as tropical eosinophilia or Löffler's pneumonia, may represent one end of the spectrum. Patients with severe endomyocardial fibrosis and no blood eosinophilia may represent the other end. Between these two extremes there may be patients who still have eosinophilia but less extensive endocardial scarring. The latter process is still active and thus eosinophilia is still present, but as the inflammatory process dies down, cardiac scar tissue remains and eosinophilia disappears.

REFERENCES

1. Ali, N., Ferrans, V. J., Roberts, W. C., and Massumi, R. A.: Clinical evaluation of transvenous catheter technique for endomyocardial biopsy. Chest, *63*:399–402, 1973.
2. Ferrans, V. J., Massumi, R. A., Shugoll, G. I., Ali, N., and Roberts, W. C.: Ultrastructural studies of myocardial biopsies in 45 patients with obstructive or congestive cardiomyopathy. *In* Bajusz, E., et al. (Editors): Recent Advances in Studies on Cardiac Structure and Metabolism: Cardiomyopathies. Baltimore, University Park Press, 1973, Vol. 2, pp. 231–272.
3. Falcone, M. E., and Roberts, W. C.: Atresia of the right atrium ostium of the coronary sinus unas-

sociated with persistence of the left superior vena cava: a clinicopathologic study of four adult patients. Am. Heart J., *83*:604–611, 1972.
4. Walsh, J. J., Burch, G. E., Black, W. C., Ferrans, V. J., and Hibbs, R. G.: Idiopathic myocardiopathy of the puerperium (post-partal heart disease). Circulation, *32*:19–31, 1965.
5. Demakis, J. G., and Rahimtoola, S. H.: Paripartum cardiomyopathy. Circulation, *44*:964–968, 1971.
6. Hibbs, R. G., Ferrans, V. J., Black, W. C., Weilbaecher, D. G., Walsh, J. J., and Burch, G. E.: Alcoholic cardiomyopathy: an electron microscopic study. Am. Heart J., *69*:766–779, 1965.
7. Bulloch, R. T., Pearce, M. B., Murphy, M. L., Jenkins, B. J., and Davis, J. L.: Myocardial lesions in idiopathic and alcoholic cardiomyopathy. Study by ventricular septal biopsy. Am. J. Cardiol., *29*:15–25, 1972.
8. Morrow, A. G., Roberts, W. C., Ross, J., Jr., Fisher, R. D., Behrendt, D. M., Mason, D. T., and Braunwald, E.: Obstruction to left ventricular outflow. Current concepts of management and operative treatment. Ann. Intern. Med., *69*:1255–1286, 1968.
9. Ewy, G. A., Marcus, F. I., Bohajalian, O., Burke, H. L., and Roberts, W. C.: Muscular subaortic stenosis. Clinical and pathologic observations in an elderly patient. Am. J. Cardiol., *22*:126–132, 1968.
10. Roberts, W. C.: Valvular, subvalvular, and supravalvular aortic stenosis: morphologic features. Cardiovas. Clin., *4*:98–126, 1973.
11. Roberts, W. C., Dangel, J. C., and Bulkley, B. H.: Nonrheumatic valvular cardiac disease: a clinicopathologic survey of 26 different conditions causing valvular dysfunction. Cardiovas. Clin., *5*:333–446, 1973.
12. Morrow, A. G., Fisher, R. D., and Fogarty, T. J.: Isolated hypertrophic obstruction to right ventricular outflow. Clinical, hemodynamic, and angiographic findings before and after operative treatment. Am. Heart J., *77*:814–817, 1969.
13. Ferrans, V. J., Morrow, A. G., and Roberts, W. C.: Myocardial ultrastructure in idiopathic hypertrophic subaortic stenosis. A study of operatively excised left ventricular outflow tract muscle in 14 patients. Circulation, *45*:769–792, 1972.
14. Abbasi, A. S., MacAlpin, R. N., Eber, L. M., and Pearce, M. L.: Echocardiographic diagnosis of idiopathic hypertrophic cardiomyopathy without outflow obstruction. Circulation, *46*:897–904, 1972.
15. Henry, W. L., Clark, C. E., and Epstein, S. E.: Asymmetric septal hypertrophy. Echocardiographic identification of the pathognomonic anatomic abnormality of IHSS. Circulation, *47*: 225–233, 1973.
16. Roberts, W. C., and Cohen, L. S.: Left ventricular papillary muscles. Description of the normal and a survey of conditions causing them to be abnormal. Circulation, *46*:138–154, 1972.
17. Perloff, J. K., and Roberts, W. C.: The mitral apparatus. Functional anatomy of mitral regurgitation. Circulation, *46*:227–239, 1972.
18. Cooley, D. A., Leachman, R. D., and Wukasch, D. C.: Diffuse muscular subaortic stenosis: surgical treatment. Am. J. Cardiol., *31*:1–6, 1973.
19. Roberts, W. C.: Operative treatment of hypertrophic obstructive cardiomyopathy. The case against mitral valve replacement. Am. J. Cardiol., *32*:377–381, 1973.
20. Buja, L. M., Khoi, N. B., and Roberts, W. C.: Clinically significant cardiac amyloidosis. Clinicopathologic findings in 15 patients. Am. J. Cardiol., *26*:394–405, 1970.
21. Buchbinder, N. A., and Roberts, W. C.: Active infective endocarditis confined to mural endocardium. A study of necropsy patients. Arch. Path., *93*:435–440, 1972.
22. Roberts, W. C., and Buchbinder, N. A.: Right-sided valvular infective endocarditis. A clinicopathologic study of twelve necropsy patients. Am. J. Med., *53*:7–19, 1972.
23. Buchbinder, N. A., and Roberts, W. C.: Left-sided valvular active infective endocarditis. A study of forty-five necropsy patients. Am. J. Med., *53*:20–35, 1972.
24. Carpenter, D. F., Golden, A., and Roberts, W. C.: Quadrivalvular rheumatoid heart disease associated with left bundle branch block. Am. J. Med., *43*:922–929, 1967.
25. Roberts, W. C., Kehoe, J. A., Carpenter, D. F., and Golden, A.: Cardiac valvular lesions in rheumatoid arthritis. Arch. Intern. Med., *122*: 141–146, 1968.
26. Roberts, W. C., and Eibin, E. A.: Idiopathic panaortitis, supra-aortic arteritis, granulomatous myocarditis and pericarditis. A cause of pulseless disease and possibly left ventricular aneurysm in the African. Am. J. Med., *41*:453–461, 1966.
27. Ghosh, P., Fleming, H. A., Gresham, G. A., and Stovin, P. G. I.: Myocardial sarcoidosis. Brit. Heart J., *34*:769–773, 1972.
28. Ferrans, V. J., Hibbs, R. G., Black, W. C., Walsh, J. J., and Burch, G. E.: Myocardial degeneration in cardiac sarcoidosis: histochemical and electron microscopic studies. Am. Heart J., *69*: 159–172, 1965.
29. Roberts, W. C., Bodey, G. P., and Wertlake, P. T.: The heart in acute leukemia. A study of 420 autopsy cases. Am. J. Cardiol., *21*:388–412, 1968.
30. Roberts, W. C., Glancy, D. L., and Devita, V. T., Jr.: Heart in malignant lymphoma (Hodgkin's disease, lymphosarcoma, reticulum cell sarcoma and mycosis fungoides). A study of 196 autopsy cases. Am. J. Cardiol., *22*:85–107, 1968.
31. Glancy, D. L., and Roberts, W. C.: The heart in malignant melanoma. A study of 70 autopsy cases. Am. J. Cardiol., *21*:555–571, 1968.
32. Terman, D. S., Alfrey, A. C., Hammond, W. S., Donndelinger, T., Ogden, D. A., and Holmes, J. H.: Cardiac calcification in uremia. A clinical, biochemical and pathologic study. Am. J. Med., *50*:744–755, 1971.
33. Roberts, W. C., and Morrow, A. G.: Causes of early postoperative death following cardiac valve replacement. Clinico-pathologic correlations in 64 patients studied at necropsy. J. Thorac. Cardiovasc. Surg., *54*:422–437, 1967.
34. Buja, L. M., Levitsky, S., Ferrans, V. J., Souther,

S. G., Roberts, W. C., and Morrow, A. G.: Acute and chronic effects of normothermic anoxia on canine hearts. Light and electron microscopic evaluation. Suppl. to Circulation *43* & *44*:I-44-I-50, 1971.

35. Testelli, M. R., and Pilz, C. G.: Massive calcification of the myocardium. A report of two cases, one associated with nephrocalcinosis. Am. J. Cardiol., *14*:407–414, 1964.
36. Buja, L. M., and Roberts, W. C.: Iron in the heart. Etiology and clinical significance. Am. J. Med., *51*:209–221, 1971,
37. Howell, R. R.: The glycogen storage diseases. *In* Stanbury, J. B., Wyngaarden, J. B., and Fredrickson, D. S. (Editors): The Metabolic Basis of Inherited Disease. Ed. 3. New York, McGraw-Hill Book Company, 1972, pp. 149–173.
38. Garancis, J. C.: Type II glycogenosis. Biochemical and electron microscopic study. Am. J. Med., *44*:289–300, 1968.
39. Bordiuk, J. M., Legato, M. J., Lovelace, R. E., and Blumenthal, S.: Pompe's disease. Electronmyographic, electron microscopic, and cardiovascular aspects. Arch. Neurol., *23*:113–119, 1970.
40. Ruttenbert, H. D., Steidl, R. M., Carey, L. S., and Edwards, J. E.: Glycogen-storage disease of the heart. Hemodynamic and angiocardiographic features in 2 cases. Am. Heart J., *67*:469–480, 1964.
41. Ehlers, K. H., Hagstron, J. W. C., Lukas, D. S., Redo, S. F., and Engle, M. A.: Glycogen-storage disease of the myocardium with obstruction to left ventricular outflow. Circulation, *25*:96–109, 1962.
42. Reed, G. B., Dixon, J. F. T., Neustein, H. B., Donnell, G. N., and Landing, B. H.: Type IV glycogenosis. Patient with absence of a branching enzyme α-1, 4-glucan; α-1, 4-glucan 6-glycosyl transferase. Lab. Invest., *19*:546–557, 1968.
43. Rosai, J., and Lascano, E. F.: Basophilic (mucoid) degeneration of myocardium. A disorder of glycogen metabolism. Am. J. Path., *61*:99–116, 1970.
44. Kosek, J. C., and Angell, W.: Fine structure of basophilic myocardial degeneration (BMD). Arch. Path., *89*:491–499, 1970.
45. Hudson, R. E. B.: Cardiovascular Pathology. Baltimore, The Williams & Wilkins Co., 1965, pp. 1581–1586.
46. Auger, C., and Chenard, J.: Quebec beer-drinkers' cardiomyopathy; ultrastructural changes in one case. Can. Med. Assoc. J., *97*:916–921, 1967.
47. Alexander, C. S.: Cobalt-beer cardiomyopathy. A clinical and pathologic study of twenty-eight cases. Am. J. Med., *53*:395–417, 1972.
48. Battersby, E. J., and Glenner, G. G.: Familial cardiomyopathy. Am. J. Med., *30*:382–391, 1961.
49. Buja, L. M., Ferrans, V. J., and Levitsky, S.: Occurrence of intramitochondrial glycogen in canine myocardium after prolonged anoxic cardiac arrest. J. Molec. Cell. Cardiol., *4*:237–254, 1972.
50. Ferrans, V. J., Hibbs, R. G., and Burda, C. D.: A histochemical and electron microscopic study of the heart in Fabry's disease. Am. J. Cardiol., *24*:95–110, 1969.
51. Roberts, W. C., Liegler, D. G., and Carbone, P. P.: Endomyocardial disease and eosinophilia. A clinical and pathologic spectrum. Am. J. Med., *46*:28–42, 1969.
52. Roberts, W. C., Buja, L. M., and Ferrans, V. J.: Löffler's fibroplastic parietal endocarditis, eosinophilic leukemia, and Davies' endomyocardial fibrosis: the same disease at different stages? Path. Microbiol., *35*:90–95, 1970.
53. Conner, D. H., Somers, K., Hutt, M. S. R., Manion, W. C., and D'Arbela, P. G.: Endomyocardial fibrosis in Uganda (Davies' disease). An epidemiologic, clinical, and pathologic study. Am. Heart J., *74*:687–709, 1967; *75*:107–124, 1968.
54. Löffler, W.: Endocarditis parietalis fibroplastica mit Bluteosinophile. Schweiz. Med. Wschr., *66*: 817–820, 1936.
55. Bousser, J.: Eosinophilie et leucémie. Sang, *28*: 553–580, 1957.
56. Odeberg, B.: Eosinophilic leukemia and disseminated eosinophilic collagen disease—a disease entity. Acta Med. Scand., *177*:129–144, 1965.
57. Davies, J. N. P.: Endocardial fibrosis in Africans. East Afr. Med. J., *25*:10–14, 1948.
58. Ive, F. A., Willis, A. J. P., Ikeme, A. C., and Brockington, I. F.: Endomyocardial fibrosis and filariasis. Quart. J. Med., *36*:495–516, 1967.

Section of Pathology
National Heart and Lung Institute
Building 10A, Room 3E-30
National Institutes of Health
Bethesda, Maryland 20014 (Dr. Roberts)

Asymmetric Septal Hypertrophy in Childhood

BARRY J. MARON, M.D., WALTER L. HENRY, M.D., CHESTER E. CLARK, M.D., DAVID R. REDWOOD, M.D., WILLIAM C. ROBERTS, M.D., AND STEPHEN E. EPSTEIN, M.D.

SUMMARY Although considerable information is available concerning the clinical features and natural history of asymmetric septal hypertrophy (ASH) in adults, little is known of this disease in children. The clinical characteristics and course of 46 children with ASH, who were evaluated at the National Heart and Lung Institute, have been analyzed. Twenty-four children had obstruction to ventricular outflow; 22 children had no obstruction to ventricular outflow, including 11 patients without overt manifestations of cardiac disease other than echocardiographic evidence of ASH. Thirty-five of the 46 children have been followed for one to 16 years (average 7.4 years). These latter children represent that subgroup of patients with ASH referred to the National Heart and Lung Institute and diagnosed prior to the general availability of echocardiography. The clinical course of these patients was variable. Fourteen (40%) of the 35 patients improved or remained stable, including four patients who received propranolol. Ten (29%) of the 35 patients deteriorated clinically and 11 (31%) of the 35 patients died suddenly (4% mortality per year). Two of the patients who died suddenly had previously undergone operation (six and 13 years previously) with resultant abolition of the outflow gradient; four others were taking propranolol. Neither symptomatology, electrocardiographic abnormalities, heart size, left ventricular ejection or upstroke time, magnitude of outflow gradient, or left ventricular end-diastolic pressure proved predictive of sudden death. Excluding patients who had previous operation, eight (40%) of 20 patients with obstruction who were followed long term and one (9%) of 11 patients without outflow obstruction died suddenly. Thus, the clinical and hemodynamic spectrum of ASH in childhood is broad. However, deterioration in clinical condition or sudden death has been relatively common in children with overt signs of cardiac disease.

□ ASYMMETRIC SEPTAL HYPERTROPHY (ASH) is a genetically transmitted[1] disease of cardiac muscle characterized by disproportionate thickening of the ventricular septum with respect to the left ventricular free wall.[2-10] Although ASH is a well-recognized cause of morbidity and mortality in adults,[6, 11-16] the clinical, hemodynamic, echocardiographic and pathologic features as well as the natural history of ASH in children have not been well defined. Previous detailed reports of ASH in children or infants[17-32] were limited to single cases or descriptions of only a few patients; other studies concerned with the natural history of this disease have included children, but generally have not given detailed information about this specific subgroup of patients.[12-16]

During the past 16 years, 46 children with ASH have been studied at the National Heart and Lung Institute (NHLI). In the present investigation a detailed analysis of the findings in these children is presented with particular attention directed to the progression of clinical findings and the incidence and circumstances of sudden death.

Methods

Selection of Patients

The case records of the NHLI were analyzed retrospectively and 41 patients were included in the study group by virtue of meeting our criteria for ASH, i.e., echocardiographic or necropsy documentation of ASH with a ventricular septal to posterobasal left ventricular free wall thickness ratio of ≥1.3. Five additional patients, in whom neither echocardiographic nor necropsy measurements of ventricular wall thicknesses were available, were nevertheless included in the study group because of 1) clinical findings of a nondilated cardiomyopathy in addition to the documented familial occurrence of ASH, 2) typical hemodynamic, angiographic, or operative findings of obstructive ASH,[6, 9-11, 33] or both.

All 46 study patients had an initial cardiac evaluation at the NHLI prior to 15 years of age, or had onset of cardiovascular symptoms prior to 15 years of age with subsequent cardiac evaluation at the NHLI within five years. Of the 46 patients, 31 were male and 15 were female; 43 were white and three were black. Eighteen of the 46 patients had been included in a previous study from this institution.[12] Seven additional patients with ASH were excluded from the study group including two patients lost to follow-up, one patient who died of postoperative complications after left ventricular myotomy-myectomy and four patients with associated cardiac malformations.

All patients were divided into two subgroups according to the degree of ventricular outflow tract obstruction (as determined by cardiac catheterization or echocardiography) present at initial evaluation: 1) obstructed — pressure gradient present under basal conditions, and 2) nonobstructed — no pressure gradient under basal conditions and either no gradient or a gradient of <30 mm Hg after provocation with isoproterenol infusion or Valsalva maneuver. None of the patients included in this report had a gradient of more than 30 mm Hg after provocation and no gradient present under basal conditions. The clinical and hemodynamic data for all 46 patients are summarized in tables 1 and 2.

Analysis of Patients

GROUP 1

Group 1 (table 1) consists of 35 patients who had clinical evidence of heart disease and were referred for evaluation to the NHLI (with the suspected diagnosis of idiopathic hypertrophic subaortic stenosis [IHSS] in 18 patients, cardiomyopathy in six patients and congenital heart disease in 11

From the Cardiology Branch and Section of Pathology, National Heart and Lung Institute, National Institutes of Health, Bethesda, Maryland.

Address for reprints: Dr. Barry J. Maron, Cardiology Branch, National Heart and Lung Institute, Building 10, Room 7B-15, Bethesda, Maryland 20014.

Received March 31, 1975; revision accepted for publication August 12, 1975.

TABLE 1. *Clinical and Hemodynamic Data in 35 Children with ASH (Group 1)*

Patient		Age (yr) I	Age (yr) II	Age (yr) Died	Sex	FC I	FC II	Age onset symptoms (yr)	Treatment with propranolol (no. of yr)	CI (L/min/m
										Survivo
Obstructive ASH										
M.R.		4	20	—	F	1	2	16	0	—
R.T.		5	7	—	M	1	1	asym	1	4.9
G.M.		6	17	—	M	1	1	asym	0	4.8
I.R.	(pre-op)	7	—	—	F	2+	—	2	0	2.7
		Left ventricular myotomy-myectomy (age 8 years)								
	(post-op)		13			—	2			2.7
M.S.		8	14	—	M	1	2	11	6	—
B.M.	(pre-op)	9	—	—	F	2+	—	12	1	3.8
		Left ventricular myotomy-myectomy (age 13 years)								
	(post-op)		16			—	1			1.9
T.B.		10	18	—	M	1	2	15	3	3.3
M.C.		13	15	—	M	2	1	13	0	4.4
B.G.		13	20	—	M	3	2	3	7	4.9
C.R.		13	22	—	M	1	(2)	21	0	4.2
G.Y.		13	21	—	M	1	2	16	8	2.3
T.O.		13	27	—	M	1	1	asym	0	4.2
L.P.		15	27	—	F	3	3	14	0	2.1
M.K.		16	24	—	M	2	3	13	5	3.8
Nonobstructive ASH										
C.W.		8	9	—	F	2	2	7	0	2.2
G.S.		9	20	—	M	2	1	4	0	—
K.D.		10	12	—	F	2	2	3	0	—
K.Y.		10	20	—	M	2	1	10	5	—
W.M.		13	18	—	F	1	1	asym	0	—
J.B.		13	25	—	M	2	1	10	0	3.3
B.P.		14	24	—	M	1	3	19	0	—
W.Y.		15	25	—	M	2	1	12	5	—
V.H.		16	18	—	F	2	3	14	2	3.8
J.M.		18	26	—	M	2	2	13	0	2.4
										Nonsurvivor
Obstructive ASH										
R.B.**		5	8	10	M	2	2	5	3	—
L.Pen.		7	—‡	8	M	2	—‡	7	0	—
L.M.		7	9	11	M	1	1	asym	0	3.9
J.P.		7	16	16	M	1	(2)	15	0	4.4
D.Pen.	(pre-op)	7	17	—	M	3	—	12	0	4.1
		Left ventricular myotomy-myectomy (age 13 years)								
	(post-op)		19			—	1			4.1
R.P.		10	14	14	M	2	2	8	0	3.1
C.F.	(pre-op)	10	22	—	M	2+	—	2	0	—
		Left ventricular myotomy (age 10 years)								
	(post-op)		23			—	1			3.6
S.C.		13	26	27	F	2	3	13	3	1.7
B.L.		14	19	21	F	2	2	11	3	3.9
D.C.		16	19	19	F	2	2	13	3	—
Nonobstructive ASH										
J.T.		8	9	9	M	3	4	7	0	1.6

*Highly variable gradient.

**Patient had documented cardiac arrest (ventricular fibrillation) at 10 years of age and was successfully resuscitated, but is include as a non-survivor for purposes of analysis.

†Measured at third cardiac catheterization; patient had previously recorded right ventricular outflow gradients of 25 mm Hg and 4 mm Hg, at four and eight years of age, respectively.

‡No second cardiac evaluation made; patient died 10 months after initial cardiac evaluation.

§Gradient measured during normal sinus rhythm; the gradient measured during junctional rhythm was 250.

[ ]Pulmonary capillary wedge pressure.

+Progressed to functional class 3 after the initial evaluation and prior to the time of operation.

patients) and were followed for one to 16 years (average, 7.4). Although seven of the 35 patients were known to have a family history of cardiomyopathy or IHSS at the time of their initial evaluation, no patient was referred for cardiac evaluation solely because of the family history of heart disease.

Thirteen symptomatic patients received propranolol (20–320 mg/day) for one to eight years (average, four); ten had obstructive ASH and three had nonobstructive ASH. Four of the 35 patients (each with obstruction to ventricular outflow) underwent septal myotomy-myectomy (three patients) or myotomy (one patient) because of marked func-

Hemodynamics at initial evaluation							Echo data (latest evaluation)			
		Pressures (mm Hg)								
					LV-SA PSG		LV outflow gradient			
RV S/D	PA-RV PSG	LA (mean)	LVS	LVEDP	Basal	Provocable	(mm Hg)	VS (mm)	PW (mm)	VS-PW ratio
20/4	—	[7]	—	—	—	—	110	16	11	1.5
25/8	0	—	200	15	100	—	40	17	10	1.7
26/9	0	17	107	19	17	—	90	28	12	2.3
18/6	0	[8]	240	7	150	—	—	—	—	—
28/9	0	[11]	90	13	0	100	—	—	—	—
25/8	0	[12]	185	11	82	160	50	18	10	1.8
32/7	0	23	172	28	105	125	—	20	12	1.7
—	—	—	120	21	20	48	—	—	—	—
30/5	11	[4]	185	16	65	—	105§	24	18	1.3
22/5	0	[6]	170	10	10–100*	110	40	20	12	1.7
57/4	25	8	169	14	74	105	25	40	12	3.3
35/7	9	—	165	20	50	64	60	25	15	1.7
28/5	10	—	145	10	35	60	40	31	15	2.1
24/6	0	15	220	14	88	—	70	22	16	1.4
30/6	5	7	118	25	40	—	0	18	9	2.0
30/4	5	6	230	18	120	—	130	27	19	1.4
32/12	0	[14]	95	16	0	—	0	13	9	1.4
25/6	5	—	85	15	0	—	20	16	12	1.3
—	—	—	—	—	—	—	0	17	10	1.7
28/7	5	—	140	17	0	0	105	20	12	1.7
40/7	10	[14]	110	15	0	—	0	22	11	2.0
24/5	2	8	102	8	0	—	0	28	11	2.5
22/7	3	[10]	—	—	—	—	0	20	10	2.0
25/7	0	—	126	16	0	5	—	—	—	—
40/12	0	[22]	118	14	0	0	0	22	16	1.4
31/7	0	20	110	16	0	0	0	25	12	2.1
23/5	0	—	180	20	70	—	70	15	10	1.5
—	—	14	103	16	15	—	—	—	—	—
27/8	0	17	92	29	18	34	—	—	—	—
30/3	0	12	175	20	75	—	—	—	—	—
135/7	118†	5	108	4	0	—	—	—	—	—
28/8	0	[8]	—	—	—	—	—	—	—	—
38/7	0	[18]	132	15	30	—	—	—	—	—
29/3	2	—	250	16	175	—	—	—	—	—
—	—	11	123	15	0	21	—	—	—	—
80/5	55	[10]	190	20	100	—	—	—	—	—
40/7	—	10	158	10	41	57	—	—	—	—
26/8	0	—	125	20	38	—	20	19	14	1.4
90/27	0	22	90	34	0	—	—	—	—	—

– Data not obtained or not applicable.
Patients with initials in *italics* are siblings from four different families.
(2)Considered to be in functional class 2 on the basis of a recent single syncopal episode.
Abbreviations: Asym = asymptomatic; CI = cardiac index; D = diastolic; Echo = echocardiographic; FC = functional class (New York Heart Association classification); L/min/m² = liters per minute per square meter of body surface area; LA = left atrial; LV = left ventricular; LVED = left ventricular end-diastolic; LVS = left ventricular systolic; mm = millimeters; mm Hg = millimeters of mercury; no. = number; PA = pulmonary arterial; PSG = peak systolic gradient; PW = posterobasal left ventricular free wall thickness; RV = right ventricular; S = systolic; SA = systemic arterial; VS = ventricular septal thickness; I = initial cardiac evaluation; II = latest cardiac evaluation; Post-op = postoperative evaluation; pre-op = preoperative evaluation.

tional limitation despite an adequate trial of propranolol. The remaining 18 patients received no therapy during the period of observation.

Clinical data from two cardiac evaluations were analyzed for each of the patients in group 1. The initial evaluation was at the patient's first in-patient admission to the NHLI; ages ranged from four to 18 years (average, 11). The ages at the latest evaluation ranged from seven to 27 years (average, 18). History and physical examination, electrocardiogram and chest radiographs were obtained at both the initial and the most recent cardiac evaluation. Left and right heart hemodynamic studies, left ventricular angiography or both

TABLE 2. *Clinical Data in 11 Children with ASH (Group 2)*

Patient	Age (yr)	Sex	FC	Echocardiographic data: LV outflow gradient	VS (mm)	PW (mm)	VS:PW ratio
R.M.*	3	M	1	0	6	4	1.5
T.M.	5	M	1	0	10	7	1.4
R.S.†	6	F	1	0	15	8	1.9
M.A.	10	M	1	0	12	8	1.5
E.L.	10	F	1	0	13	9	1.4
J.K.	11	M	1	0	17	10	1.7
A.P.‡	11	M	1	0	15	10	1.5
K.C.	12	F	1	0	14	10	1.4
M.L.	12	F	2	0	12	9	1.3
D.W.	12	M	1	0	15	11	1.4
J.D.	14	M	1	0	14	10	1.4

*Offspring of patient J.M. in table 1.
†Offspring of patient L.P. in table 1.
‡Sibling of patients L.P. and R.P. in table 1.
Abbreviations: FC = functional class (New York Heart Association classification); LV = left ventricular; PW = posterobasal left ventricular free wall thickness; VS = ventricular septal thickness.

were performed in 32 of the 35 patients at initial evaluation. Phonocardiograms and indirect carotid pulse tracings were also obtained in 23 patients at the initial evaluation; echocardiography was performed in 24 patients at the most recent evaluation.

GROUP 2

Group 2 (table 2) consists of 11 children (3–14 years old, average 10) who were observed for less than two years. In each patient the diagnosis of ASH was made only by echocardiography. Ten patients in group 2 were asymptomatic and one patient was mildly symptomatic; none of the 11 patients underwent cardiac catheterization. The 11 children were members of families in which a relative was known to have ASH. Each child was not referred to the NHLI for cardiac evaluation, but rather, at our request, participated in an echocardiographic study designed to determine the genetic transmission of ASH.[1]

Echocardiographic Evaluation

The echocardiographic technique employed in this study has been described previously.[8] All studies were performed in the resting, supine position with a modified Ekoline-20 ultrasound unit and an Aerotech gamma transducer. The thickness of the ventricular septum was measured below the tips of the mitral valve leaflets before atrial systole; the posterobasal left ventricular wall thickness was measured at the level of the tips of the mitral valve leaflets during the same phase of the cardiac cycle. The left ventricular outflow gradient (in mm Hg) was estimated from the echocardiogram by a method described elsewhere,[34] using a revised formula: gradient = (1.8 × obstruction index) − 53.

Necropsy Studies

Detailed necropsy studies were performed in seven patients, aged 8–27 years. Four of these patients had obstruction to ventricular outflow and three had no outflow obstruction (including two patients in whom a previously documented gradient was abolished by operation) at the latest cardiac evaluation. Measurements were made of the thickness of the ventricular septum, the posterobasal left ventricular free wall (directly behind the posterior mitral leaflet), the left ventricular free wall in the area of maximum thickness, and the right ventricular free wall.

Multiple blocks of myocardium were taken from the ventricular septum and left ventricular free wall in each heart. The tissue specimens were fixed, processed, embedded in paraffin, sectioned at 6 μ thickness and stained with hematoxylin and eosin. In addition, in one patient (R. B., who had had a cardiac arrest and was successfully resuscitated four months previously) myocardium was resected from the ventricular septum and a myocardial biopsy was taken from the left ventricular posterior wall at the time of left ventricular myotomy-myectomy; the specimens obtained at operation were prepared for histologic study by methods previously described.[35, 36] The severity and extent of disorganization of cardiac muscle cells was assessed by light microscopy in each tissue block.

Electrocardiographic Evaluation

Criteria employed for the electrocardiographic diagnosis of left ventricular hypertrophy were those of Ziegler[37] for patients 18 years old or less or those of Romhilt and Estes[38] for patients over 18 years. Q-T intervals (measured in standard lead II) were corrected for heart rate and compared with normal standards.[39, 40]

Survival Curve Analysis and Statistical Methods

A survival curve for the study population was constructed using the life-table method.[41] Data were analyzed statistically by Student's t-test for unpaired data.

Results

Group 1 (35 patients)

CLINICAL CONDITION

At the time of initial evaluation, 13 patients were asymptomatic (New York Heart Association functional class I), 18 patients were in class II and four patients were in classes III or IV (fig. 1). The most common symptoms were dyspnea or excessive fatigue on exertion (15 patients), presyncope (10 patients), syncope (7 patients), palpitations (2 patients) and chest pain (11 patients). The chest pain in seven of the 11 patients was considered to be typical angina pectoris. Two patients (J. T. and C. W.) with nonobstructive ASH had evidence of congestive heart failure (i.e., dyspnea, tachypnea and hepatomegaly). Otherwise, patients with and patients without obstruction to ventricular outflow did not differ in regard to the nature of their symptoms.

Of the 35 patients in group 1, 31 were or became symptomatic or died, including 21 of 24 with obstructive ASH and 10 of 11 with nonobstructive ASH. The age at onset of symptoms for these 31 patients ranged from two to 21 years (average, 11) and did not differ significantly between patients with and patients without obstruction. Changes in clinical status of the 35 patients with follow-up studies are depicted in figures 1 and 2. Surviving patients were classified as either stable, improved or deteriorated depending on their clinical state at the initial and most recent cardiac evaluations. The two surviving patients who underwent operation (and who progressed from functional class II to class III prior to operation) were classified as deteriorated even though one (patient B. M.) was improved and one (patient I. R.) was unchanged following operation.

PHYSICAL AND PHONOCARDIOGRAPHIC FINDINGS

Thirty-three (94%) of the 35 patients had systolic ejection murmurs, usually loudest at the lower left sternal border or apex; in 26 the intensity of the murmur was grade III/VI or louder, including 23 of the 24 patients with obstruction to ventricular outflow under basal conditions. Nine of the 35 patients either had no murmur or a murmur of grade I-II/VI, including eight of the 11 patients without obstruction. The second heart sound split normally with the respiratory cycle in 29 patients, split paradoxically in four patients and was single in two patients. Phonocardiograms recorded a third heart sound in 13 patients (37%) and a fourth heart sound in 18 patients (51%).

Left ventricular ejection times (corrected for heart rate) were measured in 23 patients and are summarized in figure 3. Prolonged ejection time[42, 43] was present in eight of 15 patients with obstructive ASH and in only one of eight patients with nonobstructive ASH. Upstroke times (corrected for heart rate) ranged from 30 to 120 msec (mean 82 ± 5 msec) and were abnormally short[42] (<60 msec) in three (14%) of 23 patients, all of whom had obstructive ASH.

HEMODYNAMIC DATA

Of the 35 patients in group 1, 24 had obstructive ASH (outflow gradient under basal conditions ranging from 15 to 175 mm Hg); eleven patients had nonobstructive ASH. Three of the 35 patients had either no or incomplete hemodynamic data obtained at the initial evaluation and were placed in either the obstructed or nonobstructed group according to the degree of outflow obstruction estimated by subsequent echocardiographic study. In one (D. Pen.) of the 24 patients with an outflow gradient, the obstruction was confined to the right ventricular outflow tract (pressure gradient of 118 mm Hg).[44]

Hemodynamic measurements in the 35 patients with follow-up studies are summarized in table 1. Patients with and patients without obstruction to outflow did not differ significantly in regard to systolic pulmonary arterial

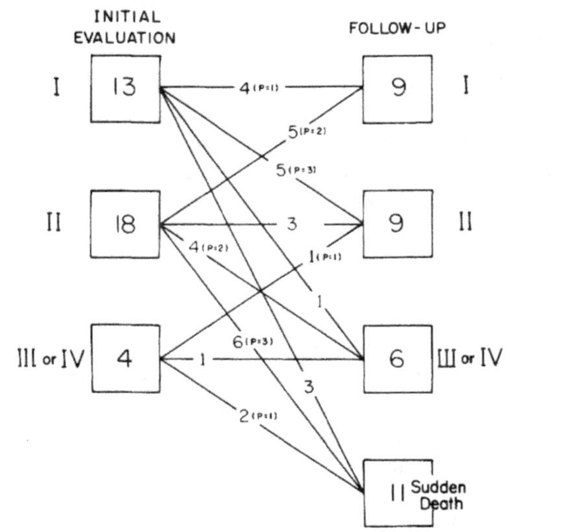

FIGURE 1 *Changes in the clinical condition of 35 children with ASH (group 1). On the left is the New York Heart Association functional classification for each patient at the initial cardiac evaluation (the most recent cardiac evaluation is used for nonsurvivors). On the right is the functional status for each patient at the latest cardiac evaluation (the last preoperative evaluation is used for surviving patients who had operation). P = number of patients treated with propranolol for at least one year.*

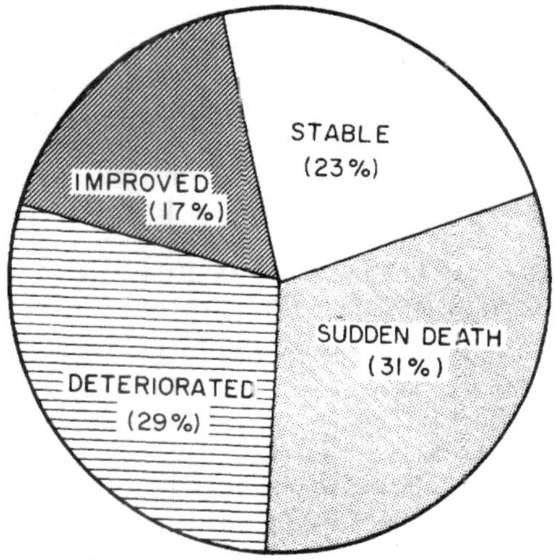

FIGURE 2 *Clinical course of 35 children with ASH (group 1).*

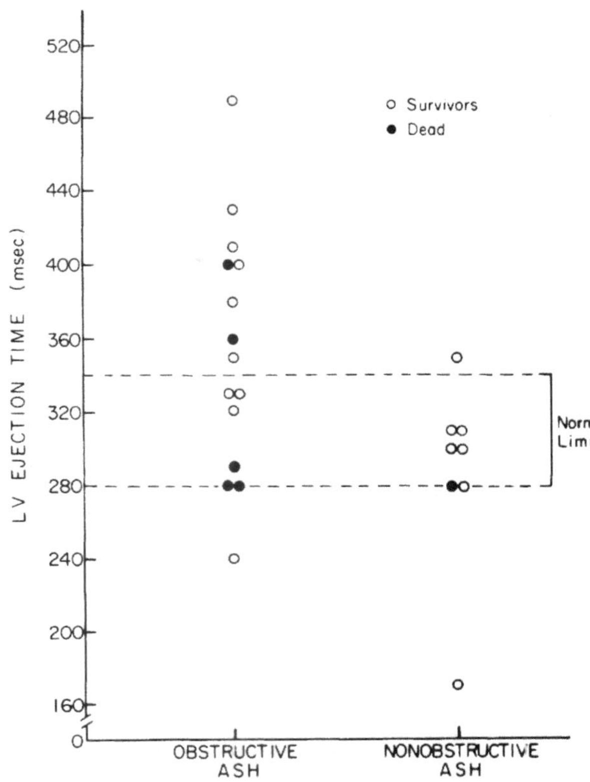

FIGURE 3 *Left ventricular ejection times (corrected for heart rate) in children with ASH (group 1), compared to normal values.*[42, 43]

pressure or left ventricular end-diastolic pressure. Right ventricular end-diastolic pressure was significantly greater in patients without obstruction (10 ± 2 [SEM] mm Hg) compared to patients with obstruction (6 ± 0.4 mm Hg; $P < 0.02$). Cardiac index was significantly less in patients without obstruction (2.7 ± 0.3 L/min/m²) compared to patients with obstruction (3.7 ± 0.2 L/min/m²; $P < 0.05$).

CHANGE IN LEFT VENTRICULAR OUTFLOW OBSTRUCTION DURING THE FOLLOW-UP PERIOD

In order to determine whether changes in the degree of outflow obstruction occurred during the period of follow-up, the left ventricular outflow gradient was estimated by echocardiography at the most recent cardiac evaluation and compared with the maximum gradient recorded at cardiac catheterization under basal conditions during the initial evaluation in 20 of 35 group 1 patients. During the period of follow-up, the magnitude of outflow obstruction did not change appreciably in 13 patients, and small increases or decreases in the degree of outflow obstruction occurred in five. In two patients (K. Y. and G. M.), however, a significant increase in gradient was demonstrated. At 10 years of age patient K. Y. was mildly symptomatic and no outflow gradient was measured at cardiac catheterization (even with provocative maneuvers); at 20 years of age, he was asymptomatic and a gradient of 105 mm Hg was estimated from the echocardiogram. At six years of age, patient G. M. was asymptomatic and had a small outflow gradient of 17 mm Hg measured at cardiac catheterization under basal conditions (no provocative maneuvers were attempted); at 17 years of age, a gradient of 90 mm Hg was estimated from the echocardiogram, although his clinical status had not changed.

ELECTROCARDIOGRAPHIC FINDINGS

The electrocardiogram was normal in only three (9%) of 35 patients. Electrocardiographic abnormalities in the remaining 32 patients are summarized in table 3. No electrocardiographic pattern was characteristic of patients with ASH, nor was the electrocardiogram helpful in distinguishing patients with obstruction from patients without obstruction. Furthermore, electrocardiographic abnormalities were not related to age of the patient, degree of functional impairment, or magnitude of outflow obstruction.

Eight patients without conduction defects initially had developed conduction abnormalities by the most recent examination, including two with left bundle branch block, two with first degree atrioventricular block, two with intraventricular conduction defect (after operation in one), one with right bundle branch block (after operation) and one with left anterior hemiblock. Prolongation of the Q-T interval was present in 14 patients (in whom conduction defects were not evident) at either the initial or follow-up evaluation. In three patients abnormal Q or QS waves that were present at initial evaluation were absent at the most recent evaluation; in seven other patients abnormal Q or QS waves were present only at the latest evaluation.

TABLE 3. *Electrocardiographic Abnormalities at Initial Cardiac Evaluation in 46 Children with ASH*

	Group 1 (35 pts)	Group 2 (11 pts)
Normal	3	8
Left ventricular hypertrophy	18	2
Right ventricular hypertrophy	4	0
Combined ventricular hypertrophy	1	0
Left axis deviation	8	0
Right axis deviation	5	0
Abnormal Q or Q-S waves (≥ 4 mm in depth) (in one or more leads)	17	1
ST segment and T wave abnormalities	20	1
Left atrial enlargement	5	0
Right atrial enlargement	3	0
WPW	2	1
Short P-R interval	2	0
RBBB	1	0
First degree atrioventricular block	2	0
IVCD	1	0
Q-T interval prolongation	14	2
Poor R wave progression in precordial leads	3	0

Abbreviations: pts = patients; WPW = Wolff-Parkinson-White syndrome; RBBB = right bundle branch block; IVCD = intraventricular conduction defect.

RADIOGRAPHIC FINDINGS

Cardiothoracic ratios ranged from 0.41 to 0.70 (average 0.50). Heart size was normal (cardiothoracic ratio <0.55) in 25 (72%) of 35 patients and enlarged in 10 (28%) of 35 patients. Pulmonary venous markings were prominent in two patients. There was no relation between the degree of cardiac enlargement and the age of the patient, severity of symptoms or magnitude of outflow obstruction.

A significant change in heart size between the initial and latest cardiac evaluation was evident in six (17%) of the 35 patients. In three patients the heart size decreased and in three others it increased. The increase in heart size in two patients was associated with clinical deterioration (T. B.) or preceded sudden death (J. T.).

SUDDEN DEATH

Eleven (31%) of the 35 patients in group 1 experienced a cardiac arrest during the period of follow-up (figs. 1 and 2). Ten of these patients died and one patient (R. B.) had a documented episode of ventricular fibrillation and was resuscitated. The age at death ranged from eight to 27 years (mean 16). The survival curve of patients during the period of follow-up is depicted in figure 4.

Death was sudden (instantaneously or within a few minutes) and occurred without warning in each of the 11 patients; none of the patients was hospitalized at the time. Death was unrelated to exertion (occurred while standing, sitting, lying, sleeping) in eight patients, occurred during vigorous physical activity in one patient and while resting after vigorous activity in two patients. At the time of sudden death, three patients were asymptomatic, six patients were in class II and two patients were in class III or IV. One patient (J. P.) was considered to be in functional class II because of a single syncopal episode that occurred 16 months prior to his death; he was otherwise asymptomatic. Only three patients (J. P., S. C. and J. T.) showed evidence of clinical deterioration just prior to death.

If the four of 24 patients with obstructive ASH who were operated upon are excluded from analysis, then 8 (40%) of the 20 patients with obstruction and one (9%) of the 11 patients without obstruction died suddenly during the course of the study (fig. 5). No significant difference in mean outflow gradient was present, however, between those patients with obstructive ASH who died and those who survived (48 ± 11 mm Hg versus 70 ± 10 mm Hg, respectively) (fig. 5).

Two of the 11 sudden deaths occurred in patients who had prior myotomy-myectomy or myotomy; operation was performed six years prior to death in one (D. Pen.) and 13 years prior to death in the other (C. F.). Preoperatively, patient D. Pen. had marked right ventricular outflow tract obstruction (118 mm Hg pressure gradient) and patient C. F. had severe left ventricular outflow obstruction (175 mm Hg pressure gradient). Both patients were asymptomatic at the time of their death; operation had completely abolished the outflow gradient in each. Four other patients were receiving propranolol at the time of their death. The dosage of propranolol was considered adequate (> 2 ml/kg/day) in three patients (S. C., B. L. and D. C.) and inadequate in one (R. B.).

No clinical data at the initial cardiac evaluation, such as age at onset of symptoms, functional status, left ventricular ejection or upstroke time, left ventricular end-diastolic pressure, heart size or electrocardiographic abnormalities proved a reliable predictor of death. In particular, of the 19 patients with a conduction defect at some time during the duration of study, five died suddenly and 14 survived; of the 14 patients with prolonged Q-T interval, five died and nine survived. Thus, death occurred as frequently in those patients with conduction abnormalities or Q-T interval prolongation as in those without such abnormalities. Furthermore, the duration of follow-up did not differ significantly between surviving and nonsurviving patients. Finally, although eight (67%) of the 11 sudden deaths occurred in males, this incidence does not differ significantly from the percentage of males in the study population as a whole (72%).

NECROPSY FINDINGS

The gross pathologic and histologic data are summarized in table 4. Each of the seven hearts available for detailed examination showed disproportionate thickening of the ventricular septum with respect to the posterobasal left ventricular free wall (septal-free wall ratio of ≥1.3).[45] One patient (B. L.) had a large transmural myocardial infarct (documented clinically three months before her death) despite widely patent extramural and intramural coronary arteries. None of the other six hearts studied at necropsy had areas of myocardial necrosis (although patient R. B., who had a cardiac arrest and was resuscitated, had an apical myocardial infarct noted at the time of myotomy-myectomy four months later).

Cardiac muscle cells in the ventricular septum of all seven patients were greatly hypertrophied. Numerous cardiac muscle cells in the ventricular septum of each patient showed the characteristic disorganized arrangement previously described,[35, 36] in which adjacent cells are arranged obliquely

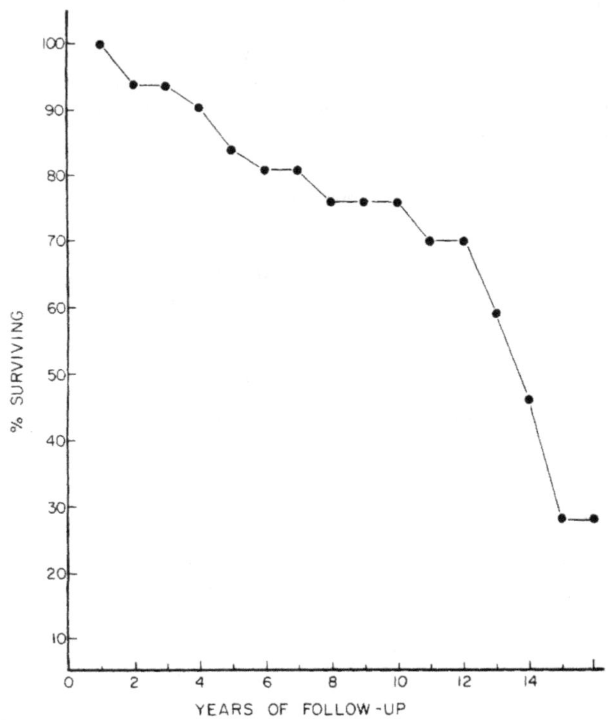

FIGURE 4 *Percent survival of the 35 patients with ASH (group 1) plotted as a function of time in the study. The marked decrease in survival occurring after the twelfth year is due to the small numbers of patients that were followed for 13 or more years. One patient (R. B.), who experienced a cardiac arrest and was resuscitated, is included as a nonsurvivor.*

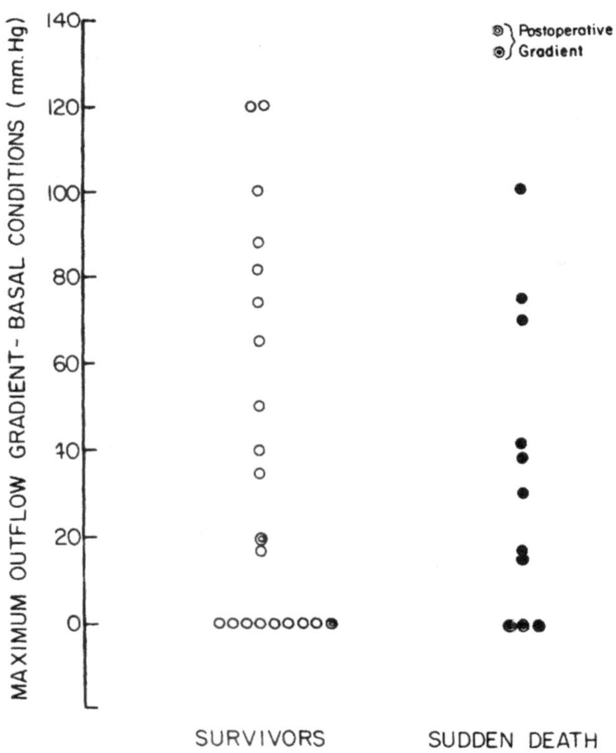

FIGURE 5 *Outflow gradients in surviving patients and patients experiencing sudden death (group 1). The most recent postoperative gradient (measured at cardiac catheterization) was used for the four patients who underwent myotomy-myectomy or myotomy. In all other patients the gradient recorded at the initial evaluation by cardiac catheterization was used.*

TABLE 4. *Necropsy Data in Seven Patients with ASH*

Patient	Age (yr)	Sex	LV-SA PSG (mm Hg)	Heart weight (g)	Ventricular wall thicknesses (mm) VS	PBLV	Max LVFW	RV	VS:PBLV ratio
J.T.	9	M	0	260	15	8	18	7	1.9
D.Pen.	19	M	0†	660	40	19	19	5	2.1
L.Pen.	8	M	15	300	30	20	20	5	1.5
D.C.	19	F	38	340	24	15	15	6	1.6
B.L.	21	F	41	1250	45	32	32	11	1.4
S.C.	27	F	100	640	32	22	22	6	1.5
C.F.	23	M	175*	840	40	20	20	6	2.0

*Represents preoperative left ventricular outflow gradient; postoperative gradient was zero under basal conditions.
**Grading system: 0 = normal cellular arrangement; 1+ = mild cellular disorganization; 2+ = moderate disorganization; 3+ = severe disorganization.
†Preoperative right ventricular outflow tract gradient of 118 mm Hg; postoperative right ventricular outflow gradient was zero.
+ = present; − = absent.
Abbreviations: g = grams; LA = left atrium; LV = left ventricle; LVFW = left ventricular free wall; LVPM = left ventricular papillary muscles; LVOT = left ventricular outflow tract; mm = millimeters; mm Hg = millimeters of mercury; MV = mitral valve; PBLV = posterobasal left ventricular free wall; PSG = peak systolic gradient; RA = right atrium; RV = right ventricle; SA = systemic artery; S.E. = subendocardial; T.M. = transmural; VS = ventricular septum.

and perpendicularly to each other. Cardiac muscle cells in the left ventricular free wall were hypertrophied and normally arranged in the four patients who had had a preoperative left ventricular outflow gradient of at least 30 mm Hg under basal conditions. In the three patients with no or minimal obstruction to left ventricular outflow, disorganized cardiac muscle cells were present in both the ventricular septum and the left ventricular free wall. In addition, operatively obtained tissue from patient R. B. showed numerous hypertrophied, disorganized cardiac muscle cells in the ventricular septum; cells with these features were present but less common in the left ventricular posterior wall. With the exception of this patient, the distribution of disorganized cardiac muscle cells in the hearts of patients with ASH in this study is similar to that described previously.[35]

Group 2 (11 Patients)

Each of the 11 patients in group 2 had either no murmur or a soft grade I-II/VI systolic ejection murmur, loudest at the lower left sternal border or apex. The electrocardiogram was normal in eight (73%) of the 11 patients. Electrocardiographic evidence of left ventricular hypertrophy was present in two patients (including one with Wolff-Parkinson-White syndrome) and abnormal Q waves were present in another patient. Prolongation of the Q-T interval was present in two of these patients. The heart size on chest radiograph was within normal limits (cardiothoracic ratio <0.55) in all 11 patients.

Echocardiographic Assessment of Ventricular Wall Thickness in Group 1 and Group 2 Patients

Thicknesses of the ventricular septum and posterobasal left ventricular free wall and the septal-free wall ratios, as assessed by echocardiography in 24 group 1 patients and the 11 group 2 patients, are shown in table 5 and figure 6. Two patients (K. Y. and G. M.) who did not have obstruction to outflow initially but who subsequently developed obstruction were included in the obstructive group only for this analysis. Mean septal thickness, posterobasal left ventricular free wall thickness and septal-free wall ratio were significantly greater in group 1 compared to group 2 patients. Similar significant differences were also present when only those patients in group 1 without outflow obstruction were compared to group 2 patients (all of whom had nonobstructive ASH). It should be noted, however, that the patients in group 1 (with or without obstruction) were older at the time of echocardiographic study than patients in group 2 (average 18 years of age compared to 10 years of age).

Discussion

This investigation demonstrates that the clinical and hemodynamic features of ASH in children, as in adults, comprise a broad spectrum. Some children with ASH have

TABLE 5. *Echocardiographic Assessment of Ventricular Wall Thicknesses in Children with ASH*

Patient group	No. of patients	Mean age (yr)	VS (mm)	PW (mm)	VS:PW ratio
Group 1	24	18	22 ± 1	12 ± 1	1.8 ± 0.1
Group 2	11	10	13 ± 1	8 ± 1	1.5 ± 0.1
			$P < .001$	$P < .001$	$P < .05$
Group 1 (Nonob.)	9	18	20 ± 2	11 ± 1	1.8 ± 0.1
Group 2	11	10	13 ± 1	8 ± 1	1.5 ± 0.1
			$P < .001$	$P < .02$	$P < .05$
Group 1 (Obst.)	15	18	18 ± 2	13 ± 1	1.8 ± 0.1
Group 1 (Nonob.)	9	18	20 ± 2	11 ± 1	1.8 ± 0.1
			NS	NS	NS

Abbreviations: Nonob. = nonobstructive; NS = not statistically significant; Obst. = obstructive; PW = posterobasal left ventricular free wall thickness; VS = ventricular septal thickness.

Cavity dilatation				MV thickening	Endocardial plaque LVOT	Disorganization of cardiac muscle cells**		Gross fibrosis		
LV	RV	LA	RA			VS	LVFW	VS	LVFW	LVPM
+	+	+	+	0	0	3+	3+	–	–	–
0	+	+	+	+	+	3+	1+	+ (S.E.)	–	+
0	0	+	+	0	0	3+	1+	+ (S.E.)	–	+
0	0	+	+	+	+	3+	0	+ (T.M.)	+ (S.E.)	+
+	+	+	+	0	0	3+	0	+ (S.E.)	+ (T.M.)	+
0	0	+	+	+	+	3+	0	+ (S.E.)	–	+
0	0	+	+	+	+	3+	0	+ (S.E.)	--	+

obstruction to ventricular outflow under basal conditions and demonstrate the typical physical, hemodynamic and angiographic features associated with outflow obstruction in this disease.[6, 9-11, 33] Most of these children with obstructive ASH either were symptomatic at initial evaluation or subsequently developed symptoms; only three of the 24 patients with obstruction did not have cardiovascular symptoms at some time during the period of observation. Many children with ASH, however, have no or little obstruction to ventricular outflow under basal conditions or with provocative maneuvers.

Although the majority of the children with nonobstructive ASH referred to us for study (prior to the application of echocardiography to the diagnosis of this disease) were symptomatic, such patients are undoubtedly highly selected and probably not representative of the entire cohort of children with nonobstructive ASH. This conclusion seems likely since it is now appreciated that the nonobstructive form of ASH is more common than originally suspected; many patients, for example, have no or minimal evidence of cardiac disease and diagnosis is difficult, if not impossible, without echocardiography.[1, 3, 6, 8, 45] Thus, if all patients eventually identified as having ASH (with the aid of echocardiography) are considered, it is possible that the majority of children with nonobstructive ASH will be found to be asymptomatic.[1] The finding that septal thickness was less in the group 2 patients (all of whom had nonobstructive ASH diagnosed by echocardiography) than in the group 1 patients without obstruction suggests that the echocardiographic studies led either to earlier detection of the disease or to detection of a less affected subgroup of patients with nonobstructive ASH.

Given the broad clinical and hemodynamic spectrum of ASH, it was not surprising to find the course of children with ASH to be extremely variable. However, it was alarming to discover that in the subgroup of 35 children referred to the NHLI because of overt manifestations of cardiac disease, less than one-half (40%) demonstrated either improvement or no change in their functional capacity; 60% of the patients showed clinical deterioration or died. Most of the 35 patients with long-term follow-up showed little or no change in the magnitude of outflow obstruction during the period of observation. Two patients, however, did demonstrate unequivocal progression of obstruction in which the outflow gradient under basal conditions increased from zero to 105 mm Hg in one and from 17 mm Hg to 90 mm Hg in the other.

The most striking finding of this investigation was that sudden death occurred in 31% of the 35 patients in group 1. Since the average follow-up period was 7.4 years, the annual mortality rate was approximately 4%. This figure is in general agreement with that reported in studies consisting primarily of adult patients,[14, 15] but is somewhat higher than that reported in children by other investigators.[13, 15, 46] An additional disconcerting feature of our data is that three of the patients who died suddenly were completely asymptomatic at the time of death, and another patient was asymptomatic except for a single syncopal episode that had occurred 16 months before death. Although little direct data are available, the circumstances of death in our patients

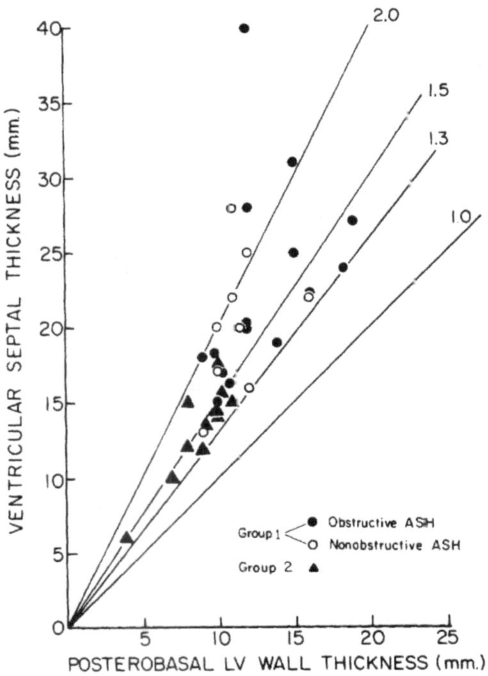

FIGURE 6 *Echocardiographic assessment of ventricular wall thicknesses in children with ASH (groups 1 and 2). Identity lines define ventricular septal to posterobasal left ventricular wall thickness ratios of 1.0, 1.3, 1.5 and 2.0.*

suggest that the terminal event was probably a ventricular arrhythmia. This contention is supported by the fact that ventricular fibrillation was documented in one patient (R. B.) who was eventually resuscitated.

Although previous investigators have suggested that elevation in left ventricular end-diastolic pressure is a poor prognostic sign in patients with ASH,[16] we found no significant difference in left ventricular end-diastolic pressure between surviving patients and patients dying suddenly. Moreover, the occurrence of sudden death did not correlate with age at onset of symptoms, functional status, electrocardiographic abnormalities or left ventricular ejection or upstroke time. However, we found that of the 20 children with obstructive ASH (i.e., defined as the presence of any gradient under basal conditions) who did not undergo operation, eight (40%) died during the course of our study. Therefore, it appears that patients with obstructive ASH are at risk of dying suddenly, regardless of the magnitude of obstruction. Of interest, only one of the 11 children with nonobstructive ASH in group 1 died during follow-up. These data suggest that the risk of sudden death in children without obstruction is small; however, we believe that it is not uncommon for patients with clinically unsuspected ASH to die suddenly and that at least some of these deaths occur in patients without obstruction. For example, we have knowledge of three other children (siblings of patients in this study but themselves never evaluated at the NHLI) who died suddenly without any previous evidence of cardiac disease. The diagnosis of ASH was confirmed at necropsy in each of these children.

Likewise, we must emphasize that the alarmingly high annual mortality rate observed in this study is based on observations confined to a rather specific subgroup of patients with ASH (those who were referred to the NHLI because of some overt manifestation of cardiac disease). Thus, a very different prognosis may apply to the broader cohort of patients with ASH currently coming to attention by virtue of echocardiographic diagnosis. Nevertheless, it would appear that the risk of sudden death in children with overt evidence of disease (i.e., similar to our group 1 patients), is great and that more aggressive therapy may be indicated. Unfortunately, neither propranolol nor myotomy-myectomy completely protected against sudden death in our patients. Four of the eight nonoperated patients with obstructive ASH who died were receiving propranolol at the time of their death, although in one of these patients the dose of propranolol was not considered adequate. Furthermore, two of the four symptomatic children with obstructive ASH who were operated upon died (six and 13 years postoperatively) despite complete relief of their obstruction. Thus, the role of prophylactic propranolol therapy or myotomy-myectomy in children with obstructive ASH remains to be determined.

Acknowledgment

We wish to express our gratitude to Ms. Cora Burn, R.N., and Mrs. Joyce McKay, R.N., for their fine technical assistance and to Mr. Joel Verter for his assistance in the statistical analyses.

References

1. Clark CE, Henry WL, Epstein SE: Familial prevalence and genetic transmission of idiopathic hypertrophic subaortic stenosis. N Engl J Med **289:** 709, 1973
2. Teare D: Asymmetrical hypertrophy of the heart in young adults. Br Heart J **20:** 1, 1958
3. Henry WL, Clark CE, Epstein SE: Asymmetric septal hypertrophy: Echocardiographic identification of the pathognomonic anatomic abnormality of IHSS. Circulation **47:** 225, 1973
4. Roberts WC: Valvular, subvalvular and supravalvular aortic stenosis: Morphologic features. Cardiovasc Clin **5:** 104, 1973
5. Menges H, Brandenburg RO, Brown AL: The clinical, hemodynamic and pathologic diagnosis of muscular subvalvular aortic stenosis. Circulation **24:** 1126, 1961
6. Epstein SE, Henry WL, Clark CE, Roberts WC, Maron BJ, Ferrans VJ, Redwood DR, Morrow AG: Asymmetric septal hypertrophy. Ann Intern Med **81:** 650, 1974
7. Abbasi AS, MacAlpin RN, Eber LM, Pearce ML: Left ventricular hypertrophy diagnosed by echocardiography. N Engl J Med **289:** 118, 1973
8. Abbasi AS, MacAlpin RN, Eber LM, Pearce ML: Echocardiographic diagnosis of idiopathic hypertrophic cardiomyopathy without outflow obstruction. Circulation **46:** 897, 1972
9. Goodwin JF, Hollman A, Cleland WP, Teare D: Obstructive cardiomyopathy simulating aortic stenosis. Br Heart J **22:** 403, 1960
10. Wigle ED, Heimbecker RO, Gunton RW: Idiopathic ventricular septal hypertrophy causing muscular subaortic stenosis. Circulation **26:** 325, 1962
11. Braunwald E, Lambrew CT, Rockoff SD, Ross J, Morrow AG: Idiopathic hypertrophic subaortic stenosis. I. A description of the disease based upon an analysis of 64 patients. Circulation **29** (suppl IV): IV-1, 1964
12. Frank S, Braunwald E: Idiopathic hypertrophic subaortic stenosis. Clinical analysis of 126 patients with emphasis on the natural history. Circulation **37:** 759, 1968
13. Adelman AG, Wigle ED, Ranganathan N, Webb GD, Kidd BSL, Bigelow WG, Silver MD: The clinical course in muscular subaortic stenosis. A retrospective and prospective study of 60 hemodynamically proved cases. Ann Intern Med **77:** 515, 1972
14. Shah PM, Adelman AG, Wigle ED, Gobel FL, Burchell HB, Hardarson T, Curiel R, De La Calzada C, Oakley CM, Goodwin JF: The natural (and unnatural) course of hypertrophic obstructive cardiomyopathy. A multicenter study. Circ Res **34** and **35** (suppl II): II-179, 1973
15. Hardarson T, De La Calzada CS, Curiel R, Goodwin JF: Prognosis and mortality of hypertrophic obstructive cardiomyopathy. Lancet **2:** 1462, 1973
16. Swan DA, Bell B, Oakley CM, Goodwin JF: Analysis of the symptomatic course and prognosis and treatment of hypertrophic obstructive cardiomyopathy. Br Heart J **33:** 671, 1971
17. Tafur E, Guntheroth WG, Baum D, Blackmon JR: The development of outflow obstruction of the left ventricle in idiopathic myocardial hypertrophy. Circulation **30:** 569, 1964
18. Raghib C, Adams P Jr, Wang Y, Amplatz K, Lillehei CW, Edwards JE: Clinical pathologic conference. Am Heart J **68:** 254, 1964
19. Daoud G, Gallaher ME, Kaplan S: Muscular subaortic stenosis. Am J Cardiol **7:** 860, 1961
20. Rudhe U, Zetterqvist P, Wallgren G: Angiocardiography of hypertrophic obstructive cardiomyopathy in infancy and childhood. Ann Radiol **9:** 185, 1966
21. Wood RS, Taylor WJ, Wheat MW, Schiebler GL: Muscular subaortic stenosis in childhood. Report of occurrence in three siblings. Pediatrics **30:** 749, 1962
22. Walther RJ, Madoff IM, Zinner K: Cardiomegaly of unknown cause occurring in a family. N Engl J Med **263:** 1105, 1960
23. Moes CAF, Peckham GB, Keith JD: Idiopathic hypertrophy of the interventricular septum causing muscular subaortic stenosis in children. Radiology **83:** 283, 1964
24. Williams RG, Ellison RC, Nadas AS: Development of left ventricular outflow obstruction in idiopathic hypertrophic subaortic stenosis. N Engl J Med **288:** 868, 1973
25. Shand DG, Sell CG, Oates JA: Hypertrophic obstructive cardiomyopathy in an infant — propranolol therapy for three years. N Engl J Med **285:** 843, 1971
26. Pernot C, Hoeffel JC, Henry M, Worms AM, Rothhahn G: Radiological patterns of obstructive cardiomyopathy of the left ventricle in childhood. Am Heart J **86:** 462, 1973
27. Soulie P, Joly F, Carlotti J: Les stenoses idiopathiques de la chambre de chasse du ventricule gauche (a propos de 10 observations). Acta Cardiol (Brux) **17:** 335, 1962
28. Lundquist CB, Amplatz K, Palma SP, Raghib G: Angiocardiographic findings in idiopathic myocardial hypertrophy with right and left ventricular outflow tract obstruction. Am J Roentgenol **93:** 315, 1965
29. Barr PA, Celermajer JM, Bowdler JD, Cartmill TB: Idiopathic hypertrophic obstructive cardiomyopathy causing severe right ventricular outflow tract obstruction in infancy. Br Heart J **35:** 1109, 1973
30. Neufeld HN, Ongley PA, Edwards JE: Combined congenital subaortic stenosis and infundibular pulmonary stenosis. Br Heart J **22:** 686, 1960
31. Maron BJ, Edwards JE, Henry WL, Clark CE, Bingle G, Epstein SE:

Asymmetric septal hypertrophy (ASH) in infancy. Circulation **50:** 809, 1974
32. Nasser WK, Williams JF, Mishkin ME, Childress RH, Helmen C, Merritt AD, Genovese PD: Familial myocardial disease with and without obstruction to left ventricular outflow. Clinical, hemodynamic, and angiographic findings. Circulation **35:** 638, 1967
33. Goodwin JF: Congestive and hypertrophic cardiomyopathies. A decade of study. Lancet **1:** 731, 1970
34. Henry WL, Clark CE, Glancy DL, Epstein SE: Echocardiographic measurement of the left ventricular outflow gradient in idiopathic hypertrophic subaortic stenosis. N Engl J Med **288:** 989, 1973
35. Maron BJ, Ferrans VJ, Henry WL, Clark CE, Redwood DR, Roberts WC, Morrow AG, Epstein SE: Differences in distribution of myocardial abnormalities in patients with obstructive and nonobstructive asymmetric septal hypertrophy (ASH): Light and electron microscopic findings. Circulation **50:** 436, 1974
36. Ferrans VJ, Morrow AG, Roberts WC: Myocardial ultrastructure in idiopathic hypertrophic subaortic stenosis. A study of operatively excised left ventricular outflow tract muscle in 14 patients. Circulation **45:** 769, 1972
37. Electrocardiography in Infants and Children, edited by Cassel DE, Ziegler RF. New York, Grune and Stratton, 1966, p 355
38. Romhilt DW, Estes EH: A point score system for the ECG diagnosis of left ventricular hypertrophy. Am Heart J **75:** 752, 1968
39. Mc Cammon RW: A longitudinal study of electrocardiographic intervals in healthy children. Acta Paediatr Scand (Uppsala) suppl 126, 1961
40. Simonson E, Cady LD Jr, Woodbury M: The normal Q-T interval. Am Heart J **63:** 747, 1962
41. Cutler SJ, Ederer F: Maximum utilization of the life table method in analyzing survival. J Chron Dis **8:** 699, 1958
42. Benchimol A, Dimond EG, Shen Y: Ejection time in aortic stenosis and mitral stenosis. Comparison between the direct and indirect arterial tracings with special reference to pre- and postoperative findings. Am J Cardiol **6:** 728, 1960
43. Golde D, Burstin L: Systolic phases of the cardiac cycle in children. Circulation **42:** 1029, 1970
44. Morrow AG, Fisher RD, Fogarty TJ: Isolated hypertrophic obstruction to right ventricular outflow. Am Heart J **77:** 814, 1969
45. Henry WL, Clark CE, Roberts WC, Morrow AG, Epstein SE: Differences in distribution of myocardial abnormalities in patients with obstructive and nonobstructive asymmetric septal hypertrophy (ASH): Echocardiographic and gross anatomic findings. Circulation **50:** 447, 1974
46. Tajik AJ, Giuliani ER, Weidman WH, McGoon DC, Brandenburg RO, Ritter DG: Idiopathic hypertrophic subaortic stenosis (IHSS) in children. Circulation **47** and **48:** (suppl IV): IV-222, 1973

A discussion on hypertrophic cardiomyopathy

Thomas L. Spray, M.D.
Barry J. Maron, M.D.
Andrew G. Morrow, M.D.
Stephen E. Epstein, M.D.
William C. Roberts, M.D.
Bethesda, Md.

Dr. Roberts: The purpose of this conference is to discuss certain clinical, operative, and morphologic features of hypertrophic cardiomyopathy as exemplified in one patient. Dr. Spray will present the patient.

Dr. Spray: R. H. (11-65-60-4), a 56-year-old white woman, was not suspected of having heart disease until she was 30 years old, when a precordial murmur was heard. She was in good health until age 40 when she developed angina pectoris and palpitations. From age 51 on her symptoms increased in frequency and severity. In addition, she developed orthopnea and paroxysmal nocturnal dyspnea. During the year before death, occasional syncopal and presyncopal episodes occurred. In February, 1976, she was admitted to a local hospital where an electrocardiogram showed left ventricular hypertrophy with the strain pattern. A treadmill exercise tolerance test was attempted but it was stopped when she developed paroxysmal atrial tachycardia. Cardiac catheterization disclosed the following pressures (in mm. Hg): right ventricle (body), 50/3; right ventricle (subpulmonic area), 21/3; pulmonary trunk, 21/17 (mean 12); pulmonary arterial wedge mean, 7; left ventricle (body) 235/0-25; left ventricle (subaortic area), 105/12, and aorta, 105/60 (mean 80). The peak systolic pressure gradient between left ventricle and aorta was 130 mm. Hg. The cardiac output was 4.7 liters per minute and the cardiac index, 3.0 liters/minute/$M.^2$ She was begun on propranolol (160 mg. per day) and quinidine.

In May, 1976, she was admitted to a local hospital for treatment of severe headache, at which time diastolic blood pressures to 130 mm. Hg were noted. Diazoxide therapy resulted in marked hypotension which required intravenous metaraminol for stabilization. She was admitted to the National Heart, Lung, and Blood Institute 19 days before death.

On examination, the blood pressure was 120/80 mm. Hg, heart rate, 56 per minute, and respiratory rate, 12 per minute. The jugular venous pulse was normal. The carotid arterial upstroke was judged to be rapid. The lung fields were clear to auscultation. The point of maximal cardiac impulse was in the sixth left intercostal space in the anterior axillary line and the apical beat had a triple character. The first and second heart sounds were normal; a fourth heart sound was present at the apex. A Grade 4/6 systolic, ejection type murmur was heard, loudest at the apex and it radiated to the base. The murmur increased in intensity on standing but did not change with Valsalva maneuver. Neither liver nor spleen were palpated but mild pedal edema was noted.

Dr. Roberts: Dr. Maron, could you describe the electrocardiogram, chest roentgenogram and echocardiogram.

Dr. Maron: The *electrocardiogram* shows left ventricular hypertrophy with strain pattern (Fig. 1). In addition, the T waves in Leads I and aV_L are deeply inverted in a symmetric fashion; ST segments are elevated in Leads V_1 and V_2 and depressed in Leads V_5 and V_6. Left atrial enlargement also is evident. The *chest radiograph* shows pectus excavatum, left ventricular enlargement,

From the Pathology, Cardiology and Surgery Branches, National Heart, Lung, and Blood Institute, National Institutes of Health, Bethesda, Md.

Received for publication May 3, 1977.

Reprint requests: William C. Roberts, M.D., Bldg. 10A, Room 3E-30, NIH, Bethesda, Md. 20014.

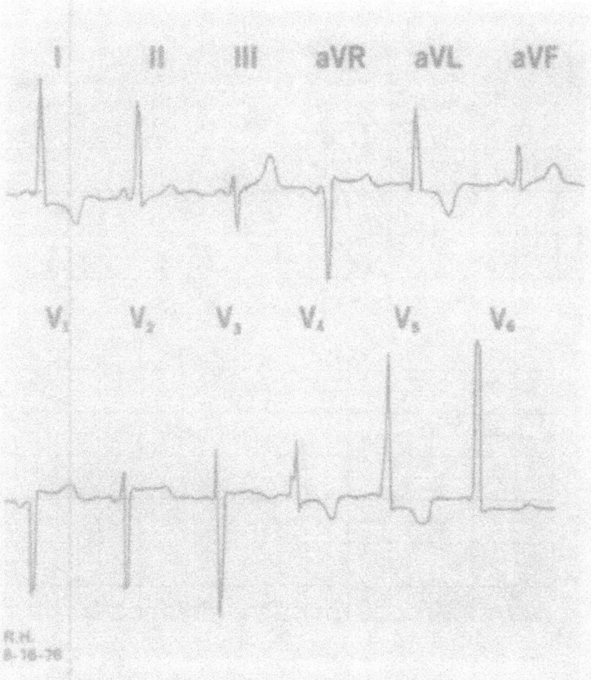

Fig. 1. Preoperative electrocardiogram of present patient showing left ventricular hypertrophy with strain pattern, left atrial enlargement, and ST segment and T wave abnormalities.

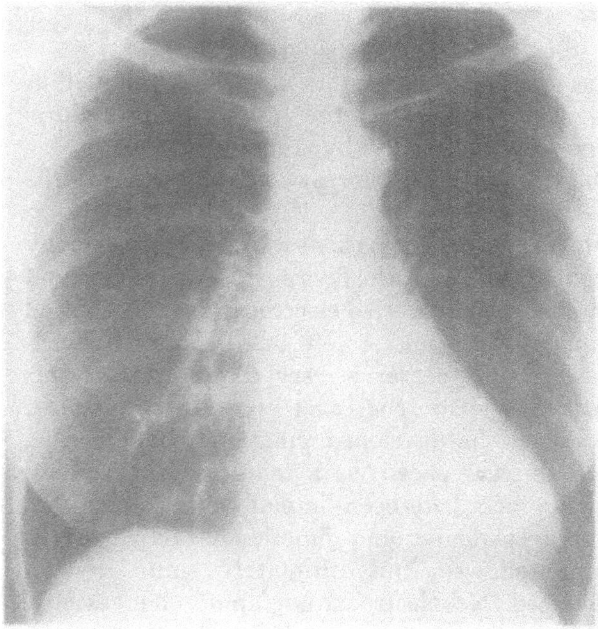

Fig. 2. Posteroanterior chest radiograph in present patient showing mild cardiac enlargement and normal pulmonary vascular markings.

and normal pulmonary vascular markings (Fig. 2). *Echocardiogram* shows (in diastole) ventricular septal thickness of 24 mm., posterobasal left ventricular wall thickness of 16 mm., and a septal-to-free wall ratio of 1.5. When wall thicknesses are measured in systole, however, the ventricular septum is 26 mm., the posterobasal left ventricular wall is 29 mm., and hence, the septal-to-free wall ratio in systole is 0.9 (Fig. 3). In addition, marked systolic anterior motion of the anterior mitral leaflet, indicative of severe obstruction to left ventricular outflow, is evident (Fig. 4). The transverse internal dimensions of the left ventricular (43 mm.) and left atrial (38 mm.) cavities and the aortic "root" (32 mm.) were within normal limits.

DR. ROBERTS: Dr. Epstein, what were your *reasons for recommending operation* in this patient.

DR. EPSTEIN: This patient was considered an ideal candidate for septal myotomy–myectomy for the following reasons: (1) she was severely limited (New York Heart Association, Functional Class III) by extreme fatigue and dyspnea with exertion, and in addition, she had numerous episodes of syncope and lightheadedness; (2) these symptoms were not lessened significantly by treatment with propranolol; (3) a marked (130 mm. Hg) peak systolic pressure gradient was present in the left ventricular outflow tract under basal conditions; (4) there was evidence by echocardiography of a markedly thickened ventricular septum that would permit an adequate myectomy to be performed; and (5) no other major medical problems were identified that would contraindicate a major cardiac operation.

DR. ROBERTS: Dr. Morrow, could you *describe what you found at operation* in this patient and the operative procedure you performed.

DR. MORROW: The operation performed was the ventricular myotomy and myectomy which has been used in this institution, with minor modifications, for 17 years.[1] With the patient on cardiopulmonary bypass, the aorta was opened. After gently retracting the aortic valve cusps, the thickened ventricular septum was observed. Two longitudinal, parallel incisions were made in the ventricular septum. The incisions extended caudally from just below the commissure between the right and left aortic valve cusps. The incisions were then joined transversely and the resulting wedge of myocardium was excised. After this procedure, the ventricular septum was palpated and noted to be somewhat thinner than in most patients after this operation. The aortotomy incision was closed. No aortic regurgitation was noted, and no systolic thrill was palpated in the right ventricle at the end of the procedure. The patient came off bypass easily.

DR. ROBERTS: Dr. Morrow, *what occurred in the postoperative period?*

DR. MORROW: The patient was hemodynamically stable throughout the first postoperative day, and the first postoperative electrocardiogram showed sinus rhythm and a left bundle branch block pattern. The latter is very common after this operation. On the first postoperative day, however, she developed junctional bradycardia, and she was paced via a temporary pacemaker wire which had been implanted at operation. Supraventricular and junctional tachyarrhythmias followed, but ultimately sinus rhythm returned. No electrocardiographic changes suggestive of acute myocardial infarct occurred. Because of the supraventricular irritability, propranolol was reinstituted. On the following day a new precordial murmur, with an accompanying thrill, was noted at the apex and left sternal border. It was holosystolic and Grade 4/6 in intensity. On the following day, her ventricular rate suddenly decreased to less than 40 beats per minute. The pacemaker failed to capture the ventricle and she died.

DR. ROBERTS: Dr. Spray, could you describe the *findings at necropsy.*

DR. SPRAY: At necropsy the heart weighed 680 grams (Figs. 5 and 6). (The patient weighed 54.5 kilograms). Considerable hemorrhage was present in the atrial septum. The tricuspid valve was normal, except that its anterior leaflet appeared more elongated than usual. The wall of the right ventricle measured up to 1.3 cm. in thickness. The pulmonic valve was normal. Both atria were quite dilated. Both mitral valve leaflets were thickened by fibrous tissue. The left ventricular cavity was small. Measurements of the thickness of the left ventricular myocardium were made at the level at which the ultrasound beam would theoretically pass during life, i.e., between the papillary muscles at the level of the distal margins of the mitral leaflets and at the midpoint of the posterior mitral leaflet. At this level (the "echo area"), the ventricular septum measured 25 mm. and the posterobasal left ventricular free wall, 25 mm. in maximal thickness. The posterobasal portion of left ventricular free wall was thick and rounded, typical of the configuration observed in patients with left ventricular outflow obstruction at rest.

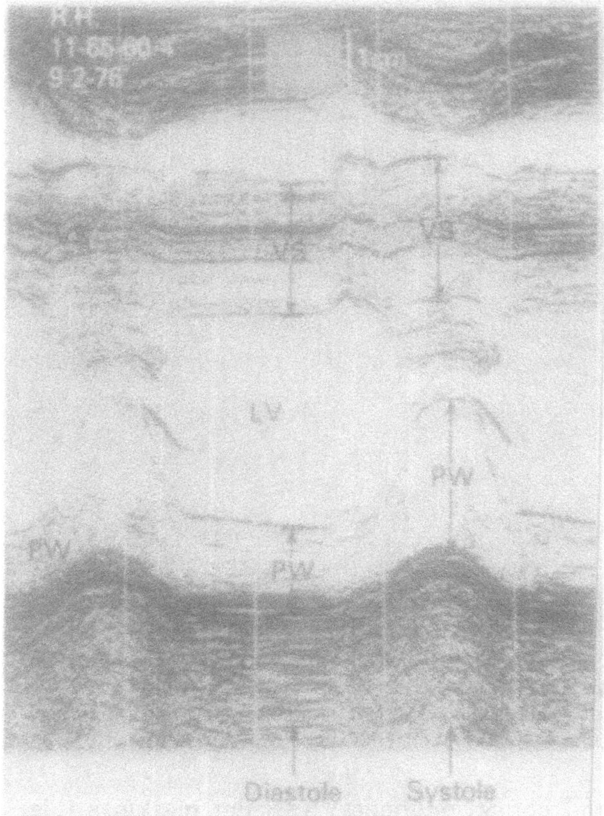

Fig. 3. Echocardiogram of present patient showing disproportionate thickening of the ventricular septum *(VS)* with respect to the posterobasal left ventricular wall *(PW)* in diastole. In contrast, concentric ventricular wall thickening is present in systole. LV = left ventricular cavity.

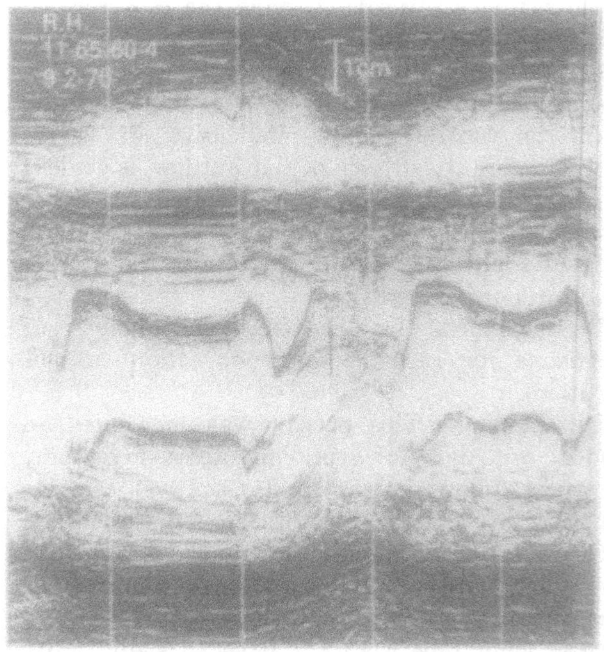

Fig. 4. Echocardiogram of present patient showing systolic anterior motion of the anterior mitral leaflet *(arrow).*

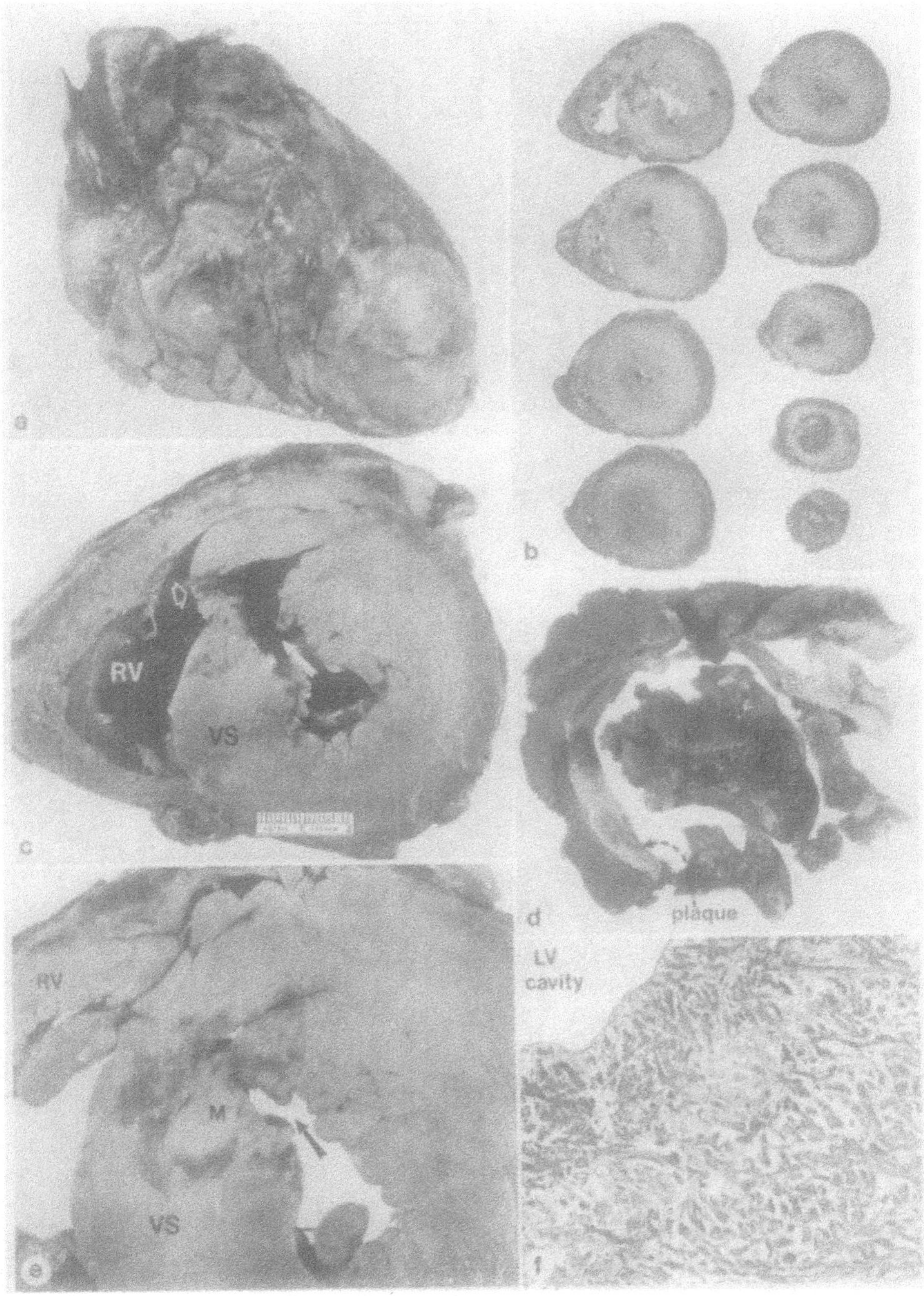

Fig. 5, a through f. *(a),* Anterior view of the heart at necropsy, showing marked left ventricular prominence. *(b),* Serial slices of the cardiac ventricles from base to apex showing severe left ventricular hypertrophy. Hemorrhagic necrosis is present in the apical slices due to its being the site of insertion of the left ventricular drain at operation. *(c),* View of the base of the heart from below showing the area of excision of muscle *(arrow)* from the left ventricular septum *(VS).* The site of rupture of the septum with creation of a ventricular septal defect *(arrow)* is shown. RV = right ventricle. *(d),* The left ventricular septal muscle excised at operation showing an endocardial fibrous plaque consistent with a contact lesion from the anterior mitral leaflet. The excised muscle weighed 4.1 grams. *(e),* Close up of a basal slice of the cardiac ventricles showing the myectomy site *(arrow)* and the surrounding area of necrosis *(M).* *(f),* Histologic section of an area of VS adjacent to the myectomy incision showing marked disorganization of myocardial cells and necrosis (Hematoxylin and eosin stain, original magnification ×80).

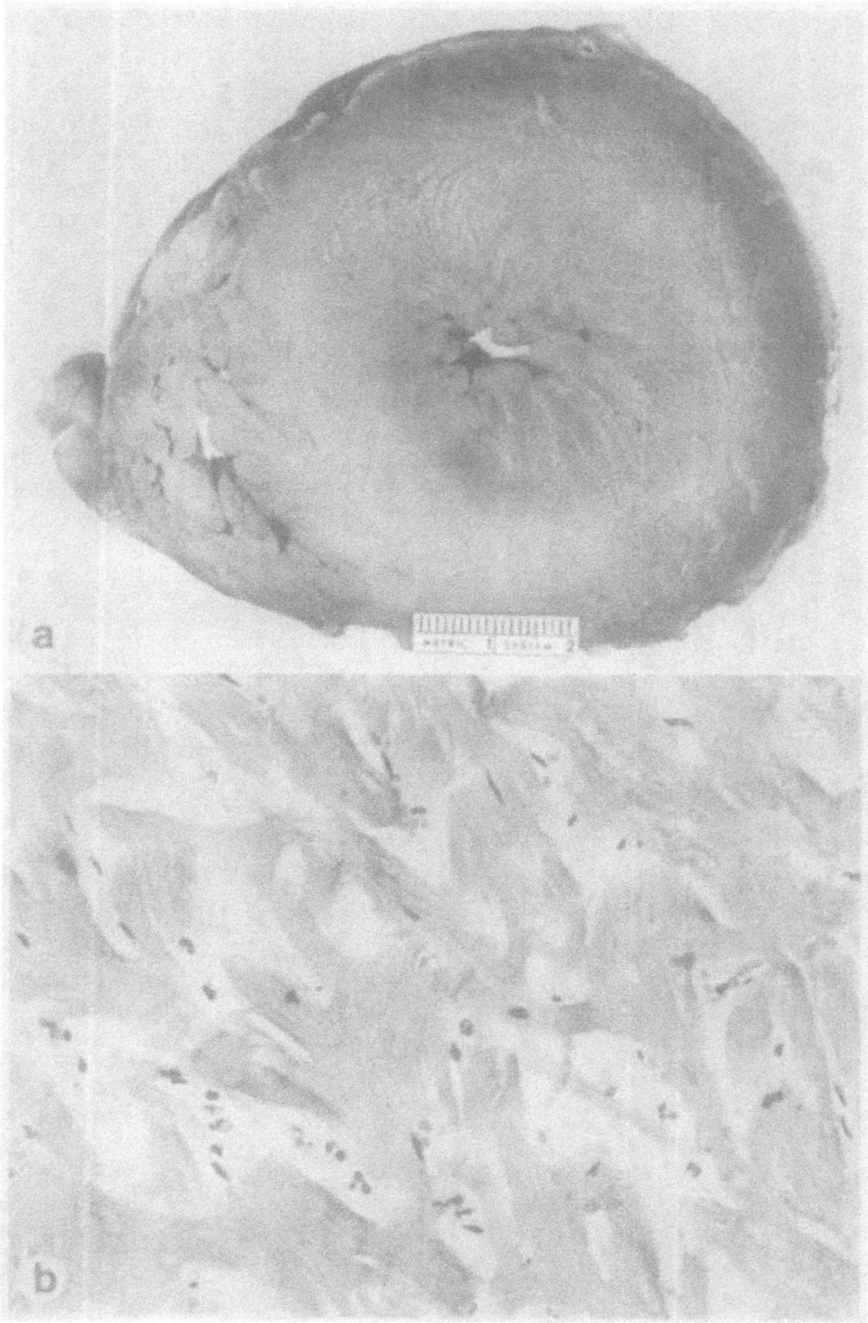

Fig. 6. *(a)*, Transverse slice of the cardiac ventricles midway from the base to the apex showing concentric left ventricular hypertrophy. *(b)*, A high power view of a portion of myocardium from ventricular septum showing marked disorganization of cells and myofibrillar elements. (Hematoxylin and eosin stain, original magnification ×330).

The myocardium adjacent to the site where the drain was inserted at operation in the apex of left ventricle was necrotic. The edges of the area of operatively excised ventricular septum were necrotic. The most cephalad aspect of this excision extended all the way through the ventricular septum, creating a slit-like ventricular septal defect 1 cm. long. There were no areas of myocardial fibrosis. The aortic valve was normal anatomically. The epicardial coronary arteries were grossly normal. Histologic examination of the left ventricular septum showed marked disorganization of myocardial fibers and coagulation necrosis of myocardium bordering the myotomy and myectomy incision (Figs. 5 and 6). The intramural coronary arteries in the ventricular septum were normal.

Dr. Roberts: Dr. Epstein, patients with hypertrophic cardiomyopathy often have *chest pain,* occasionally clear angina pectoris, just like patients with valvular aortic stenosis. What is the cause of angina pectoris in patients with hypertrophic cardiomyopathy? Do they have associated coronary arterial narrowing due to atherosclerosis or is there another cause for the angina pectoris? Or is it really angina pectoris?

Dr. Epstein: It is true that many patients with hypertrophic cardiomyopathy, or ASH, have chest pain or discomfort indistinguishable from that of typical angina pectoris. Since coronary artery disease is relatively common, it is not surprising to find that the two diseases occasionally coexist in a given patient. In such patients the coronary artery disease undoubtedly contributes to the chest pain syndrome. However, in the large majority of patients with hypertrophic cardiomyopathy, chest discomfort occurs without any coronary arterial abnormality discernible by coronary angiography or at necropsy. In patients with obstruction to left ventricular outflow (who consequently have high intraventricular pressures) angina probably occurs because of the excessively high myocardial oxygen consumption; i.e., myocardial oxygen demands outstrip the capacity of the coronary arteries to deliver oxygen, just as in patients with aortic stenosis. In patients without obstruction, the origin of the patient's chest pain is unclear. It may be that proliferation of myocardial capillaries has not kept pace with the excessive amount of hypertrophy present in these patients.

Dr. Roberts: Dr. Epstein, what is the cause of *syncope or presyncope* in patients with hypertrophic cardiomyopathy? Is syncope more frequent in the patients with obstruction to left ventricular outflow at rest or is it just as frequent in patients without obstruction either at rest or with provocation?

Dr. Epstein: Syncope and presyncope occur commonly in patients with obstruction to left ventricular outflow as well as in patients without obstruction to left ventricular outflow. This fact suggests that while syncope in patients with hypertrophic cardiomyopathy may be due to an abrupt increase in the magnitude of left ventricular outflow obstruction in some patients, other mechanisms also must be operative. One such mechanism that can lead to syncope and presyncope in patients with hypertrophic cardiomyopathy is a ventricular arrhythmia. Supportive evidence for this conclusion is the documentation of ventricular fibrillation just after collapse in a few patients observed by us and other investigators. It should also be emphasized that although syncope and presyncope are common in patients with obstructive hypertrophic cardiomyopathy, these symptoms do not have the same alarming connotation in such patients as they would in patients with fixed valvular aortic stenosis. We have, for example, followed many patients for over 10 years with such symptoms. Such a benign course would be unheard of in a patient with syncope associated with valvular aortic stenosis. Hence, we do not recommend operation to relieve obstruction in patients with hypertrophic cardiomyopathy on the basis of syncope or presyncope alone. On the other hand, we have evaluated some patients who have died suddenly with no symptomatology before death other than a single episode of syncope or occasional presyncope. Hence, it is possible that syncope can be the first manifestation of cardiac disease before sudden death in patients with hypertrophic cardiomyopathy.

Dr. Roberts: Dr. Epstein, I understand a number of patients with hypertrophic cardiomyopathy with or without obstruction have *exertional dyspnea.* How many patients with this condition actually have overt evidence of *congestive heart failure* or, to put it another way, is congestive heart failure in the patient with hypertrophic cardiomyopathy similar to congestive heart failure in patients with other cardiac conditions? Morphologically, hypertrophic cardiomyopathy is one of the conditions in which congestive heart failure occurs, and yet, neither ventricular cavity is dilated. Among the few conditions in which congestive cardiac failure occurs and the ventricular cavities are not dilated are amyloidosis, mitral stenosis, hemochromatosis and constrictive pericarditis. Is there anything different clinically about the congestive heart failure in patients with hypertrophic cardiomyopathy compared to that occurring in patients with other cardiac conditions?

Dr. Epstein: Patients with hypertrophic cardiomyopathy may demonstrate many of the clinical manifestations we interpret as indicative of congestive heart failure. The mechanism of "failure", however, is probably different in this condition than in patients with acquired valvular heart disease, for example. Patients with hypertrophic cardiomyopathy have a poorly compliant left ventricle. This is due presumably to the markedly thickened ventricular walls. This stiffened ventricle results in restriction to left ventricular filling, i.e., left ventricular inflow obstruction. As a result, left atrial and pulmonary venous pressures increase and consequently may lead to clinical manifestations of left- and right-sided heart failure. This occurs despite preservation of systolic function, at least as assessed at rest. Many patients with either the obstructive or the non-obstructive form of the disease may manifest these findings. In fact, in the latter stages of non-obstructive hypertrophic cariomyopathy, patients may present with a picture very similar to that of congestive or dilated cardiomyopathy with the exception that the ventricular cavities do not dilate. On the other hand: (1) we and others have observed a small number of patients with non-obstructive hypertrophic cardiomyopathy who, in the end stages of their disease, manifest impaired systolic function (normal end-diastolic volume with decreased ejection fraction); and (2) a very few patients have shown mild enlargement of the left ventricular cavity in end–diastole. The most characteristic picture of end–stage disease in non-obstructive hypertrophic cardiomyopathy, however, is inflow obstruction with normal left ventricular end-diastolic volume and preservation of systolic function.

Dr. Roberts: The present patient had historical evidence of *systemic hypertension* on one or more occasions, although the blood pressure recordings at NIH were normal. Dr. Maron, how often does systemic hypertension occur in patients with hypertrophic cardiomyopathy and how often do patients with systemic hypertension have echocardiographic or morphologic evidence of hypertrophic cardiomyopathy?

Dr. Maron: One of the first concepts of hypertrophic cardiomyopathy was that the subaortic muscular stenosis was due to preexisting systemic hypertension, probably because some of the first patients described with this condition nearly 20 years ago just happened to have coexistent systemic hypertension. Subsequently, we have come to realize that hypertension is not common in patients with hypertrophic cardiomyopathy. Hence, there is very little evidence for a causal relation between the two conditions. Looking at this question in another way, we have studied by echocardiography and at necropsy over 300 patients with systemic hypertension and found disproportionate septal thickening in about 5 per cent. Furthermore, the disporportionate septal thickening in patients with systemic hypertension does not appear to be genetically transmitted, but rather secondary to the patient's particular hemodynamic state—i.e., systemic hypertension. Hence, systemic hypertension is uncommon in patients with hypertrophic cardiomyopathy and disproportionate septal thickening is uncommon in patients with systemic hypertension.

Dr. Roberts: The present patient had a loud *precordial murmur* and most patients with hypertrophic cardiomyopathy, I understand, have a precordial murmur. Dr. Maron, do any patients with hypertrophic cardiomyopathy not have a murmur and when a murmur is present what is it due to?

Dr. Maron: Actually in our experience, loud precordial murmurs are rare in the over-all population of patients whom we see with hypertrophic cardiomyopathy. This is due principally to the fact that about 75 per cent of the patients who we evaluate with this condition do *not* have obstruction to left ventricular outflow. If outflow obstruction is absent, then a loud murmur (Grade 3/6 or more) rarely, if ever, is present. In patients with obstruction to left ventricular outflow (such as the patient discussed here) a loud systolic ejection murmur is almost invariably present along the left sternal border and at the apex. These statements, however, have to be tempered by the fact that the left ventricular outflow gradient in hypertrophic cardiomyopathy is extremely labile and may be present or absent from beat to beat, hour to hour, or day to day. Therefore, the presence or absence of a precordial murmur or its intensity at any one point in time cannot be used as definitive evidence of obstruction to outflow.

Dr. Roberts: Thus, a patient with a loud precordial systolic murmur and hypertrophic cardiomyopathy, with rare exception, has obstruction to left ventricular outflow. What happens to the *systolic precordial murmur after adequate myotomy or myectomy?*

DR. MARON: The precordial murmur in patients with hypertrophic cardiomyopathy is mainly related to systolic anterior motion of the mitral valve, which results in outflow obstruction and often mitral regurgitation. Since myotomy-myectomy almost invariably obliterates the resting gradient in these patients, the murmur either disappears or is markedly diminished in intensity.

DR. ROBERTS: Although a few patients with hypertrophic cardiomyopathy have obstruction not only to left ventricular outflow but also to right ventricular outflow, I wonder, Dr. Maron, what the explanation for the *right ventricular outflow obstruction* really is. For example, I am not aware that the ventricular septum is any thicker in patients with right ventricular outflow obstruction than in patients with no obstruction to right ventricular outflow but considerable left ventricular outflow obstruction. Why is not the right ventricular outflow obstruction more common, and what is your explanation for the obstruction when it does occur?

DR. MARON: About 20 per cent of our patients with hypertrophic cardiomyopathy and obstruction to left ventricular outflow also have right ventricular outflow tract gradients (usually less than 40 mm. Hg). However, a rare patient manifests marked obstruction to right ventricular outflow which is occasionally greater than, or present in the absence of, obstruction to left ventricular outflow. Although the explanation for right ventricular outflow gradients in patients with hypertrophic cardiomyopathy is unclear, it is perhaps most likely that the markedly hypertrophied ventricular septum and/or crista supraventricularis impinges on the right ventricular outflow tract and produces obstruction.

DR. ROBERTS: We have studied 65 patients with hypertrophic cardiomyopathy at necropsy and as I recall only three had obstruction to right ventricular outflow, and the largest gradient among the three was 50 mm. Hg. In that particular patient the anterior tricuspid valve leaflet was quite elongated, and it appeared possible that the excessive length of the anterior tricuspid valve leaflet located in a small right ventricular cavity was the likely explanation for the obstruction. In the present patient, the right ventricular outflow gradient was 29 mm. Hg and the anterior tricuspid valve leaflet probably was more elongated than normal. The present patient also had a very thick crista supraventricularis and an extremely small right ventricular cavity. At necropsy, for example (Figs. 5 and 6), the right ventricular free wall virtually contacts the right ventricular aspect of the ventricular septum.

Dr. Maron, there appears to be some *discrepancy between the thicknesses of the ventricular walls measured at necropsy and during life by echocardiography* in this patient. Can you explain these discrepancies?

DR. MARON: Recently, we have observed several patients with hypertrophic cardiomyopathy similar in this respect to the patient described in this report.[2] That is, the echocardiogram during life showed asymmetric septal hypertrophy but at necropsy concentric hypertrophy was present. In this patient, the echocardiogram showed a septal to free wall ratio of 1.5 in diastole, which met our diagnostic criteria of ASH. However, at necropsy the septal-to-free wall ratio was 0.9 and therefore, not diagnostic of ASH. These discrepancies may be explained as follows. First, in patients with ASH, the ventricular septum thickens less during ventricular systole than does the left ventricular free wall. As a result, septal-to-free wall ratios are greater when measurements are obtained in diastole than when they are obtained in systole. Second, hearts examined at necropsy appear to be in the systolic phase of the cardiac cycle. This conclusion is suggested by the fact that the ventricular wall thickness, septal-to-free wall ratios, and left ventricular internal transverse dimensions measured at necropsy all correlated more closely with measurements attained echocardiographically in systole than in diastole.[2] Since by convention, echocardiographic measurements of wall thicknesses are made during diastole, it becomes clear why septal-to-free wall ratios consistent with the diagnosis of hypertrophic cardiomyopathy (ASH) during life may be inconsistent with this diagnosis after death. Hence, we believe that, at least occasionally, echocardiographic measurements in diastole provide a more sensitive method than necropsy examination for documenting the presence of hypertrophic cardiomyopathy.

The implication of these findings is that in certain patients with typical genetically-transmitted hypertrophic cardiomyopathy, the diagnosis will not be established at necropsy by simple measurement of the relative thicknesses of the ventricular septum and left ventricular free wall.

In such patients, the correct diagnosis will rely on other ancillary observations, including typical hemodynamic and echocardiographic features of left ventricular outflow obstruction during life (as shown in the present patient), and the presence of a documented family history of hypertrophic cardiomyopathy. Other necropsy findings suggestive, but not diagnostic, of hypertrophic cardiomyopathy include a contact plaque on the endocardium of the ventricular septum in apposition to a thickened anterior mitral leaflet, and the presence of numerous hypertrophied and disorganized cardiac muscle cells in the ventricular septum.

DR. ROBERTS: Dr. Maron, *on the echocardiographic record* are you always sure about the *exact location of the epicardial surface of the posterior left ventricular free wall* in patients with hypertrophic cardiomyopathy? I would assume that you would be considerably pleased if patients with hypertrophic cardiomyopathy had a little pericardial effusion so that this surface of the free wall would be clearly delineated. Could you comment on how often you feel that you cannot make a precise, unequivocal measurement of the posterior free wall by echocardiogram in patients with hypertrophic cardiomyopathy.

DR. MARON: Dr. Roberts' comments about technical considerations in obtaining optimal echocardiograms is certainly well taken. A satisfactory echocardiogram can probably be obtained in 80 to 90 per cent of patients with hypertrophic cardiomyopathy. Nevertheless, there are some important technical points that should always be considered. For example, delineation of the right ventricular surface of the ventricular septum, itself, is often very difficult in some patients. Furthermore, as Dr. Roberts has pointed out, measurement of the posterobasal left ventricular wall is also frequently difficult in these patients, with regard to definition of either the endocardial or epicardial surface. In a small minority of patients with clinically evident hypertrophic cardiomyopathy, it has not been possible to make a definitive conclusion about the septal-to-free wall ratio because of these considerations.

DR. ROBERTS: Dr. Morrow, your *results with myotomy and myectomy* in patients with hypertrophic cardiomyopathy have been quite gratifying with few exceptions. The present patient, obviously, is one of those exceptions. I understand that you have operated on nearly 200 patients with hypertrophic cardiomyopathy and that the occurrence of a ventricular septal defect has been quite rare. I wonder if you could comment on your general results with this procedure and your views on the particular operative complications in this particular patient.

DR. MORROW: I have now operated upon approximately 175 patients with the obstructive form of hypertrophic subaortic stenosis. The operative mortality rate associated with the procedure is similar to that for aortic valve replacement, i.e., 5 to 7 per cent. We have had relatively few late deaths due to heart disease, and as yet I do not think we can make meaningful comparisons of the natural histories of operated and unoperated patients. Among operative survivors, symptomatic improvement has been quite satisfactory: nearly two-thirds of patients consider themselves asymptomatic, and the others, with few exceptions, are in Functional Class II. Ventricular septal defects have occurred in a total of seven patients. Several of them were created and recognized at the time of operation, but it was not considered necessary to close them. One of these patients subsequently had to have the defect closed because he developed heart failure. In the remaining patients, including the patient being discussed here, the ventricular septum ruptured after operation as a consequence of septal infarction. I assume that infarction occurred in these patients because the muscular resection was too extensive and compromised the blood supply of the septum beneath and adjacent to it. We have recently found that intraoperative measurements of the thickness of the septum, by means of an intracardiac echo transducer, are of aid in gauging the extent of resection necessary.

DR. ROBERTS: In the present patient, 4.1 Gm. of ventricular septum was excised at operation. Dr. Spray, in the other patients in whom this procedure has been performed by Dr. Morrow, how many *grams of myocardium* were *excised from ventricular septum?*

DR. SPRAY: Among 75 specimens, the excised muscle ranged in weight from 0.2 to 6.8 grams (average 1.8 Gm.).

DR. ROBERTS: One other anatomic feature of hypertrophic cardiomyopathy is the presence of wall thickening and luminal narrowing of *intramural coronary arteries* located primarily in the ventricular septum but also occasionally in right ventricular and left ventricular free walls.[4] These abnormal arteries have been observed in about 50 per cent of the 65 patients whom we have studied at necropsy. In the present patient, despite severe left ventricular outflow obstruction, the intramural coronary arteries were normal. We have been unable to correlate the abnormal intramural arteries with the degree of obstruction or the presence of chest pain or any other clinical or hemodynamic parameter. The abnormalities in these arteries, however, are more striking than are observed in any other condition we have studied at necropsy.

REFERENCES

1. Morrow, A. G., Reitz, B. A., Epstein, S. E., Henry, W. L., Conkle, D. M., Itscoitz, S. B., and Redwood, D. R.: Operative treatment in hypertrophic subaortic stenosis. Techniques, and the results of pre- and postoperative assessments in 83 patients, Circulation **52**:88, 1975.
2. Maron, B. J., Henry, W. L., Roberts, W. C., and Epstein, S. E.: Comparison of echocardiographic and necropsy measurements of ventricular wall thickness in patients with and without disproportionate septal thickening, Circulation **55**:341, 1977.
3. Roberts, W. C., and Ferrans, V. J.: Pathologic anatomy of the cardiomyopathies. Idiopathic dilated and hypertrophic types, infiltrative types, and endomyocardial disease with and without eosinophilia, Human Pathol. **6**:287, 1975.
4. McReynolds, R. A., and Roberts, W. C.: The intramural coronary arteries in hypertrophic cardiomyopathy (Abstr.), Am. J. Cardiol. **35**:154, 1975.

Sudden Death in Patients with Hypertrophic Cardiomyopathy: Characterization of 26 Patients Without Functional Limitation

BARRY J. MARON, MD*
WILLIAM C. ROBERTS, MD, FACC*
JESSE E. EDWARDS, MD, FACC†
HUGH A. McALLISTER, Jr., MD, FACC‡
DANIEL D. FOLEY, MD†
STEPHEN E. EPSTEIN, MD, FACC*

Bethesda, Maryland
St. Paul and Minneapolis, Minnesota
Washington, DC

Sudden death is a recognized complication in symptomatic patients with hypertrophic cardiomyopathy. However, its occurrence in patients with no or transient previous cardiac symptoms presents a particularly challenging diagnostic and therapeutic dilemma. Therefore, 26 patients with hypertrophic cardiomyopathy whose death was the first definitive manifestation of cardiac disease were evaluated. Their ages ranged from 8 to 49 years (mean 18) and 23 were less than 25 years of age; 19 were male and 7 female. Of the 26 patients, 13 died during or immediately after moderate or severe physical exertion. Of 12 patients with previous cardiac catheterization, 6 had no or a small left ventricular outflow tract gradient under basal conditions and 6 had an outflow gradient of 50 mm Hg or greater. Left ventricular end-diastolic pressure was elevated in nine patients, and the ventricular septum was moderately to severely thickened (17 mm or more) in all patients. The electrocardiogram was abnormal in all 19 patients studied before death. Thus, sudden death may be the first definitive manifestation of cardiac disease in some patients with hypertrophic cardiomyopathy. Although the effects of patient selection in this study group cannot be excluded, sudden death was common in children and young adults and was often related to physical exertion; each patient showed a distinctly abnormal electrocardiogram and moderate to severe ventricular septal thickening.

From the Cardiology Branch and Pathology Branch, National Heart, Lung, and Blood Institute, National Institutes of Health, Bethesda, Maryland*; Department of Pathology, United Hospitals—Miller Division, St. Paul, Minnesota; Department of Pathology, University of Minnesota, Minneapolis, Minnesota†; and Department of Cardiovascular Pathology, Armed Forces Institute of Pathology, Washington, D.C.‡ This work was supported in part by U. S. Public Health Service Research Grant 5R01 HL 05694 and Research Training Grant 5T01 HL 05570 from the National Heart, Lung, and Blood Institute, Bethesda, Maryland; and the Bremer Foundation, St. Paul, Minnesota. Manuscript received July 29, 1977; revised manuscript received November 15, 1977, accepted November 16, 1977.

Address for reprints: Barry J. Maron, MD, National Heart, Lung, and Blood Institute, Cardiology Branch, Bldg. 10, Room 7B-15, Bethesda, Maryland 20014.

Hypertrophic cardiomyopathy is a genetically transmitted disease of cardiac muscle characterized by disproportionate thickening of the ventricular septum.[1–7] Sudden and unexpected death is a recognized complication in symptomatic adults and children with this disease.[8–13] Patients with hypertrophic cardiomyopathy who were asymptomatic or experienced only rare transient symptoms before death have been described occasionally[8,10–15] but not in detail or in a manner permitting proper characterization of this subgroup. Nevertheless, identification and subsequent management of such patients with hypertrophic cardiomyopathy presents particularly difficult problems. Therefore, to define and characterize more clearly this subgroup, we analyzed the clinical and morphologic features of 26 patients with hypertrophic cardiomyopathy whose first definitive symptomatic manifestation of cardiac disease was death.

TABLE I

Clinical, Hemodynamic and Pathologic Data in 26 Cases

Case no.	Age (yr) & Sex	Electro-cardiogram	Hemodynamics: LVOT Gradient: Basal	Hemodynamics: LVOT Gradient: Provo-cation	Hemodynamics: LV Pressure	Hemodynamics: RVOT Gradient	Hemodynamics: CI	Circumstances of Death	Family History SD	Necropsy: Heart Weight (g)	Necropsy: VS	Necropsy: PW	Necropsy: VS/PW	Necropsy: Disorga-nized Cells in VS	Possible Cardiac Symptoms
1	8M	—	—	—	—	—	—	After hiking	0	350	25	13	1.9	+	0
2	10M	LVH	—	—	—	—	—	Stepped out of school bus*	+	—	Marked VS hypertrophy[d]			+	0
3	11F	—	—	—	—	—	—	After mild calisthenics	0	400	17	9	1.9	+	1 episode syncope 3 wk before death
4	11M	LAD; probable LVH; LAE; ST-T changes	5	35	92/29	0	3.9	After light play	0	—	—	—	—	—	0
5	12M	ST-T changes‡	—	—	—	6	—	Jogging**	+	270	18	10	1.8	+	0
6	13M	—	—	—	—	—	—	After recreational ball game	+	375	25	17	1.5	—	0
7	14M	LVH with "strain"§; diffuse T wave inversion; Q wave in leads II, III, aVF, V_6	13	—	110/24	0	3.0	After walking up steep hill	+	360	20	10	2.0	+	0
8	15F	LVH; Q waves in leads I, aVL, V_5V_6; S-T depressed in I, aVL	—	—	—	—	—	Sedentary activity	0	320	22	11	2.0	+	Lightheaded-ness
9	15F	LVH; marked LAD; Q waves in leads I, II, III, aVF, V_5, V_6; S-T elevated in II, III, aVF, V_6	50	95	157/20	—	6.0	Stepping out of car	0	550	34	20	1.7	—	0
10	15F	LVH with "strain"; Q waves in lead aVL; LAD; LAE; ST-T changes[a]	10-55	115	110-155/30	15	3.7	Running	+	400	38	16	2.4	+	1 episode dyspnea, lightheaded-ness during running 5 mo before death
11	15F	LVH[ф]; ST-T changes; poor progression of precordial R waves; LAE	100	—	200/24	—	3.0	Running	+	550 (est)	36	14	2.6	+	0
12	15M	—	—	—	—	—	—	During recreational basketball	+	475	—	—	—[e]	—	0

Table I (continued)

Case no.	Age (yr) & Sex	Electrocardiogram	Hemodynamics: LVOT Gradient Basal	Hemodynamics: LVOT Gradient Provocation	Hemodynamics: LV Pressure	Hemodynamics: RVOT Gradient	Hemodynamics: CI	Circumstances of Death	Family History SD	Necropsy: Heart Weight (g)	Necropsy: VS	Necropsy: PW	Necropsy: VS/PW	Necropsy: Disorganized Cells in VS	Possible Cardiac Symptoms
13	16M	LVH; LAE; Q wave in lead V_6; T wave inversion in leads II, III, aVF; P-R = 0.10	75	—	175/20	0	4.4	After light play	0	520	—	—	—	—	1 episode syncope 1 yr before death
14	16F	Deep Q wave in leads III, aVF; possible RVH	—	—	—	—	—	Jogging	+	310	21	8	2.6	+	0
15	17M	LVH[g]; LAD; T wave inversion in leads I, aVL; S-T elevated in V_1V_2	60	—	140/16	0	4.7	Sedentary	0	—	27[f]	17	1.6	—	0
16	17M	—	—	—	—	—	—	Jogging	0	530	21	12	1.8	+	0
17	17M	—	—	—	—	—	—	During competitive basketball game	0	740	—	—	—[b]	+	Lightheadedness
18	19M	LVH with "strain"[δ]; Q wave in lead V_6; S-T elevated in V_1-V_3	15	50	136/12	8	4.2	Running	0	900	55	30	1.8	—	Lightheadedness
19	21F	T wave inversion in leads III, aVF; LAE; possible LVH	—	—	—	—	—	Walking[θ]	0	400	24	9	2.7	+	1 episode syncope 3 yr before death; lightheadedness: paroxysmal AF and other SVT + PVCs
20[c]	21M	LVH; LAD; poor progression of precordial R waves; QS waves in leads III, aVF, V_1; S-T elevated in V_1-V_3; LAE	65	—	185/16	10	3.3	Mild exertion; throwing football	0	—	—	—	—	—	0
21	22M	LAD; possible LVH; Q waves in leads II, III, aVF[†]	—	—	—	—	—	Running up a grade	+	610	35	21	1.7	+	0

Table I (continued)

Case no.	Age (yr) & Sex	Electro-cardiogram	Hemodynamics: LVOT Gradient Basal	Hemodynamics: LVOT Gradient Provo-cation	Hemodynamics: LV Pressure	Hemodynamics: RVOT Gradient	Hemodynamics: CI	Circumstances of Death	Family History SD	Necropsy: Heart Weight (g)	Necropsy: VS	Necropsy: PW	Necropsy: VS/PW	Necropsy: Disorga-nized Cells in VS	Possible Cardiac Symptoms
22	23M	LVH; deep T wave inversion; VT with exertion	0	—	130/5	0	3.3	During recreational basketball game	0	500	20	15	1.3	0	0
23	23M	—	—	—	—	—	—	Sedentary activity	0	750	30	15	2.0	+	0
24	29M	Probable LVH; LAD;IVCD; 1^0 AVB (P-R =) 0.24)	0	0	110/12	0	3.7	Dived in ocean surf[Δ]	0	450	25	12	2.1	+	Lightheaded-ness; occasional palpitations
25	31M	RBBB; Q waves in lead aVL	—	—	—	—	—	During mild calisthenics	0	450	24	12	2.0	+	0
26	49M	LVH with "strain"; LAD; ST-T changes; Q waves in leads I, aVL	20	30	130/15	15	3.3	Watching television	0	—	—	—	—	—	A Fl (2:1 block) with diaphoresis and pallor 3 mo before death

Case numbers in boldface italics indicate siblings from two families; that is, Patients 2, 6 and 12 and Cases 5 and 7 are siblings.

AF = atrial fibrillation; A Fl = atrial flutter; CI = cardiac index (liters/min per m^2); est = estimated; 1^0AVB = first degree atrioventricular block; IVCD = intraventricular conduction defect; LAD = left axis deviation; LAE = left atrial enlargement; LV Pressure = left ventricular pressure (systolic/diastolic) (mm Hg); LVH = left ventricular hypertrophy; LVOT gradient = left ventricular outflow tract pressure gradient (mm Hg); MV = mitral valve; PVC = premature ventricular complexes; PW = posterior left ventricular free wall (mm); RAD = right axis deviation; RBBB = right bundle branch block; RVH = right ventricular hypertrophy; RVOT gradient = right ventricular outflow tract pressure gradient (mm Hg); SD = sudden death; SVT = supraventricular tachycardia; VS = ventricular septum (mm); VS/PW = ventricular septal to posterobasal left ventricular free wall ratio; VT = ventricular tachycardia.

* Previous cardiac arrest after mild exertion, 20 months before death; this patient died 8 days after his brother (Case 6).

† Electrocardiograms obtained at age 14 to 20 years showed right axis deviation and right ventricular hypertrophy.

‡ Electrocardiogram obtained 5 weeks after cardiac arrest; no tracing recorded before arrest.

** Ventricular fibrillation documented after collapse; patient survived in coma for 5 weeks with evidence of cerebral anoxia; transmural ventricular septal infarct present at necropsy.

Δ Previous cardiac arrest while running, 8 months before death; ventricular fibrillation documented after collapse; atrial flutter after syncopal spell, 1 month before death.

§ Appearance of "strain pattern" (left ventricular hypertrophy with secondary ST-T abnormalities) 7 months before death.

δ Appearance of "strain pattern" (left ventricular hypertrophy with secondary ST-T abnormalities) 3 1/2 years before death.

ϕ RAD present at age 12 years; normal QRS axis present at age 13 and subsequently.

θ Ventricular fibrillation documented after collapse; patient survived 2 hours.

[a] Electrocardiogram normal at age 10 years, abnormal at age 12 and subsequently.

[b] Although ventricular wall thickness data were not available in this patient, the presence of echocardiographically determined asymmetric septal hypertrophy in his mother and brother and the presence of disorganized cardiac muscle cells in his ventricular septum provide strong presumptive evidence that he had hypertrophic cardiomyopathy.

[c] Patient had documented cardiac arrest (ventricular fibrillation), was successfully resuscitated and has survived with evidence of severe cerebral anoxia.

[d] Exact wall thickness measurements not available.

[e] Wall thickness measurements not available; diagnosis of hypertrophic cardiomyopathy is a presumptive one, based on the presence of cardiac hypertrophy and a strong family history of hypertrophic cardiomyopathy.

[f] Measurements of ventricular septal and posterobasal left ventricular wall thicknesses made with echocardiography[15] 5 months before death; measurements of ventricular septal thickness with echocardiography and subsequently at necropsy usually agree closely.[20]

[g] RAD, RVH present at age 5 years; normal QRS axis, poor R wave progression and deep Q wave in lead aVL at age 9 years; normal electrocardiogram except for Q wave in lead aVL at age 10 years; left ventricular hypertrophy at age 14 and subsequently.

— Data not available.

\+ Present.

0 Absent.

Methods

Selection of patients: The study group was divided into two subgroups: Group I, 17 patients with hypertrophic cardiomyopathy who had no cardiac symptoms before death, and Group II, 9 patients who were asymptomatic except for rare transient symptoms that may have been due to hypertrophic cardiomyopathy. Group II included three patients with a single syncopal episode, one patient with an episode of mild dyspnea and lightheadedness while running, one patient with one episode of atrial flutter (2:1 block; ventricular rate 150/min) and four patients with lightheadedness. None of these nine patients were evaluated initially because of their symptoms.

Two patients in Group I had ventricular fibrillation and cardiac arrest from which they were successfully resuscitated before death; another patient in Group I experienced ventricular fibrillation. For convenience, we have equated ventricular fibrillation with actual cardiac death in these three patients.

Patients were selected from the case records of the following sources: National Heart, Lung, and Blood Institute (16 patients), Armed Forces Institute of Pathology Cardiovascular Registry (2 patients), United Hospitals-Miller Division Cardiovascular Registry (4 patients) and Children's Hospital of Pittsburgh (4 patients). The diagnosis of hypertrophic cardiomyopathy was confirmed in 23 patients at necropsy or with echocardiography (ventricular septal to left ventricular free wall thickness ratio of 1.3 or more) or on the basis of the typical clinical and hemodynamic features of hypertrophic cardiomyopathy. In the remaining three patients the diagnosis of hypertrophic cardiomyopathy was made presumptively, on the basis of presence of cardiac hypertrophy and a confirmed family history of hypertrophic cardiomyopathy.

Description of patients: The patients ranged in age from 8 to 49 years (mean 18); 23 of the 26 patients were less than 25 years old at death. Nineteen patients were male and 7 female; 24 were white and 2 black. Nineteen of the 26 patients had a cardiac evaluation before death. Right and left heart hemodynamic studies were performed in 12 of these patients from 6 months to 11 years (median 2 1/2 years) before death, usually because of the presence of a heart murmur, abnormal electrocardiogram or family history of heart disease or sudden death. Five patients were competitive athletes, including one who had competed on his varsity college basketball team for 4 years without evidence of limitation. There were two sets of siblings, two patients from one family and three from another. Four other patients had at least one first degree relative who died suddenly of hypertrophic cardiomyopathy.

Results

No differences in any of the following variables were found between the two patient groups. The clinical, hemodynamic and pathologic findings in each of the study patients are summarized in Table I.

Physical findings: Four patients had not had an adequate cardiac physical examination before death. Heart murmurs were present in 16 of the remaining 22 patients. These murmurs, first identified from birth to age 28 years, were usually grade 2 to 3/6 systolic ejection murmurs heard loudest at the lower left sternal border or apex. In the other six patients no murmur had been identified.

Chest radiographic findings: Heart size was normal in 14 of the 17 patients who had a chest radiograph taken; the remaining three patients had a cardiothoracic ratio of 0.55 to 0.60. No patient had abnormal pulmonary arterial or venous markings on X-ray examination.

TABLE II

Electrocardiographic Abnormalities in 19 Patients

	Patients (no.)	
Left ventricular hypertrophy	15	
Probable		10
Possible		2
With "strain" pattern*		4
S-T segment and T wave abnormalities	14	
Abnormal Q or QS†	10	
Left axis deviation	8	
Left atrial enlargement	5	
Right bundle branch block	1	
First degree atrioventricular block	1	
Intraventricular conduction defect	1	
Marked diffuse T wave inversion (ventricular tachycardia with exercise)	1	
Possible right ventricular hypertrophy	1	

* Tall voltages in the left precordial leads associated with secondary S-T segment and T wave changes.

† 4 or more mm in depth or 0.04 second in duration, in one or more leads.

Electrocardiographic findings: Electrocardiograms were obtained in 19 of the 26 patients and were abnormal in each (Table II). Although no electrocardiographic pattern was entirely characteristic of the study group, the most common abnormalities were left ventricular hypertrophy, S-T segment and T wave changes and deep, wide Q waves.

In six patients the electrocardiographic pattern changed 7 months to 4 years before death. A left ventricular "strain" pattern developed in three of these patients, including one with a previously normal electrocardiogram. In three other patients the electrocardiograms initially revealed right ventricular hypertrophy or right axis deviation, or both, but later were consistent with left ventricular hypertrophy.

Only one patient demonstrated premature complexes in the routine electrocardiogram; however, one other patient (Case 22) did show ventricular tachycardia (6 seconds' duration) and frequent premature ventricular complexes during the course of a routine treadmill stress test. In five patients ventricular fibrillation was documented after the patient's sudden collapse. One of these patients (Case 24) also had atrial flutter with variable block (3:1 to 6:1) after a severe syncopal episode 7 months after his initial cardiac arrest and 1 month before death. Another patient (Case 26) also demonstrated atrial flutter (with 2:1 block), associated with diaphoresis and pallor, 3 months before death.

Hemodynamic and angiographic data: *Right and left heart hemodynamic studies* were performed in 12 cases. In 6 of the 12 patients peak systolic left ventricular outflow tract pressure gradients of 50 mm Hg or greater were present under basal conditions (Fig. 1). In the remaining six patients, either no outflow gradient (two patients) or a small gradient of 20 mm Hg or less (four patients) was present. One patient with a 5 mm Hg

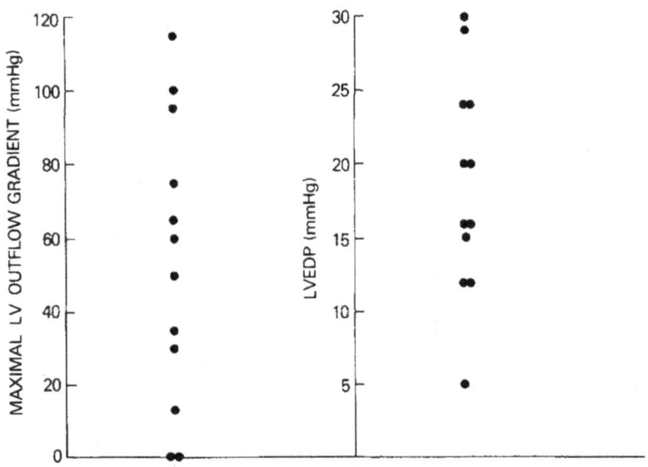

FIGURE 1. Left ventricular (LV) outflow gradients (maximal under basal conditions or with provocation) and left ventricular end-diastolic pressures (LVEDP) in the 12 patients with such measurements.

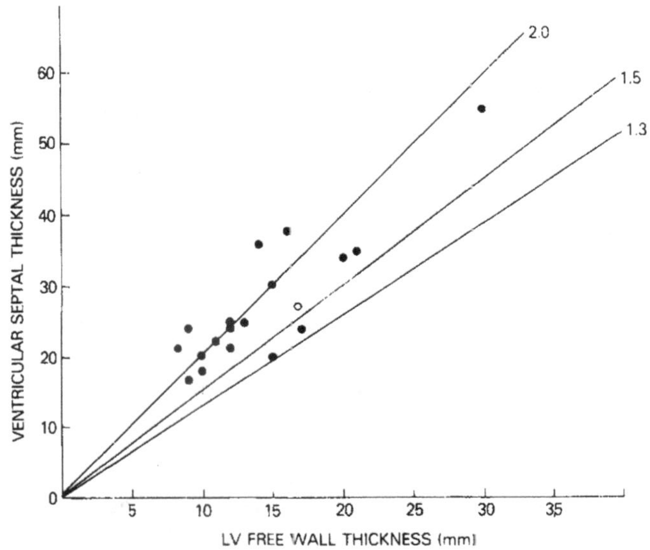

FIGURE 2. Ventricular septal and left ventricular (LV) free wall thicknesses in the 19 patients in whom such measurements were obtained. **Identity lines** define septal/free wall ratios of 1.3, 1.5 and 2.0. **Open symbol** denotes a patient whose ventricular septal and left ventricular free wall thicknesses were measured with echocardiography during diastole 5 months before death.

gradient under basal conditions had a 35 mm Hg gradient with provocation with isoproterenol infusion, and another with a 15 mm Hg gradient under basal conditions had a 50 mm Hg gradient with provocation. Five of the 12 patients had a relatively small peak systolic gradient of 6 to 15 mm Hg between the right ventricle and pulmonary artery. Left ventricular end-diastolic pressure ranged from 5 to 30 mm Hg and was elevated (more than 12 mm Hg) in 9 of the 12 patients (Fig. 1).

Left ventricular angiography was performed in nine patients. In five of these patients, the study showed obliteration of the left ventricular apex during systole, a finding considered characteristic of hypertrophic cardiomyopathy. Two other patients showed severe narrowing of the mid left ventricular cavity during systole that appeared to be due to papillary muscle encroachment. In the remaining two patients, left ventricular contraction was considered normal although deformities in the contour of the left ventricle suggested bulging of a hypertrophied ventricular septum into the left ventricular cavity.

Circumstances of death: Cardiac arrest was sudden and occurred without warning in each of the 26 patients. In 23 patients death occurred instantaneously or within a few minutes. Of the other three patients, one (Case 5) was resuscitated and survived 5 weeks after cardiac arrest with evidence of severe cerebral anoxia, and another (Case 19) survived 2 hours after cardiac arrest; the remaining patient (Case 20) had an episode of ventricular fibrillation, was successfully resuscitated and has survived to date. In 2 of the 26 patients the fatal cardiac arrest was preceded by an initial cardiac arrest that occurred 20 (Case 2) and 8 (Case 24) months earlier. None of the 26 patients were hospitalized at the time of the initial cardiac arrest.

Death occurred during sedentary or normal activities in 6 patients, during or just after mild exertion in 7 and during or just after moderate or severe exertion in 13. No patient died during sleep.

Necropsy findings: Heart weight ranged from 270 to 900 g (median 450) and was increased with respect to age in each patient.[16] In 18 patients either the heart was in suitable condition for detailed examination or sufficient pathologic information was available to assign a septal/free wall ratio. In one other patient (Case 15), in whom necropsy was not performed, measurements of ventricular septal and posterobasal left ventricular wall thicknesses were obtained with echocardiography[2] 5 months before death. Each of these 19 hearts showed disproportionate thickening of the ventricular septum with respect to the left ventricular free wall (septal/free wall ratio 1.3 or more[2,17]) (Fig. 2). Septal/free wall ratios ranged from 1.3 to 2.7 (median 1.9). Absolute ventricular septal thickness ranged from 17 to 55 mm (median 25); in all but two patients septal thickness was 20 mm or greater. The two patients in this study with a septal thickness of less than 20 mm (17 and 18 mm) were only 11 and 12 years of age, respectively (Cases 3 and 5). One patient (Case 5), who survived for 5 weeks after cardiac arrest, had a large transmural ventricular septal infarct despite widely patent extramural coronary arteries; none of the other hearts had areas of transmural scarring or evidence of coronary artery disease (more than 50 percent cross-sectional narrowing of a coronary arterial lumen).

Of the 17 hearts in which the mitral valve and endocardial surface of the left ventricular outflow tract could be studied, 8 showed an endocardial contact plaque on the ventricular septum adjacent to a thickened anterior mitral leaflet. One patient had only an endocardial plaque, one only a thickened anterior mitral leaflet and seven patients had neither an endocardial plaque nor a thickened mitral leaflet.

In 16 of the 17 patients with histologic studies, numerous cardiac muscle cells in the ventricular septum showed a disorganized arrangement characteristic of hypertrophic cardiomyopathy.[15,18,19] In another patient disorganization was only minimal. Microscopy in the remaining patient, who demonstrated the typical gross anatomic features of hypertrophic cardiomyopathy, revolved normally arranged cardiac muscle cells in the ventricular septum.

Morphologic observations regarding arrangement of cardiac muscle cells in the left ventricular free wall were made in 15 of the 17 patients. Six of the 15 had numerous disorganized cardiac muscle cells in the left ventricular free wall, 2 had mild disorganization and 7 had a normal arrangement of virtually all cardiac muscle cells in the left ventricular free wall.

Therapy: Seven of the 26 patients had been treated with propranolol. Each of these patients was under treatment at the time of death and had been taking propranolol for 3 months to 2 1/2 years. The dose of propranolol was considered adequate (2 or more mg/kg per day) in three patients and inadequate in the other four. Six of these patients were given propranolol in the hope of arresting progression of disease; the seventh was given propranolol because of an episode of atrial flutter.

Discussion

Our results indicate that sudden death is not rare in patients with hypertrophic cardiomyopathy who previously did not manifest functional limitation. Moreover, children and young adults appear to be particularly susceptible to sudden death: 23 of our 26 patients were less than 25 years of age at death.

Characteristic clinical features: Two clinical features were characteristic of this unique population of patients: (1) a distinctly abnormal electrocardiogram, and (2) a moderately to severely thickened ventricular septum. Although this latter finding is based on necropsy measurements, we have previously shown a relatively close correlation between measurements of ventricular septal thickness obtained with echocardiography and subsequently at necropsy in patients with disproportionate septal thickening.[20] Our finding of moderate to severe ventricular septal thickening in the patients in our study group has potentially important clinical implications, but one must be aware of the possible influence of patient selection. For example, it may be less likely that patients with hypertrophic cardiomyopathy and only a mildly hypertrophied septum would be systematically identified as having this disease at necropsy. Therefore, such patients may not have been referred to us. Nevertheless, our findings that a distinctly abnormal electrocardiogram and moderate to severe ventricular septal thickening were characteristic of our study group are highly relevant to any future prospective studies designed to identify the risk factors for sudden death in patients with hypertrophic cardiomyopathy.

No clinical or hemodynamic variable was an entirely reliable predictor of death in our patients. These variables included radiographically determined heart size, specific electrocardiographic abnormality and left ventricular end-diastolic pressure. Although previous investigators[12] have suggested that elevated left ventricular end-diastolic pressure is a poor prognostic sign in patients with hypertrophic cardiomyopathy, this was not true in the present study group or in our previous study[13] of children with hypertrophic cardiomyopathy. Although 6 of the 12 patients had markedly elevated left ventricular end-diastolic pressure (20 mm Hg or greater), 3 had only mildly elevated pressure (15 to 16 mm Hg) and 3 had a normal pressure (12 mm Hg or less). However, 6 of our 25 patients showed electrocardiographic evidence of increasing left ventricular overload within 4 years of the time of death. Hence, such an evolution in the electrocardiographic pattern may be an early sign of impending sudden death in some patients with hypertrophic cardiomyopathy even though there may be no symptomatic evidence of disease.

Therapeutic implications: Treatment with propranolol did not appear to be entirely protective against sudden death in our patients. Seven patients had been taking propranolol before and at the time of death; but the dosage could be considered adequate (2 or more mg/kg per day) in only three. Moreover, we do not know the role that patient selection played in these data, that is, how many patients at risk of sudden death did not die *because* they were taking propranolol. Hence, the available data are inconclusive regarding the potential efficacy of propranolol administered prophylactically in asymptomatic or mildly symptomatic patients with hypertrophic cardiomyopathy.

Mechanisms of sudden death: Although the exact mechanism of sudden death in patients with hypertrophic cardiomyopathy is not known, ventricular arrhythmias have been suggested as the terminal event.[13] Our finding that four patients had ventricular fibrillation immediately after their collapse supports this contention. It also is not uncommon to observe frequent ventricular premature complexes in such patients.[21] However, our data also raise the possibility that atrial arrhythmias play an etiologic role in the precipitation of ventricular fibrillation in some patients with hypertrophic cardiomyopathy. For example, one patient (Case 26) was completely asymptomatic until age 49 years, when he experienced an episode of atrial flutter; he died suddenly 3 months later. Another patient (Case 24), who experienced two cardiac arrests, had atrial flutter documented immediately after a syncopal spell 1 month before his death. Thus, it is possible (but purely speculative) that rapid supraventricular tachycardias lead to inadequate ventricular filling (particularly in hearts with diminished compliance) that then results in hypotension and subsequent cardiac arrest. Alternatively, it is possible that abnormally rapid atrioventricular transmission can occur in patients with hypertrophic cardiomyopathy through accessory conduction pathways and that the extremely rapid ventricular response may ultimately deteriorate into ventricular fibrillation.

Family history: About one third of our 26 patients had a family history of sudden cardiac death in a first degree relative (including siblings in two instances). This finding suggests that sudden death is more prevalent in some families with hypertrophic cardiomyopathy and that a history of sudden death in a closely related relative may be a poor prognostic factor for patients with hypertrophic cardiomyopathy. Although about 75 percent of our study patients were male, this prevalence rate does not differ significantly from that of male subjects in the overall population of patients with hypertrophic cardiomyopathy (67 percent).[10]

Acknowledgments

We thank Drs. J. R. Zuberbuhler and Frank Sherman of Children's Hospital of Pittsburgh, Dr. Robert A. Miller of Children's Memorial Hospital, Chicago and Dr. David Bialostozky, Mexico City, for providing some of the clinical and pathologic data.

References

1. **Clark CE, Henry WL, Epstein SE:** Familial prevalence and genetic transmission of idiopathic hypertrophic subaortic stenosis. N Engl J Med 289:709–714, 1973
2. **Henry WL, Clark CE, Epstein SE:** Asymmetric septal hypertrophy (ASH): echocardiographic identification of the pathognomonic anatomic abnormality of IHSS. Circulation 47:225–233, 1973
3. **Epstein SE, Henry, WL, Clark CE, et al:** Asymmetric septal hypertrophy. Ann Intern Med 81:650–680, 1974
4. **Abbasi AS, MacAlpin RN, Eber LM, et al:** Left ventricular hypertrophy diagnosed by echocardiography. N Engl J Med 289:118–121, 1973
5. **Menges H, Brandenburg RO, Brown AL:** The clinical, hemodynamic and pathologic diagnosis of muscular subvalvular aortic stenosis. Circulation 24:1126–1136, 1961
6. **Roberts WC:** Valvular, subvalvular and supravalvular aortic stenosis: morphologic features. Cardiovasc Clin 5: 104–126, 1973
7. **Abbasi AS, MacAlpin RN, Eber LM, et al:** Echocardiographic diagnosis of idiopathic hypertrophic cardiomyopathy without outflow obstruction. Circulation 46:897–904, 1972
8. **Hardarson T, De La Calzada CS, Curiel R, et al:** Prognosis and mortality of hypertrophic obstructive cardiomyopathy. Lancet 2: 1462–1467, 1973
9. **Shah PM, Adelman AG, Wigle ED, et al:** The natural (and unnatural) course of hypertrophic obstructive cardiomyopathy. A multicenter study. Circ Res 34, 35:Suppl II:II-179–II-195, 1973
10. **Frank S, Braunwald E:** Idiopathic hypertrophic subaortic stenosis. Clinical analysis of 126 patients with emphasis on the natural history. Circulation 37:759–788, 1968
11. **Adelman AG, Wigle ED, Ranganathan N, et al:** The clinical course in muscular subaortic stenosis. A retrospective and prospective study of 60 hemodynamically proved cases. Ann Intern Med 77: 515–525, 1972
12. **Swan DA, Bell B, Oakley CM, et al:** Analysis of the symptomatic course and prognosis and treatment of hypertrophic obstructive cardiomyopathy. Br Heart J 33:671–685, 1971
13. **Maron BJ, Henry WL, Clark CE, et al:** Asymmetric septal hypertrophy in childhood. Circulation 53:9–18, 1976
14. **Folger GM, Harper DT, Mehrizi A:** Asymmetrical hypertrophy of the heart in childhood. J Pediatr 67:204–213, 1965
15. **Teare D:** Asymmetrical hypertrophy of the heart in young patients. Br Heart J 20:1–18, 1958
16. **Gould SE:** Pathology of the Heart and Blood Vessels, third edition. Springfield, IL, Charles C Thomas, 1968, p 1139
17. **Henry WL, Clark CE, Roberts WC, et al:** Differences in distribution of myocardial abnormalities in patients with obstructive and nonobstructive asymmetric septal hypertrophy (ASH): echocardiographic and gross anatomic findings. Circulation 40:447–455, 1974
18. **Ferrans VJ, Morrow AG, Roberts WC:** Myocardial ultrastructure in idiopathic hypertrophic subaortic stenosis. A study of operatively excised left ventricular outflow tract muscle in 14 patients. Circulation 45:769–792, 1972
19. **Maron BJ, Ferrans VJ, Henry WL, et al:** Differences in distribution of myocardial abnormalities in patients with obstructive and nonobstructive asymmetric septal hypertrophy (ASH): light and electron microscopic findings. Circulation 50:436–446, 1974
20. **Maron BJ, Henry WL, Roberts WC, et al:** Comparison of echocardiographic and necropsy measurements of ventricular wall thicknesses in patients with and without disproportionate septal thickening. Circulation 55:341–345, 1977
21. **Lever HM, Shah PM, Reeves WC, et al:** The relation of left ventricular outflow obstruction to ventricular arrhythmias in hypertrophic subaortic stenosis (abstr). Circulation 53, 54:Suppl II:II-105, 1976

"Malignant" Hypertrophic Cardiomyopathy: Identification of a Subgroup of Families With Unusually Frequent Premature Death

BARRY J. MARON, MD
LEWIS C. LIPSON, MD
WILLIAM C. ROBERTS, MD, FACC
DANIEL D. SAVAGE, MD
STEPHEN E. EPSTEIN, MD, FACC

Bethesda, Maryland

Eight families were identified in which premature cardiac death due to hypertrophic cardiomyopathy occurred with unusual frequency. A total of 69 first degree relatives in the eight families were studied; 41 relatives had evidence of hypertrophic cardiomyopathy and 31 (75 percent) died of their heart disease. Eighteen of these 31 patients were less than 25 years of age at the time of death. Death was sudden and unexpected in 23 of the 31 patients; in 15 of these 23 patients sudden death was the initial manifestation of cardiac disease. The remaining eight patients (seven were from two families) died after a chronic cardiac illness characterized by congestive heart failure, atrial fibrillation or thromboembolic events.

Hence, premature cardiac death occurs frequently in certain families with hypertrophic cardiomyopathy. Such deaths are usually sudden, often occur in previously asymptomatic subjects and are common in children and young adults. These findings suggest that some families may manifest an unusually virulent expression of hypertrophic cardiomyopathy. Although this study cannot establish the precise prevalence with which "malignant" hypertrophic cardiomyopathy occurs, such families appear to be uncommon.

Premature death is a recognized complication in symptomatic[1-7] and asymptomatic[1-3,5-8] patients with hypertrophic cardiomyopathy. However, specific subgroups of patients at high risk of death have not previously been identified. Recently we have observed that premature cardiac death occurred frequently in certain families with hypertrophic cardiomyopathy. This investigation is an analysis of eight families with hypertrophic cardiomyopathy in which the number of cardiac deaths was much greater than in the vast majority of families with this disease.

Methods

Selection of families: The case records of the Cardiology Branch, National Heart, Lung, and Blood Institute from 1960 to 1972 were reviewed and the family histories of 198 index patients with hypertrophic cardiomyopathy (exclusive of those operated upon) were analyzed. In four of these families (C., P., F. and S.) with hypertrophic cardiomyopathy the occurrence of multiple premature cardiac deaths was documented. Members of four other families (Mo., B., M. and Ba.) were initially identified at other medical centers and because of the unusual family history of sudden death the National Heart, Lung, and Blood Institute subsequently became involved in evaluation of the family.

These eight families constitute the present study group by virtue of meeting the following criteria: (1) two or more first degree relatives (the designated propositus or parents, siblings and offspring of the propositus) had died of hypertrophic cardiomyopathy; (2) documentation of hypertrophic cardiomyopathy was possible in the majority of patients who died, either on clinical evaluation or at necropsy; (3) deaths were premature, that is, occurred before 50 years of

From the Cardiology and Pathology Branches, National Heart, Lung, and Blood Institute, National Institutes of Health, Bethesda, Maryland. Manuscript received November 15, 1977; revised manuscript received January 24, 1978, accepted January 25, 1978.

Address for reprints: Barry J. Maron, MD, Cardiology Branch, National Heart, Lung, and Blood Institute, National Institutes of Health, Building 10, Room 7B-15, Bethesda, Maryland.

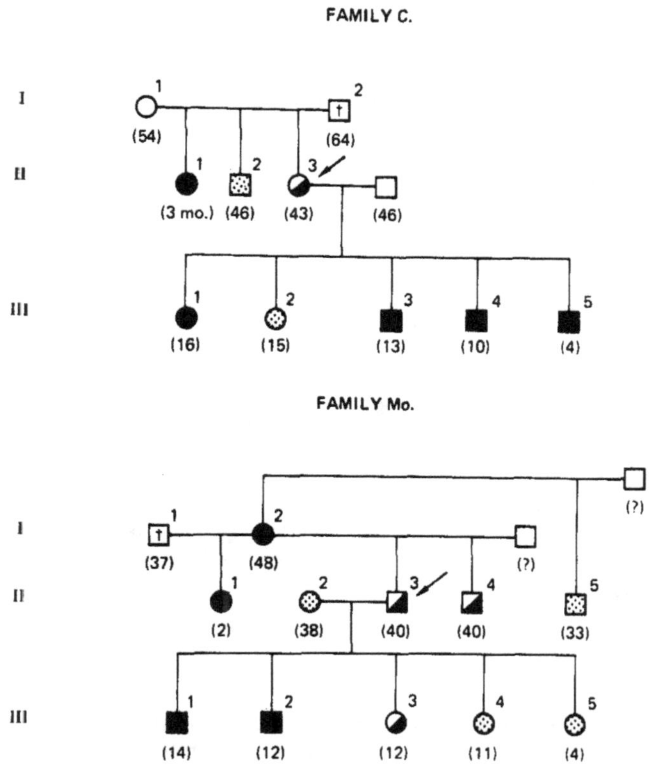

FIGURE 1. Pedigrees of Families C. and Mo. **Arrow** = propositus; **solid symbols** = death probably or definitely due to hypertrophic cardiomyopathy; **half-filled symbols** = alive with an echocardiogram that was diagnostic of asymmetric septal hypertrophy; **clear symbols** = echocardiogram not obtained; † = dead of noncardiac cause or cardiac disease other than hypertrophic cardiomyopathy; **stippled symbols** = alive, but asymmetric septal hypertrophy not evident in the echocardiogram; **circles** = female subjects; **squares** = male subjects. Only first degree relatives of the propositus are shown. Patients' ages (yr) are shown in parentheses below the symbols; patient identification numbers are to the upper right of the symbols. Patient II.2. in Family Mo., the mate of the propositus, is shown in the pedigree because echocardiographic data were available; however, she is not considered part of the family unit for purposes of data analysis. Although Patient I.2. of Family Mo. had three mates, for simplicity only Patient I.1. is included in the data analysis.

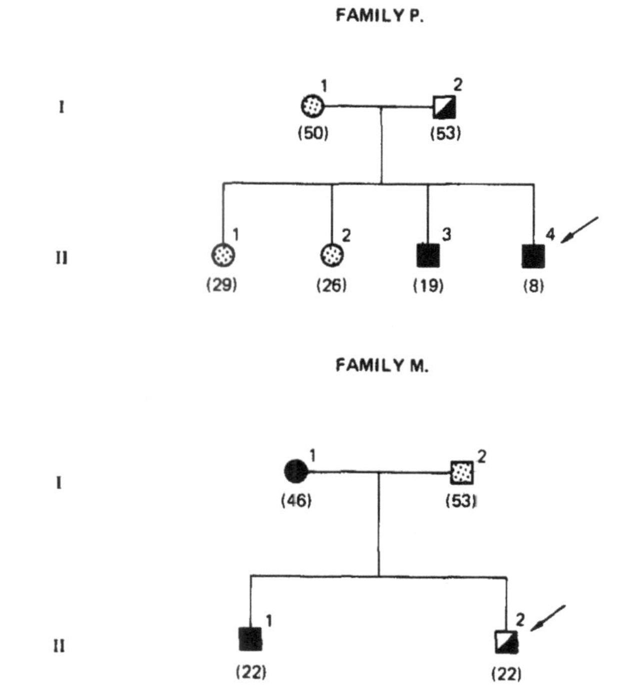

FIGURE 2. Pedigrees of Families P. and M. **Solid symbols** = death definitely due to hypertrophic cardiomyopathy. Other symbols as in Figure 1.

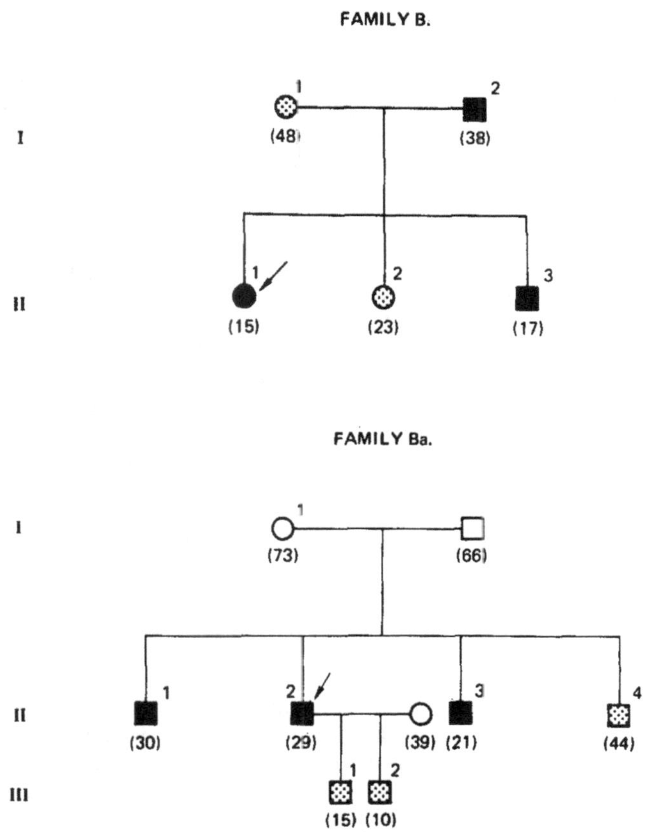

FIGURE 3. Pedigrees of Families B. and Ba. Symbols as in Figure 1. Four offspring of Patients II.1. and II.4. in Family Ba. had a normal septal-free wall ratio on echocardiography; one 20 year old son of Patient II.1. had a septal-free wall ratio of 1.3. These five patients are not shown here or included in the data analysis.

age; and (4) surviving members of the families were available for echocardiographic studies.

Identification of cause of death in family members: Thirty-one of the 69 relatives in the eight families died prematurely (before 50 years of age). In each of the 31 patients the available clinical or pathologic information (either from the National Institutes of Health or other institutions) or the circumstances of death indicated or strongly suggested that death was cardiac in origin. In 25 of the 31 patients coronary artery disease and other cardiac or noncardiac diseases capable of causing death were excluded at necropsy. Three patients who did not undergo necropsy examination were less than 25 years old and hence, it is unlikely that they had coronary artery disease. In two other patients (aged 47 and 48 years, respectively) coronary artery disease could not be excluded definitively because necropsy examination was not performed; however, neither of these two patients had angina pectoris and their clinical course was consistent with hypertrophic cardiomyopathy. The remaining patient had two

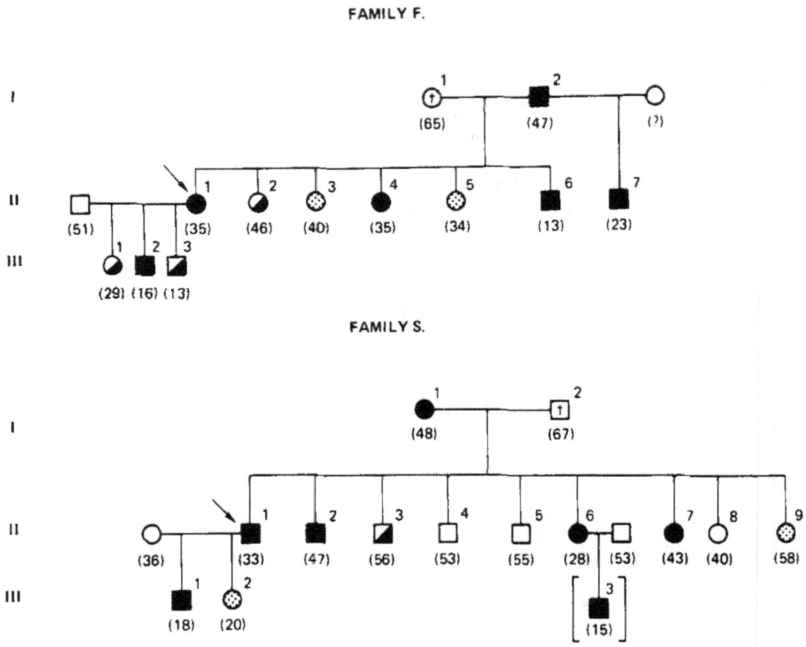

FIGURE 4. Pedigrees of Families F. and S. **Clear symbols** = no echocardiogram or a technically unsatisfactory echocardiogram obtained. Other symbols as in Figure 1. Patient III.3. in Family S., although not a first degree relative of the propositus and therefore not included in the data analysis, is also shown (in **brackets**) because he represents another instance of sudden death probably due to hypertrophic cardiomyopathy. Two children (aged 21 and 24 years) of Patient II.3. in Family S. have hypertrophic cardiomyopathy and are symptomatic. Two cousins of the propositus of Family F. also died suddenly of hypertrophic cardiomyopathy at age 13 and 20 years, respectively. These latter four patients are not shown here or included in the data analysis.

vessel coronary artery disease documented at necropsy, but death was clearly related to hypertrophic cardiomyopathy (that is, atrial fibrillation and thromboemboli).

The diagnosis of hypertrophic cardiomyopathy was considered certain in 20 of the 31 patients because of the presence of one or more of the following: (1) the typical clinical, operative or hemodynamic features of this disease, including left ventricular outflow tract obstruction under basal conditions or with provocation (11 patients); (2) documentation on echocardiography or at necropsy of increased ventricular septal thickness and a septal-free wall ratio of 1.3 or more (14 patients)[9]; in three other patients actual measurements of the ventricular walls were not available, but the qualitative description of marked septal hypertrophy at necropsy was considered supportive of the diagnosis of hypertrophic cardiomyopathy; and (3) the presence of other characteristic gross anatomic or histologic features of hypertrophic cardiomyopathy, that is, either numerous disorganized cardiac muscle cells in the ventricular septum[7,10,11] or an endocardial contact plaque on the ventricular septum in apposition to a thickened anterior mitral leaflet,[12] or both (11 patients).

In 11 other patients the diagnosis of hypertrophic cardiomyopathy was considered probable. In these patients death was usually sudden and unexpected (seven had been asymptomatic). Available clinical and hemodynamic data were insufficient to identify unequivocally hypertrophic cardiomyopathy, and no quantitative or qualitative assessment of ventricular septal thickness was available. However, cardiac hypertrophy was present in four of the five patients in this subgroup who had necropsy examination. In none of the six patients without necropsy examination did there appear to be another obvious explanation for death. Eight of the 11 patients considered to have probable hypertrophic cardiomyopathy died before 1958, when the initial pathologic description[7] of this disease was made; therefore, necropsy descriptions of these hearts could not have been expected to identify the gross anatomic features of hypertrophic cardiomyopathy. For analysis of our data, we considered all deaths of patients with a certain or probable diagnosis of hypertrophic cardiomyopathy as being deaths related to this disease.

Echocardiographic techniques: Echocardiograms were performed in 34 relatives in the eight families (including 2 relatives who subsequently died). Echocardiograms were obtained with a 2.25 megahertz, 1.2 cm diameter Aerotech transducer connected to either a modified Ekoline 20A or a Hoffrel 201 ultrasound unit employing methods previously described.[9] The ultrasonic signal was connected by means of a custom-built video amplifier to a Honeywell 1856 Visicorder and recorded continuously on light-sensitive paper. The thickness of the ventricular septum was measured below the tips of the mitral valve leaflets just before atrial systole; posterobasal left ventricular wall thickness was measured at the level of the tips of the mitral valve leaflets during the same phase of the cardiac cycle.

In 31 of the 34 relatives studied, the echocardiograms were of sufficient technical quality to permit accurate measurements of ventricular wall thickness; in the other three relatives, they were not adequate for such measurements.

Results

Cardiac Status and Circumstances of Death

Pedigrees for each of the eight families studied and summaries of clinical and morphologic data in each of the 69 first degree relatives are shown in Figures 1 to 4 and Tables I and II. Pedigrees include the propositus and siblings, offspring and both parents of the propositus; mates of the propositus are not considered part of the family unit for purposes of data analysis.

Sudden death: The 31 patients who died of hypertrophic cardiomyopathy (Fig. 5) ranged in age (Fig. 6) from 3 months to 48 years (median 19); 18 of these patients were less than 25 years of age and 5 were 10 years old or younger. Twenty-three of the 31 patients died suddenly. In 20 of these 23 patients death occurred instantaneously or within a few minutes. Two other patients were resuscitated after cardiac arrest; one survived for 1 day and the other for 5 weeks. Neither pa-

TABLE I

Summary of Clinical Data in Members of Eight Families With "Malignant" Hypertrophic Cardiomyopathy

	First Degree Relatives (no.)							Circumstances of Death and NYHA Functional Class			
								Sudden Death			Chronic CHF
Family	Total Subjects*	Total Affected Subjects	Death Due to Hypertrophic Cardiomyopathy	Surviving Affected Subjects§	Prevalence of Death in Affected Subjects	Surviving Unaffected Subjects	Uncertain Whether Affected	I	II	III	III or IV
C.	10	6	5	1	5/6	2	2	5	0	0	0
Mo.	11	7	4	3	4/7	3	1	4	1	0	0
P.	6	3	2	1	2/3	3	0	1	1†	0	0
M.	4	3	2	1	2/3	1	0	1	1	0	0
B.	5	3	3	0	3/3	2	0	1	1†	0	1
Ba.	8	3	3	0	3/3	3	2	2	1	0	0
F.	12	9	6	3	6/9	2	1	2	1	1‡	2
S.	13	7	6	1	6/7	2	4	0	1	0	5
Total	69	41	31	10	31/41 (75%)	18	10	16	7	1	8

* Propositus and siblings (or half-siblings), offspring and both parents of propositus.
† Each died 6 years after operation for obstructive hypertrophic cardiomyopathy.
‡ In functional class III due to angina pectoris; no clinical evidence of congestive heart failure.
§ As determined with echocardiography (septal-free wall ratio 1.3 or greater).
CHF = congestive heart failure; NYHA = New York Heart Association.

tient regained consciousness after the initial episode. The remaining patient (Patient I.2. in Family Mo.), who had previously been asymptomatic, experienced sudden onset of congestive heart failure after a retrograde pyelogram and died 2 days later; she is considered to have died suddenly for the purposes of our data analysis. Two of the 20 patients in whom death occurred instantaneously had experienced a previous cardiac arrest from which they were successfully resuscitated (Patients III.3. in Family C. and I.1. in Family M.). In these two patients the interval between the initial cardiac arrest and the second (fatal) arrest was 20 and 25 months, respectively.

Of the 23 patients who died suddenly, 8 were symptomatic at the time of death (7 patients in New York Heart Association[13] functional class II and one in class III); the remaining 15 patients were asymptomatic and therefore sudden death was the initial symptomatic manifestation of hypertrophic cardiomyopathy.[8] Death occurred during minimal or sedentary activities in 12 patients, during or just after mild exertion in 2 patients and during or just after moderate or severe exertion in 7 patients; 1 patient died during sleep. The exact activity at the time of death was unknown in one patient. In two families the sudden death of two siblings occurred within a short time interval; that is, 7 days for Patients III.3. and III.4. in Family C. and 9 1/2 months for Patients III.1. and III.2. in Family Mo. Also, in Family M. a son (Patient II.1.) and mother (Patient I.1.) had a cardiac arrest within 9 weeks of each other; the mother survived but nevertheless died suddenly 2 years later.

Cardiac murmur: A cardiac examination was performed in 32 of the 41 affected relatives in this study. In 13 of the 32 patients a grade 3/6 or louder systolic ejection murmur was present along the left sternal border or at the apex, or both. In the remaining 19 patients no murmur or a systolic ejection murmur less than grade 3/6 was present.

TABLE II

Clinical Findings in Affected Surviving and Nonsurviving Members of Families With "Malignant" Hypertrophic Cardiomyopathy

	Survivors (no. = 10)	Nonsurvivors (no. = 31)
Asymptomatic	2	15
Cardiac symptoms		
Dyspnea on exertion/fatigue	3	7
Angina	3	7
Syncope	1	8
Lightheadedness	4	4
Palpitations	1	0
Signs of severe CHF	1	7
CVA/thromboemboli	0	5
Arrhythmias		
Atrial fibrillation	0	3
Ventricular	1	1

CHF = congestive heart failure; CVA = cerebrovascular accident.

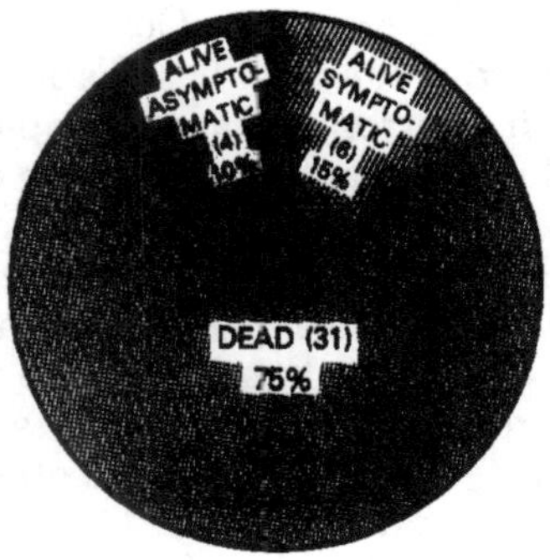

FIGURE 5. Diagram summarizing the clinical outcome of 41 affected first degree relatives in the eight families with "malignant" hypertrophic cardiomyopathy. The number of patients in each subgroup is shown in parentheses.

Previous operation: Two patients who died suddenly had had previous operations. Patient II.3. in Family P. underwent myotomy-myectomy at age 13 years for relief of severe right ventricular outflow tract obstruction (pressure gradient 120 mm Hg); no obstruction to left ventricular outflow was present.[14] Although operation obliterated the gradient and eliminated cardiac symptoms in this patient, he died suddenly 6 years after operation. Patient II.3. in Family B. underwent septal myotomy-myectomy at age 11 years for relief of severe left ventricular outflow tract obstruction (pressure gradient 100 mm Hg) and mitral anuloplasty for mitral regurgitation secondary to ruptured chordae tendineae. Subsequently, this patient continued to have mild functional limitation and died suddenly 6 years after operation.

Previous cardiac catheterization: Hemodynamic data had been obtained in 6 of the 21 patients not operated on who died suddenly. Marked obstruction to left ventricular outflow, with a peak systolic pressure gradient under basal conditions of 50 mm Hg or more, was present in three of these patients; the remaining three patients had a gradient of less than 50 mm Hg under basal conditions or with provocation. Two other patients who did not undergo cardiac catheterization had an echocardiographic study that demonstrated absence of systolic anterior motion of the anterior mitral leaflet.

Chronic congestive heart failure: Eight patients died of chronic cardiac decompensation (6 months to 15 years in duration) and each was in functional class III or IV just before death. The clinical profile of these patients was that of marked functional limitation (dyspnea and fatigue with exertion), often associated with paroxysmal atrial fibrillation and thromboembolic events, and physical findings of congestive heart failure. Of the four patients who underwent cardiac catheterization, two had a peak systolic pressure gradient under basal conditions or with provocation of more than 50 mm Hg; the remaining two patients had a gradient of 10 mm Hg or less under basal conditions or with provocation. The eight patients with chronic congestive cardiac failure died later in life (mean age 40 years) than the 22 patients who died suddenly (mean age 19 years; $P < 0.001$) (Fig. 6).

Interfamily differences: Considered from the standpoint of individual families (Table I), all but one death due to hypertrophic cardiomyopathy occurred suddenly and unexpectedly in six of the eight families studied (C., Mo., P., M., B. and Ba.). In contrast, in the other two families (S. and F.), relatives died either suddenly or in the course of chronic congestive heart failure. For example, in Family S., five relatives who died of hypertrophic cardiomyopathy had experienced chronic cardiac failure. However, two other relatives in this family died suddenly at age 15 and 18 years, respectively; both were offspring of patients who died with congestive heart failure. In Family F., four relatives died suddenly and two others died after chronic cardiac illnesses.

No consistent predilection was evident in the eight families for either the obstructive or nonobstructive form of hypertrophic cardiomyopathy. For example, each of the affected relatives in Families M. and B. (in whom the magnitude of outflow obstruction was measured) had marked obstruction. On the other hand, the relatives in other families (F. and S.) had either outflow obstruction or no obstruction.

Mitral valve prolapse: Members of two families (M. and Ba.) with hypertrophic cardiomyopathy also had evidence of mitral valve prolapse. Patient I.1. in Family M. with hypertrophic cardiomyopathy demonstrated "floppy mitral valve" at necropsy. In addition, four surviving offspring or nieces of the propositus (Patient II.2.) of Family Ba. manifested either mitral valve prolapse on echocardiography or midsystolic clicks on physical examination, or both; each of these latter patients was asymptomatic or minimally symptomatic and none had abnormal septal-free wall ratios or increased ventricular wall thicknesses on echocardiography.

Necropsy Findings

Heart weight, assessed in 23 hearts, ranged from 35 to 940 g (median 420 g in the 20 patients 12 or more years of age); in all but one patient (Patient II.1. in

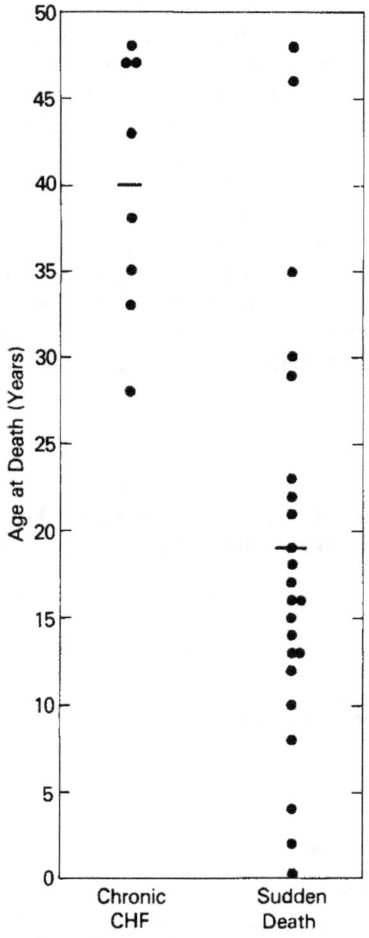

FIGURE 6. Comparison of age at death of patients who died with chronic congestive heart failure (CHF) and of patients who died suddenly.

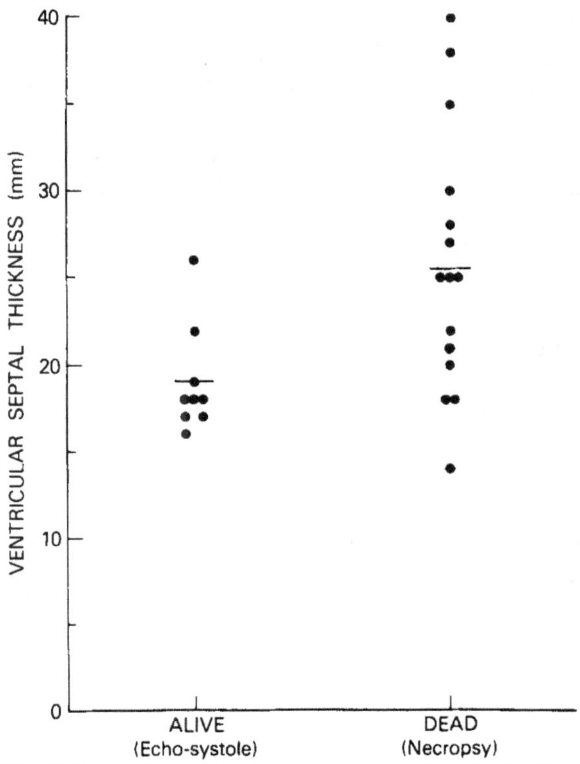

FIGURE 7. Ventricular septal thickness measurements obtained in nine surviving affected family members with echocardiography (Echo) compared with those obtained at necropsy in 15 relatives who had died. The echocardiographic measurements shown were obtained during systole (see Results for explanation). Patient II.2. in Family M. was excluded from this analysis (even though alive) because he underwent a "prophylactic" septal myotomy-myectomy 1.5 years before this report was prepared.

Family C.) heart weight was increased with respect to age.[15] In 15 patients either the heart was in suitable condition for detailed examination or sufficient pathologic information was available to assign a septal-free wall thickness ratio. Septal-free wall ratio ranged from 0.9 to 2.8 (median 1.8) and was more than 1.3 in 13 of the 15 hearts. Although the septal-free wall ratio obtained at necropsy in the other two patients (Patients II.7. and III.1. in Family S.) was not indicative of disproportionate septal thickening, the ratio obtained in both of these patients with echocardiography (in diastole) was 1.3 or greater and, therefore, diagnostic of disproportionate septal thickening.[16] Absolute ventriclar septal thickness (Fig. 7) ranged from 14 to 40 mm (median 25 mm); in all but three patients septal thickness was 20 mm or greater. One patient (Patient III.2. in Family Mo.) had a large transmural ventricular septal infarct despite widely patent extramural coronary arteries.

Mitral valve and endocardium: Of 12 hearts in which the mitral valve and endocardium of the left ventricular outflow tract could be studied, 5 showed an endocardial contact plaque on the ventricular septum in apposition to a thickened anterior mitral leaflet. One patient had only an endocardial plaque, one had only a thickened anterior mitral leaflet and three had neither an endocardial plaque nor a thickened mitral leaflet.

Histology: Histologic observations regarding arrangement of cardiac muscle cells in the ventricular septum were made in 10 hearts. In each of these hearts the septum had numerous disorganized cells, characteristic of patients with hypertrophic cardiomyopathy.[7,10,11]

Cardiac Status of Surviving Relatives

Ten surviving relatives in six of the eight families were identified as affected by hypertrophic cardiomyopathy through echocardiographic documentation of asymmetric septal hypertrophy (septal-free wall ratio 1.3 or greater).[9] Six of these patients were symptomatic (four patients in functional class II and two in class III), and four other patients were asymptomatic (Fig. 5). With the exception of Patient II.2. in Family M., who underwent "prophylactic" myotomy-myectomy (preoperative outflow gradient under basal conditions of 100 mm Hg), none of the other three surviving affected relatives who had cardiac catheterization had a left ventricular outflow gradient of 50 mm Hg or more. In addition, none of the other six surviving patients had marked systolic anterior motion of the anterior mitral leaflet on echocardiographic study, suggesting that there was no significant outflow obstruction under basal conditions.

In four of the eight families (Mo., P., M. and B.), echocardiographic studies were performed in both parents of either the propositus or another relative who had died of hypertrophic cardiomyopathy. In each instance one member of the parental pair had a normal heart and the other had asymmetric septal hypertrophy. These findings excluded the possibility that the virulent expression of hypertrophic cardiomyopathy in these families could be explained by the fact that two persons with this disease had coincidentally mated.

Comparison of Surviving and Nonsurviving Family Members

Ventricular septal thickness: Mean ventricular septal thickness was significantly greater in those family members who died (and in whom septal thickness measurements were obtained at necropsy; mean 25.4 ± 2.0 [standard error] mm) than in the surviving family members with an abnormal septal-free wall ratio (in whom septal thickness was measured during systole[15] with echocardiography; mean 19.0 ± 1.0, $P < 0.05$) (Fig. 7). Eleven of 13 subjects with a ventricular septal thickness of 20 mm or more had died, and the remaining 2 surviving subjects were symptomatic. Conversely, only 4 of 11 relatives with a septal thickness of less than 20 mm had died. In two of these four patients the relatively small septal thickness could be explained on the basis of young age or small body surface area. Although values for ventricular septal thickness at necropsy may be greater than those obtained during life with echocardiography during diastole,[16] septal thickness during systole during life corresponds closely to that at necropsy.[16] For this reason, we compared our necropsy measurements of septal thickness with those obtained with echocardiography during systole.

Electrocardiography: Electrocardiograms were obtained in nine surviving relatives with asymmetric septal hypertrophy and in 19 relatives who subsequently died, either suddenly or with chronic congestive heart failure. No electrocardiographic pattern was characteristic of either survivors or nonsurvivors, and there were no consistent differences in the severity of electrocardiographic abnormalities between these two groups of patients. However, although four of the surviving patients with asymmetric septal hypertrophy had either normal or only mildly abnormal electrocardiograms, two patients who died also had an electrocardiogram that showed only mild abnormalities. The specific electrocardiographic abnormalities in these two groups of patients are summarized in Table III.

Outflow tract obstruction: The magnitude of left ventricular outflow tract obstruction was compared in nine surviving affected relatives who were not operated on and 19 family members who died without operation. Evidence taken as indicating marked outflow obstruction under basal conditions included one or more of the following: hemodynamic documentation of a gradient of 50 mm Hg or more, marked systolic anterior motion of the anterior mitral leaflet on echocardiographic study, grade 3/6 or louder systolic ejection murmur, rounded posterobasal segment of the left ventricular free wall,[17] and numerous disorganized cardiac muscle cells present in the ventricular septum but rare or absent in the left ventricular free wall.[11] With use of these criteria, marked outflow obstruction under basal conditions was less common in surviving affected relatives who were not operated on (0 of 9) than in patients who died of hypertrophic cardiomyopathy without operation (7 of 19; 37 percent). This difference did not achieve statistical significance.

TABLE III

Electrocardiographic Abnormalities in Affected Surviving and Nonsurviving Members of Families With "Malignant" Hypertrophic Cardiomyopathy

	Survivors (no. = 9)*	Nonsurvivors (no. = 19)†
Normal	2	0
Left ventricular hypertrophy	1	5
Left axis deviation	2	4
Right axis deviation	0	1
Left atrial enlargement	0	2
Abnormal Q or QS waves‡	4	5
S-T segment and T wave abnormalities	6	10
Left bundle branch block	1	1
Right bundle branch block	0	0
Atrial fibrillation	1	3
First degree atrioventricular block	0	3
Bifascicular block	0	1

* Excluded from this analysis is one patient with "prophylactic" myotomy-myectomy (II.2. in Family M.).

† Excluded are two patients who died after operation and one patient in whom only a post-cardiac arrest electrocardiogram was obtained; electrocardiograms were not available in nine other patients who died of hypertrophic cardiomyopathy.

‡ 4 mm or more in depth or 0.04 second in duration, in one or more leads.

Discussion

Prevalence of "malignant" hypertrophic cardiomyopathy: These data demonstrate that in certain families with hypertrophic cardiomyopathy premature cardiac death occurs with alarming frequency. Because of the potential bias introduced by the selection of our patient population, this study cannot establish the precise prevalence with which "malignant" hypertrophic cardiomyopathy occurs. Nevertheless, it seems reasonable to conclude that such families are relatively uncommon.

Our definition of a "malignant" family—one with two or more first degree relatives who died of hypertrophic cardiomyopathy before 50 years of age—is necessarily arbitrary. Hence, it is possible that our relatively few selected families with multiple deaths represent chance occurrences at the extreme end of the distribution curve rather than a distinctly different and more virulent form of hypertrophic cardiomyopathy. However, to discriminate between these two possibilities would require knowledge of the probability of survival for the overall population of patients with hypertrophic cardiomyopathy. This statistic depends upon the identification and follow-up of a large otherwise unselected cohort of patients with hypertrophic cardiomyopathy in the general population. Obtaining such data is unfortunately impractical, if not impossible.

Role of propranolol prophylaxis: If the frequent deaths of first degree relatives of certain families represent a more virulent form of hypertrophic cardiomyopathy, surviving members of such "malignant" families present difficult therapeutic decisions. Although definitive data concerning the efficacy of propranolol in preventing sudden death in patients with hypertrophic cardiomyopathy are not yet available, the possibility of prophylactic treatment with propranolol must be considered in asymptomatic or mildly symptomatic affected members of "malignant" families, whether or not they have obstruction to left ventricular outflow.

Role of prophylactic septal myotomy-myectomy: Of the patients with evidence regarding the presence or absence of left ventricular outflow obstruction, all those who had marked outflow obstruction had died by the time this study was completed; that is, none of the nine surviving affected relatives who were not operated on had evidence of marked outflow obstruction. In contrast, obstruction had been present in 7 of the 19 nonoperated patients who died. Although this difference is not statistically significant, these findings do suggest that members of "malignant" families with marked outflow obstruction, if not at definitively greater risk of dying prematurely than those with no or mild obstruction, are certainly not at lesser risk. However, the advisability of "prophylactic" septal myotomy-myectomy is uncertain, because the effects of operation on long-term survival of patients with hypertrophic cardiomyopathy are currently unsubstantiated. Hence, we continue to recommend operation to patients in "malignant" families only if marked outflow obstruction is present (gradient of 50 mm Hg or more under basal conditions or with provocation) and if symptoms are incapacitating despite propranolol therapy.

Prognostic significance of increased septal thickness: Another finding of potential importance was that ventricular septal thickness was significantly greater in affected family members who died than in those who survived. In another study we found that moderate to severe ventricular septal thickening was also characteristic of patients with hypertrophic cardiomyopathy who died suddenly and who were asymptomatic before death[8] (most of these patients were not members of "malignant" families). Hence, it is possible that moderate to marked ventricular septal thickening (20 mm or more during systole during life or at necropsy) may identify a subgroup of patients with hypertrophic cardiomyopathy who are at relatively high risk of sudden death. However, such a risk factor analysis is obviously not all inclusive. This is illustrated by the two patients designated III.1. in Families S. and C., who were mildly symptomatic or asymptomatic and died suddenly at age 18 and 16 years, respectively. At necropsy, these patients had a ventricular septal thickness of only 14 mm and 16 mm, respectively. Furthermore, definitive conclusions regarding the prognostic significance of increased septal thickness will require prospectively obtained data from a population of patients followed up longitudinally after echocardiographic measurement of septal thickness.

References

1. **Frank S, Braunwald E:** Idiopathic hypertrophic subaortic stenosis. Clinical analysis of 126 patients with emphasis on the natural history. Circulation 37:759–788, 1968
2. **Maron BJ, Henry WL, Clark CE, et al:** Asymmetric septal hypertrophy in childhood. Circulation 53:9–18, 1976
3. **Adelman AG, Wigle ED, Ranganathan N, et al:** The clinical course in muscular subaortic stenosis. A retrospective and prospective study of 60 hemodynamically proven cases. Ann Intern Med 77: 515–525, 1972
4. **Shah PM, Adelman AG, Wigle ED, et al:** The natural (and unnatural) course of hypertrophic obstructive cardiomyopathy. A multicenter study. Circ Res 34, 35:Suppl II: II-179–II-195, 1973
5. **Hardarson T, De La Calzada CS, Curiel R, et al:** Prognosis and mortality of hypertrophic obstructive cardiomyopathy. Lancet 2: 1462–1467, 1973
6. **Swan DA, Bell B, Oakley CM, et al:** Analysis of the symptomatic course and prognosis and treatment of hypertrophic obstructive cardiomyopathy. Br Heart J 33:671–685, 1971
7. **Teare D:** Asymmetrical hypertrophy of the heart in young adults. Br Heart J 20:1–18, 1958
8. **Maron BJ, Roberts WC, Edwards JE, et al:** Sudden death in patients with hypertrophic cardiomyopathy: characterization of 26 patients without functional limitation. Am J Cardiol 41:803–810, 1978
9. **Henry WL, Clark CE, Epstein SE:** Asymmetric septal hypertrophy: echocardiographic identification of the pathognomonic anatomic abnormality of IHSS. Circulation 47:225–233, 1973
10. **Ferrans VJ, Morrow AG, Roberts WC:** Myocardial ultrastructure in idiopathic hypertrophic subaortic stenosis: a study of operatively excised left ventricular outflow tract muscle in 14 patients. Circulation 45:769–792, 1972
11. **Maron BJ, Ferrans VJ, Henry WL, et al:** Differences in distribution of myocardial abnormalities in patients with obstructive and nonobstructive asymmetric septal hypertrophy (ASH): light and electron microscopic findings. Circulation 50:436–446, 1974
12. **Roberts WC:** Valvular, subvalvular and supravalvular aortic stenosis: morphologic features. Cardiovasc Clin 5:104–126, 1973
13. Criteria Committee of the New York Heart Association: Diseases of the Heart and Blood Vessels: Nomenclature and Criteria for Diagnosis, seventh edition. Boston, Little, Brown, 1973, p 286
14. **Morrow AG, Fisher RD, Fogarty TJ:** Isolated hypertrophic obstruction to right ventricular outflow. Am Heart J 77:814–817, 1969
15. **Gould SE:** Pathology of the Heart and Blood Vessels, third edition. Springfield, IL, Charles C Thomas, 1968, p 1139
16. **Maron BJ, Henry WL, Roberts WC, et al:** Comparison of echocardiographic and necropsy measurements of ventricular wall thicknesses in patients with and without disproportionate septal thickening. Circulation 55:341–345, 1977
17. **Epstein SE, Henry WL, Clark CE, et al:** Asymmetric septal hypertrophy. Ann Intern Med 81:650–680, 1974

Quantitative Analysis of Cardiac Muscle Cell Disorganization in the Ventricular Septum of Patients with Hypertrophic Cardiomyopathy

BARRY J. MARON, M.D. AND WILLIAM C. ROBERTS, M.D.

with the technical assistance of Thomas J. Anan and James Wolfson

SUMMARY The presence of numerous abnormally arranged cardiac muscle cells in the ventricular septum has been considered a characteristic anatomic feature of patients with hypertrophic cardiomyopathy. To determine the specificity of this histologic marker for patients with hypertrophic cardiomyopathy, we used a quantitative method to determine the area of myocardium occupied by disorganized cells. In hypertrophic cardiomyopathy, septal disorganization was present in 94% of the 54 patients studied at necropsy. Furthermore, disorganization was extensive in most of these patients, involving 5% or more of the transverse plane tissue section in 89% of the patients and 25% or more of the section in 56% of the patients. Septal disorganization was best identified in tissue sections cut perpendicular to the long axis of the left ventricle. Septal disorganization was present in only 26% of the 144 control patients with other heart diseases or normal hearts. Most important, when present in these patients, disorganization was usually limited in extent. In only 7% of the controls studied did abnormally arranged cells occupy 5% or more of the tissue section. The average area of septum disorganized was 31 ± 3% (mean ± SEM) in patients with hypertrophic cardiomyopathy and only 1.5 ± 0.6% in the controls ($p < 0.001$). Hence, while the presence of ventricular septal disorganization is not pathognomonic of hypertrophic cardiomyopathy, widespread distribution of this abnormality is a very sensitive and specific histologic marker for this disease.

IN THE INITIAL PATHOLOGIC REPORT of hypertrophic cardiomyopathy published in 1958, Teare described a bizarre and unique arrangement of cardiac muscle cells in the asymmetrically hypertrophied ventricular septum.[1] Several other investigators[2-11] have made similar observations regarding the histologic appearance of ventricular septal myocardium in this disease. However, the presence of disorganized septal architecture per se is not pathognomonic of hypertrophic cardiomyopathy, i.e., areas of disorganization, although usually small, may be present in the ventricular septum of some patients with various acquired or congenital heart diseases,[12-15] as well as in normal embryos and fetuses,[16] normal infants[16, 17] and infants who die suddenly without evidence of structural cardiac disease.[17]

Some investigators[18-21] have questioned the specificity of disordered septal architecture for patients with hypertrophic cardiomyopathy, based primarily on qualitative or semiquantitative histologic analysis of myocardium obtained from patients with heart diseases other than hypertrophic cardiomyopathy. Hence, the present study was undertaken to: 1) establish detailed morphologic criteria for cardiac muscle cell disorganization; and 2) determine, for the first time in quantitative terms, the extent of cardiac muscle cell disorganization in the ventricular septum of patients with hypertrophic cardiomyopathy compared with patients who have other forms of cardiac hypertrophy.

Selection of Case Material

Patients with Hypertrophic Cardiomyopathy

The cardiovascular registry of the Pathology Branch, National Heart, Lung, and Blood Institute, was reviewed and 64 hearts with hypertrophic cardiomyopathy were considered for inclusion in the study. Ten of these specimens were excluded because we could not obtain ventricular septal tissue suitable for histologic analysis, including two specimens that were in poor condition and five that had extensive septal scarring. Three other hearts that were particularly good examples of hypertrophic cardiomyopathy were excluded so that the pathologic specimens could be preserved intact. The remaining 54 hearts comprised the study group.

In 48 (89%) of the 54 patients the diagnosis of hypertrophic cardiomyopathy was based on the presence of asymmetric septal hypertrophy (defined as a septal-free wall ratio of 1.3 or greater), identified either at necropsy[6, 22] or by echocardiography,[23-25] in the absence of an associated valvular or congenital heart defect which itself could have produced left ventricular hypertrophy. In 37 of these 48 patients the typical clinical, hemodynamic, angiocardiographic and operative[26-30] findings of hypertrophic cardiomyopathy were also present; the 11 other patients had no cardiac evaluation during life, and sudden death was the first definitive manifestation of cardiac disease.[31]

In the other six patients with hypertrophic cardiomyopathy, concentric ventricular wall thickening

From the Cardiology and Pathology Branches, NHLBI, NIH, Bethesda, Maryland.

Address for reprints: Barry J. Maron, M.D., Senior Investigator, Cardiology Branch, NHLBI, National Institutes of Health, Building 10, Room 7B-15, Bethesda, Maryland 20014.

Received May 26, 1978; revision accepted November 14, 1978.
Circulation 59, No. 4, 1979.

TABLE 1. *Clinical and Hemodynamic Findings in 54 Patients with Hypertrophic Cardiomyopathy*

	Symptoms		LVOT - PSG (mm Hg)			LVEDP (mm Hg)			Mode of death					
	+	0	≥30 at rest	<30 at rest	Provocable*	≤12	13–20	>20	Sudden	CHF	CVA	Suicide	Cath	Op
No. of patients	38	16	26†	4	6‡	15	14	12	26	8	1	2	2	15
%	70	30	63	10	15	36	34	30	48	15	2	4	4	28

*<30 mm Hg at rest; ≥30 mm Hg with provocation (Valsalva maneuver or isoproterenol infusion).

†Includes one patient with severe (i.e., 118 mm Hg PSG) obstruction to right ventricular outflow but no LVOT obstruction.[9]

‡Provocative maneuvers not performed in five other patients with <30 mm Hg LVOT gradient at rest.

Abbreviations: Cath = cardiac catheterization; CHF = congestive heart failure; CVA = cerebrovascular accident; LVEDP = left ventricular end-diastolic pressure; LVOT = left ventricular outflow tract; Op = cardiac operation; PSG = peak systolic gradient; + = present; 0 = absent.

(septal-free wall ratio < 1.3) was present at necropsy. Although echocardiographic studies were not performed in these six patients, three were considered to have hypertrophic cardiomyopathy based on the presence of typical clinical, hemodynamic, angiographic and operative features of the disease.[26-30] The other three patients were considered to have hypertrophic cardiomyopathy because of marked cardiac hypertrophy and the presence of an endocardial contact plaque on the ventricular septum in apposition to a thickened anterior mitral leaflet.[6]

TABLE 2. *Cardiac Diseases in 144 Control Patients*

Disease	No. of patients	No. with marked septal disorganization§
Aortic valve disease	39*	5¶
Coronary heart disease	31	2
Systemic hypertension	17	1
Isolated mitral valve disease	13†	1**
Dilated (congestive) cardiomyopathy	10	0
Primary pulmonary hypertension	7	1
Combined mitral and aortic valve disease	3	0
Pulmonic valve stenosis	3	0
Mitral valve prolapse	3	0
Ventricular septal defect	3‡	0
Discrete (membranous) subaortic stenosis	2	0
Supravalvular aortic stenosis	2	0
Normal	11	1
Totals	144	11 (7%)

*Includes 28 patients with predominant aortic stenosis, eight with pure aortic regurgitation and three with combined aortic stenosis and regurgitation.

†Includes three patients with predominant mitral stenosis, seven with predominant mitral regurgitation and three with combined mitral stenosis and regurgitation.

‡Includes one patient with associated valvular pulmonic stenosis.

§Disorganized cardiac muscle cells involving ≥ 5% of the relevant areas of the tissue section.

¶Includes three patients with pure aortic regurgitation, one patient with predominant aortic stenosis and one with combined aortic stenosis and regurgitation.

**A patient with predominant mitral regurgitation.

TABLE 3. *Comparison of Clinical and Morphologic Features in Patients with Hypertrophic Cardiomyopathy and in Controls*

Parameter	Hypertrophic cardiomyopathy	Other heart diseases and normals	p
No. of patients	54	144	—
Age (years) Mean (range)	33 (11–70)	45 (5–91)	<0.001
Female:male (%)	61:39	40:60	<0.025
Heart weight (g) Mean (range)	535§ (270–1020)	532¶ (185–1360)	NS
Septal thickness (mm) Mean (range)	26 (15–44)	15 (8–34)	<0.001
Septal-free wall ratio* Mean (range)	1.7 (1.0–2.6)	1.1 (0.7–1.7)	<0.001
Septal-free wall ratio ≥ 1.3	78†	16‡	<0.001

*Ratio of maximal ventricular septal thickness (usually present one-third to one-half the distance from base to apex) to posterior left ventricular wall thickness measured at the level of the inferior margins of the mitral leaflets.

†Echocardiograms were recorded during life in seven of 12 patients with concentric hypertrophy (septal-free wall ratio <1.3) at necropsy; asymmetric septal hypertrophy was present on each of these studies. Since septal-free wall ratios during life in diastole usually exceed those obtained at necropsy,[32] it is likely that at least 49 (91%) of the 54 patients with hypertrophic cardiomyopathy would have had asymmetric septal hypertrophy during life by echocardiography.

‡Septal-free wall ratio was <1.3 in each of the 11 normal hearts; one patient with coronary heart disease had a ratio of >1.3, due primarily to scarring, loss of myocardium, and hence decreased posterior left ventricular wall thickness (in the area of the wall through which the ultrasound beam would have passed in life;[15] this patient was considered to have concentric ventricular wall thickening for the purposes of data analysis.

§Heart weight exceeded normal values[33] in all 54 patients.

¶Heart weight exceeded normal values[33] in each of 133 patients with congenital or acquired heart disease and was within normal limits in each of the 11 subjects without cardiac disease.

Abbreviation: NS = not significant.

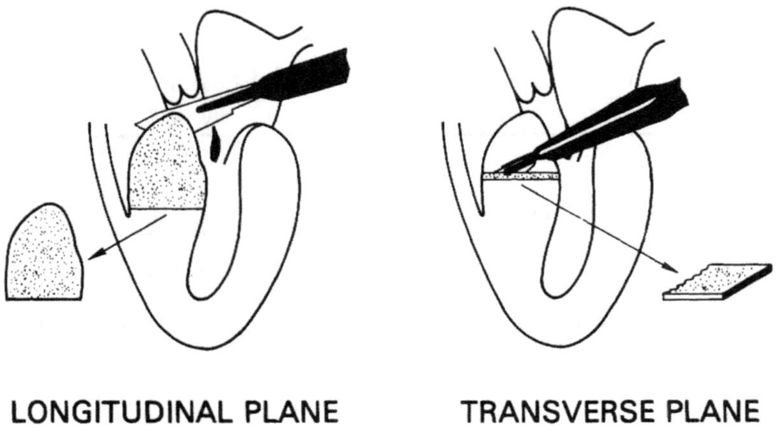

FIGURE 1. *Orientations in which sections of ventricular septum were taken. Longitudinal sections were obtained in a plane parallel to the long axis of the left ventricle; transverse sections were obtained in a plane perpendicular to the long axis of the left ventricle.*

Associated coronary artery disease (> 50% narrowing by atherosclerosis of the cross-sectional lumen of at least one major coronary artery) was present in seven of the 54 patients with hypertrophic cardiomyopathy; one of these patients also had a secundum atrial septal defect. Clinical and hemodynamic data in the 54 patients with hypertrophic cardiomyopathy are summarized in table 1.

Patients with Cardiac Diseases Other Than Hypertrophic Cardiomyopathy and Normal Hearts

The hearts of 144 patients were selected for study as controls. This group included 133 patients with a variety of congenital or acquired heart diseases and 11 subjects with structurally normal hearts who died of trauma (table 2). The 133 diseased control hearts had greater weights (mean ± SEM 555 ± 17 g vs 295 ± 12 g; $p < 0.001$) and ventricular septal thicknesses (16 ± 0.4 mm vs 12 ± 0.6 mm; $p < 0.02$) than did the 11 normal hearts; these two groups did not differ with regard to age, sex distribution or septal-free wall ratio. The normal and diseased controls were combined for convenience in data analysis. The 144 control patients and 54 patients with hypertrophic cardiomyopathy are compared with regard to clinical and anatomic parameters in table 3.

Materials and Methods

Measurement of Ventricular Wall Thicknesses

Measurements of ventricular wall thicknesses were made in the following two areas: 1) ventricular septum, at the point of maximum thickness, usually about one-half the distance between the base of the aortic valve and the apex of left ventricle; and 2) posterobasal left ventricular wall, behind the midpoint of the posterior mitral leaflet, at a level corresponding to the tips of the mitral leaflets. In making measurements of ventricular wall thicknesses, we avoided including trabeculae, papillary muscles or crista supraventricularis.

Preparation of Tissue

In each of the 198 hearts in this study (54 with hypertrophic cardiomyopathy and 144 controls) tissue blocks were taken from the full thickness of the ventricular septum, at the point of maximal thickness, and in a plane perpendicular to the long axis of the left ventricle (i.e., transverse plane) (fig. 1); in the anteroposterior axis these sections extended to the point of junction of the ventricular septum with the left and right ventricular free walls. In 25 of the 54 patients with hypertrophic cardiomyopathy and in eight control patients, additional tissue blocks (about 3 mm thick) were taken from the ventricular septum in a plane parallel to the long axis of the left ventricle (i.e., longitudinal plane) (fig. 1); these sections extended from the most cephalad aspect of the muscular septum to a point approximately three-fourths the distance from base and apex. Each tissue block was embedded in paraffin, sectioned at 6 μ and stained with hematoxylin and eosin.

Definition and Classification of Cardiac Muscle Cell Arrangement

Abnormally Arranged Cardiac Muscle Cells

In this study, cardiac muscle cell disorganization was classified into four major types (figs. 2 and 3). Type I-A disorganization was the most common, and consisted of areas of myocardium in which adjacent cardiac muscle cells were aligned perpendicularly or obliquely to each other, usually forming tangled masses or "pinwheel" configurations. Although most of these lesions were small, the size of individual foci of type I-A disorganization varied greatly. Disorganization of this type assumed a wide spectrum of morphologic appearances (fig. 4). In Type I-B disorganization relatively broad bundles of muscle cells were oriented at oblique or perpendicular angles to each other; cells within these bundles were, however, normally arranged. Both types I-A and I-B exclusively involved areas of septum in which cardiac muscle cells were cut longitudinally, i.e., appeared to be rectangularly shaped.

Type II-A disorganization consisted of relatively narrow (usually one or two cells wide), longitudinally cut bundles of cells that were interlaced in various directions among larger groups of transversely cut cells (which appeared circular). This type of disorganization gave the myocardium a swirled

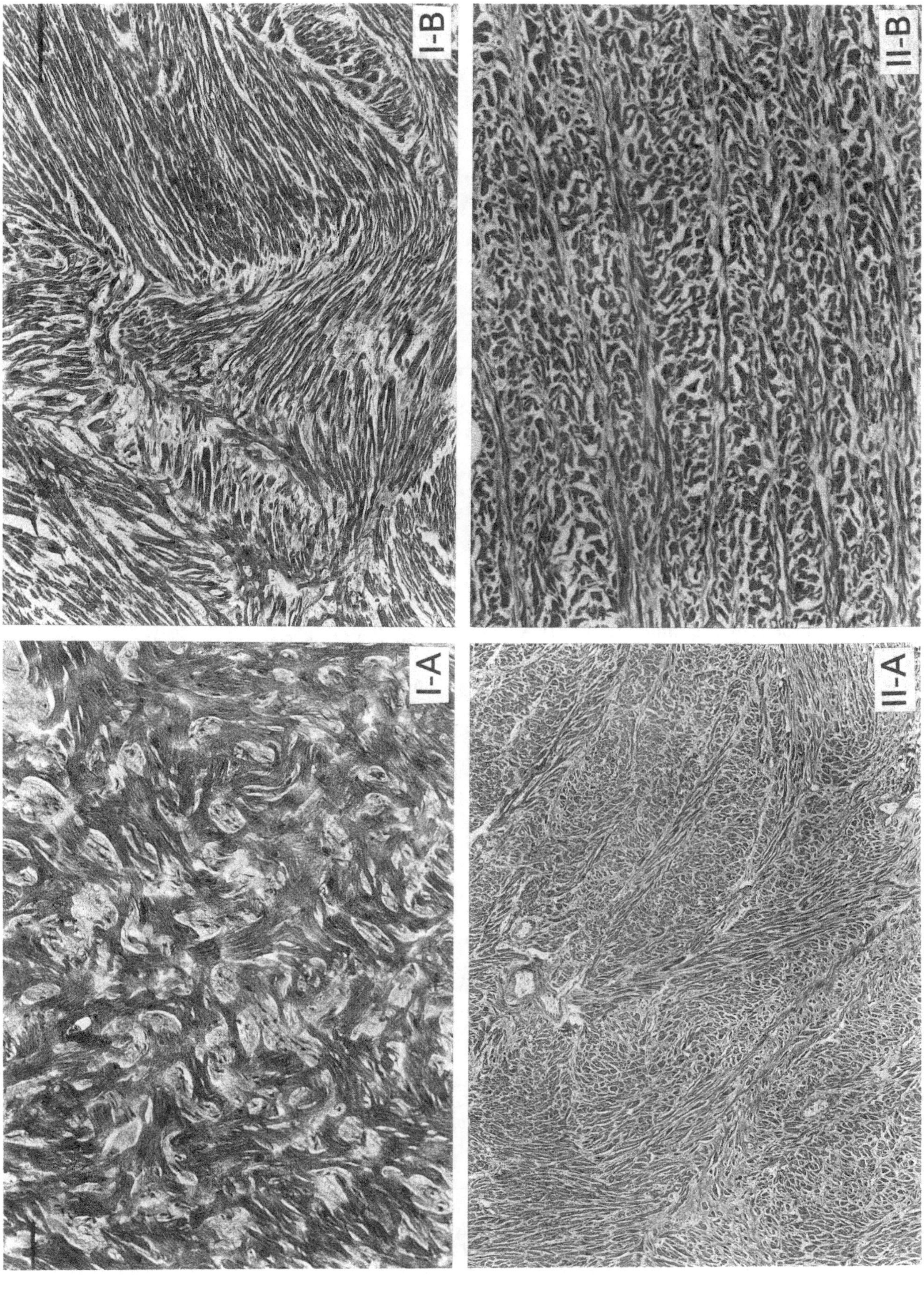
I-B
II-B
I-A
II-A

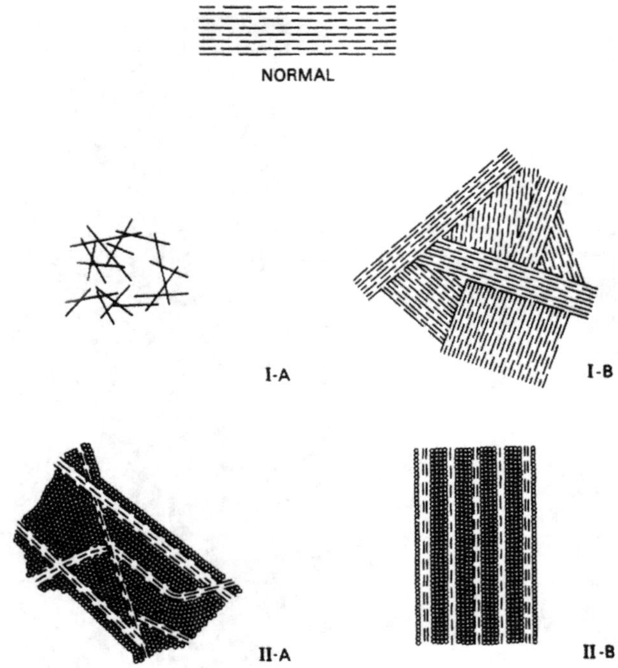

FIGURE 3. *Diagrammatic representation of four major types of cardiac muscle cell disorganization. Compare with photomicrographs in figure 2. Normal arrangement of cardiac muscle cells is shown at the top for comparison.*

appearance.[7] Type II-B was similar to type II-A disorganization, except that the narrow, longitudinally cut bundles of cells were more linear. A fifth type of cardiac muscle cell disorganization (type II-C) was identified in only three control patients; none had hypertrophic cardiomyopathy. This pattern of cardiac muscle cell malalignment showed relatively small "islands" of disorganized, longitudinally cut cells within much larger areas of transversely cut cells (fig. 5). Hence, type II-A, II-B or II-C disorganization involved both longitudinally and transversely cut cardiac muscle cells.

Abnormally arranged cardiac muscle cells were not considered to represent true disorganization if present in the following areas where cells normally converge at acute angles: 1) at or near the junction of ventricular septum with left and right ventricular free walls; 2) in trabeculations; 3) in or at the edges of areas of fibrosis; 4) at points of convergence of major muscle bundles; or 5) adjacent to interstitial spaces containing blood vessels.

Normally Arranged Cardiac Muscle Cells

A definition of cardiac muscle cell disorganization also requires a description of cardiac muscle cell arrangements *not* considered to constitute true abnormalities (fig. 6). Examples of such arrangements include, in addition to cardiac muscle cells in rigidly parallel relation to each other (fig. 6A), 1) minor deviations in alignment from the rigid parallelism shown in figure 6A, which often give cells the appearance of "branching" (fig. 6B); 2) small "fascicles" of cells in areas in which two muscle bundles converge (figs. 6C and D); and 3) artifacts of tissue preparation such as "waviness" (fig. 6E) or "buckling" (fig. 6F). The histologic appearance of "buckled" tissue is probably due to the phenomenon illustrated in figure 7.

Quantitation of Cardiac Muscle Cell Arrangement

We used a technique to assess quantitatively the extent to which cardiac muscle cell disorganization was present in tissue sections of ventricular septum from the 198 hearts. Hematoxylin and eosin-stained tissue sections were photographed and the images were enlarged to occupy 30″ × 40″ positive prints; this resulted in an average magnification of 1,200 times the original tissue section (range in magnification of × 200–5,300) (fig. 8). A transparent cellulose overlay was then placed over the print. Using a marking pen, areas of myocardium occupied by disorganized cardiac muscle cells were outlined on the transparent overlay. Although we could often make this assessment exclusively from direct examination of the print, we frequently had to reexamine the original tissue section with a light microscope to aid in localizing the disorganized area. In addition, areas in which cardiac muscle cells were cut either longitudinally or transversely were demarcated. Large areas of fibrosis (replacement or interstitial), artifacts of tissue preparation or large interstitial spaces with blood vessels also were outlined and ultimately excluded from the analysis. The transparent overlay was then removed from the print, photographed and the image reproduced (with substantial reduction) as a 5 × 7 inch positive print. Each area into which the tissue section had been divided was outlined separately with a fine-point marking pen on ordinary tablet paper. The area of each outlined silhouette was then quantitated using a video planimetry system.[34, 35] We analyzed print enlargements, usually without knowledge of whether the tissue section was from a patient with hypertrophic cardiomyopathy. Often, however, recognition of the patient's disease was unavoidable because a particularly large tissue section strongly suggested the presence of hypertrophic cardiomyopathy.

FIGURE 2. *Classification of four major types of cardiac muscle cell disorganization present in ventricular septal myocardium. Types I-A and I-B exclusively involve cardiac muscle cells cut longitudinally. Types II-A and II-B involve cardiac muscle cells cut either longitudinally or transversely. Magnifications: I-A, × 130; I-B and II-A, × 40, II-B, × 80. These and all tissue sections shown subsequently were stained with hematoxylin and eosin.*

Formulas Used in Quantitative Calculations of Cardiac Muscle Cell Arrangement

The formulas used to calculate the percent area of ventricular septum occupied by disorganized cardiac muscle cells are expressed below; the area of septum "at risk" for disorganization is in the denominator of both equations:

$$\%\text{ area of type I (I-A + I-B) disorganization} = \frac{D_I}{L + D_I} \times 100;$$

$$\%\text{ area of type II (II-A + II-B + II-C)} = \frac{D_{II}}{L + T + D_{II}} \times 100,$$

where L = area occupied by longitudinally cut but normally arranged cells, T = area occupied by transversely cut cells (excluding those incorporated into areas of type II disorganization), D_I = area occupied by type I disorganization, and D_{II} = area occupied by type II disorganization. The percent septal disorganization plotted for each patient was the value for type I or type II disorganization, whichever figure was greater.

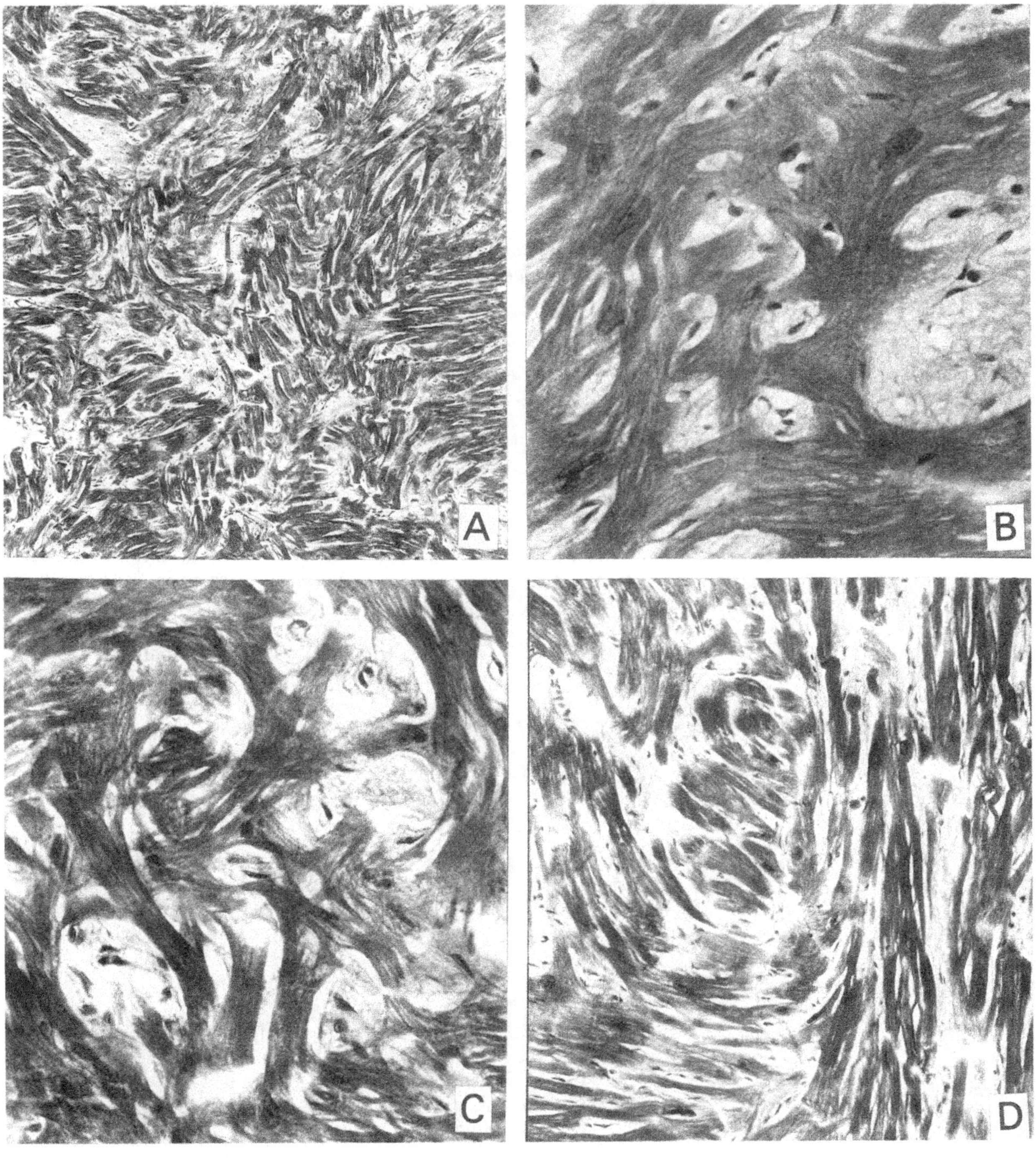

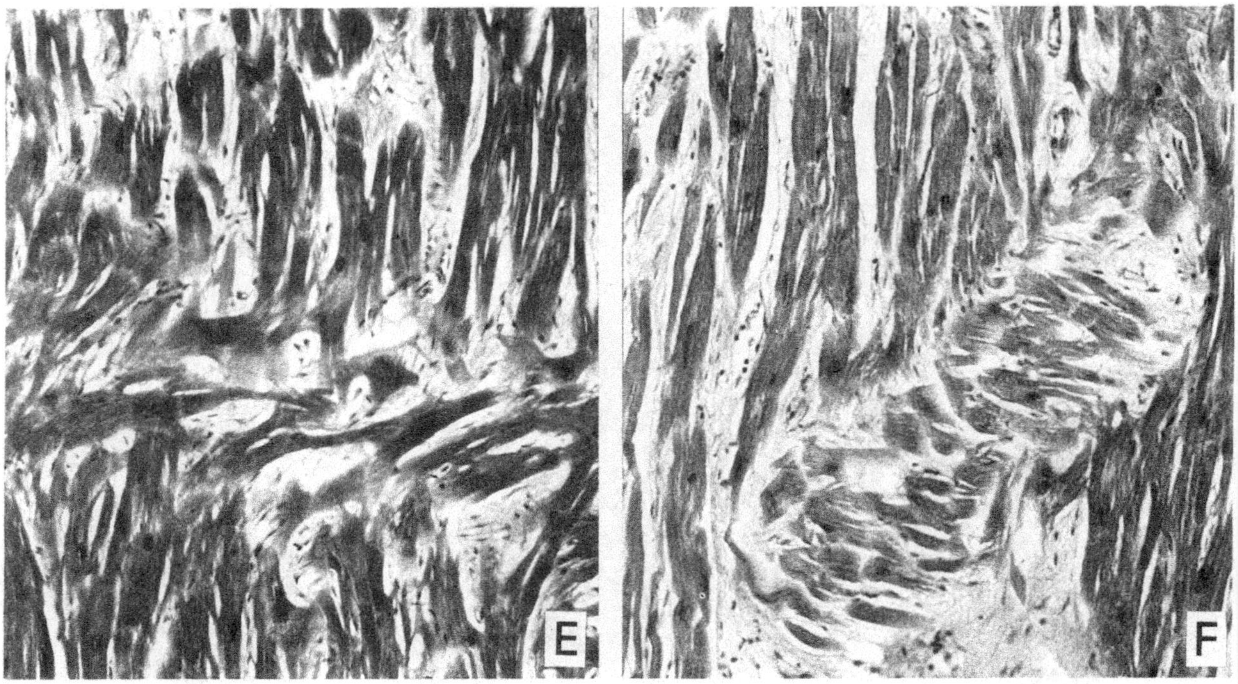

FIGURE 4. *Several examples of type I-A disorganization which illustrate the wide morphologic spectrum of this lesion. A) "Chaotic" pattern in which adjacent cells are arranged at perpendicular and oblique angles to each other (also, see upper left panel in figure 2 for similar example); magnification × 55; B) "Swiss cheese" appearance that results when adjacent cells are oriented at particularly acute angles; magnification × 350; C) Tangled arrangement of cardiac muscle cells in whorled configurations; magnification × 350. D) Whorl pattern in which some cells are oriented circumferentially to other cells; magnification × 130; E) and F) Patterns in which small groups of cells are oriented at extremely acute angles to larger groups of cells; magnification × 130.*

We could not combine values for types I and II disorganization in those patients who had both types, since this calculation often resulted in a marked underestimation of the overall extent of disorganization present in a tissue section. We did not attempt to assess the *degree* to which cells were malaligned in a given area of tissue. Rather, septal disorganization was judged only to be present or absent, and its severity was expressed in terms of extent.

Two other formulas were used to calculate the percent area of longitudinally or transversely cut cardiac muscle cells:*

$$\% \text{ area of longitudinally cut cells} = \frac{L + D_I}{To} \times 100;$$

$$\% \text{ area of transversely cut cells} = \frac{T + D_{II}}{To} \times 100,$$

where L = area occupied by longitudinally cut cells, T = area occupied by transversely cut cells, To = total area of tissue section, D_I = area occupied by type I disorganization (if present), and D_{II} = area occupied by type II disorganization (if present).

*Obliquely cut cells were classified as either longitudinally or transversely cut, depending on the degree of obliquity. Such cells were most commonly present in areas where large bundles of cells came into apposition at acute angles.

Results

Ventricular Wall Thicknesses

Ventricular septal thicknesses and septal-free wall ratios were significantly greater in the patients with hypertrophic cardiomyopathy than in control patients (table 3). In addition, asymmetric septal hypertrophy was present in 42 (78%) of the 54 patients with hypertrophic cardiomyopathy compared with 23 (16%) of the 144 controls (table 3). This latter prevalence figure is similar to that previously reported in necropsy studies of similar groups of hearts.[13, 15]

Quantitative Histologic Findings in Transverse Plane Tissue Sections

The architecture of large muscle bundles was relatively uniform in transverse plane tissue sections. Usually, a narrow bundle of longitudinally cut cardiac muscle cells was present in the center of the tissue section extending from the anterior to the posterior limits of the ventricular septum (fig. 9); this band usually comprised one-third of the overall tissue section area in both patients with hypertrophic cardiomyopathy and controls (table 4). Usually, transversely cut cells were present in the areas on either side of the central band (adjacent to the left and right ventricular cavities); each of these two areas comprised about one-third of the tissue section.

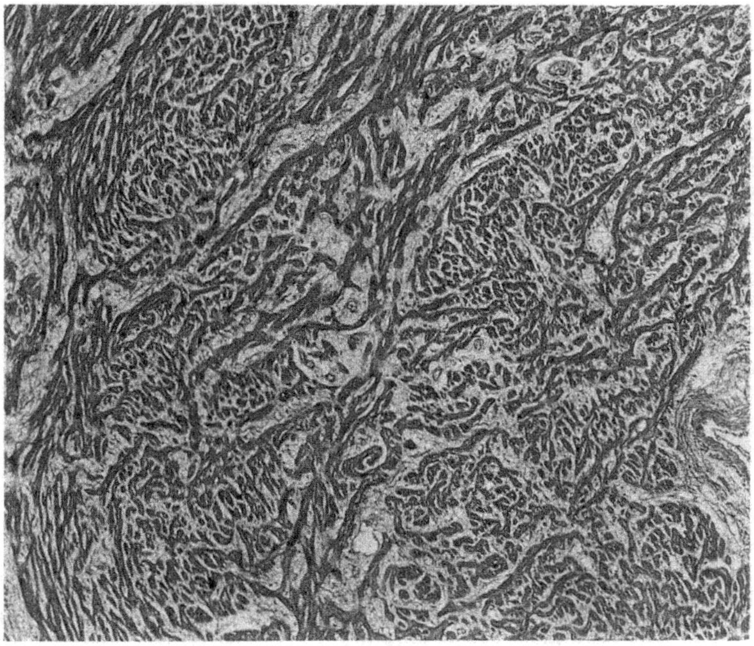

FIGURE 5. *Uncommon fifth type of cardiac muscle cell disorganization (type II-C). Consists of small "islands" of disorganized, longitudinally cut cardiac muscle cells, present within much larger areas of transversely cut cells; magnification × 80.*

Patients with hypertrophic cardiomyopathy and controls differed markedly in the extent of ventricular septal disorganization (fig. 10, table 4). In patients with hypertrophic cardiomyopathy, the percent area of septum disorganized ranged from 0–94% (mean ± SEM 31 ± 3%). In contrast, 109 (76%) of the 144 control patients showed no disorganization. While there was some overlap between control patients and

TABLE 4. *Quantitative Histologic Findings*

Parameter	Hypertrophic cardiomyopathy		Other heart diseases and normals		p
	No. of pts	Mean ± SEM	No. of pts	Mean ± SEM	
Size of septal tissue section (cm²)					
Transverse plane	54	4.7 ± 0.4	144	2.5 ± 0.1	<0.001
Longitudinal plane	25	7.2 ± 0.9	8	4.3 ± 0.9	NS
		p <0.005		p <0.005	
% area longitudinally cut cells in septum					
Transverse plane	54	32 ± 2	144	33 ± 1	NS
Longitudinal plane	25	15 ± 1	8	16 ± 4	NS
		p <0.001		p <0.005	
% area of septum disorganized (transverse plane)					
Type I-A	46	19 ± 3	31	5 ± 1	<0.001
Type I-B	25	33 ± 5	3	27 ± 22	NS
Total type I	51	33 ± 3†‡	32	7 ± 2	<0.001
Type II-A	6	8 ± 2	1	2	—
Type II-B	5	10 ± 2	2	5 ± 0.4	NS
Type II-C	0	—	3	3 ± 2	—
Total type II	10	10 ± 2†	6	3 ± 1	<0.025
Total type I or II§	54	31 ± 3*	144	1.5 ± 0.6	<0.001
% area of septum disorganized (longitudinal plane)					
Type I-A	13	5 ± 1	0	—	—
Type I-B	1	23	0	—	—
Total type I	14	6 ± 2‡	0	—	—
Type II-A	4	14 ± 2	0	—	—
Type II-B	1	8	0	—	—
Total type II	5	12 ± 2	0	—	—
Total type I or II§	25	6 ± 2*	0	—	—

*p <0.001 when these two variables are compared.
†p <0.005 when these two variables are compared.
‡p <0.001 when these two variables are compared.
§Value for % septal disorganization used for each patient was that of either type I or type II disorganization, whichever figure was greater.
Abbreviation: NS = not significant.

those with hypertrophic cardiomyopathy, the mean area of septum disorganized in controls (1.5 ± 0.6%) was significantly less than in patients with hypertrophic cardiomyopathy ($p < 0.001$).

The extent of cardiac muscle cell disorganization in patients with hypertrophic cardiomyopathy compared to patients with other cardiac diseases is illustrated in figures 11–13. Of the 54 patients with hypertrophic cardiomyopathy, 51 (94%) had some disorganization, 48 (89%) had disorganization comprising 5% or more of the relevant part of the tissue section, 30 (56%) had disorganization comprising 25% or more of the section, and 14 (26%) had particularly extensive disorganization involving 50% or more of the section. In contrast, cardiac muscle cell disorganization in the 144 control patients was much less extensive; only 7% of these patients had areas of disorganization comprising 5% or more of the tissue section, and just 1% (two patients) had 25% or more of the section involved (fig. 11). In the control group, significant septal disorganization was most common in patients with aortic valve disease (table 2). However, the percent area of septum disorganized did not differ significantly among control patients with acquired (mean 1.9 ± 0.7%) or congenital heart disease (mean 0.5 ± 0.4%) or normal hearts (mean 1.3 ± 1.2%).

At relatively high magnification (fig. 13A), the small areas of disorganization in some control patients appeared qualitatively identical to the widespread lesions in patients with hypertrophic cardiomyopathy; however, at lower magnification such areas of disorganization were barely discernible and obviously constituted only a small part of the tissue section (fig. 13B).

Each of the 51 patients with hypertrophic cardiomyopathy and septal disorganization had type I (I-A, I-B or both) lesions. Ten of these 51 patients also had type II (II-A, II-B or both) lesions, although in only one patient did the extent of type II disorganization exceed that of type I (17% vs 10%). The percent area of ventricular septum occupied by either type I or type II lesions was significantly greater in patients with hypertrophic cardiomyopathy than in controls (table 4). Furthermore, while individual foci of type I and type II disorganization varied considerably in size, they were usually larger in patients with hypertrophic cardiomyopathy than in controls. Type I-A disorganization generally manifested the greater number of individual foci of disorganization per tissue block; these foci of disordered cells were interspersed among areas of myocardium in which the cells were more normally arranged (fig. 14).

In transverse plane sections from patients with hypertrophic cardiomyopathy or controls, abnormally arranged cells were most common in the middle one-third of the septum,[10] although there was no particular localization of disorganized cells within this area (e.g., anteriorly or posteriorly). However, it is in the middle one-third of the septum that longitudinally cut cells are usually present (fig. 9). Hence, we would expect that disorganization (i.e., the common type I which can only be identified in areas of longitudinally cut cells) would be observed most frequently in the middle one-third of sections taken perpendicular to the long axis of the left ventricle. It was difficult to determine the extent to which disorganization was present in the areas of septum adjacent to the ventricular cavities. Cells in these regions were usually cut transversely, prohibiting identification of type I disorganization. However, analysis of sections taken parallel to the long axis of the left ventricle showed that relatively small foci of disorganization were frequently present (in 14 of 23 patients studied; table 4) in areas adjacent to the ventricular cavities.

Quantitative Histologic Findings in Longitudinal Plane Tissue Sections

In tissue sections obtained parallel to the long axis of the left ventricle, longitudinally cut cardiac muscle cells were located primarily in narrow strips on or near the periphery of the septum, adjacent to the ventricular cavities (fig. 15). These areas occupy a relatively small segment of the overall tissue section (about 15% in patients with hypertrophic cardiomyopathy and in controls; table 4).

The extent of septal disorganization was significantly greater in transverse plane sections (mean 32 ± 4%) than in longitudinal plane sections (6 ± 2%; $p < 0.001$) (fig. 16); in 23 of the 25 patients so analyzed, septal disorganization was more marked in the transverse plane sections. Analysis of only the *longitudinal* plane sections showed that 16 of the 25 patients had no or minimal disorganization (< 5% of the tissue section); hence, the diagnosis of hypertrophic cardiomyopathy could not have been made histologically in the majority of these patients from analysis of these sections alone. However, in 14 of these 16 patients, the *transverse* plane sections showed extensive disorganization (≥ 5%) compatible with the histologic diagnosis of hypertrophic cardiomyopathy.

Correlation of Extent of Septal Disorganization with Other Parameters

Various clinical, hemodynamic and anatomic parameters identified in the 54 patients with hypertrophic cardiomyopathy were analyzed to determine whether there was a correlation with the extent of septal disorganization (in transverse plane sections). There was no relation between extent of septal disorganization and sex, presence or absence of symptoms, duration of symptoms, presence of coronary heart disease or paroxysmal atrial fibrillation, mode of death (sudden vs chronic decompensation), magnitude of left ventricular outflow tract obstruction or left ventricular end-diastolic pressure, heart weight, ventricular septal thickness, septal-free wall ratio, or whether septal myotomy-myectomy had been performed.

However, three variables did show a statistically significant relation with the extent of septal disorganization (table 5). Septal disorganization was significantly greater in patients younger than 18 years of age at death compared with those older than 18 years, although a linear relation did not exist between percent septal disorganization and increasing age. In addition, septal disorganization was more marked in patients who were members of families with "malignant" hypertrophic cardiomyopathy,[36] but less extensive in patients with a documented history of systemic hypertension. Furthermore, no clinical or anatomic parameter appeared to be characteristic of either the six patients with hypertrophic cardiomyopathy who showed no or minimal ($\leq$ 3%) septal disorganization or the five patients with marked ($>$ 70%) disorganization.

Discussion

The findings of this quantitative morphologic study indicate that extensive cardiac muscle cell disorganization in the ventricular septum is a highly specific histologic marker of hypertrophic cardiomyopathy; hence, these data confirm our previous impression, based upon qualitative analysis of septal myocardium from patients with hypertrophic cardiomyopathy or other heart diseases.[2,6-8,12-15] Our data also emphasize that three considerations are most important in assessing the specificity of disorganized septal architecture for patients with hypertrophic cardiomyopathy: 1) well-defined, descriptive morphologic criteria for abnormal cardiac muscle cell arrangement, based on analysis of septal tissue from a wide variety of cardiac diseases, including hypertrophic cardiomyopathy; 2) assessment of the extent of cardiac muscle cell disorganization in quantitative terms; and 3) selection of the optimal tissue section for analysis.

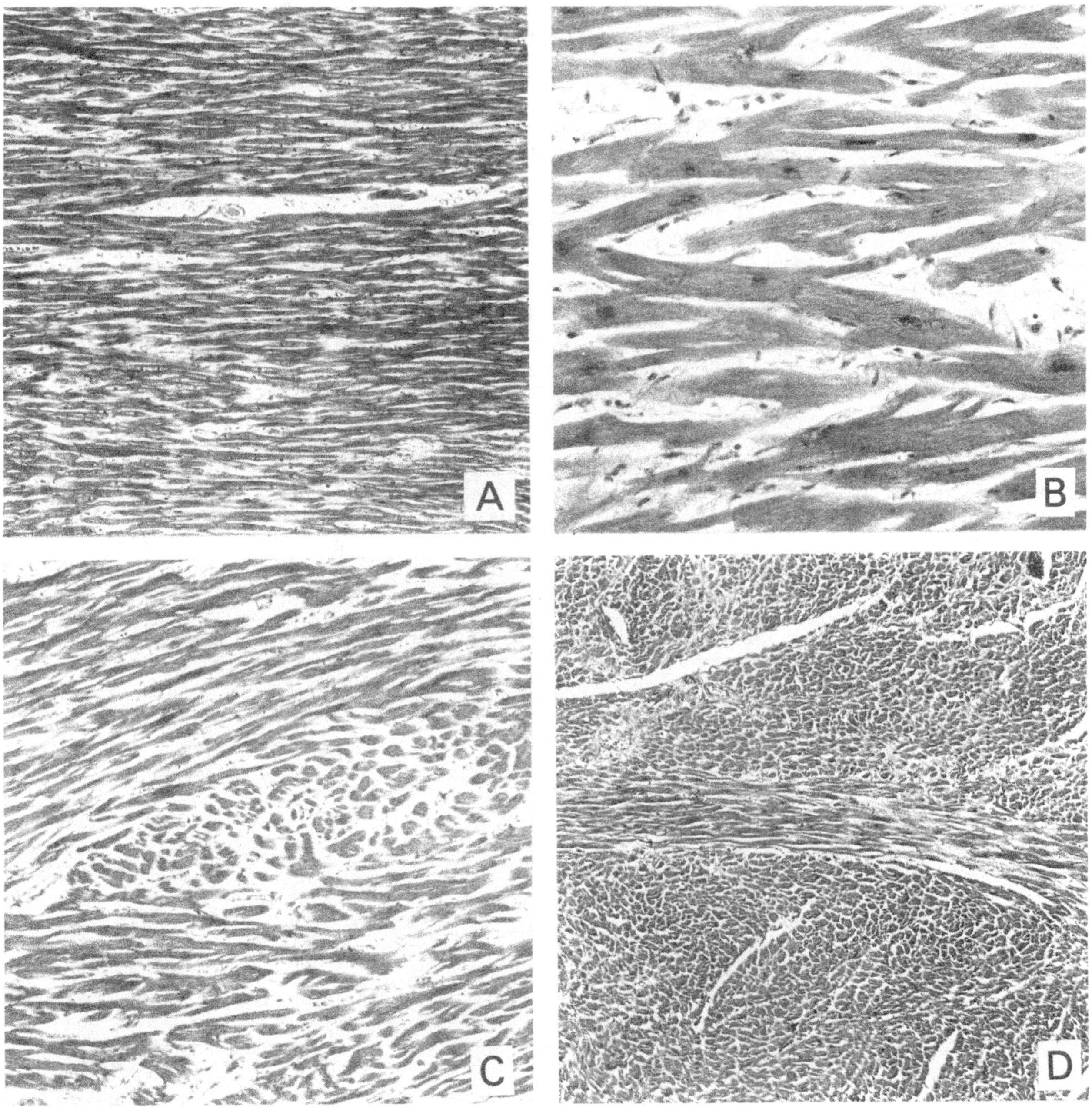

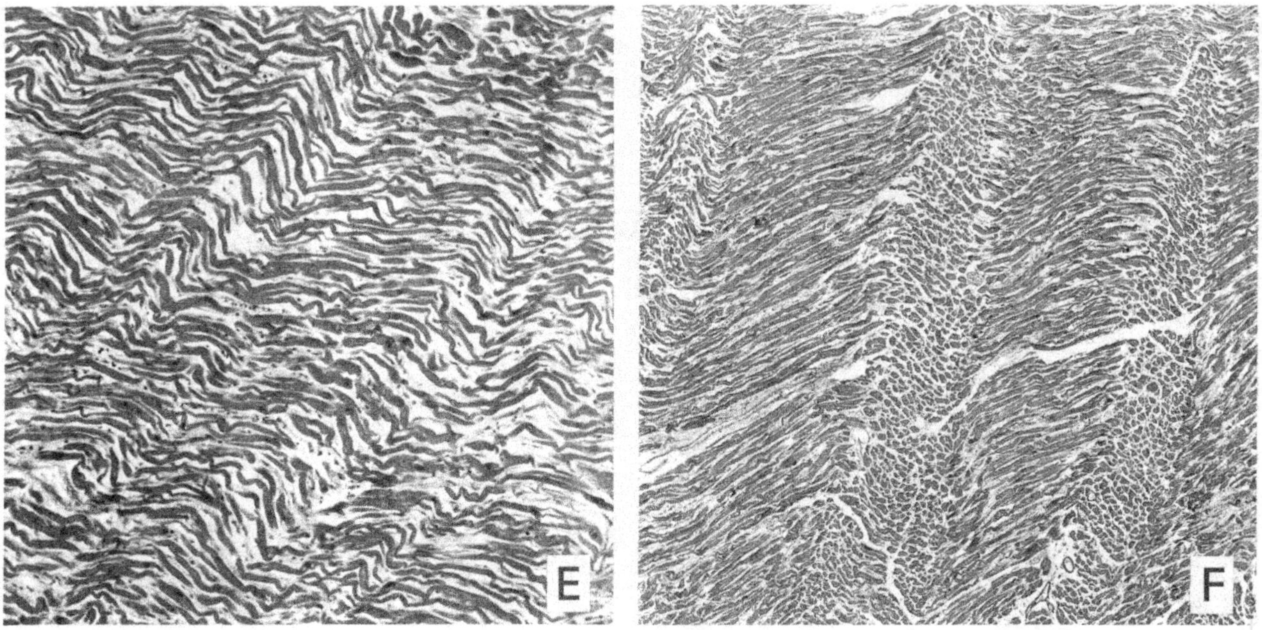

FIGURE 6. *Examples of cardiac muscle cell arrangements that were* not *considered to represent true abnormalities. C) and D) show similar cell arrangement in tissue sections cut perpendicular to each other. Magnifications: A) × 80; B) × 220; C) × 80; D) × 55; E) × 80; and F) × 40.*

First, since there has been no specific, generally accepted definition of what constitutes abnormal cardiac muscle cell arrangement, confusion has arisen among investigators in this field. Perhaps the classification proposed in this study will minimize such problems. Our definition of disorganization is confined to more obvious abnormalities of cellular arrangement, and therefore excludes minimal deviations from parallel alignment. Several recent morphologic studies have concluded that septal disorganization is not a particularly sensitive or reliable marker of hypertrophic cardiomyopathy. However, these studies were based primarily on analysis of patients with heart diseases other than hypertrophic cardiomyopathy.[18-21] Such an experimental design creates a more limited view of what constitutes cardiac muscle cell disorganization than would an analysis that also included a large number of patients with hypertrophic cardiomyopathy, many of whom demonstrate the most extensive and striking examples of cellular disorganization we have observed in septal myocardium.

Second, the quantitative method we used demonstrated that cardiac muscle cell disorganization is characteristically widespread in patients with hypertrophic cardiomyopathy. Almost 90% of our patients had disorganization occupying 5% or more of the relevant part of the tissue section, over 50% of the

TABLE 5. *Clinical Parameters Showing Positive Correlation with Percent Septal Disorganization*

	No. of patients	% septal disorganization	*p*
1. Age (years)			
<18	10	50 ± 9	<0.005
>18	44	27 ± 3	
2. Premature death in >1 family member ("malignant" HCM[36])	8	50 ± 10	<0.05
in 0 or 1 family member	46	28 ± 3	
3. Systemic hypertension*			
Absent	41	34 ± 4	<0.025
Present	5	8 ± 5	

*In eight patients the available history was inadequate to determine reliably whether or not systemic hypertension had been present.

Abbreviations: HCM = hypertrophic cardiomyopathy.

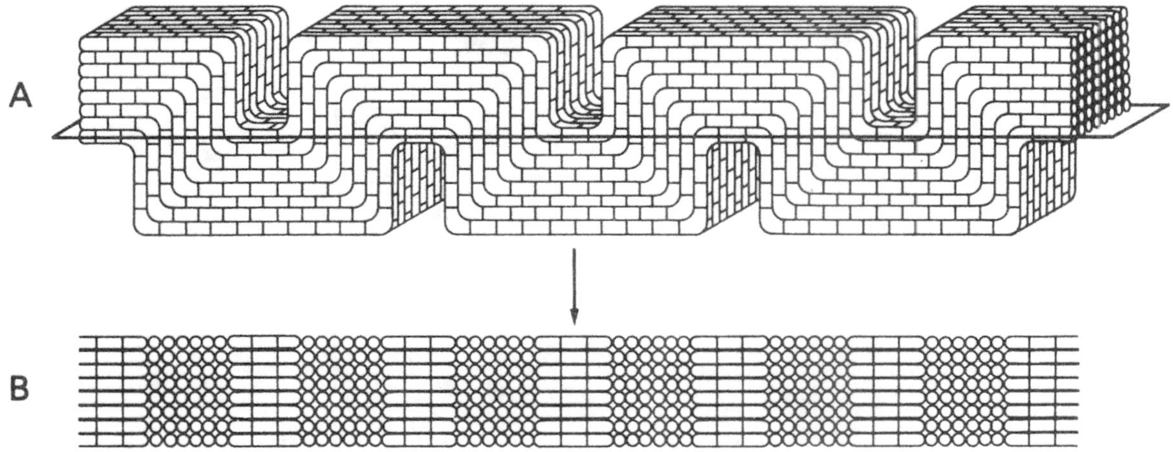

FIGURE 7. *Schematic representation of tissue section "buckling" phenomenon that results in histologic pattern shown in figure 6F. A) View of "buckled" tissue section from the side; solid line denotes the plane of section; B) Lower half of tissue section viewed from above after removal of the upper half. Hence, sectioning this tissue results in the appearance of alternating layers of transversely and longitudinally cut cells.*

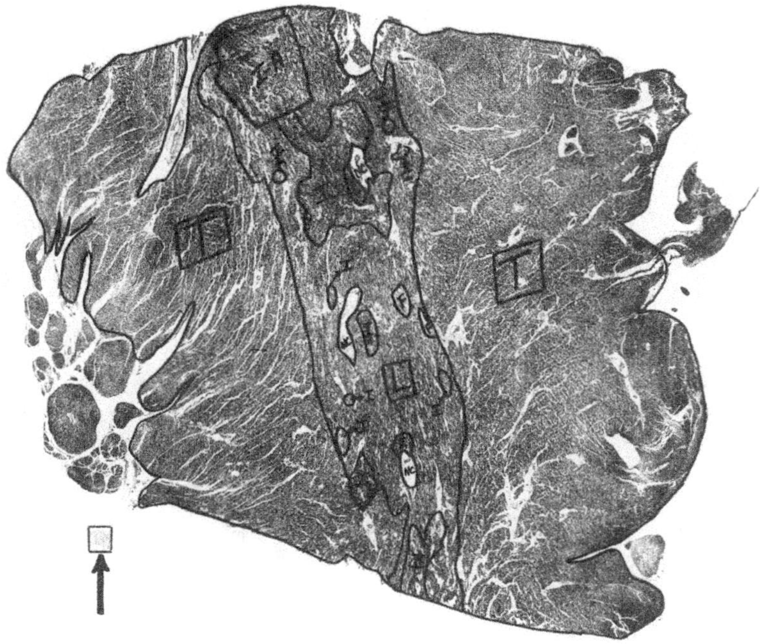

FIGURE 8. *Photographic enlargement (with transparent overlay in place) of a section of ventricular septum from a patient with hypertrophic cardiomyopathy. Actual size of tissue section is shown at lower left (arrow) for comparison. Magnification of the print relative to the original tissue section was 2,000 times.*

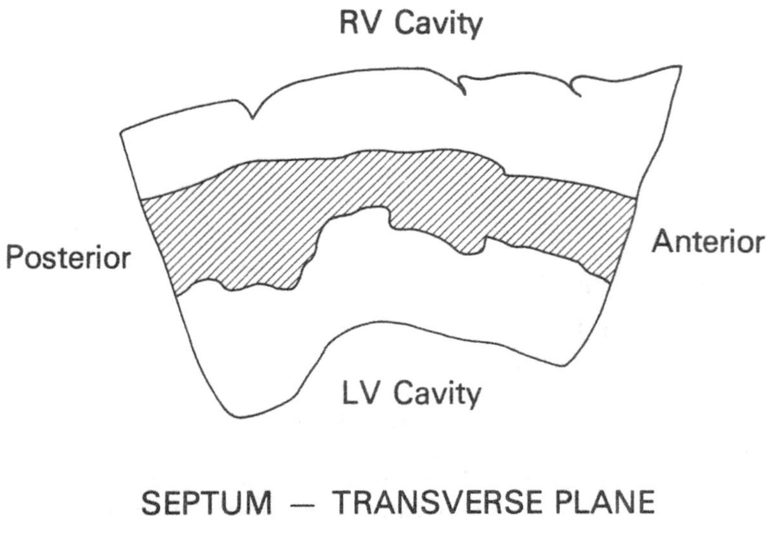

FIGURE 9. *"Map" of transverse plane tissue section from a 16-year-old girl with mitral regurgitation and concentric ventricular hypertrophy. Longitudinally cut cardiac muscle cells, all of which are normally arranged, are present in the relatively narrow striped area in the center of the section.*

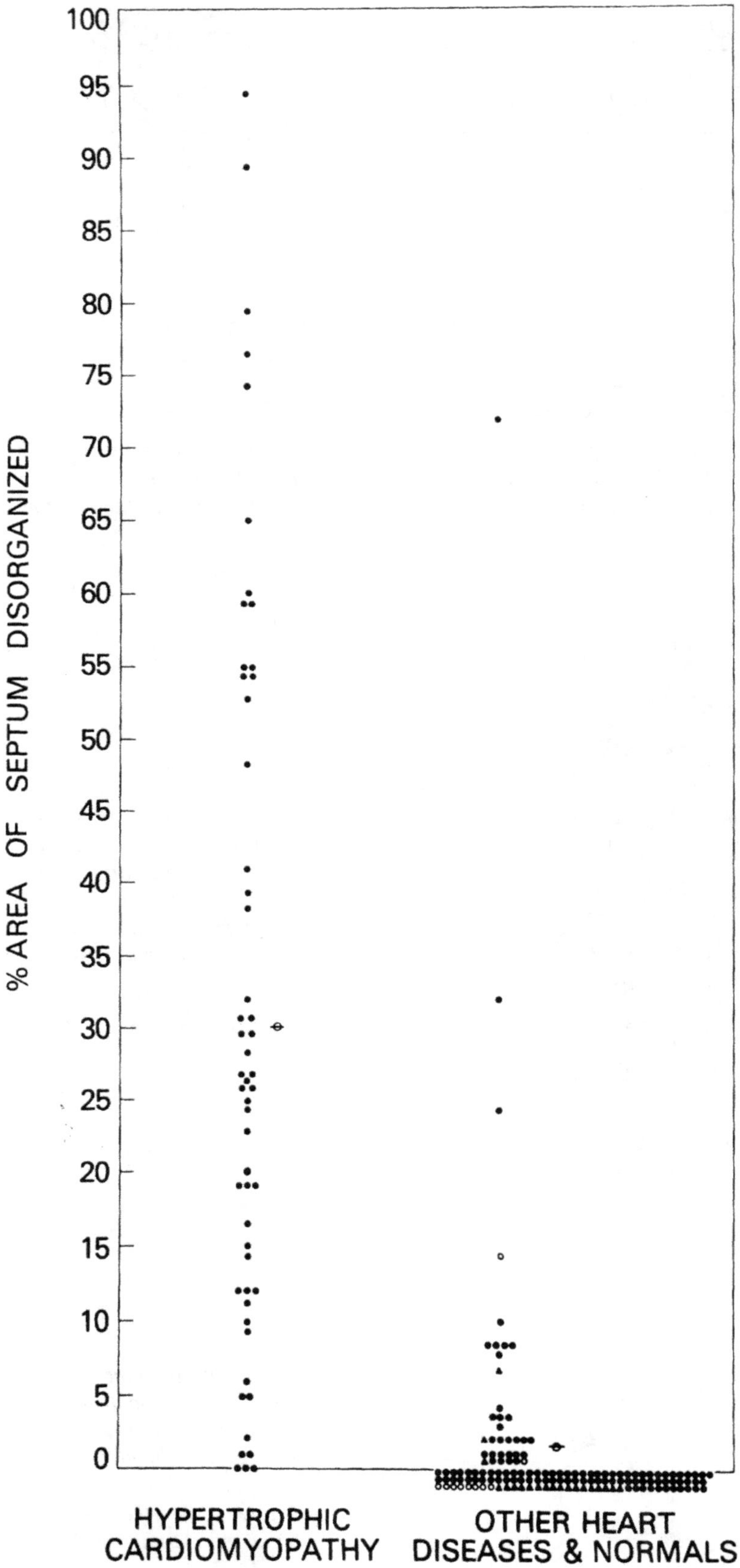

FIGURE 10. *Percent area of ventricular septum occupied by disorganized cardiac muscle cells in 54 patients with hypertrophic cardiomyopathy and 144 control patients. Control subjects with normal hearts are shown by open circles, those with congenital heart disease by triangles, and those with acquired heart disease by solid circles. θ = mean value.*

patients had ≥ 25% of the section involved and over 25% of the patients had more than 50% involved. Nevertheless, the presence per se of cellular disorganization in the ventricular septum is *not* pathognomonic of hypertrophic cardiomyopathy. About 25% of patients with cardiac diseases other than hypertrophic cardiomyopathy or normal subjects showed some disorganization in ventricular septal tissue.

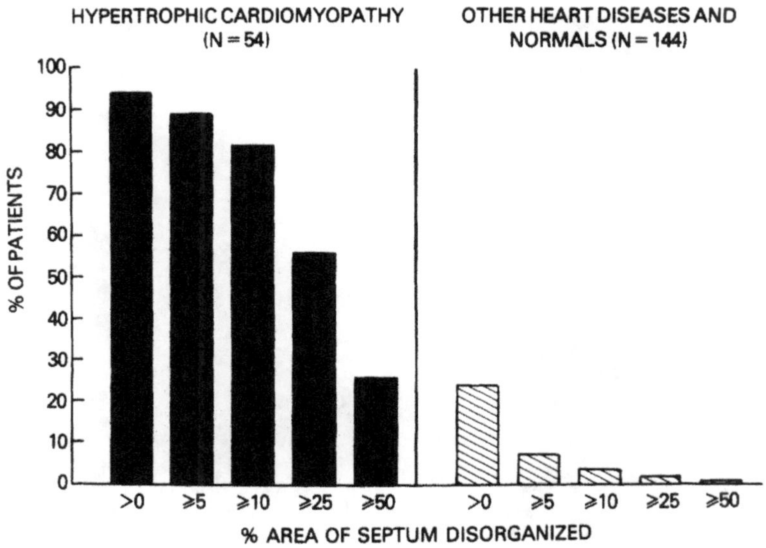

FIGURE 11. *Extent of septal disorganization in 54 patients with hypertrophic cardiomyopathy and 144 controls. Each of the comparisons achieved high statistical significance ($p < 0.001$).*

However, in almost 70% of these patients the areas of disorganization were very small (< 5% of the tissue section analyzed). Hence, it is not the presence or absence of septal disorganization that distinguishes patients with hypertrophic cardiomyopathy from those with other heart diseases histologically, but rather the extent to which disorganization is present.

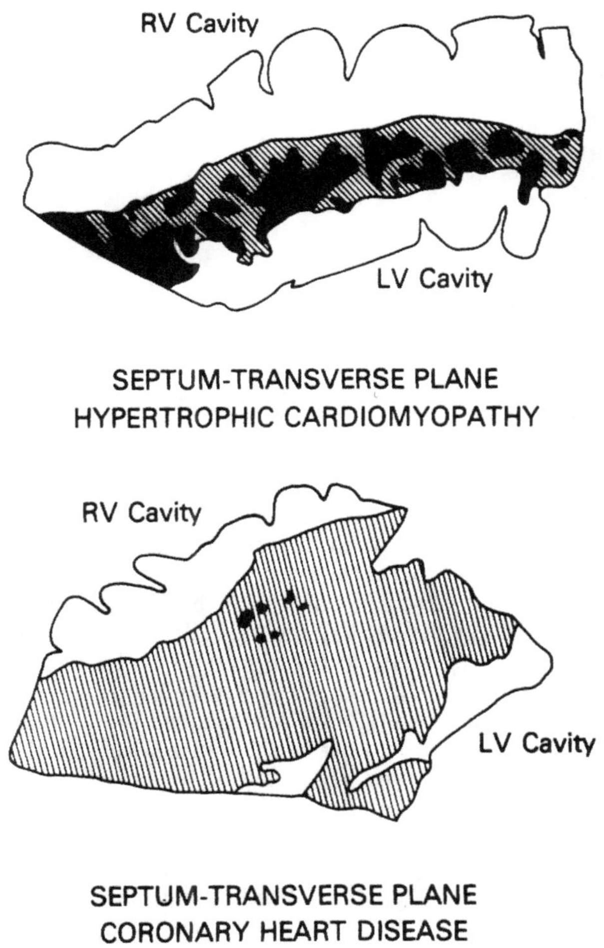

Without comprehensive echocardiographic studies in first-degree relatives, we cannot definitively exclude the possibility that some of the control patients in this study with extensive septal disorganization also had genetically transmitted hypertrophic cardiomyopathy.[13] It is possible that the sole control patient in this study with > 35% septal disorganization actually had hypertrophic cardiomyopathy, particularly since, in addition to her isolated, severe mitral regurgitation, she had marked septal thickening of 25 mm and a septal-free wall ratio of 1.5.

The cut point that appeared to best distinguish patients with hypertrophic cardiomyopathy from patients with other cardiac diseases, histologically, was septal disorganization involving 5% or more of the relevant part of the tissue section. Therefore, septal disorganization of ≥ 5% is consistent with the histologic diagnosis of hypertrophic cardiomyopathy, while septal disorganization of < 5% makes this diagnosis unlikely. Furthermore, if a patient with congenital, valvular, or coronary heart disease had < 5% septal disorganization and a septal-free wall ratio

FIGURE 12. *Representative maps of ventricular septum from two patients with type I-A disorganization. Both sections were obtained in a plane perpendicular to the long axis of the left ventricle. At the top is the septum of a 14-year-old boy with hypertrophic cardiomyopathy. Below is the septum of a 50-year-old man with coronary heart disease and concentric ventricular hypertrophy. Striped areas represent normally arranged cardiac muscle cells cut longitudinally. Clear areas adjacent to the left ventricular (LV) and right ventricular (RV) cavities contain cells cut transversely. Solid areas represent foci of disorganized cardiac muscle cells. In the patient with hypertrophic cardiomyopathy, disorganized cardiac muscle cells occupy about one-half of the relatively small striped area; in contrast, in the patient with coronary heart disease the disorganized areas are very small (both individually and in summation) and together represent less than 1% of the relatively large striped area.*

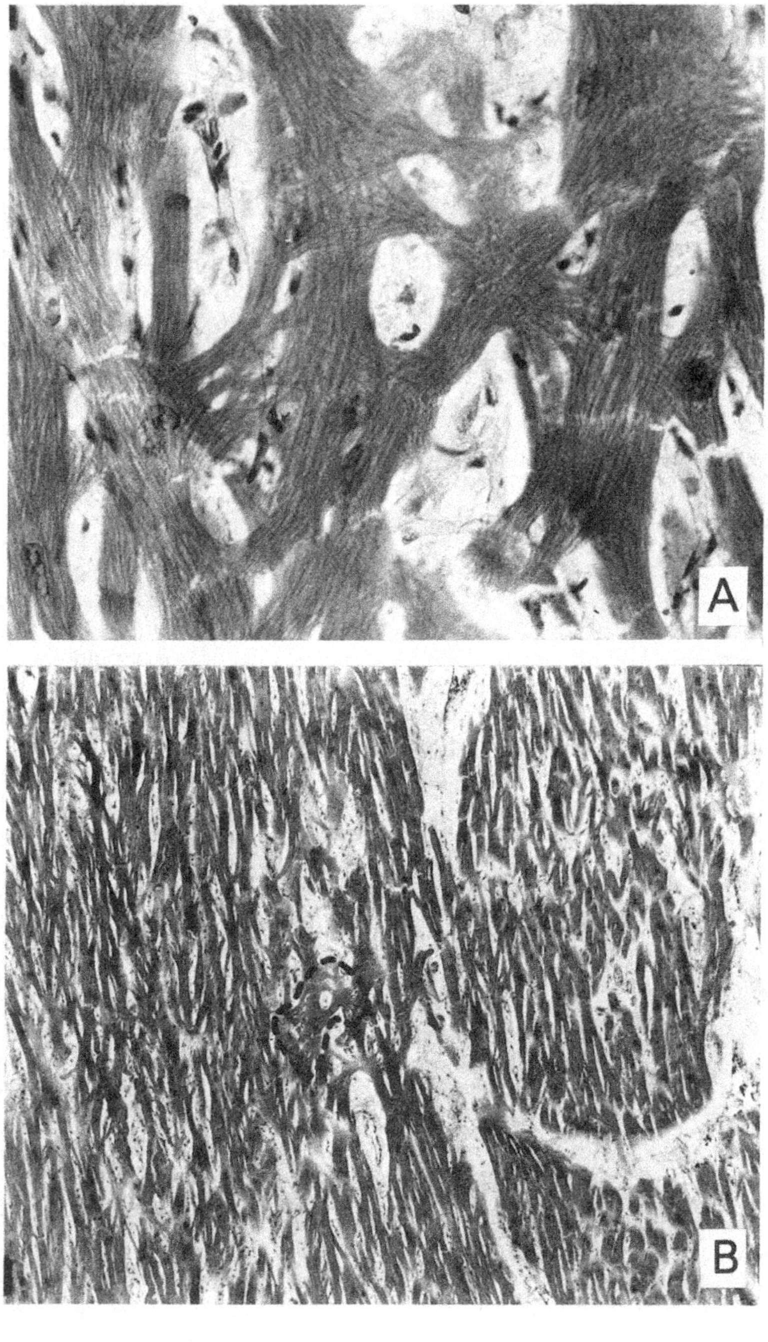

FIGURE 13. *Photomicrographs of the same area of ventricular septal myocardium from a 52-year-old woman with severe valvular aortic stenosis. A) At a relatively high magnification of × 350 an abnormal arrangement of cardiac muscle cells typical of type I-A disorganization is shown. **B)** Same area of myocardium shown at a much lower magnification of × 55; the area of disorganization (outlined by broken line), so impressive at high magnification, is barely discernible here and obviously constitutes an extremely small part of the overall tissue section.*

$<$ 1.3, the chance of hypertrophic cardiomyopathy being present would be virtually nil; only 2% of our control group had both disproportionate septal thickening and $\geq$ 5% septal disorganization.

Third, our data indicate that optimal identification of cellular disorganization depends greatly on selection of the most appropriate tissue section for analysis — i.e., that taken perpendicular to the long axis of the left ventricle. Disorganization was present both more frequently and to a greater extent in transverse plane sections than in longitudinal plane sections. This is apparently related to the fact that longitudinally cut cardiac muscle cells comprise a relatively greater area of tissue sections taken perpendicular to the long axis of the left ventricle than of sections taken parallel to the long axis;[37] hence, the more common type I disorganization, which can only be identified in longitudinally cut cardiac muscle cells, is most likely to be observed in septal tissue sections taken perpendicular to the long axis of the left ventricle.

The present investigation was confined to the study of malalignment *between cardiac muscle cells* in the ventricular septum. Disarray of myofibrils and myofilaments *in* septal muscle cells has also been described in light and electron microscopic studies of plastic embedded tissue from patients with hypertrophic cardiomyopathy. These abnormalities are most pronounced in branched, stellate-shaped and dis-

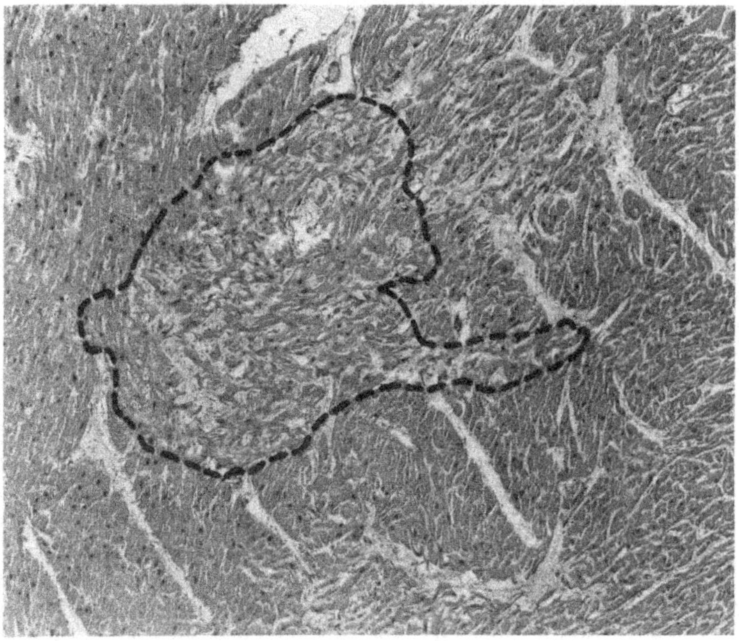

FIGURE 14. *Ventricular septum from a 14-year-old boy with hypertrophic cardiomyopathy. Broken line outlines focus of cardiac muscle cell disorganization. Note that myocardium surrounding this area is normally arranged. Magnification × 40.*

organized cells, but are also found occasionally in cells with more normal shapes and orientation. However, disarray of myofibrils and myofilaments occurs in a variety of cardiac conditions in both man and animals[2, 38-43] and hence, appears to be a relatively nonspecific morphologic alteration. For this reason, and because the histologic techniques we used did not permit reliable identification of myofibrillar and

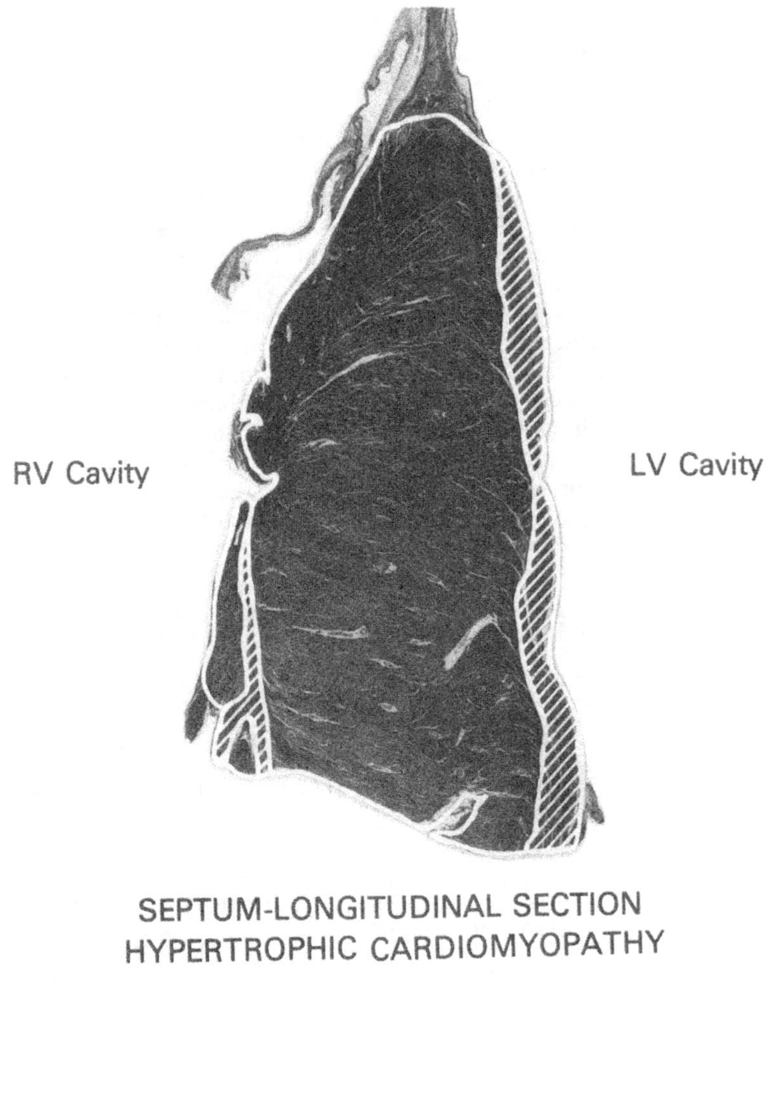

FIGURE 15. *Map of section of ventricular septum obtained parallel to the long axis of the left ventricle superimposed upon actual tissue section. Cardiac muscle cells viewed in longitudinal orientation occupy only the relatively small (striped) areas adjacent to the right ventricular (RV) and left ventricular (LV) cavities (compare with fig. 9). The section is from a 56-year-old woman with hypertrophic cardiomyopathy.*

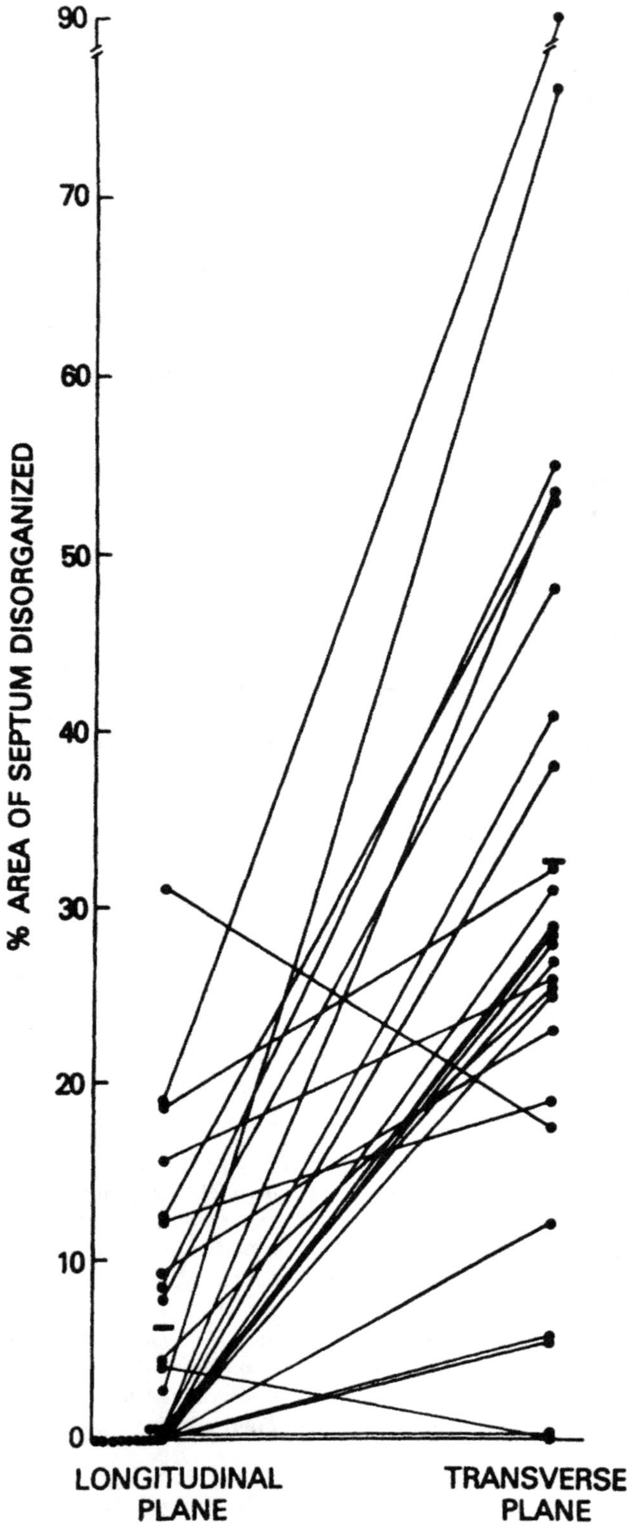

FIGURE 16. *Percent area of ventricular septum occupied by disorganized cardiac muscle cells, shown separately for tissue sections taken in the longitudinal and transverse planes from 23 patients with hypertrophic cardiomyopathy. Symbols for individual patients are connected by solid lines. Mean values are shown by short horizontal lines.*

myofilament disarray, the extent of intracellular disorganization was not analyzed. In addition, we were concerned only with disorganization of cardiac muscle cells in the ventricular septum. Although true cellular disorganization has also been reported in areas of diseased hearts other than the septum, including crista supraventricularis[43, 44] and the left and right ventricular free walls,[8] we did not study this subject in the present investigation.

The potential bias introduced into our data by tissue sample selection must also be considered. All tissue sections from patients with hypertrophic cardiomyopathy and patients with other cardiac diseases were obtained in a standardized fashion and location. However, because of practical considerations related to preservation of necropsy specimens, our data analysis was essentially limited to a single section of ventricular septum from each patient. Because the distribution of cardiac muscle cell disorganization was often "patchy" in the tissue sections analyzed, the theoretical possibility arises that the extent of disorganization might differ significantly in other areas of the ventricular septum not analyzed as part of this study. However, some of our findings suggest that significant variations in disorganization in different areas of the septum do not occur. For example, in four patients with hypertrophic cardiomyopathy and zero or ≤ 3% disorganization, a second transverse plane tissue section (taken 2 cm below the first section) showed an almost identical extent of septal disorganization as observed in the first section.

In conclusion, our data suggest that marked cellular disorganization in septal myocardium links patients within the varied clinical and pathological spectrum of hypertrophic cardiomyopathy; disorganization was present and did not differ significantly in extent in patients with or without symptoms before death, patients with asymmetric or symmetric (concentric) ventricular wall thickening at necropsy, or patients with or without obstruction to left ventricular outflow. Furthermore, the presence or extent of septal disorganization was not related to absolute heart weight; hence, disorganization cannot be considered simply a manifestation of particularly marked cardiac hypertrophy, as occurs in hypertrophic cardiomyopathy. These findings support our hypothesis[8] that extensive cardiac muscle cell disorganization is probably a morphologic manifestation of the underlying genetic defect present in hypertrophic cardiomyopathy.

Acknowledgment

We gratefully acknowledge the valuable assistance provided by Willard C. Whitehouse of the Laboratory of Applied Studies, Division of Computer Research.

References

1. Teare D: Asymmetrical hypertrophy of the heart in young patients. Br Heart J **20**: 1, 1958
2. Ferrans VJ, Morrow AG, Roberts WC: Myocardial ultrastructure in idiopathic hypertrophic subaortic stenosis: a study of operatively excised left ventricular outflow tract muscle in 14 patients. Circulation **45**: 769, 1972
3. Pomerance A, Davies MJ: Pathological features of hypertrophic obstructive cardiomyopathy (HOCM) in the elderly. Br Heart J **37**: 305, 1975
4. Pare JA, Fraser RG, Pirozynski WJ, Shanks JA, Stubington D: Hereditary cardiovascular dysplasia: a form of familial cardiomyopathy. Am J Med **31**: 37, 1961

5. Van Noorden S, Olsen EG, Pearse AG: Hypertrophic obstructive cardiomyopathy. A histological, histochemical and ultrastructural study of biopsy material. Cardiovasc Res **5**: 118, 1971
6. Roberts WC: Valvular, subvalvular and supravalvular aortic stenosis: morphologic features. Cardiovasc Clin **5**: 104, 1973
7. Maron BJ, Edwards JE, Henry WL, Clark CE, Bingle GJ, Epstein SE: Asymmetric septal hypertrophy (ASH) in infancy. Circulation **50**: 809, 1974
8. Maron BJ, Ferrans VJ, Henry WL, Clark CE, Redwood DR, Roberts WC, Morrow AG, Epstein SE: Differences in distribution of myocardial abnormalities in patients with obstructive and nonobstructive asymmetric septal hypertrophy (ASH): light and electron microscopic findings. Circulation **50**: 436, 1974
9. Maron BJ, Henry WL, Clark CE, Redwood DR, Roberts WC, Epstein SE: Asymmetric septal hypertrophy in childhood. Circulation **53**: 9, 1976
10. Wigle ED, Adelman AG, Silver MD: Pathophysiological considerations in muscular subaortic stenosis. *In* Hypertrophic Obstructive Cardiomyopathy, edited by Wolstenholme GE, O'Connor M. London, J and A Churchill, 1971, p 63
11. Knieriem H-J, Stroobandt R, Meyer H, Bouregeois M: Hypertrophic nonobstructive cardiomyopathy caused by disorder of the myofiber texture. Virchows Arch A Pathol Anat Histol **367**: 209, 1975
12. Maron BJ, Edwards JE, Ferrans VJ, Clark CE, Lebowitz EA, Henry WL, Epstein SE: Congenital heart malformations associated with disproportionate ventricular septal thickening. Circulation **52**: 926, 1975
13. Maron BJ, Clark CE, Henry WL, Fukuda T, Edwards JE, Mathews EC, Redwood DR, Epstein SE: Prevalence and characteristics of disproportionate ventricular septal thickening in patients with acquired or congenital heart diseases: echocardiographic and morphologic findings. Circulation **55**: 489, 1977
14. Maron BJ, Edwards JE, Epstein SE: Prevalence and characteristics of disproportionate ventricular septal thickening in patients with systemic hypertension. Chest **73**: 466, 1978
15. Maron BJ, Savage DD, Clark CE, Henry WL, Vlodaver Z, Edwards JE, Epstein SE: Prevalence and characteristics of disproportionate ventricular septal thickening in patients with coronary artery disease. Circulation **57**: 250, 1978
16. Maron BJ, Verter J, Kapur S: Disproportionate ventricular septal thickening in the developing normal human heart. Circulation **57**: 520, 1978
17. Maron BJ, Fisher RS: Sudden infant death syndrome (SIDS): cardiac pathologic observations in infants with SIDS. Am Heart J **93**: 762, 1977
18. Becu L, Somerville J, Gallo A: "Isolated" pulmonary valve stenosis as part of more widespread cardiovascular disease. Br Heart J **38**: 472, 1976
19. Van Der Bel-Kahn J: Muscle fiber disarray in common heart diseases. Am J Cardiol **40**: 355, 1977
20. Somerville J, Becu L: Congenital heart disease associated with hypertrophic cardiomyopathy. Johns Hopkins Med J **140**: 151, 1977
21. Bulkley BH, Weisfeldt ML, Hutchins GM: Asymmetric septal hypertrophy and myocardial fiber disarray: features of normal, developing and malformed hearts. Circulation **56**: 292, 1977
22. Menges H, Brandenburg RO, Brown AL: The clinical, hemodynamic and pathologic diagnosis of muscular subvalvular aortic stenosis. Circulation **24**: 1126, 1961
23. Henry WL, Clark CE, Epstein SE: Asymmetric septal hypertrophy (ASH): echocardiographic identification of the pathognomonic anatomic abnormality of IHSS. Circulation **47**: 225, 1973
24. Abbasi AS, MacAlpin RN, Eber LM, Pearce ML: Echocardiographic diagnosis of idiopathic hypertrophic cardiomyopathy without outflow obstruction. Circulation **46**: 897, 1972
25. Abbasi AS, MacAlpin RN, Eber LM, Pearce ML Left ventricular hypertrophy diagnosed by echocardiography. N Engl J Med **289**: 118, 1973
26. Epstein SE, Henry WL, Clark CE, Roberts WC, Maron BJ, Ferrans VJ, Redwood DR, Morrow AG: Asymmetric septal hypertrophy. Ann Intern Med **81**: 650, 1974
27. Braunwald E, Lambrew CT, Rockoff SD, Ross J, Morrow AG: Idiopathic hypertrophic subaortic stenosis. I. A description of the disease based upon an analysis of 64 patients. Circulation **29** (suppl IV): IV-1, 1964
28. Wigle ED, Heimbecker RO, Gunton RW: Idiopathic ventricular septal hypertrophy causing muscular subaortic stenosis. Circulation **26**: 325, 1962
29. Morrow AG, Fogarty TJ, Hannah H, Braunwald E: Operative treatment in idiopathic hypertrophic subaortic stenosis. Techniques and the results of preoperative and postoperative clinical and hemodynamic assessments. Circulation **37**: 589, 1968
30. Goodwin JF, Hollman A, Cleland WP, Teare D: Obstructive cardiomyopathy simulating aortic stenosis. Br Heart J **22**: 403, 1960
31. Maron BJ, Roberts WC, Edwards JE, McAllister HA, Foley DD, Epstein SE: Sudden death in patients with hypertrophic cardiomyopathy: characterization of 26 patients without previous functional limitation. Am J Cardiol **41**: 803, 1978
32. Maron BJ, Henry WL, Roberts WC, Epstein SE: Comparison of echocardiographic and necropsy measurements of ventricular wall thicknesses in patients with and without disproportionate septal thickening. Circulation **55**: 341, 1977
33. Gould SE: Pathology of the heart and blood vessels, 3rd ed. Springfield, Charles C Thomas, 1968, p 1139
34. Marcus ML, Schuette WH, Whitehouse WC, Bailey JJ, Douglas MA, Glancy DL: Use of a video system in the study of ventricular function in man. Am J Cardiol **32**: 175, 1973
35. Dvorak JA, Schuette WH, Whitehouse WC: A simple video method for the quantification of microscopic objects. J Microsc **102**: 71, 1974
36. Maron BJ, Lipson LC, Roberts WC, Savage DD, Epstein SE: "Malignant" hypertrophic cardiomyopathy: identification of a subgroup of families with unusually frequent premature deaths. Am J Cardiol **41**: 1133, 1978
37. Streeter DD, Spotnitz HM, Patel P, Ross J, Sonnenblick EH: Fiber orientation in the canine left ventricle during diastole and systole. Circ Res **24**: 339, 1969
38. Adomian GE, Beazell JW, Furmanski M, Tan KS, Laks MM: The production of myofibrillar disarray in hearts of normal dogs produced by chronic electronic pacing. (abstr) Circulation **56** (suppl III): III-204, 1977
39. Olsen EGJ: Postmortem findings and histologic, histochemical and electron microscopic findings of myocardial biopsies. *In* Cardiomyopathy and Myocardial Biopsy, edited by Kaltenbach M, Loogen F, Olsen EGJ. Berlin, Springer-Verlag, 1978, p 52
40. Knieriem H-J: Electron-microscopic findings in congestive cardiomyopathy. *In* Cardiomyopathy and Myocardial Biopsy, edited by Kaltenbach M, Loogen F, Olsen EGJ. Berlin, Springer-Verlag, 1978, p 71
41. Kunkel B, Kober G, Kaltenbach M: Ultrastructural evaluations in early and advanced congestive cardiomyopathies, *In* Cardiomyopathy and Myocardial Biopsy, edited by Kaltenbach M, Loogen F, Olsen EGJ. Berlin, Springer-Verlag, 1978, p 87
42. Hibbs RG, Ellison JP: The atrioventricular valves of the guinea pig. II. An ultrastructural study. Am J Anat **138**: 347, 1973
43. Jones M, Ferrans VJ, Morrow AG, Roberts WC: Ultrastructure of crista supraventricularis muscle in patients with congenital heart diseases associated with right ventricular outflow tract obstruction. Circulation **51**: 39, 1975
44. Maron BJ, Ferrans VJ, White RI: Unusual evolution of acquired infundibular stenosis in patients with ventricular septal defect: clinical and morphologic observations. Circulation **48**: 1092, 1973

Congenital Cardiovascular Abnormalities Usually "Silent" until Adulthood: Morphologic Features of the Floppy Mitral Valve, Valvular Aortic Stenosis, Discrete Subvalvular Aortic Stenosis, Hypertrophic Cardiomyopathy, Sinus of Valsalva Aneurysm, and the Marfan Syndrome

William C. Roberts, M.D.

Congenital heart disease most commonly consists of *defects* (absent tissue) in cardiac septa causing shunts, *obstructions* (excess tissue) at or near valvular levels, *anomalous connections* between arteries and veins or between arteries or veins and cardiac chambers, and *combinations* of these three malformations. Less commonly, a congenital cardiovascular malformation consists of an improperly formed tissue which functions normally or almost normally at birth and during the early decades of life, but later causes cardiac dysfunction. This chapter describes certain morphologic features in six of these conditions.

FLOPPY ATRIOVENTRICULAR VALVE

Delineation of the click-late systolic murmur syndrome was a major addition to cardiologic knowledge in the 1960s.[1-5] It is now apparent that the click-late systolic murmur is common, probably occurring in 5 percent or more of persons older than 15 years.[6,7] Although generally not considered as such, the click-systolic murmur syndrome, probably in the majority of persons, is a form of congenital heart disease and, therefore, is the most common congenital heart disease. The auscultatory manifestations, however, are usually not manifest until adulthood.

The click-murmur syndrome may be viewed from both auscultatory and morphologic standpoints as manifesting three stages (Fig. 1): (1) systolic click(s) only, (2) click(s) plus a mid-to-late systolic murmur, and (3) pansystolic murmur only. Although progression from stage one to stage three has been documented in relatively few patients, it appears likely that this is the natural sequence of events in some patients. In others, there may be no progression from stage 1; patients in stage 2 may revert to stage 1; patients in stage 1 may lose their click(s) altogether; and patients appearing in stage 3 (pansystolic murmur) may have had no documentation of stages 1 and 2. This condition in stages 1 and 2 is usually unassociated with symptomatic evidence of cardiac dysfunction; the rare exceptions are patients with arrhythmias and/or chest pain. Patients in stage 3 may have congestive heart failure because of the associated severe mitral regurgitation. The stage 3 floppy mitral valve appears to be a major cause, possibly the most common, of severe *pure* mitral regurgitation requiring valve replacement. As a consequence, there is considerable anatomic information available on the floppy mitral valve which produces a pansystolic murmur (stage 3) and causes severe mitral regurgitation.[8-18] In contrast, there is relatively little anatomic information available in patients with systolic click(s) only (stage 1) or those with both click(s) and late systolic murmur (stage 2).

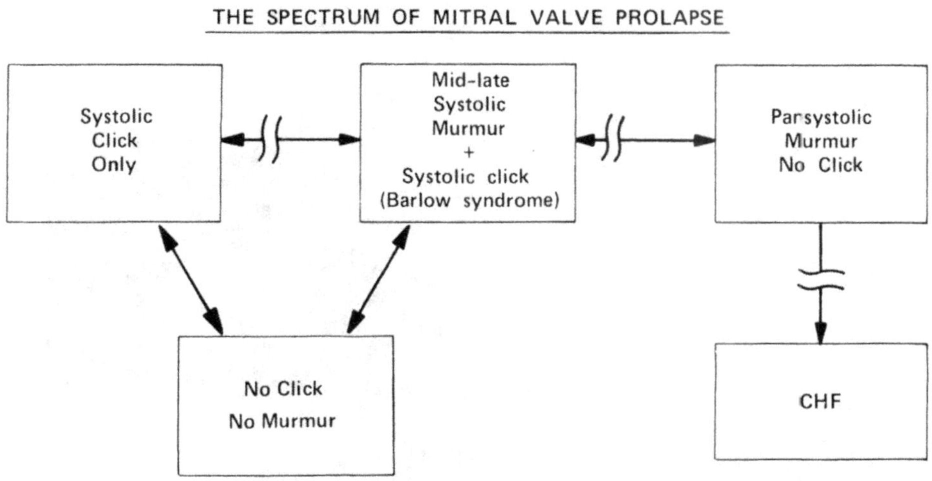

Figure 1. Diagram showing likely auscultatory progression in the prolapsing mitral valve syndrome. CHF = congestive heart failure.

Several names applied to this syndrome describe to some extent what the valve looks like anatomically; "prolapsing posterior mitral leaflet," "prolapsing mitral valve," "billowing or ballooning mitral leaflet syndrome," "overshooting or hooded mitral valve," "floppy mitral valve," and "myxomatous" or "mucinous degeneration of the mitral valve." The common anatomic denominator of the floppy mitral valve is either *excessive leaflet tissue* or *excessive length of chordae tendineae,* or both. Of these, the most common is excessive leaflet tissue. The excess most commonly results from an increase in the transverse or commissure-to-commissure dimension of the leaflet (width). This excess may be focal, involving only a portion of one or both leaflets, or it may be diffuse, involving both leaflets but not necessarily uniformly. The increase in transverse dimension causes the circumferences of the leaflets, measured on a line corresponding to the distal margin of the posterior leaflet, to be much larger than the circumference of the mitral valve anulus; in the normal valve the two are equal. The result is analogous to an accordian not fully extended, or better, a skirt gathered at the waist. The leaflets or the opened normal mitral valve are flat or smooth (like the mucosa of the ileum) whereas those of the opened floppy mitral valve are undulating (like the mucosa of the duodenum or jejunum).

Excessive leaflet tissue also results when there is an increase in the longitudinal or base-to-distal margin dimension of the leaflet (length). Again, this increase may be focal, involving portions of one or both leaflets, or diffuse when both leaflets are involved throughout, though not necessarily uniformly. In some patients there may be an increase in both the transverse and longitudinal dimensions of the leaflets.

Excessive length of chordae tendineae may be an additional cause of mitral valve prolapse. Again, all chordae may be elongated (diffuse) or just a few of them (focal). Elongation of chordae by itself is probably the least frequent mechanism of prolapse. In some patients there appears to be both excessive leaflet tissue and excessive length of chordae tendineae.

Opportunities for structural study of a mitral valve associated with click(s) only have been extremely rare. Figure 2 depicts such a valve. This child was examined while alive by Dr. John Barlow of Johannesburg, South Africa, who by auscultation heard three systolic clicks and no precordial murmur. The child had no symptoms of cardiac dysfunction and died of leukemia; necropsy revealed a perfectly competent mitral valve but three distinct foci where leaflet overlapped adjacent leaflet. The leaflets otherwise were

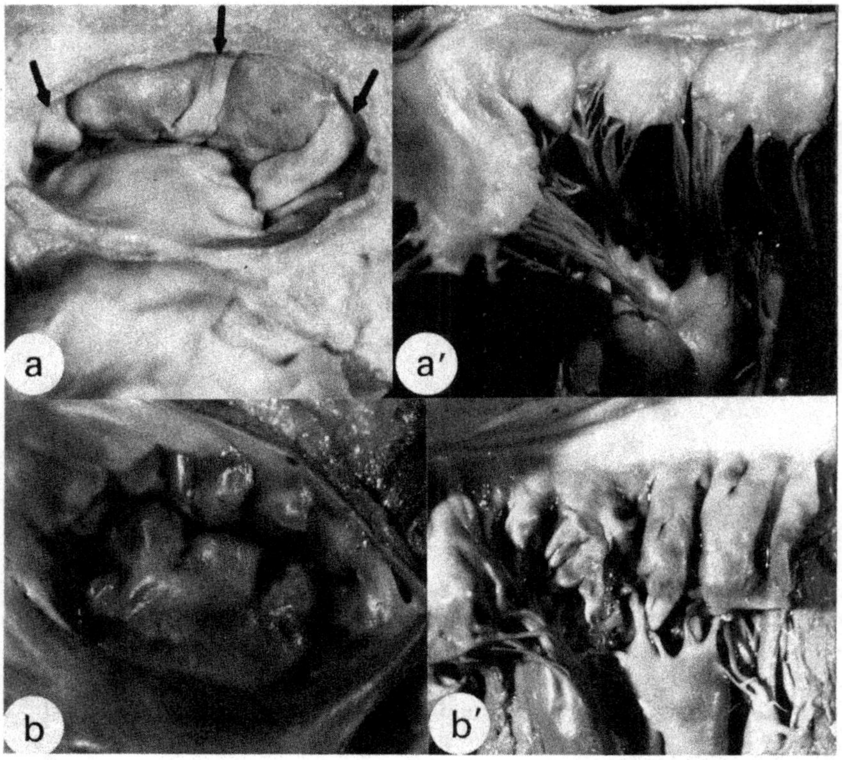

Figure 2. Mitral valves of two children, aged 9 and 13, who died of leukemia. Neither had symptoms of cardiac dysfunction. *a* and *a'*, Mitral valve as viewed from left atrium (a) and after opening (a'). Three areas of leaflet overlap (arrows) are present with the valve intact and the orifice is competent. The leaflets are devoid of scallops and relatively smooth (a'). This child had three systolic clicks during life but no precordial murmur. *b* and *b'*, Mitral valve as viewed from left atrium (b) and after opening (b'). Both leaflets of this valve, in contrast to the valve above, are highly scalloped causing the orifice to be incompetent. This child had a systolic click and a late systolic murmur. (The children whose valves are shown here were examined by Dr. John Barlow in Johannesburg, South Africa, and the auscultatory findings described above were those of Dr. Barlow. I am indebted to him for allowing me to photograph each of these hearts.)

smooth and notably devoid of so-called scallops. There are no reported anatomic descriptions, to my knowledge, of mitral valves producing one or more systolic clicks without an associated precordial systolic murmur. I recently learned, however, of a young woman in her 20s who had, on different occasions, one or more systolic clicks without murmur, associated with recurring arrhythmias. She died during an arrhythmia and a competent pathologist described the mitral valve at necropsy as "entirely normal."

The opportunity to examine the mitral valves (at necropsy) of patients who had systolic click(s) plus a mid-to-late systolic murmur (Barlow syndrome) also is infrequent since this stage is usually asymptomatic. Death in stage 2—as in stage 1—is usually from a noncardiac cause. The mitral valves of three such patients are illustrated in Figures 2 to 4. In this stage the most characteristic feature is leaflet scalloping, which represents excessive leaflet due to an increase in the transverse or commissure-to-commissure dimension of the leaflet. The mitral anulus, as in stage 1, is not dilated. The chordae tendineae may or may not be elongated and they may even be shorter than normal.

The major anatomic characteristic of stage 3 "floppiness" is dilatation of the mitral anulus.[19] Normally, the mitral anulus in adults measures about 9 cm. in circumference.

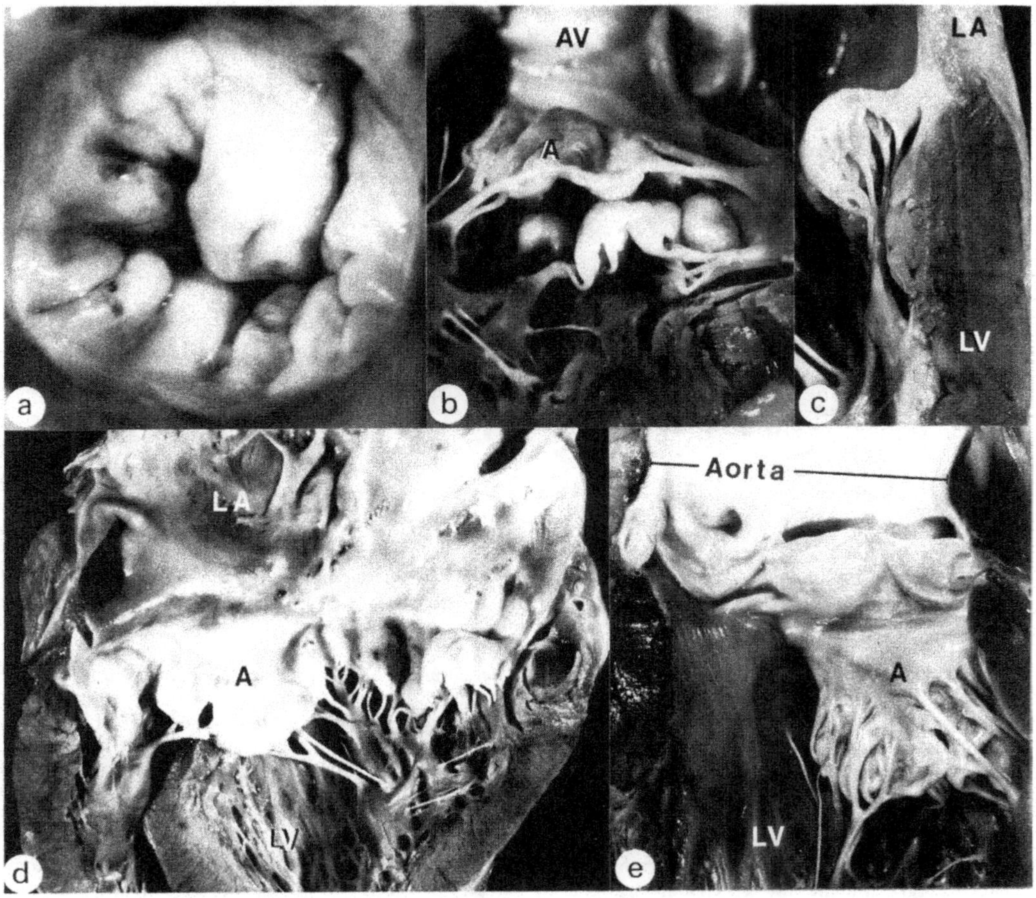

Figure 3. *Floppy mitral valve* in an 18-year-old girl who died of Ewing's sarcoma. She never had symptoms of cardiac dysfunction despite an active life. She had a mid-systolic click and a grade 3/6, ejection-type systolic murmur over the precordium, loudest over the apex. Necropsy revealed Ebstein's anomaly of the tricuspid valve. The mitral valve leaflets shown are elongated transversely, but the chordae are not elongated. *a,* Mitral valve as viewed from left atrium showing marked scalloping. *b,* Same valve as viewed from left ventricle. (A = anterior mitral leaflet; AV = aortic valve) *c,* Longitudinal section of left atrium (LA), billowing posterior mitral leaflet and left ventricle (LV). *d,* Opened mitral valve. *e,* View of anterior mitral leaflet (A) from the left ventricular (LV) aspect. The mitral leaflets and chordae tendineae contained excessive amounts of acid mucopolysaccharide material.

In patients with left ventricular dilatation from any cause with or without mitral regurgitation, the circumference of the mitral anulus usually dilates slightly, to about 11 cm. or less than 25 percent.[19] Among patients with floppy mitral valves associated with severe mitral regurgitation, the circumference of the mitral anulus generally increases by well over 50 percent of normal dimensions (15 to 18 cm.).[19] When the anulus dilates to this extent, the leaflets may "stretch" or flatten transversely, and this stretching diminishes the amount of scalloping. In addition, the left ventricular dilatation may cause longitudinal stretching of the leaflets. The amount of scalloping in the stage 3 valves, therefore, appears to be less than that observed in the stage 2 valves.

Microscopically, the floppy mitral valve leaflets contain an excessive amount of acid mucopolysaccharide material. Both the normal and the floppy mitral leaflet consists of two elements, the fibrosa and the spongiosa. The fibrosa consists of fibrous tissue (collagen), and the spongiosa, of mucoid or myxomatous material high in acid

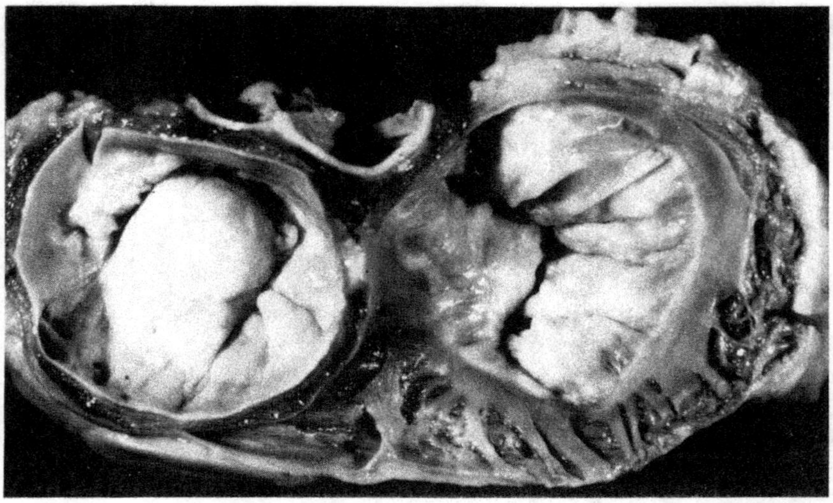

Figure 4. *Floppy mitral valve* (left) and *floppy tricuspid valve* (right) in a 51-year-old man who died suddenly at a dance. Although always asymptomatic, he was found to have a precordial systolic murmur when he was 36 years old. When evaluated about one year before death, he had a systolic murmur; echocardiogram disclosed the classic "hammocking" of the mitral leaflets during ventricular systole, and left ventricular angiography also showed "classic" mitral leaflet prolapse during ventricular systole.

At necropsy, at least one third of the posterior mitral leaflet had prolapsed toward left atrium; several chordae tendineae to this prolapsed segment were thickened and a few were absent, indicating that rupture had occurred. The anterior mitral leaflet appeared normal from the left ventricular aspect, but from the left atrial aspect it was thickened as a result of abnormal contact by the large prolapsed segment of posterior leaflet. All chordae tendineae from the anterior leaflet were elongated, whereas those from the posterior leaflet were thickened. The tricuspid-valve leaflets also were elongated but only mildly thickened compared to the mitral leaflets. There was no clinical evidence of dysfunction of the tricuspid valve. Both atria were mildly dilated. The coronary arteries were normal in course and size and free of significant luminal narrowing. The myocardial walls were free of foci of necrosis or fibrosis.

This case is an example of sudden death in a previously asymptomatic patient with classical auscultatory, echocardiographic and left ventricular angiographic features of the systolic click–late systolic murmur syndrome.

mucopolysaccharide material. In most valve diseases the fibrosa element proliferates and may entirely replace the spongiosa element. In the floppy mitral valve the spongiosa element comprises the more central portion of the leaflet, and appears to proliferate with a far less proportional increase in the fibrosa element. The resulting proliferated myxoid or myxomatous stroma, however, does not appear abnormal, i.e., degenerated, simply increased in amount. Thus, the term myxoid or myxomatous "degeneration" for this condition is not appropriate. The fibrosa element makes up the periphery of the leaflet, and is also increased focally in this condition. The fibrosa element may be subdivided into two components, the *auricularis,* which normally is a thin layer forming the atrial or contact aspect of the leaflet, and the *ventricularis,* which normally is a relatively thick layer which covers the ventricular aspect of the leaflet. The atrial aspect of the floppy mitral leaflet often is focally thickened. This change is considered secondary to abnormal friction from contact between the prolapsed segment of the leaflet and its "opposite number," i.e., the other leaflet, or between two prolapsed segments of the same leaflet.[17,18] The changes on the ventricular surface of the leaflet consist of connective tissue "pads" forming primarily in the interchordal segments. This proliferation of fibrous tissue may extend into adjacent chordae tendineae and onto ventricular endocardium behind the posterior mitral leaflet.[18] The interchordal collections of fibrous tissue are considered responses to the tension and stretching that occurs at the undersurface of prolapsed leaflet or segment of leaflet.[18] This increase in fibrous tissue,

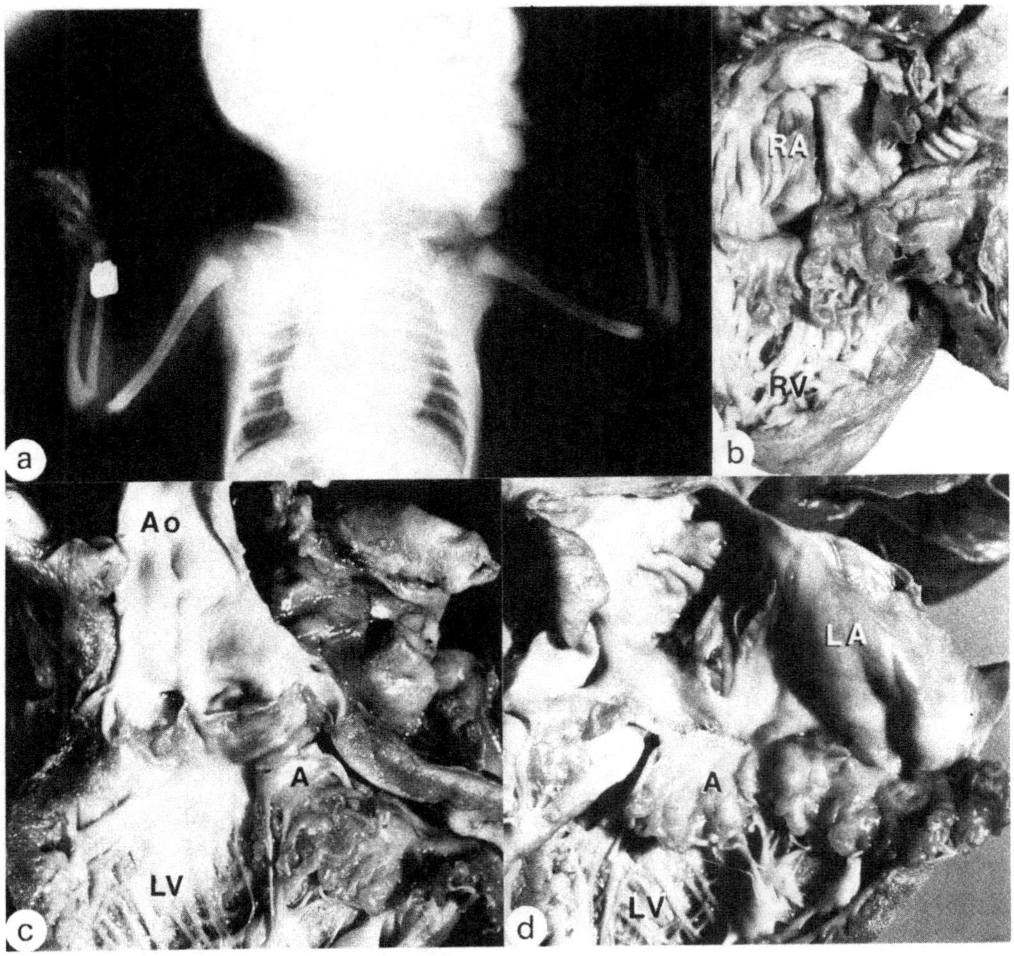

Figure 5. Congenital *floppy mitral valve* and *floppy tricuspid valve* in a 2-day-old boy who had long toes and fingers, a high-arched palate, and a grade 3/6 precordial systolic murmur typical of mitral regurgitation. The heart was enlarged *(a)* and he died of congestive cardiac failure. At necropsy, the intima of the ascending aorta (Ao) was wrinkled *(c)* suggesting that the underlying media was abnormal at this early stage. Shown here is the opened aorta, aortic valve, and left ventricle (LV) (A = anterior mitral leaflet). *(d)* Opened left atrium (LA), mitral valve, and left ventricle (LV). The mitral leaflets are considerably elongated in both longitudinal and transverse dimensions. The left atrium (LA) is dilated. *b,* The tricuspid valve leaflets also are elongated in both transverse and longitudinal dimensions (RA = right atrium; RV = right ventricle).

particularly on the ventricular surface of the valve, has, on occasion, caused this type of valve to be considered as rheumatic in origin rather than floppy.[17]

Ultrastructural studies of floppy mitral valves[20] have disclosed alterations of the collagen fibers in the leaflets and in the chordae tendineae. These changes have included fragmentation, splitting, swelling and coarse granularity of the individual collagen fibers, as well as spiraling and twisting of the fibers.[20] Also, some elastic fibers are fragmented and contain cystic spaces. These alterations in the structure of the collagen may be more important than the accumulation of the acid mucopolysaccharide material in that they lead to focal weaknesses in the leaflets. The left ventricular systolic pressure exerted against these weakened areas may lead to prolapse or focal interchordal hooding. Although the actual prolapse of the mitral valve may be acquired and a consequence of the left ventricular systolic (closing) pressure, the focally weak areas of

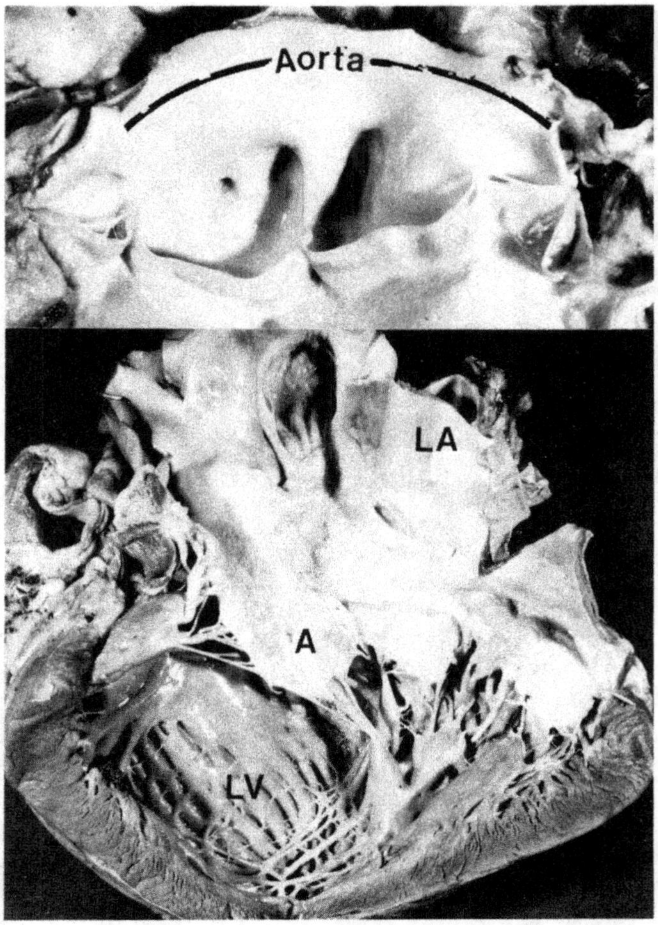

Figure 6. *Floppy mitral valve*—pure mitral regurgitation without aortic disease—in the *Marfan syndrome* in a 28-year-old man who died from severe mitral regurgitation. He had been well until age 24 when he developed exertional dyspnea and hemoptysis and was found to have cardiomegaly. Catheterization was performed at age 25 and the pressures (in mm. Hg) were: pulmonary artery, 19/10; right ventricle, 19/5; right atrial mean, 5; pulmonary arterial wedge mean, 10; and systemic artery 130/80. The cardiac output was 2.3 L./min. He remained functionally class II for the next three years but during his last year of life the congestive heart failure worsened and he became class IV. When examined seven days before his death he was quite ill. A grade 5/6 pansystolic precordial murmur, loudest over the apex, was audible. No diastolic murmur was present. The chest radiograph showed a big heart and severe kyphoscoliosis. Electrocardiogram showed sinus rhythm and left ventricular hypertrophy. He died of progressive heart failure.

At necropsy, the heart was huge (850 gm.). Although the sinuses were dilated, the aorta was entirely normal histologically (top). The mitral leaflets (bottom) were mildly thickened and elongated and the mitral anulus was severely dilated (15 cm.). Calcific deposits were present in the anulus behind the posterior mitral leaflet. The left atrium (LA) was quite dilated as was the left ventricle (LV) (A = anterior mitral leaflet).

the leaflets are probably most often congenital in origin. This focal leaflet weakness may be analogous to the berry aneurysm of the cerebral artery—the weakness in the arterial wall is almost certainly congenital in origin and the later bulging, with or without rupture, is acquired as a consequence of a high intra-arterial pressure. Mitral valve prolapse also may be higher in persons with elevated left ventricular systolic pressures than in persons with normal levels of this pressure. Certainly, calcification of the mitral anulus is more common in hypertensive than in normotensive individuals,[21] and mitral anular calcification is more common in persons with floppy mitral valves

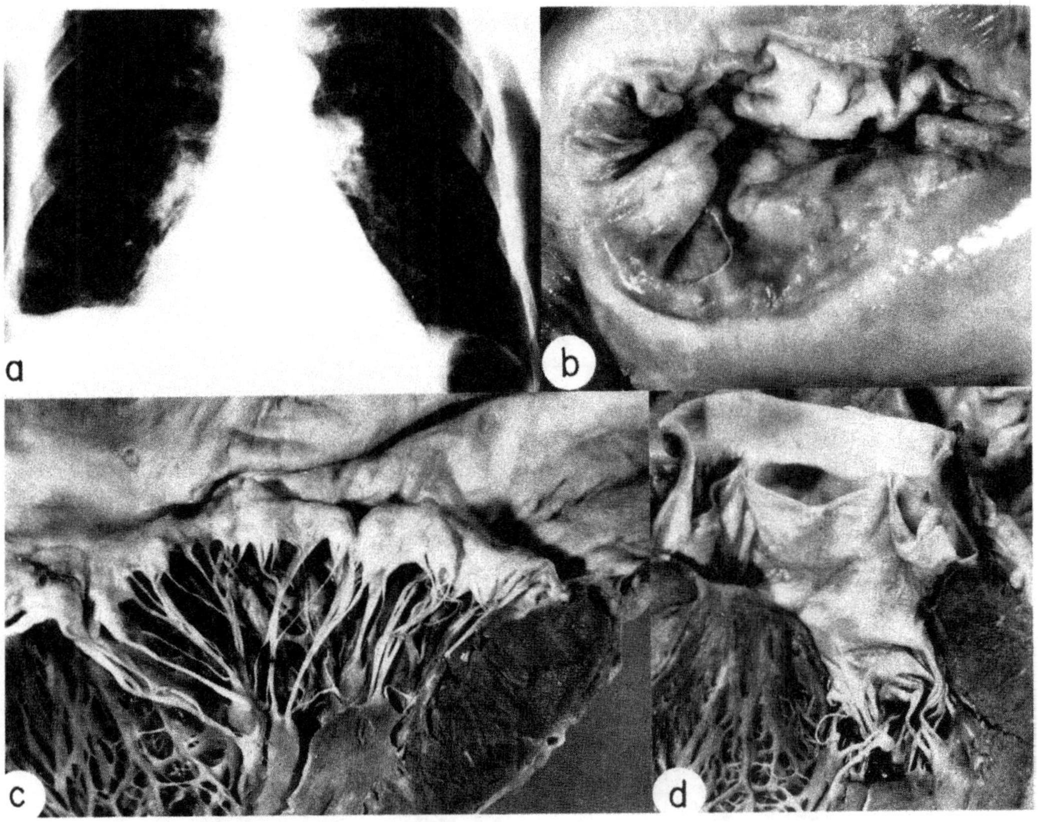

Figure 7. *Floppy mitral valve* in a 70-year-old man who died of gastric carcinoma. During life a grade 3/6 pansystolic blowing murmur was heard, loudest over the apex with radiation to the left axilla. The rhythm was atrial fibrillation. He never had symptoms of cardiac dysfunction. The heart was enlarged by radiograph *(a)*, but at necropsy it weighed only 310 gm. Both atria were quite dilated. The mitral leaflets protruded toward the left atrium *(b)* because the chordae tendineae were too long. A portion of opened mitral valve showing the elongated chordae is shown in *c*. *d*, The opened left ventricle and aortic valve show excessively long chordae. Focal calcific deposits also were present in the mitral anulus.

than it is in individuals of similar age and sex without floppy mitral valves.[21,22] Another factor supporting the concept that the underlying fault of mitral floppiness is congenital is its high frequency in patients with other congenital defects (atrial septal defect)[23–26] or deficiencies (the Marfan syndrome)[14,21,27–34] (Figs. 5–7).

Recognized complications of the floppy mitral valve are listed in Table 1. Because a valve may be floppy or prolapsed without mitral regurgitation, it appears reasonable to consider mitral regurgitation as a complication of floppiness rather than a necessary component of this syndrome. Calcification of the mitral anulus almost surely is the second most frequent complication of mitral floppiness (Fig. 8). Rupture of mitral chordae tendineae may be the consequence of infective endocarditis, or rupture may occur without evidence of infection ("spontaneous" rupture)[35-37] (Figs. 9 and 10). Chordal rupture is probably noninfective more often than infective in origin.[38] Nevertheless, because patients with systolic murmurs are at increased risk to develop infective endocarditis and because infection superimposed on a floppy valve is usually highly destructive, antibiotic prophylaxis against this valvular infection appears warranted.

The cause of the arrhythmias is unclear.[39] There is no anatomic evidence in these patients of "a myocardial factor" or abnormality in course or size of any of the major

Table 1. Complications of prolapsing mitral valve.

1. Mitral regurgitation
2. Calcification, mitral "anulus"
3. Rupture of chordae tendineae
   A. Infective endocarditis
   B. Non-infective ("spontaneous")
4. Infective endocarditis
5. Arrhythmias
6. Chest pain
7. Stroke (transient ischemic attacks)
8. Sudden death

coronary arteries. An attractive but unproven explanation is the considerable friction between chordae tendineae and the underlying left ventricular mural endocardium.[18] The cause of the chest pain which occurs occasionally in these patients is also unknown. Associated coronary arterial disease is clearly not the explanation for the chest pain in the majority of these patients. Acute nonprogressive strokes or transient cereb-

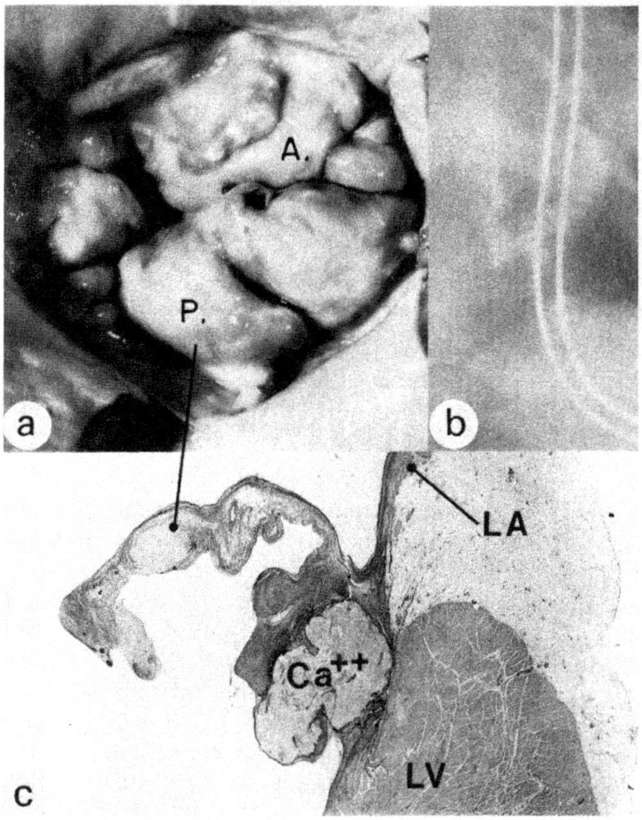

Figure 8. *Floppy mitral valve* and *calcium in the mitral anulus* of a 70-year-old woman who had a grade 3/6 murmur of mitral regurgitation, atrial fibrillation and complete heart block. *a*, Mitral valve from left atrial aspect (A., P. = anterior and posterior mitral leaflets, respectively). *b*, Radiograph taken while the patient was alive shows a C-shaped deposit of calcium in the mitral anular area. Pacing wires also are visible. *c*, Photomicrograph through wall of left atrium (LA), prolapsed posterior leaflet, and left ventricle (LV). The calcium (CA^{++}) in the anular area is apparent.

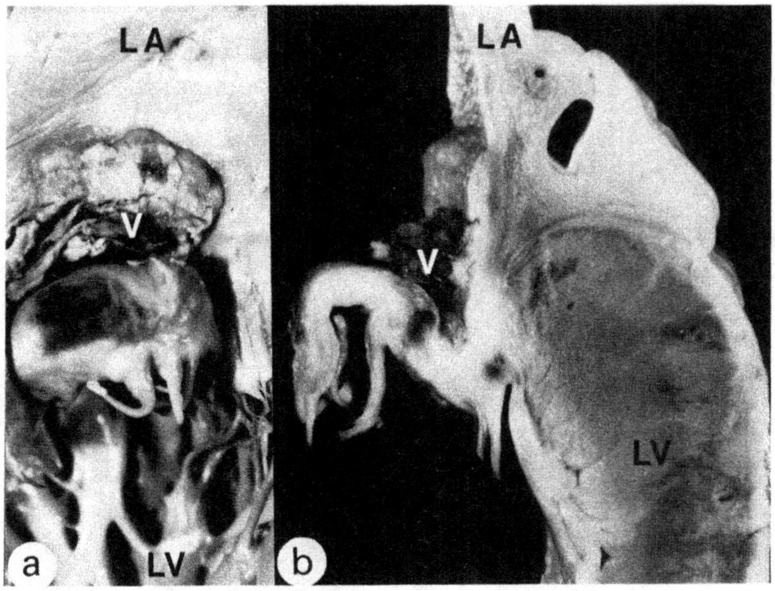

Figure 9. *Floppy mitral valve* with superimposed *Staphylococcus aureus endocarditis* in a 52-year-old man who was known to have a murmur of mitral regurgitation for 10 years. He was asymptomatic, however, until he developed typical clinical features of active infective endocarditis which caused a fatal septic cerebral embolus. Necropsy revealed a portion of posterior mitral leaflet prolapsed toward left atrium (LA) and vegetative (V) material at the acute angle formed by the hooded posterior leaflet and mural endocardium of left atrium. (This junction is a common location of fibrin-platelet deposits in patients with prolapsed posterior mitral leaflets.) *a,* Closeup of hooded segment of posterior leaflet with the superimposed vegetation. *b,* Longitudinal section through left atrium, prolapsed and thickened posterior leaflet and left ventricle (LV).

ral ischemic attacks recently have been noted to occur with increased frequency in these patients.[40] In some patients, small fibrin-platelet thrombi have been observed on the atrial aspects of the prolapsed segments of mitral leaflet at junctions with the left atrial mural endocardium.[18] It has been suggested that dislodgement of these small fibrin-platelet thrombi and their migration to the cerebral arteries is the explanation for the transient cerebral ischemia. It is also possible that these minute thrombi dislodge and embolize to the coronary arteries, triggering an arrhythmia or chest pain or both.[41]

AORTIC VALVE STENOSIS AND THE CONGENITALLY MALFORMED AORTIC VALVE

If papillary muscle dysfunction is excluded, valvular aortic stenosis (AS) is the most common fatal cardiac valve lesion; it was found in 50 percent of patients older than 15 years with valvular heart disease whom I have studied at necropsy.[42-44] Of the patients with AS (with or without aortic regurgitation), the lesion was isolated in 66 percent; in the other 34 percent the mitral valve was stenotic or incompetent or both. The evidence is substantial that the cause of AS, when associated with mitral valve disease, is rheumatic.[44] In contrast, the evidence is substantial that isolated AS (anatomically normal mitral valve) is nonrheumatic in origin.[42-44] This section focuses on patients with isolated AS.[42-50]

In contrast to what was generally believed 30 years ago[51], at least three factors indicate that anatomically isolated aortic valve disease (actually either stenosis or pure regurgitation) is nonrheumatic in origin: (1) the low frequency (about 10 percent) of a positive history of acute rheumatic fever, (2) the absence of Aschoff bodies, and, most

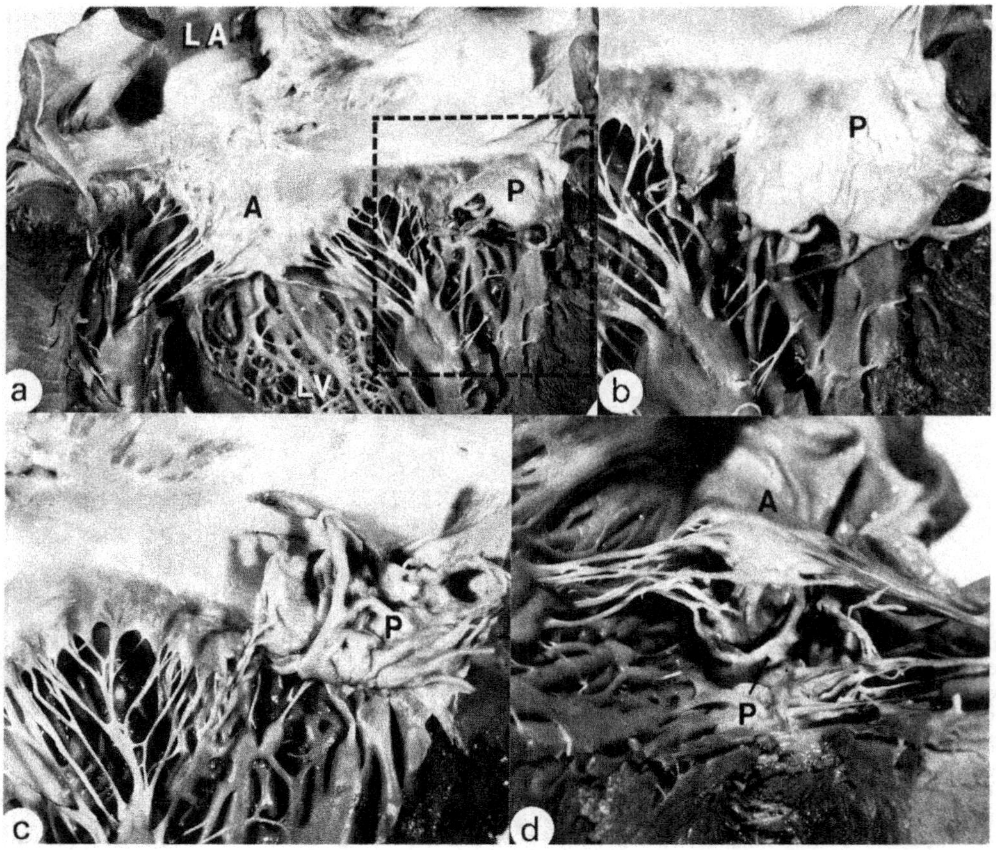

Figure 10. *Floppy mitral valve* in a 38-year-old man who had been well until three years before death, when he experienced a fairly abrupt onset of congestive heart failure. Cardiac catheterization at that time confirmed the presence of pure mitral regurgitation. His blood urea nitrogen at that time was 41 mg./dl. During the next three years he developed severe systemic hypertension (240/140 mm. Hg), severe anemia, severe azotemia (blood urea nitrogen = 230 mg./dl.), and finally, fatal hemorrhagic cardiac tamponade. Necropsy revealed a large segment of posterior mitral leaflet, elongated and prolapsed into the left atrium. Most of the chordae tendineae from this prolapsed segment were ruptured. (The patient never had evidence of infective endocarditis.) The heart weighed 620 gm.

a, Opened left atrium (LA), mitral valve, left ventricle (LV), and prolapsed segment (P). The portion outside the boxed area of mitral leaflets and chordae are normal or near normal (A = anterior mitral leaflet). *b*, Closeup of atrial aspect of the prolapsed segment. *c*, Same view showing the prolapsed segment flipped back into left atrium, exposing its ventricular aspect. *d*, View of mitral valve from left ventricle. In this case mitral prolapse may have been worsened by systemic hypertension; increased closing pressure on the mitral leaflets is created by the elevated systolic pressure.

importantly, (3) the frequency of an underlying congenital malformation of the aortic valve.

The structure of the aortic valve in AS can be correlated to some extent with the age of the patient (Table 2).[43] In patients younger than 15 years, the aortic valve most commonly (60 percent) is congenitally unicuspid and unicommissural;[45,50] in patients 15 to 65 years of age, the valve is most commonly (60 percent) congenitally bicuspid;[46,48] and in patients age older than 65 years, the valve is most commonly (90 percent) tricuspid.[49] The stenosis is either caused by or superimposed on the congenitally malformed aortic valve in virtually all the patients under 15 and in at least 70 percent—possibly as high as 85 percent—of patients between 15 and 65.[43] A congenitally mal-

Table 2. Configuration of aortic valve in isolated aortic stenosis in relation to age

	No. valve cusps	*<age 15 years*	*Age 16-65*	*>age 65 years*
1	1	60%	10%	0
2	2	20%	60%	10%
3	3	15%	25%	90%
4	Uncertain	5%	5%	0

formed (in this case congenitally bicuspid) valve appears to be the underlying condition in only about 10 percent of the patients over 65 with AS.[49]

The unicommissural valve, the only type of unicuspid valve observed in the aortic valve position, was described initially by Edwards in 1958[52] (Figs. 11 and 12). This valve, like all other congenitally malformed aortic valves, tends to become more stenotic with time,[50] in contrast to the congenitally bicuspid aortic valve. But the unicuspid aortic valve is almost certainly stenotic from the time of birth, and the fewer the number of aortic valve cusps and commissures, the greater is the likelihood that the valve is stenotic from birth.[43]

Next to the floppy mitral valve, the congenitally bicuspid aortic valve is the most frequent major congenital malformation of the heart or great vessels (Figs. 13 to 19). It is possible that the frequency of this malformation is as high as 2 percent of all human births.[48] In 1800 hearts studied personally, none of which had cardiac valvular, septal, or great vessel abnormalities causing dysfunction, 17 had normally functioning congenitally bicuspid aortic valves. This frequency of nearly 1 percent is similar to that reported by others who examined hearts for the specific purpose of determining presence or absence of congenitally bicuspid aortic valves. Osler[53] found 10 apparently normally functioning congenitally bicuspid aortic valves in 800 autopsies (750 of which were performed by him), an incidence of 1 percent. Eight additional patients had infective endocarditis involving congenitally bicuspid aortic valves. Thus, 18 of 800 (2 percent) had either normally functioning or infected congenitally bicuspid aortic valves. Grant, Wood, and Jones[54] found apparently normally functioning congenitally bicuspid aortic valves in 12 of 1350 (1 percent) necropsy patients. Osler,[53] Lewis and Grant,[55] and Grant and coworkers[54] appear not to have recognized that the bicuspid condition of this valve may underlie severe stenosis or calcification at this site. Thus, if congenitally bicuspid aortic valves that develop complications (stenosis or incompetency with or without infection) are added to those which function normally during the entire lifetime, the frequency of congenitally bicuspid aortic valves may approach 2 percent of the population.

Among the complications of the bicuspid condition of the aortic valve, stenosis is by far the most frequent; pure regurgitation is next, and the latter lesion is most frequently

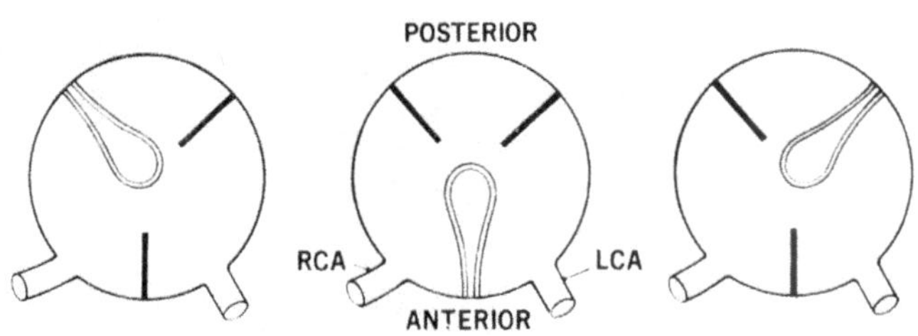

Figure 11. Location of the true commissure in congenitally unicommissural aortic valve stenosis. RCA, LCA = right and left coronary arteries, respectively.

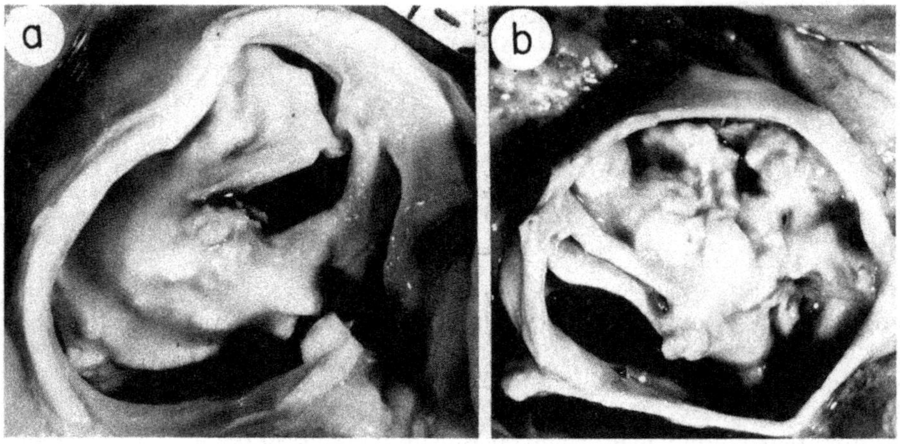

Figure 12. *Congenitally unicommissural stenotic aortic valve* in two men aged 28 *(a)* and 48 years *(b)*.

the result of its being the site of infective endocarditis.[37,38] Why one congenitally bicuspid aortic valve becomes stenotic, another incompetent, and another the site of infective endocarditis is unknown. However, it is clear that stenosis, regurgitation, and infection are complications of the bicuspid condition of the aortic valve and none of them are present at birth. It appears likely that a congenitally bicuspid aortic valve becomes stenotic only as its cusps become fibrotic and calcified; neither cusp of a congenitally bicuspid aortic valve is fibrotic or calcified at the time of birth.

The frequency of development of stenosis or incompetency at the site of a congeni-

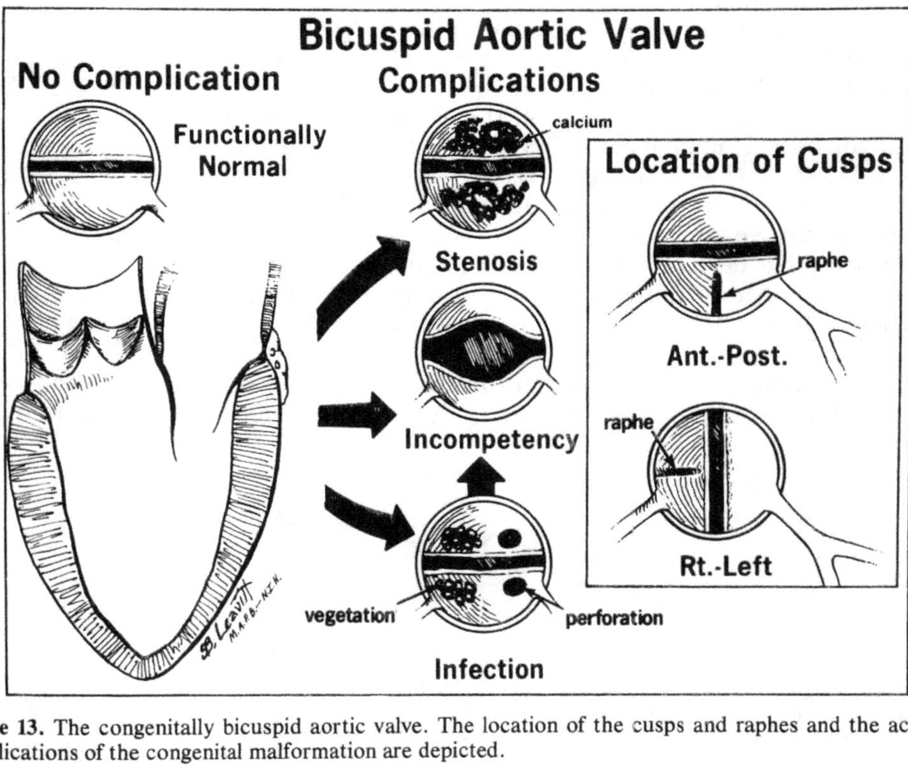

Figure 13. The congenitally bicuspid aortic valve. The location of the cusps and raphes and the acquired complications of the congenital malformation are depicted.

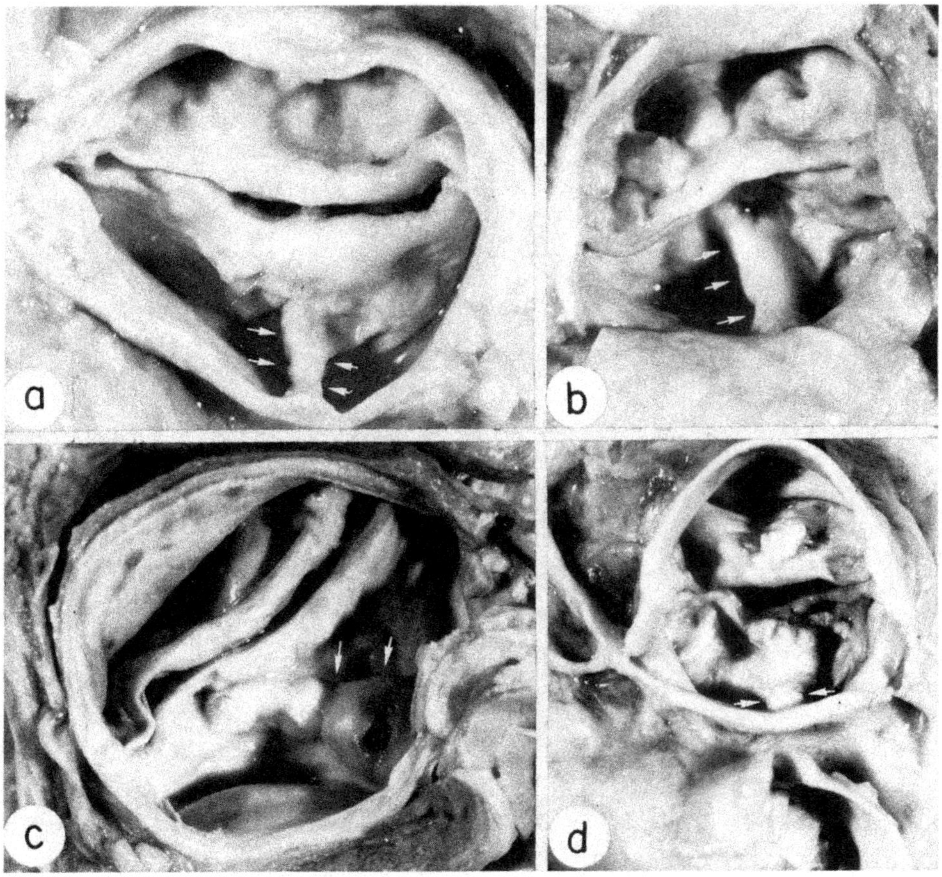

Figure 14. *Calcified, stenotic, congenitally bicuspid aortic valves* in four patients. The cusps are situated anteriorly and posteriorly and the commissures right and left, respectively. Each of the valves has a raphe (white arrows) in the anterior cusp. *a*, Valve of a 61-year-old man. At catheterization two years before his death, the peak systolic gradient (PSG) across the valve was 45 mm. Hg when the cardiac index was 2.6 l./min./m.^{2}. He had complete heart block secondary to destruction of the atrioventricular bundle by calcium. *b*, Valve of a 60-year-old man who suddenly collapsed on the street. Electrocardiogram recorded in the emergency room showed left bundle branch block. His only previous symptom of cardiac dysfunction was mild exertional dyspnea. *c*, Valve of a 75-year-old man who died after resection of an asymptomatic abdominal aortic aneurysm which had been discovered during a routine physical examination. A grade 3/6 murmur consistent with aortic stenosis had been heard, but he had no symptoms of cardiac dysfunction. *d*, Valve of a 51-year-old man. The PSG across this valve was only 18 mm. Hg but it was severely incompetent.

tally bicuspid aortic valve also is unknown. Lewis and Grant[55] concluded that vegetations develop at these sites in about 23 percent of adults (16 of 69) with congenitally bicuspid aortic valves. More information is available regarding the incidence of congenitally bicuspid valves in patients with infective endocarditis involving the aortic valve. Of 31 patients with "subacute infective endocarditis" studied at necropsy by Lewis and Grant,[55] 8 had congenitally bicuspid aortic valves. Such valves were found in 4 of 13 patients with infective endocarditis involving aortic valves studied at necropsy by Starling[56] and in 2 of 22 patients studied at necropsy by Fulton and Levine.[57] These investigators apparently were not aware of the fact that congenitally bicuspid aortic valves could become stenotic.

Of the 157 necropsy patients older than 15 years in whom I found congenitally bicuspid stenotic aortic valves, 99 percent had grossly visible extensive calcific deposits in

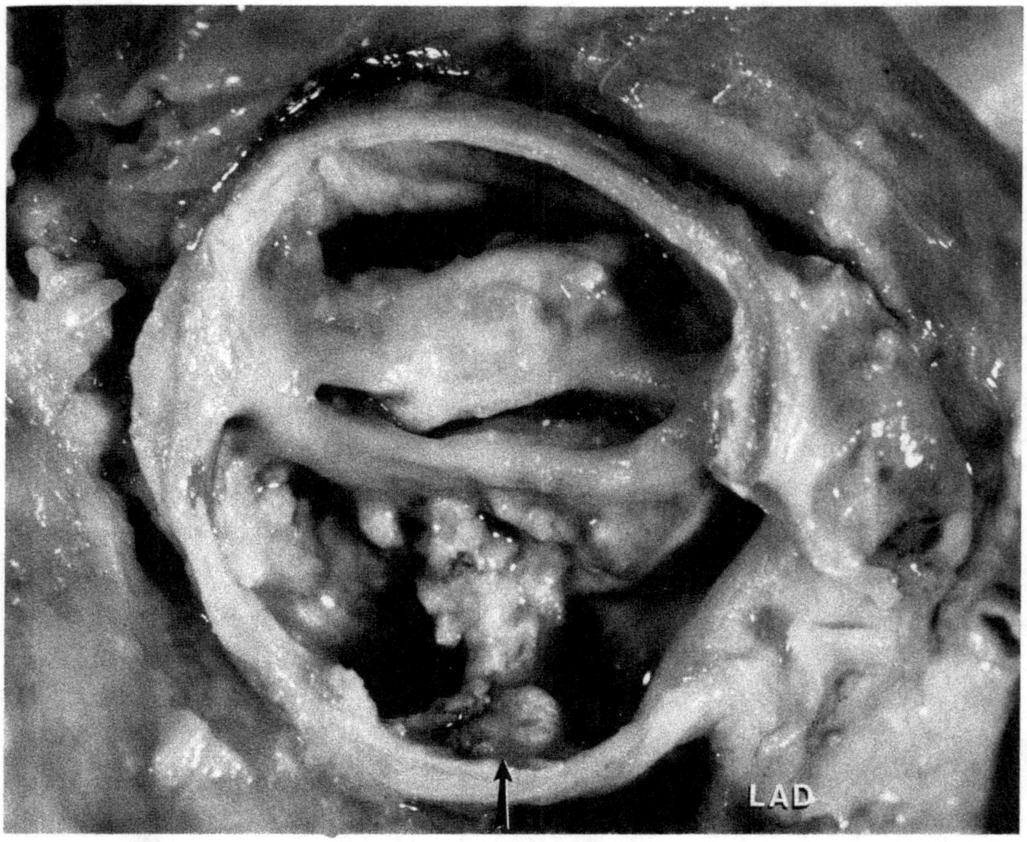

Figure 15. *Congenitally bicuspid, stenotic aortic valve* in an 87-year-old man who developed angina pectoris one year before his sudden death at home. He never had congestive heart failure or syncope. The two cusps are located anteriorly and posteriorly with a raphe (arrow), which is calcified, in the anterior cusp. In addition to the heavy deposits of calcium in the aortic valve, large calcific deposits also were present in the mitral anulus. Aortic stenosis had been diagnosed by physical examination 10 years before he died. LAD = left anterior descending coronary artery.

both cusps. The two patients without calcific deposits were under 30. In contrast, only 5 of the 22 patients with purely incompetent congenitally bicuspid aortic valves had calcific deposits which were focal and small. Calcific deposits are to be expected in adults with stenotic congenitally bicuspid aortic valves. Furthermore, heavy deposits of calcium do not occur in purely incompetent congenitally bicuspid aortic valves; valvular stenosis appears to be a prerequisite for the development of heavy deposits of calcium at this site. Development of infective endocarditis on a heavily calcified valve also is rare.[58] Infective endocarditis was found in only 13 (8 percent) of the 157 patients I studied with stenotic congenitally bicuspid aortic valves; infection was superimposed on a heavily calcified valve in only 4 of them. Of the 22 patients with purely incompetent congenitally bicuspid aortic valves, the valve was the site of vegetative endocarditis in 19 (86 percent), and this infection was the principal cause of incompetency.

The mechanism by which a congenitally bicuspid aortic valve becomes stenotic or incompetent is uncertain. There is no evidence that the valve is stenotic or incompetent at birth. Likewise, there is no evidence that superimposed rheumatic fever or rheumatic heart disease is the cause of the stenosis or incompetency. The explanation advanced by Edwards[59] is attractive. He proposed that it is not mechanically possible for a

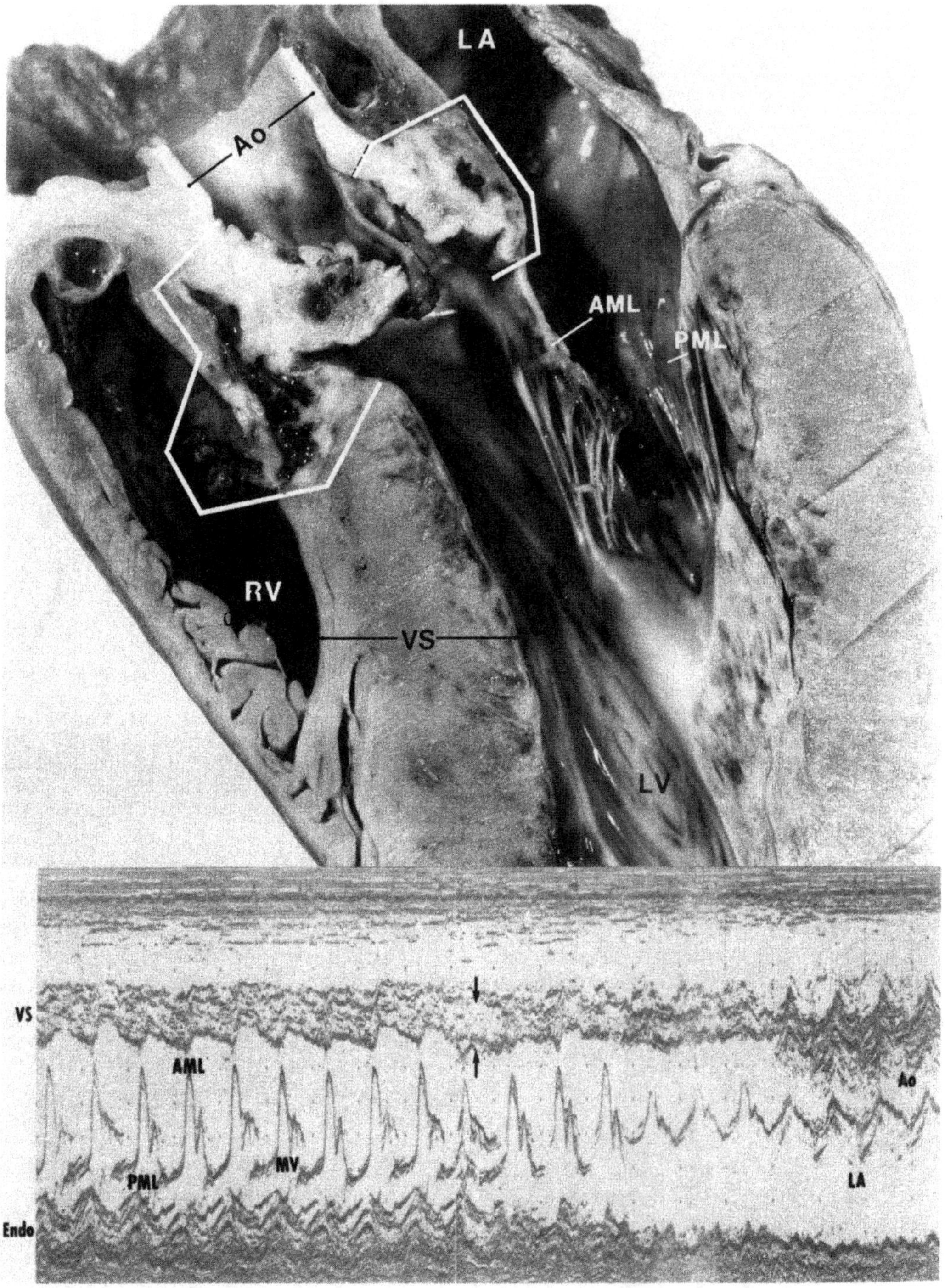

Figure 16. *Congenitally bicuspid aortic valve* with superimposed *Staphylococcus aureus endocarditis* in a 30-year-old man. Before the onset of the infective endocarditis the patient was asymptomatic but before the infection the valve was already mildly stenotic and mildly calcified. Nail biting, to the point of bleeding, apparently was the source of the infection. At necropsy the heart weighed 560 gm. The infection of the aortic valve burrowed into the adjacent soft tissues (brackets) producing large "ring abscesses." Ring abscess caused complete right bundle branch block. There was extensive subendocardial and papillary muscle necrosis of the left ventricle, presumably the result of severely diminished cardiac output. The echocardiogram was recorded several days before death. The arrows in the ventricular septum of the echocardium designate the probable ring abscess. Ao = aorta; LA = left atrium; RV = right ventricle; LV = left ventricle; AML and PML = anterior and posterior mitral leaflets; VS = ventricular septum; MV = mitral valve; Endo = endocardium.

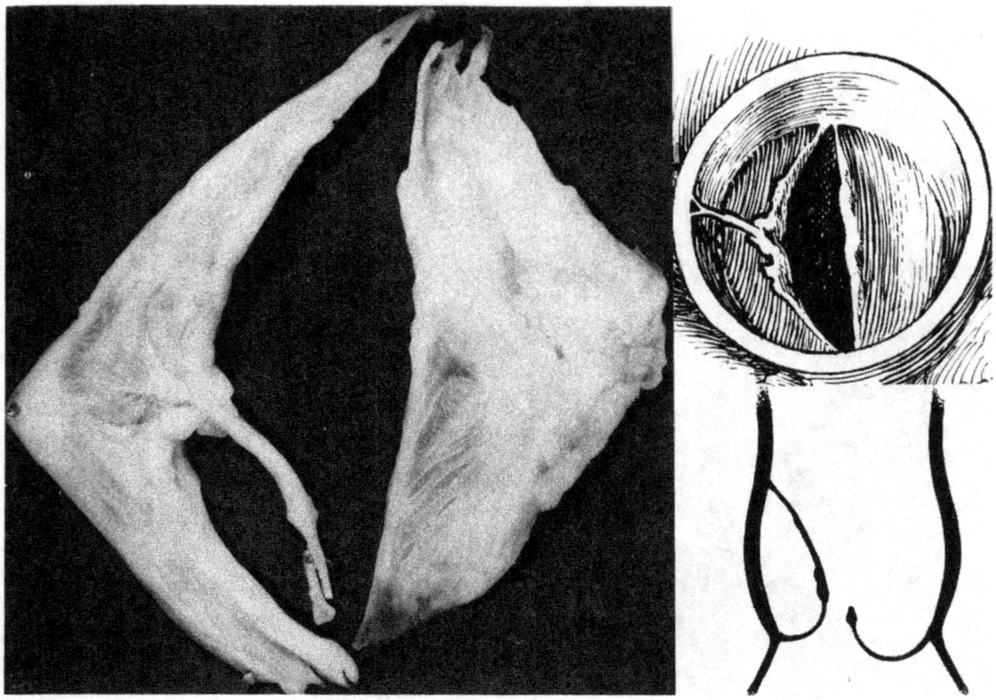

Figure 17. *Purely incompetent congenitally bicuspid aortic valve* in a 27-year-old man who was found to have aortic regurgitation at age 17; he developed exertional dyspnea at age 25. Just before valve replacement, simultaneous left ventricular and brachial arterial pressures were 125/25 and 126/54 mm. Hg, respectively, when the cardiac index was 2.2 l./min./m.^{2}. He died suddenly 13 months after valve replacement. The heart weighed 800 gm. Excised aortic valve is pictured at left. The drawing shows the supporting fibrous band that stretched from the margin in the midportion of one cusp to the aortic wall above one sinus of Valsalva (right). This patient is an example of pure severe aortic regurgitation of a congenitally bicuspid valve which was never the site of infective endocarditis.

congenitally bicuspid aortic valve to open and close properly. The distances between lateral attachments of normal aortic valvular cusps along their free margins are curved lines. The extra length allows the cusps to move freely during opening and closing of the valves. In contrast, the distances between lateral attachments of congenitally bicuspid aortic valves along their free margins are almost straight lines. (If the distances were

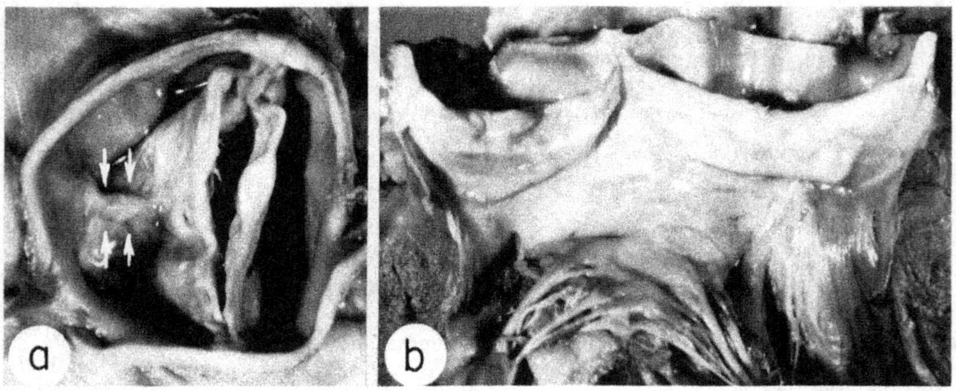

Figure 18. *Functionally normal congenitally bicuspid aortic valve. a,* The right cusp contains the raphe (arrows) and is the larger of the two cusps. *b,* Opened valve.

exactly straight, the valves could not open during ventricular systole.) Consequently, at least one cusp is larger than the other. The excessive length of one or both cusps of a congenitally bicuspid aortic valve produces abnormal contact between the cusps. This abnormal contact, in turn, causes focal fibrous thickening that becomes diffuse with time, eventually causing dystrophic calcification. Thus, stenosis of a congenitally bicuspid aortic valve may be the result of trauma to these cusps produced by their abnormal contact with each other. Although this explanation is appealing, it does not explain why one congenitally bicuspid aortic valve becomes stenotic, another becomes entirely incompetent, and another remains free of complications.

Criteria for differentiating a bicuspid valve of congenital origin from a bicuspid valve of acquired origin have been debated (Fig. 19). There is no controversy over the distinction between a congenitally bicuspid aortic valve devoid of a raphe (false commissure or ridge) and complications (stenosis, incompetency, or infection) and a tricuspid aortic valve devoid of similar complications. There was controversy about the means of differentiating a congenitally bicuspid aortic valve with a raphe from an acquired bicuspid aortic valve resulting from fusion of two cusps at one true commissure.* Osler,[53] from his study of 18 hearts (15 adults), deduced the following characteristics of a congenitally bicuspid aortic valve, all recognizable by gross observation: (1) The raphe is located where the true commissure normally would be, i.e., between the right and left anterior aortic valve cusps; (2) The length of the free margin of the cusp without a raphe is slightly shorter (by an average of 12 percent in his measurements on 7 hearts) than the length of the margin of the cusp containing a raphe, the "conjoint" cusp; (3) The free border of the conjoint cusp is straight or curled and free of nodular thickenings which would indicate bodies of Arantius; (4) The border of attachment of the conjoint cusp, as viewed from the ventricular aspect, presents either the contour of a single semilunar cusp or a shallow groove, indicative of the junction of two cusps; (5) The raphe may be located on the aortic wall alone or may extend onto the cusp for variable distances, but in either case it usually divides the sinus of Valsalva into units of equal size.

In 1923 Lewis and Grant[54] clarified several gross features of "unequivocally" congenital bicuspid aortic valves and presented histologic criteria for differentiating bicuspid valves of "congenital" origin from those of "inflammatory" origin. In contrast to Osler's findings these authors found that fusion could occur not only between right and left anterior cusps but also between right anterior and posterior cusps. A raphe, dividing one of the two cusps, was observed "in about half the cases." The two cusps could be the same size, but usually the conjoined cusp was larger, though less than twice the size of the undivided cusp; or else, "the subdivided cusp is larger than one normal cusp but smaller than two normal cusps." However, Lewis and Grant considered gross distinction between congenital and acquired bicuspid aortic valves unreliable. Elastic tissue stains of transverse sections of congenital raphes showed them to consist mainly of elastic fibers; thus, histologically the raphe was similar to the media of the aorta. In contrast, transverse sections of two fused cusps at a true commissure disclosed that the fused commissure was devoid of elastic fibers and consisted of fibrous valvular tissue. Other investigators[60,61] confirmed these histologic criteria. Koletsky[61] also pointed out that congenital raphes were devoid of vascular channels and inflammatory cells, whereas both were seen in acquired, fused commissures. Since Lewis and Grant de-

*The definition of a *commissure* differs depending on whether a semilunar or an atrioventricular (A-V) cardiac valve is under consideration. The aortic valve commissure is the space between two lateral attachments on the aortic wall. Normally each aortic valve cusp is an independent similar sized unit and adherence of one cusp to another at the narrow space (commissure) between the two cusps is abnormal. In contrast to a semilunar valve, the leaflets of an atrioventricular valve are continuous one with another. Thus, the commissures of the A-V valves are the sites of connection between the unequal sized leaflets, not the spaces between the cusps as in the case of the semilunar valves.

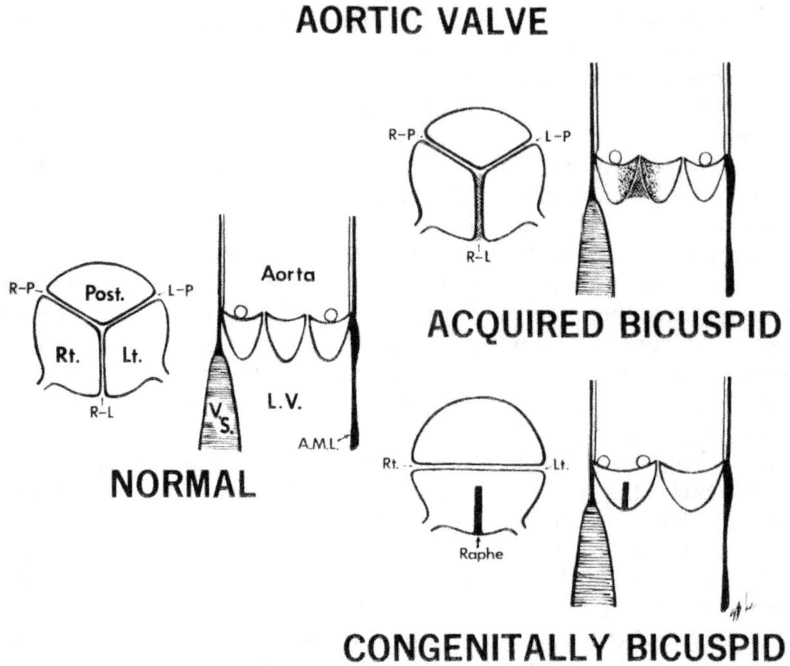

Figure 19. Diagram illustrating differences between *bicuspid aortic valves* of congenital origin as compared to the normal valve. The circumferential distances between each of the three commissures in a normally formed valve are similar. L-P = left-posterior; R-L = right-left, and R-P = right-posterior commissures; Rt., Lt., Post., = right, left, and posterior cusps, respectively; V.S. = ventricular septum; L.V. = left ventricular outflow tract; and A.M.L. = anterior mitral leaflet. In the *acquired bicuspid valve* the circumferential distance between the commissures remains equal, as in a normal valve. The fused commissure is wide, the distal margins of each of the two fused cusps are still usually visible, and the most cephalad margin of the fused commissure is on the same horizontal level as the most cephalad margins of the two nonfused commissures. In the *congenitally bicuspid valve*, the raphe is generally narrow and rarely extends to the free margin of the conjoined cusp or to the cephalad level reached by the two true commissures. The circumferential distances between the two true commissures are greater than this distance between either true commissure and the raphe. The circumferential distance between the true commissures around the conjoined cusp, i.e., the cusp with the raphe, is equal to or slightly greater than the circumferential distance between the true commissures around the cusp devoid of the raphe.

scribed these histologic features, many pathologists have been reluctant to distinguish between congenital and acquired bicuspid aortic valves without microscopic examination of raphes. But however helpful these histologic criteria may be, they are not specific. In some patients certain sections of a raphe show a structure like that of the aortic media, while other sections of the same raphe show only fibrous tissue. Also, the congenital raphe may lose its elastic fibers as the valvular cusps become fibrotic and calcified. The raphe may be the first portion of a congenitally bicuspid aortic valve to calcify, and these deposits destroy existing elastic fibers. Interestingly, Lewis and Grant and others who emphasized the importance of histologic distinction between congenital raphes and fused true commissures were unaware that calcific stenosis was a consequence of a congenitally bicuspid aortic valve. Once the valve is extensively scarred and calcified, histologic examination of the raphe is often fruitless. Furthermore, as Edwards[62] pointed out, in the patient with a bicuspid aortic valve that must be assumed to be congenital—as in infants with aortic coarctation—the raphe may not only be fibrous, but may grossly display features suggesting fusion of two distinguishable, separate cusps.

It appears that tricuspid aortic valves are rarely stenotic at birth. If stenosis is present at birth and the aortic valve has three cusps, the stenosis is usually the result of a very small aortic "anulus" rather than the result of fusion of the cusps; whereas acquired stenosis of a three-cusp aortic valve is common. Of the patients studied personally with clinically isolated AS (with or without regurgitation), aged 16 to 65 years (Table 2), 25 percent had tricuspid valves, and among those over 65, 90 percent had tricuspid valves. In the younger group, about one half of the patients with clinically isolated AS had diffuse fibrous thickening of the mitral leaflets as well. The associated diffuse mitral leaflet thickening is strong evidence that the etiology of AS in this group is rheumatic.[44] Also, nearly 75 percent of this group had positive histories of acute rheumatic fever, whereas 10 percent of the other group, i.e., those with anatomically normal mitral valves and AS, had positive histories.[42,44] The etiology of AS in the patients with anatomically normal mitral valves is unknown. Possibly, as mentioned earlier, minor abnormalities in the sizes of the aortic valve cusps from birth set the stage for abnormal contact of the leaflets with one another, resulting in fibrosis and, finally, stenosis[47] (Fig. 20).

DISCRETE SUBAORTIC STENOSIS

Like valvular AS, discrete subaortic stenosis (DSS), when isolated, usually does not produce symptoms of cardiac dysfunction until adulthood, and it is compatible with a relatively long survival. The average age of death is 35.[63] Unlike valvular AS, however, DSS is rare. In this condition the discrete obstruction is located about 1 cm. caudal to the bases of the aortic valve cusps.[43] The obstruction is on a line corresponding to the site where the atrial septum inserts into the anterior mitral leaflet. The obstruction, at

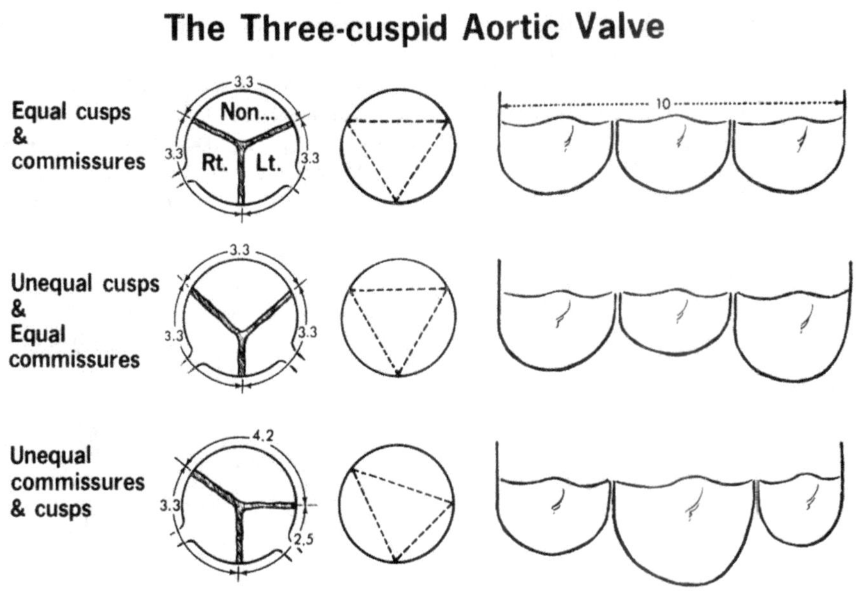

Figure 20. Diagrammatic portrayal of aortic valve cusps equal and unequal in size. *Top row,* The cusps of the aortic valve are equal in size and the circumferential distances between the commissures are equal. The straight-line distances between the commissures (as indicated by the dashed lines in the center circle) also are equal. On the right the aortic valve is opened. *Middle row,* Here the cusps are of unequal size, and they are made unequal by differing cephalocaudal lengths of the individual cusps. The distances between the commissures circumferentially around the aorta and the straight-line distances within the lumen of the aorta are similar to the normal shown in the top panel. *Bottom row,* Here the cephalocaudal lengths of the individual cusps differ and the circumferential distances around the aorta and the straight-line distances within the lumen of the aorta between the commissures (lateral attachments) are different as well.

least in adults, is produced by dense fibrous tissue—not really a "membrane"—which encircles the entire left ventricular outflow tract. The dense fibrous tissue may spread slightly cephalad, approaching the bases of the aortic valve cusps, and caudally for about a centimeter. Because in DSS the obstruction is usually severe and located just below (1 cm.) the aortic valve, the aortic valve cusps are the site of the impact of the blood ejected through the discrete obstruction. As a consequence, the aortic valve cusps become thickened and thus are ideal sites for vegetations. The consequence of cuspal thickening, with or without superimposed infective endocarditis, is development of mild aortic regurgitation. As a result, nearly all adults with DSS have precordial diastolic murmurs of aortic regurgitation in addition to the systolic murmurs of left ventricular outflow obstruction.[64,65] The absence of aortic valve calcific deposits and the absence of dilatation of the ascending aorta in adults, however, helps, before cardiac catheterization, to separate these patients from patients with valvular AS.

Although adequate data is not yet available, it is likely that DSS, on a percentage basis, is the cardiac condition most frequently complicated by infective endocarditis, being more common than that infection's association with congenitally bicuspid or unicuspid aortic valve, prolapsed aortic valve associated with ventricular septal defect, or floppy mitral valve.[58,66] The narrow jet of blood contacting one or more aortic valve cusps under high pressure and velocity provides the ideal circumstance for infective endocarditis to develop. Of five Newfoundland dogs with DSS that were dying naturally, four had active infective endocarditis, which was the cause of death, at necropsy.[66] Among seven patients with DSS whom I studied at necropsy, four had died from active infective endocarditis (Figs. 21 and 22).

Infective endocarditis complicating DSS may be difficult to diagnose clinically, at least before embolic events occur, and early diagnosis in this circumstance is essential to prevent severe damage to the aortic valve cusps. The high pressure jet ejected through the subaortic stenosis damages these cusps naturally, as already mentioned, but when infection is present this damage by the jet is markedly accelerated and the cusps are rapidly destroyed. In patients with destroyed aortic valve cusps and no subaortic stenosis, the consequence is severe aortic regurgitation with progressive left ventricular dilatation and failure. But in patients with destroyed aortic valve cusps associated with DSS, severe aortic regurgitation is prevented by the subaortic obstruc-

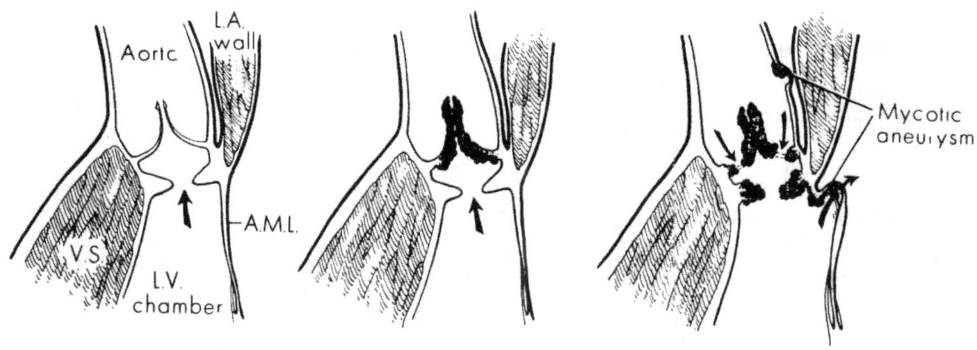

Figure 21. Diagram of aortic-valve region of the patient described in detail in Figure 22. Here the course of the pathologic process suggested by the necropsy findings is illustrated. The left diagram shows the *discrete subvalvular obstruction* before the development of *bacterial endocarditis* when the valve was traumatized by the jet of blood from below. The central diagram depicts the initial formation of bacterial vegetations, exclusively on the aortic valve cusps. As vegetations proliferated, the cusps ruptured (right diagram); the infection then extended to the discrete subvalvular fibrous band and anterior mitral leaflet (A.M.L.) where a mycotic aneurysm formed immediately below the "membrane" where systolic pressure was highest. A second aneurysm in the wall of the ascending aorta resulted from the effects of a systolic jet through the valve. L.A. = left atrium; V.S. = ventricular septum; L.V. = left ventricle.

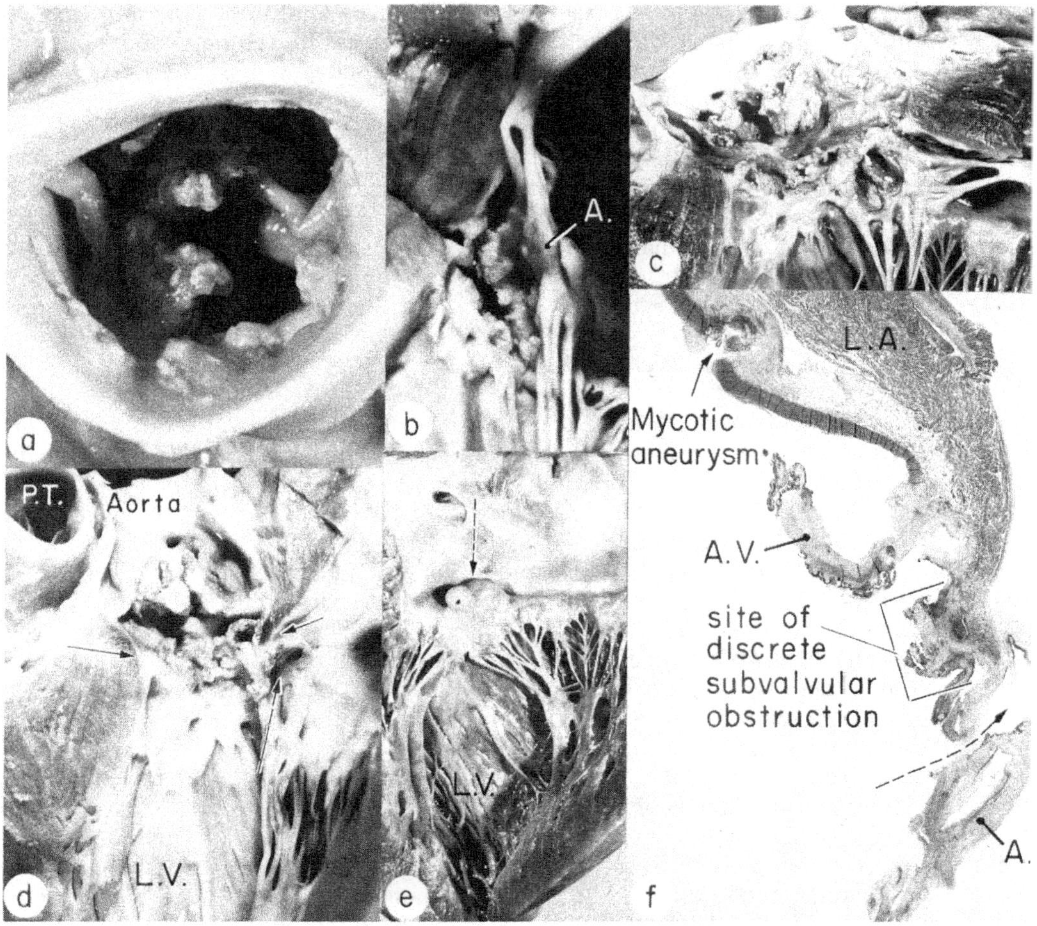

Figure 22. Alpha hemolytic streptococcus endocarditis complicating congenitally *discrete subaortic stenosis* in a 28-year-old man. The infection, which appeared about nine months before death, produced valvular aortic regurgitation. *a,* Aortic valve from above. *b,* Left ventricular outflow tract from below, showing vegetative material on the subvalvular "membrane" and adjacent anterior mitral leaflet (A.). *c,* Opened left ventricular outflow tract showing vegetations on each aortic cusp, on the subvalvular "membrane," and on the ventricular surface of anterior mitral leaflet. *d,* Longitudinal section showing the left ventricular outflow tract. The area of subaortic stenosis is apparent (between the *solid arrows*) and a mycotic aneurysm *(dashed arrow)* is seen in the anterior mitral leaflet. The mitral aneurysm is in the high-pressure portion of the left ventricle (L.V.), i.e., below the discrete subvalvular obstruction. P.T. = pulmonary trunk. *e,* Opened mitral valve showing atrial aspect of the mycotic aneurysm *(dashed arrow)* on the anterior leaflet. *f,* Photomicrograph of section through aorta, left atrium (L.A.), aortic valve (A.V.) cusp, subvalvular "membrane," and anterior mitral leaflet (A.). A mycotic aneurysm is present in the ascending aorta *(solid arrow)* as well as in the anterior mitral leaflet *(dashed arrow)*. Vegetations are present on the aortic valve cusp and on the subvalvular membrane. (Hematoxylin and eosin stain; x 2, reduced 15%)

tion; therefore, the aortic or systemic arterial diastolic pressure does not fall significantly despite an anatomically destroyed aortic valve. As a consequence, the left ventricle does not dilate and congestive cardiac failure may be absent. Because the aortic valve cusps in these patients are previously traumatized by the jet of blood traversing the subaortic stenosis, the infection is superimposed on a previously abnormal valve. In this situation the most common infecting organisms are alpha streptococci, organisms of a relatively low virulence that are compatible with active infective endocarditis over a long period (many months) without antibiotic treatment.[58]

One of the essential reasons for diagnosing DSS before adulthood is to allow operative resection of the "membrane" so that cuspal damage is prevented. When operative treatment is delayed until adulthood, aortic valve replacement is often required in addition to resection of the subaortic "membrane." Then survival becomes dependent on the "survival" of the valvular prosthesis, and anticoagulants usually are required with all of their inherent complications.

A recent anatomic observation in necropsy patients with DSS is severe thickening and luminal narrowing of the intramural coronary arteries located in the ventricular septum.[66] A similar finding has been observed in patients with hypertrophic cardiomyopathy (see next section) and in patients with tunnel subaortic stenosis.[67]

HYPERTROPHIC CARDIOMYOPATHY

In his original description,[68] Teare applied the term *asymmetrical hypertrophy of the heart* to this condition. Subsequently, terms such as *functional subaortic stenosis, diffuse muscular subaortic stenosis, idiopathic hypertrophic subaortic stenosis, hypertrophic obstructive cardiomyopathy,* and *asymmetric septal hypertrophy (ASH)* have been applied. The terms which include the words "stenosis" and "obstruction" appear inappropriate because obstruction is more often absent than present.[69] The terms which emphasize asymmetry of the walls bordering the left ventricular cavity have served a useful purpose in emphasizing a characteristic morphologic feature of this condition,[43] but the ventricular septum may be thicker than the left ventricular free wall in conditions other than hypertrophic cardiomyopathy (HC).[70–77] A few patients (about 5 percent) with HC do not have ASH (i.e., septum thicker than free wall[78,79]) and in rare cases the free wall is not thickened in HC.[78]

Study at necropsy of patients with HC[78] has demonstrated the following morphologic features: (1) greater thickening of the ventricular septum than of the left ventricular free wall (95 percent); (2) small or normal-sized left and right ventricular cavities (95 percent); (3) mural endocardial plaque, left ventricular outflow tract (75 percent, adults only); (4) thickened mitral valve (75 percent, adults only); (5) dilated atria (100 percent, adults only); (6) abnormal intramural coronary arteries (50 percent);[80] and (7) disorganization of myocardial fibers in the ventricular septum (95 percent) (Figs. 23–31; Table 3).

The chief morphologic abnormality in HC resides in the *ventricular septum.* As pointed out by Teare in 1958, the ventricular septum nearly always is thicker than the left ventricular free wall. Among our adult necropsy patients, the maximal thickness of ventricular septum averaged 3.0 cm. and the maximal thickness of left ventricular free wall, 1.8 cm. The thickest portion of the septum is that part located about midway between aortic valve and left ventricular apex. This level corresponds approximately to the apex of right ventricle. Although in all our necropsy patients the ventricular septum was thicker than normal, the left ventricular free wall was usually, though not always, thicker than normal.

Although *ventricular asymmetry* (i.e., a significant difference in maximal thickness of ventricular septum and left ventricular free wall) is a characteristic morphologic feature of HC, about 5 percent of our patients with this condition showed *ventricular symmetry* at necropsy (i.e., equal maximal thickness of the ventricular septum and left ventricular free wall). Thus, although asymmetric septal hypertrophy (ASH) is a highly sensitive marker for HC,[69] it is not specific for this condition. Ventricular septa thicker than left ventricular free walls have been reported in conditions causing thinning of the left ventricular free wall relative to the septum and in conditions causing thickening of the septum relative to the free wall. The most common cause of preferential free wall

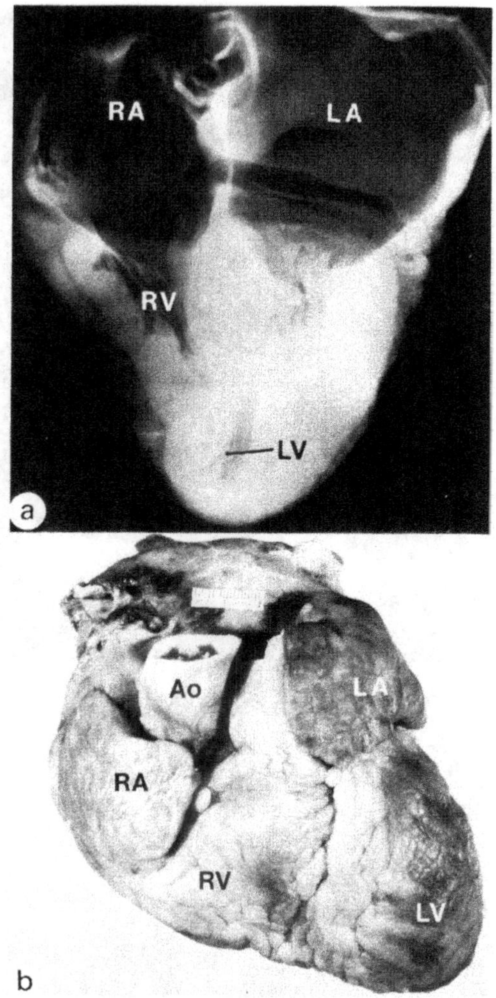

Figure 23. *a*, Radiograph of heart specimen and *b*, the heart itself in a 43-year-old woman with *hypertrophic cardiomyopathy*. Eleven years before she died the peak systolic pressure gradient between left ventricle and aorta was 54 mm. Hg at rest. She had periodic atrial fibrillation, chronic congestive cardiac failure, and an event compatible with cerebral embolus. The radiograph shows very dilated right (RA) and left (LA) atria, small-sized right (RV) and left (LV) ventricular cavities and a ventricular septum thicker than the left ventricular free wall. The exterior view of the specimen also shows very prominent atria. Ao = aorta.

Table 3. Idiopathic dilated (DC) and hypertrophic (HC) cardiomyopathies: morphologic differences

	DC	HC
1. Dilated ventricular cavities	+	0
2. Intracardiac thrombi	+	0
3. Asymmetric septal hypertrophy	0	+
4. Myocardial fiber disorientation	0	+
5. Endocardial plaque, LV outflow tract	0	+
6. Thickened mitral valve	0	+
7. Abnormal intramural coronary arteries	0	+
8. Ventricular scarring (gross)	0 – +	+
9. Thickened ventricular walls	0 – +	+
10. Increased cardiac weight	+	+
11. Dilated atrial cavities	+	+

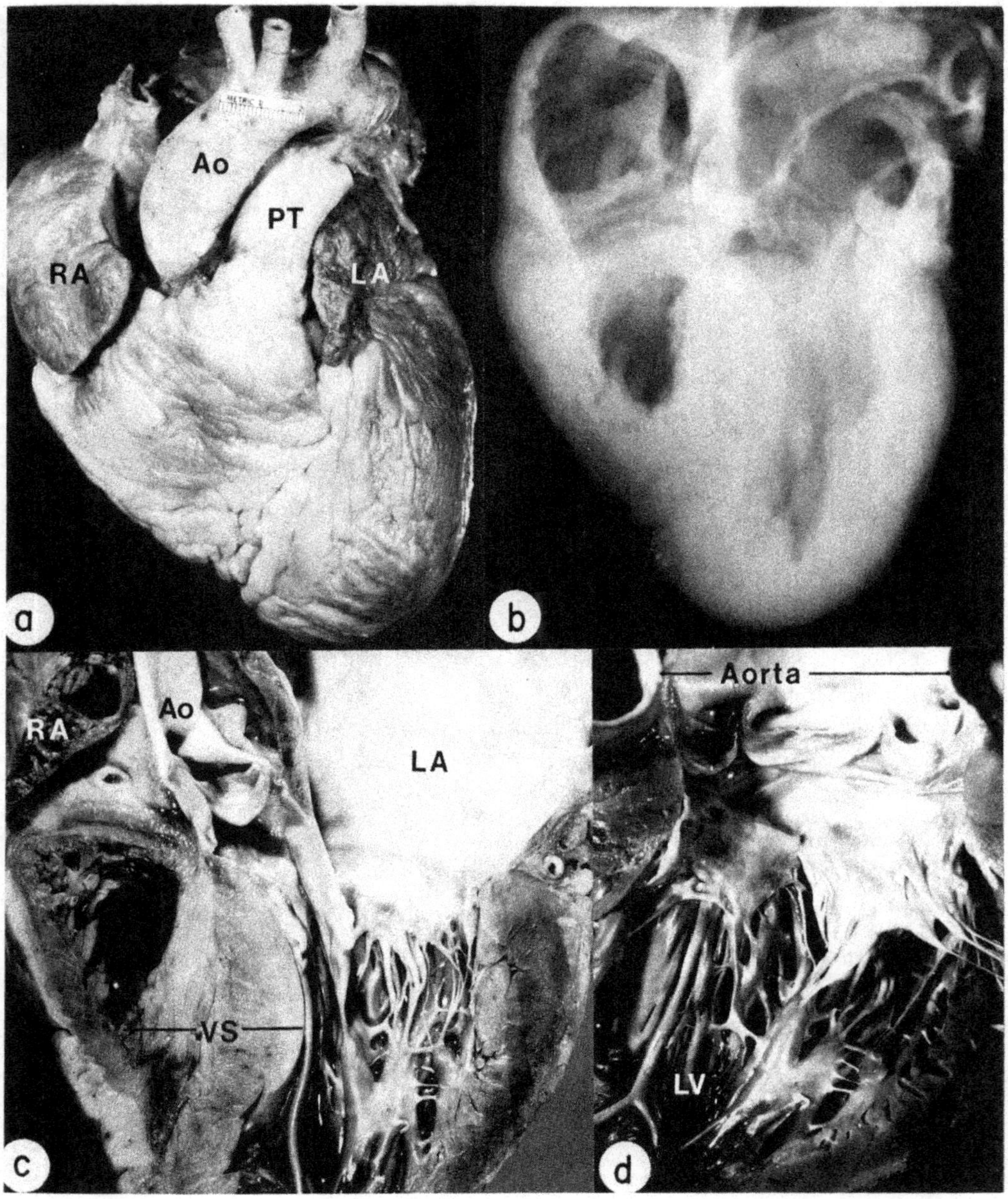

Figure 24. Heart of a 26-year-old man with *hypertrophic cardiomyopathy.* At catheterization three years before his death, a peak systolic pressure gradient of 30 mm. Hg was present between left ventricle and brachial artery and the gradient increased to 85 mm. Hg with provocation (ouabain). The cardiac index was 2.1 l./min./m.^{2}. At another catheterization done only six days before his sudden death, the gradient at rest was zero and it rose to only 33 mm. Hg when provoked (isoproterenol). The cardiac index was 2.0 l./min./m.^{2}. The anatomic features of hypertrophic cardiomyopathy are demonstrated in these photographs. *a,* Exterior view; both right (RA) and left (LA) atria are dilated. Ao = aorta; PT = pulmonary trunk. *b,* Radiograph of specimen showing the ventricular septum to be thicker than left ventricular free wall. *c,* Coronal section; the septum (VS) is clearly thicker than the left ventricular free wall, and an endocardial mural plaque is present in the left ventricular outflow tract in apposition to the anterior mitral leaflet. *d,* A closer view of the plaque and the thickened anterior mitral leaflet.

thinning is myocardial infarction; the most common cause of preferential septal thickening is right ventricular systolic hypertension from any of a variety of conditions.

Among patients with HC, the thickness of the ventricular septum is not dependent on the presence of left ventricular outflow tract obstruction at rest, and, indeed, the thickness of the septum is similar in patients with outflow obstruction at rest and in those without outflow obstruction at rest. Although examination of the septum in patients with HC is not helpful in separating the patients *with* from those *without* left ventricular outflow obstruction at rest, examination of the basal portion of the left ventricular free wall (posterior or posterolateral portion) does permit delineation between these two groups of patients.[81,82] In the patients with the obstructive type of HC, this posterobasal portion of left ventricular free wall represents the thickest portion of free wall, whereas in the patients with the nonobstructive type of HC, this posterobasal portion is thinner than normal and often pointed like a bird's bill (Fig. 25). In the patients with obstruction at rest, the thickest portion of the left ventricular free wall is about midway between the base of posterior mitral leaflet and apex of left ventricle.

Another abnormality in the ventricular septum in patients with HC is focal *myocardial fiber disarray* or disorganization[68,78,81-83] (Fig. 30). This abnormality also was described by Teare in 1958, and occurs in 90 to 100 percent of these patients depending on how "septal disorganization" is defined.[83] Small foci of myocardial fibers not parallel to one another in the ventricular septum are common in normal hearts. When, however, the definition of "septal disorganization" is rigid and quantitation of the amount of disorganization is introduced, about 90 percent of the patients with HC can be clearly delineated from persons with normal hearts or from patients with cardiac conditions other than HC.[83] Studies by Maron and associates[83] have shown that among patients

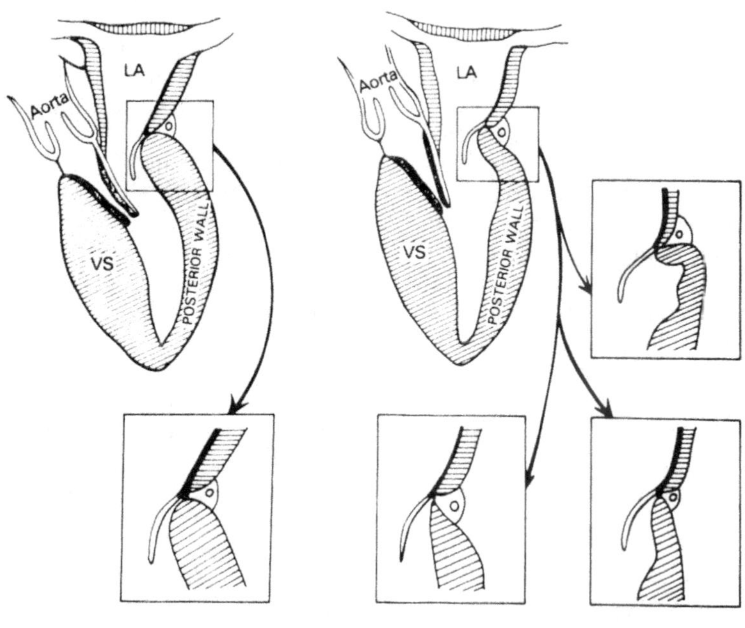

Figure 25. Diagram depicting the configuration and thickness of the posterolateral left ventricular free wall just behind the posterior mitral leaflet in the obstructive and nonobstructive types of *hypertrophic cardiomyopathy.* In the obstructive form, the most basal portion of free wall is rounded and thick. In the nonobstructive form, the most basal portion of left ventricular free wall is pointed and thin. In each type the ventricular septum is much thicker than the left ventricular free wall. The mural endocardium in the left ventricular outflow tract and the anterior mitral leaflet in apposition to it is thickened.

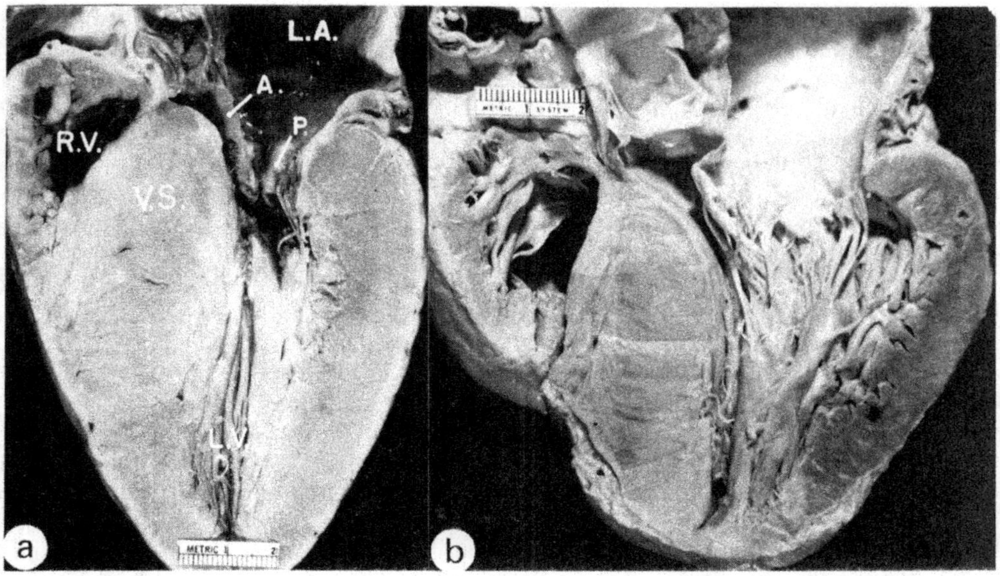

Figure 26. *Hypertrophic cardiomyopathy* in two patients. *a*, Left ventricular outflow obstruction in patient whose gradient at rest was 77 mm. Hg. *b*, Patient with no gradient at rest. The posterobasal portion of left ventricular (L.V.) free wall in the first patient is rounded and thick; this portion of free wall in the second patient is more pointed and thin. The result is a larger left ventricular cavity in the basal portion in *b* than in *a* and, consequently, more room for the mitral valve. The ventricular septum (V.S.) in both patients, however, is severely thickened. A., P. = anterior and posterior mitral leaflets, respectively; R.V. = right ventricle.

with HC nearly 90 percent had 5 percent or more of the area of the ventricular septum showing myocardial fiber disorganization. In contrast, among persons with normal hearts or heart conditions other than HC, less than 5 percent of the area of the ventricular septum showed such disorganization.

Although "septal disorganization" of greater than 5 percent of the area of the ventricular septum occurs in about 90 percent of the patients with HC, about 10 percent of these patients have less than 5 percent of the area of the septum showing disarray and of them a few patients have absolutely no disarray at all.[83] Thus, like ventricular asymmetry, "septal disorganization" of greater than 5 percent of the area of the septum occurs in most patients with HC, but this abnormality may involve a smaller area of the septum, or, rarely, may be entirely absent.

Not only does disorganization of *myocardial fibers* occur; ultrastructural studies have shown disarray of *myofibrils* and *myofilaments* within individual cells.[84] Again, the abnormalities of myofibrils and myofilaments are not absolutely specific for HC, but when disorganization of these subcellular components is found in other cardiac conditions, the abnormal cells are in small numbers. The individual septal myocardial cells in HC also frequently show increased amounts of Z-band material and nonspecific changes of cellular hypertrophy and degeneration.[84]

Myocardial fiber disarray in the left and right ventricular free walls is more difficult to determine by light microscopy than that in the ventricular septum. Ultrastructural examination of the left and right ventricular free walls, however, has disclosed many bizarrely shaped, disorganized cells in the ventricular free walls of patients *without* obstruction whereas the bizarrely shaped and disorganized myocardial fibers are virtually entirely absent from the ventricular free walls in the patients *with* obstruction.[81,82] Thus, the disorientation of groups of myocardial cells and the disarray of myofibrils and myofilaments within individual myocardial cells is not the result of left ventricular outflow obstruction or high intraventricular systolic pressures.

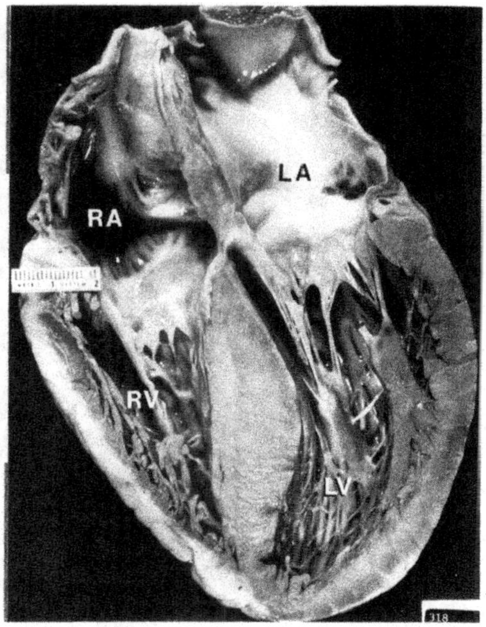

Figure 27. *Hypertrophic cardiomyopathy* (HC) in a 16-year-old girl who was always asymptomatic and died suddenly while jogging. Her mother had HC and three of her four siblings died suddenly. HC had been demonstrated clinically in each of them. The present patient by echocardiograms had systolic anterior motion of the anterior mitral leaflet, an ejection fraction of 87 percent, and no evidence of left ventricular outflow obstruction. She had no precordial murmur. The electrocardiogram had shown narrow Q waves in II, III, and AVF. The heart weighed 310 gm. and the ventricular septum was twice as thick as the left ventricular free wall (19 to 9 mm.). The left ventricular free wall was actually of normal thickness. RA = right atrium; RV = right ventricle; LA = left atrium; LV = left ventricle.

The functional or clinical significance of "septal disorganization" among patients with HC is not entirely clear. Among the patients studied at necropsy by Maron and associates,[83] those with high percentages of disorganization in the septal area were younger, had a higher frequency of premature deaths involving more than one member of the same family,[85,86] and thicker ventricular septa than those with lower percentages. A comparison of the presence or degree of left ventricular outflow obstruction, length of symptoms of cardiac dysfunction, mode of death, arrhythmias, etc., revealed no significant difference between the patients with high percentages and those with low percentages of septal area disorganization.[83]

Another abnormality of ventricular septum with HC is the presence of *abnormal intramural coronary arteries,* found in about one half of the patients[80] (Fig. 31). The abnormalities observed in the intramural coronary arteries in these patients are striking and consist of increased number and size of arteries with thickened walls and narrowed lumens. The thickening results from proliferation of smooth-muscle cells and collagen in both the media and the intima. Also, mucoid deposits (acid mucopolysaccaride material) are more numerous. Like disproportionate septal thickening (causing ventricular asymmetry) and septal disorganization, however, abnormality of the intramural coronary arteries is not specific for HC, though it is certainly more striking in HC than in most other conditions. Similar abnormality of the intramural coronary arteries may be observed in patients and in Newfoundland dogs with discrete subaortic stenosis,[66] in patients with tunnel subaortic stenosis,[67] and in newborns with aortic-valve atresia.[87]

The significance of the changes in the intramural coronary arteries in patients with HC is unknown. Their presence or absence does not correlate with any analyzed clinical parameter including age, sex, presence or degree of left ventricular outflow tract obstruction, presence of cardiac dysfunction including chest pain, or length of symptoms of cardiac dysfunction.

The cause of the striking abnormalities of the intramural coronary arteries also is uncertain. In each of the four conditions in which this degree of abnormality have been observed, namely, HC, discrete and tunnel subaortic stenosis and aortic-valve atresia, the septum is extremely thick and movement of the septum during life as shown by

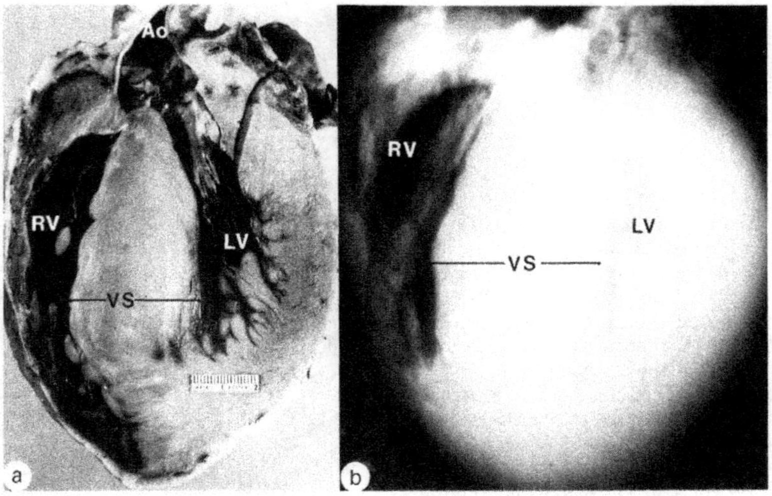

Figure 28. *Hypertrophic asymmetric obstructive* (right-sided) *cardiomyopathy.* This 18-year-old boy described in detail in the text was first studied when he was asymptomatic at age eight; his brother had died suddenly at age nine from idiopathic hypertrophic subaortic stenosis (left-sided obstruction). At catheterization no systolic pressure gradient was observed between the left ventricle and the systemic artery, but a systolic pressure gradient of 35 mm. Hg was recorded between the right ventricle (56/5) and the pulmonary artery (21/9). An electrocardiogram showed right axis deviation, right ventricular hypertrophy, and a right ventricular conduction delay. The child remained asymptomatic until age 12, when he developed chest pain while playing football. Precordial pain recurred frequently thereafter and was precipitated by exertion of decreasing intensity so that he was forced to limit his activities to a sedentary level. When he was restudied at age 13, a grade 1/6 systolic ejection-type precordial murmur was heard which was loudest along the left sternal border. Electrocardiography now showed more severe right ventricular hypertrophy. Cardiac catheterization showed a peak systolic pressure gradient of 118 mm. Hg between the right ventricle (135/7) and pulmonary artery (17/7) and there was no systolic gradient between the left ventricle (108/4) and the brachial artery (108/63 mm. Hg). Resection of the right ventricular outflow myocardium with insertion of a patch at the right ventriculuotomy was performed, and catheterization seven months postoperatively showed virtually no systolic pressure gradient between the right ventricle (30/4 mm. Hg) and the pulmonary artery (28/12). He was asymptomatic. Electrocardiograms now showed a right bundle branch block. This boy apparently remained asymptomatic until the day of death, when he felt faint while driving a car. He pulled over to the side of the road and collapsed. No anatomic explanation for death was revealed at necropsy. His heart weighed 660 gm. The right ventricular (RV) outflow tract was wide open. The ventricular septum (VS) was much thicker than the left ventricular (LV) free wall (1.0 compared to 1.9 cm.), and the right ventricular wall was of normal thickness. The endocardium of the left ventricular outflow tract was not thickened and the mitral valve was normal. Mild interstitial fibrosis involved the ventricular septum. *a,* A longitudinal section of the ventricles shows the disproportionate ventricular septal hypertrophy. The right ventricular cavity is larger than the left. Ao = Aorta. *b,* The radiograph of the heart was taken before it was opened.

echocardiogram is extremely limited. It is possible that the severe septal thickening prevents adequate expansion of these vessels during ventricular diastole and thus reduces flow. The fibrous-smooth muscle cell response, in turn, may serve to obliterate the unused lumen. However, this explanation does not explain the large size of these arteries. It is possible that the proliferation of the smooth-muscle cells in the walls of these arteries represents a response to the same stimulus which is causing severe hypertrophy and abnormal configuration of many striated myocardial cells.

A fourth abnormality of the ventricular septum in adults with HC is the occurrence of a fibrous plaque on the mural endocardium of the outflow portion of the septum[77] (Fig. 24). This fibrous thickening is located in direct apposition to the ventricular aspect of the anterior mitral leaflet and is the result of contact between the valvular and mural endocardium. The mural plaque, in other words, is the anatomic equivalent of the "systolic anterior motion" (SAM) of the anterior mitral leaflet observed on echocar-

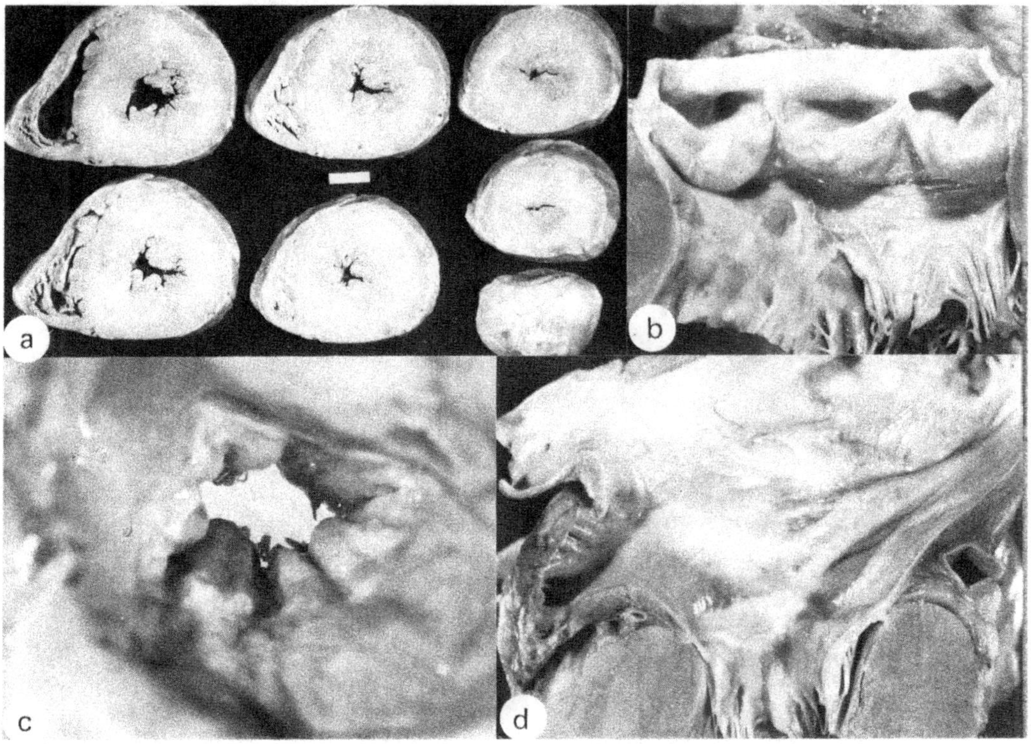

Figure 29. *Hypertrophic cardiomyopathy* in a 53-year-old man who died suddenly at home six weeks after onset of atrial fibrillation. Catheterization when he was asymptomatic (but had cardiomegaly) at age 46 disclosed a left ventricular to systemic arterial peak systolic gradient of 8 mm. Hg at rest, and a gradient of 69 mm. Hg with provocation (isoproteronol). Thereafter, he developed exertional dyspnea, dizziness, and angina. *a,* "Bread loaf" slices of cardiac ventricles. Although the echocardiogram had shown the ventricular septum to be thicker than left ventricular free wall during ventricular diastole, both were of similar thickness at necropsy (25 mm.). *b,* Opened aortic valve showing thickening of the mural endocardium in apposition to the thickened anterior mitral leaflet. *c,* View of mitral valve from left atrium. Thickening of its leaflets is typical of hypertrophic cardiomyopathy. *d,* Opened left atrium and thickened mitral valve. The basal portion of left ventricular wall is rounded and thick.

diogram in patients with HC and occasionally in other conditions.[76] When present in HC, the obstruction almost certainly begins at a level corresponding to the distal margin of the anterior mitral leaflet and with the caudal margin of the septal endocardial plaque. The mural endocardial septal plaque is present more frequently and is thicker in the patients with obstruction at rest compared to those without obstruction at rest.

It appears that HC is primarily a disease of the ventricular septum and that the morphologic abnormalities in it are apparent at the gross, microscopic, and ultrastructural levels. Other portions of the heart, however, are affected in HC but it seems likely that these other abnormalities are secondary to the abnormalities of the ventricular septum. These other abnormalities include *decreased ventricular cavity size* or, at least, lack of ventricular cavity dilatation, *increased atrial cavity size,* varying degrees of interstitial and replacement *myocardial fibrosis* (particularly in the ventricular septum), thickening of the posterior as well as the anterior mitral leaflet and, in elderly patients, calcification of the mitral anulus.[77,88,89]

The cause of the relatively small size of ventricular cavities in HC is unclear. The septum, being on the average about twice normal thickness, surely occupies space normally represented by cavity. The ventricular free walls are, on the average, about a

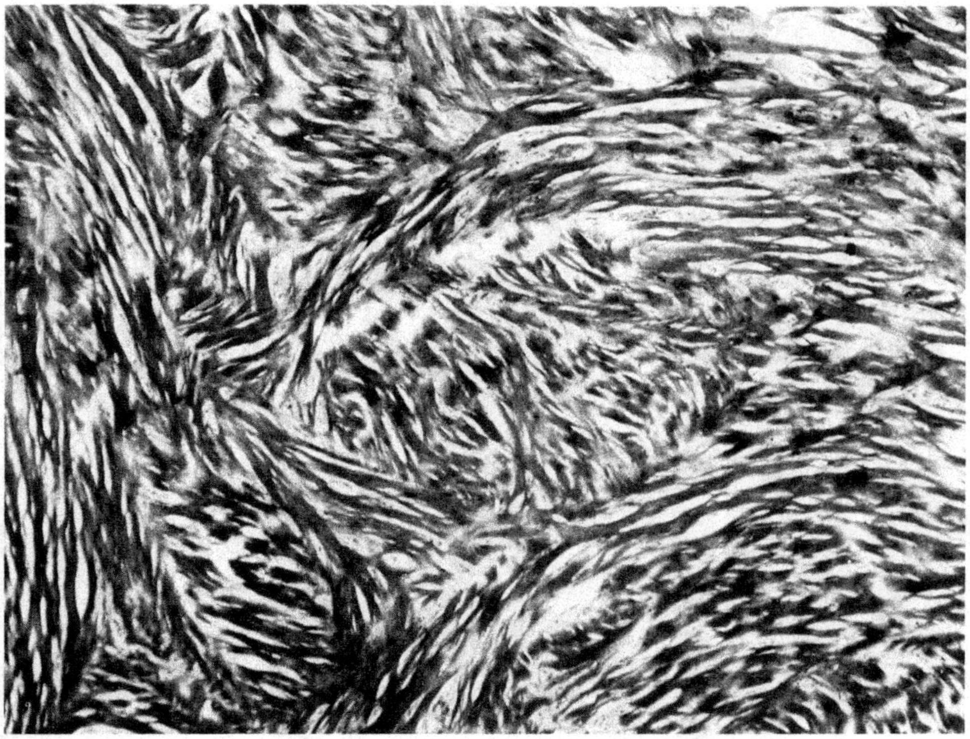

Figure 30. Photomicrograph of portion of ventricular septum in a 19-year-old man with *hypertrophic cardiomyopathy* showing the myocardial fiber disarray typical of this condition. (Masson stain; x 60 magnification)

third thicker than normal; this probably compromises slightly the intracavitary space even further. The greater thickness of the septum makes it relatively noncompliant (as demonstrated by its absent or minimal movement on echocardiogram). Although the left ventricular free wall in HC (by echocardiogram) usually contracts vigorously (in contrast to the septum), it appears to have little capacity to distend outwardly. Whatever the explanation, ventricular cavity size is rarely enlarged in these patients. The patients I have studied with dilated ventricular cavities at necropsy (4 of 65 with HC) have either nonscarred left and/or right ventricular free walls of normal thickness or scarred ventricular free walls of less than normal thickness. Dilatation may occur after operative septotomy-septectomy in HC.[90]

The impression of ventricular cavity size as observed at necropsy in patients with HC may be somewhat misleading because the cavity at necropsy in patients with HC represents the size at the end of ventricular systole.[91] This information was derived by comparing the left ventricular free wall thickness at necropsy to that measured by echocardiogram during life.[91] The thickness at necropsy corresponds to the thickness during ventricular systole, not diastole, which is observed by echocardiogram.

In contrast to the ventricular cavities, the atrial cavities in HC, at least in adults, are always dilated. The dilatation appears to be a response to difficulty in filling the relatively small ventricular caivities.

Not only is the anterior mitral leaflet thickened, but often (more frequently in the patients with obstruction) the posterior mitral leaflet too is thickened. The thickening of both leaflets is probably the consequence of the small left ventricular cavity. It is important to recall that the mitral valve resides in the left ventricle, which because of its

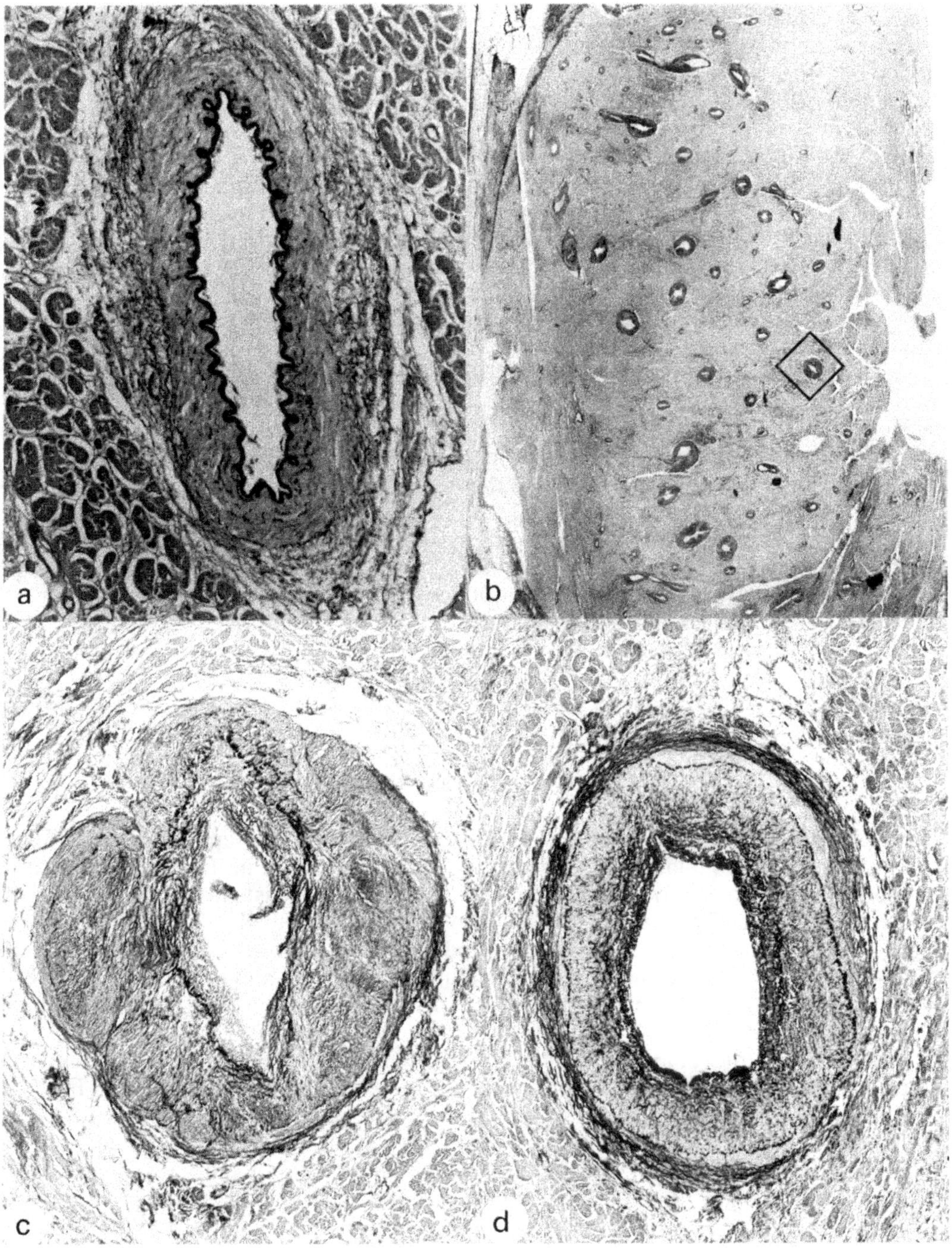

Figure 31. *Intramural coronary arteries in ventricular septum in hypertrophic cardiomyopathy* (HC) in three different patients. *a,* A normal artery (in a patient with HC) x 140. *b,* Low-power (x 4) photomicrograph of portion of ventricular septum showing marked prominence of the intramural coronary arteries in another patient. The arteries appear to be increased in number, size, and wall thickness. *c,* The artery enclosed by the box in *b* is shown here x 90. *d,* This artery, from another patient, has marked intimal thickening by fibroelastic proliferation, in contrast to the artery shown in *c,* which shows no delineation between intima and media. (Elastic van Gieson stains.) (Reduced 18%.)

small size, causes abnormal contact of the leaflets with themselves and also causes the anterior one to contact the septum. In the patients without obstruction, the basal portion of the left ventricular cavity is larger than in the patients with obstruction because of the thinning of the basal portion of free wall posteriorly and laterally. The focal fibrous thickening of the posterior mitral leaflet probably results from abnormal contact during ventricular systole since there is not enough room in the ventricular cavity to easily accommodate the leaflets and chordae. In this respect the ventricle and mitral leaflets mimic the movement of an accordion. The mitral leaflet thickening in HC is somewhat analogous to that which occurs normally as a consequence of aging. With aging, the left ventricular cavity becomes smaller, presumably in response to the lowered cardiac output; the mitral leaflets thicken; the left ventricular muscle becomes less compliant; and the left atrium dilates in response to increased work required to fill the small left ventricle. The same mechanisms appear to be accelerated in HC.

Most patients with HC have some degree of mitral regurgitation. It is not related to anular dilatation because the mitral anulus in this condition is not dilated.[78] Furthermore, the leaflet thickening in and of itself is not extensive enough to cause valvular regurgitation. The most likely explanation appears to be abnormal bending of the papillary muscles, particularly the anterolateral one.[69] These structures may be bent abnormally by the bulging ventricular septum with resulting excessive tension on the chordae tendineae preventing closure of the mitral orifice. Although they are usually present in the papillary muscles in HC, focal scars cannot account for the regurgitation. Although it is usually mild in HC, mitral regurgitation may be the predominant clinical feature of this condition. Despite advocacy by some investigators,[92,93] mitral valve replacement in HC is hazardous and unwarranted for a number of reasons.[94] The small left ventricular cavity is rarely capable of freely accommodating a prosthesis, and the mitral regurgitation in patients with HC nearly always either disappears or is strikingly lessened by adequate partial septectomy-septotomy.

SINUS OF VALSALVA ANEURYSM

Dilatation of each of the three sinuses of Valsalva is a normal consequence of aging and this "senile-type dilatation" appears to be more common in hypertensive than in normotensive persons.[21] In addition to aging, there are at least three other causes of dilatation of each of the three sinuses of Valsalva; these are the Marfan and Marfan-like syndromes,[14] syphilis,[95] and ankylosing spondylitis.[96,97] A congenital type of dilatation of all three aortic sinuses unassociated with other congenital anomalies of the heart or great vessels also has been recorded,[98] but its occurrence, if indeed of congenital origin, must be unique.

In contrast to the common occurrence of dilatation of all three aortic sinuses, aneurysmal dilatation of only one or two of the three sinuses is quite unusual (Figs. 32 to 34). The most common cause is probably infective endocarditis with spread of the infective process into adjacent structures and formation of one or more ring abscesses.[99] Aneurysmal dilatation of only one aortic sinus unassociated with infective endocarditis is extremely rare. In this circumstance the localized aneurysmal dilatation is generally attributed to a congenital absence of media in the wall of the aorta behind the sinus of Valsalva[100] (Fig. 35). The wall of aorta behind the sinus may rupture, and when this occurs, aortic regurgitation into either right ventricle or right atrium is the usual consequence (Fig. 33). Less commonly, the sinus aneurysm may obstruct right ventricular outflow or cause a conduction disturbance.[101]

The basic defect in patients with aneurysms involving only one or two of the three aortic valve sinuses is an absence of a portion or all of the media in the wall of aorta behind the sinus. Just because the media is deficient, however, does not assure the

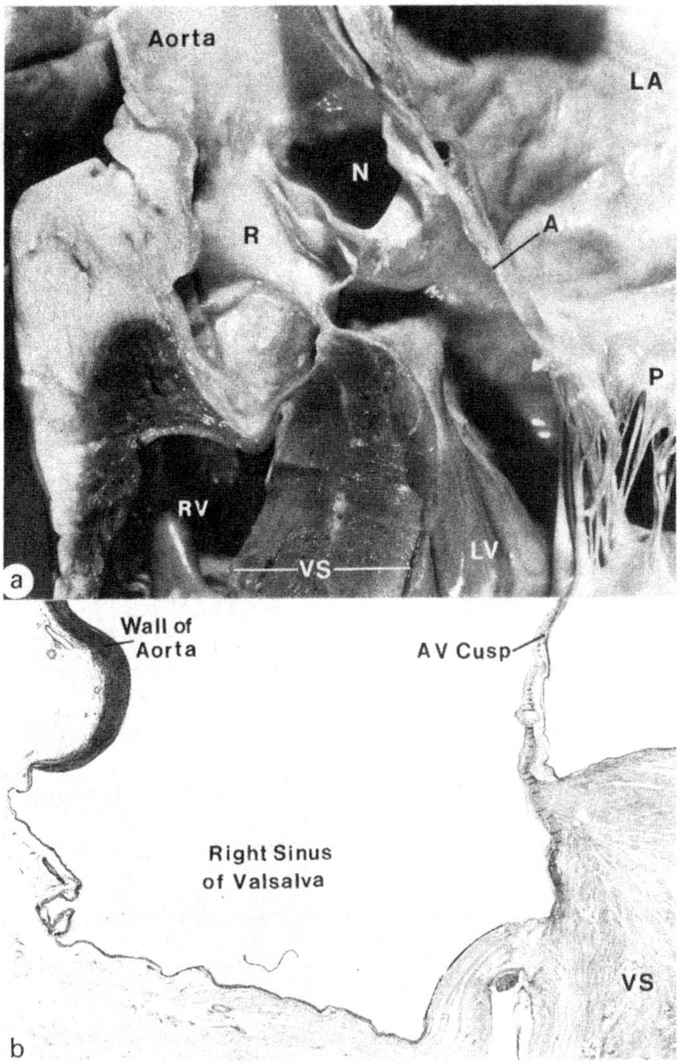

Figure 32. *Unruptured sinus of Valsalva aneurysm* in an 82-year-old man who died of cancer. An unexpected finding at necropsy was aneurysmal dilatation of the right sinus of Valsalva. The right sinus was 2.5 cm. deep and held 15 ml. of fluid, while the left and noncoronary sinuses of Valsalva were only 1.5 cm. deep and held only 5 ml. of fluid.

a, Longitudinal section of heart showing the aneurysmal dilatation of the right (R) sinus of Valsalva. N = noncoronary sinus of Valsalva; A, P = anterior and posterior mitral leaflets, respectively; LA = left atrium; LV = left ventricle; VS = ventricular septum. *b,* Histologic section of wall of right sinus of Valsalva showing the absence of aortic media in the caudal portion of the aneurysm. AV = aortic valve.

appearance of an aortic sinus aneurysm. When a deficiency of aortic media occurs, the wall involved most commonly is that behind the right anterior cusp (about 70 percent of patients); occasionally it is the portion behind the noncoronary (posterior) cusp (about 29 percent); it rarely (< 1%) involves that portion behind the left anterior cusp.[102] The explanation for these differences is uncertain.

Whether or not a sinus of Valsalva aneurysm is ever present from birth is uncertain; most likely the aneurysm is acquired, presumably the result of the aortic pressure. The higher the aortic pressure (for example, in patients with coarctation of the aortic

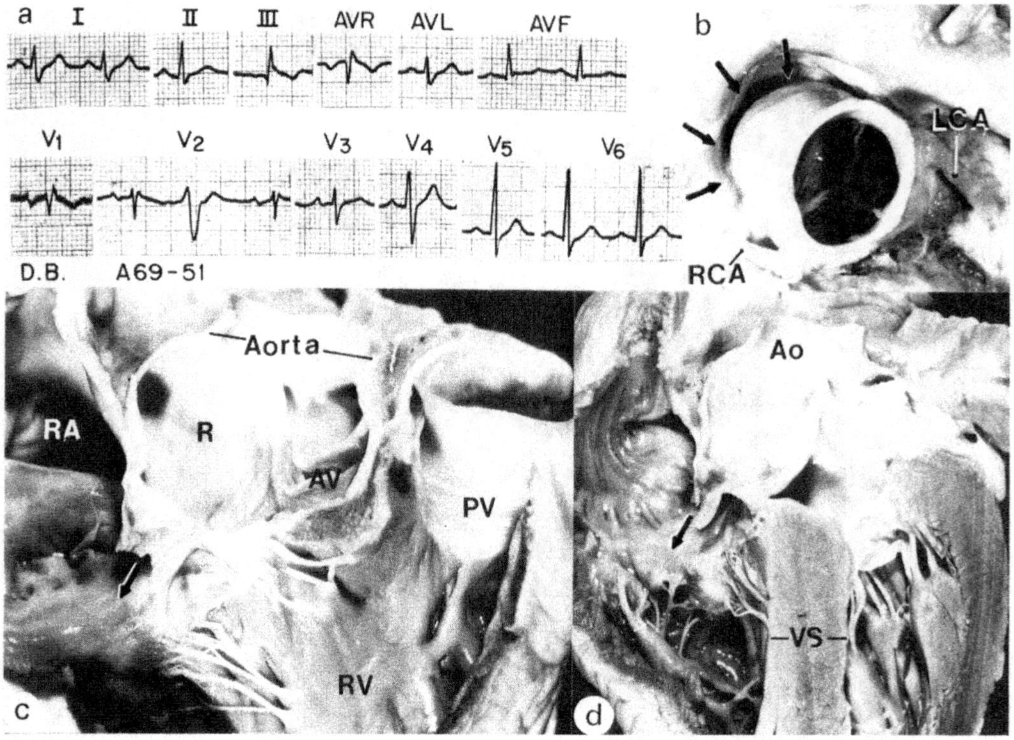

Figure 33. *Rupture of right (R) sinus of Valsalva aneurysm into right ventricle* (RV) in a 31-year-old woman who had been well until about 60 days before death when exertional dyspnea appeared. Eighteen days before death, she developed acute pulmonary edema and a murmur of aortic regurgitation. She died of progressive congestive cardiac failure. *a*, An electrocardiogram taken several days before her death. At necropsy the heart weighed only 300 gm. *b*, An aneurysm of the right sinus of Valsalva was present and bulged to the right (arrows). LCA, RCA = left and right coronary arteries, respectively. *c*, Opened right ventricle (RV) and wall of aorta behind right (R) sinus of Valsalva showing the aneurysm which had ruptured (arrow) into the right atrium (RA) anatomically and into right ventricle functionally. AV = aortic valve; PV = pulmonic valve. *d*, In this view the anterior half of the heart has been removed; the ruptured (arrow) aneurysm's relation to the right side of the heart and to the ventricular septum (VS) is apparent. Ao = aorta.

isthmus), the more likely is the possibility that an aortic sinus aneurysm will develop. The youngest child described with isolated sinus of Valsalva aneurysm was four years old.[103] Although the aneurysm itself may or may not be congenital, the deficiency in aortic media behind the sinus must be congenital.[101]

Both the natural history and the frequency of media-deficient aortic sinus wall are uncertain. The number of persons with a media-deficient aortic sinus wall in whom a sinus aneurysm developed is uncertain, as is the frequency of rupture of a developed sinus aneurysm. Among 78 cases of sinus of Valsalva aneurysm collected from previous publications by Kieffer and Winchell,[104] 59 (76 percent) had ruptured and 19 (24 percent) had not. In some of these cases, however, the aneurysms involved all three sinuses and were therefore probably associated with the Marfan syndrome. Among seven hearts with aneurysm of one aortic sinus studied at necropsy by Edwards and Burchell,[100] four aneurysms had ruptured and three had not. Of six single (one of three sinuses involved) aortic sinus aneurysms which I studied at necropsy, five had ruptured and only one[101] was unruptured. The latter patient was 82 years old; the five patients with ruptured aneurysms ranged in age from 31 to 49 years (average, 38). These figures indicate that among reported cases of aortic sinus aneurysm, rupture is more common than nonrupture. These data are probably considerably biased in favor of ruptured aneurysms;

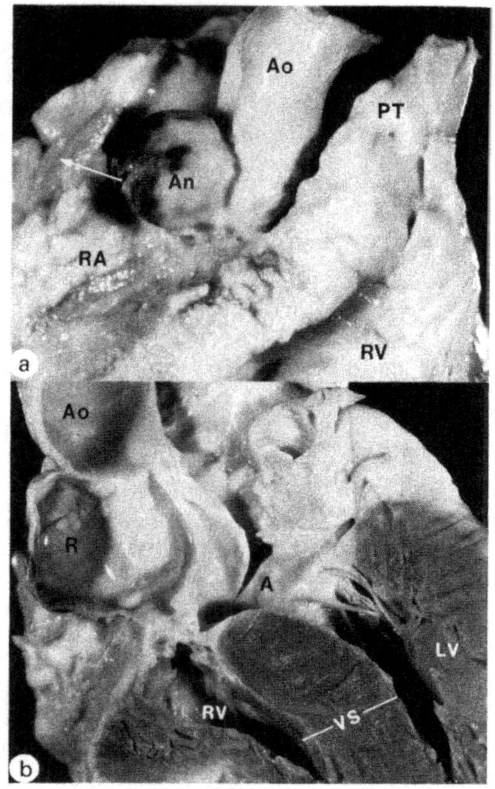

Figure 34. *Rupture of right sinus of Valsalva aneurysm into pericardial sac* in a 33-year-old woman who had been well until she died suddenly while house cleaning. At necropsy the pericardial sac was filled with blood. *a,* The right sinus of Valsalva is exteriorly round and a rupture (arrow) is visible in its right lateral wall. Extravasation was into the pericardial space only and not into a cardiac chamber. An = aneurysm; Ao = aorta; PT = pulmonary trunk; RA = right atrium; RV = right ventricle. *b,* The anterior portion of the heart has been removed again showing the right (R) sinus of Valsalva aneurysm. A = anterior mitral leaflet; LV = left ventricle; VS = ventricular septum.

nonruptured sinus aneurysm may be missed at necropsy, while the nonruptured aneurysm, with few exceptions, produces no evidence of cardiac dysfunction. Therefore, at necropsy there may be no clinical sign or symptom to alert the pathologist to the presence of an aortic sinus aneurysm. Furthermore, incidental necropsy findings, which an aortic sinus aneurysm usually represents, are infrequently reported. Thus, it

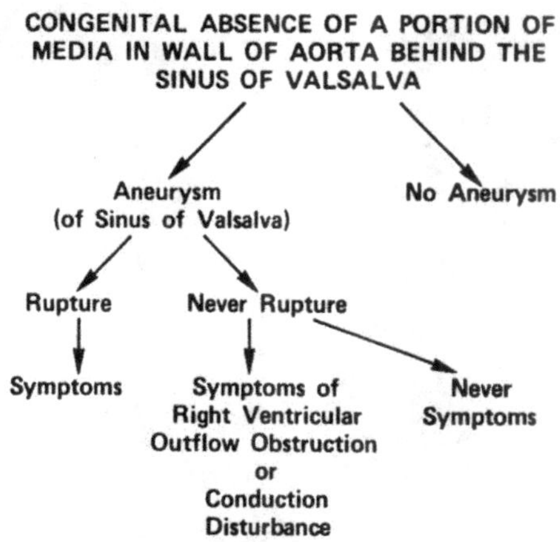

Figure 35. Diagram showing possible outcome in patients with *congenital absence of a portion of media in aortic wall behind sinus of Valsalva.* If no aneurysm occurs, the congenital defect will go unrecognized. If an aneurysm does occur it may or may not rupture. Rupture will virtually always produce clinical symptoms and signs of cardiac dysfunction. If rupture does not occur, symptoms will usually be present only if there is right ventricular outflow obstruction or conduction disturbances.

is likely that the frequency of unruptured aortic sinus aneurysm is considerably greater than has been reported.

On rare occasion an unruptured single aortic sinus aneurysm may produce evidence of cardiac dysfunction. Kerber and associates[105] described clinical and operative findings in a 62-year-old man who had evidence of right ventricular outflow obstruction as the result of an aortic sinus aneurysm's bulging into the crista supraventricularis. Complete heart block has also been described in a patient with unruptured aortic sinus aneurysm.[106] The latter patient, however, also had calcific aortic stenosis, and thus it is not certain that the sinus aneurysm was responsible for the conduction defect.

Rupture of the sinus of Valsalva aneurysm is clearly the most frequent complication of aneurysm involving only one of the three aortic sinuses. Rupture rarely occurs before adulthood. Like all conditions affecting the aorta and the aortic valve, it is more common in males than females (about 4 to 1). Death occurs suddenly if the rupture is into the pericardial space rather than into a cardiac cavity (Fig. 34). Death usually occurs, however, within a year after rupture with regurgitation into a cardiac chamber. Death most commonly is the result of congestive cardiac failure.

THE MARFAN SYNDROME

This inheritable disorder may involve the bones, joints, eyes, heart, and blood vessels. The extremities are long and thin (dolichostenomelia), the ligaments and joint capsules are redundant, the lenses may be dislocated (ectopia lentis), the ascending aorta often is dilated, and one or both left-sided cardiac valves usually are incompetent. Cardiovascular disease is by far the most common cause of death in patients with the Marfan syndrome. Of 18 patients that I studied at necropsy, all fulfilled McKusick's rigid criteria for this syndrome,[107] and all died prematurely from cardiovascular disease (average age, 34; range, 15 to 52). Of 56 decreased patients with this syndrome studied by Murdoch and associates,[108] cardiovascular disease was the cause of death in 52 (93 percent) and the average age at death was 32 years.

A variety of cardiovascular lesions have been observed in the aorta and heart of patients with the Marfan syndrome.[107] The 18 necropsy patients with this syndrome just

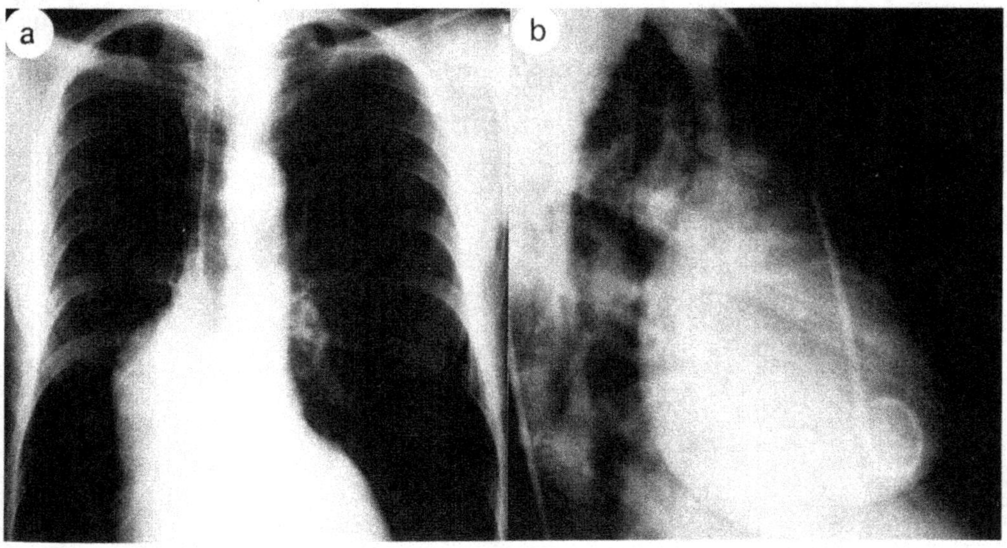

Figure 36. Chest radiograph *(a)* and aortogram *(b)* in a 38-year-old man with *Marfan syndrome*. A large aortic "root" aneurysm is present. (see Figure 37 for additional findings in this patient)

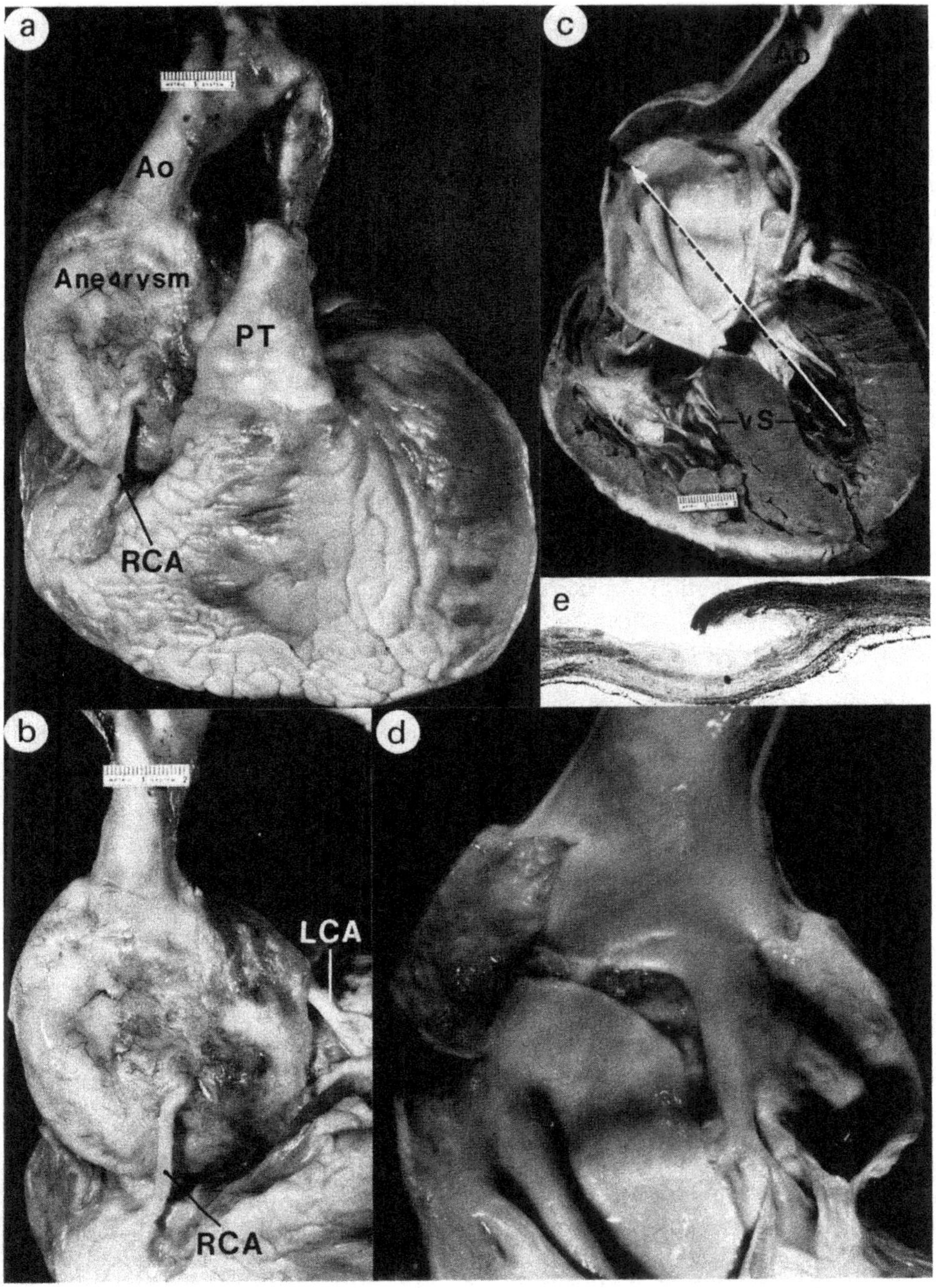

Figure 37. *The Marfan syndrome with rupture of ascending aortic aneurysm* in a 38-year-old black man. The patient was known to have a murmur of aortic regurgitation (aortic pressure 115/55 mm. Hg) but there was no evidence of congestive heart failure. He died suddenly at home and at necropsy the pericardial space was filled with blood and a tear was present in a large aneurysm involving all three sinuses of Valsalva and the proximal tubular portion of ascending aorta. *a*, View of heart shows the size of the aneurysm in comparison to the sizes of other structures. Ao = aorta; PT = pulmonary trunk; RCA = right coronary artery. *b*, A closer view of the large aneurysm with the coronary arteries arising from it. LCA = left coronary artery. *c*, The anterior half of the heart and aorta have now been removed. The dashed line depicts the direction of the blood ejected from the left ventricle. The arrow points to the rupture site in the wall of the aneurysm. The right lateral wall is the site of the rupture. VS = ventricular septum. *d*, Closeup of interior lining of aortic aneurysm at site of rupture. Several healed incomplete tears are present in the wall of the aneurysm and these have been confused with aortic dissections. *e*, Photomicrograph through one of the aortic tears showing massive degeneration of elastic fibers.

mentioned were readily separated into three distinct groups on the basis of their cardiovascular lesions. Group 1 included 12 patients with *saccular aneurysms of ascending aorta* (Figs. 36 to 38). All 12 patients had aortic regurgitation and 6 of them also had associated mitral regurgitation. Their aneurysms involved the sinus portion and the proximal tubular portion of ascending aorta, and two also had saccular aneurysms in the descending thoracic aorta. Histologic study of the wall of the ascending aorta disclosed the typical lesion of this syndrome, i.e., massive degeneration of elastic fibers and increase in mucoid material in the media (Fig. 38).

Group 2 included three patients with *dissection of the entire aorta* (Fig. 39). Before dissection, the aorta was of normal size in all three patients, and histologic study of the aortic wall disclosed that the typical lesion of this syndrome was absent; in fact, except for the dissection itself, the wall of aorta was histologically normal save for some aging changes.[109,110] Only one of the three patients had aortic regurgitation and then only after the dissection; one had mitral regurgitation and two had systemic hypertension before the aortic dissection.

Group 3 included two patients *without aortic saccular aneurysm or aortic disease* but with *pure mitral regurgitation* with floppy mitral leaflets and markedly dilated mitral anuli (Fig. 6). The aorta was of normal size and its wall was histologically normal in both.

Thus, the major lesions in the aorta in patients with this syndrome are saccular root aneurysms and dissection. In contrast to that described clinically by others,[111] our study of 18 necropsy patients suggests that the two rarely go together, since none of these patients had both a saccular aortic aneurysm and aortic dissection. These two aortic lesions may be mutually exclusive. None of the 12 patients with saccular aortic root aneurysms had evidence of dissection, although 9 of the 12 had focal intimal and medial tears in the wall of the saccular aneurysms (Figs. 37 and 38). These aortic tears have been mistakenly called "dissections" in a number of reports. None of the three with aortic dissection had saccular aneurysms of the aorta which was of normal size before the dissection. Histologically, the wall of the aorta varies with the type of lesion. In all 12 patients with aortic root saccular aneurysms, there was massive degeneration of the elastic fibers associated with increased amounts of collagen and mucoid material in the media of the aneurysmal wall. The increased amount of collagen in the aortic wall in these patients may actually prevent longitudinal dissection. In each of the three patients with aortic dissection, the wall of the aorta appeared histologically "normal," i.e., as it does in patients with aortic dissection who do not have the Marfan syndrome,[112] with no changes other than aging. Interestingly, two of the three patients with aortic dissection had evidence of diastolic systemic hypertension, whereas none of the other 16 patients had diastolic hypertension.

The term applied to the characteristic histologic lesion in the aorta in patients with the Marfan syndrome has been "cystic medial necrosis," a term first used by Erdheim in 1929[113] and an outgrowth of the term "medionecrosis" coined by Gsell[114] a year earlier. This term, however, is not ideal because "cysts" as such are infrequent and "necrosis," to my knowledge, has never been observed in the aortic media in this condition. Gsell used the term "medionecrosis" to designate areas in the aortic media with a diminished number of nuclei. Becker[109] recently showed that these areas devoid of nuclei actually consisted of large amounts of fibrous tissue and were a regular feature of the normal, aging aorta. Furthermore, the striking histologic aortic lesion in the Marfan syndrome is *massive degeneration of elastic fibers* in the media and this feature is ignored by the term "cystic medial necrosis." When Erdheim coined this term, stains for elastic fibers were poor or rarely used, and loss or degeneration of elastic fibers are difficult to appreciate on hematoxylin-eosin stained sections. Thus, he apparently could not appreciate this histologic feature of this condition.

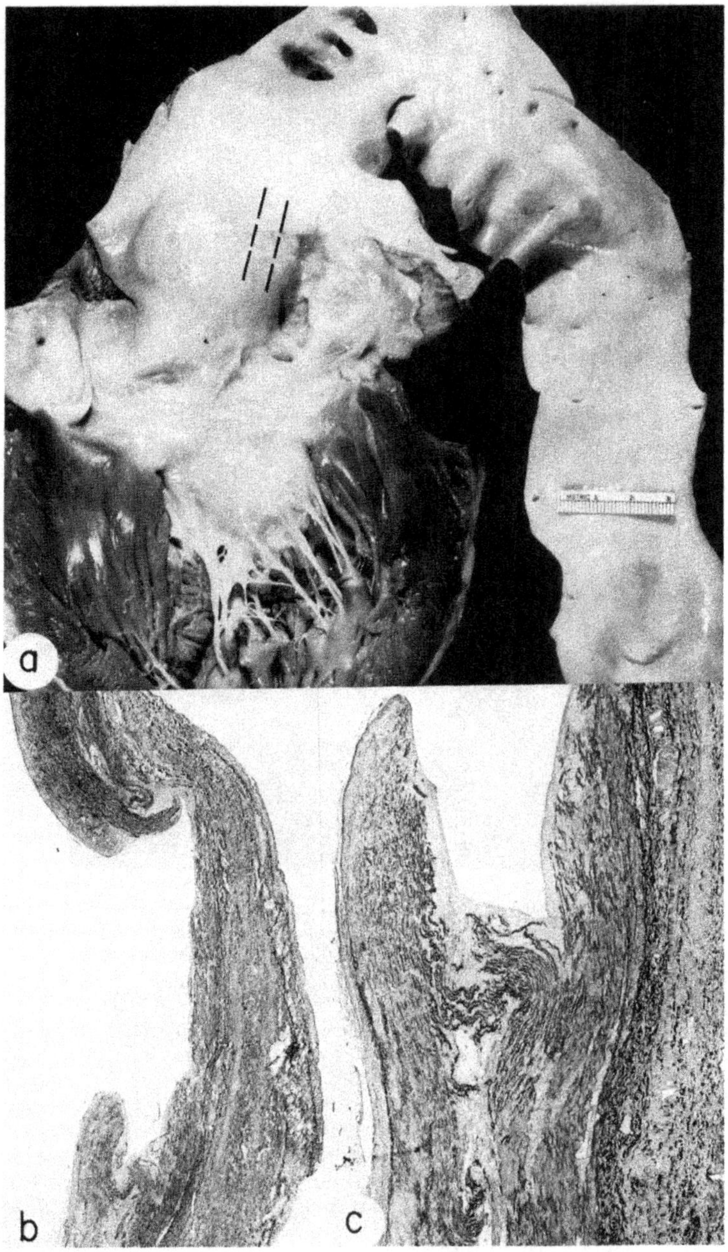

Figure 38. *The Marfan syndrome.* This 21-year-old man had the typical skeletal and optic features of this syndrome but had always been asymptomatic. He was found dead in his parked car after playing in a band for several hours. At necropsy the pericardial sac was filled with blood. *a,* Evidence of a through-and-through rupture is visible in the ascending aorta just above the aortic valve. In addition, several partial ruptures or tears are also present in the ascending aorta. *b,* A histologic section of one tear (shown between dashed lines in *a*). *c,* A closeup of an adjacent section of *b* reveals severe degeneration of elastic fibers of the media. (Elastic tissue stains; *b,* x 7 and *c,* x 18 magnification)

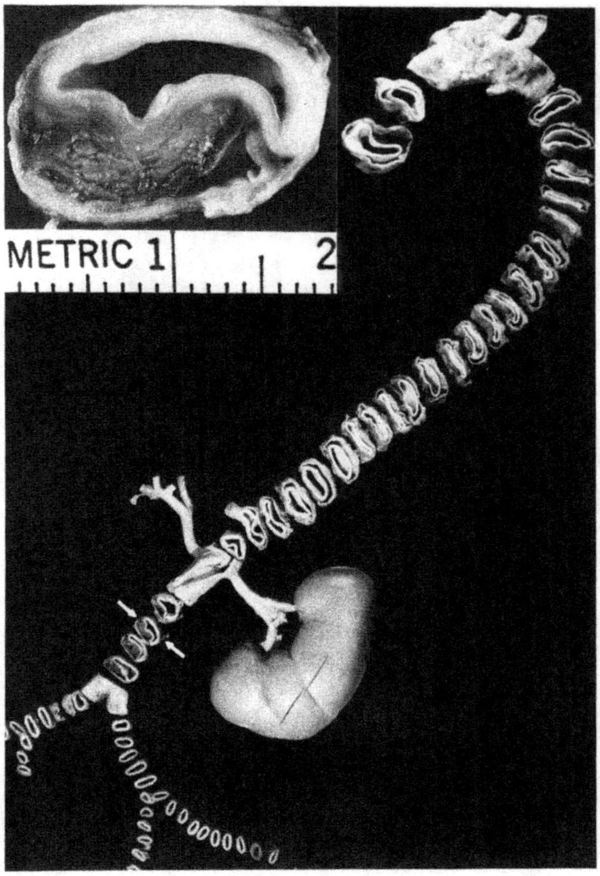

Figure 39. *Aorta* in a 43-year-old man known to have *Marfan syndrome*. He died 15 days after the sudden onset of typical clinical features of *aortic dissection*. Before the aortic dissection there was no precordial murmur. At necropsy, except for the acute dissection, there was no enlargement of the aorta, and except at the site of the entrance into the false channel, there were no tears in the aorta. Shown here is the complete aorta with both true and false channels and a hematoma in the false channel of the abdominal portion. A closeup of the transverse section indicated by the arrows is shown in the upper left. Histologically, there was no evidence of elastic fiber degeneration in the media of aorta. The heart weighed 500 gm. and neither ventricle was dilated. Thus, although this patient had both aortic dissection and Marfan syndrome, the typical histologic aortic medial lesion of this syndrome was absent. Therefore, it is more likely that the systemic hypertension was a more important contributing factor to the aortic dissection.

When elastic fibers disappear from the aortic wall in this condition, the space previously occupied by them appears to be replaced by collagen fibrils and mucoid material. Although the increased acid mucopolysaccharide material has been considered an inherent defect in this condition, it is just as reasonable to believe that this material serves simply as "a filler" for the lost elastic fibers and even smooth muscle cells. It is not clear whether or not the numbers of the elastic lamellae are normal or decreased at the time of birth in patients with the Marfan syndrome; however, aortic root aneurysm, with or without tears, has not been described in newborns with this syndrome. Thus, it appears that although the composition of the aortic media may be defective at birth, the aneurysms form later, presumably as a consequence of intra-aortic pressure on an inherently weak wall. The possible consequences of the inherently or congenitally weakened aortic media is shown diagrammatically in Figure 40.

Aortic regurgitation in patients with the Marfan syndrome is usually the result of

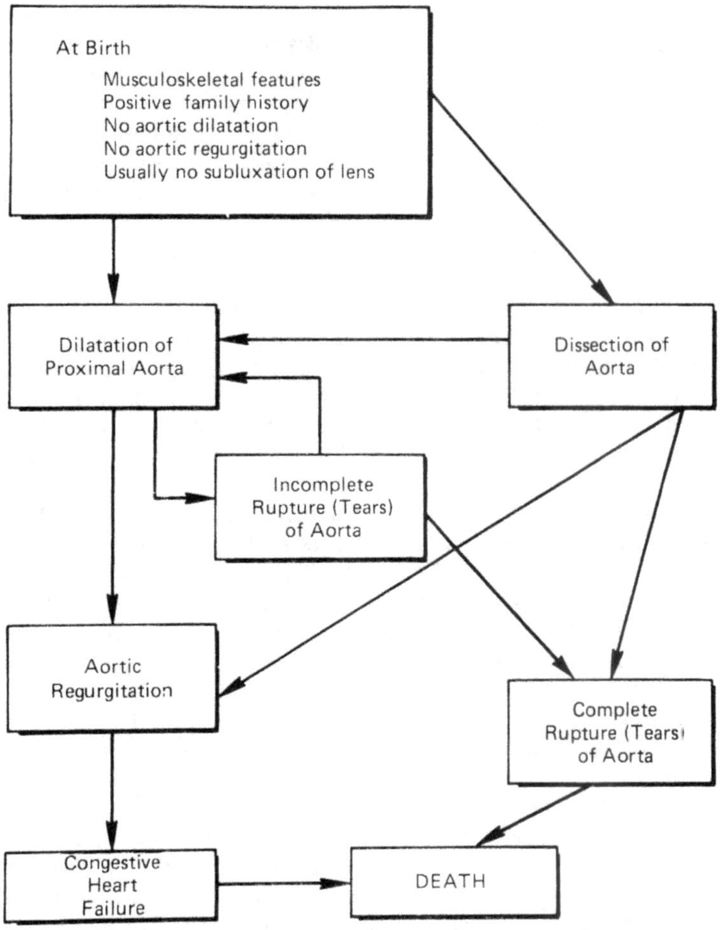

Figure 40. *The Marfan syndrome.* Schema of development of the aortic complications.

severe dilatation of the aortic "root" by the saccular aneurysm. The amount of regurgitation may not, however, correlate directly with the size of the aortic root aneurysm.[111] The aortic regurgitation is the consequence of aortic dissection even less commonly. The aortic valve cusps in patients with the Marfan syndrome appear to have an increased amount of mucoid material (acid mucopolysaccharide), irrespective of the presence of aortic regurgitation.

Mitral regurgitation also is frequent. At least five factors may be important in causing mitral regurgitation in patients with this syndrome. These are (1) floppiness of the mitral leaflets and/or chordae tendineae, (2) dilatation of the mitral anuli, (3) calcification of the mitral anuli, (4) rupture of mitral chordae tendineae, and (5) papillary muscle dysfunction. Of these factors, the first three appear to cause the most severe mitral regurgitation. Of the necropsy patients mentioned, 9 had mitral regurgitation: it was isolated in two and combined with aortic regurgitation in seven. Six of the nine with mitral regurgitation had floppy mitral valves and none of the nine without mitral regurgitation had floppy valves. The "floppiness" involved the posterior mitral leaflet in all six patients. Furthermore, of the nine patients with mitral regurgitation, the circumference of the mitral anulus ranged from 10 to 17 cm. (average, 15 cm.; normal, 9 cm.); of the nine patients without mitral regurgitation this circumference ranged from 9 to 12.5 cm. (average, 11 cm.). In the six patients with floppy mitral valves, the mitral circumference ranged from 14 to 17 cm. (average, 16 cm.). Thus, the average circumference of the mitral anulus in the nine patients with mitral regurgitation (15 cm.) was dilated 67 percent over normal (9 cm.) and in the nine patients without mitral regurgitation it was only 22 percent over normal (12 cm.). It therefore seems reasonable to conclude that both mitral leaflet floppiness and anular dilatation play significant roles in causing mitral regurgitation in these patients. Calcification of the mitral anulus is known to cause or at least be associated with mitral regurgitation.[21] The degree of regurgitation produced by this mechanism alone, however, is nearly always mild or minimal, and the mitral anuli in non-Marfan patients with mitral anular calcification is nearly always of normal or near-normal circumference. Of the 18 patients seen, four had mitral anular calcific deposits with associated mitral regurgitation; three also had floppy mitral leaflets. All four showed a mitral anulus which was quite dilated (range, 13 to 17 cm.; average, 15 cm.). Evidence for rupture of mitral chordae tendineae was found in four of the nine patients with mitral regurgitation. Two of these four patients had histories of infective endocarditis which had healed.[38] All four patients with evidence of mitral chordae rupture had floppy mitral leaflets and dilated mitral anuli (range, 15 to 17 cm.; average, 16 cm.).

The role played by "papillary muscle dysfunction" in causing mitral regurgitation in these patients is less clear.[115] All our 18 patients had dilated left ventricles and all had increased left ventricular masses. The hearts of the 18 patients ranged in weight from 375 to 850 gm. (average, 654 gm.). In 13 of the 18 patients the mitral leaflets were elongated from their basal attachments to their distal margins. This "stretching" probably was the result of the elongation (apex to base) of the left ventricular cavities, resulting primarily from the associated aortic regurgitation. The resulting left ventricular dilatation may have altered the normal angulation between the papillary muscles and the mitral leaflets. Whether or not mitral regurgitation was increased by this mechanism is uncertain.

Although the foregoing discussion concerns only patients with typical features of the Marfan syndrome, the cardiovascular features described in them also occur in patients without the skeletal or ocular manifestations of this syndrome or with histories of this syndrome in other family members. In addition, the characteristic histologic features in the wall of ascending aorta also have been observed in the aorta of patients with congenitally malformed aortic valves, particularly the bicuspid condition, and in patients with aortic stenosis when superimposed on congenitally malformed valves.[116,117] In individuals with the characteristic ascending aortic root aneurysms and histologic evidence of massive elastic-fiber degeneration of aortic media, features of the Marfan syndrome are more often absent than present.

REFERENCES

1. Barlow, J. B., Pocock, W. A., Marchand, P., et al.: *The significance of late systolic murmurs*. Am. Heart J. 66:443,1963.
2. Barlow, J. B., and Bosman, C. K.: *Aneurysmal protrusion of the posterior leaflet of the mitral valve: an auscultatory-electrocardiographic syndrome*. Am. Heart J. 71:166,1965.
3. Criley, J. M., Lewis, K. B., Humphries, J. O., et al.: *Prolapse of the mitral valve: clinical and cine-angiocardiographic findings*. Br. Heart J. 28:488,1966.
4. Stannard, M., Sloman, J. G., Hare, W. S., et al.: *Prolapse of the posterior leaflet of the mitral valve. A clinical, familial and cineangiographic study*. Br. Med. J. 3:71,1967.
5. Barlow, J. B., Bosman, C. K., Pocock, W. A., et al.: *Late systolic murmurs and non-ejection ('mid-late') systolic clicks: An analysis of 90 patients*. Br. Heart J. 30:203,1968.
6. Markiewicz, W., Stoner, J., London, E., et al.: *Mitral valve prolapse in one hundred presumably healthy young females*. Circulation 53:464,1976.
7. Procacci, P. M., Savran, S. V., Schreiter, S. L., et al.: *Prevalence of clinical mitral-valve prolapse in 1169 young women*. N. Engl. J. Med. 294:1086,1976.

8. Promerance, A.: *Ballooning deformity (mucoid degeneration) of atrioventricular valves.* Br. Heart J. 31:343,1969.
9. Sherman, E. B., Char, F., Dungan, W. T., et al.: *Myxomatous transformation of the mitral valve producing mitral insufficiency. Floppy valve syndrome.* Am. J. Dis. Child. 119:171,1970.
10. McCarthy, L. J., and Wolf, P. L.: *Mucoid degeneration of heart valves: Blue valve syndrome.* Am. J. Clin. Pathol. 54:582,1970.
11. Davis, R. H., Schuster, B., Knoebel, S. B., et al.: *Myxomatous degeneration of the mitral valve.* Am. J. Cardiol. 28:449,1971.
12. Edwards, J. E.: *Mitral insufficiency resulting from "overshooting" of leaflets.* Circulation 43:606,1971.
13. Kern, W. H., and Tucker, B. L.: *Myxoid changes in cardiac valves: pathologic, clinical, and ultrastructural studies.* Am. Heart J. 84:294,1972.
14. Roberts, W. C., Dangel, J. C., and Bulkley, B. H.: *Non-rheumatic valvular cardiac disease: a clinicopathologic survey of 27 different conditions causing valvular dysfunction.* Cardiovasc. Clin. 5(2):333,1973.
15. Ranganathan, N., Silver, M. D., Robinson, T. I., et al.: *Angiographic-morphologic correlation in patients with severe mitral regurgitation due to prolapse of the posterior mitral valve leaflet.* Circulation 48:514,1973.
16. Marshall, C. E., and Shappell, S. D.: *Sudden death and the ballooning posterior leaflet syndrome: detailed anatomic and histochemical investigation.* Arch. Pathol. 98:134,1974.
17. Guthrie, R. B., and Edwards, J. E.: *Pathology of the myxomatous mitral valve: nature, secondary changes and complications.* Minn. Med. 59:637,1976.
18. Shrivastava, S., Guthrie, R. B., and Edwards, J. E.: *Prolapse of the mitral valve.* Mod. Concepts Cardiovasc. Dis. 46:57,1977.
19. Bulkley, B. H., and Roberts, W. C.: *Dilatation of the mitral anulus. A rare cause of mitral regurgitation.* Am. J. Med. 59:457,1975.
20. Renteria, V. G., Ferrans, V. J., Jones, M., et al.: *Intracellular collagen fibrils in prolapsed ("floppy") human atrioventricular valves.* Lab. Invest. (in press).
21. Roberts, W. C., and Perloff, J. K.: *Mitral valvular disease. A clinicopathologic survey of the conditions causing the mitral valve to function abnormally.* Ann. Intern. Med. 77:939,1972.
22. Jeresaty, R. M.: *Etiology of the mitral valve prolapse-click syndrome.* Am. J. Cardiol. 36:110,1974.
23. McDonald, A., Harris, A., Jetterson, K., et al.: *Association of prolapse of posterior cusp of mitral valve and atrial septal defect.* Br. Heart J. 33:383,1971.
24. Pocock, W. A., and Barlow, J. B.: *An association between billowing posterior mitral leaflet syndrome and congenital heart disease, particularly atrial septal defect.* Am. Heart J. 81:720,1971.
25. Betriu, A., Wigle, E. D., Felderhof, C. H., et al.: *Prolapse of the posterior leaflet of the mitral valve associated with secundum atrial septal defect.* Am. J. Cardiol. 35:363,1975.
26. Leachman, R. D., Cokkinos, D. V., and Cooley, D. A.: *Association of ostium secundum atrial septal defects with mitral valve prolapse.* Am. J. Cardiol. 38:167,1976.
27. Edynak, G. M., and Rawson, A. J.: *Ruptured aneurysm of the mitral valve in a Marfan-like syndrome.* Am. J. Cardiol. 11:674,1963.
28. Ragib, G., Jue, K. L., Anderson, R. C., et al.: *Marfan's syndrome with mitral insufficiency.* Am. J. Cardiol. 16:127,1965.
29. Read, R. C., Thal, A. P., and Vernon, E. W.: *Symptomatic valvular myxomatous transformation (the floppy valve syndrome); a possible forme fruste of the Marfan syndrome.* Circulation 32:897,1965.
30. Shankar, K. R., Hultgren, M. K., Laver, R. M., et al.: *Lethal tricuspid and mitral regurgitation in Marfan's syndrome.* Am. J. Cardiol. 20:122,1967.
31. Dietzman, R. H., Peter, E. T., Wang, Y., et al.: *Mitral insufficiency in Marfan's syndrome. A case report of surgical correction.* Dis. Chest 51:650,1967.
32. Crocker, D. W.: *Marfan's syndrome confined to the mitral valve region: two cases in siblings.* Am. Heart J. 76:538,1968.
33. Grossman, M., Knott, A. P., Jr., and Jacoby, W. J., Jr.: *Calcified annulus fibrosis with mitral insufficiency with Marfan's syndrome.* Arch. Intern. Med. 121:561,1968.
34. Jortner, R., Shahin, W., Eshkol, D., et al.: *Cardiovascular manifestations and surgery for Marfan's syndrome.* Dis. Chest 56:24,1969.
35. Goodman, D., Kimbiris, D., and Linhart, J. W.: *Chordae tendineae rupture complicating the systolic click-late systolic murmur syndrome.* Am. J. Cardiol. 33:681,1974.
36. Lachman, A. S., Bramwell-Jones, D. M., Lakier, J. B., et al.: *Infective endocarditis in the billowing mitral leaflet syndrome.* Br. Heart J. 37:326,1975.

37. ARNETT, E. N., AND ROBERTS, W. C.: *Active infective endocarditis: a clinicopathologic analysis of 137 necropsy patients*. Curr. Probl. Cardiol. 1(7):1,1976.

38. ROBERTS, W. C., AND BUCHBINDER, N. A.: *Healed left-sided infective endocarditis. A clinicopathologic study of 59 patients*. Am. J. Cardiol. 40:876,1977.

39. DEMARIA, A. N., AMSTERDAM, E. A., VISMARA, L. A., ET AL.: *Arrhythmias in the mitral valve prolapse syndrome. Prevalence, nature and frequency*. Ann. Intern. Med. 84:656,1976.

40. BARNETT, H. J., JONES, M. W., BOUGHNER, D. R., ET AL.: *Cerebral ischemic events associated with prolapsing mitral valve*. Arch. Neurol. 33:777,1976.

41. ROBERTS, W. C.: *Coronary embolism. A review of causes, consequences and diagnostic considerations*. Cardiovasc. Med. 3:699,1978.

42. ROBERTS, W. C.: *Anatomically isolated aortic valvular disease. The case against its being of rheumatic etiology*. Am. J. Med. 49:151,1970.

43. ROBERTS, W. C.: *Valvular, subvalvular, and supravalvular aortic stenosis: morphologic features*. Cardiovasc. Clin. 5(1):97,1973.

44. ROBERTS, W. C., AND VIRMANI, R.: *Aschoff bodies at necropsy in valvular heart disease. Evidence from an analysis of 543 patients over 14 years of age that rheumatic heart disease, at least anatomically, is a disease of the mitral valve*. Circulation 57:803,1978.

45. ROBERTS, W. C., AND MORROW, A. G.: *Congential aortic stenosis produced by a unicommissural valve*. Br. Heart J. 27:505,1965.

46. ROBERTS, W. C., AND ELLIOTT, L. P.: *Lesions complicating the congenitally bicuspid aortic valve. Anatomic and radiographic features*. Radiol. Clin. North Am. 6:409,1968.

47. ROBERTS, W. C.: *The structure of the aortic valve in clinically-isolated aortic stenosis. An autopsy study of 162 patients over 15 years of age*. Circulation 42:91,1970.

48. ROBERTS, W. C.: *The congenitally bicuspid aortic valve. A study of 85 autopsy cases*. Am. J. Cardiol. 26:72,1970.

49. ROBERTS, W. C., PERLOFF, J. K., AND COSTANTINO, T.: *Severe valvular aortic stenosis in patients over 65 years of age. A clinicopathologic study*. Am. J. Cardiol. 27:497,1971.

50. FALCONE, M. W., ROBERTS, W. C., MORROW, A. G., ET AL.: *Congenital aortic stenosis resulting from unicommissural valve. Clinical and anatomic features in twenty-one adult patients*. Circulation 44:272,1971.

51. KARSNER, H. T., AND KOLETSKY, S.: *Calcific Disease of the Aortic Valve*. J. B. Lippincott, Philadelphia, 1947.

52. EDWARDS, J. E.: *Pathologic aspects of cardiac valvular insufficiencies*. Arch. Surg. 77:634,1958.

53. OSLER, W.: *The bicuspid condition of the aortic valves*. Trans. Assoc. Am. Physicians 2:185,1886.

54. GRANT, R. T., WOOD, J. E., AND JONES, T. D.: *Heart valve irregularities in relation to subacute bacterial endocarditis*. Heart 14:247,1928.

55. LEWIS, T., AND GRANT, R. T.: *Observations relating to subacute infective endocarditis. Part 1. Notes on the normal structure of the aortic valve. Part 2. Bicuspid aortic valves of congenital origin. Part 3. Bicuspid aortic valves in subacute infective endocarditis*. Heart 10:21,1923.

56. STARLING, H. J.: *Endocarditis lenta*. Q. J. Med. 16:263,1923.

57. FULTON, M. N., AND LEVINE, S. A.: *Subacute bacterial endocarditis, with special reference to the valvular lesions and previous history*. Am. J. Med. Sci. 183:60,1932.

58. ROBERTS, W. C.: *Characteristics and consequences of infective endocarditis (active or healed or both) learned from morphologic studies*. In Rahimtoola, S. H. (ed.): *Infective Endocarditis*, Grune & Stratton, New York, 1978, pp. 55–123.

59. EDWARDS, J. E.: *The congenital bicuspid aortic valve*. Circulation 23:485,1961.

60. BISHOP, L. F., JR., AND TRUBEK, M.: *Bicuspid aortic valve. A differential study between inflammatory and congenital origin*. J. Tech. Meth. 15:111,1936.

61. KOLETSKY, S.: *Congenital bicuspid aortic valves*. Arch. Intern. Med. 67:129,1941.

62. EDWARDS, J. E.: *Congenital malformations of the heart and great vessels: C. Malformations of the valves*. In Gould, S. E. (ed.): *Pathology of the Heart and Blood Vessels*, ed. 3. Charles C Thomas, Springfield, Ill., 1968, p. 341.

63. FONTANA, R. S., AND EDWARDS, J. E.: *Congenital Cardiac Disease. A Review of 357 Cases Studied Pathologically*. W. B. Saunders, Philadelphia, 1962.

64. MORROW, A. G., FORT, L., III, ROBERTS, W. C., ET AL.: *Discrete subaortic stenosis complicated by aortic valvular regurgitation. Clinical, hemodynamic, and pathologic studies and the results of operative treatment*. Circulation 20:1003,1959.

65. REIS, R. L., PETERSON, L. M., MASON, D. T., ET AL.: *Congenital fixed subvalvular aortic stenosis. An anatomical classification and correlations with operative results*. Circulation 43,44(Suppl. I):11,1971.

66. MUNA, W. F. T., FERRANS, V. J., PIERCE, J. E., ET AL.: *Discrete subaortic stenosis in Newfoundland dogs: association of infective endocarditis.* Am. J. Cardiol. 41:746,1978.

67. MARON, B. J., REDWOOD, D. R., ROBERTS, W. C., ET AL.: *Tunnel subaortic stenosis. Left ventricular outflow tract obstruction produced by fibromuscular tubular narrowing.* Circulation 54:404,1976.

68. TEARE, D.: *Asymmetrical hypertrophy of the heart in young adults.* Br. Heart J. 20:1,1958.

69. EPSTEIN, S. E., HENRY, W. L., CLARK, C. E., ET AL.: *Asymmetric septal hypertrophy.* Ann. Intern. Med. 81:650,1974.

70. MARON, B. J., EDWARDS, J. E., FERRANS, V. J., ET AL.: *Congenital heart malformations associated with disproportionate ventricular septal thickening.* Circulation 52:926,1975.

71. MARON, B. J., CLARK, C. E., HENRY, W. L., ET AL.: *Prevalence and characteristics of disproportionate ventricular septal thickening in patients with acquired or congenital heart disease: echocardiographic and morphologic findings.* Circulation 55:489,1977.

72. MARON, B. J., SAVAGE, D. D., CLARK, C. E., ET AL.: *Prevalence and characteristics of disproportionate ventricular septal thickening in patients with coronary artery disease.* Circulation 57:250,1978.

73. MARON, B. J., VERTER, J., AND KAPUR, S.: *Disproportionate ventricular septal thickening in the developing normal human heart.* Circulation 57:520,1978.

74. MARON, B. J., EDWARDS, J. E., AND EPSTEIN, S. E.: *Disproportionate ventricular septal thickening in patients with systemic hypertension.* Chest 73:466,1978.

75. SPRAY, T. L., MARON, B. J., MORROW, A. G., ET AL.: *A discussion on hypertrophic cardiomyopathy.* Am. Heart J. 95:511,1978.

76. MARON, B. J., GOTTDIENER, J. S., ROBERTS, W. C., ET AL.: *Disproportionate ventricular septal thickening (ASH) with systolic anterior motion of the anterior mitral leaflet secondary to valvular heart disease.* Br. Heart J. (in press).

77. ISNER, J. M., FALCONE, M. W., VIRMANI, R., ET AL.: *Cardiac sarcoma causing "ASH" and simulating coronary heart disease.* Am. J. Med. (in press).

78. ROBERTS, W. C., AND FERRANS, V. J.: *Pathologic anatomy of the cardiomyopathies. Idiopathic dilated and hypertrophic types, infiltrative types, and endomyocardial disease with and without eosinophilia.* Hum. Pathol. 6:287,1975.

79. MARON, B. J., GOTTDIENER, J. S., ROBERTS, W. C., ET AL.: *Left ventricular outflow tract obstruction due to systolic anterior motion of the anterior mitral leaflet in patients with concentric left ventricular hypertrophy.* Circulation 57:527,1978.

80. MCREYNOLDS, R. A., AND ROBERTS, W. C.: *The intramural coronary arteries in hypertrophic cardiomyopathy.* Am. J. Cardiol. 35:120,1975.

81. MARON, B. J., FERRANS, V. J., HENRY, W. L., ET AL.: *Differences in distribution of myocardial abnormalities in patients with obstructive and nonobstructive asymmetric septal hypertrophy (ASH). Light and electron microscopic findings.* Circulation 50:436,1974.

82. HENRY, W. L., CLARK, C. E., ROBERTS, W. C., ET AL.: *Differences in distribution of myocardial abnormalities in patients with obstructive and non-obstructive asymmetric septal hypertrophy (ASH). Echocardiographic and gross anatomic findings.* Circulation 50:447,1974.

83. MARON, B. J., EPSTEIN, S. E., AND ROBERTS, W. C.: *Cardiac muscle cell disorganization in the ventricular septum: evidence from quantitative histology that it is a highly sensitive marker of hypertrophic cardiomyopathy.* Am. J. Cardiol. 41:435,1978.

84. FERRANS, V. J., MORROW, A. G., AND ROBERTS, W. C.: *Myocardial ultrastructure in idiopathic hypertrophic subaortic stenosis. A study of operatively excised left ventricular outflow tract muscle in 14 patients.* Circulation 45:769,1972.

85. MARON, B. J., ROBERTS, W. C., EDWARDS, J. E., ET AL.: *Sudden death in patients with hypertrophic cardiomyopathy. Characterization of 26 patients without functional limitation.* Am. J. Cardiol. 41:803,1978.

86. MARON, B. J., LIPSON, L. C., ROBERTS, W. C., ET AL.: *"Malignant" hypertrophic cardiomyopathy. Identification of a subgroup of families with unusually frequent premature deaths.* Am. J. Cardiol. 41:1133,1978.

87. ROBERTS, W. C., PERRY, L. W., CHANDRA, R. S., ET AL.: *Aortic valve atresia: a new classification based on necropsy study of 73 cases.* Am. J. Cardiol. 37:753,1976.

88. EWY, G. A., MARCUS, F. I., BOHJALIAN, O., ET AL.: *Muscular subaortic stenosis. Clinical and pathologic observations in an elderly patient.* Am. J. Cardiol. 22:126,1968.

89. ROBERTS, W. C.: *Cardiomyopathy and myocarditis: morphologic features.* Adv. Cardiol. 22:184,1978.

90. MERRILL, W. H., HENRY, W. L., MARON, B. J., ET AL.: *Echocardiographic assessment of the left ventricle following myotomy and myectomy for idiopathic hypertrophic subaortic stenosis (IHSS).* Am. J. Cardiol. 41:435,1978.

91. Maron, B. J., Henry, W. L., Roberts, W. C., et al.: *Comparison of echocardiographic and necropsy measurements of ventricular wall thicknesses in patients with and without disproportionate septal thickening.* Circulation 55:341,1977.

92. Cooley, D. A., Leachman, R. D., and Wukasch, D. C.: *Diffuse muscular subaortic stenosis: surgical treatment.* Am. J. Cardiol. 31:1,1973.

93. Cooley, D. A., Grace, R. R., Wukasch, D. C., et al.: *Replacement and/or repair of the mitral valve as treatment of idiopathic hypertrophic subaortic stenosis.* Cardiovasc. Dis. Bull. Texas Heart Inst. 3:381,1976.

94. Roberts, W. C.: *Operative treatment of hypertrophic obstructive cardiomyopathy. The case against mitral valve replacement.* Am. J. Cardiol. 32:377,1973.

95. Roberts, W. C.: *Left ventricular outflow tract obstruction and aortic regurgitations.* In Edwards, J. E., Lev, M., and Abell, M. R. (eds.): *The Heart.* Williams & Wilkins, Baltimore, 1974, pp. 110–175.

96. Bulkley, B. H., and Roberts, W. C.: *Ankylosing spondylitis and aortic regurgitation. Description of the characteristic cardiovascular lesion from study of eight necropsy patients.* Circulation 48:1014,1973.

97. Roberts, W. C., Hollingsworth, J. F., Bulkley, B. H., et al.: *Combined mitral and aortic regurgitation in ankylosing spondylitis. Angiographic and anatomic features.* Am. J. Med. 56:237,1974.

98. Pomerance, A., and Davies, M. J.: *Congenital aneurysms of all three sinuses of Valsalva.* J. Pathol. Bacteriol. 89:607,1965.

99. Arnett, E. N., and Roberts, W. C.: *Valve ring abscess in active infective endocarditis. Frequency, location, and clues to clinical diagnosis from the study of 95 necropsy patients.* Circulation 54:140,1976.

100. Edwards, J. E., and Burchell, M. B.: *Specimen exhibiting the essential lesion in aneurysm of the aortic sinus.* Mayo Clin. Proc. 31:407,1956.

101. Fishbein, M. C., Obma, R., and Roberts, W. C.: *Unruptured sinus of Valsalva aneurysm.* Am. J. Cardiol. 35:918,1975.

102. Sakakibara, S., and Konno, S.: *Congenital aneurysm of the sinus of Valsalva. Anatomy and classification.* Am. Heart J. 63:405,1962.

103. Fowler, R. E. L., and Bevel, H. H.: *Aneurysms of the sinus of Valsalva.* Pediatrics 8:340,1951.

104. Kieffer, S. A., and Winchell, P.: *Congenital aneurysms of the aortic sinuses with cardioaortic fistula.* Dis. Chest 38:79,1960.

105. Kerber, R. W., Ridges, J. D., Kriss, J. P., et al.: *Unruptured aneurysm of the sinus of Valsalva producing right ventricular outflow obstruction.* Am. J. Med. 53:775,1972.

106. Duras, P. F.: *Heart block with aneurysm of the aortic sinus.* Br. Heart J. 6:61,1944.

107. McKusick, V. A.: *Heritable Disorders of Connective Tissue.* C. V. Mosby Co., St. Louis, 1972, pp. 61–223.

108. Murdoch, J. L., Wlaker, B. A., Halpern, B. L., et al.: *Life expectancy and causes of death in the Marfan syndrome.* N. Engl. J. Med. 286:804,1972.

109. Becker, A. E.: *Medionecrosis aortae.* Pathol. Microbiol. (Basel) 43:124,1975.

110. Schlatmann, T. J. M., and Becker, A. E.: *Histologic changes in the normal aging aorta: implications for dissecting aortic aneurysm.* Am. J. Cardiol. 39:13,1977.

111. Lemon, D. K., and White, C. W.: *Anuloaortic ectasia: angiographic, hemodynamic and clinical comparison with aortic valve insufficiency.* Am. J. Cardiol. 41:482,1978.

112. Schlatmann, T. J. M., and Becker, A. E.: *Pathogenesis of dissecting aneurysm of aorta. Comparative histopathologic study of significance of medial changes.* Am. J. Cardiol. 39:21,1977.

113. Erdheim, J.: *Medionecrosis aortae idiopathica.* Virchows Arch. (Pathol. Anat.) 273:454,1929.

114. Gsell, O.: *Wandnekrosen der Aorta als selbstandige Erkrankung und ihre Beziehung zur Spontanruptur.* Virchows Arch. (path. Anat.) 270:1,1928.

115. Roberts, W. C., and Cohen, L. S.: *Left ventricular papillary muscles. Description of the normal and a survey of conditions causing them to be abnormal.* Circulation 46:138,1972.

116. McKusick, V. A., Logue, R. B., and Bahnson, H. T.: *Association of aortic valvular disease and cystic medial necrosis of the ascending aorta. Report of four instances.* Circulation 16:188,1957.

117. Fukuda, T., Tadavarthy, S. M., and Edwards, J. E.: *Dissecting aneurysm of aorta complicating aortic valvular stenosis.* Circulation 53:169,1976.

Hypertrophic Cardiomyopathy and Transmural Myocardial Infarction Without Significant Atherosclerosis of the Extramural Coronary Arteries

BARRY J. MARON, MD, FACC
STEPHEN E. EPSTEIN, MD, FACC
WILLIAM C. ROBERTS, MD, FACC

Bethesda, Maryland

Clinical and morphologic features of transmural myocardial infarction (associated with insignificant or absent atherosclerosis of the extramural coronary arteries) are described in seven patients with hypertrophic cardiomyopathy. Marked chronic congestive heart failure associated with supraventricular arrhythmias occurred in six of the seven patients, each of whom had no or mild left ventricular outflow tract obstruction under basal conditions. No patient had typical angina pectoris, and only one patient had clinically evident acute myocardial infarction. Infarction may have caused cardiac arrest in one other patient, but was "silent" in the remaining five patients.

At necropsy, six of the seven patients had extensive myocardial scarring involving the ventricular septum, left ventricular free wall and one or both left ventricular papillary muscles; in four patients portions of the right ventricular wall were also scarred. Six patients had dilated ventricular cavities, including two who were known to have nondilated ventricular cavities earlier in their clinical course.

It is concluded that transmural myocardial infarction in the absence of significant coronary atherosclerosis is a not uncommon finding (prevalence rate 15 percent) in a population of patients who had died from hypertrophic cardiomyopathy. Although transmural infarction is possibly a secondary event, it more likely contributes causally to the clinical deterioration of some patients with hypertrophic cardiomyopathy, leading to ventricular dilatation and progressive fatal cardiac failure.

Patients with hypertrophic cardiomyopathy often complain of chest pain (which may be typical or atypical of classic angina pectoris) and have electrocardiograms suggesting myocardial damage or ischemia.[1-7] Some of these patients have associated coronary arterial atherosclerosis[8-13] that may cause acute myocardial infarction.[14] In addition, previous necropsy studies[15-17] of hearts of adult patients with hypertrophic cardiomyopathy have shown that relatively small areas of interstitial or replacement fibrosis are commonly present in the left ventricular wall (particularly the subendocardial region and papillary muscles). However, it has not been appreciated that transmural myocardial infarction may occur in patients with hypertrophic cardiomyopathy who do *not* have significant coronary atherosclerosis or that it may play a role in the natural history of such patients with hypertrophic cardiomyopathy. This report describes the clinical and morphologic features of seven patients with hypertrophic cardiomyopathy and transmural myocardial infarction unassociated with significant atherosclerotic narrowing of the extramural coronary arteries.

From the Cardiology and Pathology Branches, National Heart, Lung, and Blood Institute, National Institutes of Health, Bethesda, Maryland. Manuscript received October 30, 1978; revised manuscript received January 12, 1979, accepted January 17, 1979.

Address for reprints: Barry J. Maron, MD, Cardiology Branch, National Heart, Lung, and Blood Institute, Bldg. 10, Room 7B-15, Bethesda, Maryland 20014.

Methods

Selection of patients: The necropsy records of the National Heart, Lung, and Blood Institute from 1958 to 1978 were reviewed. Eighty-two patients over the age of 10 years whose hemodynamic, angiographic, echocardiographic and necropsy findings were consistent with the diagnosis of hypertrophic cardiomyopathy[3–5,18–21] were identified. Thirty-two patients who had undergone septal myotomy-myectomy, one patient who had cardiac transplantation and one patient who had mitral valve replacement were excluded from the analysis. Of the remaining 48 patients who had not undergone operation, 7 (15 percent) were judged by gross inspection of the heart to have *transmural* myocardial scarring (that is, a healed myocardial infarct) of the left ventricle, and they constitute the study group. None of these seven patients had significant atherosclerosis of any of the four major extramural coronary arteries. The patients ranged in age from 12 to 60 years (median 33).

Echocardiographic studies: Echocardiograms were performed with a 2.25 megahertz, 1.2 cm diameter Aerotech transducer connected to either a modified Ekoline-20A or a Hoffrel 201 ultrasonic unit employing methods previously described.[18] The thickness of the ventricular septum was measured below the tips of the mitral valve leaflets just before atrial systole; posterior left ventricular wall thickness was measured at the level of the tips of the mitral valve leaflets during the same phase of the cardiac cycle. End-diastolic and end-systolic left ventricular transverse dimensions were taken as the maximal and minimal dimensions, respectively, with the ultrasonic beam passing through the left ventricle slightly below the tips of the mitral valve leaflets.

Necropsy studies: *The location of myocardial scars* was assessed by gross inspection of the heart. The location of the left ventricular free wall scars was designated as either anterior or posterior, either apical or basal and either transmural or nontransmural[22] (Fig. 1).

Measurements were made of the maximal thickness of the ventricular septum, left and right ventricular free walls and the posterior left ventricular free wall at a level corresponding with the distal margin of the posterior mitral leaflet.[23] These measurements were obtained, when possible, in areas of the ventricular walls relatively free of scarring. The size of the ventricular and atrial cavities was judged by visual inspection to be either normal or dilated.

The coronary arteries were excised *intact* in four patients, and sectioned by a method described elsewhere.[24] Briefly, the excised arteries were cut at 5 mm intervals at right angles to the longitudinal axes of the vessels, and each 5 mm long segment was processed, embedded in paraffin and cut. A single Movat-stained histologic section was examined from each 5 mm segment. In the other three patients, the extramural coronary arteries were studied in the intact specimen by making multiple cross sections of the vessels (about 5 mm apart) and viewing the lumens grossly.

Results

Clinical findings and course (Table I): None of the seven patients had typical angina pectoris. Two patients (Cases 3 and 4) experienced occasional chest discomfort that was probably of cardiac origin but was not typical of angina pectoris; Patient 3 had a 5 year history of retrosternal pain precipitated by palpitations, and Patient 4 had a 7 year history of periodic, prolonged retrosternal discomfort. Only Patient 3 had a clinical episode consistent with acute myocardial infarction; 3 months before death this patient experienced severe substernal chest pain that lasted for 1 hour, radiated to both arms and was associated with diaphoresis, nausea, vomiting and fine rales in the left lung and marked elevations in serum myocardial enzyme levels (glutamic oxaloacetic

DEFINITION OF MYOCARDIAL INFARCTS

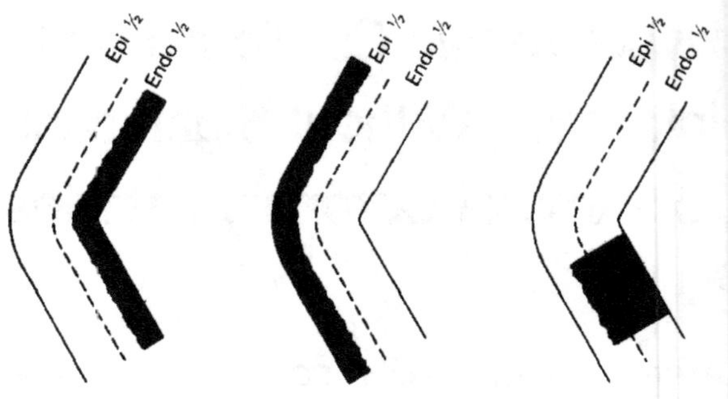

FIGURE 1. Definition of myocardial infarcts. *Subendocardial* infarcts involve no more than the inner one-half of the ventricular wall. *Subepicardial* infarcts involve no more than the outer one-half of the ventricular wall. *Transmural* infarcts involve more than the inner one-half of the ventricular wall. Endo ½ and Epi ½ = endocardial and epicardial one-half of the ventricular wall thickness, respectively.

transaminase 630, lactic dehydrogenase 3,580 and creatine kinase 2,475 units; a pericardial friction rub and paroxysmal atrial tachycardia were present on the following day.

In six of the seven patients the clinical course was characterized by profound chronic congestive heart failure with cardiac enlargement (Fig. 2a, 2b, 3b and 4a) and supraventricular arrhythmias. Two of these patients (Cases 5 and 6) experienced progressive and steady clinical deterioration over a period of several years. Two patients (Cases 3 and 4) manifested rapid symptomatic deterioration 1 week before death; two other patients (Cases 2 and 7) had marked changes in their clinical condition 3 months before death. The remaining patient (Case 1) was asymptomatic before experiencing a cardiac arrest at age 12 years; he subsequently survived for 6 weeks with evidence of severe cerebral anoxia. The transmural myocardial scarring was significantly more common in our patients who died of congestive heart failure (6 of 14 [43 percent]) than in those who died suddenly (1 of 22 [4 percent]; $P < 0.025$) (Fig. 5).

Two patients (Cases 2 and 6) (Table II) had marked congestive heart failure and ventricular dilatation in the latter stages of their illness (as assessed with echocardiography or at necropsy) but had a nondilated heart by angiography 8 and 9 years earlier, respectively (Fig. 4, b and c). This evolution from a nondilated hyperdynamic left ventricle to a dilated poorly contractile ventricle was associated with symptomatic deterioration.

Physical findings: One patient (Case 1) had not had an adequate cardiac physical examination before death. Systolic ejection murmurs were present under basal conditions in each of the other six patients; these murmurs were heard loudest at the lower left sternal border and apex. In two patients (Cases 3 and 5) the murmur was grade 3/6, suggesting the presence of marked left

TABLE I

Hypertrophic Cardiomyopathy and Transmural Myocardial Infarction: Clinical Findings

	Case 1	Case 2	Case 3	Case 4	Case 5	Case 6	Case 7
Age (yr) & sex	12M	19F	20F	33M	41F	50F	60M
NYHA class*	1	IV[‖]	II	III	IV	III	IV[‖]
Chest pain	0	0	+	+	0	0[c]	0[e]
Duration of illness (yr)[†]	0	7 mo	10	7	3	25[d]	11
AMI	0	0	+	0	0	0	0
Pressures (mm Hg)							
LVOT (PSG)							
Basal	—	0	40	0	0	0	—[f]
Provoked	—	60	55	0	—	7	—
LV S/D	—	130/-	160/10	100/16	85/26	110/23	—
SA S/D	—	130/90	120/60	120/80	90/55	115/65	—
PA S/D	—	—	40/-	28/10	50/25	27/11	—
Other cardiac findings	None	A Fl	SVT; sev MR	SVT (occ); CVA age 28	AF; sev MR	AF	AF
Treatment with propranolol (no. of yr. before death)	0	8	3	6	0	0	0
Mode of death							
CHF		+[¶]	+[a]	+[a]	+[b]	+	+[g]
Sudden	+[‡]						
Family history of premature cardiac death	+[§]	+	0	0	0	+[§]	+

* Assessment made arbitrarily 1 month before death.
[†] From the time symptoms were first noted consistently.
[‡] Collapsed while jogging; ventricular fibrillation documented; patient survived 6 weeks with anoxic brain damage.
[§] "Malignant" hypertrophic cardiomyopathy.[26]
[‖] Rapid clinical deterioration occurred 3 months or less before death (from functional class II to class IV).
[¶] Patient's terminal illness was characterized by left ventricular failure, fever, nausea, diarrhea, abdominal pain, weakness, dyspnea, atrial flutter and hyponatremia.
[a] Acute deterioration due to congestive heart failure 3 days before death.
[b] History of marked congestive heart failure thought to be due to severe rheumatic mitral regurgitation; however, at operation the mitral valve was noted to be normal; the patient died 1 day after operation because of pulmonary embolus with infarction.
[c] Brief stabbing left precordial pain not thought to be cardiac in origin.
[d] Including a 10 year period (between age 30 and 40 years) during which there was a spontaneous loss of symptoms.
[e] Chest pain occurred before but not after age 43.
[f] However, absence of systolic anterior motion of the anterior mitral leaflet on echocardiography (under basal conditions) and absence of a cardiac murmur (under basal conditions or with provocative maneuvers) indicated that obstruction to left ventricular outflow was not present in this patient.
[g] Patient's terminal illness (during last 10 weeks of life) was characterized by left ventricular failure with pulmonary edema, paroxysmal atrial fibrillation, hypotension, periods of bradycardia and renal failure; pulmonary arterial wedge pressure was 28 mm Hg; pressor agents were required to maintain systolic blood pressure at 90–110/60–75 mm Hg.
+ = present; 0 = absent; — = data not available.
AF = atrial fibrillation; A Fl = atrial flutter; AMI = acute myocardial infarct; CHF = congestive heart failure; CVA = cerebrovascular accident; 1° AVB = first degree atrioventricular block; LV = left ventricle; LVOT = left ventricular outflow tract; MR = mitral regurgitation; NYHA class = New York Heart Association functional class; occ = occasional; PA = pulmonary artery; PSG = peak systolic gradient; RVH = right ventricular hypertrophy; SA = systemic artery; S/D = systolic/diastolic; sev = severe; SVT = supraventricular tachycardia.

TABLE II

Serial Clinical Data in Two Patients With Hypertrophic Cardiomyopathy and Transmural Myocardial Infarction: Progression From Nondilated to Dilated Left Ventricle

	Patient 2		Patient 6	
	I	II	I	II
Age (yr)	11	19	41	50
NYHA class	II	IV	II	III
Systolic ejection murmur (grade)	2/6	2/6*	2/6	None*
Cardiothoracic ratio (X-ray)	0.53	0.63	0.50	0.62
LVOT gradient (mm Hg) (basal/provoked)	0/60	0*	0/7	0*
$LVID_S/LVID_D$ (mm)	—	50/57[†]	—	61/67[†]
Ejection fraction (%)	90 (angio)	30 (echo)	65 (angio)	25 (echo)

* Absence of systolic anterior motion of the anterior mitral leaflet on echocardiography (under basal conditions) and absence of a loud cardiac murmur (grade 3/6 or higher) under basal conditions or with provocative maneuvers indicated that obstruction to left ventricular outflow was not present.
[†] This patient died within 1 year of the most recent cardiac evaluation and showed ventricular dilatation at necropsy.
— = data not available.
Angio = angiography; I = initial cardiac evaluation; II = most recent cardiac evaluation; echo = echocardiography; $LVID_D$ and $LVID_S$ = left ventricular internal dimension in diastole and systole, respectively (as assessed with echocardiography); LVOT = left ventricular outflow tract; NYHA class = New York Heart Association functional class.

ventricular outflow obstruction. In four patients the murmur was grade 1-2/6, suggesting minimal obstruction to outflow. The second heart sound was single in two patients and was physiologically split in four patients. A third heart sound was heard in two patients, a fourth heart sound in two patients and both third and fourth heart sounds in two patients.

Echocardiographic findings: The echocardiographic data obtained in four of the seven patients are summarized in Table III. In each patient both the diastolic and systolic left ventricular internal dimensions were increased over normal. Hence, left ventricular ejection fraction (as well as percent fractional shortening) was abnormally decreased in each patient (Fig. 6).

Electrocardiographic findings: The electrocardiograms were abnormal in each of the six patients whose tracings were obtained (Table IV) (Fig. 3c, 4d, 7, 8a and 9c). Analysis of the electrocardiograms obtained in the latter stages of each patient's illness (within 1 year of death) disclosed that the most consistent abnormality was diffuse T wave alterations (usually symmetric T wave inversion). Deep (more than 4 mm) or wide (more than 0.04 second) Q waves were present in each of the six patients, primarily in "lateral" electrocardiographic leads (that is, leads I, aVL, V_5 and V_6) and were usually associated with abnormally small R waves in the left precordial leads. Conduction abnormalities (intraventricular conduction defect, left anterior hemiblock or first degree atrioventricular block) were also present in five patients. Of 25 patients in the original study group *without* transmural myocardial scars or significant coronary arterial narrowing (and whose electrocardiograms were available for analysis), 10 also showed deep wide Q waves in one or more leads. However, the prevalence of Q waves in these patients was significantly less than that in patients with transmural scarring ($P < 0.05$).

Electrocardiographic evidence of left ventricular hypertrophy was present in only one patient (Case 6),

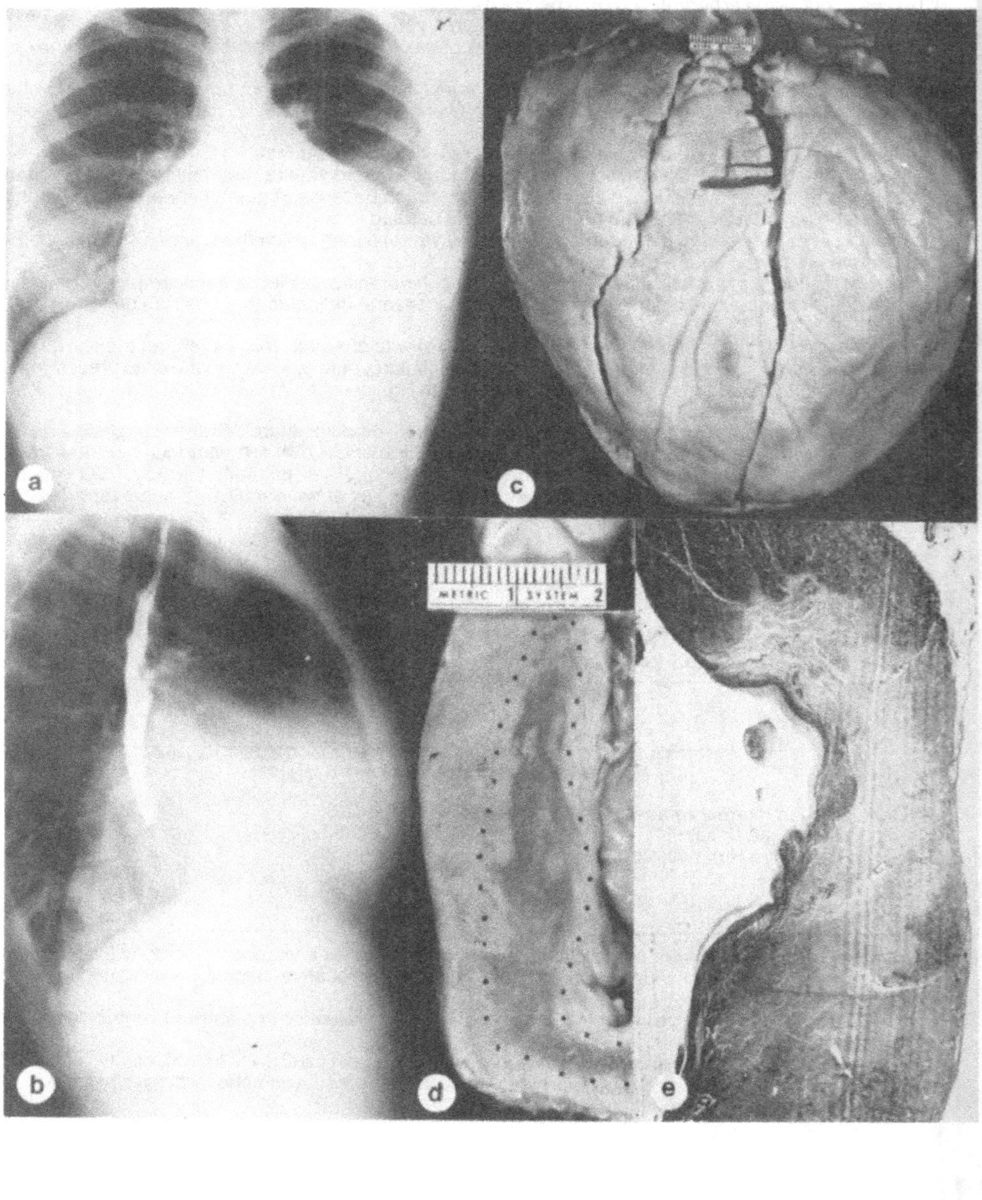

FIGURE 2. Case 3. Radiographic and necropsy findings. **a** and **b**, posteroanterior and lateral chest radiographs, respectively, taken 5 years before death and showing marked cardiac enlargement (cardiothoracic ratio = 0.73). **c**, exterior view of heart showing massive cardiomegaly (heart weight = 1,250 g). **d**, longitudinal cut of ventricular septum showing extensive scarring (**outlined by dots**); **e**, longitudinal section of basal left ventricular free wall showing an extensive scar that involves the entire thickness of the wall.

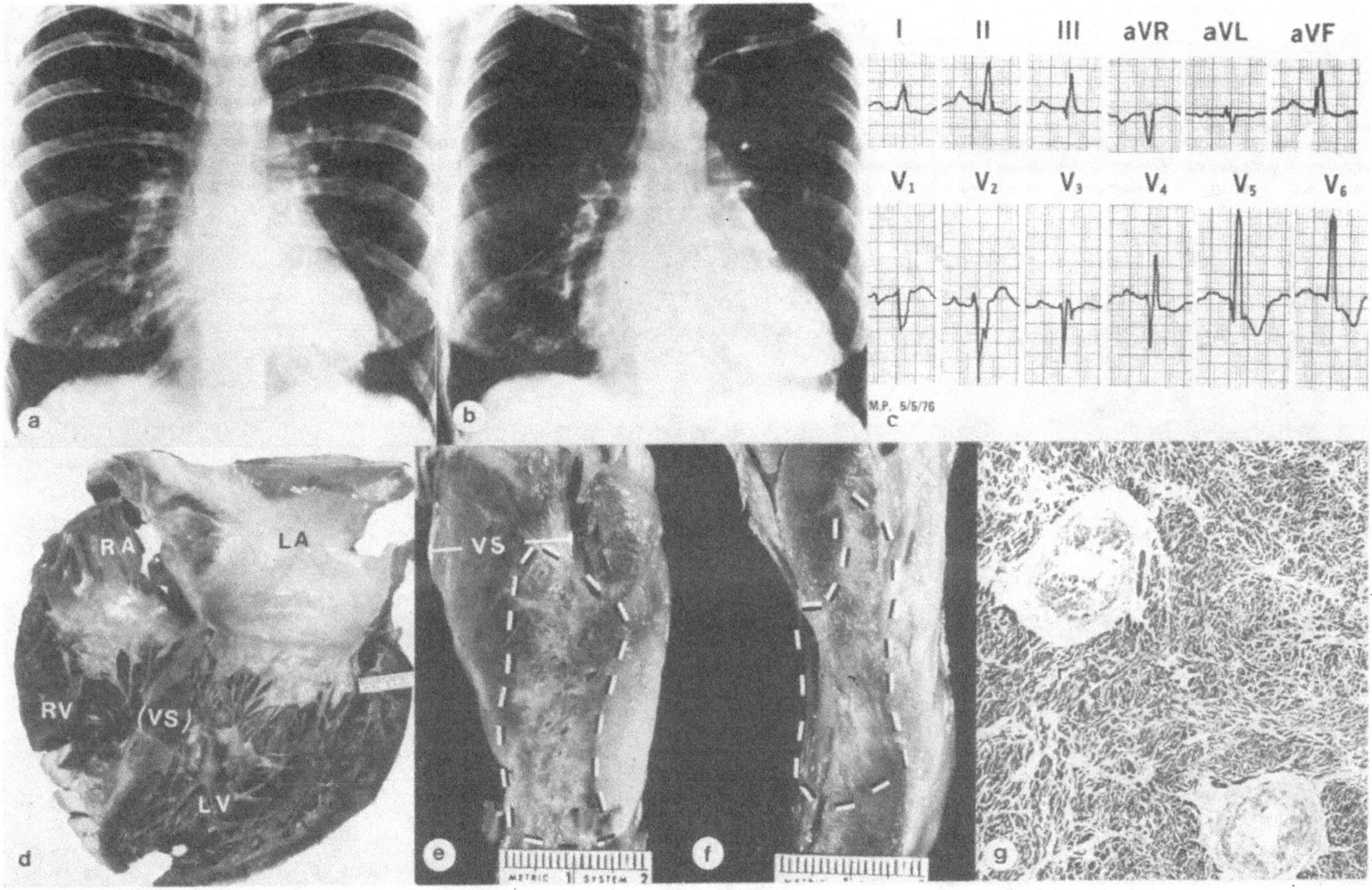

FIGURE 3. Case 6. Radiographs, electrocardiogram and necropsy findings. **a,** posteroanterior chest radiograph obtained at age 41 years showing a normal-sized heart (cardiothoracic ratio = 0.50). **b,** posteroanterior chest radiograph obtained 9 years later showing a marked increase in heart size (cardiothoracic ratio = 0.62). **c,** electrocardiogram showing left ventricular hypertrophy with "strain," left atrial abnormality, intraventricular conduction defect, first degree atrioventricular block, Q wave in lead V_5, "poor R wave progression" across the anterior precordium and diffuse S-T segment and T wave abnormalities. **d,** longitudinal section of the heart showing dilatation of left ventricle (LV), right ventricle (RV), left atrium (LA) and right atrium (RA); the ventricular septum (VS) is disproportionately thickened with respect to the left ventricular free wall. **e,** longitudinal cut of ventricular septum (VS) showing extensive transmural scarring (**outlined by broken line**). **f,** longitudinal cut of left ventricular free wall showing a transmural scar (**outlined by broken line**). **g,** section of a portion of ventricular septum showing abnormal intramural coronary arteries with thickened walls and narrowed lumens (hematoxylin-eosin ×35, reduced by 25 percent).

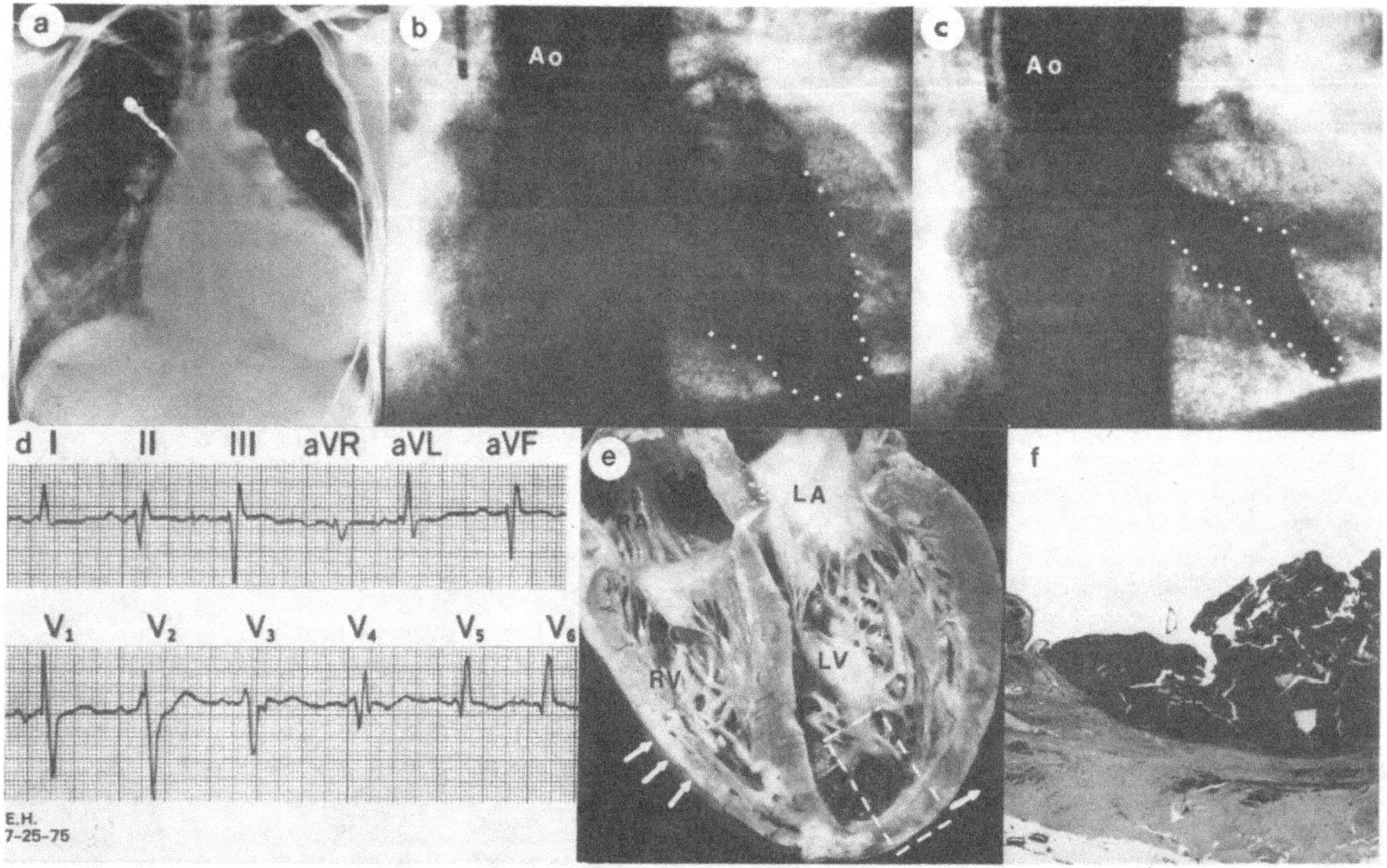

FIGURE 4. Case 2. Chest radiograph, angiocardiograms, electrocardiogram and necropsy findings. **a,** posteroanterior chest radiograph obtained 1 month before death shows marked cardiac enlargement (cardiothoracic ratio = 0.64). **b,** left ventricular angiocardiogram in end-diastole (obtained 8 years before death) showing normal ventricular volume and marked thickening of the ventricular wall; the **dotted line** outlines left ventricular cavity; Ao = aorta. **c,** left ventricular angiocardiogram in end-systole showing small ventricular volume; the **dotted line** outlines the left ventricular cavity. **d,** electrocardiogram shows the left atrial abnormality and T wave abnormalities; the tall R wave in lead V_1 reflects hypertrophy of either the ventricular septum or the right ventricular wall. **e,** longitudinal section of the heart with the anterior half removed showing considerable dilatation of both the right (RV) and the left ventricular (LV) cavities and concentric (symmetric) ventricular hypertrophy; transmural scarring of the left ventricular apex and right ventricular wall (**arrows**) is evident; LA = left atrium; RA = right atrium. **f,** extensive transmural scarring of left ventricular apex with superimposed thrombus; from the portion of apical scarring outlined by broken line in **e,** but shown at higher magnification (hematoxylin-eosin ×3, reduced by 25 percent).

although Patients 2 and 3 had shown this abnormality earlier in their clinical course. In particular, the changes in electrocardiographic pattern demonstrated by Patient 3 suggested progressive ventricular scarring over a 5 year period (Fig. 7); however, the possibility also exists that these abnormalities (deep Q waves in the lateral precordial leads and tall R waves in the right precordial leads) were due to increased forces of depolarization in the greatly thickened ventricular septum.[1]

Hemodynamic findings: Five patients underwent cardiac catheterization, 6 months to 10 years before death (Table I). A left ventricular outflow gradient of 40 mm Hg was present under basal conditions in one patient (Case 3); gradients were absent under basal conditions in the other four patients (although one of these had a 60 mm Hg gradient with isoproterenol infusion). One additional patient (Case 7), who had not undergone hemodynamic study, had an echocardiogram recorded 3 months before death that showed no systolic anterior motion of the anterior mitral leaflet under basal conditions, a finding consistent with the absence of outflow obstruction.[21] In two patients without outflow obstruction who had undergone hemodynamic study more than 5 years before death an echocardiogram recorded within 18 months of death showed no evidence of systolic anterior motion of the anterior mitral leaflet. This finding suggested the continued absence of outflow obstruction in these patients.

Genetic transmission: Genetic transmission of hypertrophic cardiomyopathy was demonstrated in first degree relatives of each of the seven patients. In four of these patients at least one first degree relative died prematurely of hypertrophic cardiomyopathy; in two of these families premature death occurred unusually frequently (that is, "malignant" hypertrophic cardiomyopathy[26] appeared to be present). In the families of the other three patients, at least one surviving relative had clinically evident hypertrophic cardiomyopathy. The only patient (Case 2) with concentric ventricular hypertrophy (demonstrated both with echocardiography and at necropsy) had a brother with hypertrophic cardiomyopathy whose sudden death at age 13 years was the first definitive manifestation of cardiac disease[27]; also, the patient's mother manifested asymmetric septal hypertrophy (septal-free wall thickness ratio of 1.7) on echocardiography. In addition, two patients (Cases 1 and 5) had the marked disorganization of cardiac muscle cells in the ventricular septum (involving 5 percent or more of the tissue section) that is characteristic of patients with hypertrophic cardiomyopathy[28]; in the other five patients a reliable assessment of the extent of septal disorganization could not be made because of widespread replacement fibrosis.

Necropsy Findings (Table V)

Gross pathology: Heart weights were increased compared with normal values[31] in each patient. In five of the seven hearts the ventricular septum was asymmetrically thickened with respect to the left ventricular

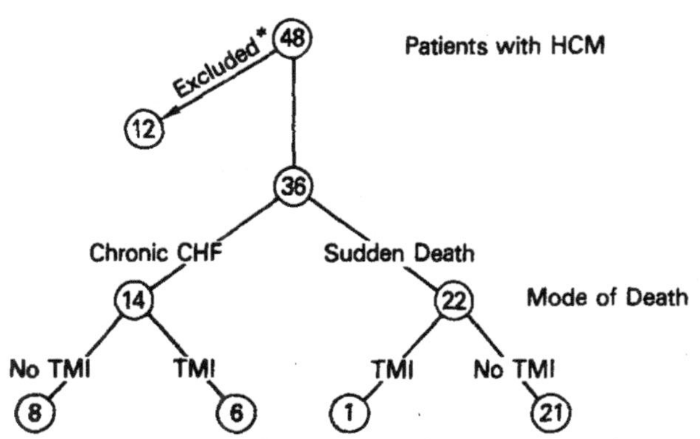

FIGURE 5. Diagram showing prevalence of transmural myocardial infarction (TMI) among patients with hypertrophic cardiomyopathy (HCM) who died suddenly and those who experienced chronic congestive heart failure (CHF). * = patients with hemodynamically significant narrowing of at least one major coronary artery and patients who died of noncardiac causes.

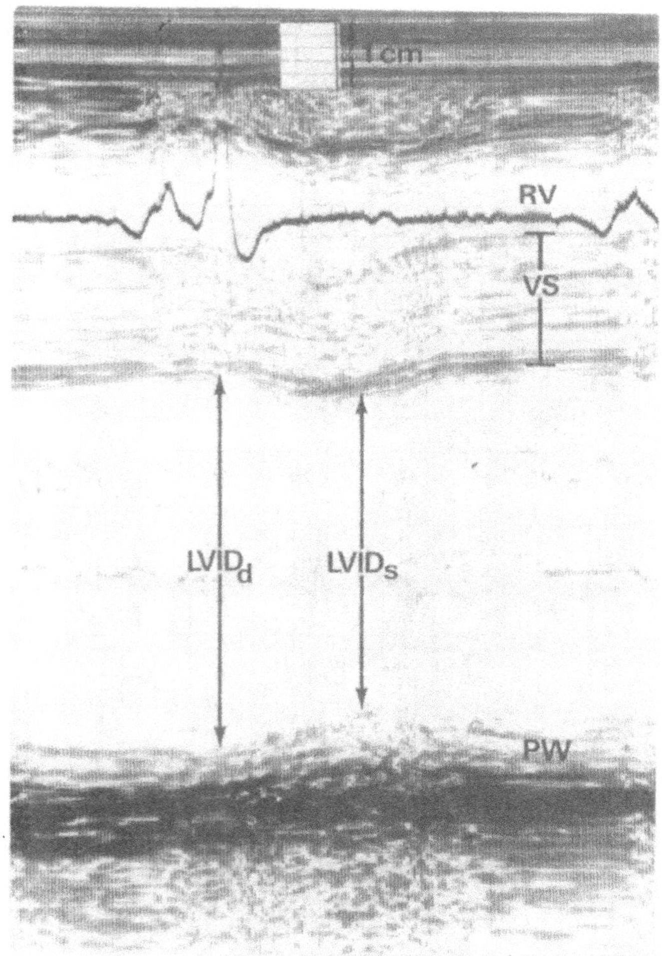

FIGURE 6. Case 7. Echocardiogram recorded inferior to the level of the mitral leaflets. The left ventricular internal dimensions in both diastole (LVID$_d$) and systole (LVID$_s$) are increased. Other portions of the tracing showed somewhat greater internal dimensions. The ventricular septum (VS) is disproportionately thickened with respect to the posterior left ventricular free wall (PW). RV = right ventricle.

free wall (septal-free wall thickness ratio greater than or equal to 1.3) (Fig. 3d and 9b).[18,21] In the remaining two patients (Cases 2 and 4) the ventricular septum and left ventricular free wall were of equal thickness at necropsy (Fig. 4f). However, in Patient 4 the septal-free wall thickness ratio calculated during life with echocardiography was abnormal (1.4), thus confirming the diagnosis of hypertrophic cardiomyopathy (with asymmetric septal hypertrophy). Such discrepancies between septal-free wall thickness ratios obtained during life and at necropsy have been explained previously.[32] In Patient 2 (whose mother had a septal-free wall thickness ratio of 1.7 on echocardiography) the echocardiographic septal-free wall thickness ratio was 1.0; this patient therefore had genetically transmitted hypertrophic cardiomyopathy with concentric (symmetric) ventricular hypertrophy.[33]

The left and right ventricular cavities were dilated in six of the seven patients (Fig. 3d and 4f) and very extensively in two of these patients. Only Patient 5, who had a relatively discrete myocardial scar, had ventricular cavities of normal size. Thrombi were present in the

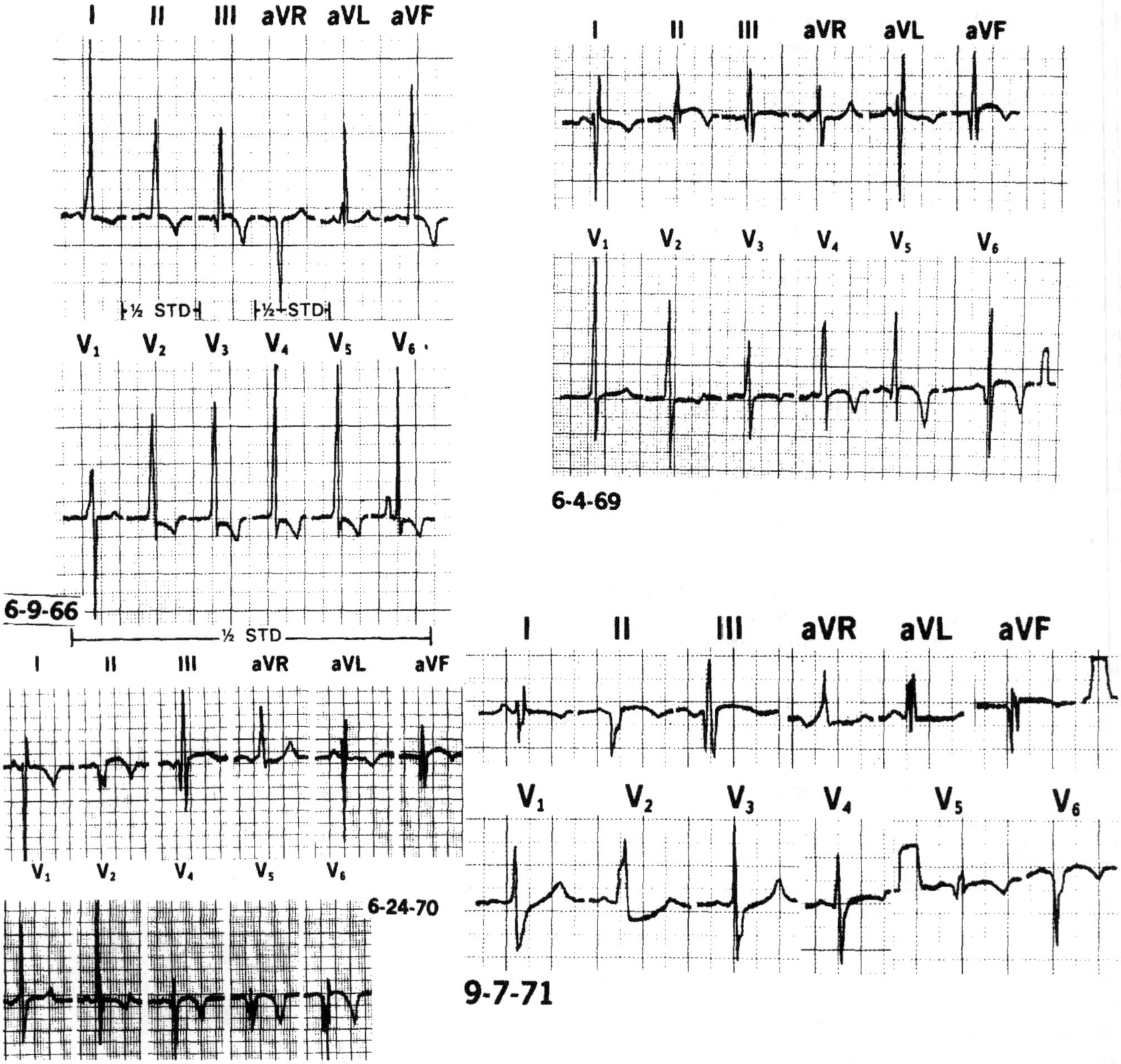

FIGURE 7. Case 3. Electrocardiograms obtained over a 5 year period. The changes suggest progressive ventricular scarring. **6-9-66,** recorded at age 16 years, showing strikingly increased precordial voltages (up to 82 mm), left ventricular "strain" pattern and diffuse T wave inversion. **6-4-69,** the tracing recorded at age 19 has changed substantially and now shows right axis deviation, a tall R wave in right precordial leads (suggestive of right ventricular or ventricular septal hypertrophy), greatly diminished left precordial R wave voltages, Q waves in leads II, III, aVF and V_6 and more marked T wave inversion in leads V_5 and V_6. **6-24-70,** in the tracing recorded at age 20, the left precordial R wave voltages are virtually absent and Q waves are more prominent in leads II, III, aVF, V_5 and V_6. **9-7-71,** the tracing recorded at age 21 (1 month after an acute myocardial infarction), the R wave in lead V_1 is diminished and left or "unusual" axis deviation is present. STD = standardization.

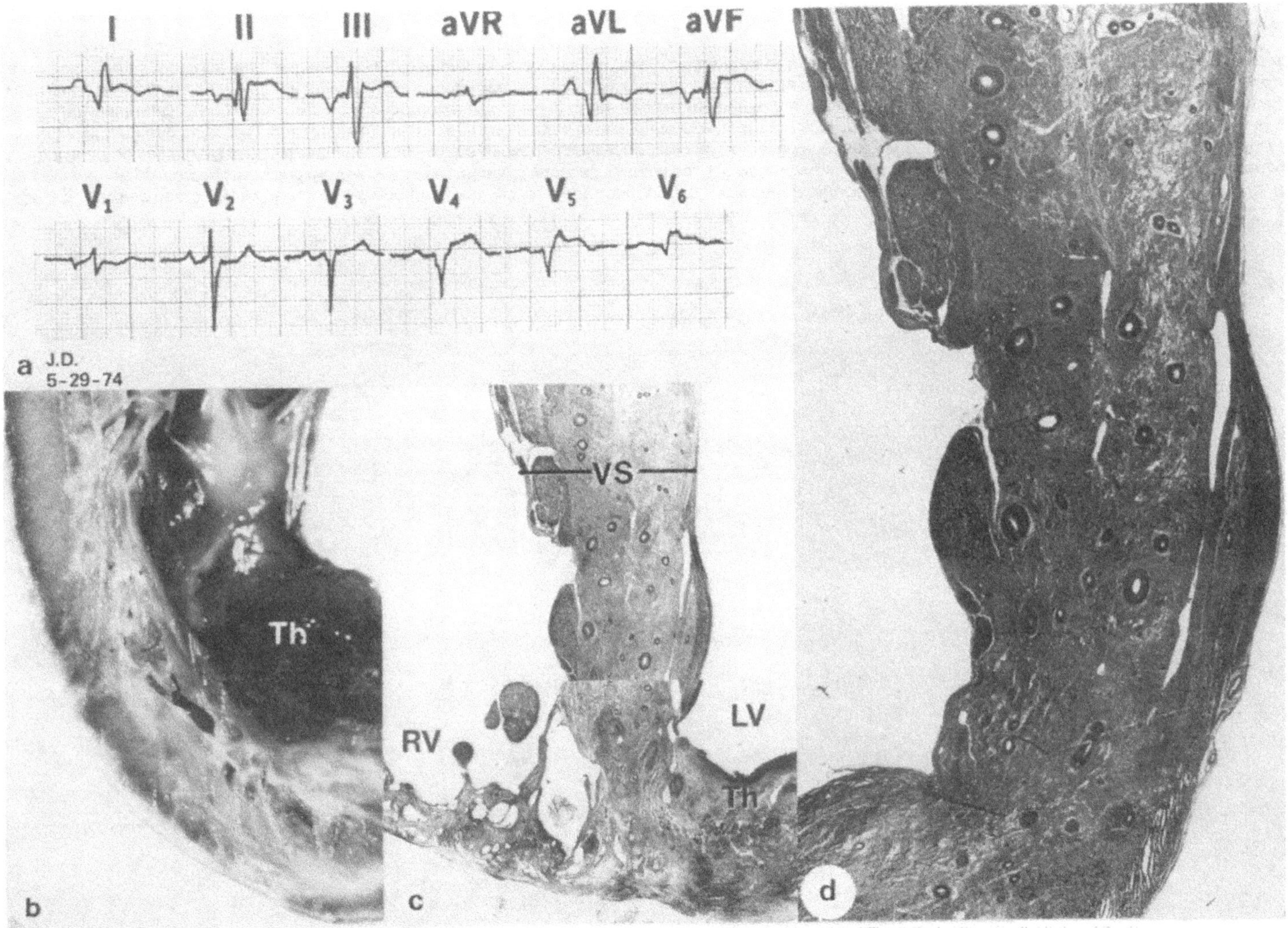

FIGURE 8. Case 4. Extensive transmural myocardial scarring. **a,** the electrocardiogram shows Q waves in leads I and aVL, diminished R wave voltage in the left precordial leads, an intraventricular conduction defect and diffuse T wave abnormalities. **b,** extensive scarring of the full thickness of the left ventricular free wall with superimposed mural thrombus (Th). **c,** composite microphotograph of a longitudinal section near the apex of the ventricular septum (VS) and contiguous areas of the right (RV) and left (LV) ventricular walls showing marked transmural scarring of both free walls and the septum; numerous abnormal intramural coronary arteries are present in the ventricular septum (elastic van Gieson stain ×3, reduced by 25 percent). **d,** the area of ventricular septum shown in **c,** but at higher magnification; extensive scarring even involves areas adjacent to prominent abnormal intramural coronary arteries (elastic van Gieson stain ×3, reduced by 25 percent).

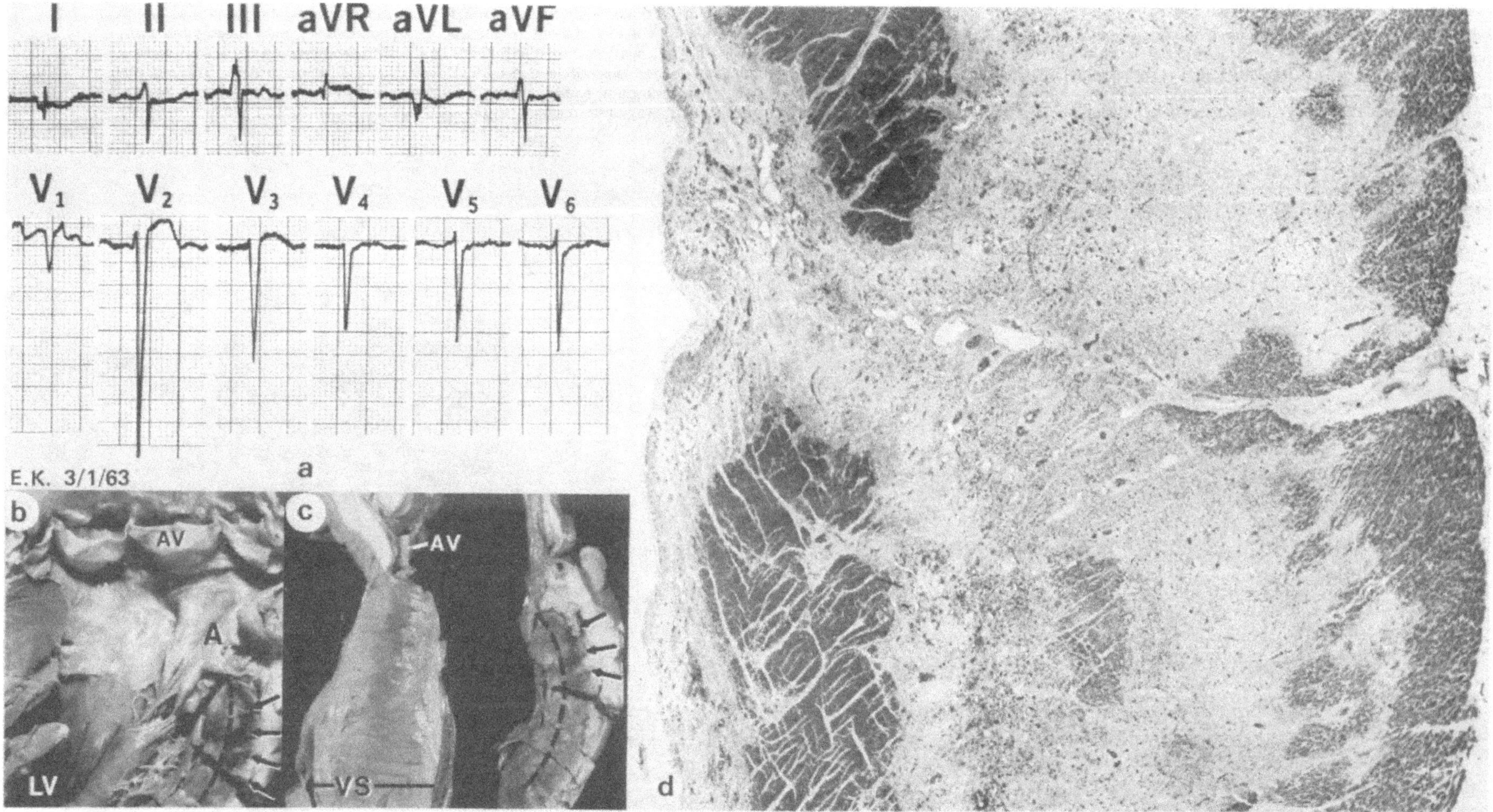

FIGURE 9. Case 5. Cardiac necropsy and electrocardiographic findings. **a,** electrocardiogram shows a left anterior hemiblock pattern, Q waves in leads I and aVL, diminished R wave voltage in the left precordial leads and diffuse S-T segment and T wave abnormalities. **b,** close-up view of left ventricular (LV) outflow tract showing endocardial mural plaque beneath the aortic valve (AV) and in direct apposition to the thickened anterior mitral leaflet (A), findings typical of hypertrophic cardiomyopathy; a subepicardial infarct is evident in the basal left ventricular free wall (**arrows**); the **broken line** serves to divide the inner from the outer halves of the ventricular wall. **c,** longitudinal cuts of ventricular septum (VS) and left ventricular free wall showing disproportionate thickening of the septum relative to the left ventricular free wall; an infarct in the basal subepicardial region of the left ventricular free wall (**arrows**) also is evident; the **broken line** serves to divide the inner from the outer halves of the ventricular wall; AV = aortic valve. **d,** histologic section of a portion of left ventricular free wall showing transmural replacement fibrosis (from an area of left ventricular free wall not shown in **b** or **c**) (hematoxylin-eosin ×21, reduced by 34 percent).

TABLE III

Hypertrophic Cardiomyopathy and Transmural Myocardial Infarction: Echocardiographic Findings*

Case no.	Age (yr) & sex	VS (mm)	PW (mm)	VS/PW	$LVID_d$ (mm)	97.5% Prediction Limit[†] $LVID_D$ (mm)	$LVID_s$ (mm)	97.5% Prediction Limit[†] $LVID_s$ (mm)	EF[‡] (%)	FS[§] (%)
2	19F	14	14	1.0	57	52	50	35	32	12
4	33M	16	13	1.2[‖]	55	54	42	36	55	24
6	50F	15	10	1.5	67	53	61	35	25	9
7	60M	19	9	2.1	58	52	50	34	36	14

* Includes data from only the echocardiogram obtained closest to the time of death.

† That value below which about 97.5 percent of the normal population lies; both $LVID_D$ and $LVID_s$ are a linear function of age and body surface area.[25]

‡ The 2.5 percent prediction limit (that value above which about 97.5 percent of the normal population lies) was 67 percent for each patient because ejection fraction is not a function of age or body surface area.[25]

§ The 2.5 percent prediction limit was 30 percent for each patient because percent fractional shortening is not a function of age or body surface area.[25]

‖ Another echocardiogram recorded 9 months earlier showed asymmetric septal hypertrophy (ventricular septal thickness 18 mm, posterior left ventricular free wall thickness 13 mm and septal-free wall thickness ratio 1.4).

EF = left ventricular ejection fraction; FS = percent fractional shortening; $LVID_D$ and $LVID_s$ = left ventricular internal dimension in diastole and systole, respectively; PW = posterior left ventricular free wall thickness; VS = ventricular septal thickness; VS/PW = ventricular septal to posterior left ventricular free wall thickness ratio.

ventricular cavities of four patients (left ventricle in one, right ventricle in one and both ventricles in two) (Fig. 4f and 8b); there was no evidence of ventricular thrombi in the three other patients with transmural scarring or in the 41 nonsurgically treated patients without transmural scarring.

Coronary arterial anatomy: At necropsy, none of the seven patients had atherosclerotic luminal narrowing greater than 75 percent of cross-sectional area[24] of any of the four major *extramural* coronary arteries. Most arteries were either free of atherosclerotic plaques or were narrowed less than 25 percent by plaques (Fig. 10 and 11). Patient 5 had an organizing clot (most likely an embolus) completely occluding the right coronary artery for a length of 3.5 cm; minimal atherosclerosis was present in the artery (Fig. 12, a to c).

In contrast, marked abnormalities of the *intramural* coronary arteries[34] were present in six of the seven patients (Fig. 3g and 8, c and d). These abnormal vessels had thickened walls (due to intimal proliferation or

TABLE IV

Hypertrophic Cardiomyopathy and Transmural Myocardial Infarction: Electrocardiographic Findings*

	Case 1	Case 2	Case 3	Case 4	Case 5	Case 6	Case 7
Age (yr) & sex	12M	19F	20F	33M	41F	50F	60M
Ventricular hypertrophy	–	R[†]	0[‡]	0	0	L	0
Diffuse T wave abnormalities	–	+	+	+	+	+	+
Q waves in leads							
I, aVL	–	0	0	+	+	0	+
V_5, V_6	–	+	+	+	0	+[¶]	+
II, III, aVF	–	0	+	0	0	0[‖]	0
IVCD	–	0[†]	0	+	0	+	0
LAH	–	0	+[§]	0	+	0	+
1°AVB	–	0	0	0	0	+	0
↓ R wave in left precordium	–	0	+	+	+	0	0
LAE	–	+	0	0	0	+	+

* The electrocardiogram recorded closest to the time of death (with the patient in a relatively stable clinical state) was used.

† The electrocardiographic pattern was also consistent with ventricular septal hypertrophy; left ventricular hypertrophy with "strain" and Wolff-Parkinson-White pattern were present 5 years previously.

‡ The patient showed substantial changes in the electrocardiographic pattern over an 11 year period (see Fig. 7); initially the electrocardiogram showed marked left ventricular hypertrophy with "strain" and subsequently a pattern consistent with either right ventricular or ventricular septal hypertrophy.

§ Left axis deviation only.

‖ Lead V_5 only.

¶ Marked decrease in prominence of Q waves in leads II, III and aVF was noted 4 years before death.

+ = present; 0 = absent; – = data not available; ↓ = decreased.

1°AVB = first degree atrioventricular block; IVCD = intraventricular conduction defect; L = left; LAH = left anterior hemiblock; LAE = left atrial enlargement; R = right.

TABLE V

Hypertrophic Cardiomyopathy and Transmural Myocardial Infarction: Necropsy Findings

	Case 1 (A105-75)	Case 2 (A75-209)	Case 3 (A72-197)	Case 4 (A74-216)	Case 5 (A63-77)	Case 6 (A77-32)	Case 7 (A76-108)
Age (yr) & sex	12M	19F	20F	33M	41F	50F	60M
Heart weight (g)	270	530	1250[b]	580	530	550	530
Location of transmural infarcts							
VS	+	+	+	+	+	+[f]	+
LV free wall							
Anterior	0	+	+	+	0	+	+
Posterior	+	+	+	+	+	0	+
Basal	+	+	+	0	+	+	+
Apical	+	+	+	+	0	+	+
RV							
Anterior	+	+	+	+	0	0	0
Posterior	0	+	+	+	0	0	0
Basal	0	+	+	0	0	0	0
Apical	+	+	+	+	0	0	0
LV pap infarct							
AL	0	+	+	+	0	+	+
PM	+	+	+	+	+	+	0
Subepicardial infarct	0	0	+	0	+	0	+
Histologic age of infarcts[29,30]							
<1 mo	0	0	0	0	+	0	0
1–2 mo	0	0	+[c]	0	+	0	0
>2 mo	+	+	+	+	+	+	+
Coronary arteries							
Extramural*							
LAD	0–25%	26–50%	0–25%[d]	51–75%	0–25%	0–25%[d]	0–25%[d]
LCx	0–25%	0–25%	0–25%	0–25%	0–25%	0–25%	0–25%
LMCA	0–25%	0–25%	0–25%	0–25%	0–25%	0–25%	0–25%
RCA	0–25%	0–25%	0–25%	26–50%	0–25%	0–25%	0–25%
Intramural†							
VS	+	0	+	+	+	+	+
LV	0	0	+	0	+	+	+
RV	0	0	0	+	0	0	0
Ventricular wall thickness							
VS	18	13	42	15	25	15	14
Post LVFW‡	10	13	10	15	9	10	10
Max LFVW	13	14	19	15	13	10	12
RV	5	6	11	5	6	3	6
VS/Post LVFW	1.8	1.0[§]	4.2	1.0[e]	2.8	1.5	1.4
Cavity size							
LV	↑	↑[‖]	↑	↑	0	↑[‖]	↑
RV	↑	↑[‖]	↑	↑	0	↑[‖]	↑
LA	0	↑	↑	↑	↑	↑	↑
RA	0	↑	↑	↑	↑	↑	↑
VS plaque	0	+[a]	0	0	+	+[g]	0
Thickened AML	0	0	0	0	+	+	0
Thrombus							
LV	0	+	+	+	0	0	0
RV	0	+	+	0	0	+	0

* Percent cross-sectional area narrowing by atherosclerosis; narrowing of any extramural coronary artery that was greater than 75 percent of the vessel lumen was considered abnormal.[24]

† Intramural coronary arteries with thickened walls (evidenced by intimal proliferation, medial hypertrophy or both) and luminal narrowing.

‡ Measured behind the mid point of the posterior mitral leaflet at the level of the inferior margins of the mitral leaflets.

§ Echocardiogram recorded 1 month before death showed concentric ventricular wall thickening (ventricular septal and posterior left ventricular free wall thicknesses were each 14 mm); no earlier echocardiograms were available for analysis.

‖ Marked dilatation similar in magnitude to that present in dilated cardiomyopathy.

a In the form of a discrete linear ridge.

b The patient weighed only 47 kg (103 pounds).

c Papillary muscles only.

d Examined by gross inspection only (that is, by making multiple cross sections of the vessels [3 to 5 mm apart] in the intact specimen, and then viewing the arterial lumens grossly).

e Echocardiogram recorded 1 1/2 years before death showed asymmetric septal hypertrophy (ventricular septal thickness 18 mm, posterior left ventricular free wall thickness 13 mm and septal-free wall thickness ratio 1.4).

f Septal infarct was present predominantly in the region of the left ventricular apex.

g Extensive endocardial fibrosis, but not a typical discrete plaque.

\+ = present; 0 = absent; ↑ = increased.

AL = anterolateral papillary muscle; AML = anterior mitral leaflet, LA = left atrium; LAD = left anterior descending coronary artery; LCx = left circumflex coronary artery; LMCA = left main coronary artery; LV = left ventricle; Max LVFW = maximal left ventricular free wall; pap = papillary muscles; Post LVFW = posterior left ventricular free wall (behind posterior mitral leaflet at the level of the inferior margins of mitral leaflets); PM = posteromedial papillary muscle; RA = right atrium; RCA = right coronary artery; RV = right ventricle; VS = ventricular septum.

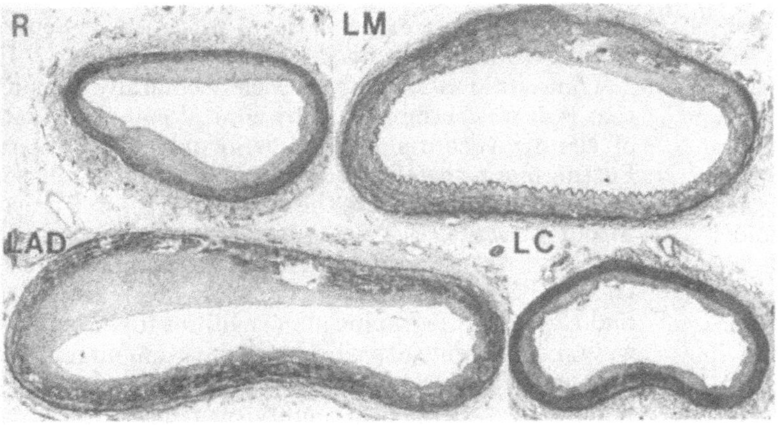

FIGURE 10. Case 2. Sections of the major extramural coronary arteries at sites of maximal narrowing. Each artery is free of significant narrowing (Movat stain ×16, reduced by 37 percent). LAD = left anterior descending, LC = left circumflex, LM = left main and R = right coronary artery, respectively.

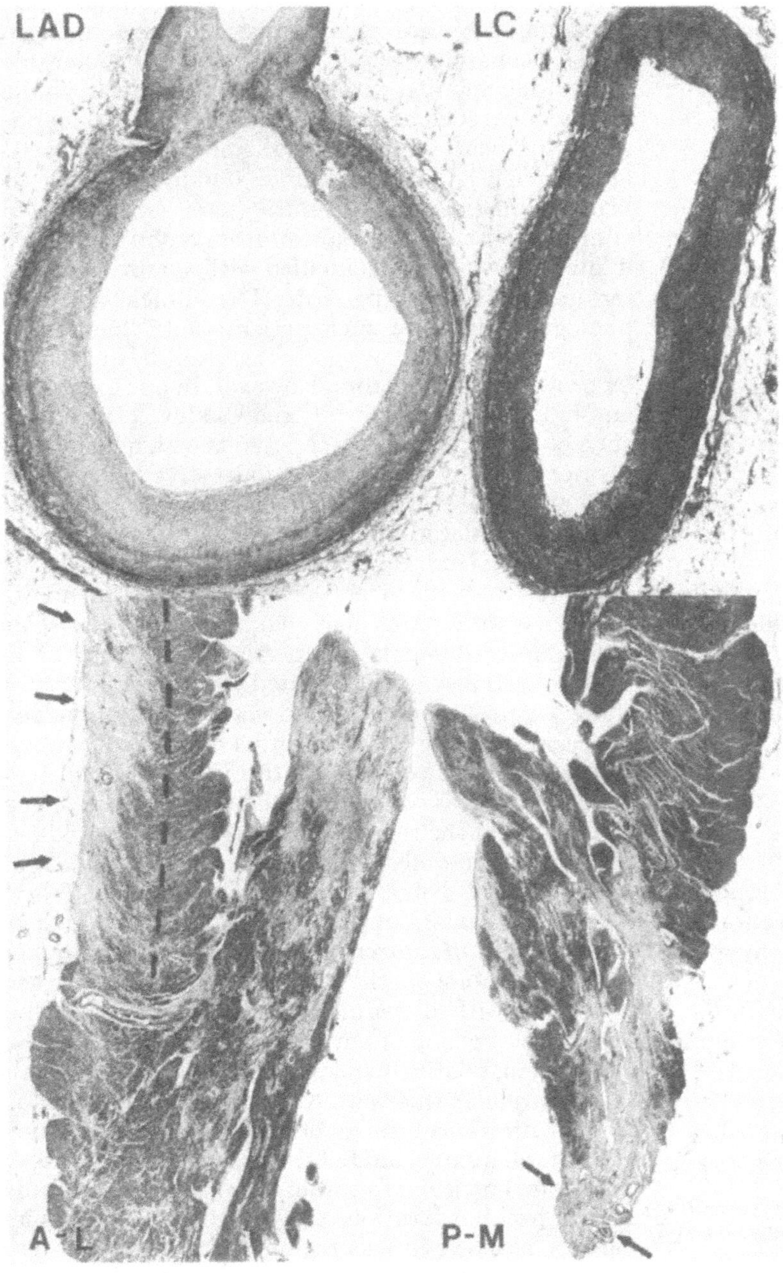

FIGURE 11. Case 7. Sections of the left anterior descending (LAD) and left circumflex (LC) coronary arteries (**top**) and of the left ventricular free wall and papillary muscles (**bottom**). Both coronary arteries are free of significant narrowing (Movat stains ×25, reduced by 20 percent). **Lower left,** section of left ventricular free wall and anterolateral papillary muscle (A-L); the scarring is localized to the subepicardial region of the left ventricular free wall (**arrows**) and to the distal half of the papillary muscle; the **broken line** serves to divide the inner from the outer halves of the ventricular wall (phosphotungstic acid-hematoxylin stain, ×3, reduced by 20 percent). **Lower right,** section of the left ventricular free wall and posteromedial papillary muscle (P-M) showing a transmural scar at the base of and caudal to the papillary muscle (**arrows**); focal scars also are present in the papillary muscle (phosphotungstic acid-hematoxylin stain ×3, reduced by 20 percent).

medial hypertrophy, or both) and narrowed lumens. Abnormal intramural coronary arteries were most common in the ventricular septum and in areas of scarring.

Myocardial infarcts: One or more foci of transmural left ventricular scarring (that is, replacement fibrosis) were present in each of the seven patients. One of these patients had an acute infarction manifested histologically by coagulation necrosis (loss of contractile elements, granularity of the cytoplasm and nuclear pyknosis or karyolysis) as well as healed myocardial infarcts (Fig. 12). The scars usually involved greater than 75 percent of the overall ventricular wall thickness.

Extensive transmural scars were present in the left ventricular free wall of six of the seven hearts (Fig. 2e, 3f, 8b, 9d, 10, 11 and 12, d and e). In each patient extensive scarring or necrosis of either one or both left ventricular papillary muscles was also evident (Fig. 11 and 12d). In addition, each of these patients had transmural scarring of the ventricular septum (Fig. 2d, 3e, 8c and 13).

The size of the left ventricular scars varied considerably. Three patients (Cases 2, 3 and 7) had particularly extensive transmural scarring involving the anterior, posterior, basal and apical regions of the left ventricular free wall and also contiguous areas of the ventricular septum. In contrast, Patient 5 (who had an occluding clot of the right coronary artery) had a relatively discrete transmural scar of the left ventricle that was limited to the posterobasal regions of the left ventricular free wall and septum (Fig. 12). The origin of the coronary clot in this patient, who also had pulmonary and renal infarcts due to emboli, is uncertain.

Four patients also had transmural scars involving the right ventricular wall (Fig. 8c). In three patients the scar was extensive and involved both the anterior and posterior right ventricular walls, and in the other patient (Case 1) the scar was relatively small and involved only a portion of the anterior right ventricular wall.

In addition to the transmural scars *subendocardial areas* often showed scarring (Fig. 13d). Three patients (Cases 3, 5 and 7) also had scarring in the *subepicardial* region of the basal left ventricular free wall (Fig. 9, a and b, 11, and 12f).

Discussion

Prevalence and clinical findings: Our study demonstrates that transmural myocardial infarction* may occur in patients with hypertrophic cardiomyopathy in the absence of significant atherosclerosis of the extramural coronary arteries. Furthermore, transmural infarction was present in 15 percent of our sizable group of nonsurgically treated patients who died of hypertrophic cardiomyopathy.

Transmural infarction was usually clinically "silent" that is, it was accompanied by clinical manifestations of acute myocardial infarction in only one patient. Furthermore, the electrocardiogram was generally of little value in identifying the site of necrosis or fibrosis in our patients. Because 10 of 25 patients who did not have transmural infarction (or significant extramural coronary arterial narrowing) at necropsy also had electrocardiographic abnormalities (deep, wide Q waves) consistent with a healed myocardial infarct, the presence of such electrocardiographic changes was not reliably predictive of transmural scarring.

Clinical course: Six of our seven patients had a relatively unusual clinical course for patients with hypertrophic cardiomyopathy—that is, one characterized by supraventricular arrhythmias and profound progressive congestive heart failure with ventricular dilatation (documented with echocardiography and at necropsy). Two such patients (Cases 2 and 6) with marked congestive heart failure and a dilated poorly contractile left ventricle had shown a nondilated hypercontractile heart on angiography 8 and 9 years earlier in their clinical course. This evolution from a nondilated to a dilated left ventricle coincided with symptomatic deterioration in these patients. The clinical and morphologic features of such patients with "end-stage" hypertrophic cardiomyopathy have not been reported by previous investigators. However, in our experience and in that of Goodwin[35-37] and Oakley,[38] the clinical state of the large majority of patients with hypertrophic cardiomyopathy and chronic congestive heart failure does not usually evolve into one characterized by left ventricular dilatation.

Necropsy findings: Areas of the ventricular septum and left ventricular free wall involved by transmural infarction were particularly large in six of the seven patients. In four patients, portions of the right ventricular wall also were infarcted. The large infarcts in these patients usually occurred without clinical evidence of accompanying acute myocardial infarction. However, the extent of transmural infarcts in the left and right ventricular walls was not related to the age of the patient, nor did the regions of the left ventricle involved by infarcts generally correspond to any particular coronary arterial distribution (as noted, Patient 5 is an exception to this).

The extent of infarction in our patients with hypertrophic cardiomyopathy exceeded that usually present in patients with idiopathic dilated cardiomyopathy.[15-17] In the latter group of patients transmural infarcts are uncommon, relatively small and usually confined to the left ventricular free wall. Also, three of our seven patients with transmural myocardial infarction had nontransmural infarcts limited to the *subepicardium* of the basal left ventricular free wall. Although the significance of this peculiar location of myocardial scarring is uncertain, scarring in this region of the left ventricle is unique, and we have not observed it in patients with

---

* The term "myocardial infarct" (or "infarction") is used in this paper to describe extensive myocardial cell necrosis that has undergone healing (that is, shows extensive replacement fibrosis). Although coagulation necrosis was present in the heart of only one of our seven patients it is our presumption that necrosis must have preceded the *extensive* scarring (replacement fibrosis) identified in the other six patients.

coronary or valvular heart disease or dilated cardiomyopathy.

Left and right ventricular dilatation was present in six (86 percent) of our seven patients with hypertrophic cardiomyopathy and transmural infarction. In two patients the ventricular dilatation was marked, similar to that present in dilated cardiomyopathy.[15–17] In contrast, only four (10 percent) of our 41 nonsurgically treated necropsy patients with hypertrophic cardiomyopathy but without transmural myocardial infarction had ventricular dilatation ($P < 0.001$). Hence, transmural infarction appears to predispose to ventricular dilatation in patients with hypertrophic cardiomyopathy.

Mural thrombi (similar to those present in about 70 percent of patients with dilated cardiomyopathy[15–17]) occurred in four of our seven patients. Because ven-

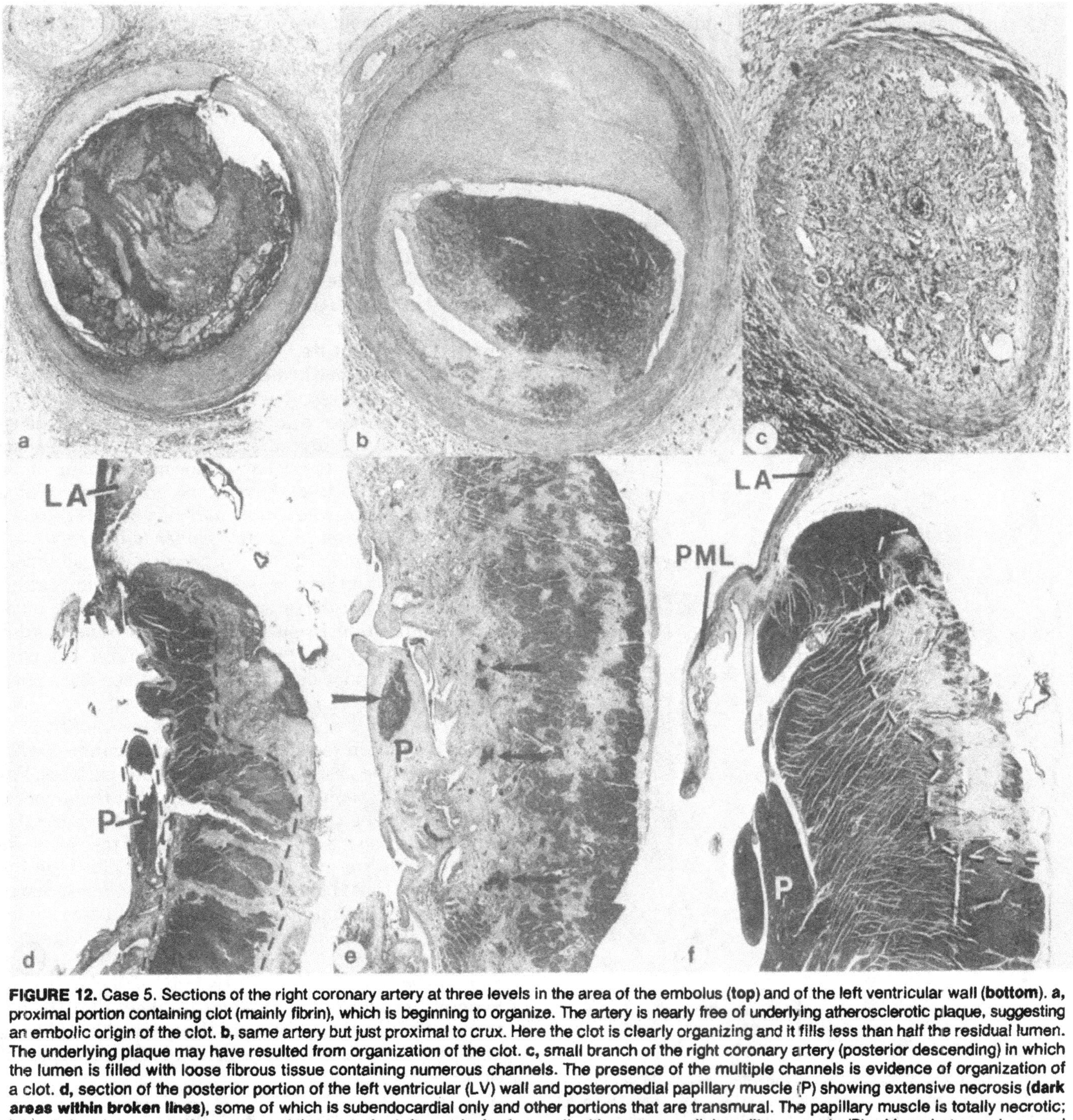

FIGURE 12. Case 5. Sections of the right coronary artery at three levels in the area of the embolus (**top**) and of the left ventricular wall (**bottom**). **a,** proximal portion containing clot (mainly fibrin), which is beginning to organize. The artery is nearly free of underlying atherosclerotic plaque, suggesting an embolic origin of the clot. **b,** same artery but just proximal to crux. Here the clot is clearly organizing and it fills less than half the residual lumen. The underlying plaque may have resulted from organization of the clot. **c,** small branch of the right coronary artery (posterior descending) in which the lumen is filled with loose fibrous tissue containing numerous channels. The presence of the multiple channels is evidence of organization of a clot. **d,** section of the posterior portion of the left ventricular (LV) wall and posteromedial papillary muscle (P) showing extensive necrosis (**dark areas within broken lines**), some of which is subendocardial only and other portions that are transmural. The papillary muscle is totally necrotic; LA = left atrium. **e,** another portion of the posterior left ventricular free wall with posteromedial papillary muscle (P) midway between base and apex. Here there is considerable fibrous scarring (light areas) with only small islands of necrosis (**arrows**). **f,** basal portion of the left ventricular free wall in another area showing only subepicardial scarring (light areas demarcated by broken line); PML = posterior mitral leaflet; LA = left atrium. **a, b,** and **c;** Movat stain ×16, 25 and 65, respectively, reduced by 20 percent; **d,** phosphotungstic acid-hematoxylin stain (×2.5, reduced by 20 percent); **e, f,** hematoxylin-eosin ×5, reduced by 20 percent.

tricular thrombi usually occur in the setting of markedly diminished cardiac output it is not surprising that they have not been observed in patients with hypertrophic cardiomyopathy and nondilated ventricles.

Etiology of transmural infarction: The etiology of transmural myocardial infarction in patients with hypertrophic cardiomyopathy and without significant coronary atherosclerosis is unclear. Several causes appear to be possible. *First, the cardiac mass may have been too great for the existent coronary blood supply and its capacity to deliver oxygen to the myocardium.* This possibility is suggested by the findings in Patient 3, who had a massive heart weighing 1,250 g (although the patient weighed only 47 kg). However, this explanation is untenable for the other six patients with transmural infarction because their heart weight did not exceed 580 gs. *Second, myocardial infarction could have been due to an occluding embolus of a major coronary artery,* which subsequently lysed.[39-42] In Patient 5 a partially organizing embolus (of unknown origin) was present in the right coronary artery. However, this patient had a relatively discrete transmural infarct of the ventricular septum and the posterobasal region of the left ventricular wall; hence, if an embolus to a single coronary artery had been responsible for infarction in any of the other study patients, the resultant areas of scarring would probably not have been as extensive as those observed. Although we cannot rule out the possibility that multiple, small coronary emboli were responsible for our findings, the lack of clinical evidence of systemic emboli elsewhere in the other six patients makes this hypothesis unlikely.

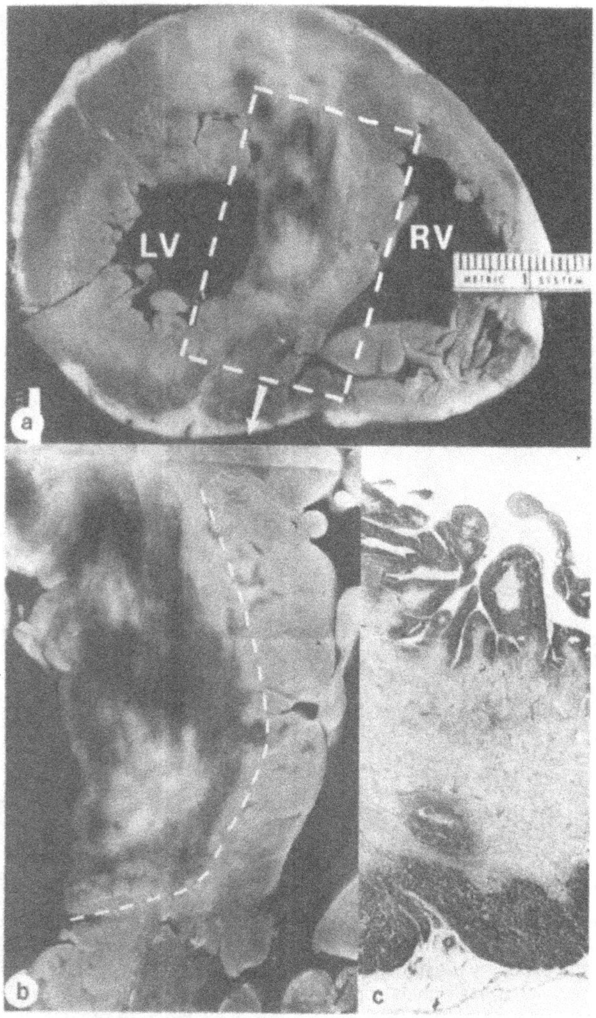

FIGURE 13. Case 1. Transmural myocardial fibrosis in ventricular septum. **a,** in a transversely cut section of the heart, an extensive septal infarct is demarcated by the **broken line;** LV and RV = left and right ventricle, respectively. **b,** area of infarction (outlined by **broken line**) shown at higher magnification. **c,** histologic section of the transmural infarct showing extensive replacement fibrosis; taken from area shown in **a** and **b** (phosphotungstic acid-hematoxylin ×3, reduced by 35 percent).

Third, it is possible that infarction in our patients was related, at least in part, to narrowing of the intramural coronary arteries. Particularly marked thickening of the walls and narrowing of the lumens of numerous intramural coronary arteries was present in the left ventricular myocardium in six of the seven patients with transmural infarction. Although abnormalities of the intramural coronary arteries have been reported in a wide variety of cardiac or systemic diseases,[43] the arterial alterations identified in the patients with hypertrophic cardiomyopathy and transmural infarction constitute, in our experience, the most widespread and marked example of "small vessel disease." Nevertheless, because abnormal intramural coronary arteries were not present in one of our patients with transmural myocardial infarction, the causal relation between these two abnormalities cannot be considered definitive. *Fourth, recent studies have shown that myocardial infarction may be precipitated by coronary spasm in vessels either with or without atherosclerotic plaques.*[44-48] Although it is possible that vasospasm (of either the extramural or abnormal intramural coronary arteries) was responsible for myocardial infarction in our patients with hypertrophic cardiomyopathy and "normal" extramural coronary arteries, we cannot be definitive about such a mechanism.

Finally, brief periods of hypoxia or hypotension might have been responsible for the transmural myocardial scarring observed in certain of our patients. For example, in Patient 1 it is most likely that the myocardial infarction either preceded or caused the cardiac arrest (based on a histologic assessment of the age of the infarct). However, we cannot definitively exclude the possibilities that the patient had a cardiac arrest due to a primary arrhythmia and that the infarct was a consequence of hypoxia or resuscitative efforts, or both, at the time of arrest. Ten weeks before death, Patient 7 had a severe episode of bradycardia associated with hypotension. However, it seems unlikely that the extensive myocardial scarring in this patient could have been due to this relatively brief period of hypotension.

Acknowledgment

We thank Dr. Dennis E. Chenowith, Department of Pathology, University of California Irvine Medical Center, Irvine, California for making one of the heart specimens available to us.

References

1. **Braudo M, Wigle ED, Keith JD:** Distinctive electrocardiogram in muscular subaortic stenosis due to ventricular septal hypertrophy. Am J Cardiol 14:599–607, 1964
2. **Bahl OP, Walsh TJ, Massie E:** Electrocardiography and vectorcardiography in idiopathic hypertrophic subaortic stenosis. Am J Med Sci 259:262–271, 1970
3. **Goodwin JF, Hollman A, Cleland WP, Teare D:** Obstructive cardiomyopathy simulating aortic stenosis. Br Heart J 22:403–414, 1960
4. **Braunwald E, Morrow AG, Cornell WP, Aygen MM, Hilbish TF:** Idiopathic hypertrophic subaortic stenosis. Am J Med 29:924–945, 1960
5. **Wigle ED, Heimbecker RO, Gunton RW:** Idiopathic ventricular septal hypertrophy causing muscular subaortic stenosis. Circulation 26:325–340, 1962
6. **Estes EH Jr, Whalen RE, Roberts SR Jr, McIntosh HD:** The electrocardiographic and vectorcardiographic findings in idiopathic hypertrophic subaortic stenosis. Am Heart J 65:155–161, 1963
7. **Prescott R, Quinn JS, Littmann D:** Electrocardiographic changes in hypertrophic subaortic stenosis which simulate myocardial infarction. Am Heart J 66:43–48, 1963
8. **Walston A, Behar VS:** Spectrum of coronary artery disease in idiopathic hypertrophic subaortic stenosis. Am J Cardiol 38:12–16, 1976
9. **Gulotta SJ, Hamby RI, Aronson AL, Ewing K:** Coexistent idiopathic hypertrophic subaortic stenosis and coronary arterial disease. Circulation 46:890–896, 1972
10. **Giuliani ER, Tajik AJ, Frye RL, Davis GD, Brandenburg RO:** Idiopathic hypertrophic subaortic stenosis (IHSS) and associated coronary artery disease (abstr). Circulation 45, 46:Suppl II:II–156, 1972
11. **Marcus GB, Popp RL, Stinson ED:** Coronary artery disease with idiopathic hypertrophic subaortic stenosis. Lancet 1:901–903, 1974
12. **Lardani H, Serrano JA, Villamil RJ:** Hemodynamics and coronary arteriography in idiopathic hypertrophic subaortic stenosis. Am J Cardiol 41:476–481, 1978
13. **Maron BJ, Savage DD, Clark CE, Henry WL, Vlodaver Z, Edwards JE, Epstein SE:** Prevalence and characteristics of disproportionate ventricular septal thickening in patients with coronary artery disease. Circulation 57:250–256, 1978
14. **Kossowsky WA, Mohr B, Dardashti I, Gabor GE:** Acute myocardial infarction in idiopathic hypertrophic subaortic stenosis. Chest 64:529–532, 1973
15. **Roberts WC, Ferrans VJ:** Morphologic observations in the cardiomyopathies. In, Myocardial Disease (Fowler NO, ed). New York, Grune & Stratton, 1973, p 59–115
16. **Roberts WC, Ferrans VJ:** Pathologic anatomy of the cardiomyopathies. Idiopathic dilated and hypertrophic types, infiltrative types and endomyocardial disease with and without eosinophilia. Human Pathol 6:287–342, 1975
17. **Roberts WC, Ferrans VJ:** Pathological aspects of certain cardiomyopathies. Circ Res 34, 35:Suppl II:II-128–II-144, 1974
18. **Henry WL, Clark CE, Epstein SE:** Asymmetric septal hypertrophy (ASH): Echocardiographic identification of the pathognomonic anatomic abnormality of IHSS. Circulation 47:225–233, 1973
19. **Braunwald E, Lambrew CT, Rockoff SD, Ross J Jr, Morrow AG:** Idiopathic hypertrophic subaortic stenosis. I. A description of the disease based upon an analysis of 64 patients. Circulation 30:Suppl IV:IV-3–IV-217, 1964
20. **Roberts WC:** Valvular, subvalvular and supravalvular aortic stenosis: morphologic features. Cardiovasc Clin 5:104–126, 1973
21. **Epstein SE, Henry WL, Clark CE, Roberts WC, Maron BJ, Ferrans VJ, Redwood DR, Morrow AG:** Asymmetric septal hypertrophy. Ann Intern Med 81:650–680, 1974
22. **Roberts WC, Gardin JM:** Location of myocardial infarcts. A confusion of terms and definitions. Am J Cardiol 42:868–872, 1978
23. **Maron BJ, Clark CE, Henry WL, Fukuda T, Edwards JE, Mathews EC, Redwood DR, Epstein SE:** Prevalence and characteristics of disproportionate ventricular septal thickening in patients with acquired or congenital heart diseases. Echocardiographic and morphologic findings. Circulation 55:489–496, 1977
24. **Roberts WC, Buja LM:** The frequency and significance of coronary arterial thrombi and other observations in fatal acute myocardial infarction. A study of 107 necropsy patients. Am J Med 52:425–443, 1972
25. **Gardin JM, Henry WL, Savage DD, Ware JH, Burn C, Borer JS:** Echocardiographic measurements in normal subjects: evaluation of an adult population without clinically apparent heart disease. J Clin Ultrasound, in press
26. **Maron BJ, Lipson LC, Roberts WC, Savage DD, Epstein SE:** "Malignant" hypertrophic cardiomyopathy: identification of a subgroup of families with unusually frequent premature deaths. Am J Cardiol 41:1133–1140, 1978
27. **Maron BJ, Roberts WC, Edwards JE, McAllister HA, Foley DD, Epstein SE:** Sudden death in patients with hypertrophic cardiomyopathy: Characterization of patients without previous functional limitation. Am J Cardiol 41:803–810, 1978
28. **Maron BJ, Roberts WC:** Quantitative analysis of cardiac muscle cell disorganization in the ventricular septum of patients with hypertrophic cardiomyopathy. Circulation, in press
29. **Mallory GK, White PD, Salcedo-Salgar J:** The speed of healing of myocardial infarction: a study of the pathologic anatomy in 72 cases. Am Heart J 18:647–671, 1939
30. **Fishbein MC, MacLean D, Maroko PR:** The histopathologic evolution of myocardial infarction. Chest 73:843–849, 1978
31. **Gould SE:** Pathology of the Heart and Blood Vessels, third edition. Springfield, IL, Charles C Thomas, 1968, p 1139
32. **Maron BJ, Henry WL, Roberts WC, Epstein SE:** Comparison of echocardiographic and necropsy measurements of ventricular wall thicknesses in patients with and without disproportionate septal thickening. Circulation 55:341–345, 1977
33. **Maron BJ, Gottdiener JS, Roberts WC, Henry WL, Epstein SE:** Left ventricular outflow tract obstruction due to systolic anterior motion of the anterior mitral leaflet in patients with concentric left ventricular hypertrophy. Circulation 57:527–533, 1978
34. **McReynolds RA, Roberts WC:** The intramural coronary arteries in hypertrophic cardiomyopathy (abstr). Am J Cardiol 35:154, 1975
35. **Goodwin JF:** Congestive and hypertrophic cardiomyopathies. A decade of study. Lancet 1:731–739, 1970
36. **Goodwin JF, Oakley CM:** The cardiomyopathies. Br Heart J 34: 545–552, 1972
37. **Goodwin JF:** Prospects and predictions for the cardiomyopathies. Circulation 50:210–219, 1974
38. **Oakley CM:** Hypertrophic obstructive cardiomyopathy—patterns of progression. In, Ciba Foundation Study Group No. 37: Hypertrophic Obstructive Cardiomyopathy. (Wolstenholme GEW, O'Connor M, ed). London, Churchill, 1971, p 9–29
39. **Richardson PM, Gotsman MS:** Angiographic evidence of coronary embolism and resolution. S Afr Med J 45:805–809, 1971
40. **O'Reilly RJ, Spellberg RD:** Rapid resolution of coronary arterial emboli. Myocardial infarction and subsequent normal coronary arteriograms. Ann Intern Med 81:348–350, 1974
41. **Rosenblatt A, Selzer A:** The nature and clinical features of myocardial infarction with normal coronary arteriogram. Circulation 55:578–580, 1977
42. **Roberts WC:** Coronary embolism: a review of causes, consequences, and diagnostic considerations. Cardiovasc Med 3: 699–706, 1978
43. **Arnett EN, Roberts WC:** Acute myocardial infarction and angiographically normal coronary arteries. Circulation 53:395–400, 1976
44. **Maseri A, L'Abbate A, Baroldi G, Chierchia S, Marzilli M, Ballestra AM, Severi S, Parodi O, Biagini A, Distante A, Pesola A:** Coronary vasospasm as a possible cause of myocardial infarction. A conclusion derived from the study of "preinfarction" angina. N Engl J Med 299:1271–1277, 1978
45. **Johnson AD, Detwiler JH:** Coronary spasm, variant angina and recurrent myocardial infarctions. Circulation 55:947–950, 1977
46. **Oliva PB, Potts DE, Pluss RG:** Coronary arterial spasm in prinzmetal angina. N Engl J Med 288:745–751, 1973
47. **Cheng TO, Bashour T, Kelser GA Jr, Weiss L, Bacos J:** Variant angina of Prinzmetal with normal coronary arteriograms. A variant of the variant. Circulation 47:476–485, 1973
48. **Cheng TO, Bashour T, Singh BK, Kelser GA:** Myocardial infarction in the absence of coronary arteriosclerosis. Result of coronary spasm (?). Am J Cardiol 30:680–682, 1972

Quantitative Analysis of Cardiac Muscle Cell Disorganization in the Ventricular Septum

Comparison of Fetuses and Infants with and Without Congenital Heart Disease and Patients with Hypertrophic Cardiomyopathy

BARRY J. MARON, M.D., NORIKO SATO, M.D., WILLIAM C. ROBERTS, M.D., JESSE E. EDWARDS, M.D., AND ROMA S. CHANDRA, M.D.

SUMMARY The presence of numerous abnormally arranged cardiac muscle cells in the ventricular septum has been considered a characteristic anatomic feature of hypertrophic cardiomyopathy. However, it has been suggested that the ventricular septum of infants with certain congenital cardiac diseases (such as aortic or pulmonic valve atresia) contains disorganized cardiac muscle cells similar to those in patients with hypertrophic cardiomyopathy. To test the validity of this concept and the true specificity and sensitivity of septal disorganization for hypertrophic cardiomyopathy, sections of ventricular septum were obtained at necropsy from 276 patients and the extent of ventricular septal disorganization was determined quantitatively. Disorganization was most marked in infants, children and adults with hypertrophic cardiomyopathy (i.e., present in 95% of 60 patients); the mean area of septum disorganized was 31 ± 3%. Although disorganized cells were present in 64% of 33 infants with aortic or pulmonic valve atresia, these cells occupied extremely small areas of ventricular septum (mean area of septum disorganized 2.8 ± 0.7%; $p < 0.001$). Furthermore, the minimal septal disorganization present in aortic or pulmonic valve atresia was similar to that found in 91 infants with other congenital heart malformations and in 92 normal fetuses or infants (mean area of septum disorganized was 1.4 ± 0.6 and 0.3 ± 0.1%, respectively). Hence, extensive ventricular septal disorganization is a highly sensitive and specific finding for hypertrophic cardiomyopathy, although small areas of disorganization may occur in infants with other heart diseases, including aortic or pulmonic valve atresia.

IN THE INITIAL REPORT of hypertrophic cardiomyopathy, Teare[1] described a bizarre arrangement of cardiac muscle cells in the asymmetrically hypertrophied ventricular septum. Subsequently, other investigators made similar observations regarding the histologic appearance of ventricular septal myocardium in this disease.[2-9] A recent report, based on a qualitative histologic analysis, emphasized that the ventricular septum of infants with aortic or pulmonic valve atresia contains disorganized cardiac muscle cells similar to those in patients with hypertrophic cardiomyopathy.[10] Recent experience with a quantitative method for assessing the extent of cellular disorganization in the ventricular septum has shown that it is not the presence or absence but rather the extent of septal disorganization that distinguishes patients with hypertrophic cardiomyopathy from those with other heart diseases histologically.[11] Hence, we undertook the present study to determine the relative extent of cardiac muscle cell disorganization in the ventricular septum of infants with congenital heart disease (including those with aortic or pulmonic valve atresia) compared with that of patients with hypertrophic cardiomyopathy.

From the Cardiology Branch, NHLBI, NIH, Bethesda, Maryland; the Department of Pathology, United Hospitals-Miller Division, St. Paul, Minnesota; the Department of Pathology, University of Minnesota School of Medicine, Minneapolis, Minnesota; and the Department of Pathology, Children's Hospital Medical Center, Washington, DC.

Supported in part by Public Health Service research grant 5R01 HL 05694 from the NHLBI, and by the Bremer Foundation, St. Paul, Minnesota.

Address for reprints: Barry J. Maron, M.D., National Institutes of Health, NHLBI, Bldg. 10, Room 7B-15, Bethesda, Maryland, 20014.

Received August 11, 1978; revision accepted March 15, 1979.
Circulation 60, No. 3, 1979.

Selection of Case Material

We reviewed the cardiovascular registries of the Pathology Branch, National Heart, Lung, and Blood Institute, United Hospitals-Miller Division, and the Children's Hospital Medical Center and selected 276 hearts for study. The following subgroups of hearts were included:

1) 23 infants with aortic valve atresia, hypoplastic left ventricle and intact ventricular septum (The mitral valve was hypoplastic in 20 patients and atretic in the other three.);[12]

2) 10 infants with pulmonic valve atresia, hypoplastic right ventricle, intact ventricular septum and nonatretic tricuspid valve. Because the ventricular wall thicknesses and histologic findings in patients with aortic or pulmonic valve atresia (with or without atretic mitral valve) did not differ appreciably, these two groups of patients were combined for convenience in data analysis;

3) 91 infants with a variety of congenital heart malformations other than aortic or pulmonic valve atresia, in which the ventricular cavities were not hypoplastic;

4) 29 fetuses (10–22 weeks gestation), without evidence of structural cardiac disease, obtained from therapeutic abortions;[13]

5) 14 live-born premature infants of 23–35 weeks gestation who died in the first 4 days of life due to septicemia or intracranial hemorrhage, and five stillborn infants,[13] none of whom had evidence of structural cardiac disease;

6) 44 live-born term infants, without evidence of structural cardiac disease, who died from 1 day to 20 months of age due to trauma, septicemia, diaphragmatic hernia, or complications of delivery.[13] For the purposes of data analysis, the fetuses, live-born premature infants, stillborns and live-born term infants were combined as a group of normal fetuses and infants;

7) 60 patients with hypertrophic cardiomyopathy, including six infants (stillborn to 11 months of age), 10 children[11] (11–17 years of age), and 44 adults[11] (18–70 years of age).

In the infants with congenital heart disease, death resulted from complications of cardiac catheterization, operative or postoperative complications, congestive heart failure, or sudden death, presumably due to ventricular arrhythmia (in nonoperated patients). Patients with hypertrophic cardiomyopathy, infants with congenital heart disease, and normal fetuses and infants are compared with regard to clinical and morphologic parameters in table 1.

Materials and Methods

Measurement of Ventricular Wall Thicknesses

Measurements of ventricular wall thicknesses were made in two areas: 1) in the ventricular septum, at the point of maximum thickness, usually about one-half the distance between the base of the aortic valve and the apex of the left ventricle; and 2) in the posterior left ventricular wall, behind the midpoint of the posterior mitral leaflet, at a level corresponding to the tips of the mitral leaflets. These measurements were made perpendicular to the endocardial surface of the ventricular walls (with calipers in infants and with a light microscope and calibrated micrometer eyepiece in fetuses). Trabeculations, papillary muscles, crista supraventricularis and mitral and tricuspid valve structures were not included in the measurements of ventricular wall thickness.

Tissue Preparation

In each patient in this study, tissue blocks were taken from the full thickness of ventricular septum, at the point of maximal thickness, about one-half the distance between the base of the aortic valve and the apex of the left ventricle, and in a plane perpendicular to the long axis of the left ventricle (i.e., the transverse

TABLE 1. *Clinical and Morphologic Data in Four Subgroups of Patients*

Parameter	Hypertrophic cardiomyopathy (n = 60)	Aortic or pulmonic atresia** (n = 33)	Other congenital heart diseases§ (n = 91)	Normal fetuses and infants (n = 92)
Median age (range)	27 years (stillborn–70 years)	3 days (1–60 days)	1 month (1 day – 2 years)	Fetuses:¶ 24 weeks gestation (10–35 weeks) Infants: 6 weeks (1 day – 20 months)
Sex (% male:female)	43:57	76:24	57:43	54:46*
VS thickness (mm)	25 ± 1	5 ± 0.3	6 ± 0.2	Fetuses:¶ 2 ± 0.1 Infants: 5 ± 0.1
VS/PW	1.7 ± 0.06	1.0 ± 0.04	1.1 ± 0.03	Fetuses:¶ 1.5 ± 0.05 Infants: 1.1 ± 0.03
VS/PW ≥ 1.3 (%)	90‡	9	25	Fetuses:¶ 69 Infants: 25
Patients with disorganization (%)	95	64	12	8†
Area of VS disorganized (%)	31 ± 3	2.8 ± 0.7	1.4 ± 0.3	0.3 ± 0.1

Values are mean ± SEM.

*Data included for only 44 live-born term infants.

†Of the seven patients in this subgroup with disorganization, four were fetuses and three were term infants.

‡In each of the 60 patients, the diagnosis of hypertrophic cardiomyopathy was based on the presence of a hypertrophied, nondilated left ventricle (in the absence of a cardiac or systemic disease that itself could produce left ventricular hypertrophy). In 54 (90%) of the 60 patients, asymmetric septal hypertrophy (defined as a septal-free wall thickness ratio of ≥ 1.3) was identified either at necropsy[14, 19] or by echocardiography.[15] In the remaining six patients with hypertrophic cardiomyopathy, concentric ventricular wall thickening (septal-free wall ratio < 1.3) was present at necropsy.

§Congenital heart malformations included the following: complete (−D) transposition of the great vessels (n = 14), coarctation of the aorta (n = 11), truncus arteriosus (n = 11), ventricular septal defect (n = 7), total anomalous pulmonary return (n = 7), valvular aortic stenosis (n = 6), Ebstein's malformation of the tricuspid valve (n = 6), double outlet right ventricle (n = 5), valvular pulmonic stenosis with intact ventricular septum (n = 5), tetralogy of Fallot (n = 5), tricuspid atresia (n = 5), ventricular septal defect and pulmonic stenosis (n = 4), cor triatriatum (n = 3), congenital mitral stenosis and ventricular septal defect (n = 1), and primary pulmonary hypertension (n = 1).

¶Includes 29 fetuses, 14 premature infants and five stillborn infants.

**Infants with aortic valve atresia did not differ significantly from those with pulmonic valve atresia with regard to each of the parameters in the table.

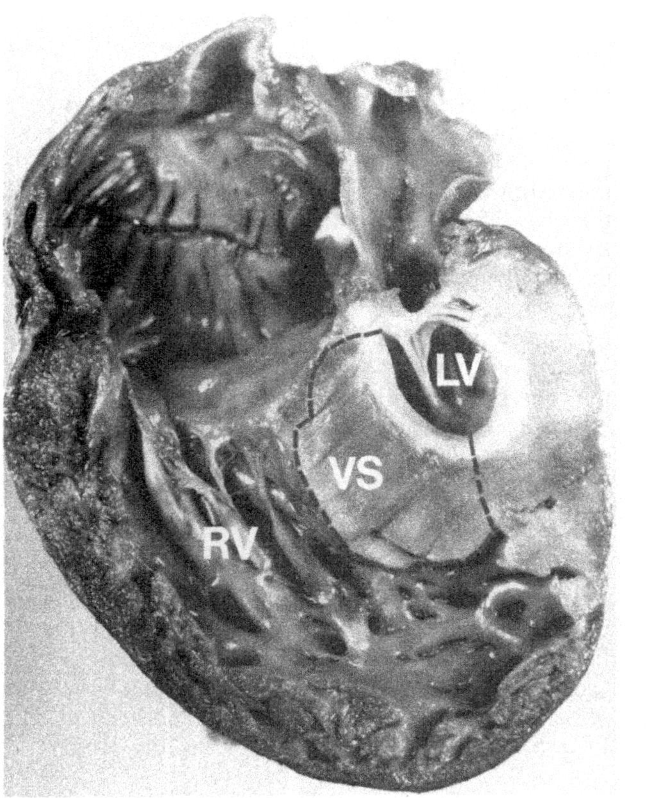

FIGURE 1. *Heart of an infant with aortic valve atresia (and hypoplastic mitral valve) cut in a plane parallel to the long axis of the left ventricle, with the anterior half removed. The left ventricular cavity (LV) is markedly hypoplastic and the right ventricular cavity (RV) is enlarged. The ventricular septum (VS) is small (and demarcated by broken lines). The left ventricular endocardium is markedly thickened.*

plane). In the anteroposterior axis, these sections extended to the point of junction of the ventricular septum with the left and right ventricular free walls. (We have previously shown that transverse plane tissue sections are the most appropriate for identifying cardiac muscle cell disorganization.[11]) In hearts with aortic or pulmonic valve atresia, we defined the ventricular septum as the segment of ventricular myocardium between the endocardium of the hypoplastic ventricular cavity and the endocardium of the dilated ventricular cavity (fig. 1). All tissue specimens were embedded in paraffin, sectioned at a thickness of 6 μ and stained with hematoxylin and eosin.

Definition and Classification of Cardiac Muscle Cell Disorganization

In contrast to normal cellular arrangement[11] (figs. 2 and 3), the cardiac muscle cell disorganization observed in the infants, children and adults in this study assumed five different forms, which have been described in detail previously[11] (fig. 4). Type I-A disorganization, the most common form encountered, consisted of areas of myocardium in which adjacent cardiac muscle cells were aligned perpendicularly or obliquely to each other, usually forming tangled masses or "pinwheel" configurations. Although most of these lesions were small, individual foci of type I-A disorganization varied greatly in size (particularly in patients with hypertrophic cardiomyopathy). In Type I-B disorganization, relatively broad bundles of muscle cells were oriented at oblique or perpendicular angles to each other; cells within these bundles were, however, normally arranged. Types I-A and I-B exclusively involved areas of ventricular septum where cardiac muscle cells were cut longitudinally, i.e., appeared to be rectangularly shaped.

Type II-A disorganization consisted of relatively narrow (usually one or two cells wide), longitudinally cut bundles of cells that were interlaced in various directions among larger groups of transversely cut cells (i.e., appeared circular). This type of disorganization gave the myocardium a swirled appearance. Type II-B was similar to type II-A disorganization, except that the narrow, longitudinally cut bundles of cells were more linear. Type II-C consisted of relatively small "islands" of disorganized, longitudinally cut cells within much larger areas of transversely cut cells. The three forms of type II disorganization involved both longitudinally and transversely cut cardiac muscle cells.

Nonparallel arrangements of cardiac muscle cells were not considered to represent disorganization if present in the following areas where cells normally converge at acute angles: 1) at or near the junction of ventricular septum with the left and right ventricular free walls; 2) in trabeculations; 3) in or at the edges of scarred areas; 4) at points of convergence of major muscle bundles; or 5) adjacent to interstitial spaces containing blood vessels.

Quantitation of Cardiac Muscle Cell Arrangement

We used a technique, previously described in detail,[11] to quantitatively assess the extent of cardiac muscle cell disorganization in tissue sections of ventricular septum from the 276 hearts studied. In brief, tissue sections (in which cardiac muscle cell disorganization was judged to be present qualitatively) were photographed and the images enlarged to occupy 30″ × 40″ positive prints, resulting in an average magnification of about 5000 times the original tissue section. A transparent cellulose overlay was then placed over the print, and the areas of myocardium occupied by disorganized cardiac muscle cells were outlined with a marking pen on the transparent overlay. Although we could often make this assessment exclusively from direct examination of the print, we frequently had to reexamine the original tissue section with a light microscope to localize the disorganized area. We also demarcated areas in which cardiac muscle cells were cut either longitudinally or transversely. Large areas of fibrosis (replacement or interstitial), artifacts of tissue preparation or large interstitial spaces with blood vessels also were outlined and excluded from the analysis. The transparent overlay was then removed from the print, photo-

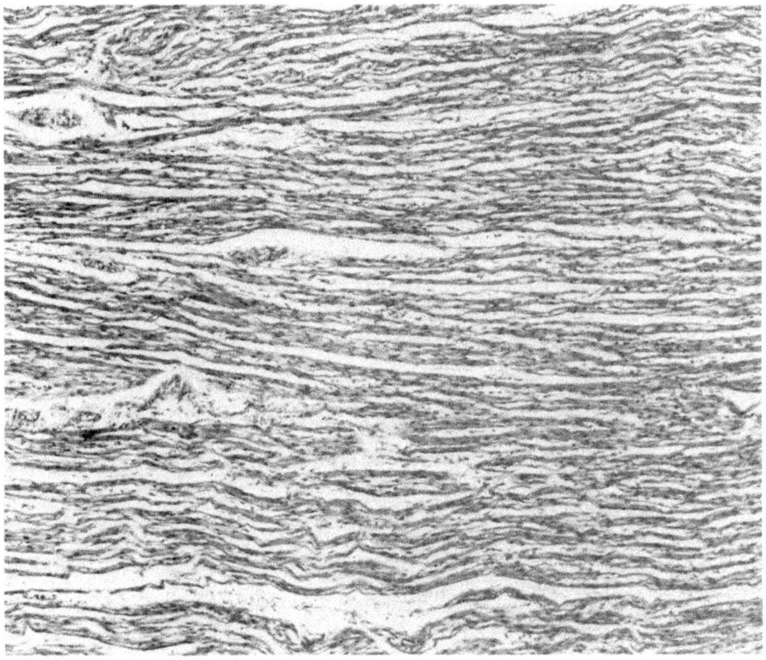

FIGURE 2. *Example of normal cellular arrangement in the ventricular septum of a 3-day-old infant with aortic valve atresia. Adjacent cardiac muscle cells are in a rigidly parallel relation to each other (magnification × 80; hematoxylin and eosin stain).*

graphed and the image reproduced (with substantial reduction) as a 5 × 7-inch positive print. Each area into which the tissue section had been divided was outlined separately with a fine-point marking pen on ordinary tablet paper, and quantitated using a video planimetry system. Two investigators independently analyzed the print enlargements, usually without knowledge of whether the tissue section was from a patient with hypertrophic cardiomyopathy. Often, however, recognition of the patient's disease was unavoidable because a particularly large tissue section strongly suggested hypertrophic cardiomyopathy.

Formulas Used in Quantitative Calculations of Cardiac Muscle Cell Arrangement

The formulas used to calculate the percent area of ventricular septum occupied by disorganized cardiac muscle cells are given below; the area of septum "at risk" for disorganization appears in the denominator of both equations:

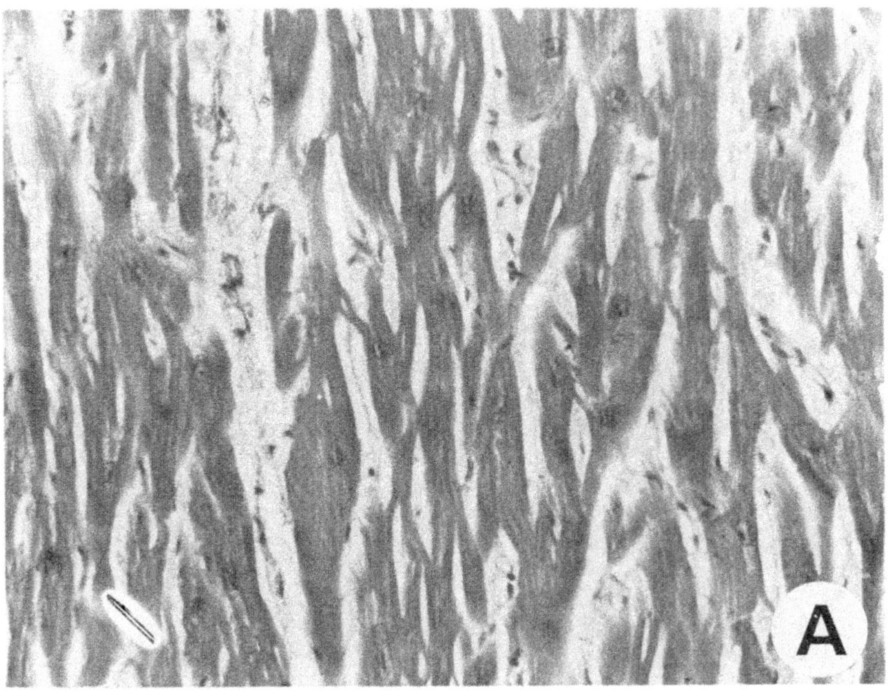

% area of type I (I-A + I-B) disorganization =

$$\frac{D_I}{L + D_I} \times 100;$$

% area of type II (II-A + II-B + II-C) disorganization =

$$\frac{D_{II}}{L + T + D_{II}} \times 100;$$

where L = area occupied by longitudinally cut but normally arranged cells, T = area occupied by transversely cut cells (excluding those incorporated into areas of type II disorganization), D_I = area occupied by type I disorganization, and D_{II} = area occupied by type II disorganization.

We could not combine values for types I and II disorganization in patients who had both types, because this calculation often resulted in a marked underestimation of the overall extent of disorganization in a tissue section. Hence, the percent septal disorganization plotted for each patient was the value for type I or type II disorganization, whichever value was greater. We did not attempt to assess the degree of cel-

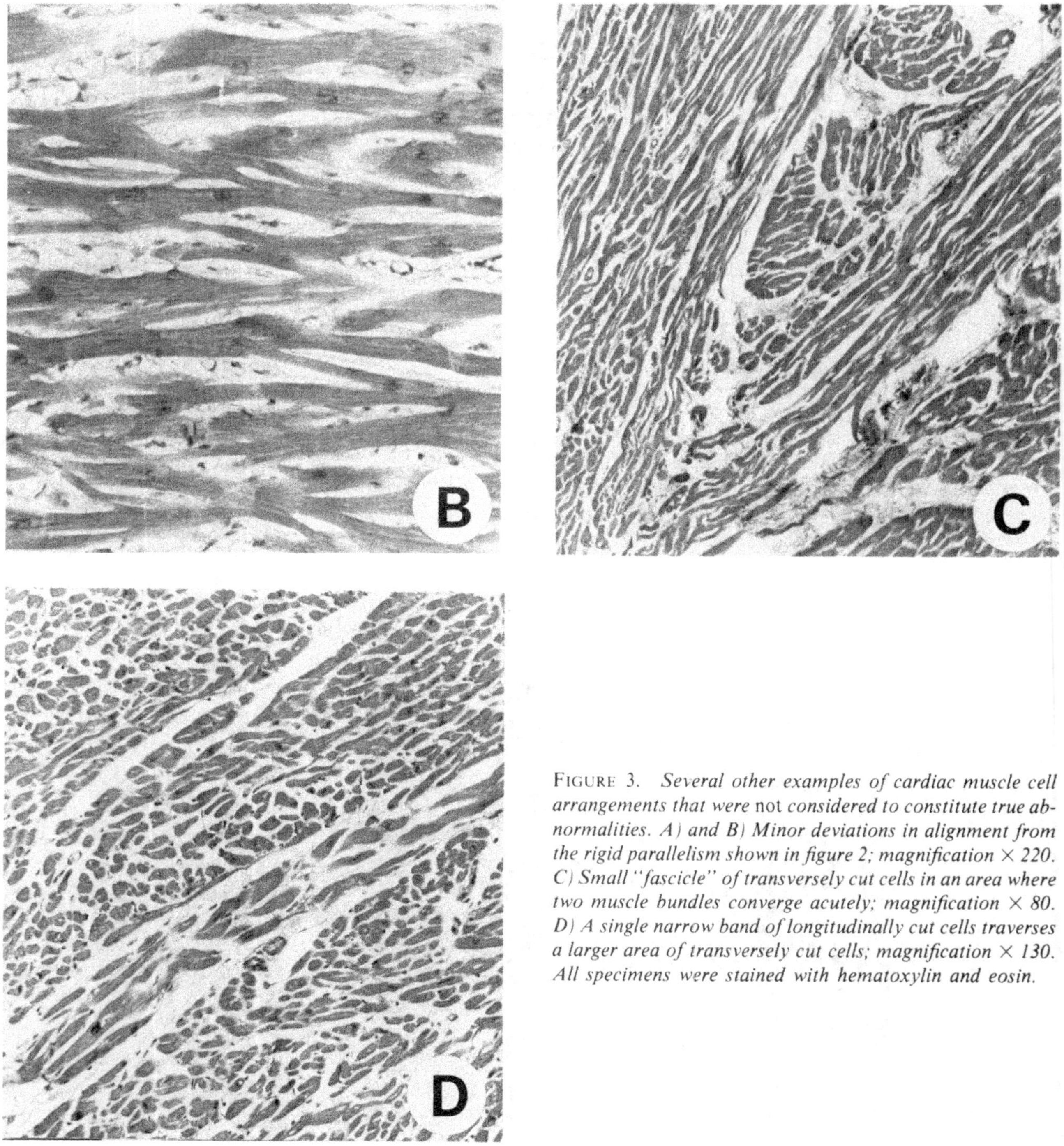

FIGURE 3. *Several other examples of cardiac muscle cell arrangements that were* not *considered to constitute true abnormalities. A) and B) Minor deviations in alignment from the rigid parallelism shown in figure 2; magnification × 220. C) Small "fascicle" of transversely cut cells in an area where two muscle bundles converge acutely; magnification × 80. D) A single narrow band of longitudinally cut cells traverses a larger area of transversely cut cells; magnification × 130. All specimens were stained with hematoxylin and eosin.*

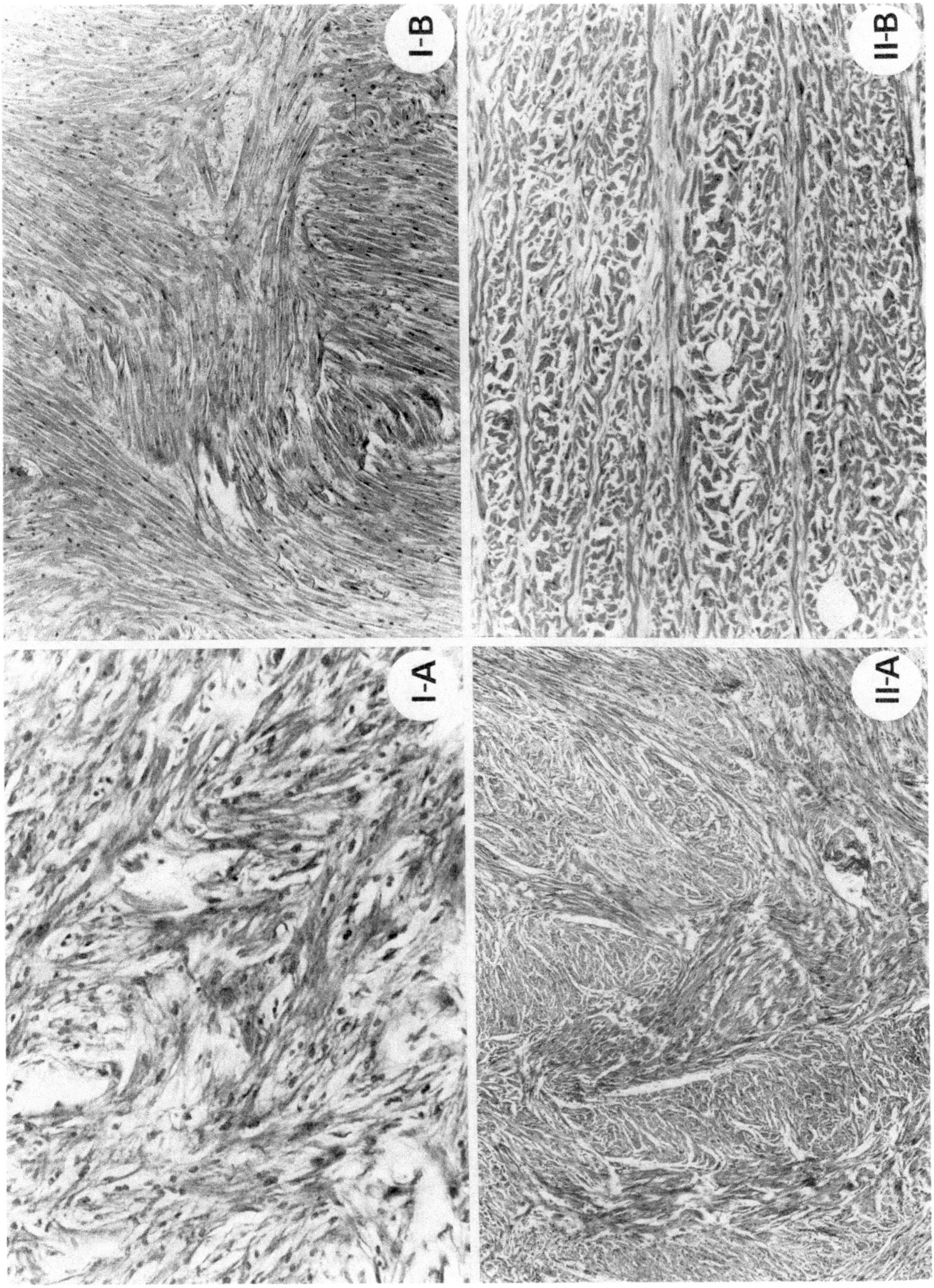
I-B
II-B
I-A
II-A

lular malalignment in a given area of tissue. Rather, septal disorganization was judged only to be present or absent, and its severity was expressed in terms of extent (as discussed above).

Results

Ventricular Wall Thicknesses

Ventricular septal thicknesses and septal-free wall ratios for each of the four subgroups of patients are summarized in table 1. Disproportionate septal thickening (septal-free wall ratio $\geq$ 1.3[14-17]) was significantly more prevalent in patients with hypertrophic cardiomyopathy (48 of 60 patients or 80%) than in any other patient group ($p < 0.001$), and was least common in the infants with aortic or pulmonic valve atresia (three of 33 patients or 9%; $p < 0.001$). The septal-free wall ratios in patients with aortic or pulmonic valve atresia (mean 1.0 $\pm$ 0.04 mm) ($\pm$ SEM) were also significantly less than in patients with other congenital heart diseases or in normal term infants ($p < 0.01$).

Morphologic Appearance of the Ventricular Septum

The architecture of large muscle bundles in the ventricular septum was relatively uniform in the vast majority of patients studied. A narrow bundle of longitudinally cut cardiac muscle cells was usually present in the center of the tissue section extending from the anterior to the posterior limits of the ventricular septum; this band usually comprised one-third (in adult patients) to one-half (in fetuses and infants) of the overall tissue section area (table 2). Transversely cut cells were present, for the most part, in the areas on either side of the central band (adjacent to the left and right ventricular cavities).

In infants with aortic or pulmonic valve atresia, the ventricular septum was particularly small because of the diminutive size of either the left or right ventricular cavity (fig. 1). In 19 of the 23 hearts with aortic valve atresia (none of the four with associated mitral valve atresia), the endocardium was diffusely thickened. In 16 of these 19 patients, the endocardial thickening was particularly marked, and the endocardium comprised at least 10% of the overall septal thickness, and more than 40% of septal thickness in three (fig. 5). In 15 of these 16 patients with aortic valve atresia and markedly thickened endocardium, one or more of the following structural alterations were present at the interface between endocardium and myocardium: cardiac muscle cells with evidence of degeneration (resembling myocytolysis[18]), calcific deposits, or foci of disorganized cardiac muscle cells.

A relatively small endocardial fibrous plaque[19] was

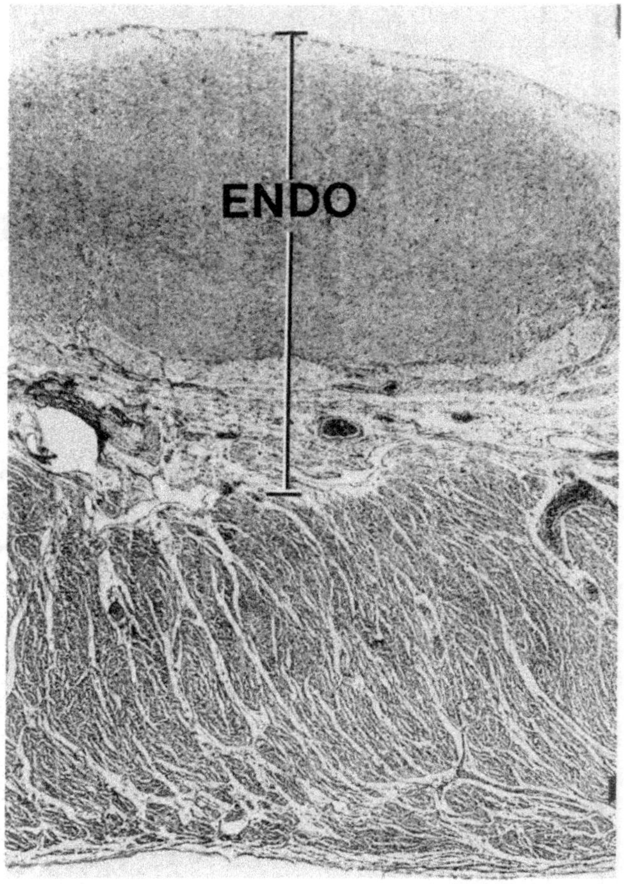

FIGURE 5. *Ventricular septum of a 2-day-old infant with aortic valve atresia. The marked thickening of the endocardium (ENDO) comprises more than one-half the overall septal thickness; magnification × 40 (hematoxylin and eosin stain).*

present on the left ventricular septal surface in sections from 10 patients with hypertrophic cardiomyopathy. These plaques were quite localized in extent compared with those seen in aortic valve atresia.

Quantitative Histologic Findings

Patients with hypertrophic cardiomyopathy and fetuses or infants in the other three subgroups differed markedly with respect to both the occurrence and extent of ventricular septal disorganization (tables 1 and 2). Disorganization was significantly more common in patients with hypertrophic cardiomyopathy (57 of 60, or 95%; $p < 0.001$) than in any of the other three subgroups of fetuses and/or infants studied. Of the three subgroups, the prevalence of septal disorganization was highest in infants with aortic or pulmonic valve

FIGURE 4. *Classification of the four major types of cardiac muscle cell disorganization in ventricular septal myocardium, shown in patients with hypertrophic cardiomyopathy. Types I-A and I-B exclusively involve cardiac muscle cells cut longitudinally. Types II-A and II-B involve cardiac muscle cells cut either longitudinally or transversely. I-A) From a stillborn infant (magnification × 220); I-B) from a 33-year-old woman (magnification × 40); II-A) from a 5-month-old infant (magnification × 55); II-B) from a 33-year-old man (magnification × 80). All specimens were stained with hematoxylin and eosin.*

atresia (21 of 33, or 64%); overall, only 39 (18%) of the 216 infants with congenital heart disease or normals showed disorganization.

Most importantly, patients with hypertrophic cardiomyopathy and the three subgroups of fetuses and/or infants differed markedly with respect to the extent of ventricular septal disorganization (figs. 6–8). The mean percent area of septum disorganized in patients with hypertrophic cardiomyopathy was 31 ± 3% (range 0–94%); the extent of disorganization in infants with hypertrophic cardiomyopathy did not differ significantly from that in children or adults with this disease. Furthermore, 90% of the patients with hypertrophic cardiomyopathy had disorganization occupying 5% or more of the relevant areas of the tissue section, 56% of the patients had ≥ 25% of the section involved and 25% of the patients had more than 50% involved. In contrast, only 16 (7%) of the 216 infants with congenital heart disease or normals had disorganization involving more than 5% of the relevant areas of the septal tissue section; in nine other fetuses or infants, the area of septum disorganized was < 1% of the tissue section. Only one infant with congenital heart disease (tricuspid atresia) had > 25% of the section involved by disorganization.

The cut point that appeared to best distinguish patients with hypertrophic cardiomyopathy from infants with other diseases, histologically, was septal disorganization involving 5% or more of the relevant parts of the tissue section. Therefore, septal disorganization of ≥ 5% is consistent with the histologic diagnosis of hypertrophic cardiomyopathy, while sep-

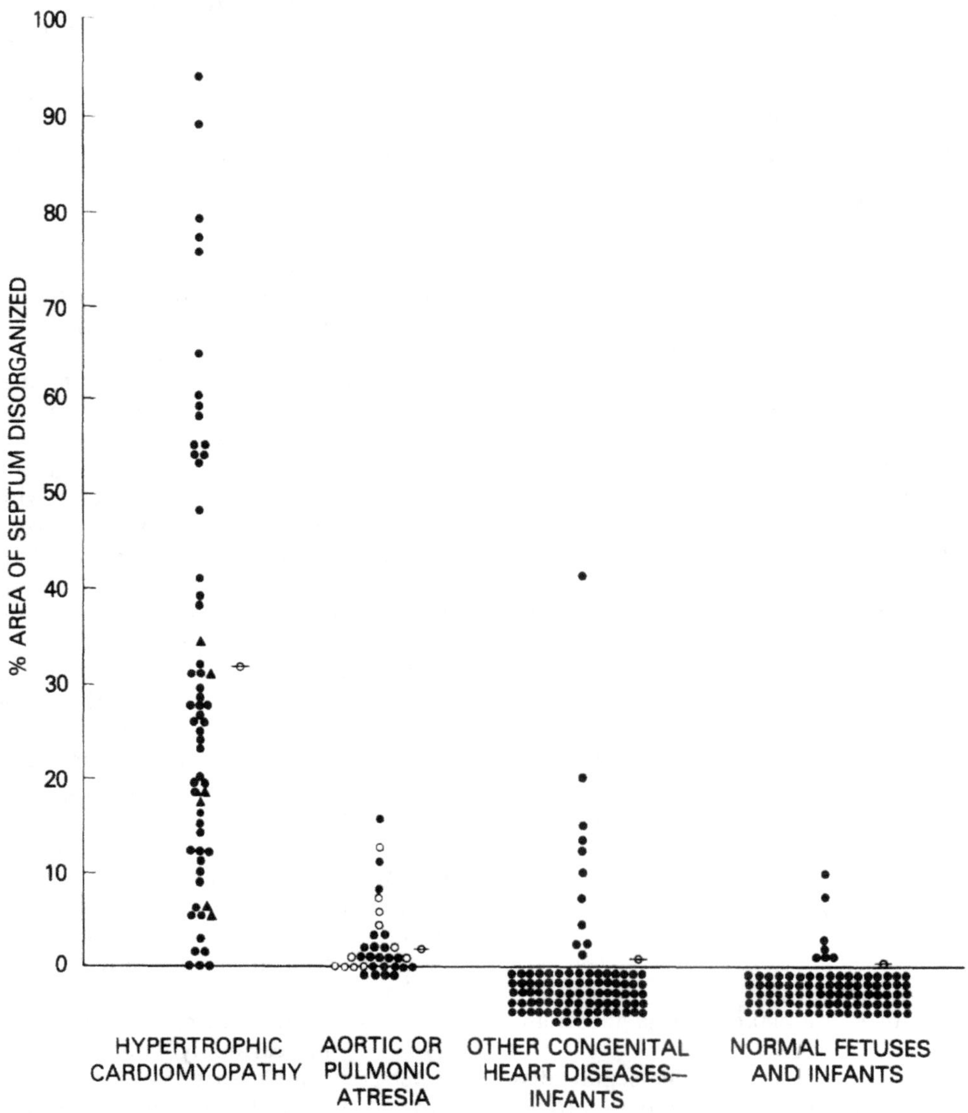

FIGURE 6. *Percent area of ventricular septum occupied by disorganized cardiac muscle cells in 60 patients with hypertrophic cardiomyopathy (six infants are designated by triangles), 33 infants with aortic or pulmonic valve atresia (patients with pulmonic atresia are designated by open circles), 91 infants with other congenital heart diseases associated with normal-sized or dilated ventricular cavities, and 92 normal fetuses or infants. θ = mean value.*

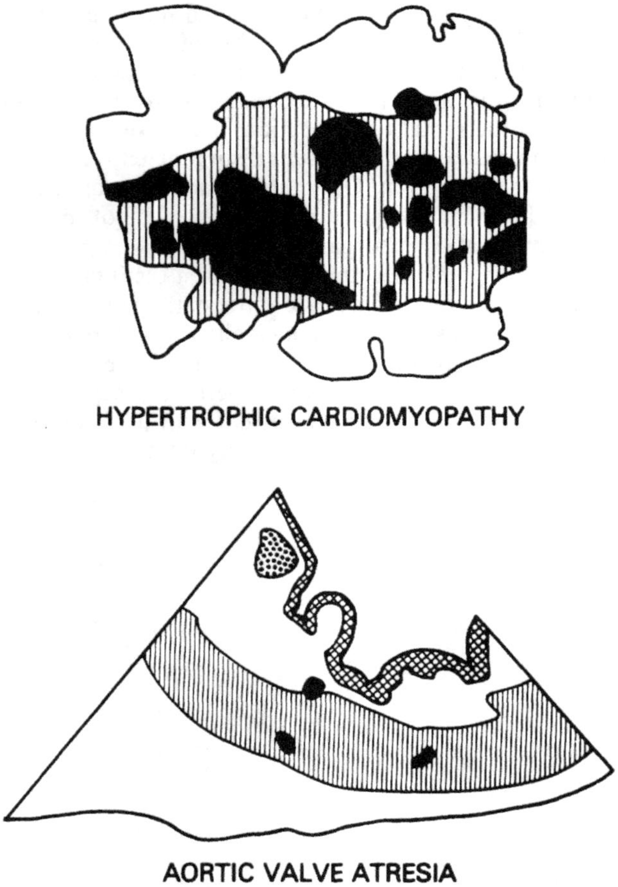

FIGURE 7. *Representative "maps" of ventricular septum from two infants with type I-A disorganization. Both sections were obtained in a plane perpendicular to the long axis of the left ventricle. The septum of a 5-month-old infant with hypertrophic cardiomyopathy is shown above. The septum of a 4-day-old infant with aortic valve atresia and concentric ventricular hypertrophy is shown below (see figure 2 for photomicrograph from the same patient). The striped areas represent normally arranged cardiac muscle cells cut longitudinally; the clear areas adjacent to the left (LV) and right ventricular (RV) cavities contain cells cut transversely. The solid areas represent foci of type I disorganization; the stippled area represents a focus of type II disorganization. In the patient with hypertrophic cardiomyopathy, disorganized cardiac muscle cells occupy about 33% of the relatively small striped area; in contrast, the disorganized areas are very small (both individually and in summation) in the patient with aortic valve atresia, and together represent only 2% of the relevant parts of the tissue section.*

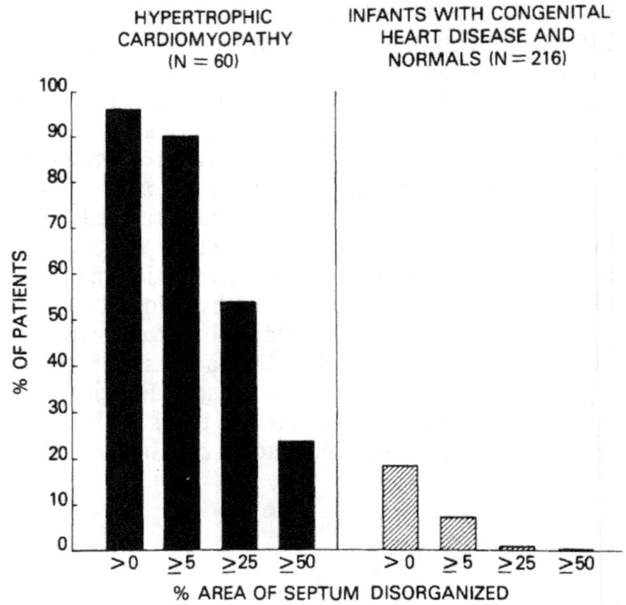

FIGURE 8. *Extent of septal disorganization in 60 patients with hypertrophic cardiomyopathy and 216 control fetuses and infants. Each of the comparisons achieved high statistical significance* ($p < 0.001$).

tal disorganization of < 5% makes this diagnosis unlikely.

Some overlap in terms of percent septal disorganization was present between the four subgroups of patients studied; however, the mean area of septum disorganized in each of the three groups of fetuses and/or infants was quite small (< 3%), and when the three groups were combined, the mean value was only 1.2 ± 0.3%. In each subgroup of fetuses and/or infants, the extent of disorganization was significantly less than that found in patients with hypertrophic cardiomyopathy ($p < 0.001$; fig. 6).

At relatively high magnification, the small areas of disorganization present in some infants with aortic or pulmonic valve atresia, as well as in those with other congenital heart malformations or normal hearts (fig. 9A), appeared qualitatively identical to the widespread lesions present in patients with hypertrophic cardiomyopathy. However, at lower magnification such areas of disorganization were barely discernible and obviously constituted only a small part of the tissue section (fig. 9B).

Abnormally arranged cardiac muscle cells were most common in the middle one-third of the ventricular septum (in hearts with and without hypertrophic cardiomyopathy). However, it is in the middle one-third of the septum that longitudinally cut cells are usually present in tissue sections taken perpendicular to the long axis of the left ventricle.[11] Hence, it would be expected that the common type I disorganization, which can only be identified in areas of longitudinally cut cells, would be observed most frequently in the middle one-third of the transverse plane sections obtained in this study.

Type I disorganization (in particular type I-A) was the most common form encountered in patients with hypertrophic cardiomyopathy and in infants with other congenital heart diseases (table 2). In contrast, type II disorganization predominated in the normal fetuses and infants.

In 15 of the infants with congenital heart diseases other than hypertrophic cardiomyopathy, alterations in cardiac muscle cell arrangement were present in the area of ventricular septum adjacent to a markedly

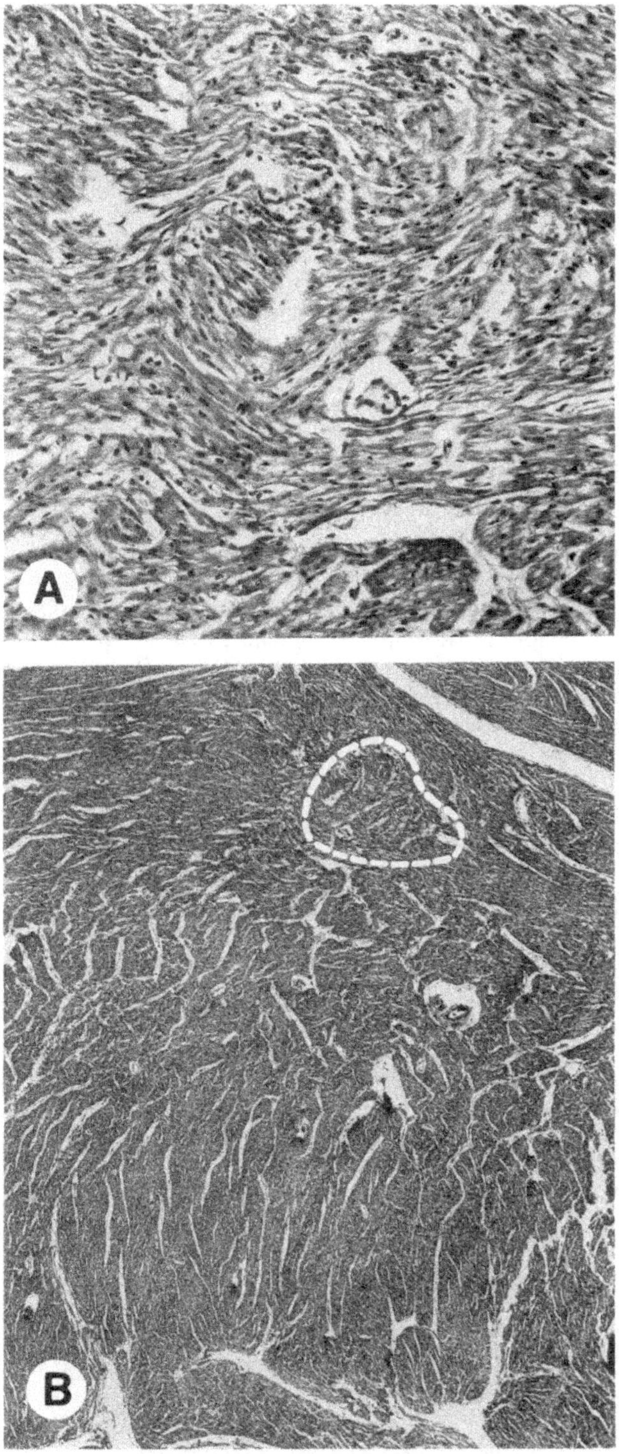

FIGURE 9. *Two photomicrographs of the same area of ventricular septal myocardium from a 3-day-old infant with a normal heart. A) An area of type I-B disorganization is shown at relatively high magnification (× 350); B) same area of myocardium shown at a much lower magnification (× 55). The area of disorganization (outlined by broken line), so impressive at higher magnification, is barely discernible here and obviously constitutes an extremely small part of the overall tissue section. Each specimen was stained with hematoxylin and eosin.*

thickened endocardium (≥ 10% of the total septal thickness) (fig. 10). This phenomenon was most common in infants with aortic valve atresia (10 patients), but it also occurred in three patients with normal-sized left ventricular cavities and either aortic valve stenosis or coarctation of the aorta, in one patient with pulmonic valve atresia and small right ventricular cavity, and in one patient with Ebstein's anomaly of the tricuspid valve. The areas of subendocardial disorganization in these patients were relatively small (mean 5 ± 1%) and did not differ significantly in size from areas of disorganization present in other regions of the septum in eight of the patients (mean 3 ± 1%). Alterations in cellular arrangement in the subendocardial region of the septum were of the type II variety in 14 patients and type I in the other patient.

Discussion

The findings of this quantitative morphologic study indicate that while small areas of cardiac muscle cell disorganization may occasionally occur in the ventricular septum of normal fetuses or infants or of infants with a variety of congenital heart diseases, extensive septal disorganization is exceedingly uncommon. For example, while 18% of the 216 patients with normal hearts or with diseases other than hypertrophic cardiomyopathy had some disorganization in the ventricular septum, only 7% of the 216 patients had disorganization occupying more than 5% of the relevant areas of the septal tissue section (our criterion for extensive disorganization).[11] Furthermore, the mean area of septum disorganized in these 216 patients was minimal (1.2 ± 0.3%). Indeed, the specificity of extensive septal disorganization in our necropsy population of 216 patients without hypertrophic cardiomyopathy was high (93%). These findings were similar to those of a previous quantitative histologic analysis of ventricular septum in 144 older children and adults with normal hearts or hearts with a variety of congenital or acquired heart defects, in which only 7% of the patients had extensive septal disorganization and the mean area of septum disorganized was 1.5 ± 0.6%.[11]

In contrast, 90% of the 60 patients with hypertrophic cardiomyopathy (including infants, children and adults) had disorganization occupying 5% or more of the tissue section, over 50% of the patients had ≥ 25% of the section involved, and about 25% of the patients had more than 50% involved. Of the 60 patients with hypertrophic cardiomyopathy, the mean area of septum disorganized was substantial (31 ± 3%). Indeed, the sensitivity of extensive septal disorganization in our necropsy population of 60 patients with hypertrophic cardiomyopathy was also high (90%).

The quantitative histologic findings in infants with aortic or pulmonic valve atresia showed that cellular disorganization in the ventricular septum of these hearts was relatively common; however, the disorganization generally involved extremely small areas of myocardium, in contrast to the widespread septal

TABLE 2. *Quantitative Histologic Findings*

Parameter	Hypertrophic cardiomyopathy n	Mean ± SEM	Aortic or pulmonic valve atresia n	Mean ± SEM	Other congenital heart diseases n	Mean ± SEM	Normal fetuses and infants n	Mean ± SEM
Size of septal tissue section (cm^2)	60	4.4 ± 0.4	33	0.4 ± 0.04	91	0.5 ± 0.04	92	0.7 ± 0.1
Area of longitudinally cut cells in septum (%)	60	34 ± 2	15*	50 ± 4	10*	50 ± 6	7*	44 ± 7
Area of septum disorganized (%) Type I (I-A + I-B)	57	31 ± 3	15	3 ± 1	10	9 ± 4	1	1
Type II (II-A + II-B + II-C)	12	8 ± 2	17	2 ± 1	9	7 ± 2	6	4 ± 1
Type I or II†	60	31 ± 3	33	2.8 ± 0.7	91	1.4 ± 0.6	92	0.3 ± 0.1

*Determined only in patients with cardiac muscle cell disorganization.

†Value for percent area of septum disorganized used for each patient was that of either type I or type II disorganization, whichever was greater.

disorganization usually present in patients with hypertrophic cardiomyopathy. For example, disorganization was trivial (≤ 1% of the tissue section) in one-third of the hearts with aortic or pulmonic valve atresia that had disorganization. Most importantly, the extent of septal disorganization in infants with aortic or pulmonic valve atresia did not differ significantly from that in infants with a variety of other congenital cardiac malformations associated with nonatretic ventricles. Hence, histologically, aortic or pulmonic atresia are no more similar to hypertrophic cardiomyopathy than are other congenital heart malformations.

The ventricular septum of hearts with aortic valve

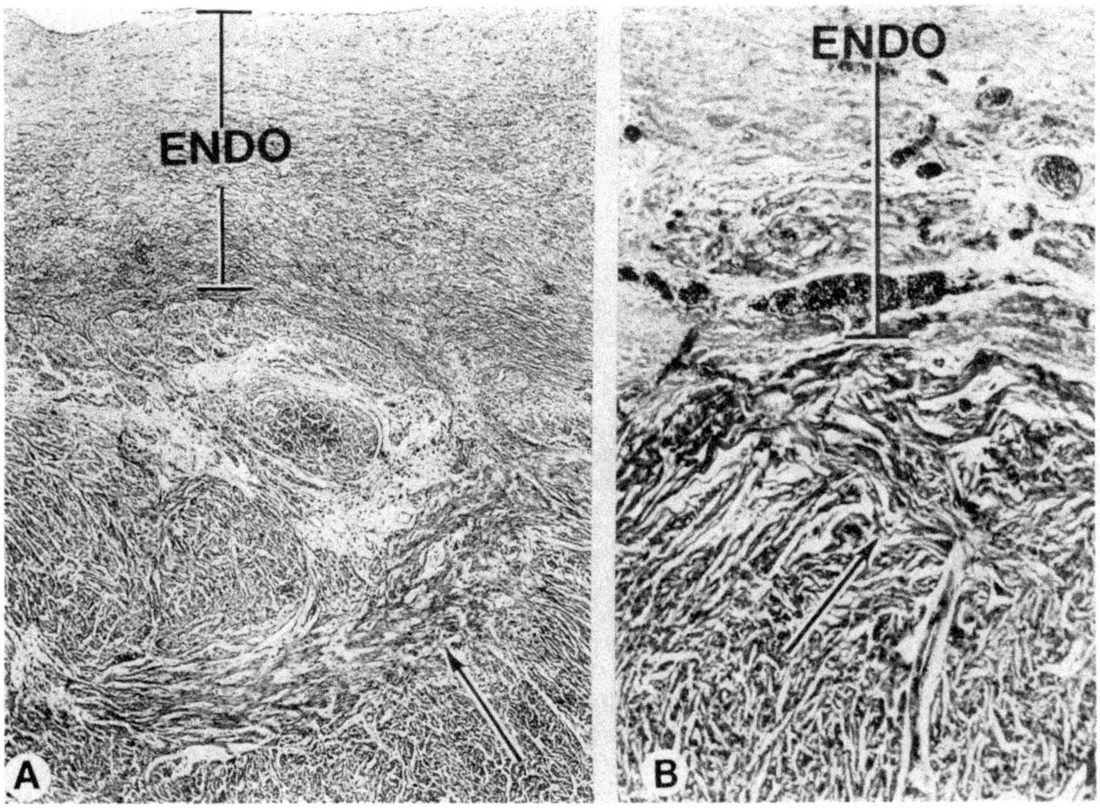

FIGURE 10. *Areas of ventricular septum directly adjacent to a markedly thickened endocardium (ENDO) in two infants with aortic valve atresia. A) Alteration in cellular arrangement of the Type II-A variety; magnification × 55. B) Small area of type I-A disorganization; magnification × 80. Both were stained with hematoxylin and eosin. Arrows denote disorganized cardiac muscle cells.*

atresia commonly showed alterations in cellular arrangement directly beneath a markedly thickened endocardium (overlying the left septal surface). Nonparallel cellular arrangement at this interface between endocardium and myocardium is probably created by the severely malformed anatomy apparent in this area of the heart and probably should not be considered to be true disorganization. However, even with such alterations in cellular arrangement in the subendocardial region included in our data analysis as true abnormalities of septal architecture, disorganization was still much more extensive in patients with hypertrophic cardiomyopathy than in infants with aortic valve atresia or other congenital heart diseases. If subendocardial cellular alterations were excluded from the analysis, the mean area of septum disorganized in patients with aortic or pulmonic valve atresia would be reduced from 2.8 ± 0.7% to 1.3 ± 0.5%.

Therefore, we found no consistent morphologic similarities in the extent of septal disorganization or the prevalence of disproportionate septal thickening between hearts with aortic or pulmonic valve atresia and hearts with hypertrophic cardiomyopathy. These findings differ appreciably from those recently reported in a similar group of infants[10] (in which quantitative analysis of septal disorganization was not undertaken) and do not support the contention that hypertrophic cardiomyopathy and aortic or pulmonic valve atresia have similar morphologic characteristics because of the theoretical possibility that hearts with these diseases each undergo a prolonged period of isometric contraction during ventricular systole.[10] Hence, the findings presented in this report further support our previous hypothesis,[7, 11] based on both qualitative[7, 16, 17] and quantitative[11] histologic analysis, that extensive cardiac muscle cell disorganization in ventricular septal myocardium is a highly sensitive and specific marker for hypertrophic cardiomyopathy, even though the presence per se of septal disorganization is not pathognomonic of hypertrophic cardiomyopathy.

Acknowledgments

We gratefully acknowledge the valuable assistance provided by Willard C. Whitehouse of the Laboratory of Applied Studies, Division of Computer Research, as well as that provided by James Wolfson.

References

1. Teare D: Asymmetrical hypertrophy of the heart in young patients. Br Heart J **20:** 1, 1958
2. Ferrans VJ, Morrow AG, Roberts WC: Myocardial ultrastructure in idiopathic hypertrophic subaortic stenosis: a study of operatively excised left ventricular outflow tract muscle in 14 patients. Circulation **45:** 769, 1972
3. Pomerance A, Davies MJ: Pathological features of hypertrophic obstructive cardiomyopathy (HOCM) in the elderly. Br Heart J **37:** 305, 1975
4. Pare JA, Fraser RG, Pirozynski WJ, Shanks JA, Stubington D: Hereditary cardiovascular dysplasia: a form of familial cardiomyopathy. Am J Med **31:** 37, 1961
5. Van Noorden S, Olsen EG, Pearse AG: Hypertrophic obstructive cardiomyopathy. A histological, histochemical and ultrastructural study of biopsy material. Cardiovasc Res **5:** 118, 1971
6. Maron BJ, Edwards JE, Henry WL, Clark CE, Bingle GJ, Epstein SE; Asymmetric septal hypertrophy (ASH) in infancy. Circulation **50:** 809, 1974
7. Maron BJ, Ferrans VJ, Henry WL, Clark CE, Redwood DR, Roberts WC, Morrow AG, Epstein SE: Differences in distribution of myocardial abnormalities in patients with obstructive and nonobstructive asymmetric septal hypertrophy (ASH): light and electron microscopic findings. Circulation **50:** 436, 1974
8. Maron BJ, Henry WL, Clark CE, Redwood DR, Roberts WC, Epstein SE: Asymmetric septal hypertrophy in childhood. Circulation **53:** 9, 1976
9. Wigle ED, Adelman AG, Silver MD: Pathophysiological considerations in muscular subaortic stenosis. *In* Hypertrophic Obstructive Cardiomyopathy, edited by Wolstenholme GE, O'Connor M. London, J and A Churchill, 1971, p 63
10. Bulkley BH, Weisfeldt ML, Hutchins GM: Isometric cardiac contraction. A possible cause of the disorganized myocardial pattern of idiopathic hypertrophic subaortic stenosis. N Engl J Med **296:** 135, 1977
11. Maron BJ, Roberts WC: Quantitative analysis of cardiac muscle cell disorganization in the ventricular septum in patients with hypertrophic cardiomyopathy. Circulation **59:** 689, 1979
12. Roberts WC, Perry LW, Chandra RS, Myers GE, Shapiro SR, Scott LP: Aortic valve atresia: a new classification based on necropsy study of 73 cases. Am J Cardiol **37:** 753, 1976
13. Maron BJ, Verter J, Kapur S: Disproportionate ventricular septal thickening in the developing normal human heart. Circulation **57:** 520, 1978
14. Menges H, Brandenburg RO, Brown AL: The clinical, hemodynamic and pathologic diagnosis of muscular subvalvular aortic stenosis. Circulation **24:** 1126, 1961
15. Epstein SE, Henry WL, Clark CE, Roberts WC, Maron BJ, Ferrans VJ, Redwood DR, Morrow AG: Asymmetric septal hypertrophy. Ann Intern Med **81:** 650, 1974
16. Maron BJ, Edwards JE, Ferrans VJ, Clark CE, Lebowitz EA, Henry WL, Epstein SE: Congenital heart malformations associated with disproportionate ventricular septal thickening. Circulation **52:** 926, 1975
17. Maron BJ, Clark CE, Henry WL, Fukuda T, Edwards JE, Mathews EC, Redwood DR, Epstein SE: Prevalence and characteristics of disproportionate ventricular septal thickening in patients with acquired or congenital heart disease: echocardiographic and morphologic findings. Circulation **55:** 489, 1977
18. Schlesinger MJ, Reiner L: Focal myocytolysis of the heart. Am J Pathol **31:** 443, 1955
19. Roberts WC: Valvular, subvalvular and supravalvular aortic stenosis: morphologic features. Cardiovasc Clin **5:** 104, 1973

Comparison of Amount of Myocardial Cell Disorganization in Operatively Excised Septectomy Specimens With Amount Observed at Necropsy in 18 Patients With Hypertrophic Cardiomyopathy

JEFFREY M. ISNER, MD, FACC
BARRY J. MARON, MD, FACC
WILLIAM C. ROBERTS, MD, FACC

Bethesda, Maryland

The extent of cardiac muscle cell disorganization in excised septectomy specimens in 18 patients was compared morphometrically with that observed at necropsy when these patients died after operation. Disorganization was present in all 18 patients at necropsy and was extensive (5 percent or greater) in 16 of the 18. In contrast, there was no disorganization in the operative specimens of three patients and only a trivial amount (less than 1 percent) in five others. Disorganization extensive enough (5 percent or greater) to suggest hypertrophic cardiomyopathy was present in the operative specimens of only 6 of the 18 patients. The mean (± standard error of the mean) area of disorganization at necropsy was 20 ± 3 percent compared with 7 ± 2 percent in the operative specimens (p <0.001). Thus, histologic examination of operatively excised septectomy specimens is of limited value in confirming the diagnosis of hypertrophic cardiomyopathy.

Widespread cardiac muscle cell disorganization in the ventricular septum has been demonstrated on quantitative necropsy examination to be a sensitive and specific histologic marker of hypertrophic cardiomyopathy.[1,2] In patients with typical features of hypertrophic cardiomyopathy[3–5] undergoing partial septotomy or septectomy, the absence of cardiac muscle cell disorganization in the excised myocardium has been interpreted as evidence that the patient may not, in fact, have had hypertrophic cardiomyopathy. This study of 18 patients who died after partial septotomy-septectomy sought to establish whether such an interpretation is valid.

Methods

Study patients: From 1960 until April 1978 at the National Heart, Lung, and Blood Institute, partial septotomy-septectomy was performed in 210 patients with hypertrophic cardiomyopathy. Of these, 41 (20 percent) died intra- or postoperatively (17, early of consequences of the operation; 24, late from consequences of hypertrophic cardiomyopathy (13) or from noncardiac causes (11). This study concerns 18 of these 41 patients—all of those in whom both operatively obtained and necropsy-obtained septectomy specimens were available for both gross and histologic examination.

Pertinent clinical and necropsy findings in the 18 patients are summarized in Table I. Each patient was severely symptomatic at the time of cardiac operation. Each had both clinical and necropsy evidence of hypertrophic cardiomyopathy.[3,4,6] In 11 patients, asymmetric septal hypertrophy (ventricular septal to left ventricular free wall thickness ratio 1.3 or greater) was present at necropsy; of the other 7 patients, 4 (22 percent) had echocardiographic evidence of asymmetric septal hypertrophy during life. Eleven patients died within 1 month of septotomy-septectomy and seven at later periods, up to 156 months (average 46) postoperatively.

From the Pathology and Cardiology Branches, National Heart, Lung, and Blood Institute, National Institutes of Health, Bethesda, Maryland. Manuscript received December 5, 1979; revised manuscript received January 29, 1980, accepted January 30, 1980.

Address for reprints: William C Roberts, MD, Building 10A, Room 3E-30, National Heart, Lung, and Blood Institute, the National Institutes of Health, Bethesda, Maryland 21205.

Pathologic examination: At necropsy, in each patient, tissue blocks were taken from the full thickness of the ventricular septum, at the point of maximal thickness, usually at a site one third to one half the distance from the base to apex, in a plane perpendicular to the long axis of the left ventricle. Operatively obtained septectomy specimens from each patient were fixed in either 10 percent buffered formalin or 3 percent buffered glutaraldehyde solution after removal at operation. Tissue blocks were taken from each septectomy specimen either perpendicular to its cephalad-caudad orientation or parallel to this orientation. Each tissue block was embedded in paraffin, sectioned at 6 μ and stained with hematoxylin-eosin.

Four types of myocardial cell disorganization were observed in the necropsy and septectomy specimens and were classified according to criteria outlined previously[1] *(Fig. 1).* Abnormally arranged cardiac muscle cells were not considered to represent true disorganization if they were present in the following areas where cells normally converge at acute angles: (1) at or near the junction of ventricular septum with left and right ventricular free walls; (2) in trabeculae; (3) in or at the edge of areas of scars; (4) at points of convergence of major muscle bundles; or (5) adjacent to interstitial spaces containing blood vessels. The extent of myocardial cell disorganization in both operatively obtained and necropsy-obtained specimens of ventricular septum was quantified using a method described elsewhere.[1] Briefly, hematoxylin-eosin-stained tissue sections were photographed and the images enlarged to occupy positive prints measuring 30 by 40 inches (76 by 102 cm). This enlargement resulted in an average magnification of about 1,200 times the original tissue section. A transparent cellulose overlay was then placed over the print. With use of a marking pen, areas of myocardium occupied by disorganized cardiac muscle cells were outlined on the transparent overlay (Fig. 2). A light microscope was used to localize the disorganized area. Those areas in which cardiac muscle cells were oriented longitudinally and those areas in which these cells were oriented in cross section also were demarcated. The transparent overlay was then removed from the print, photographed, and the image reproduced as a 5 by 7 inch (13 by 18 cm) positive print. Each area into which the tissue section had been divided was outlined separately with a fine-point marking pen on ordinary tablet paper. The area of each outlined silhouette was then quantified using a video planimetry system.[7,8]

The percent area of myocardium occupied by disorganized muscle cells was calculated in the following manner: Because type IA and IB disorganization can only be recognized among

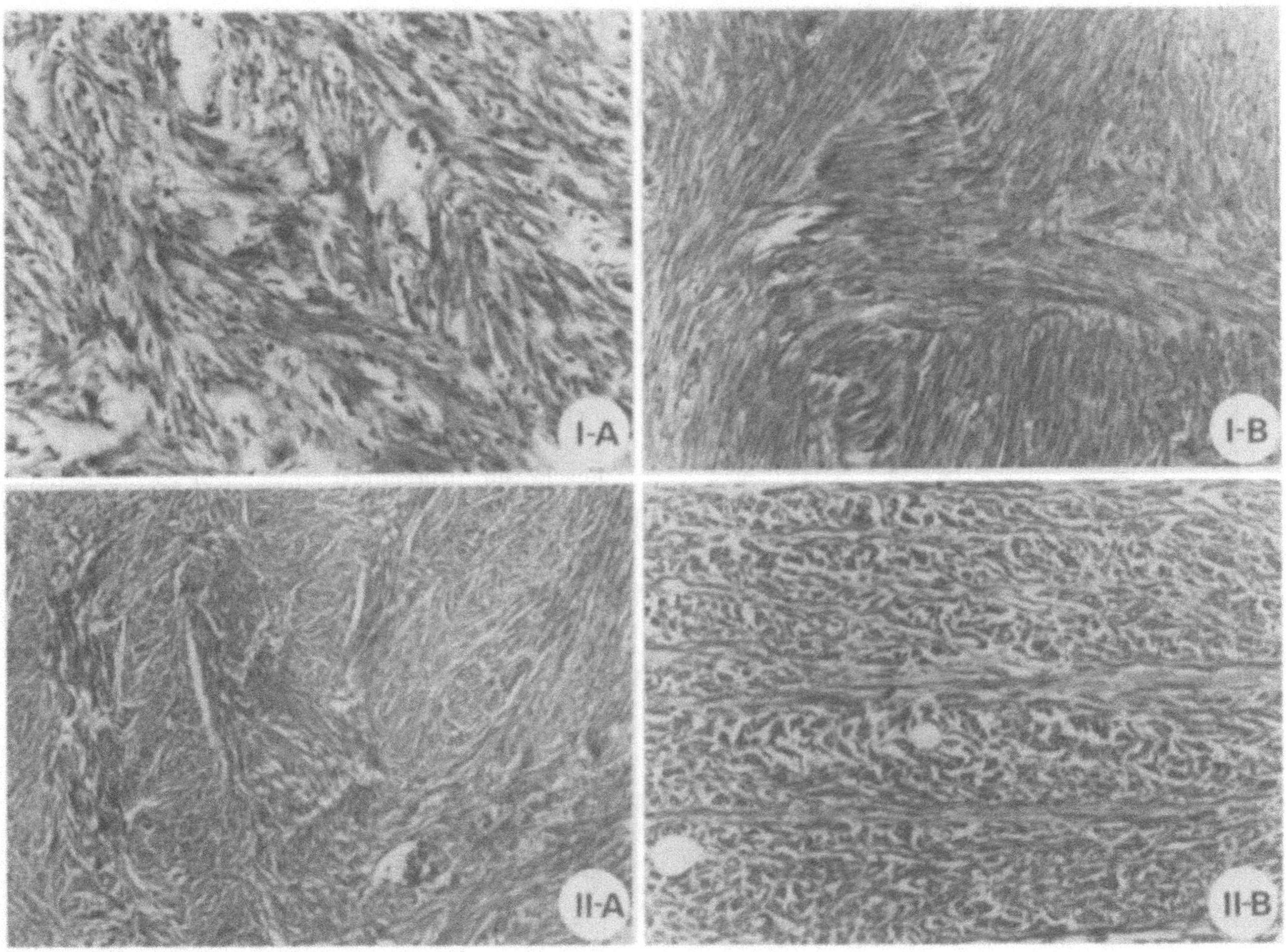

FIGURE 1. Classification of four major types of cardiac muscle cell disorganization present in ventricular septal myocardium. Types 1-A and 1-B exclusively involve cardiac muscle cells cut longitudinally. Types II-A and II-B involve cardiac muscle cells cut either longitudinally or transversely. Magnifications: I-A, ×130; I-B and II-A, ×40; II-B, ×80, all reduced by 23 percent. These and all tissue sections shown subsequently were stained with hematoxylin-eosin.

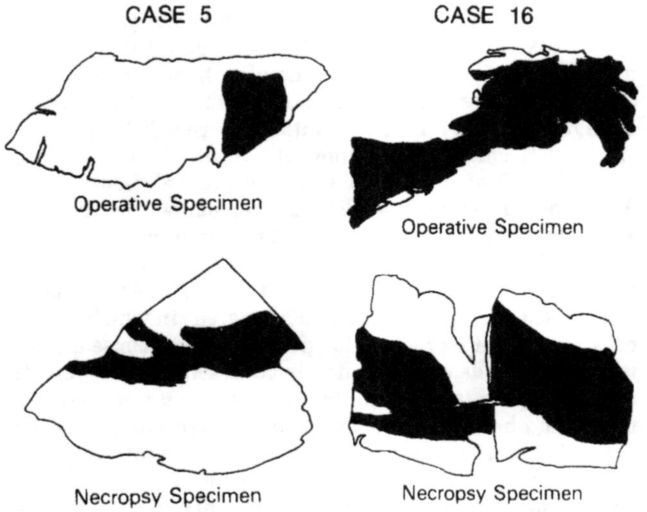

FIGURE 2. Examples of maps of disorganized muscle cells from operative and necropsy specimens of Patients 5 and 16 (Table I). The **black area** represents that portion of the histologic section in which the myocardial cells are oriented longitudinally. The **stippled areas** within the black areas indicate foci of disorganized cardiac muscle cells. In Case 5 the operative specimen contained no foci of disorganization, despite extensive disorganization in the necropsy specimen. In Case 16, two small foci of disorganized cells are present in the operative specimen, multiple larger foci in the necropsy specimen. (Although the histologic sections of the operative specimen are smaller than the histologic sections of the necropsy specimens, the positive prints from which the maps are made are in each case 30 by 40 inch [76 by 102 cm] enlargements).

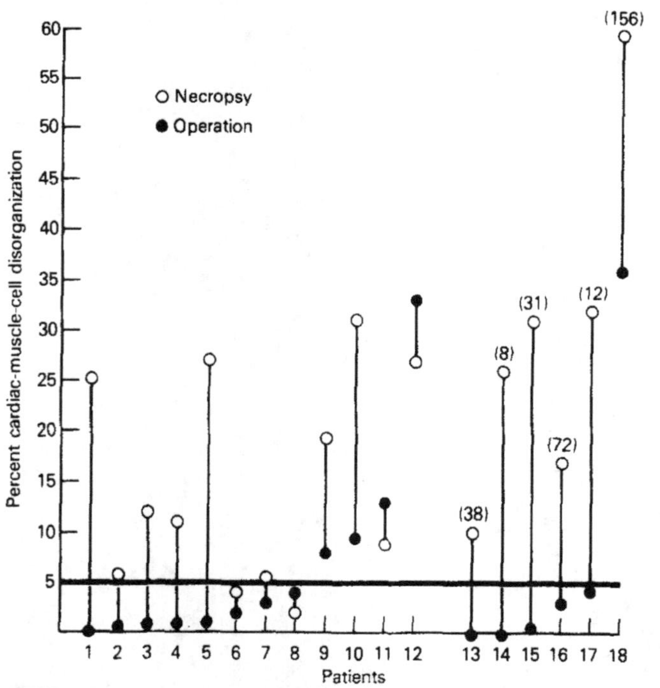

FIGURE 3. Comparison of the extent of cardiac muscle cell disorganization in histologic sections from the necropsy and operative septectomy specimens in each of the 18 patients with hypertrophic cardiomyopathy. The **horizontal line** at 5 percent indicates the minimal extent of disorganized cardiac muscle cells generally present at necropsy in patients with hypertrophic cardiomyopathy. Patients 13 through 18 died late postoperatively; the **numbers in parentheses** indicate the survival time (in months) after operation.

longitudinally oriented cells, type I disorganization was calculated as a percent of the total area of longitudinally oriented cells:

$$\% \text{ area of type I (A + B) disorganization} = \frac{D_I}{L + D_I} \times 100,$$

where D_I = area occupied by type I disorganized cells, and L = area occupied by longitudinally cut but normally arranged cells. Identification of types IIA and IIB disorganization involves examination of muscle fibers oriented in cross section as well. Therefore, type II disorganization is calculated as a percent of cells oriented both longitudinally and in cross-section:

$$\% \text{ area of type II (A + B)} = \frac{D_{II}}{L + T + D_{II}} \times 100,$$

where D_{II} = area occupied by type II disorganization and T = area occupied by transversely (cross section) oriented but normally arranged cells. The percent septal disorganization listed in Table I for each patient was the value for type I or type II disorganization, whichever figure was greater. In addition, each operatively obtained and necropsy-obtained specimen was examined qualitatively for the presence of foci of fibrosis, cell hypertrophy, thickened intramural coronary arteries and adipose tissue cells.

Results

Quantitative Assessment of Myocardial Cell Disorganization

Necropsy specimens: Muscle cell disorganization in the ventricular septum was present at necropsy in all 18 patients (Table I): In 18 patients the pattern of disorganization was type I (IA in 13, IA + IB in 5) and in 5 patients type II disorganization also was present (IIA in 3, IIB in 2). The area of muscle cell disorganization at necropsy ranged from 1 to 59 percent (mean ± standard error of the mean = 20 ± 3 percent) of the relevant area of tissue section examined. In 16 patients (89 percent) the area of disorganization was equal to or in excess of 5 percent.

Operative specimens: Examination of the operatively obtained septectomy specimens disclosed foci of muscle cell disorganization in 15 of the 18 patients (Table I). The area of disorganization in the operative specimens ranged from 0 to 36 percent (mean 7 ± 2 percent); this value was significantly less than the extent of disorganization observed in the ventricular septum of these patients at necropsy ($p < 0.001$). In addition to the three patients whose operative septectomy specimen manifested no foci of cardiac muscle disorganization, there were five other patients whose operative specimens manifested only a trivial (1 percent or less) amount of disorganization. In only six patients was the extent of disorganization present in the operative specimens 5 percent or greater. Comparisons of the extent of disorganization in the necropsy specimen versus that in the operative specimen in the 18 patients (Fig. 3) showed that in 15 (83 percent) the extent of disorganization in the necropsy specimens exceeded that observed in the operative specimens. The type I pattern of disorganization was observed in all 15 operative specimens with disorganization (type IA in 11,

TABLE I

Clinical and Morphologic Features in the 18 Patients Who Died After Septotomy-Septectomy for Hypertrophic Cardiomyopathy

Case	Age (yr) & Sex	SH	LV-SA psg (mm Hg)	Survival Postop	Specimen Wt (g)	Heart Weight (g)	Ventricular Wall Thickness VS (mm)	FW (mm)	VS/FW	% D (S)	% D (N)
1	19F	0	160	9 days	5.0	730	28	25	1.1	3	5
2	19M	0	118*	72 mo	5.0	660	32	15	2.1	3	17
3	23M	0	175	156 mo	—	840	39	20	1.9	36	59
4	25F	0	0	0	—	400	25	15	1.7	8	19
5	27M	0	70	3 days	—	950	34	27	1.2‡	0	25
6	28F	0	82	21 days	2.0	580	28	17	1.6	1	11
7	41M	0	100†	0	1.7	700	27	17	1.6	4	2
8	42M	+	120†	38 mo	—	580	20	15	1.3	0	10
9	42M	0	55	0	8.5	650	30	15	2.0	1	27
10	46F	0	70	12 mo	—	475	19	19	1.0‡	5	32
11	49F	0	80	50 days	0.5	545	25	12	2.1	10	31
12	50F	0	128	31 mo	—	450	20	19	1.1	0.5	31
13	52F	0	90†	3 days	1.4	470	25	21	1.2‡	13	9
14	56F	+	40	1 days	1.7	310	15	15	1.0	33	27
15	58F	+	100	7 days	1.0	490	30	22	1.4	2	4
16	61F	0	70	0	1.4	500	20	15	1.3	1	12
17	61F	0	100†	8 mo	1.3	500	22	14	1.6	0	26
18	65F	0	100	2 days	1.0	410	27	25	1.1‡	0.1	5

* RVOT peak systolic gradient = 118 mm Hg at rest; no LV-SA peak systolic gradient.
† Provokable (no resting gradient).
‡ VS/FW 1.3 or greater on echocardiography.
d = days; D = cardiac muscle cell disorganization; FW = left ventricular free wall; LV = left ventricle; mo = months; N = necropsy; psg = peak systolic gradient; RVOT = right ventricular outflow tract; S = septectomy specimen; SA = systemic artery; SH = systemic hypertension; VS = ventricular septum. 0 = absent; + = present.

type IA + IB in 4); type II disorganization also was present in the operative specimens of 2 patients (type IIA in 1, type IIB in the other). The type of disorganization observed in the operative specimen was always present in the necropsy specimen as well; however, in three of the five patients with type II disorganization in the necropsy specimen, this type was not observed in the respective operative specimen.

Qualitative Assessment of Necropsy and Operative Specimens

The operative and necropsy specimens also were evaluated qualitatively for histologic features other than cardiac muscle cell disorganization (Table II). Marked *endocardial fibrosis* (involving the septum in the left ventricular outflow tract in apposition to the anterior mitral leaflet) and myocardial cell hypertrophy were observed in both the operative and necropsy specimens of all 18 patients. Foci of *interstitial fibrosis* occurred in 14 operative (78 percent) and in all 18 necropsy specimens. *Adipose tissue cells,* located immediately below the site of endocardial thickening, were present in 10 operative (55 percent) and in 13 necropsy (72 percent) specimens. *Thickened intramural coronary arteries* were found in 12 necropsy specimens (67 percent) ($p < 0.007$) and in three operative specimens (17 percent).

Discussion

Diagnostic sensitivity of operative septectomy specimen examination: Previous studies have demonstrated that the finding of extensive muscle cell disorganization in the ventricular septum at necropsy is a highly sensitive marker for hypertrophic cardiomyopathy.[1,2] In nearly 90 percent of patients with hypertrophic cardiomyopathy there was disorganization of 5 percent or greater (mean 33 ± 3 percent) of the relevant areas of muscle cells in the ventricular septum. Indeed, among our 18 patients, disorganization was present in the ventricular septum at necropsy of all 18, and in 16 (89 percent) it was 5 percent or greater (mean 20 percent). In contrast, disorganization involving 5 percent or more of the relevant areas of cardiac muscle cells was present in the operative septectomy specimen of only 6 of the 18 patients; in the remaining 12, disorganization was either absent or insufficient to suggest hypertrophic cardiomyopathy. Therefore, examination of septectomy

TABLE II

Comparison of Certain Morphologic Features of Operative and Necropsy Septectomy Specimens in 18 Patients

	Operative Specimens (n)	Necropsy Specimens (n)
Muscle cell disorganization		
Present	15	18
≥5%	3	16
Hypertrophied cells	18	18
Thickened intramural coronary arteries	3	12
Interstitial fibrosis	14	18
Discrete endocardial fibrosis	18	18
Adipose cells	10	13

specimens from patients undergoing septotomy-septectomy is not a sensitive means of confirming the diagnosis of hypertrophic cardiomyopathy.

Causes of discrepancy in operative versus autopsy septal specimens: There are several possible explanations for the discrepancy between the generally widespread disorganization observed in the septum at necropsy and the trivial amount observed in portions of the same septum excised at operation. First, one might expect that those patients with the most widespread disorganization at necropsy would be more likely to have disorganization present in that portion of the septum from which the septectomy specimen was excised and, conversely, that patients with less extensive disorganization at necropsy might be less likely to have disorganization present at the septectomy site, purely on the basis of statistical sampling. The five patients whose operative specimens had the most extensive disorganization also had extensive disorganization at necropsy (greater than 15 percent in four of the five). There were four patients in whom no or trivial disorganization was present in the septectomy specimens, although at necropsy the extent of disorganization ranged from 25 to 35 percent. Extensive disorganization in the septum at necropsy, then, appeared to improve, though not guarantee, the finding of disorganization in the operative specimen.

An alternative explanation is that the amount of disorganization observed at necropsy was simply a function of the amount of operatively excised tissue available for examination. Two indexes used to assess the amount of tissue available for examination were the weight of the septectomy specimen and the absolute area of the histologic section taken from the operative specimen. The weight of the specimen is an index of the *total* amount of operatively excised tissue available for

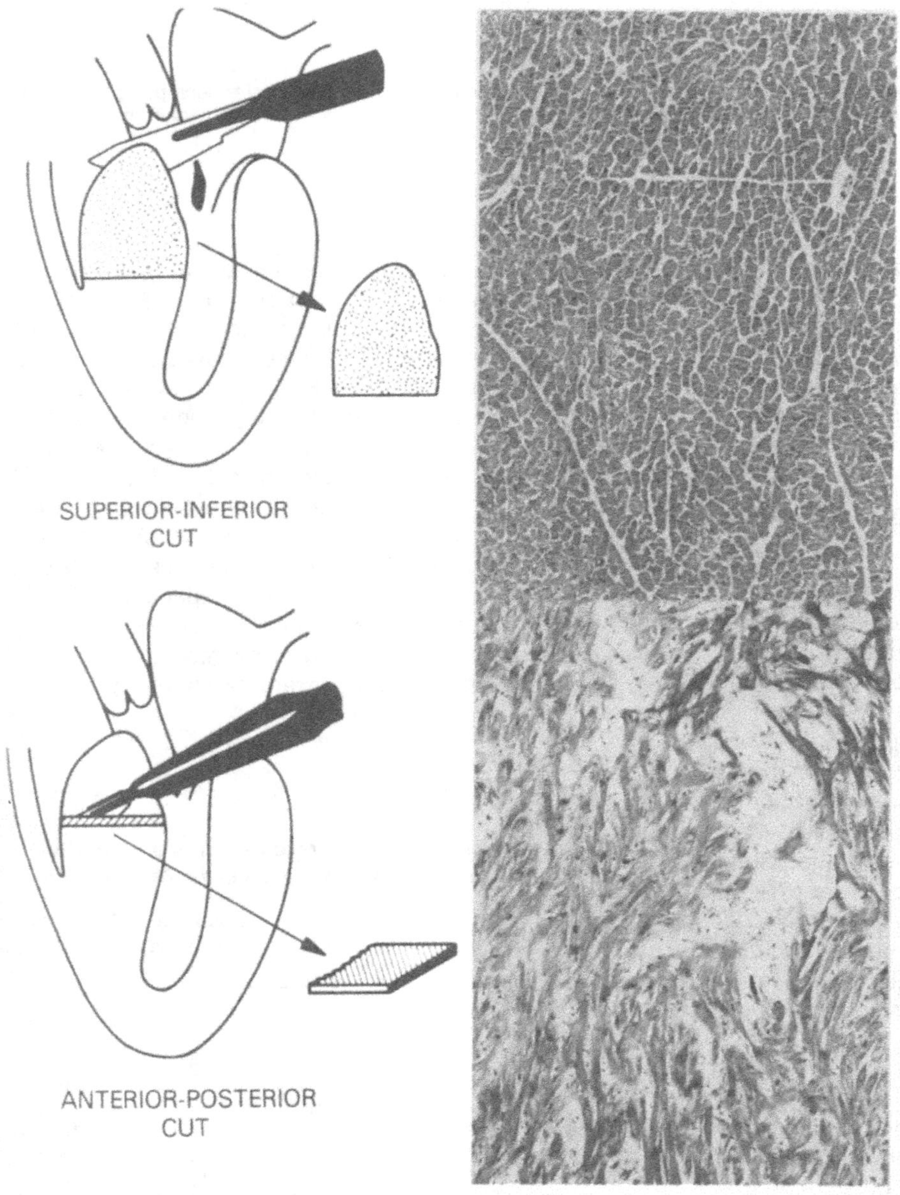

FIGURE 4. Schematic drawings and photomicrographs showing that the orientation of cells in histologic sections of myocardium is a function of the manner in which the section is cut. An anterior-posterior (cephalad-caudad) cut yields longitudinally oriented cells; type I disorganization (**lower right**) can only be recognized when the cells are oriented in this way. The result of a superior-inferior (cephalad-caudad) cut is that the cells are seen in cross section (**top right**). (Hematoxylin-eosin ×130, reduced by 23 percent.)

examination, regardless of how the histologic section was cut from the operative specimen; the absolute area of the histologic section could (and did) vary, depending on how the histologic section was cut (parallel, perpendicular or oblique to the long axis of the operative specimen). Neither the weight of the operative specimen nor the absolute area of the histologic section correlated with the extent of disorganization observed in the operatively excised septectomy specimens. Finally, because the most common type of disorganization (type I) can be identified only by inspection of areas of longitudinally oriented cells, the histologic section taken from each septectomy specimen was evaluated to determine if those sections with the most extensive disorganization had the largest areas of longitudinally oriented cells. Such was not the case.

Although none of these three variables—the weight of the operative specimen, the area of the histologic section taken from the operative specimen or the area of longitudinally oriented cells in the operative specimen—distinguished the 5 operative specimens with extensive disorganization from the group of 18 as a whole, the magnitude of each variable was significantly less for each of the operative specimens than for the respective necropsy specimens. This finding is not unexpected in view of the consistent discrepancy in absolute size between the operative specimen and the respective portion of septum excised at necropsy. The operative specimen constitutes what is, in effect, a relatively large myocardial biopsy sample. Although it provides more tissue than is obtained by closed chest biopsy, the limitations inherent in the morphometric analysis of closed chest biopsy specimens also apply to the evaluation of septectomy specimens.[9] The sampling problem is further complicated by the fact that the most common type of disorganization (type I) can be identified only in those sections of tissue in which cardiac muscle cells are oriented in a longitudinal fashion. The fiber orientation of the ventricular myocardium is such that a greater proportion of longitudinally oriented fibers is obtained on tissue sections taken perpendicular to the long axis of the heart (Fig. 4). The operatively excised specimen unfortunately represents the result of a cephalad-caudad cut; that is, the septectomy specimen is removed by incisions made in the ventricular septum parallel to the long axis of the heart.[10] A histologic section of the septectomy specimen taken parallel to its long axis thus results in relatively few longitudinally oriented cells. Although the yield of longitudinally oriented cells theoretically may be increased by sectioning the operative specimen perpendicular to its own long axis, this potential gain is offset by the considerable reduction in the resultant tissue area available for morphometric examination.

Associated pathologic findings: The operative specimens from the 18 patients also were evaluated qualitatively for other morphologic features that might be helpful in establishing the diagnosis of hypertrophic cardiomyopathy. All 18 specimens contained a white plaque of fibrous tissue on their endocardial surfaces. This endocardial plaque, also present in the septum of all 18 patients at necropsy, was in direct apposition to a thickened anterior mitral leaflet. This plaque represents the site of contact of the anterior mitral leaflet and the ventricular septum.[6] The endocardial plaque is a sensitive marker for hypertrophic cardiomyopathy. Thickened intramural coronary arteries located in the ventricular septum are characteristic, when present, of hypertrophic cardiomyopathy.[11] However, this finding was observed in only 3 (17 percent) of the 18 operative specimens (and in 12 of the necropsy specimens). In the operative specimens of 10 patients there was a shallow layer, usually 2 to 3 cell layers thick, of subendocardial adipose cells. This finding also was present in a similar number (13) of necropsy specimens. The significance and etiology of these subendocardial adipose cells is unclear. Although all 18 operative specimens contained hypertrophied cardiac muscle cells and 14 of 18 contained foci of interstitial fibrosis, the nonspecificity of these two histologic findings limits their utility in confirming the diagnosis of hypertrophic cardiomyopathy.

References

1. **Maron BJ, Roberts WC.** Quantitative analysis of cardiac muscle cell disorganization in the ventricular septum of patients with hypertrophic cardiomyopathy. Circulation 1979;59:689–706.
2. **Maron BJ, Sato N, Roberts WC, Edwards JE, Chandra RS.** Quantiative analysis of cardiac muscle cell disorganization in the ventricular septum. Comparison of fetuses and infants with and without congenital heart disease and patients with hypertrophic cardiomyopathy. Circulation 1979;60:685–96.
3. **Braunwald E, Lambrew CT, Rockoff SD, Ross J, Morrow AG.** Idiopathic hypertrophic subaortic stenosis. I. A description of the disease based upon an analysis of 64 patients. Circulation 1964;29:Suppl IV:IV-1–64.
4. **Epstein SE, Henry WL, Clark, CE, et al.** Asymmetric septal hypertrophy. Ann Intern Med 1974;81:650–80.
5. **Maron BJ, Epstein SE.** Hypertrophic cardiomyopathy: a discussion of nomenclature. Am J Cardiol 1979;43:1242–4.
6. **Roberts WC.** Valvular, subvalvular, and supravalvular aortic stenosis: morphologic features. Cardiovasc Clin 1973;5:97–126.
7. **Marcus ML, Schuette WH, Whitehouse WC, Bailey JJ, Douglas MA, Glancy DL.** Use of a video system in the study of ventricular function in man. Am J Cardiol 1973;32:175–9.
8. **Dvorak JA, Schuette WH, Whitehouse WC.** A simple video method for the quantification of microscopic objects. J Microscopy 1974;102:71–8.
9. **Ferrans VJ, Roberts WC.** Myocardial biopsy: a useful diagnostic procedure or only a research tool? Am J Cardiol 1978;41:965–7.
10. **Morrow AG.** Hypertrophic subaortic stenosis. Operative methods utilized to relieve left ventricular outflow obstruction. J Thorac Cardiovasc Surg 1978;76:423–30.
11. **McReynolds RA, Roberts WC.** The intramural coronary arteries in hypertrophic cardiomyopathy (abstr). Am J Cardiol 1975;35: 154.

Quantitative Analysis of the Distribution of Cardiac Muscle Cell Disorganization in the Left Ventricular Wall of Patients with Hypertrophic Cardiomyopathy

BARRY J. MARON, M.D., THOMAS J. ANAN, B.A., AND WILLIAM C. ROBERTS, M.D.

SUMMARY The distribution of cardiac muscle cell disorganization in different regions of the left ventricular wall was studied quantitatively in 52 patients with hypertrophic cardiomyopathy. Cellular disorganization in the ventricular septum was both common and extensive (mean area of septal tissue section disorganized, 35 ± 4%). Disorganization was also substantial (24 ± 3%) in the left ventricular free wall of these patients, although less marked than in the ventricular septum ($p < 0.05$). Anterior left ventricular free wall disorganization was particularly extensive (32 ± 4%) and did not differ significantly from that present in the ventricular septum. Marked cardiac muscle cell disorganization (≥ 5% of the tissue section) was diffusely distributed in the ventricular septum and left ventricular free wall in 33 of the 52 patients (63%).

Particularly marked left ventricular free wall and combined free wall and septal disorganization was present in 14 patients without functional limitation in whom sudden death occurred early in life (≤ 25 years of age) and was the initial manifestation of cardiac disease. In contrast, although abnormally arranged cardiac muscle cells were identified in the left ventricular free wall in 47% of patients with other congenital or acquired heart diseases or normal hearts, this disorganization was usually limited in extent (mean area of section disorganized, 2 ± 0.5%).

Hence, in a large population of patients with hypertrophic cardiomyopathy, cellular disorganization was widely distributed throughout both the ventricular septum and left ventricular free wall. No definitive conclusions can be made regarding the significance of this distribution of cellular disorganization; however, our data suggest that this pattern may represent a diffuse cardiomyopathic process and be a determinant of clinical outcome in certain patients with hypertrophic cardiomyopathy.

HYPERTROPHIC CARDIOMYOPATHY is a disease of cardiac muscle that is characterized by a hypertrophied, nondilated left ventricle[1] and, in most patients, asymmetric septal hypertrophy.[2-6] Marked disorganization of cardiac muscle cells in the ventricular septum[7-10] has also been shown by quantitative histologic analysis to be a highly specific and sensitive anatomic hallmark of hypertrophic cardiomyopathy.[11-13] Qualitative histologic studies have shown that cellular disorganization may also be present in the left ventricular free wall of patients with hypertrophic cardiomyopathy.[14-19] In this study, we quantitated, for the first time, the extent of cellular disorganization in both the ventricular septum and left ventricular free wall of patients with hypertrophic cardiomyopathy compared with patients with other forms of cardiac hypertrophy; we also determined whether the distribution and extent of the cellular disorganization in patients with hypertrophic cardiomyopathy has significance with regard to clinical course or hemodynamic state.

Selection of Case Material

Patients with Hypertrophic Cardiomyopathy

The cardiovascular registry of the Pathology Branch of the National Heart, Lung, and Blood Institute was reviewed and 52 hearts with hypertrophic cardiomyopathy were considered to be in suitable condition for inclusion in the study.

In each, the diagnosis of hypertrophic cardiomyopathy was based on the presence of a hypertrophied, nondilated left ventricle.[1] In 41 of the 52 patients (79%), asymmetric septal hypertrophy (septal–free wall thickness ratio ≥ 1.3) was present at necropsy. In 40 of the 52 patients, the typical clinical, hemodynamic, angiocardiographic or operative findings of hypertrophic cardiomyopathy were also present; the 12 other patients had no cardiac evaluation during life and sudden death was the initial manifestation of cardiac disease.[20]

Associated coronary heart disease (> 75% cross-sectional area narrowing by atherosclerotic plaque of at least one of the four major extramural coronary arteries) was present in eight of the 52 patients with hypertrophic cardiomyopathy; one of these patients also had a secundum atrial septal defect and one had systemic hypertension; three other patients also had systemic hypertension. The 11 patients with associated cardiac lesions were included because the degree of left ventricular hypertrophy present was greater than would be expected in patients having these abnormalities alone. Clinical and hemodynamic data in the 52 patients with hypertrophic cardiomyopathy are summarized in table 1.

Patients with Normal Hearts or with Cardiac Diseases other than Hypertrophic Cardiomyopathy

The hearts of 83 patients were selected for study as controls. This group included 72 patients with a variety of congenital or acquired heart diseases other

From the Cardiology and Pathology Branches, National Heart, Lung, and Blood Institute, National Institutes of Health, Bethesda, Maryland.

Address for correspondence: Barry J. Maron, M.D., National Heart, Lung, and Blood Institute, National Institutes of Health, Building 10, Room 7B-15, Bethesda, Maryland 20205.

Received March 11, 1980; revision accepted August 5, 1980.

Circulation 63, No. 4, 1981.

TABLE 1. *Clinical and Hemodynamic Findings in 52 Patients with Hypertrophic Cardiomyopathy*

	No. of pts	%
Functional limitation		
Present	36§	56
Absent	16	44
LVOT-PSG (mm Hg)		
≥ 30 at rest	24	63‡
< 30 at rest		
≥ 30 with provocation*	5	13‡
< 30 with provocation†	5	13‡
Provocation not done	4	11‡
LVEDP (mm Hg)		
< 12	10	26‡
13–20	16	42‡
> 20	12	32‡
Mode of death		
Sudden¶	27	52
Congestive heart failure	9**	17
CVA	1	2
Suicide	2	4
Cardiac catheterization	1	2
Operative	12	23

*Provocable outflow tract obstruction.
†Nonobstructive hypertrophic cardiomyopathy.
‡Percentage calculated on the basis of 38 patients who underwent cardiac catheterization; 14 patients with hypertrophic cardiomyopathy did not have cardiac catheterization.
§Includes one patient who became asymptomatic after ventricular septal myotomy-myectomy.[23]
¶Death was virtually instantaneous in 24 patients; the remaining patient survived 2 months after her initial cardiac arrest.
**Includes three patients with previous septal myotomy-myectomy.[23]
Abbreviations: CVA = cerebrovascular accident; LVEDP = left ventricular end-diastolic pressure; LVOT = left ventricular outflow tract; PSG = peak systolic gradient.

than hypertrophic cardiomyopathy and 11 subjects with structurally normal hearts who died of trauma (table 2). The normal and diseased controls were similar with regard to age, sex distribution and septal–free wall thickness ratio and therefore were combined in the data analysis. The 83 control patients and the 52 patients with hypertrophic cardiomyopathy are compared with regard to clinical and anatomic variables in table 3.

Materials and Methods

Measurement of Ventricular Wall Thicknesses

Ventricular wall thicknesses were measured in two areas: in the ventricular septum at the point of maximal thickness, usually about one-half the distance between the aortic valve and the apex of the left ventricle, and in the posterior* left ventricular wall, behind the midpoint of the posterior mitral leaflet, at a level corresponding to the caudal margins of the mitral leaflets. These measurements were made perpendicular to the endocardial surfaces of the ventricular walls. Trabeculations, papillary muscles, and the crista supraventricularis were not included in the measurement of ventricular wall thickness.

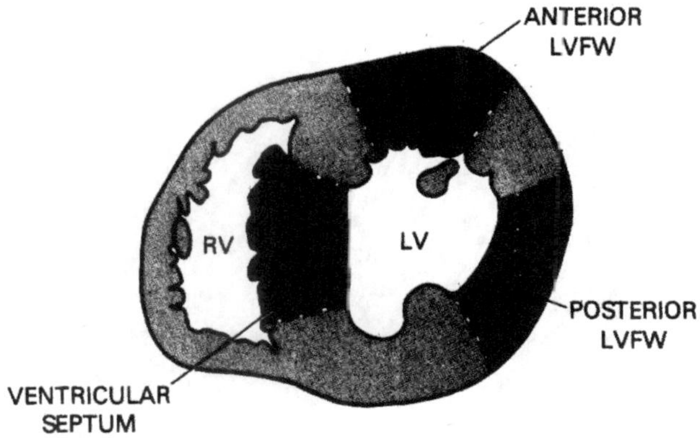

FIGURE 1. *Section of a heart in the anteroposterior (transverse) plane about one-half the distance between left ventricular base and apex, showing the location of the three tissue sections that were analyzed quantitatively in each patient. LV = left ventricle; RV = right ventricle; LVFW = left ventricular free wall.*

Tissue Preparation

In each of the 135 hearts in this study (52 with hypertrophic cardiomyopathy and 83 controls), three tissue blocks were taken from the full thickness of the ventricular wall in a plane perpendicular to the long axis of the left ventricle (i.e., transverse plane), about one-half the distance between the aortic valve and left ventricular apex. In the anteroposterior plane, the tissue sections were obtained from three locations: the ventricular septum, the anterior left ventricular free wall about 2 cm lateral to the left anterior descending coronary artery, and the posterior left ventricular free wall between the papillary muscles (fig. 1). All tissue specimens were embedded in paraffin, sectioned at a thickness of 6 μ and stained with hematoxylin-eosin.

Definition and Classification of Cardiac Muscle Cell Disorganization

In contrast to normal cellular arrangement, cardiac muscle cell disorganization observed in the patients in this study usually assumed four different forms (fig. 2), which have been described in detail.[11] Type I-A disorganization, the most common form, consisted of areas of myocardium in which adjacent cardiac mus-

*The term "posterior" left ventricular wall is used to describe the region of the free wall between the papillary muscles, directly behind the posterior mitral leaflet. This area is often described by pathologists as the "lateral" or "posterolateral" left ventricular free wall.

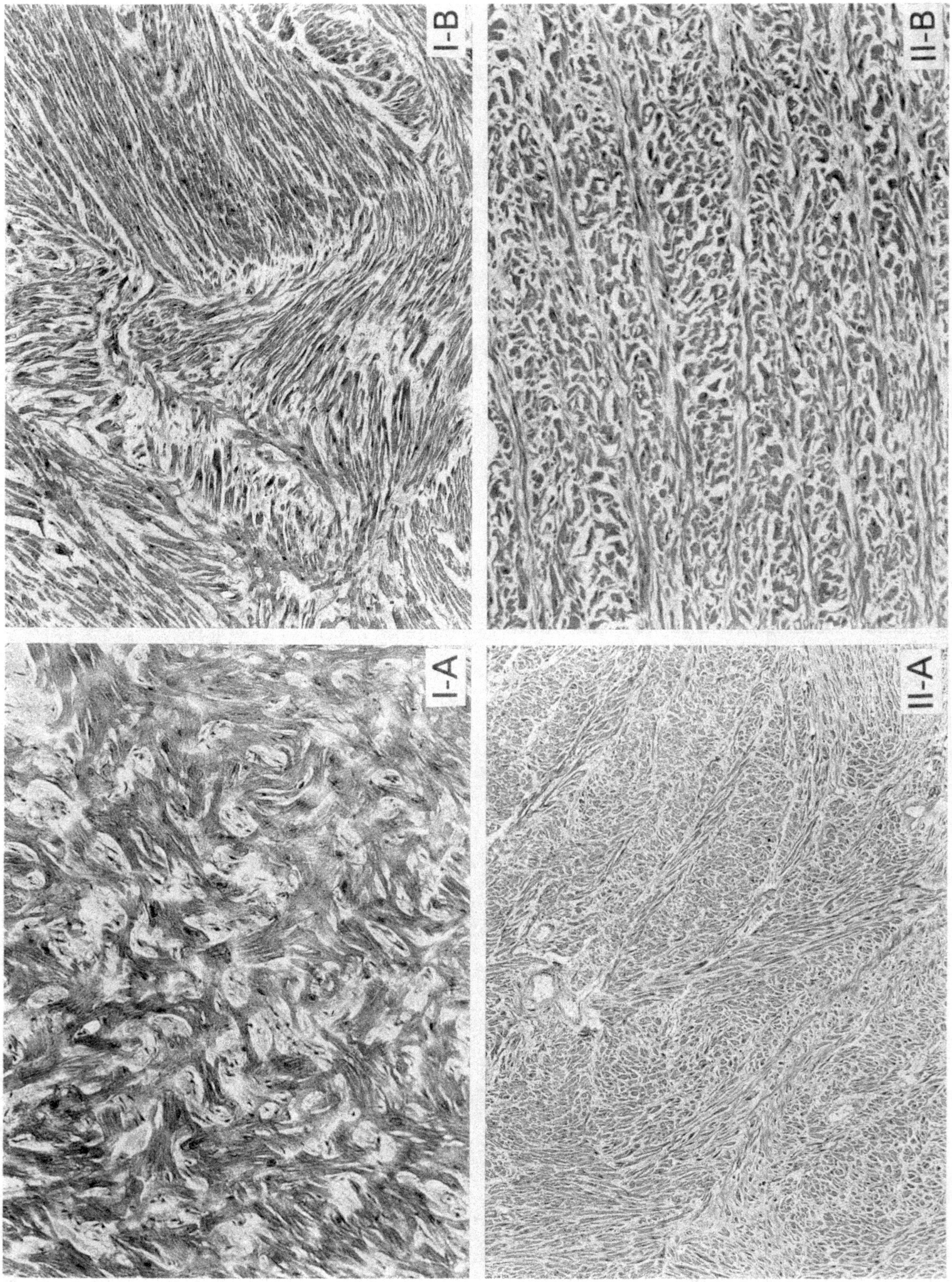
I-B
II-B
I-A
II-A

TABLE 2. *Cardiac Diseases in 83 Control Patients*

Disease	No. of pts	No. of pts with marked VS disorganization*	No. of pts with marked LVFW disorganization*
Aortic valve disease	17†	1	3
Coronary heart disease	15	2	1
Mitral valve disease	10‡	1	5
Systemic hypertension	8	1	1
Idiopathic dilated cardiomyopathy	6	0	1
Primary pulmonary hypertension	6	1	3
Pulmonic valve stenosis	3	0	0
Combined aortic and mitral valve disease	2	0	0
Supravalvular aortic stenosis	2	0	1
Ventricular septal defect	2	0	1
Discrete subaortic stenosis	1	0	0
Normal	11	1	0
Total	83	7 (8%)	16 (19%)

*Involving at least 5% of the relevant areas of the tissue section.

†Includes 12 patients with predominant aortic stenosis, three with pure aortic regurgitation and two with combined aortic stenosis and regurgitation.

‡Includes three patients with predominant mitral stenosis, six with predominant mitral regurgitation, and one with combined mitral stenosis and regurgitation.

Abbreviations: LVFW = left ventricular free wall; VS = ventricular septal.

TABLE 3. *Comparison of Clinical and Morphologic Features in Patients with Hypertrophic Cardiomyopathy and in Controls*

Variable	Hypertrophic cardiomyopathy (n = 52)	Other heart diseases and normals (n = 83)	*p*
Mean age (years) (range)	31 (11–65)	43 (5–80)	< 0.001
Female:male (%)	52:48	39:61	NS
Mean heart weight (g) (range)	547† (270–1020)	510‡ (185–1360)	NS
Mean ventricular septal thickness (mm) (range)	26 (15–44)	15 (8–26)	< 0.001
Mean posterior LV free wall thickness (mm) (range)	17 (9–27)	14 (7–23)	< 0.001
Mean septal–free wall ratio (range)	1.6 (0.8–2.7)	1.1 (0.8–1.6)	< 0.001
Septal–free wall ratio ≥ 1.3 (%)	79*	17	< 0.001

*Echocardiograms were recorded during life in seven of the 11 patients with concentric hypertrophy (septal–free wall ratio < 1.3) at necropsy; asymmetric septal hypertrophy was present in each of those patients. Because diastolic septal–free wall ratios during life usually exceed those obtained at necropsy,[24] it is likely that at least 48 (92%) of the 52 patients with hypertrophic cardiomyopathy would have had asymmetric septal hypertrophy identified if echocardiography had been performed during life.

†Heart weight exceeded normal values[25] in all 52 patients.

‡Heart weight exceeded normal values[25] in each of the 72 patients with congenital or acquired heart disease and was normal in each of the 11 subjects without cardiac disease.

Abbreviation: LV = left ventricular.

FIGURE 2. *Classification of four major types of cardiac muscle cell disorganization present in ventricular septal myocardium. Magnifications: I-A, × 130; I-B and II-A, × 40; II-B, × 80. Each tissue section was stained with hematoxylin and eosin.*

cle cells were aligned perpendicularly or obliquely to each other, usually forming tangled masses or "pinwheel" configurations. Although most of these lesions were relatively small, individual foci of type I-A disorganization varied greatly in size. In type I-B disorganization, relatively broad bundles of muscle cells were oriented at oblique or perpendicular angles to each other; cells within these bundles were, however, normally arranged. Types I-A and I-B disorganization exclusively involved areas of myocardium where cardiac muscle cells were cut longitudinally (i.e., appeared rectangular).

Type II-A disorganization consisted of relatively narrow (usually one or two cells wide) longitudinally cut bundles that were interlaced in various directions among larger groups of transversely cut cells (i.e., appeared circular). This type of disorganization gave the myocardium a swirled appearance. Type II-B was similar to type II-A disorganization, except that the narrow, longitudinally cut bundles of cells were more linear. Type II-C disorganization consisted of relatively small "islands" of disorganized, longitudinally cut cells within much larger areas of transversely cut cardiac muscle cells. Types II-A, II-B and II-C disorganization involved areas of myocardium that included both longitudinally and transversely cut cardiac muscle cells. Nonparallel arrangements of cardiac muscle cells were not considered to represent disorganization if present in the following areas where cells normally converge at acute angles: (1) at or near the junction of ventricular septum with the left and right ventricular free walls, (2) within trabeculations, (3) within or at the edges of scarred areas, (4) at points of convergence of major muscle bundles, or (5) adjacent to interstitial spaces containing blood vessels.

Quantitation of Cardiac Muscle Cell Disorganization

A technique that has been described in detail[11] was used to assess quantitatively the extent of cardiac muscle cell disorganization in the 405 tissue sections studied. We studied only transverse plane tissue sections because this orientation is most appropriate for identifying cardiac muscle cell disorganization.[11] Tissue sections were photographed and the images enlarged to occupy 30 × 40-inch positive prints, resulting in a magnification of about 1500 times the original tissue section. A transparent cellulose overlay was then placed over the print, and the areas of myocardium occupied by disorganized cardiac muscle cells were outlined with a marking pen. Although this assessment could sometimes be made exclusively from direct examination of the print, frequently the original tissue section had to be reexamined with a light microscope to localize the disorganized area. Areas in which cardiac muscle cells were either cut longitudinally or transversely were also demarcated. Large areas of fibrosis (replacement or interstitial), artifacts of tissue preparation or large interstitial spaces containing blood vessels were excluded from the analysis. The transparent overlay was then removed from the print, photographed and reproduced (with substantial reduction) as a 5 × 7-inch positive print. Each area into which the tissue section had been divided was outlined separately with a fine-point marking pen on ordinary tablet paper and quantitated using a video planimetry system.

Formulas Used in Quantitative Calculations of Cardiac Muscle Cell Arrangement

The formulas used to calculate the percentage of the tissue section occupied by disorganized cardiac muscle cells are given below; the area of myocardium "at risk" for disorganization appears in the denominator of both equations:

$$\%\text{ area of type I (I-A + I-B) disorganization} = \frac{D_I}{L + D_I} \times 100;$$

$$\%\text{ area of type II (II-A + II-B + II-C) disorganization} = \frac{D_{II}}{L + T + D_{II}} \times 100,$$

where L = area occupied by longitudinally cut but normally arranged cells, T = area occupied by transversely cut cells (excluding those incorporated into areas of type II disorganization), D_I = area occupied by type I disorganization, and D_{II} = area occupied by type II disorganization.

Values for type I and type II disorganization could not be combined in patients who had both types, because this calculation often resulted in a marked underestimation of the overall extent of disorganization in a tissue section. Therefore, the percentage of disorganization plotted for each patient was the value for type I or type II disorganization, whichever value was greater. We did not attempt to assess the severity of cellular malalignment in a given area of tissue, but judged disorganization only as present or absent. For the purposes of certain analyses, quantitative data regarding cellular arrangement in the anterior and posterior left ventricular free wall sections were combined and the sum was expressed as representing the "left ventricular free wall." Ventricular septal and left ventricular free wall tissue sections were also combined for an analysis of "total left ventricular wall" disorganization.

Statistical Methods

Data were compared and analyzed using the *t* test or chi-square test.

Results

Ventricular Wall Thicknesses

Ventricular septal thicknesses, posterior left ventricular free wall thicknesses and septal–free wall ratios were significantly greater in patients with hypertrophic cardiomyopathy than in control patients (table 3). In addition, the septal–free wall thickness ratio was 1.3 or greater[2, 5, 13] in 41 of the 52 patients (79%) with hypertrophic cardiomyopathy and in only 14 of the 83 controls (17%) ($p < 0.001$).

Morphologic Appearance of the Ventricular Walls

The architecture of large muscle bundles appeared relatively uniform[21] in tissue sections from the ventricular septum and anterior and posterior left ventricular free wall in patients with hypertrophic cardiomyopathy and in controls. A bundle of longitudinally cut cardiac muscle cells was usually present in the center of the tissue section, oriented parallel to the endocardial or epicardial surfaces. This band usually comprised about one-third of the area of the overall tissue section. Transversely cut cells were present, for the most part, in the areas on either side of the central band; each of these latter two areas comprised about one-third of the tissue section.

Quantitative Histologic Findings in the Ventricular Septum

Cardiac muscle cell disorganization was common and extensive in the ventricular septum of patients with hypertrophic cardiomyopathy (figs. 3 and 4). Of the 52 patients with hypertrophic cardiomyopathy, 50 (96%) had some septal disorganization, 45 (87%) had disorganization in 5% or more of the relevant areas of the tissue section, 31 (60%) had disorganization comprising 25% or more of the section and 16 (31%) had particularly extensive disorganization involving 50% or more of the section (figs. 3 and 4). In the patients with hypertrophic cardiomyopathy, the mean percentage area of ventricular septum disorganized was substantial (35 ± 4% [SEM], range 0–95%).

In contrast, septal disorganization was much less common and extensive in control patients. Although 25 of the 83 controls (30%) showed some septal disorganization, only seven (8%) had areas of disorganization comprising 5% or more of the tissue section and only one patient had more than 25% of the section involved. The mean area of ventricular septal tissue section disorganized in control patients (2 ± 1%) was significantly less than that in patients with hypertrophic cardiomyopathy (35 ± 4%, $p < 0.001$). Type I (particularly type I-A) was most often the predominant form of disorganization in a given ventricular septal tissue section. In 72 (95%) of the 76 control patients or patients with hypertrophic cardiomyopathy who showed septal disorganization, type I was the predominant form of disorganization identified (table 4).

Quantitative Histologic Findings in the Left Ventricular Free Wall

Cardiac muscle cell disorganization was also common and extensive in the left ventricular free wall of patients with hypertrophic cardiomyopathy (figs. 3–8). Of the 52 patients with hypertrophic cardiomyopathy, 47 (90%) had some disorganization in the left ventricular free wall (i.e., in the combined anterior and posterior free wall sections), 33 (63%) had disorganization comprising 5% or more of the free wall sections, 20 (39%) had disorganization comprising 25% or more of the sections and 11 (21%) had particularly extensive disorganization involving 50% or

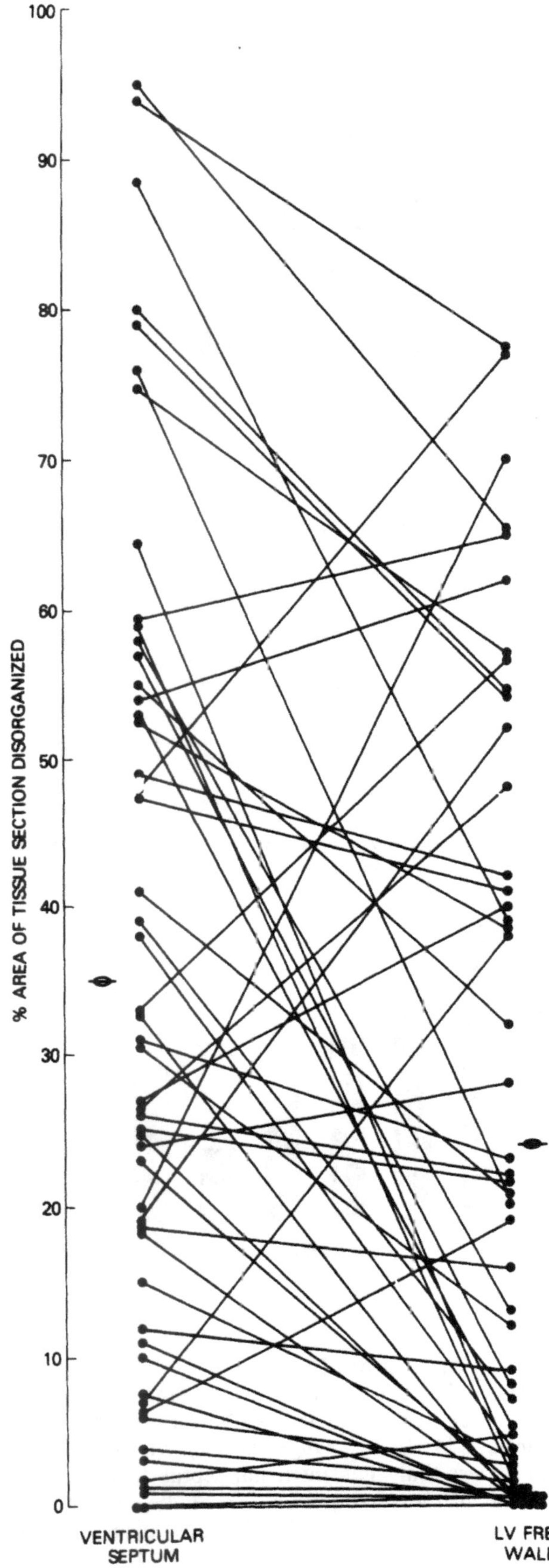

FIGURE 3. *Comparison of the extent of ventricular septal and left ventricular (LV) free wall disorganization in 52 patients with hypertrophic cardiomyopathy. Values for each patient are connected by a solid line. Mean values are indicated by the symbol Θ.*

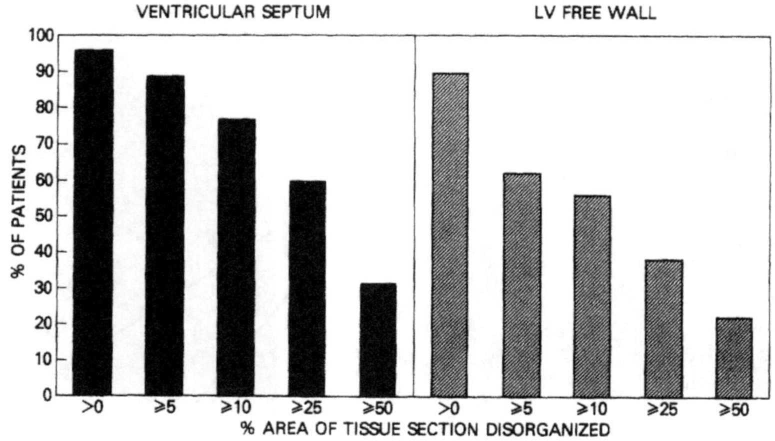

FIGURE 4. *Extent of cardiac muscle cell disorganization in the ventricular septum and in left ventricular (LV) free wall of 52 patients with hypertrophic cardiomyopathy.*

TABLE 4. *Predominant Types of Cellular Disorganization in Patients with Hypertrophic Cardiomyopathy and in Controls*

Region of left ventricle	Hypertrophic cardiomyopathy				Other heart diseases and normals					
	No. of pts	Type I-A	Type I-B	Type II-B	No. of pts	Type I-A	Type I-B	Type II-A	Type II-B	Type II-C
Ventricular septum	50	31	19	0	26	19	3	0	2	2
Anterior LV free wall	44	29	15	0	30	26	2	2	0	0
Posterior LV free wall	39	25	13	1	19	13	4	1	1	0

Abbreviation: LV = left ventricular.

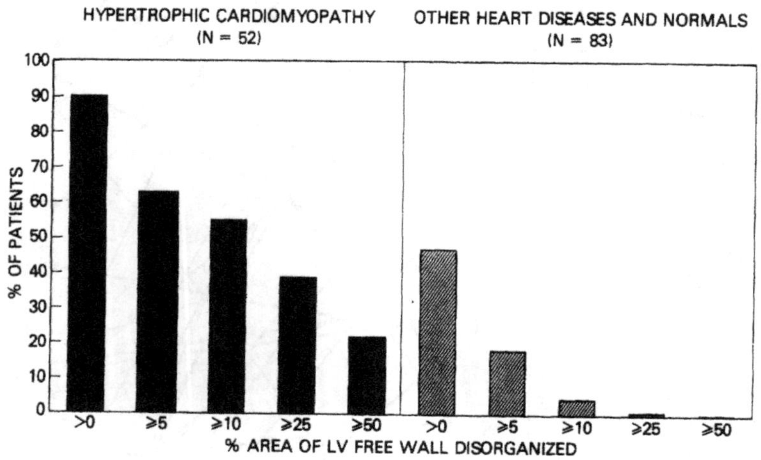

FIGURE 5. *Extent of left ventricular (LV) free wall disorganization in 52 patients with hypertrophic cardiomyopathy and in 83 controls. Comparisons of the respective bars from patients with hypertrophic cardiomyopathy and control patients each achieved high statistical significance ($p < 0.001$).*

more of the sections (figs. 4 and 5). In patients with hypertrophic cardiomyopathy, the mean percentage area of left ventricular free wall disorganized was substantial (24 ± 3%, range 0–77%), although significantly less than the ventricular septal disorganization present in the same patients (35 ± 4%, $p < 0.05$).

Of the 45 patients with at least 5% disorganization in the ventricular septal tissue sections, 33 also had more than 5% disorganization in the sections of left ventricular free wall. Each of the seven patients with no or less than 5% disorganization in the septum also had no or less than 5% disorganization in the free wall.

As in the ventricular septum, type I (particularly I-A) was most commonly the predominant form of disorganization in the left ventricular free wall of patients with hypertrophic cardiomyopathy and controls (table 4).

The anterior left ventricular free wall section in patients with hypertrophic cardiomyopathy showed significantly more disorganization (32 ± 4%) than the posterior free wall section (15 ± 3%, $p < 0.005$) (fig. 8). The extent of disorganization in the anterior free wall (32 ± 4%) did not differ significantly from that in the ventricular septum (35 ± 4%); however, there was

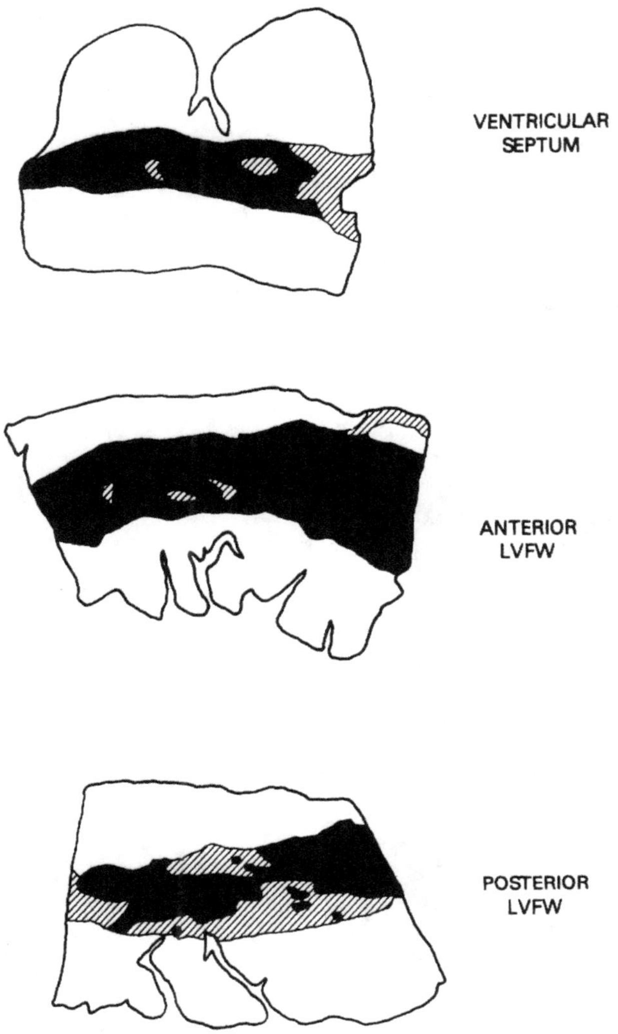

FIGURE 6. *Histologic "maps" of sections of left ventricular wall from a 12-year-old boy with hypertrophic cardiomyopathy in whom sudden death was the initial manifestation of cardiac disease. Particularly marked and diffuse disorganization is present in the three sections. Solid areas contain type I cellular disorganization. Striped areas represent normally arranged cardiac muscle cells that have been cut longitudinally. Clear areas contain cells cut transversely. Tissue sections are oriented with the left ventricular endocardium toward the bottom of the page. LVFW = left ventricular free wall.*

significantly less disorganization in the posterior free wall (15 ± 3%) than in the ventricular septum ($p < 0.001$). In patients with hypertrophic cardiomyopathy, the overall left ventricular wall disorganization (combined ventricular septal and free wall tissue sections) (28 ± 3%) significantly exceeded that in the control patients (2 ± 0.5%, $p < 0.001$) (fig. 9).

In contrast, left ventricular free wall disorganization was less common and less extensive in control patients than in patients with hypertrophic cardiomyopathy (figs. 5, 9 and 10), although there was some overlap between the two groups. Although 39 of the 83 controls (47%) showed some left ventricular free wall disorganization, only 16 of the patients (19%) had areas of disorganization comprising 5% or more of the tissue section, and only one patient had more than 25% of the section involved (fig. 5). The mean percentage area of left ventricular free wall disorganized in control patients (2 ± 0.5%) was also considerably less than that in patients with hypertrophic cardiomyopathy (24 ± 3%, $p < 0.001$). In the 83 control patients, cellular disorganization occurred more often in the free wall (39 of 83, 47%) than in the septum (25 of 83, 30%; $p < 0.05$); however, in controls, the percentage of disorganization in the ventricular septum (2 ± 1%), anterior (3 ± 1%) and posterior free wall (1.5 ± 0.5%) did not differ significantly.

Correlation of Extent of Disorganization with Other Variables

Clinical, hemodynamic and anatomic variables identified in the 52 patients with hypertrophic cardiomyopathy were analyzed to determine whether there was a correlation with the extent of left ventricular free wall or combined ventricular septal and free wall disorganization. There was no relation between the extent of disorganization and sex distribution, duration of symptoms, presence of coronary heart disease or paroxysmal atrial fibrillation, magnitude of left ventricular end-diastolic pressure, heart weight, ventricular septal thickness, or septal–free wall thickness ratio. The two patients who showed no septal disorganization did not differ from the 50 patients who had septal disorganization with regard to these clinical and anatomic variables.

Other variables did show a statistically significant relation with the extent of disorganization. Disorganization in tissue sections from left ventricular free wall and combined ventricular septal and free wall was most marked in the younger patients and patients without functional limitation, particularly in the subgroup of 14 patients (25 years of age or younger) without functional limitation, in whom sudden death was the initial manifestation of cardiac disease[20] (table 5). Nine of these 14 patients had more than 35% disorganization in each of the three regions of left ventricular wall sampled.

Five patients who died late after operation (9 months to 17 years) of causes related to hypertrophic cardiomyopathy or showed no improvement postoperatively did not differ from other patients with regard to free wall (28 ± 14%) or combined septal and free wall disorganization (25 ± 11%).

The extent of free wall and combined septal and free wall disorganization was also greater in five patients with nonobstructive hypertrophic cardiomyopathy than in 24 patients with obstruction to left ventricular outflow under basal conditions; however, this difference did not achieve statistical significance (table 5). Free wall and combined septal and free wall disorganization was absent or particularly focal in four patients with associated systemic hypertension (mean area disorganized, only 0.5%).

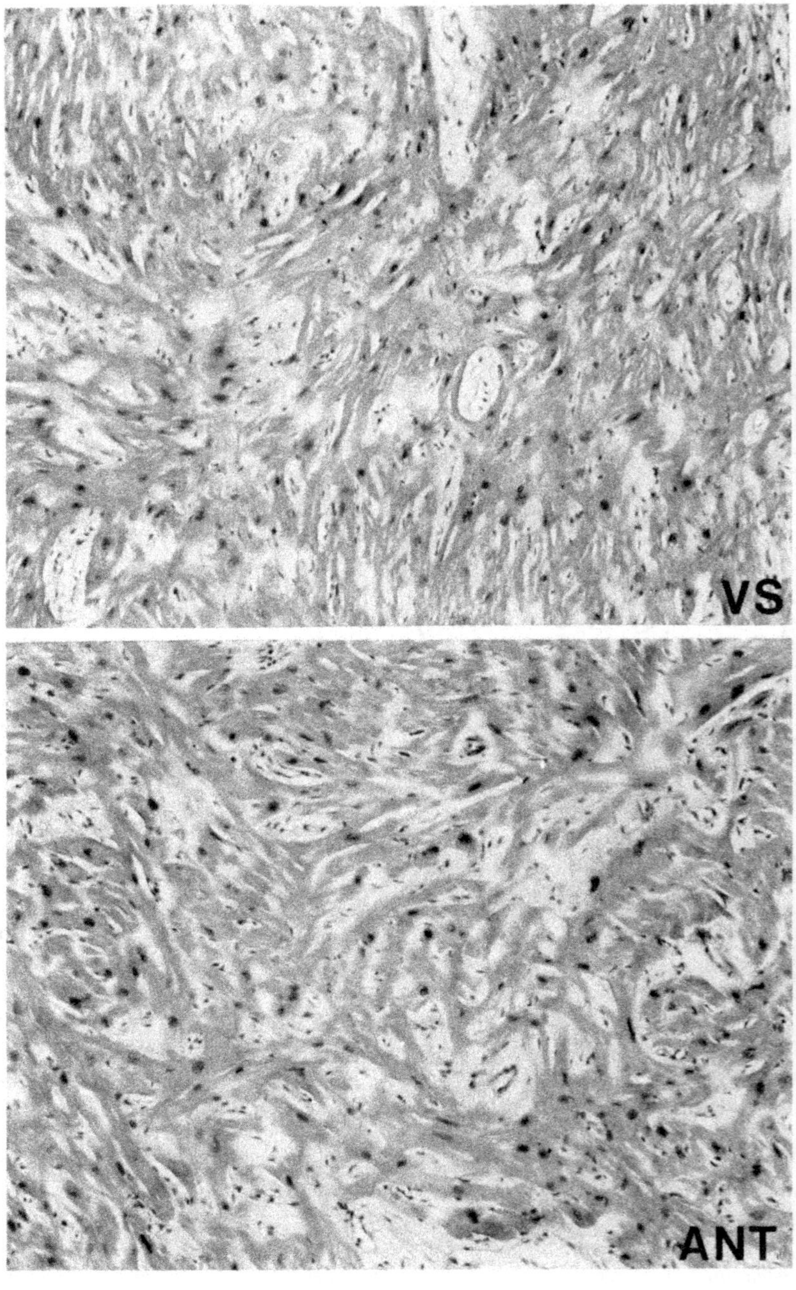

Discussion

The results of this quantitative histologic study confirm our previous observation that marked ventricular septal disorganization involving at least 5% of the relevant areas of the tissue section is a highly sensitive (86%) and specific (92%) marker for hypertrophic cardiomyopathy.[11-13] In addition, in the large population of patients with hypertrophic cardiomyopathy studied, cellular disorganization commonly and extensively involved regions of the left ventricular free wall.[14] Ninety percent of the 52 patients had some disorganization in the free wall and 63% of the patients had at least 5% disorganization in the free wall tissue sections. In the patients with hypertrophic cardiomyopathy, the mean area of free wall tissue section disorganized was substantial (24 ± 3%), although less marked than that in the septum (35 ± 4%). However, the extent of septal and free wall disorganization in many patients was similar. Of 45 patients with marked disorganization in the ventricular septum, 33 also had marked disorganization in the free wall. Conversely, in each of the seven patients with minimal or absent septal disorganization, the extent of cellular disorganization was similar (less than 5%) in the free wall.

Left ventricular free wall disorganization was also common (i.e., 47%) in the 83 patients with normal hearts or cardiac diseases other than hypertrophic cardiomyopathy. However, foci of left ventricular free wall disorganization in these patients usually involved extremely small areas of myocardium (less than 5%), in contrast to the widespread disorganization present in most patients with hypertrophic cardiomyopathy.

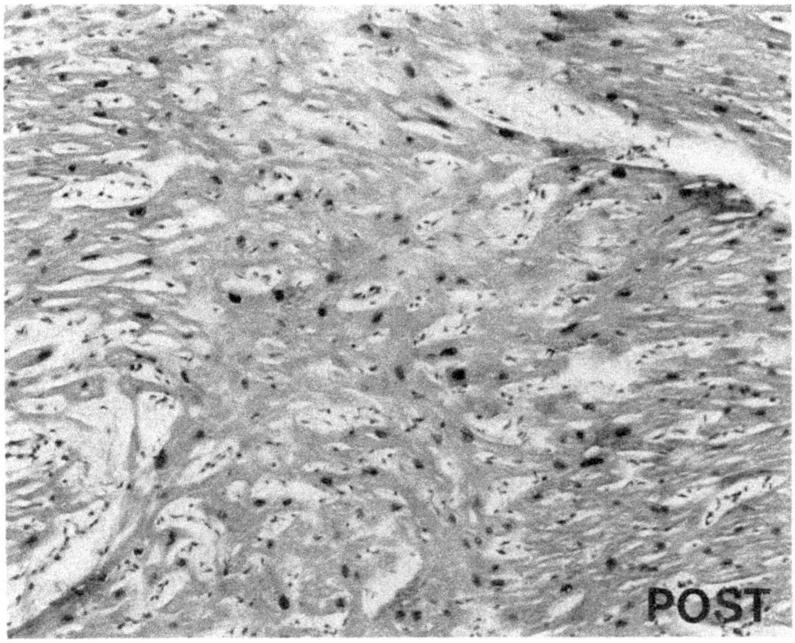

FIGURE 7. *Histologic sections of ventricular septum (VS) and anterior (ANT) and posterior (POST) left ventricular free wall from the patient with hypertrophic cardiomyopathy shown in figure 6. Marked type I disorganization of cardiac muscle cells is present in each of the three tissue sections. Hematoxylin and eosin stain; magnification × 105.*

On the other hand, the specificity of marked left ventricular free wall disorganization (involving 5% or more of the tissue section) in our necropsy population of 83 patients without hypertrophic cardiomyopathy was relatively high (82%).

A potentially important question is whether the distribution and extent of cardiac muscle cell disorganization in the left ventricular wall of patients

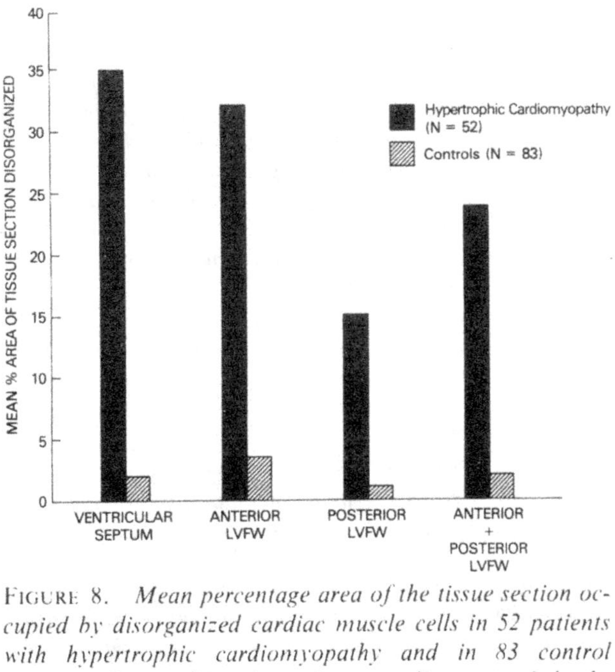

FIGURE 8. *Mean percentage area of the tissue section occupied by disorganized cardiac muscle cells in 52 patients with hypertrophic cardiomyopathy and in 83 control patients. For each region of myocardium sampled, the percentage of disorganization in patients with hypertrophic cardiomyopathy significantly exceeded that in control patients* ($p < 0.001$). *LVFW = left ventricular free wall.*

with hypertrophic cardiomyopathy has any relation to clinical course or hemodynamic state. Our data show that left ventricular free wall and combined septal and free wall disorganization was most extensive in the younger (25 years of age or younger) and least symptomatic patients studied, particularly those who had no functional limitation before their sudden and unexpected death. Hence, in patients in whom cellular disorganization is extensive and distributed widely throughout the left ventricular wall, this pattern may represent a diffuse cardiomyopathic process and be a determinant of clinical outcome. The mechanism by which particularly marked and diffuse cardiac muscle cell disorganization may increase the likelihood of premature sudden death is unknown. However, it is possible that the disorganized arrangement of adjacent cardiac muscle cells in the ventricular walls of these patients may be very inefficient in producing an orderly pattern of electrical depolarization or repolarization and could provide the substrate for ventricular ectopy.

The distribution and extent of cardiac muscle cell disorganization in the left ventricular wall in five patients without obstruction to left ventricular outflow under basal conditions or with provocation was compared with that in patients with obstruction. Although disorganization was greater in the patients without left ventricular outflow tract obstruction, the difference was not statistically significant. Hence, in this quantitative study we could not definitively confirm our previous impression, based upon qualitative histologic analysis of ventricular myocardium,[15] that patients with nonobstructive hypertrophic cardiomyopathy have more widespread distribution of cellular disorganization in the left ventricular free wall than patients with outflow obstruction. There are certain possible explanations for the differences between

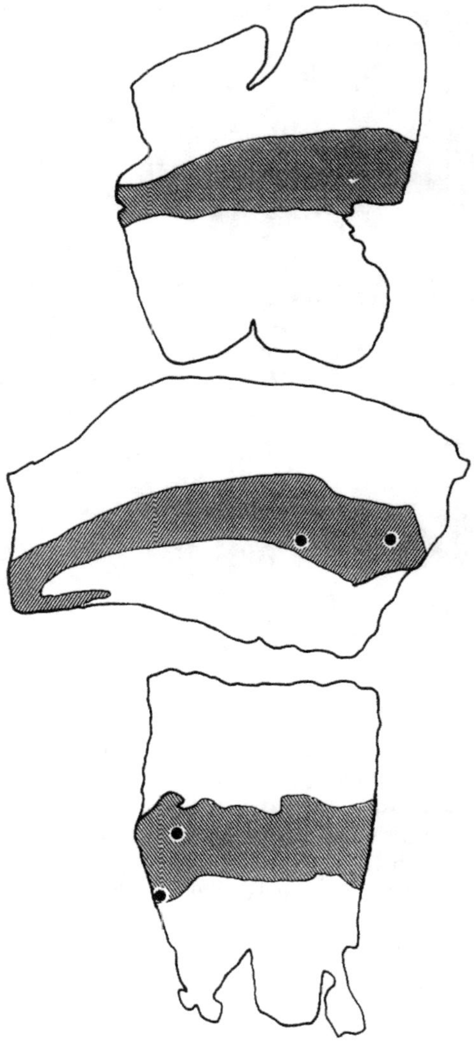

FIGURE 10. *Histologic "maps" of the three sections of left ventricular wall from a subject with a structurally normal heart. Solid areas in anterior and posterior left ventricular free wall sections represent small foci of type I cellular disorganization. Striped areas represent normally arranged cardiac muscle cells cut longitudinally. Clear areas contain cells cut transversely. Tissue sections are oriented with the left ventricular endocardium toward the bottom of the page. LVFW = left ventricular free wall.*

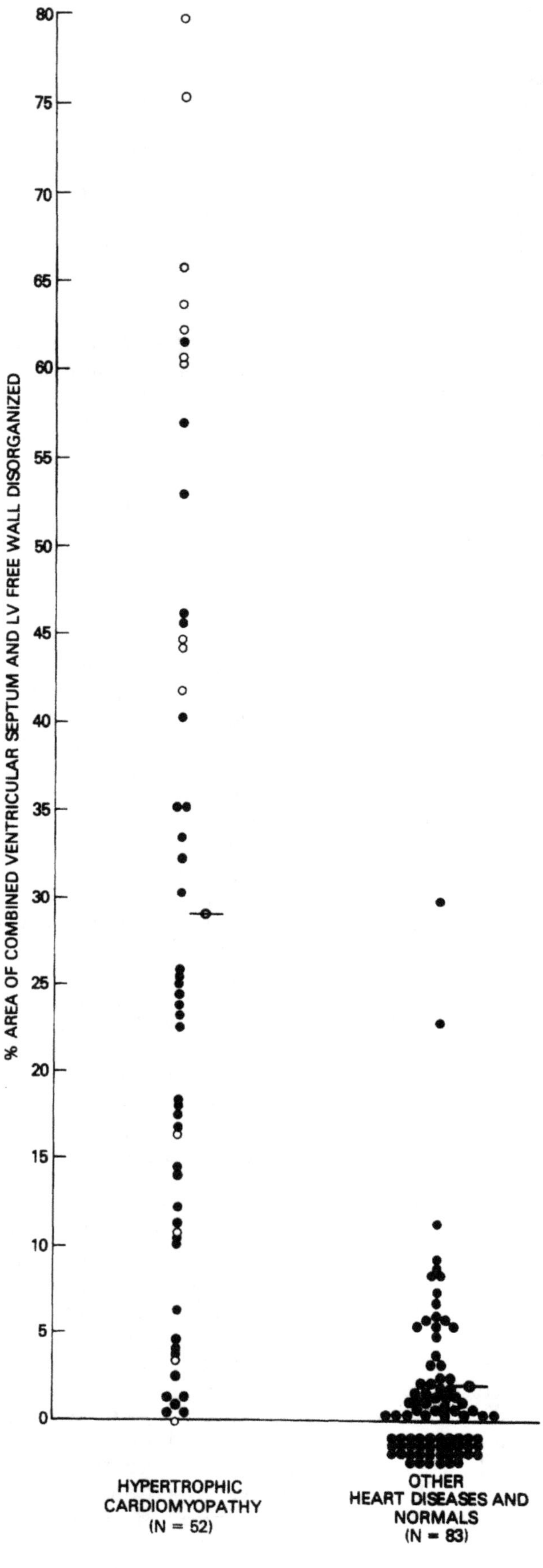

FIGURE 9. *Percentage area of combined ventricular septal and left ventricular (LV) free wall tissue sections occupied by disorganized cardiac muscle cells in 52 patients with hypertrophic cardiomyopathy and in 83 control patients. Patients 25 years of age or younger in whom sudden death was the initial manifestation of hypertrophic cardiomyopathy are indicated by open symbols. Mean values are indicated by the symbol* Θ.

TABLE 5. *Correlation of Extent of Cellular Disorganization with Clinical Variables*

Variable	No. of pts	% area LVFW disorganized (mean ± SEM)		% area of combined VS and LVFW disorganized (mean ± SEM)	
Age at death (years)					
≤ 25	24	37 ± 6	$p < 0.001$	39 ± 5	$p < 0.001$§
> 25	28	13 ± 3		17 ± 3	
Functional limitation (symptoms)					
Absent*	16¶	41 ± 6	$p < 0.005$	43 ± 6	$p < 0.005$§
Present**	28¶	19 ± 4		24 ± 3	
Functional state and age					
No functional limitation,* ≤ 25 years	14¶	43 ± 7	$p < 0.001$	45 ± 7	$p < 0.005$§
Functional limitation,** > 25 years	19¶	15 ± 3		19 ± 3	
Obstruction to LV outflow					
Absent† (basal and provoked)	5	22 ± 10	NS	33 ± 7	NS
Present‡ (basal)	24	18 ± 5		21 ± 4	

*Patients in whom sudden death was the first definitive manifestation of cardiac disease.[20]
†< 30 mm Hg.
‡≥ 30 mm Hg.
§These differences in combined ventricular septal and left ventricular free wall disorganization were due primarily to the differences in extent of free wall disorganization; the extent of ventricular septal disorganization alone did not differ significantly between the two subgroups analyzed.
¶Patients with associated coronary heart disease were excluded from these analyses.
**New York Heart Association functional classes II and III.
Abbreviations: LV = left ventricular; LVFW = left ventricular free wall; VS = ventricular septum.

our qualitative study[15] and the present quantitative investigation. First, the qualitative study included morphologic data from needle biopsies obtained at operation in 14 patients with obstructive hypertrophic cardiomyopathy. Such biopsy specimens are necessarily small and cellular disorganization in hypertrophic cardiomyopathy is often "patchy" in distribution.[11] Hence, sampling bias[22] implicit in the biopsy technique may have contributed to the differences between the two studies with regard to the presence and extent of disorganization. Second, the qualitative method used in our first study for both biopsy and necropsy specimens may not have permitted as accurate an assessment of the *extent* of cardiac muscle cell disorganization as did the quantitative histologic technique used in the second study. It is likely that future quantitative histologic analyses of larger numbers of patients with nonobstructive hypertrophic cardiomyopathy will permit more definitive conclusions to be drawn regarding the distribution and extent of cellular disorganization in this subgroup of patients.

Acknowledgment

We gratefully acknowledge the valuable assistance provided by Willard C Whitehouse, Laboratory of Applied Studies, Division of Computer Research, and by James Wolfson.

References

1. Maron BJ, Epstein SE: Hypertrophic cardiomyopathy: a discussion of nomenclature. Am J Cardiol **43:** 1242, 1979
2. Menges H, Brandenburg RO, Brown AL: The clinical, hemodynamic and pathologic diagnosis of muscular subvalvular aortic stenosis. Circulation **24:** 1126, 1961
3. Abbasi AS, MacAlpin RN, Eber LM, Pearce ML: Echocardiographic diagnosis of idiopathic hypertrophic cardiomyopathy without outflow obstruction. Circulation **46:** 897, 1972
4. Abbasi AS, MacAlpin RN, Eber LM, Pearce ML: Left ventricular hypertrophy diagnosed by echocardiography. N Engl J Med **289:** 118, 1973
5. Henry WL, Clark CE, Epstein SE: Asymmetric septal hypertrophy (ASH): echocardiographic identification of the pathognomonic anatomic abnormality of IHSS. Circulation **47:** 225, 1973
6. Roberts WC: Valvular, subvalvular and supravalvular aortic stenosis: morphologic features. Cardiovasc Clin **5:** 104, 1973
7. Teare D: Asymmetrical hypertrophy of the heart in young patients. Br Heart J **20:** 1, 1958
8. Van Noorden S, Olsen EG, Pearse AG: Hypertrophic obstructive cardiomyopathy. A histological, histochemical and ultrastructural study of biopsy material. Cardiovasc Res **5:** 118, 1971
9. Ferrans VJ, Morrow AG, Roberts WC: Myocardial ultrastructure in idiopathic hypertrophic subaortic stenosis: a study of operatively excised left ventricular outflow tract muscle in 14 patients. Circulation **45:** 769, 1972
10. Knieriem H-J, Stroobandt R, Meyer H, Bouregeois M: Hyper-

trophic nonobstructive cardiomyopathy caused by disorder of the myofiber texture. Virchows Arch [Pathol Anat] **367:** 209, 1975

11. Maron BJ, Roberts WC: Quantitative analysis of cardiac muscle cell disorganization in the ventricular septum of patients with hypertrophic cardiomyopathy. Circulation **59:** 689, 1979
12. Maron BJ, Sato N, Roberts WC, Edwards JE, Chandra RS: Quantitative analysis of cardiac muscle cell disorganization in the ventricular septum: comparison of fetuses and infants with and without congenital heart disease and patients with hypertrophic cardiomyopathy. Circulation **60:** 685, 1979
13. Maron BJ, Epstein SE: Hypertrophic cardiomyopathy. Recent observations regarding the specificity of three hallmarks of the disease: asymmetric septal hypertrophy, septal disorganization and systolic anterior motion of the anterior mitral leaflet. Am J Cardiol **45:** 141, 1980
14. Wigle ED, Adelman AG, Silver MD: Pathophysiological considerations in muscular subaortic stenosis. *In* Hypertrophic Obstructive Cardiomyopathy, edited by Wolstenholme GE, O'Connor M. London, Churchill, 1971, p 63
15. Maron BJ, Ferrans VJ, Henry WL, Clark CE, Redwood DR, Roberts WC, Morrow AG, Epstein SE: Differences in distribution of myocardial abnormalities in patients with obstructive and nonobstructive asymmetric septal hypertrophy (ASH): light and electron microscopic findings. Circulation **50:** 436, 1974
16. Maron BJ, Edwards JE, Henry WL, Clark CE, Bingle GJ, Epstein SE: Asymmetric septal hypertrophy (ASH) in infancy. Circulation **50:** 809, 1974
17. Maron BJ, Henry WL, Clark CE, Redwood DR, Roberts WC, Epstein SE: Asymmetric septal hypertrophy in childhood. Circulation **53:** 9, 1976
18. Sutton MSJ, Anderson KR, Lie JT, Frye RL: Specificity and topography of myocardial fiber disarray and fibrosis in hypertrophic obstructive cardiomyopathy (HOCM). (abstr) Circulation **56** (suppl III): III-205, 1977
19. Fujiwara H, Kawai C, Hamashima Y: Myocardial fascicle and fiber disarray in 25-micron-thick sections. Circulation **59:** 1293, 1979
20. Maron BJ, Roberts WC, Edwards JE, McAllister HA, Foley DD, Epstein SE: Sudden death in patients with hypertrophic cardiomyopathy: characterization of 26 patients without previous functional limitation. Am J Cardiol **41:** 803, 1978
21. Lev M, Simkins CS: Architecture of the human ventricular myocardium. Technic for study using a modification of the Mall-MacCallum method. Lab Invest **5:** 396, 1956
22. Isner JM, Maron BJ, Roberts WC: Comparison of amount of cardiac-muscle-cell disorganization in operatively excised septectomy specimens to amount observed at necropsy in the same 18 patients with hypertrophic cardiomyopathy. Am J Cardiol **46:** 42, 1980
23. Morrow AG: Hypertrophic subaortic stenosis: operative methods utilized to relieve left ventricular outflow obstruction. J Thorac Cardiovasc Surg **76:** 423, 1978
24. Maron BJ, Henry WL, Roberts WC, Epstein SE: Comparison of echocardiographic and necropsy measurements of ventricular wall thicknesses in patients with and without disproportionate septal thickening. Circulation **55:** 341, 1977
25. Gould SE: Pathology of the Heart and Blood Vessels, 3rd ed. Springfield, Charles C Thomas, 1968, p 1139

Transmural Myocardial Infarction in Hypertrophic Cardiomyopathy

A Cause of Conversion from Left Ventricular Asymmetry to Symmetry and from Normal-Sized to Dilated Left Ventricular Cavity

Bruce F. Waller, M.D.; Barry J. Maron, M.D.; Stephen E. Epstein, M.D.; and William C. Roberts, M.D., F.C.C.P.

Herein we will discuss a woman with hypertrophic cardiomyopathy who had an acute myocardial infarction which healed.

Case Report

A 30-year-old woman who died on Oct 8, 1978, first had a precordial murmur noted at age 15 years (1963). At age 17, she was studied at the National Heart Institute. Her mother and father were healthy and free of known cardiac disease. Each of three brothers had precordial murmurs of apparently undetermined etiology, but none had symptoms of cardiac dysfunction. The peripheral arterial pulse had a rapid upstroke and downstroke. A loud fourth heart sound (S_4), an intermittent third heart sound (S_3), and a grade 3/6 systolic ejection-type murmur, which was loudest along the left sternal border and which increased in intensity with the Valsalva maneuver, were audible. The ECG (Fig 1) disclosed sinus rhythm, QRS axis of about −35°, and voltage changes indicative of severe left ventricular hypertrophy. Chest roentgenogram disclosed an enlarged cardiac silhouette and cardiac catheterization (Table 1), a 12-mm Hg peak left ventricular-to-brachial arterial systolic pressure gradient at rest and a 32-mm Hg gradient with the Valsalva maneuver. Left ventricular angiography disclosed a small- to normal-sized left ventricular cavity.

At age 18 years, mild exertional dyspnea and fatigue appeared, and a second cardiac catheterization was performed (Table 1). At age 21, the dyspnea and fatigue worsened, and the pulmonary vascular markings on roentgenogram were more prominent. Propranolol, digoxin, and diuretic therapy was begun, and the dyspnea lessened. Electrocardiogram (Fig 1) now disclosed sinus rhythm, QRS axis of about −40°, and left ventricular hypertrophy with a "strain" pattern. At age 22, she noted exertional substernal chest pain that disappeared quickly with rest, and the pain recurred intermittently during the next eight years. Now on ECG, the QRS axis was about −60°; the P-R interval, 0.16 sec.

At age 26, she had two episodes of dizziness. Precordial examination now disclosed a grade 5/6 systolic ejection murmur with a thrill over the left sternal border. Chest roentgenogram (Fig 2) showed an increased cardiothoracic ratio. The ECG (Fig 1) was unchanged from four years earlier. Intracardiac electrophysiologic studies disclosed a normal H-V interval. On M-mode echocardiogram (Fig 3 [9-3-

Table 1—*Hemodynamic Data on Patient Studied**

	Age 17 (1965)	Age 18 (1966)
Left ventricle, s/d	112/28	95/20
Brachial artery, s/d	100/66 (70)	95/57 (65)
LV-BA peak systolic gradient, Rest×Valsalva	12×32	0×20
Left atrium, a:v:m	–	13:20:15
Pulmonary arterial wedge, m	18	–
Pulmonary artery, s/d	40/22	26/13
Right ventricle, s/d	40/22	32/3
Right atrium, a:v:m	–	5:2:2
Cardiac index, L/min/m²	2.8	2.4

*Pressure measurements in mm Hg.

*From the Pathology and Cardiology Branches, National Heart, Lung, and Blood Institute, National Institutes of Health, Bethesda, Md.
Reprint requests: Dr. Roberts, Building 10A, Room 3E30, National Institutes of Health, Bethesda 20205

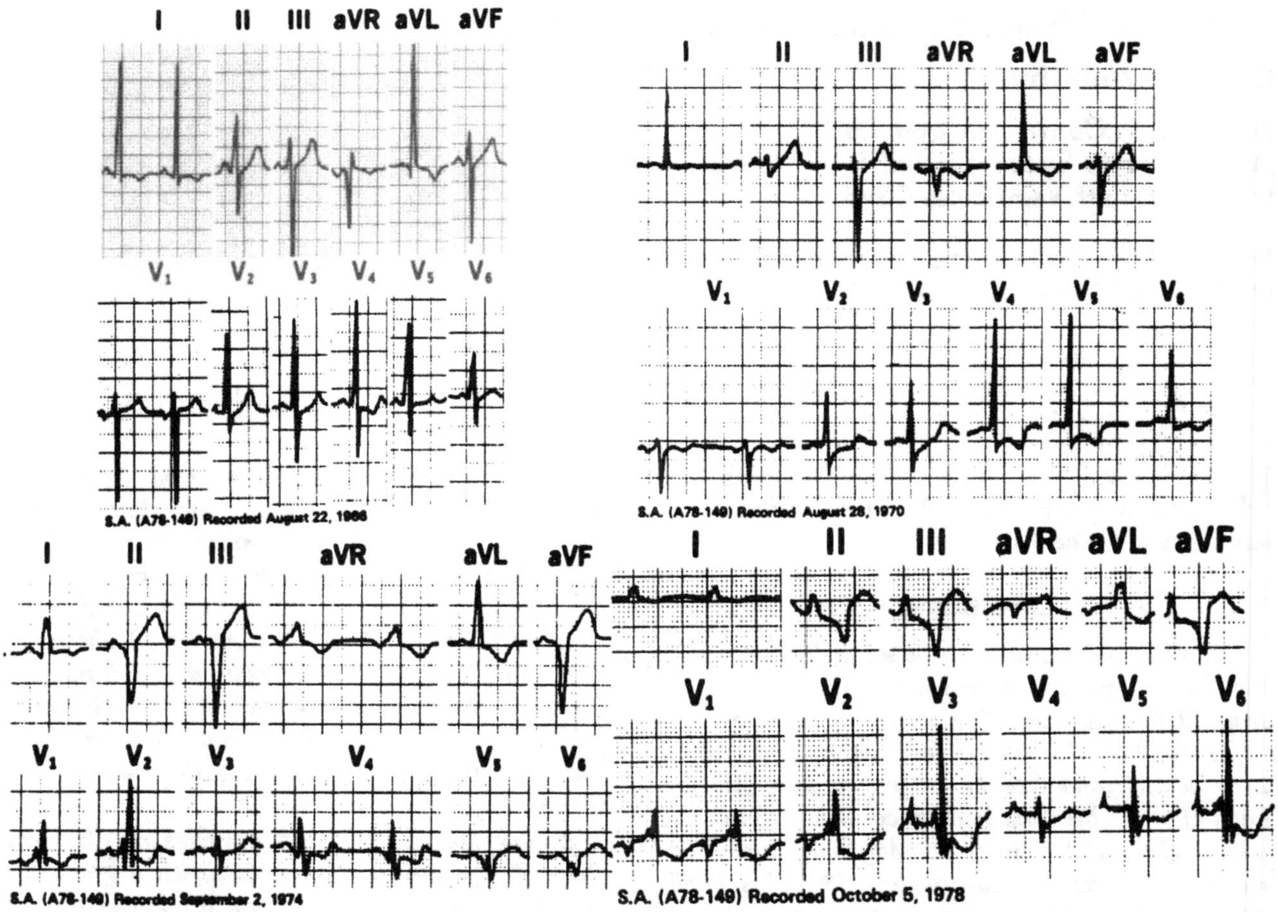

FIGURE 1. Four ECGs from our patient recorded over a 14-year period. During this time, the P-R interval lengthened, the QRS axis became more leftward, the QRS duration widened, and the QRS voltage lessened.

74]), the ventricular septum was 23 mm in thickness in both diastole and peak systole; the left ventricular free wall measured up to 13 mm in thickness in diastole and 27 mm in peak systole; the left ventricular cavity was about 38 mm in transverse dimension in end-diastole and 23 mm in peak systole. The left ventricular ejection fraction was 50 percent.

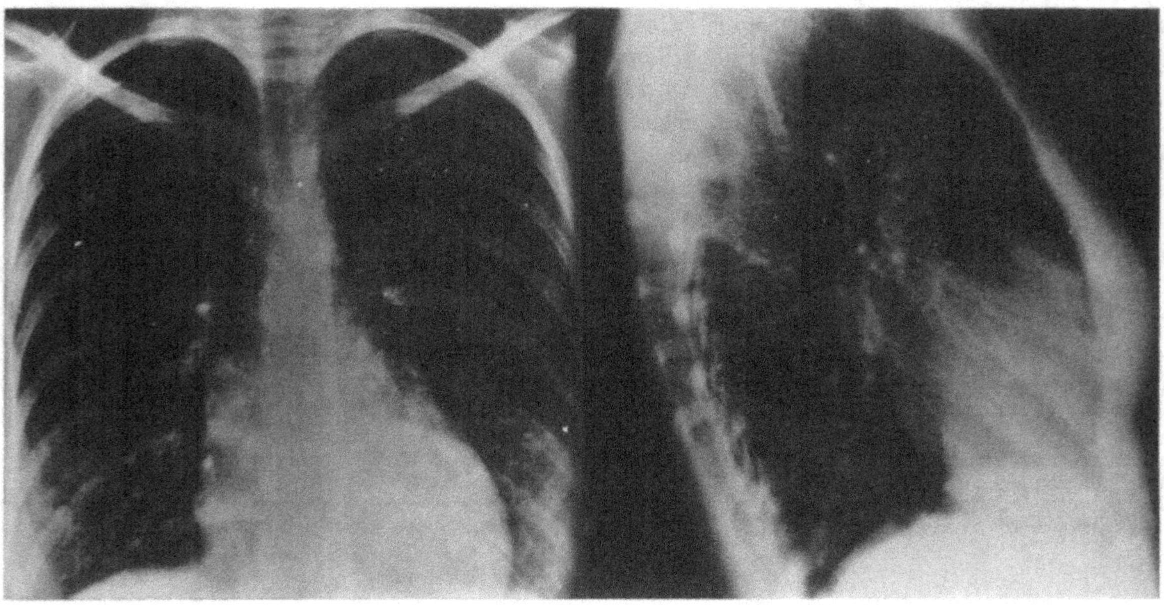

FIGURE 2. Posteroanterior and lateral chest roentgenograms obtained September 1974. The cardiac silhouette is enlarged.

At age 30 (nine months before death), in January 1978, the exertional chest pain became more frequent, and the patient had the first of three episodes of sudden severe dyspnea diagnosed as acute pulmonary edema. In July 1978, an episode of hemoptysis prompted another hospitalization, and repeated ECG disclosed atrial fibrillation. On Sept 9, 1978, while sitting, she had chest pain associated with nausea and sweating. After about two hours of progressive worsening of the pain, she arose and collapsed. The rescue squad arrived a few minutes later and began cardiopulmonary resuscitation, which continued until arrival at the local hospital about 20 minutes later. On ECG after arrival at the hospital, no R waves were present in the precordial leads. Her heart contractions shortly thereafter were adequate to sustain adequate pressure. Later that day, an episode of ventricular tachycardia was documented. During the 20 days in the local hospital, she gradually regained consciousness, and although able to speak, she was unable to speak in sentences or recall past events. Cardiac enzymes were elevated.

On Sept 28, 1978, she was transferred to the National Heart Institute. Her mental status was unchanged. The systemic blood pressure was 90/62 mm Hg, and the jugular veins were mildly distended. Now no precordial murmur was audible at rest; with straining, a grade 2/6 systolic ejection murmur was heard along the left sternal border. An S_3 also was present. No subcutaneous edema was present, and the liver was not palpable. Chest roentgenogram showed bilateral pleural effusions and a left basilar pulmonary infiltrate, which prevented evaluation of cardiac size. On M-mode echocardiogram (Fig 3 [9-28-78]), the ventricular septum was about 13 mm in thickness in both diastole and peak systole; the left ventricular free wall measured up to 10 mm in thickness in diastole and 14 mm in peak systole; the left ventricular cavity was 50 mm in transverse dimension in diastole and 46 mm in peak systole. The left ventricular ejection fraction was about 10 percent. On Sept 29, 1978, Mobitz II heart block was noted, and a temporary pacemaker

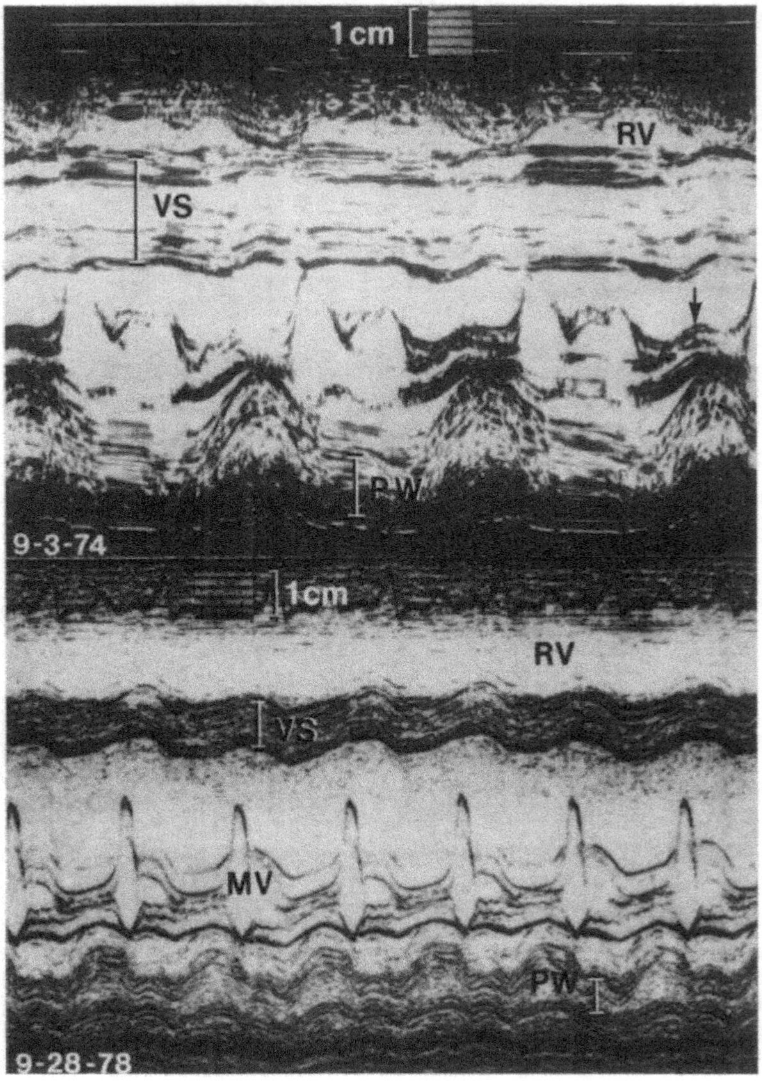

FIGURE 3. M-mode echocardiograms. The ventricular septum (VS) is much thicker than left ventricular free wall (PW); anterior mitral leaflet moves slightly anteriorly (*arrow*) during ventricular systole, and right (RV) and left ventricular cavities are of normal size. On 9-28-78, VS and PW are of similar thickness, and both are much thinner than on 9-3-74. Anterior mitral leaflet (MV) no longer moves anteriorly during ventricular systole, and left ventricular (LV) cavity is dilated.

was inserted. During the next two days, she became hypotensive, acidotic, febrile, and was intubated. Ventricular fibrillation occurred six days before death, and she was resuscitated. An ECG obtained three days before death (Fig 1) showed a QRS axis of about —75°, widened QRS complexes, and a P-R interval of 0.20 sec. Fatal ventricular fibrillation occurred on Oct 8, 1978.

At necropsy (A78-149), the heart weighed 510 g (Fig 4 and 5). A healed transmural infarct involved the left ventricular free wall and ventricular septum (Fig 4). The ventricular septum measured up to 15 mm in thickness, and the left ventricular free wall up to 20 mm in thickness. Both ventricular and both atrial cavities were dilated. A small fibrous plaque was present in the left ventricular outflow tract in apposition to the anterior mitral leaflet. The lumens of the major epicardial coronary arteries were narrowed less than 25 percent in cross-sectional area (Fig 5). Some intramural coronary arteries in the ventricular septum had thickened walls and a few had narrowed lumens (Fig 5). On quantitative examination by a method described elsewhere,[1] 53 percent of the area of the ventricular septum (where a transverse section was examined) and 5 percent of the area of the left ventricular free wall were occupied by disorganized myocardial fibers.

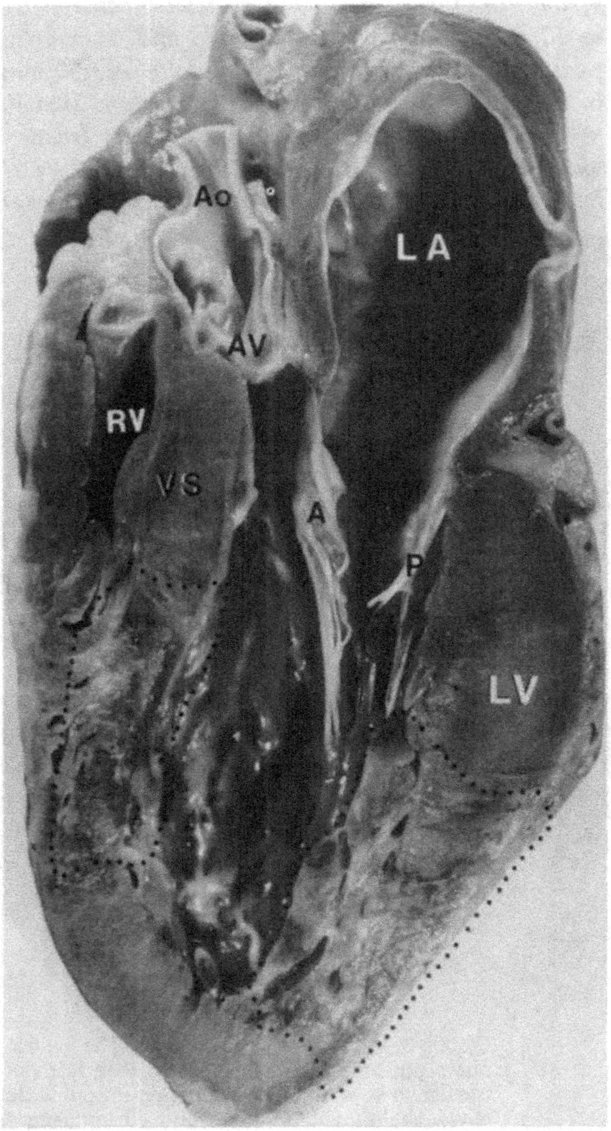

FIGURE 4. Anteroposterior healed transmural infarct (*dotted area*) present in left ventricular free wall (LV) and ventricular septum (VS). Both left ventricular and left atrial (LA) cavities dilated. A = anterior and P = posterior mitral valve leaflets; Ao = ascending aorta; AV = aortic valve; RV = right ventricular cavity.

COMMENTS

The 30-year-old patient described converted from a nondilated (hypertrophic cardiomyopathy) to a dilated type of cardiomyopathy, and this conversion probably took place about two months before death. When first seen at age 17, she had left

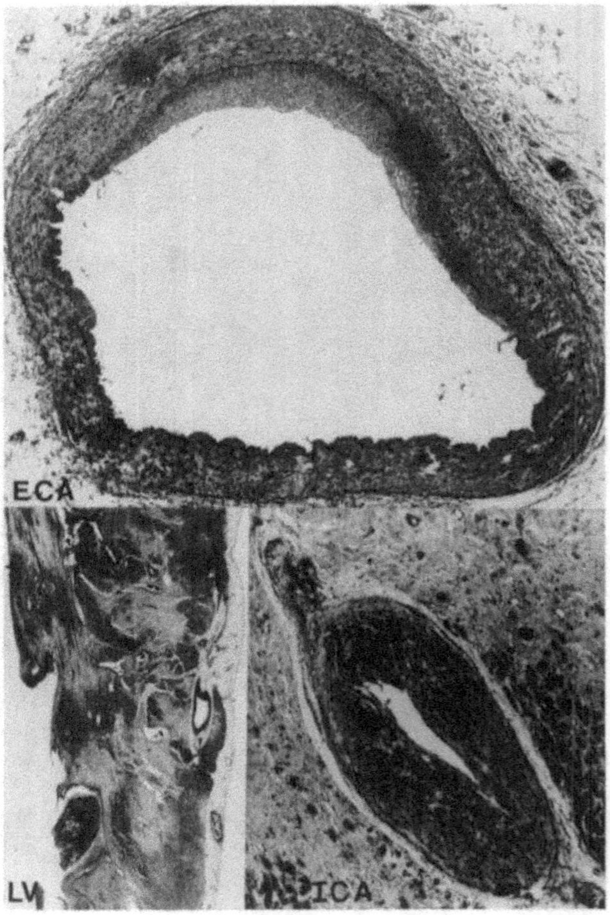

FIGURE 5. The lumens of the major epicardial (E) coronary arteries were virtually normal. (*Upper*): Left anterior descending coronary artery (CA) (original magnification × 14). (*Lower left*): Longitudinal section of wall of left ventricle (LV) which has a transmural scar partially covered by thrombus (original magnification × 4). (*Lower right*): An intramural (I) CA from infarcted ventricular septum has thickened walls and a narrowed lumen (original magnification × 150; all Movat stains).

ventricular hypertrophy by ECG and a normal- to small-sized left ventricular cavity by angiography. At age 26 the left ventricular cavity was still of normal size by echocardiogram, but by age 30 it was considerably dilated. From ages 17 to 30, the intensity of the precordial murmur, ECG findings, and ventricular wall thicknesses also changed. At age 17, the systolic precordial murmur was of grade 2-3/6 in intensity; at age 26, it was grade 5/6 and associated with a thrill, and by age 30 it was absent. The ventricular septum by echocardiogram at age 26 during both peak systole and end-diastole measured about 23 mm in thickness, but at age 30 was only 15 mm in thickness; the left ventricular free wall at age 26 was 27 mm in thickness during peak systole and 14 mm four years later. The left ventricular ejection fraction (by echocardiogram) diminished from 50 percent at age 26 to 10 percent at age 30.

The cause of the transformation of the left ventricular cavity from a nondilated to a dilated one appears to have been the occurrence of transmural left ventricular infarction. Two months before death this patient had severe substernal chest pain associated with nausea and sweating, and approximately two hours after onset, the heart arrested. Although cardiac resuscitation was successful, the mental processes thereafter were slowed. At necropsy, a considerable portion of left ventricular free wall and ventricular septum was transmurally scarred, yet the epicardial coronary arteries were virtually free of atherosclerotic plaques. Thus, hypertrophic cardiomyopathy is a cause of transmural myocardial infarction in the absence of significant narrowing of the epicardial coronary arteries. Although the occurrence of myocardial infarction in hypertrophic cardiomyopathy is established,[2] the cause of the infarction usually is not discernible. Although usually not apparent clinically, transmural myocardial infarction appears to be the most common cause of ventricular cavity dilation in patients with hypertrophic cardiomyopathy. We have previously studied seven patients with hypertrophic cardiomyopathy in whom transmural left ventricular scars were present at necropsy.[2] Severe chronic congestive heart failure and supraventricular arrhythmias were present in six, left ventricular outflow obstruction under basal conditions was absent or minimal in all seven, angina pectoris was absent in all seven, clinical evidence of acute myocardial infarction was present in only one, and significant narrowing of the major epicardial coronary arteries was present in only one. Transmural myocardial infarction has been present at necropsy in 15 percent of the patients with hypertrophic cardiomyopathy we studied.[2]

Summary

Transmural myocardial infarction in the absence of epicardial coronary arterial narrowing is fairly common at necropsy in patients with hypertrophic cardiomyopathy. Although difficult to diagnose clinically in patients with hypertrophic cardiomyopathy, acute myocardial infarction occasionally has a typical presentation, as in the patient presented in this report. More often, however, transmural acute myocardial infarction in patients with hypertrophic cardiomyopathy is not associated with classic signs and symptoms, but leads to production of, or worsening of, congestive cardiac failure which thereafter usually rapidly progresses. Thus, transmural myocardial infarction is a major complication of hypertrophic cardiomyopathy.

References

1 Maron BJ, Roberts WC. Quantitative analysis of cardiac muscle cell disorganization in the ventricular septum of patients with hypertrophic cardiomyopathy. Circulation 1979; 59:689-706

2 Maron BJ, Epstein SE, Roberts WC. Hypertrophic cardiomyopathy and transmural infarction without significant atherosclerosis of the extramural coronary arteries. Am J Cardiol 1979; 43:1086-1102

Hypertrophic cardiomyopathy and complete heart block in infancy*

Barry J. Maron, M.D., Thomas M. Connor, M.D., Capt. (MC), USNR, and William C. Roberts, M.D. *Bethesda, Md.*

Hypertrophic cardiomyopathy (HCM) is a congenital malformation that usually does not present clinically until adulthood.[1,2] However, HCM may be identified during the first year of life[3-5] when it often manifests marked congestive heart failure (CHF).[5] While complete heart block (CHB) due to congenital conducting tissue disorder[6,7] may occur during the first few weeks of life, it is not usually associated with clinical deterioration during infancy.[8,9] This communication describes the unusual association of HCM and congenital CHB in an infant.

A 2-month-old girl had weighed 2.8 kg at term birth by a noninsulin-dependent diabetic mother; CHB with heart rate 40 beats/minute (bpm) (Fig. 1) was known since the first day of life. Severe CHF developed by 3 days of age and an epicardial pacemaker was implanted at a ventricular rate of 100 bpm; digitalis and furosemide were begun. Cardiac catheterization showed left ventricular (LV) pressure 95/12 mm Hg without systolic gradient or mitral regurgitation; LV contractile pattern was normal with an ejection fraction of 0.70. CHF worsened, respiratory failure ensued, and her last month of life was further complicated by disseminated intravascular coagulation.

Necropsy heart weight was 62 gm (normal 23 gm).[10] The ventricular septum was disproportionately thickened relative to LV free wall[11,12] (Fig. 2); septal thickness was 8 mm and LV free wall thickness was 3 mm (ratio 2.7). The coronary arteries were normal and there was no myocardial fibrosis or associated malformations. Marked disorganization of cardiac muscle cells was present in the ventricular septum (Fig. 3); longitudinal cut muscle fibers oriented at oblique and perpendicular angles to each other occupied 17% of myocardium analyzed.[13] LV free wall

From the Cardiology and Pathology Branches, National Heart, Lung and Blood Institute, National Institutes of Health, and the Pediatric Cardiology Section, Department of Pediatrics, National Naval Medical Center and United States Uniformed Health Services Medical School.

Received for publication Feb. 20, 1981; accepted Feb. 27, 1981.

Reprint requests: Barry J. Maron, M.D., Cardiology Branch, NHLBI, Bldg. 10, Room 7B-15, Bethesda, MD 20205.

*The opinions and assertions expressed are those of the authors and do not reflect the official position of the Navy.

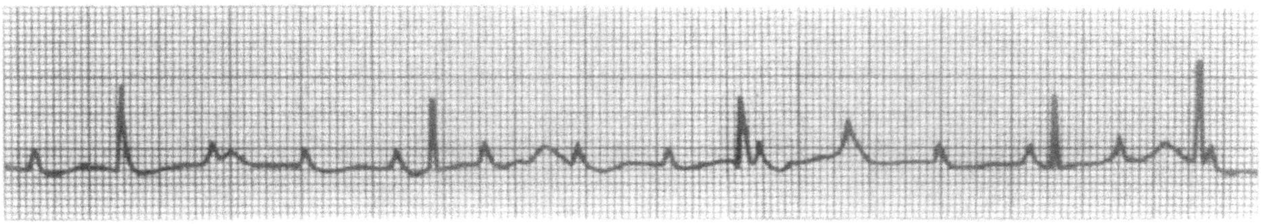

Fig. 1. Rhythm strip showing complete atrioventricular block with ventricular rate of 40 bpm and atrial rate of 120 bpm.

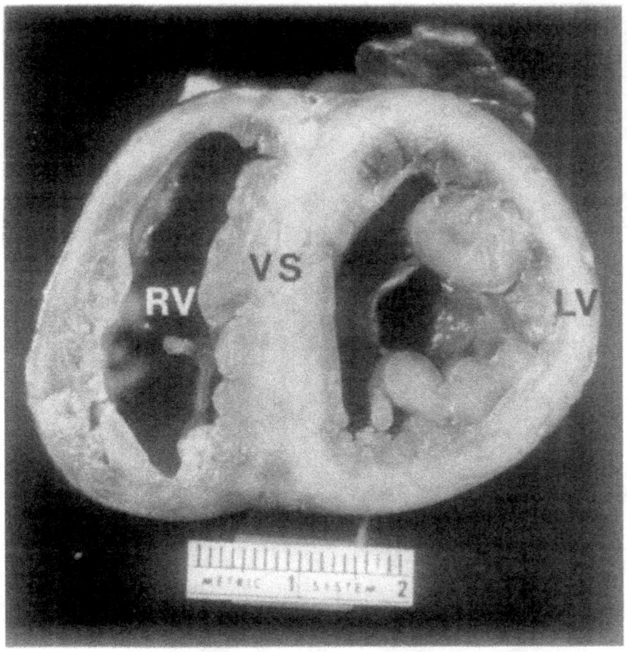

Fig. 2. Heart of the patient with hypertrophic cardiomyopathy and congenital complete heart block. The ventricular septum *(VS)* is substantially thicker than the left ventricular free wall *(LV)*. Note the large left ventricular papillary muscles. *RV* = right ventricular cavity.

cardiac fibers were normally arranged. The AV node area was serially sectioned at 6 μm thickness and every tenth section was stained with hemotoxylin and eosin or elastic van Gieson. AV nodal tissue was normal; however, continuity of the conduction system was interrupted in the penetrating portion of the AV bundle (bundle of His) as it coursed through the central fibrous body (Fig. 4). Distal to this area of discontinuity the conducting tissue was normal and the AV bundle divided normally into left and right bundle branches. Because of necropsy findings, M-mode and two-dimensional echocardiograms were obtained in the infant's parents. The mother's echogram was normal but the father had asymmetric hypertrophy of the ventricular septum; septal thickness was 18 mm and LV free wall thickness was 10 mm (ratio 1.8).

Congenital CHB most commonly occurs in structurally normal hearts, but 30% to 50% of such CHB is associated with a variety of congenital cardiovascular malformations.[6-8] Our patient demonstrates the previously undescribed association of congenital CHB and HCM. CHB has been reported previously in a few patients with HCM[14-21]; however, since the age at which CHB was identified in those patients ranged from 10 to 71 years, it is unlikely that CHB was congenital.

Our patient appears to have the typical genetically transmitted form of HCM[22]: (1) disproportionate ventricular septal thickening,[23, 24] (2) marked disorganization of cardiac muscle cells in the ventricular septum,[13] and (3) echocardiographic identification of asymmetric hypertrophy of the ventricular septum in the patient's father.[22] CHB in our patient appears to have emanated from a developmental defect in the conduction system—discontinuity in the AV bundle at the level of the central fibrous body. This anatomic abnormality of conducting tissue has not been reported in HCM,[25] but has been described in infants with congenital CHB and other congenital heart malformations.[6] Whether the conduction system defect in our patient is a morphologic component of HCM or an etiologically independent abnormality can not be determined with certainty at this time.

The patient's clinical course suggests that CHB and slow ventricular rate may not have contributed substantially to her clinical deterioration and eventual death. The patient's CHF progressed markedly even after ventricular pacemaker insertion. The probability that our patient's clinical deterioration was due primarily to the underlying cardiomyopathic process is supported by our previous experience that HCM commonly presents with CHF in the first year of life and leads to death in a substantial percentage of such patients.[5] This patient emphasizes the broad morphologic spectrum of HCM and suggests that HCM should be considered in an infant with CHB and CHF.

REFERENCES

1. Frank S, Braunwald E: Idiopathic hypertrophic subaortic stenosis. Clinical analysis of 126 patients with emphasis on the natural history. Circulation **37**:759, 1968.
2. Shah PM, Adelman AG, Wigle ED, Gobel FL, Burchell HB, Hardarson T, Curiel R, De la Calzada C, Oakley CM, Goodwin JF: The natural (and unnatural) course of hypertrophic obstructive cardiomyopathy. A multicenter study. Circ Res **34** and **35**(suppl II):II-179, 1973.
3. Barr PA, Celermajer JM, Bowdler JD, Cartmill TB: Idiopathic hypertrophic obstructive cardiomyopathy causing severe right ventricular outflow tract obstruction in infancy. Br Heart J **35**:1109, 1973.
4. Maron BJ, Edwards JE, Henry WL, Clark CE, Bingle GJ,

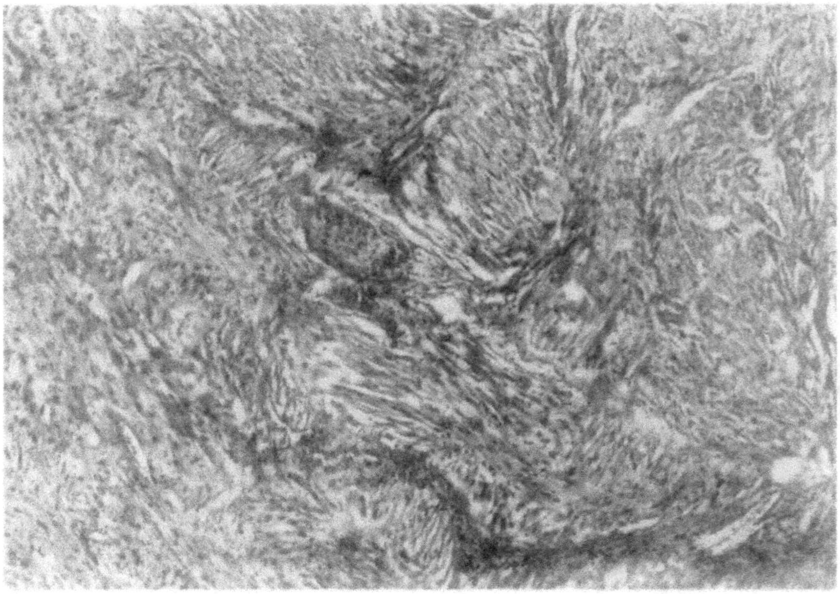

Fig. 3. Area of ventricular septum showing disorganized arrangement of the cardiac muscle cells. Bundles of longitudinally cut cardiac muscle cells are oriented obliquely and perpendicularly to each other. (Hematoxylin and eosin stain; original magnification ×100).

Epstein SE: Asymmetric septal hypertrophy (ASH) in infancy. Circulation **50:**809, 1974.

5. Maron BJ, Tajik AJ, Ruttenberg HD, Graham TP, Atwood GF, Victorica BE, Lie JT, Roberts WC: Hypertrophic cardiomyopathy in infants: Clinical features and natural history. Circulation (In press)
6. Lev M: Pathogenesis of congenital atrioventricular block. Progr Cardiovasc Dis **15:**145, 1973.
7. James TN, McKone RC, Hudspeth AS: De Subitaneis Mortibus X. Familial congenital heart block. Circulation **51:**379, 1975.
8. Nakamura FF, Nadas AS: Complete heart block in infants and children. N Engl J Med **270:**1261, 1964.
9. Michaëlsson M, Engle MA: Congenital complete heart block: An international study of the natural history. Cardiovasc Clin **4:**86, 1972.
10. Gould SE: Pathology of the heart and blood vessels. 3rd ed. Springfield, Ill., 1968, Charles C Thomas, p 1139.
11. Menges H, Brandenburg RO, Brown AL: The clinical, hemodynamic and pathologic diagnosis of muscular subvalvular aortic stenosis. Circulation **24:**1126, 1961.
12. Henry WL, Clark CE, Epstein SE: Asymmetric septal hypertrophy (ASH): Echocardiographic identification of the pathognomonic anatomic abnormality of IHSS. Circulation **47:**225, 1973.
13. Maron BJ, Sato N, Roberts WC, Edwards JE, Chandra RS: Quantitative analysis of cardiac muscle cell disorganization in the ventricular septum: Comparison of fetuses and infants with and without congenital heart disease and patients with hypertrophic cardiomyopathy. Circulation **60:**685, 1979.
14. Luisada AA: Subaortic muscular stenosis and complete heart block in an adolescent. Chicago Med School Q **25:**169, 1965.
15. Matlof HJ, Zener JC, Harrison DC: Idiopathic hypertrophic subaortic stenosis and heart block. Cycle-to-cycle variation as a function of alterations in preload and afterload. Am J Cardiol **32:**719, 1973.
16. Johnson AD, Daily PO: Hypertrophic subaortic stenosis complicated by high degree heart block: Successful treatment with an atrial synchronous ventricular pacemaker. Chest **67:**491, 1975.

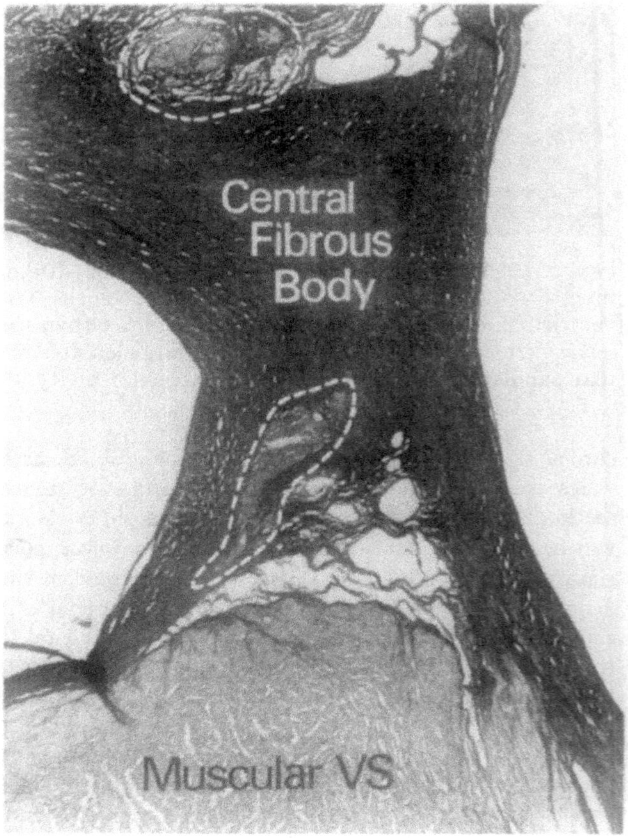

Fig. 4. A section of the atrioventricular bundle area showing interruption in the penetrating portion of the bundle at the level of the central fibrous body. The two unconnected portions of conducting tissue are outlined by *broken lines. VS* = ventricular septum.

17. Spilkin S, Mitha AS, Matisonn RE, Chesler E: Complete heart block in a case of idiopathic hypertrophic subaortic stenosis. Noninvasive correlates with the timing of atrial systole. Circulation **55:**418, 1977.
18. Chmielewski CA, Riley RS, Mahendran A, Most AS: Complete heart block as a cause of syncope in asymmetric septal hypertrophy. AM HEART J **93:**91, 1977.
19. Tajik AJ, Guiliani ER, Frye RL, McGoon DC, Nunn SL: Muscular subaortic stenosis with complete heart block. Am J Cardiol **31:**101, 1973.
20. Gavrilescu S, Gavrilescu M, Streian C, Luca C: Hypertrophic obstructive cardiomyopathy associated with complete heart block. Pathologic correlations in a case studied with His bundle electrography. Acta Cardiol (Brux) **29:**241, 1974.
21. Gilgenkrantz JM, Cherrier F, Petitier H, Dodinot B, Houplon M, Legoux J: Cardiomyopathie obstructive du ventricule gauche avec bloc auriculo-ventriculaire complet; Considerations thérapeutiques. Arch Mal Coeur **61:**439, 1968.
22. Clark CE, Henry WL, Epstein SE: Familial prevalence and genetic transmission of idiopathic hypertrophic subaortic stenosis. N Engl J Med **289:**709, 1973.
23. Maron BJ, Henry WL, Roberts WC, Epstein SE: Comparison of echocardiographic and necropsy measurements of ventricular wall thicknesses in patients with and without disproportionate septal thickening. Circulation **55:**341, 1977.
24. Henry WL, Ware J, Gardin JM, Hepner SI, McKay J, Weiner M: Echocardiographic measurements in normal subjects. Growth-related changes that occur between infancy and early adulthood. Circulation **57:**278, 1978.
25. James TN, Marshall TK: De Subitaneis Mortibus XII. Asymmetric hypertrophy of the heart. Circulation **51:**1149, 1975.

Hypertrophic cardiomyopathy and cardiac muscle cell disorganization revisited: Relation between the two and significance

Barry J. Maron, M.D., and William C. Roberts, M.D. *Bethesda, Md.*

The disorganized arrangement of cardiac muscle cells in left ventricular (LV) myocardium of patients with hypertrophic cardiomyopathy (HCM) was first described by Teare in his initial report on this condition in 1958.[1] Teare described eight patients with "asymmetric hypertrophy or muscular hamartoma of the heart" and a "bizarre and disorganized arrangement of muscle bundles" in the asymmetrically hypertrophied ventricular septum (IVS). During the ensuing several years a number of reports based on analysis of tissue obtained at necropsy, operation, or biopsy confirmed the observations of Teare and concluded that a disorganized arrangement of cardiac muscle cells in the IVS was a characteristic and consistent morphologic feature of patients with HCM.[2-18] Electron microscopic analysis showed that the disorganized cells often had highly irregular shapes and large branches that extended in several directions and formed intercellular junctions with several adjacent cells.[5]

Subsequently, however, bizarre cellular architecture was identified in the LV wall of patients with congenital or acquired cardiac diseases other than HCM.[19-30] This finding led some investigators to dispute the usefulness of IVS disorganization as a marker of HCM.[19, 24-26] The present report reexamines the issue of cardiac muscle cell disorganization in the LV wall of patients with HCM and discusses the potential significance of this morphologic alteration.

SOURCES OF CONTROVERSY

Several considerations explain the lack of consensus among investigators regarding the sensitivity and specificity of cardiac muscle cell disorganization for HCM: (1) Lack of generally accepted or standardized histologic criteria for what constitutes abnormal cellular arrangement; as a consequence each investigator has necessarily created his or her own concept and definition of cellular disorganization. (2) No standard guidelines have been established regarding the *extent* of cellular malalignment in the IVS that is necessary to constitute a histologic diagnosis of HCM; most assessments of disorganization in these patients have only been qualitative or semiquantitative estimates. (3) Reports suggesting that IVS disorganization is an unreliable marker for HCM have been based on analysis of extremely small numbers of patients with HCM or were virtually limited to patients with cardiac diseases other than HCM.[24-27] (4) Most studies of IVS architecture in HCM have been made without selecting tissue sections from a standard location and orientation. As will be discussed, optimal identification of cellular disorganization depends greatly on analyzing sections obtained *perpendicular to the long-axis of the LV* (i.e., in the transverse plane)[13] (Fig. 1).

DEFINITION OF CARDIAC MUSCLE CELL DISORGANIZATION

Over the past 10 years we have assessed the presence and extent of cardiac muscle cell disorganization in a large number of patients with HCM or with other cardiac diseases.[6, 7, 10, 13, 14, 16, 20-23, 28, 31] Based upon this experience, a classification of cardiac muscle cell disorganization has been proposed that emphasizes more obvious abnormalities of cellular arrangement and excludes minimal deviations from normal parallel alignment.[13] The types of cellular disorganization in this classification are illustrated in Fig. 2. *Type I disorganization* (Figs. 2 and 3) is most common and consists of cardiac muscle cells (or bundles of cells) which are aligned perpendicularly and obliquely to each other, usually forming tangled masses or "pinwheel" configura-

From the Cardiology and Pathology Branches, National Heart, Lung and Blood Institute, National Institutes of Health.

Received for publication Feb. 26, 1981; accepted March 11, 1981.

Reprint requests: Barry J. Maron, M.D., Bldg. 10, Room 7B-15, National Heart, Lung and Blood Institute, Bethesda, MD 20205.

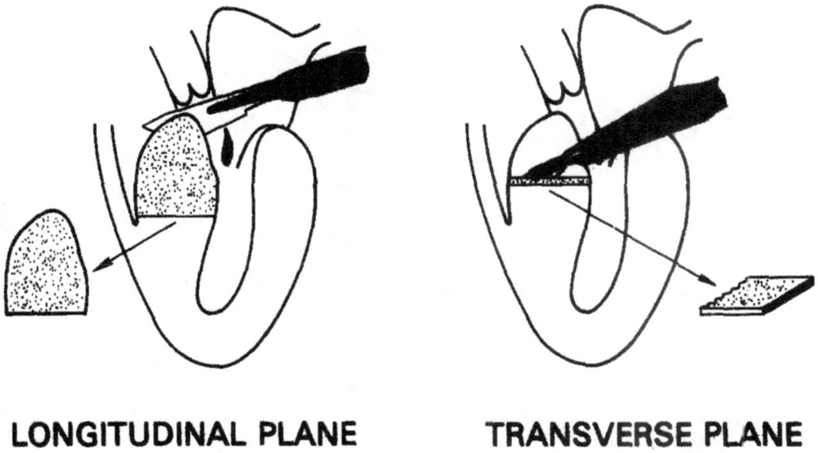

Fig. 1. Orientations in which sections of ventricular septum may be taken at necropsy. *Transverse* sections were obtained in a plane perpendicular to the long-axis of the left ventricle; *longitudinal* sections were obtained in a plane parallel to the long axis of the left ventricle.

tions. This abnormal arrangement can only be identified in those areas of myocardium in which the cells are cut longitudinally (i.e., appear to be rectangularly shaped). Thus type I disorganization can not be observed in regions of myocardium consisting of transversely cut cardiac muscle cells. *Type II disorganization* (Fig. 2) is relatively uncommon and consists of interlacing bundles of cells; cardiac muscle cells within these bundles are normally arranged. Abnormally arranged cardiac muscle cells within or at the edges of areas of fibrosis are generally not considered to be examples of "true" disorganization, nor are disoriented cells within trabeculations, at points of convergence of major muscle bundles, or adjacent to interstitial spaces containing blood vessels.

IVS disorganization, as described herein, pertains specifically to intercellular abnormalities (i.e., the malalignment *between cardiac musle cells*). Disarray of myofibrils and myofilaments within individual muscle cells also has been described by light and electron microscopic studies of plastic embedded tissue from patients with HCM[5, 7] (Fig. 4). These intracellular abnormalities are most pronounced in branched, stellate-shaped, and disorganized cells (Figure 4, *A*), but are found occasionally in cells with more normal shapes and orientation. However, since disarray of myofibrils and myofilaments also commonly occurs in a variety of other cardiac conditions in both humans and animals, it must be considered to be a nonspecific morphologic alteration.[5, 25, 32-34] In addition to the chracteristic cellular changes, the myocardium of patients with HCM shows nonspecific ultrastructural changes of interstitial fibrosis, cellular hypertrophy, and cellular degeneration similar to those present in patients with long-standing hypertrophy of other causes.[7, 32]

QUANTITATIVE HISTOLOGIC ANALYSIS OF SEPTAL DISORGANIZATION

Recently, we devised a quantitative histologic method[13] that permits a more critical assessment of the relative area of myocardium occupied by disorganized cells, and which thereby obviates many of the aforementioned problems. In brief, hematoxylin and eosin stained tissue sections are photographed and the images enlarged sufficiently to occupy 30- by 40-inch positive prints; this enlargement results in a magnification of as much as 5,000 times the original tissue section. A transparent cellulose overlay is then placed over the print and areas of myocardium occupied by disorganized cardiac muscle cells are demarcated on the overlay (Fig. 5). Each area into which the tissue section has been divided is then quantitated utilizing a video-planimetry system.

In developing this quantitative method we found that cardiac muscle cell disorganization was present more frequently and to a significantly greater extent in tissue sections obtained in an orientation perpendicular to the LV long-axis (Figs. 1 and 6) in the region of maximum IVS thickening. This is true primarily because tissue sections taken perpendicular to the long-axis are comprised of relatively large areas of longitudinally cut cardiac muscle cells. Since the most common form of disorganization (type I) can only be viewed in areas of myocardium where cells are cut longitudinally, analysis of tissue sections taken in this plane affords an enhanced opportunity to identify cellular disorganization. In

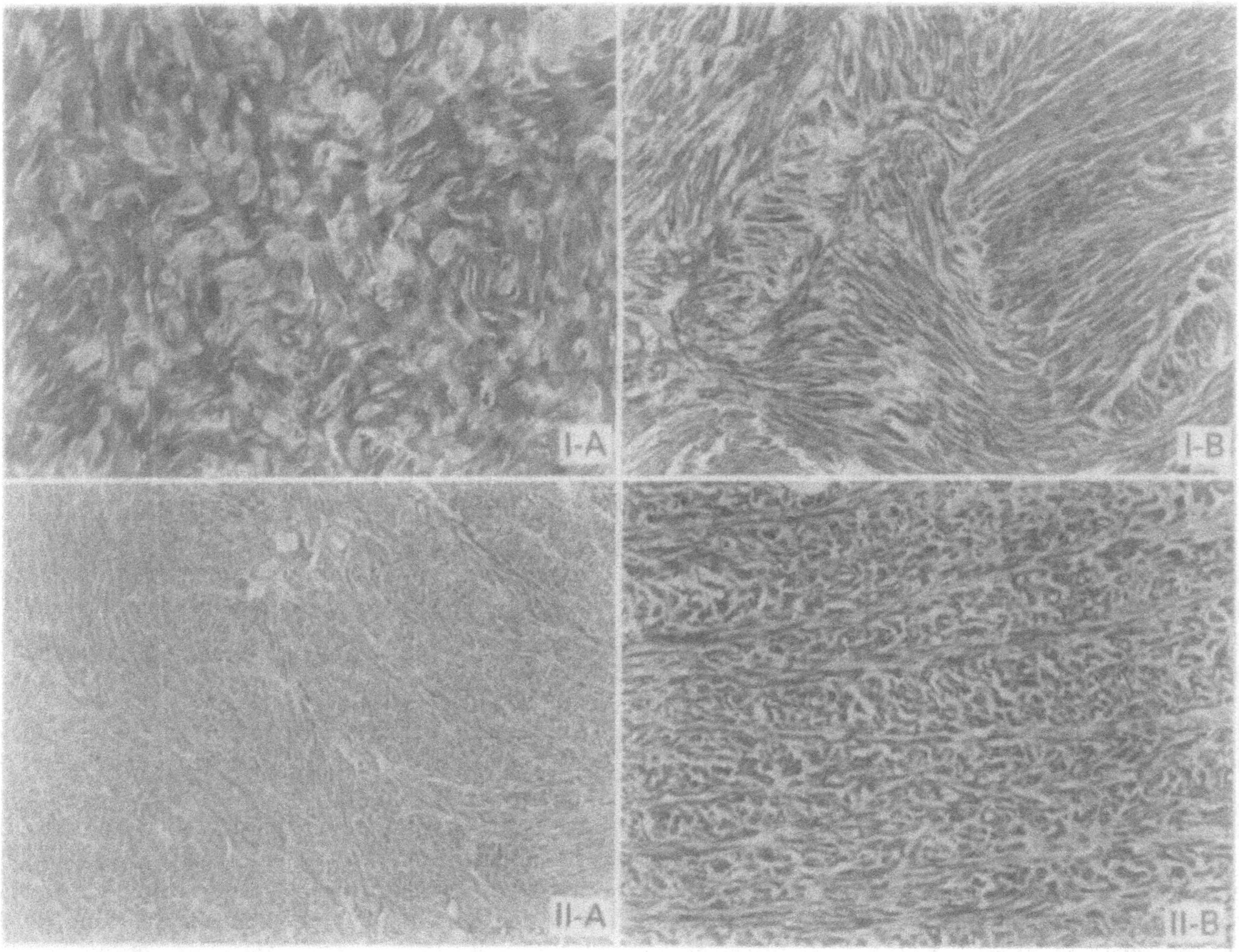

Fig. 2. Classification of four major types of cardiac muscle cell disorganization present in ventricular septal myocardium. *Type I-A (upper left)* consists of areas of myocardium in which adjacent cardiac muscle cells were aligned perpendicularly and obliquely to each other. *Type I-B (upper right)* consists of relatively broad bundles of muscle cells that are oriented at oblique and perpendicular angles to each other; cells within these bundles are, however, normally arranged. *Type II-A (lower left)* consists of relatively narrow (usually one or two cells wide), longitudinally cut bundles of cells that are interlaced in various directions among larger groups of transversely cut cells (which appear circular). This type of disorganization gave the myocardium a "swirled" appearance. *Type II-B (lower right)* is similar to type II-A disorganization, except that the narrow, longitudinally cut bundles of cells are more linear. (Original magnifications: I-A, ×130; I-B and II-A, ×40; II-B, ×80; all hematoxylin and eosin stain.)

contrast, tissue sections taken parallel to the long-axis of the LV contain relatively few longitudinally cut cells (Fig. 7), thereby restricting the opportunity to observe the most common variety of cellular disorganization (type I). Most importantly, by using this quantitative method we found that it was possible to *reliably distinguish at necropsy patients with HCM from patients with normal hearts or other cardiac diseases (congenital, coronary or valvular) based on the extent of cellular disorganization present in the IVS.*

Disorganization is common and usually widespread in the IVS of patients with HCM (Figs. 8 and 9). Of the 78 patients with HCM that we have now studied quantitatively, 94% had some IVS disorganization; in 86% of the 78 patients disorganized cells occupied 5% or more of the tissue section. Cellular disorganization may be remarkably extensive in the IVS of these patients, as is evidenced by the fact that 55% had ≥25% of the section involved and 24% had ≥50% of the section occupied by disorganized cells. The mean area of IVS disorganized for the 78 patients was 32% (Fig. 8).

The presence of marked cellular disorganization

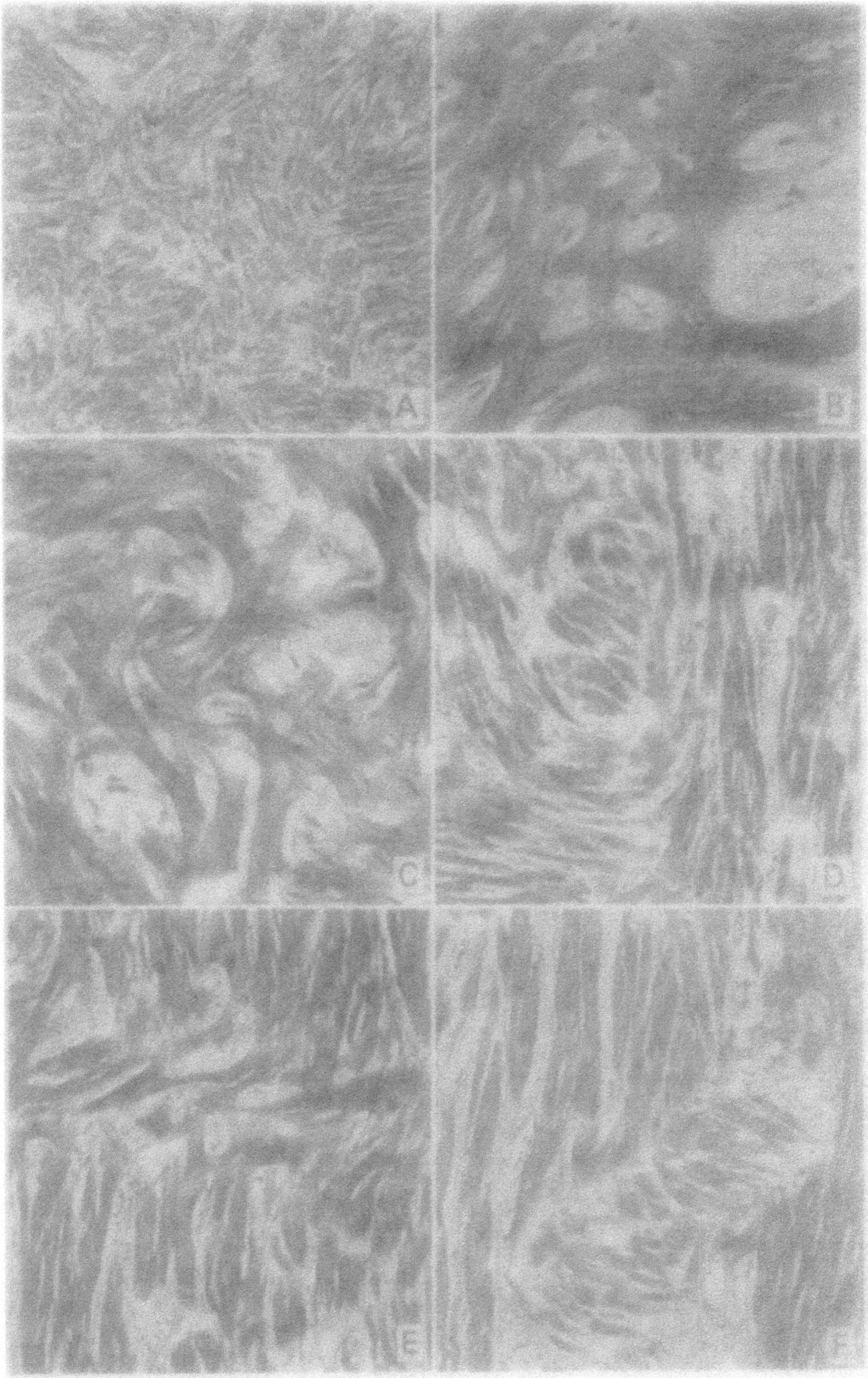

Fig. 3. Examples of the most common form of cellular disorganization (type I-A). The wide morphologic spectrum of this lesion is illustrated. *A,* "Chaotic" pattern in which adjacent cells are arranged at perpendicular and oblique angles to each other (Original magnification ×55). *B,* "Swiss cheese" appearance that results when adjacent cells are oriented at particularly acute angles, (Original magnification ×350). *C,* Tangled arrangement of cardiac muscle cells in whorled configurations (Original magnification ×350). *D,* "Whorl" pattern in which some cells are oriented circumferentially to other cells (Original magnification ×130). *E* and *F,* Patterns in which small groups of cells are oriented at extremely acute angles to larger groups of cells (Original magnification ×130). All hematoxylin and eosin stain.

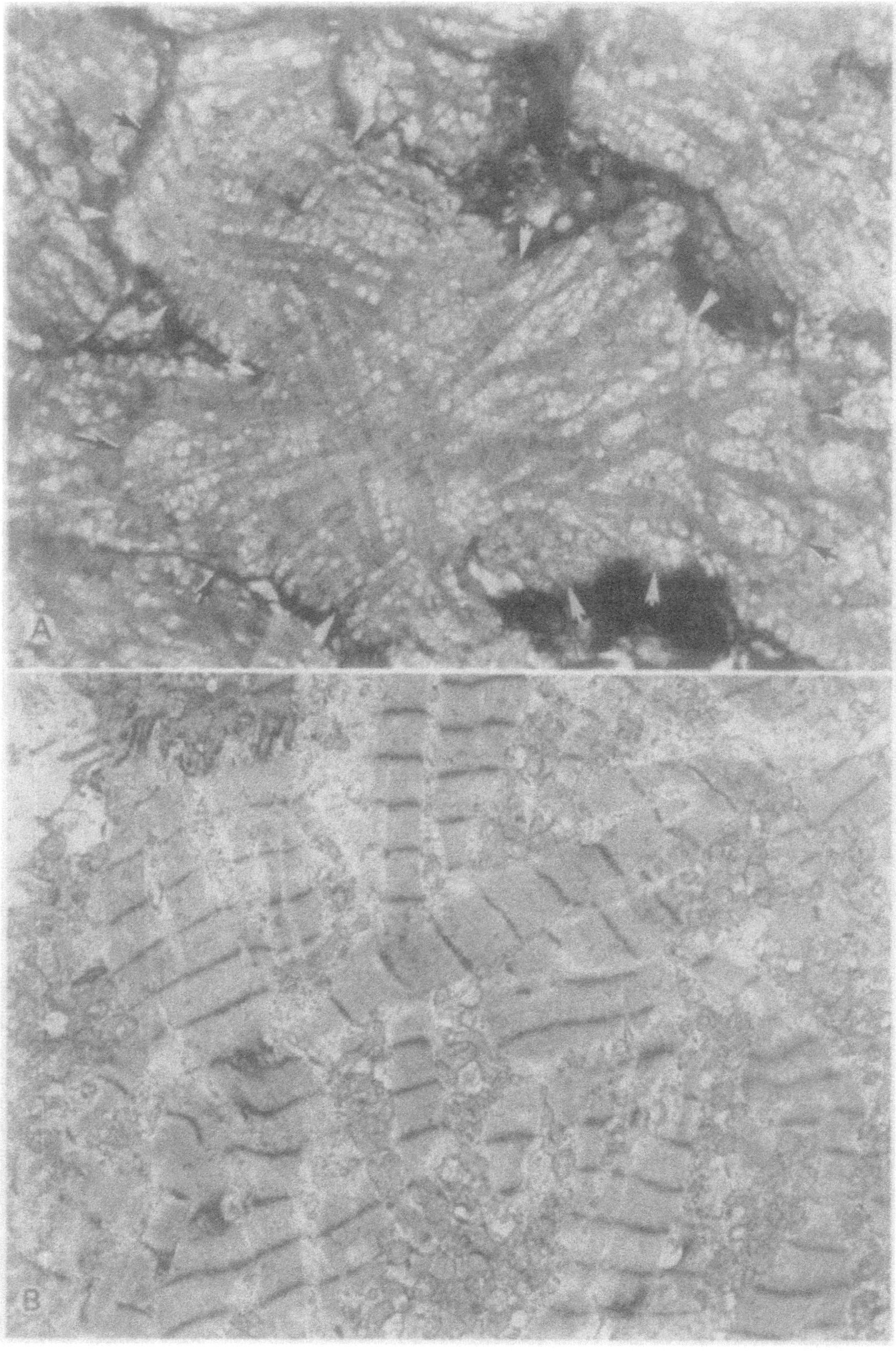

Fig. 4. Photomicrographs of plastic embedded tissue from the ventricular septum of a patient with HCM. *A,* A hypertrophied, stellate-shaped muscle cell having intercellular connections with several adjacent cells. Obliquely and transversely oriented myofibrils are shown in the center. The boundaries of the cell are outlined by arrowheads. (Alkaline toluidine blue stain; Original magnification ×675.) *B,* Electron micrograph of part of a similar cardiac muscle cell showing an area of myofibrillar disarray. (Original magnification ×5,900.)

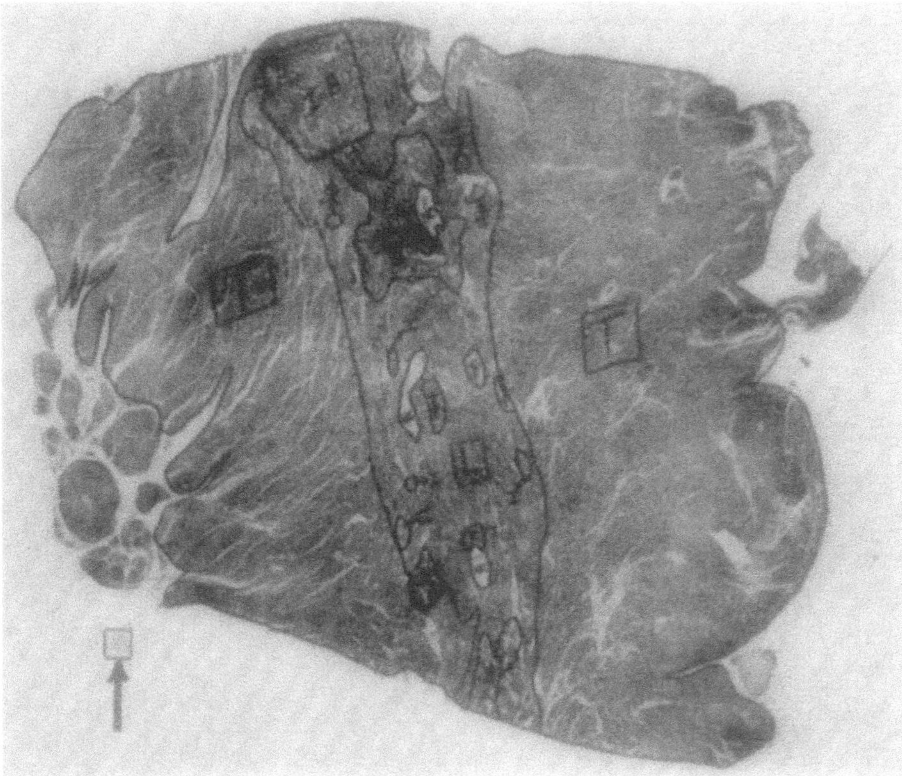

Fig. 5. Photographic enlargement (with transparent overlay in place) of a section of ventricular septum from a patient with HCM. Actual size of tissue section is shown at lower left *(arrow)* for comparison. Magnification of the print relative to the original tissue section is ×2,000.

in the IVS also links patients within the broad clinical and pathologic spectrum of HCM. For example, marked IVS disorganization is present in patients with *and* patients without obstruction to LV outflow, indicating that disorganization does not result secondarily from elevation in LV systolic pressure. The extent of disorganization also does not differ appreciably between patients with or without symptoms and, indeed, extensive IVS disorganization may even occur in patients with HCM who never experienced a symptomatic manifestation of the disease but subsequently died of noncardiac causes[8] (personal observations in four patients, mean age 66 years; mean IVS disorganization 18%). Also, no relation exists between the extent of IVS disorganization and heart weight, indicating that disorganization is not simply a manifestation of marked cardiac hypertrophy.

The absence of IVS disorganization, however, does not exclude the diagnosis of HCM (Figs. 8 and 9). Of our 78 patients, 6% showed no IVS disorganization in the tissue section analyzed; these patients were similar clinically or in other morphologic respects from those patients with IVS disorganization. Conversely, the presence *per se* of malaligned cardiac muscle cells in the IVS is *not* pathognomonic of HCM. About 20% of 360 infants, children, and adults with cardiac diseases other than HCM (or with normal hearts) studied by our quantitative method had some disorganized cells in the IVS tissue section. However, in almost two thirds of these patients the areas of disorganization were small (Figs. 10 and 11) (involving <5% of the tissue section analyzed) and the mean area of IVS disorganized for the 360 controls was only about 1%. The "cut-point" that appears to best distinguish HCM from other cardiac diseases, histologically, is IVS disorganization involving 5% or more of the relevant parts of the tissue section. IVS disorganization of ≥5% is a highly specific (93%) as well as sensitive (89%) histologic marker of HCM. *Hence, it is not the presence or absence of IVS disorganization that distinguishes patients with HCM from those with other heart diseases (or normal hearts), but rather the extent to which disorganization is present.*

DISTRIBUTION OF CELLULAR DISORGANIZATION IN THE LV WALL

While cardiac muscle cell disorganization is present extensively in the IVS of most patients with

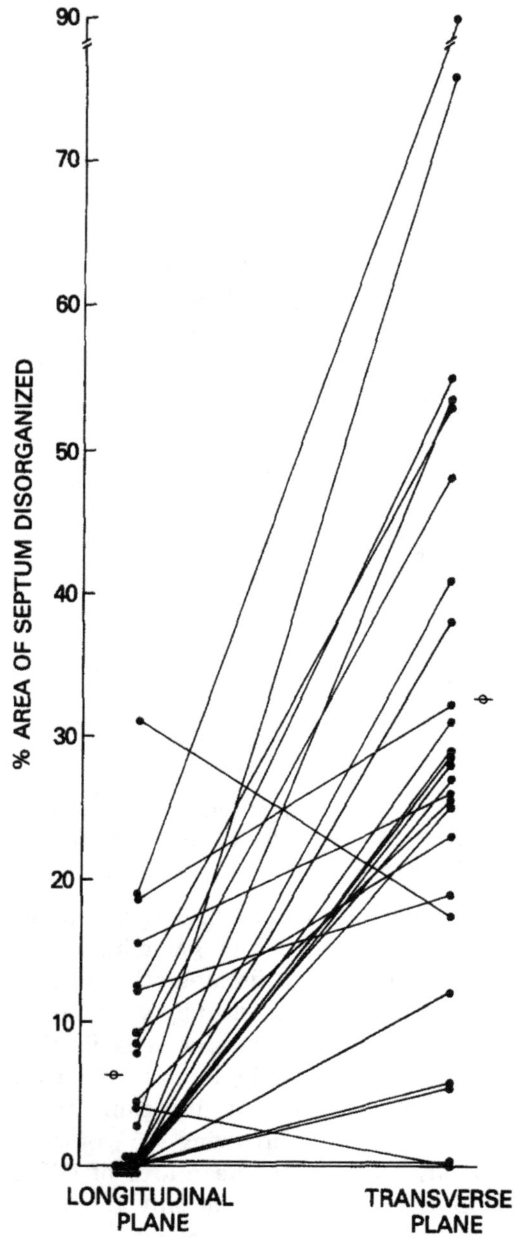

Fig. 6. Percent area of ventricular septum occupied by disorganized cardiac muscle cells, shown separately for tissue sections taken in the transverse and longitudinal planes from 25 patients with HCM. Symbols for individual patients are connected by *solid lines.* θ = mean values.

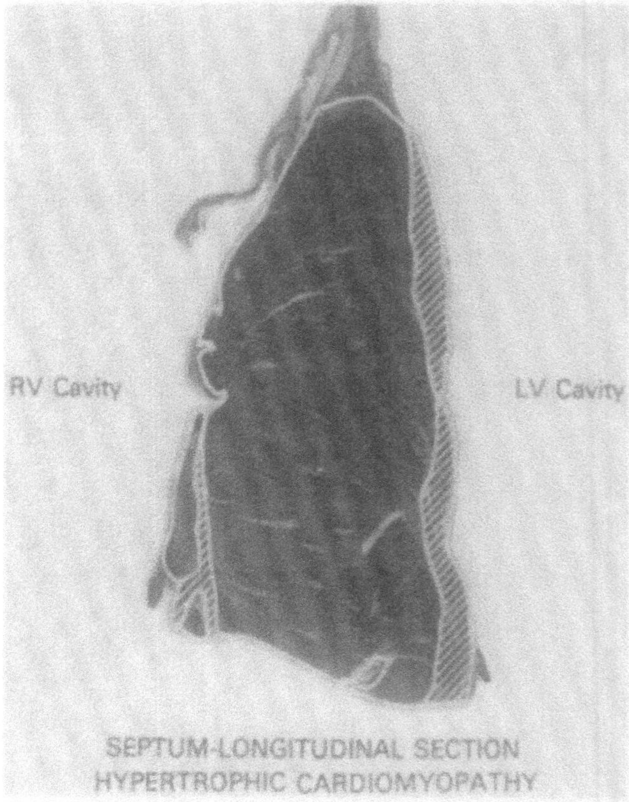

Fig. 7. "Map" of section of ventricular septum obtained parallel to the long-axis of the left ventricle superimposed on actual tissue section. Longitudinally cut cardiac muscle cells occupy only the small (*striped*) areas adjacent to the right ventricular *(RV)* and left ventricular *(LV)* cavities. The section is from a 56-year-old woman with HCM.

HCM, this distortion of myocardial architecture is also often present in other regions of the LV.[16, 17, 19] A recent quantitative study (of tissue sections taken in the transverse plane) in 52 patients with HCM[16] showed a considerable amount of disorganization to be present in the LV free wall (mean 24 ± 3%), although somewhat less than in the IVS (35 ± 4%) (Fig. 12). The extensive degree to which cellular disorganization is present in the LV wall of patients with HCM is evidenced by the fact that the mean LV wall disorganization (combined IVS and free wall tissue sections) in 52 patients was 28 ± 3%.

LV free wall disorganization is also common in patients with acquired or congenital heart diseases other than HCM (ie., in 47%). However, when present in such patients, cellular disorganization is usually limited in extent (mean area of section involved only 2%). Hence, small foci of cardiac muscle cell disorganization are: (1) not uncommon in LV myocardium from patients with cardiac diseases other than HCM but (2) are more commonly present in the LV free wall than in the IVS (Fig. 13).

UTILITY OF MYOCARDIAL BIOPSY FOR HISTOLOGIC DIAGNOSIS OF HCM

Confirmation from necropsy studies that marked cardiac muscle cell disorganization in LV myocar-

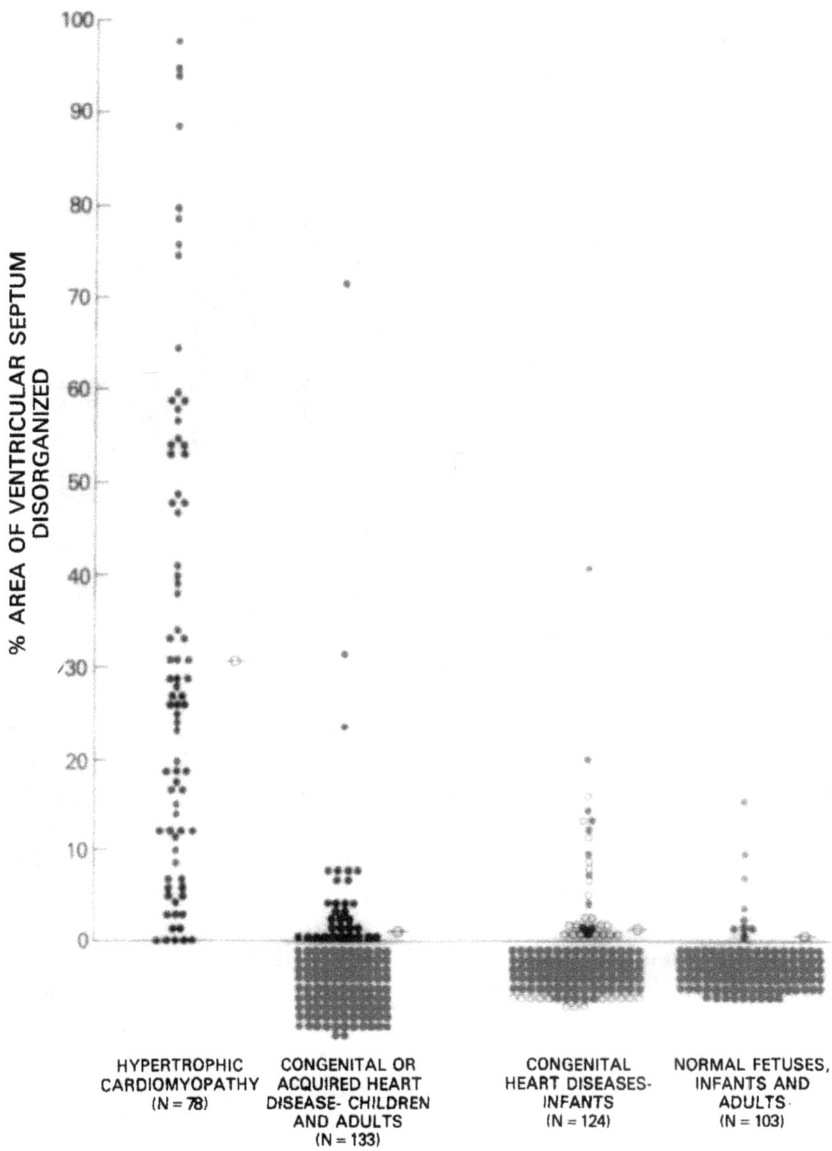

Fig. 8. Percent area of ventricular septum occupied by disorganized cardiac muscle cells in 78 patients with HCM, 133 children and adults with other congenital or acquired heart diseases, 124 infants with a variety of other congenital heart diseases, and 103 normal fetuses, infants, and adults studied at necropsy. Thirty-three infants with aortic or pulmonic valve atresia and a hypoplastic ventricular cavity are indicated by *open circles.* All 78 patients (38 males and 40 females) with HCM had experienced cardiac symptoms during life or died suddenly before the onset of symptoms; ages ranged from stillborn to 70 years (mean 28 years). θ = mean values.

dium is both a highly sensitive and specific histologic marker for HCM raises the attractive possibility that closed chest endomyocardial biopsy of the right side of the IVS septum[18, 35-39] might be useful in establishing the diagnosis of HCM during life. While some investigators have suggested that myocardial biopsy (with electron microscopic analysis of the tissue) is reliable in making the histologic diagnosis of HCM,[18] others have not found such biopsies to be useful in this regard.[38] Since the distribution of cardiac muscle cell disorganization is usually "patchy" (ie., nonhomogeneous) (Fig. 14) in the IVS, it is unlikely that the sampling of only a limited region of IVS by biopsy will provide a reliable estimate of overall myocardial disorganization in patients with HCM.

Also, it is not possible to evaluate the arrangement of large *groups* of cells (Fig. 2) in small tissue samples obtained by biopsy. For example, the patterns of type I-B and type II disorganization constitute malalignment between muscle bundles and can only be appreciated in larger tissue sections. Tissue artifacts related to the biopsy technique and preparation of the tissue may further complicate histologic interpretation of small biopsy specimens. The limitation of analyzing small tissue samples to make the histologic diagnosis of HCM is illustrated by a comparative study of IVS tissue resected at the time of operation (myotomy-myectomy) and subsequently at necropsy in the same 18 patients (Fig. 15).[40] At necropsy, disorganization was present in all 18 patients and was extensive (≥5%) in 16. Disorganization extensive enough to suggest the diagnosis of HCM (≥5%) was present in the operative specimens of only six (33%) of the 18 patients.

CELLULAR DISORGANIZATION IN ANIMALS WITH HCM

Spontaneously occurring primary myocardial disease, with pathologic and clinical features resembling in many respects that of hypertrophic cardiomyopathy in man, has also been described in dogs and cats.[41, 42] Cardiac muscle cell disorganization in the IVS, similar in appearance and extent to that characteristically present in patients with HCM, not uncommonly occurs in these feline and canine forms of the disease. IVS disorganization involving ≥ 5% of the tissue section was observed in 15 (30%) of 51 cats and in 2 of 10 dogs with HCM (each of which showed an abnormal IVS-LV free wall ratio).

Hence this histologic abnormality is not confined to the human variety of the disease, but appears to represent an anatomic linkage between different species in which HCM occurs. Furthermore, marked IVS disorganization is distinctly uncommon in dogs and cats with normal hearts or with cardiac diseases other than HCM (present in only about 2% of 160 control animals studied) and therefore is a highly specific finding (98%) for feline or canine HCM.

ETIOLOGY OF CARDIAC MUSCLE CELL DISORGANIZATION

In patients with HCM, cellular disorganization (like asymmetric LV hypertrophy) is probably a congenital, developmental alteration of the heart.[6, 43] The number of patients less than 1 year of age with this disease that have been studied at necropsy is still relatively small. Nevertheless, marked IVS disorganization appears to be common and usually extensive in infants with HCM (Figs. 16 and 17),[6, 43] although not a feature of the normal developing (embryonic or fetal) and neonatal heart.[24, 44] The extent of IVS disorganization in infants with HCM does not differ substantially from that present in adults (Fig. 17), and the qualitative appearance of disorganization in infants and older patients with HCM is usually similar (i.e., type I) (Fig. 16,*A*).

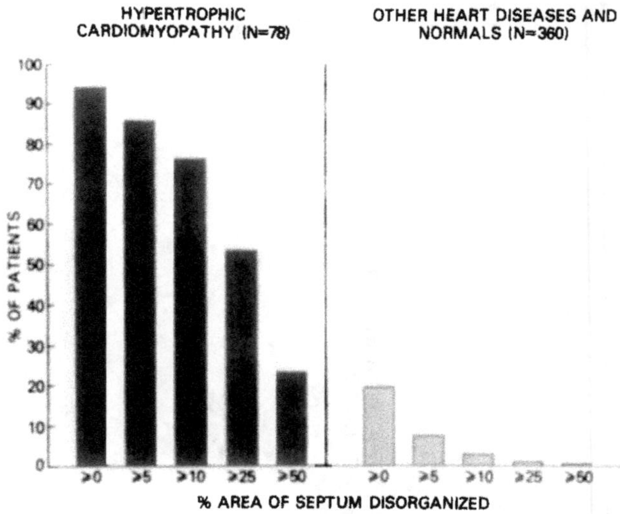

Fig. 9. Extent of septal disorganization at necropsy in 78 patients with HCM and 360 controls with congenital or acquired heart diseases other than HCM (or normal hearts). Each of the comparisons achieved high statistical significance ($p < 0.001$).

In the majority of instances, HCM appears to be a disease that is genetically transmitted as an autosomal dominant trait.[45, 46] Since marked cardiac muscle cell disorganization may be congenital, it is reasonable to postulate that this bizarre cellular architecture represents a morphologic manifestation of the underlying genetic defect present in HCM. However, absolute confirmation of this hypothesis must await demonstration that those patients with marked cellular disorganization studied at necropsy indeed have the genetically transmitted form of HCM and that those patients with no or minimal disorganization have a nongenetic (and presumably etiologically distinct) form of the disease.

Some investigators have maintained that cellular disarray in HCM results secondarily from unique mechanical stresses to which the LV is exposed (e.g., the prolonged period of isometric contraction during mid and late ventricular systole).[24] Cited as support for this theory is the presence of disorganized cardiac muscle cells in the diminutive IVS of infants who have died of complex congenital heart diseases associated with a hypoplastic ventricular cavity (i.e., aortic or pulmonic valve atresia), in which prolonged isometric contraction may also theoretically occur

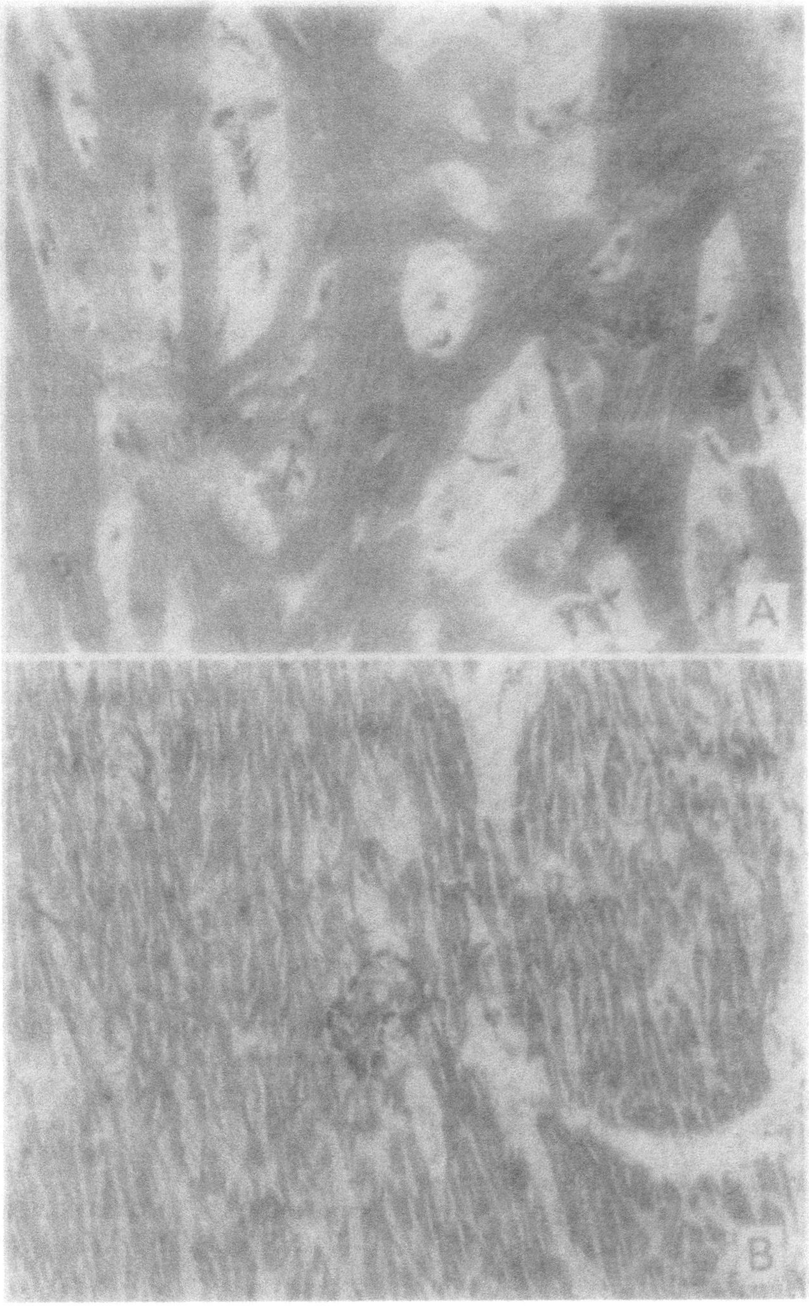

Fig. 10. Photomicrographs of the same area of ventricular septal myocardium from a 52-year-old woman with severe valvular aortic stenosis. *A,* At a relatively high magnification of ×350 an abnormal arrangement of cardiac muscle cells typical of HCM is shown. *B,* Same area of myocardium shown at a much lower magnification of ×55. The area of disorganization (outlined by ***broken line***) impressively abnormal at higher magnification in *A* is barely discernible in *B* and constitutes only an extremely small part of the overall tissue section. (Hematoxylin and eosin stain.)

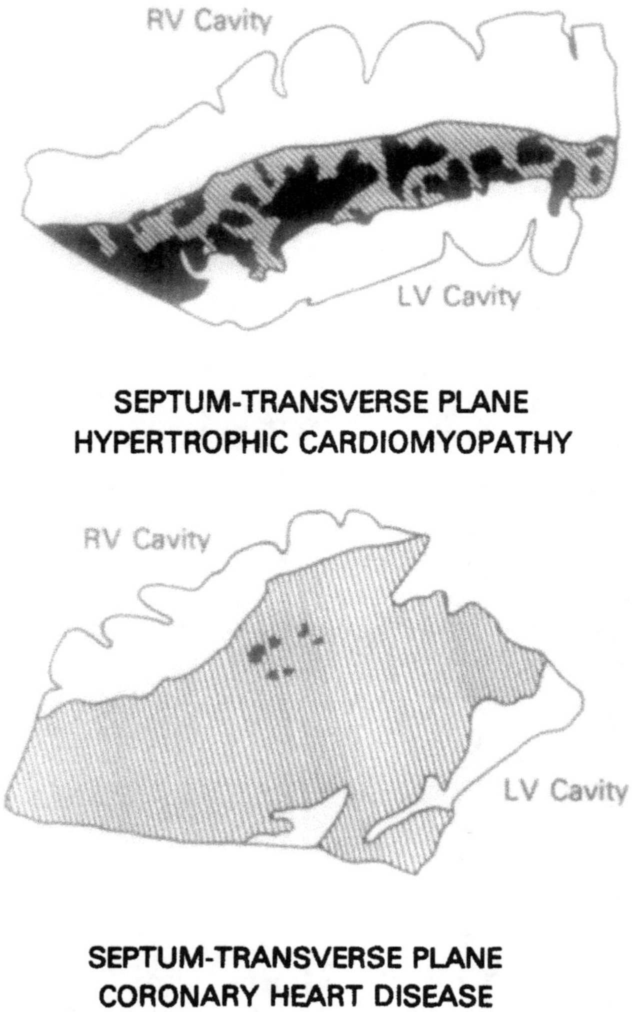

Fig. 11. Representative "maps" of ventricular septal tissue sections in the transverse plane from two patients with cardiac muscle cell disorganization. At the *top* is a 14-year-old boy with HCM. *Below* is a 50-year-old man with coronary heart disease and concentric ventricular hypertrophy. *Striped areas* represent cut and normally longitudinally arranged cardiac muscle cells. *Clear areas* adjacent to the left ventricular *(LV)* and right ventricular *(RV)* cavities contain muscle cells cut transversely. *Solid areas* represent foci of disorganized cardiac muscle cells. In the patient with HCM, disorganized cardiac muscle cells occupy about 50% of the relatively small striped area; in contrast, in the patient with coronary heart disease the disorganized areas are very small and together represent less than 1% of the relatively large striped area.

during life. We have found no quantitative morphologic evidence, however, to support this hypothesis.[14] Our histologic analysis of 33 infants with aortic or pulmonic valve atresia showed that the extent of IVS disorganization was: (1) extremely limited (mean area of IVS disorganized about 2%), (2) did not differ substantially from that present in infants

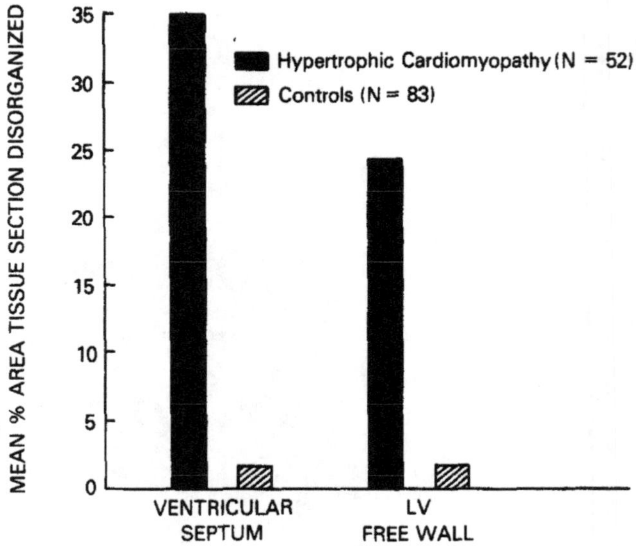

Fig. 12. Extent of cardiac muscle cell disorganization at necropsy in the ventricular septum and left ventricular (LV) free wall of 52 patients with HCM, compared to 83 control patients. For both the septum and free wall, the percent disorganization in patients with HCM significantly exceeded that in control patients ($p < 0.001$). Percent disorganization shown for the free wall represents a combination of the anterior and posterior free wall tissue sections.

with other congenital heart diseases associated with normal-sized or dilated ventricular cavities, and (3) was significantly less than that present in infants, children, or adults with HCM (mean area of IVS disorganized 32%; $p < 0.001$) (Fig. 8).

Nevertheless, it is probably possible for cardiac muscle cell disorganization to be "acquired." For example, relatively small areas of abnormal cellular orientation have been identified in operatively resected right ventricular muscle from patients with congenital heart malformations other than HCM.[34] These disorganized cells were in areas of interstitial fibrosis and were most common in older patients (particularly those ≥ 30 years of age). Most studies of cardiac muscle cell disorganization, however, have excluded from analysis myocardium in or near regions of fibrosis.[13-15]

CLINICAL AND FUNCTIONAL SIGNIFICANCE OF CARDIAC MUSCLE CELL DISORGANIZATION

The relevance of bizarre myocardial architecture to clinical course in patients with HCM is unclear. However, certain speculations may be warranted. First, sudden death in patients with HCM probably results from a primary ventricular arrhythmia.[47-49] It is possible that the disorganized myocardial cells dispersed throughout the LV wall of these patients

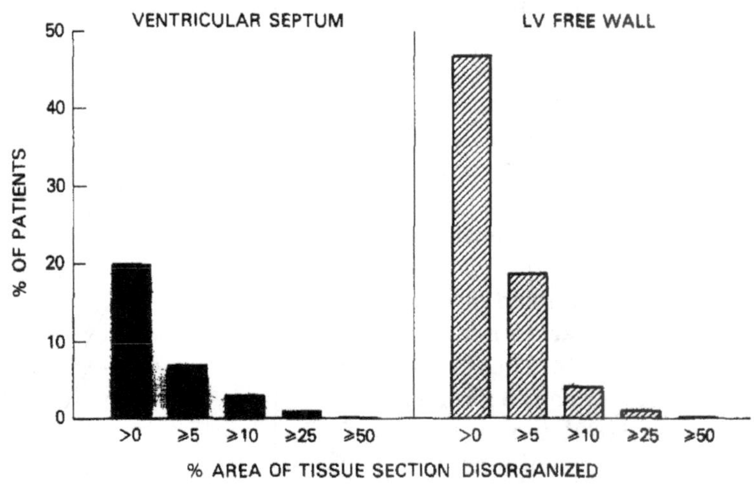

Fig. 13. Extent of cardiac muscle cell disorganization in the left ventricular myocardium of patients *with cardiac diseases other than HCM (or normal hearts)*. Shown separately are the ventricular septum (360 patients) and left ventricular free wall (83 patients).

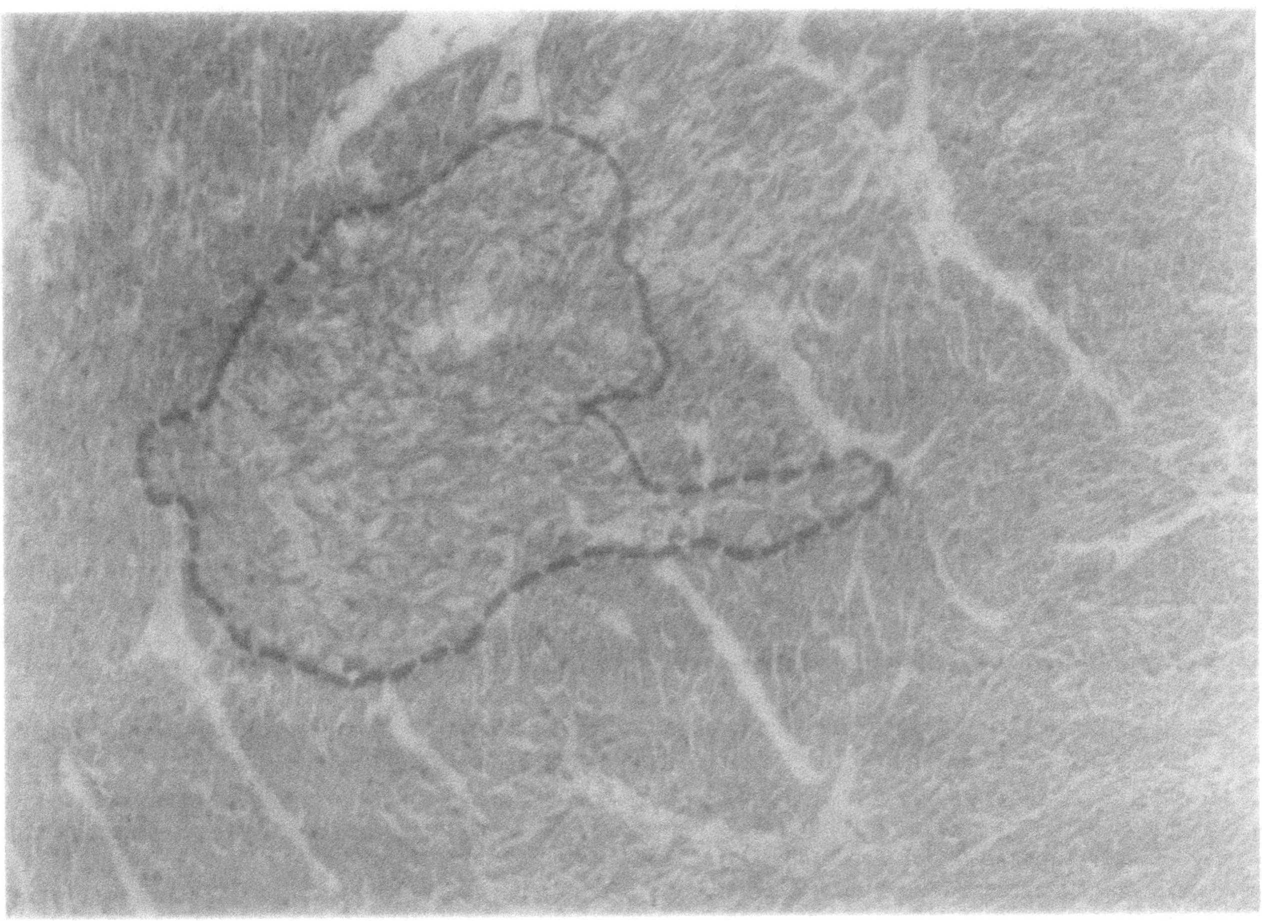

Fig. 14. Portion of ventricular septum from a 14-year-old boy with HCM. *Broken line* demarcates a focus of cardiac muscle cell disorganization. Note that myocardium surrounding this area is normally arranged. (Original magnification ×40.)

may be inefficient in producing an orderly pattern of electrical depolarization and repolarization, impair the transmission of normal electrophysiologic impulses, and thereby serve as a nidus for primary, fatal ventricular arrhythmias. In support of this hypothesis is the fact that the most extensive LV wall disorganization found at necropsy in patients with HCM has been in those young patients (≤ 25 years of age) in whom sudden and unexpected death was the first definitive manifestation of cardiac disease.[16]

Second, it has been suggested that abnormally arranged cardiac muscle cells probably do not produce an efficient pattern of contractility and may be responsible for the occurrence of marked functional limitation in those patients with HCM who do not have obstruction to LV outflow.[7] While the number of patients with nonobstructive HCM (no or small LV outflow gradient under basal conditions and after provocative maneuvers) that have been studied at necropsy is relatively small, such patients appear to have somewhat greater amounts of combined IVS and LV free wall disorganization than do patients with obstruction. Certainly, greater numbers of patients with the nonobstructive form of HCM will have to be studied in this fashion to determine definitively whether the extent and distribution of cellular disorganization can explain their unfavorable clinical course.

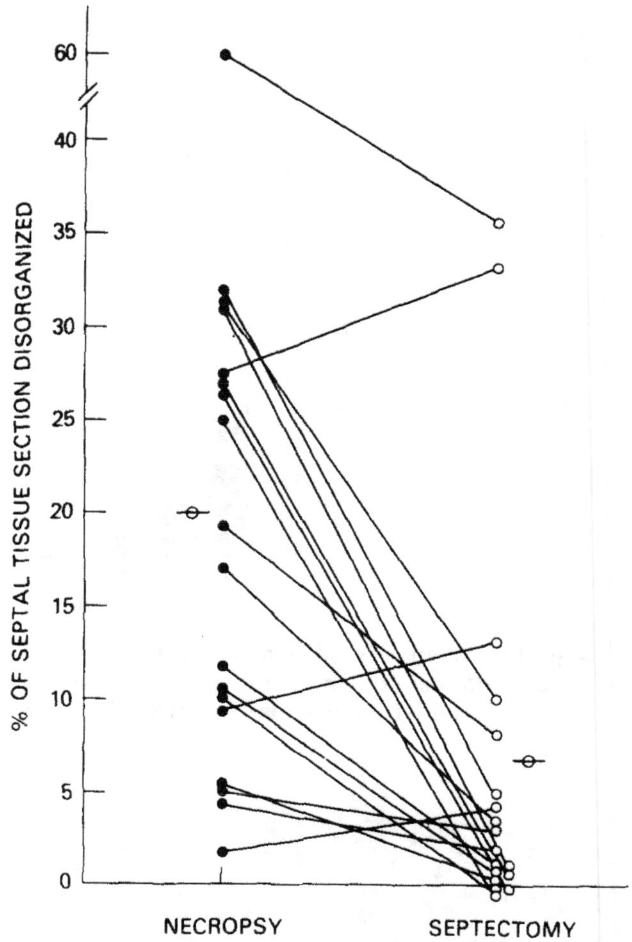

Fig. 15. Comparison of the extent of cardiac muscle cell disorganization in histologic sections obtained at operation (septal myotomy–myectomy) and at necropsy in 18 patients with HCM. Values for extent of disorganization found at necropsy and at operation are connected by a *solid line* for each patient.

CONCLUSIONS

The presence of abnormally arranged cardiac muscle cells in the IVS is not pathognomic or unique to patients with HCM. However, disorganization is characteristically common and widespread in the IVS of such patients and it is possible to reliably distinguish at necropsy patients with HCM from patients with other cardiac diseases (or normal hearts), based on the *extent* of cellular disorganization present in the IVS.

Quantitative histologic studies have demonstrated that marked disorganization (≥ 5% of a IVS tissue section) is both a highly sensitive (89%) and specific (93%) histologic marker for HCM, while disorganization involving < 5% of a section makes this diagnosis unlikely. The extensive nature of the bizarre distortion of IVS architecture in patients with HCM is illustrated by the fact that the mean area of tissue section disorganized in 78 patients was 32%, compared to about 1% in 360 patients with a variety of other congenital or acquired heart diseases or normal hearts. Furthermore, marked IVS disorganization is commonly present in patients showing a variety of clinical, hemodynamic, and morphologic manifestations of HCM, including those with and those without obstruction to LV outflow.

Substantial cardiac muscle cell disorganization is not limited to the IVS in HCM, but in most patients it is also widely distributed in the LV free wall (mean area of section disorganized, 24%). The presence of cellular disorganization in both IVS and LV free wall supports the view that this histologic lesion may represent a diffuse cardiomyopathic process in most patients with HCM.

IVS disorganization probably represents a primary (congenital) derangement of myocardial architecture since marked cellular disorganization is characteristic of infants with HCM (and is absent in the normal developing heart). The high frequency

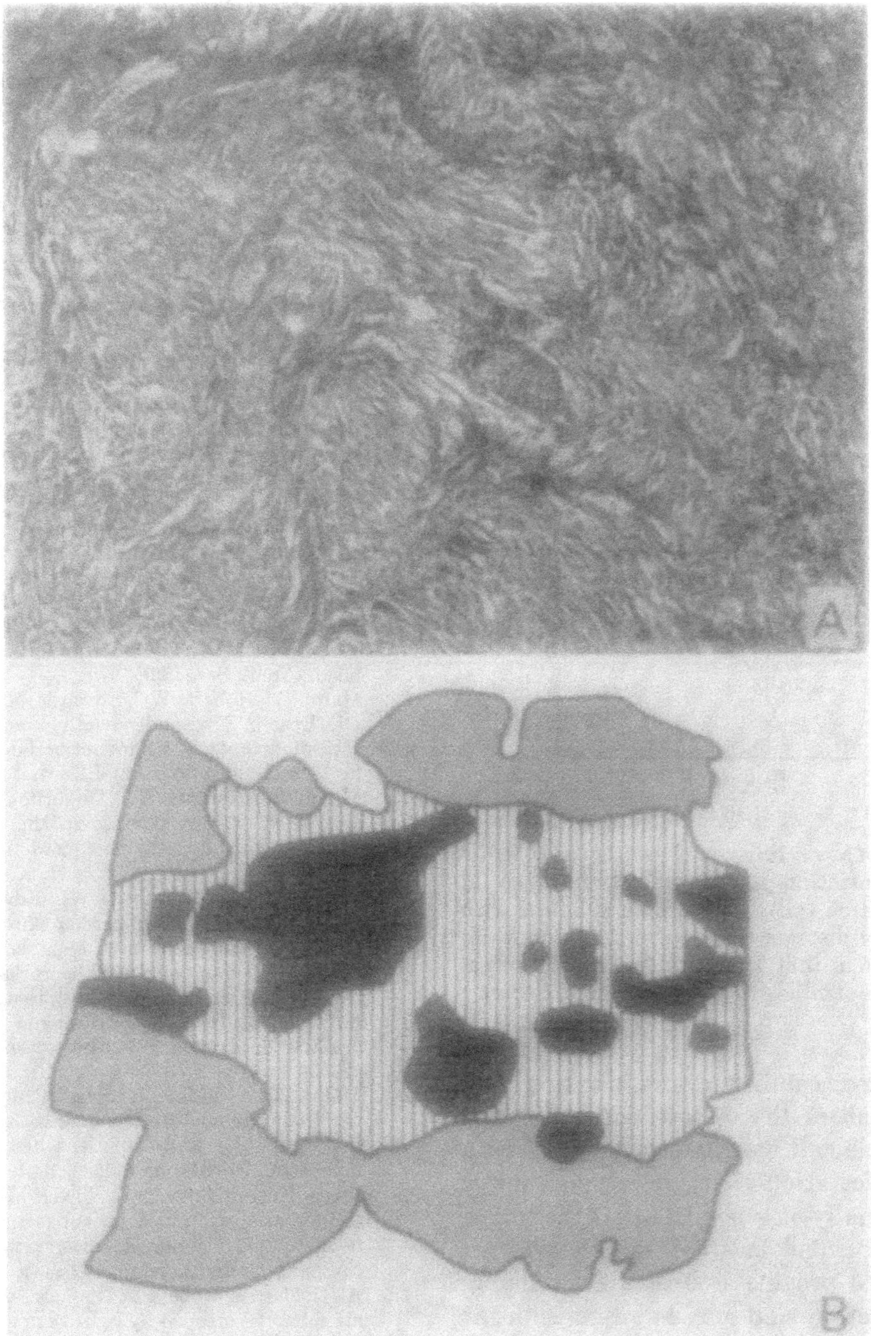

Fig. 16. *A,* Histologic section of ventricular septum in the transverse plane from a 2-month-old infant with HCM. Abnormally arranged bundles of cardiac muscle cells are oriented obliquely and perpendicularly to each other. (Hematoxylin and eosin stain; original magnification ×100.) *B,* Histologic "map" of the ventricular septal tissue section showing extensive distribution of cellular disorganization *(solid areas)* within the area of longitudinally cut cardiac muscle cells *(striped area);* the *outer dotted areas* are muscle cells cut transversely.

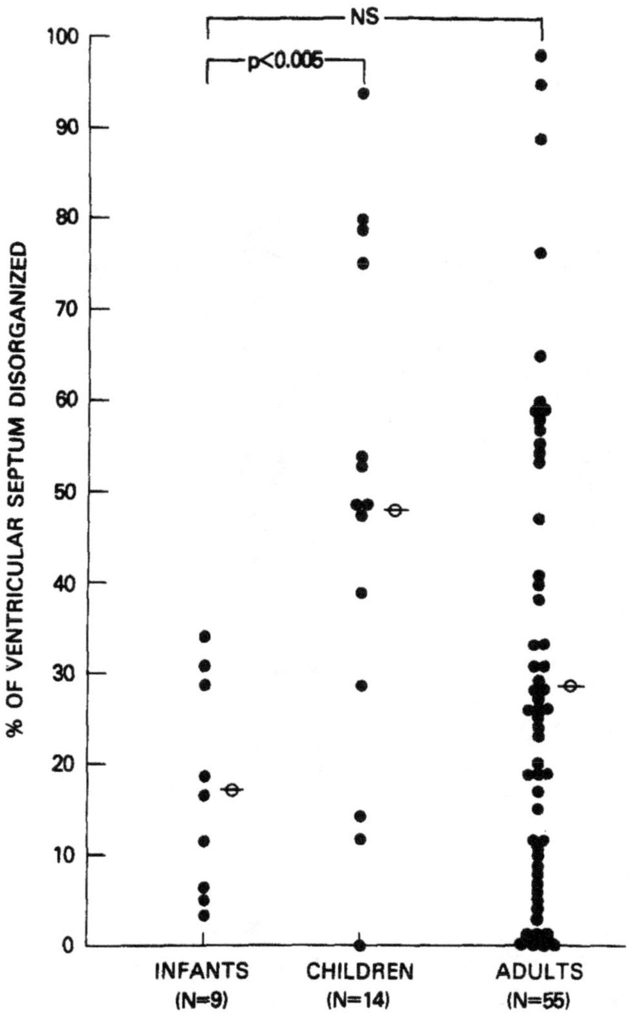

Fig. 17. Comparison at necropsy of the extent of ventricular septal disorganization in infants (stillborn to 11 months of age), children (11 to 17 years), and adults with HCM. The extent of disorganization in infants does not differ significantly from that in adults; however, disorganization in infants is significantly less than in children.

with which marked cellular disorganization and genetic transmission of the disease occur suggests that cardiac muscle cell disorganization may be a morphologic manifestation of an underlying genetic defect in HCM. Finally, it is possible that the foci of disorganized myocardial cells in the LV wall of patients with HCM provide a substrate for malignant ventricular ectopy and may be responsible, at least in part, for the occurrence of premature sudden death in such patients.

REFERENCES

1. Teare D: Asymmetrical hypertrophy of the heart in young patients. Br Heart J **20**:1, 1958.
2. Pare JA, Fraser RG, Pirozynski WJ, Shanks JA, Stubington D: Hereditary cardiovascular dysplasia: A form of familial cardiomyopathy. Am J Med **31**:37, 1961.
3. Van Noorden S, Olsen EG, Pearse AG: Hypertrophic obstructive cardiomyopathy. A histological, histochemical and ultrastructural study of biopsy material. Cardiovasc Res **5**:118, 1971.
4. Snijder J, DeJong J, Meyer A: Light microscopical, ultrastructural and histochemical aspects of hypertrophic obstructive cardiomyopathy (subaortic stenosis). J Mol Cell Cardiol **3**:81, 1971.
5. Ferrans VJ, Morrow AG, Roberts WC: Myocardial ultrastructure in idiopathic hypertrophic subaortic stenosis: A study of operatively excised left ventricular outflow tract muscle in 14 patients. Circulation **45**:769, 1972.
6. Maron BJ, Edwards JE, Henry WL, Clark CE, Bingle GJ, Epstein SE: Asymmetric septal hypertrophy (ASH) in infancy. Circulation **50**:809, 1974.
7. Maron BJ, Ferrans VJ, Henry WL, Clark CE, Redwood DR, Roberts WC, Morrow AG, Epstein SE: Differences in distribution of myocardial abnormalities in patients with obstructive and nonobstructive asymmetric septal hypertrophy (ASH): Light and electron microscopic findings. Circulation **50**:436, 1974.
8. Pomerance A, Davies MJ: Pathological features of hypertrophic obstructive cardiomyopathy (HOCM) in the elderly. Br Heart J **37**:305, 1975.
9. Knierium H-J, Stroobandt R, Meyer H, Bouregeois M: Hypertrophic nonobstructive cardiomyopathy caused by disorder of the myofiber texture. Virchows Arch (Pathol Anat) **367**:209, 1975.
10. Roberts WC, Ferrans VJ: Pathologic anatomy of the cardiomyopathies. Idiopathic dilated and hypertrophic types, infiltrative types, and endomyocardial disease with and without eosinophilia. Human Pathol **6**:288, 1975.
11. Maron BJ, Henry WL, Clark CE, Redwood DR, Roberts WC, Epstein SE: Asymmetric septal hypertrophy in childhood. Circulation **53**:9, 1976.
12. Maron BJ, Roberts WC, Edwards JE, McAllister HA, Foley DD, Epstein SE: Sudden death in patients with hypertrophic cardiomyopathy: Characterization of 26 patients without functional limitation. Am J Cardiol **41**:803, 1978.
13. Maron BJ, Roberts WC: Quantitative analysis of cardiac muscle cell disorganization in the ventricular septum of patients with hypertrophic cardiomyopathy. Circulation **59**:689, 1979.
14. Maron BJ, Sato N, Roberts WC, Edwards JE, Chandra RS: Quantitative analysis of cardiac muscle cell disorganization in the ventricular septum: Comparison of fetuses and infants with and without congenital heart disease and patients with hypertrophic cardiomyopathy. Circulation **60**:685, 1979.
15. Fujiwara H, Kawai C, Hamashima Y: Myocardial fascicle and fiber disarray in 25 μ-thick sections. Circulation **59**:1293, 1979.
16. Maron BJ, Anan TJ, Roberts WC: Quantitative analysis of the distribution of cardiac muscle cell disorganization in the left ventricular wall of patients with hypertrophic cardiomyopathy. Circulation **63**:882, 1981.
17. Wigle ED, Adelman AG, Silver MD: Pathophysiological considerations in muscular subaortic stenosis. *In* Wolstenholme GE, O' Connor M, editors: Hypertrophic obstructive cardiomyopathy. London, 1971, J & A Churchill, p 63.
18. Alexander CS, Gobel FL: Diagnosis of idiopathic hypertrophic subaortic stenosis by right ventricular septal biopsy. Am J Cardiol **34**:142, 1974.
19. Sutton MSJ, Lie JT, Anderson KR, O'Brien PC, Frye RL: Histopathological specificity of hypertrophic obstructive cardiomyopathy. Myocardial fibre disarray and myocardial fibrosis. Br Heart J **44**:433, 1980.
20. Maron BJ, Ferrans VJ, White RI: Unusual evolution of acquired infundibular stenosis in patients with ventricular septal defect: Clinical and morphologic observations. Circulation **48**:1092, 1973.
21. Maron BJ, Edwards JE, Ferrans VJ, Clark CE, Lebowitz

EA, Henry WL, Epstein SE: Congenital heart malformations associated with disproportionate ventricular septal thickening. Circulation **52**:926, 1975.

22. Maron BJ, Clark CE, Henry WL, Fukuda T, Edwards JE, Mathews EC, Redwood DR, Epstein SE: Prevalence and characteristics of disproportionate ventricular septal thickening in patients with acquired or congenital heart diseases: Echocardiographic and morphologic findings. Circulation **55**:489, 1977.
23. Maron BJ, Fisher RS: Sudden infant death syndrome: Cardiac pathologic observations in infants with SIDS. AM HEART J **93**:762, 1977.
24. Bulkley BH, Weisfeldt ML, Hutchins GM: Isometric cardiac contraction. A possible cause of the disorganized myocardial pattern of idiopathic hypertrophic subaortic stenosis. N Engl J Med **296**:135, 1977.
25. Dingemans KP, Becker AE: Specificity of cellular and myofibrillar disorientation in hypertrophic obstructive cardiomyopathy. Arch Pathol Lab Med **101**:493, 1977.
26. Bulkley BH, Weisfeldt ML, Hutchins GM: Asymmetric septal hypertrophy and myocardial fiber disarray: Features of normal, developing and malformed hearts. Circulation **56**:292, 1977.
27. Van der Bel-Kahn J: Muscle fiber disarray in common heart diseases. Am J Cardiol **40**:355, 1977.
28. Maron BJ, Edwards JE, Moller J, Epstein SE: Prevalence and characteristics of disproportionate ventricular septal thickening in infants with congenital heart disease. Circulation **59**:126, 1979.
29. Becu L, Somerville J, Gallo A: "Isolated" pulmonary valve stenosis as part of more widespread cardiovascular disease. Br Heart J **38**:472, 1976.
30. Somerville J, Becu L: Congenital heart disease associated with hypertrophic cardiomyopathy. Johns Hopkins Med J **140**:151, 1977.
31. Maron BJ, Epstein SE: Hypertrophic cardiomyopathy. Recent observations regarding the specificity of three hallmarks of the disease: Asymmetric septal hypertrophy, septal disorganization and systolic anterior motion of the anterior mitral leaflet. Am J Cardiol **45**:141, 1980.
32. Maron BJ, Ferrans VJ: Ultrastructural features of hypertrophied human ventricular myocardium. Progr Cardiovasc Dis **21**:207, 1978.
33. Jones M, Ferrans VJ, Morrow AG, Roberts WC: Ultrastructure of crista supraventricularis muscle in patients with congenital heart diseases associated with right ventricular outflow tract obstruction. Circulation **51**:39, 1975.
34. Jones M, Ferrans VJ: Myocardial ultrastructure in children and adults with congenital heart disease. *In* Roberts WC, editor: Congenital heart disease in adults. Philadelphia, 1979, FA Davis Co, p 501.
35. Sekiguchi M, Konno S: Diagnosis and classification of primary myocardial disease with the aid of endomyocardial biopsy. Jpn Circ J **35**:737, 1971.
36. Sekiguchi M: Electron microscopical observations of the myocardium in patients with idiopathic cardiomyopathy using endomyocardial biopsy. J Molec Cell Cardiol **6**:111, 1974.
37. Kuhn H, Breithardt G, Knieriem H-J, Loogen F: Endomyocardial catheter biopsy in heart disease of unknown etiology. *In* Kaltenbach M, Loogen F, Olsen EGJ, editors: Cardiomyopathy and myocardial biopsy. Berlin, 1978, Springer-Verlag, p 121.
38. Ferrans VJ, Roberts WC: Myocardial biopsy: A useful diagnostic procedure or only a research tool? Am J Cardiol **41**:965, 1978.
39. Olsen EGJ: Postmortem findings and histologic, histochemical and electron microscopic findings of myocardial biopsies. *In* Kaltenbach M, Loogen F, Olsen EGJ, editors: Cardiomyopathy and myocardial biopsy. Berlin, 1978, Spring-Verlag, p 52.
40. Isner JM, Maron BJ, Roberts WC: Comparison of amount of myocardial cell disorganization in operatively excised septectomy specimens with amount observed at necropsy in 18 patients with hypertrophic cardiomyopathy. Am J Cardiol **46**:42, 1980.
41. Liu S-K, Maron BJ, Tilley LP: Hypertrophic cardiomyopathy in the dog. Am J Pathol **94**:497, 1979.
42. Liu S-K, Maron BJ, Tilley LP: Feline hypertrophic cardiomyopathy: Gross anatomic and quantitative histologic features. Am J Pathol **102**:388, 1981.
43. Maron BJ, Tajik AJ, Ruttenberg HD, Graham TP, Atwood GF, Victorica BE, Lie JT, Roberts WC: Hypertrophic cardiomyopathy in infants: Clinical features and natural history. Circulation (In press)
44. Maron BJ, Verter J, Kapur S: Disproportionate ventricular septal thickening in the developing normal human heart. Circulation **57**:520, 1978.
45. Clark CE, Henry WL, Epstein SE: Familial prevalence and genetic transmission of idiopathic hypertrophic subaortic stenosis. N Engl J Med **289**:709, 1973.
46. ten Cate FJ, Hugenholtz PG, van Dorp WG, Roelandt J: Prevalence of diagnostic abnormalities in patients with genetically transmitted asymmetric septal hypertrophy. Am J Cardiol **43**:731, 1979.
47. Savage DD, Seides SF, Maron BJ, Meyers DJ, Epstein SE: Prevalence of arrhythmias during 24-hour electrocardiographic monitoring and exercise testing in patients with obstructive and non-obstructive hypertrophic cardiomyopathy. Circulation **59**:866, 1979.
48. McKenna WJ, England D, Oakley CM, Goodwin JF: Detection of arrhythmia in hypertrophic cardiomyopathy: Prospective study (abstr). Circulation **62**(Suppl III):III-187, 1980.
49. Maron BJ, Savage DD, Wolfson J, Epstein SE: Prognostic significance of 24-hour ambulatory electrocardiographic monitoring in patients with hypertrophic cardiomyopathy: A prospective study. Am J Cardiol. (In press)

Cardiac lymphoma mimicking hypertrophic cardiomyopathy

Henry Scott Cabin, M.D., Ralph M. Costello, M.D., Gopalan Vasudevan, M.D., Barry J. Maron, M.D., and William C. Roberts, M.D. *Bethesda, Md., and Greensburg, Pa.*

Among patients with lymphoma, about 25% at autopsy have the neoplasm in the heart.[1] The cardiac involvement, however, infrequently causes cardiac dysfunction, and when cardiac dysfunction does occur it rarely is the initial manifestation of the lymphoma.[1,2] Such was the case, however, in a 62-year-old man who had been well until 6 weeks before death when exertional dyspnea and substernal discomfort appeared, followed in several days by subcutaneous edema and nonexertional (nocturnal) dyspnea. Examination 19 days before death disclosed overt evidence of congestive cardiac failure (CHF), a blood pressure of 130/180 mm Hg, and a grade 1/6 systolic murmur at the left sternal border and apex. ECG (Fig. 1) disclosed changes consistent with posterior wall damage and chest roentgenogram (Fig. 2) showed an enlarged cardiac silhouette and pleural effusions. Despite treatment with digoxin and furosemide, CHF worsened and the intensity of the precordial systolic murmur increased to grade 4/6. On echocardiogram (Fig. 3), the left ventricular (LV) cavity was not dilated, the mitral leaflets moved anteriorly during ventricular systole (SAM), the ventricular septum and LV free wall were thickened, and the left

From the Pathology and Cardiology Branches, National Heart, Lung and Blood Institute, National Institutes of Health; and the Departments of Pathology and Medicine, Westmoreland Hospital Association.

Received for publication May 7, 1981; accepted May 13, 1981.

Reprint requests: William C. Roberts, M.D., Pathology Branch, NHLBI–NIH, Bldg. 10A, Room 3E-30, Bethesda, MD 20205.

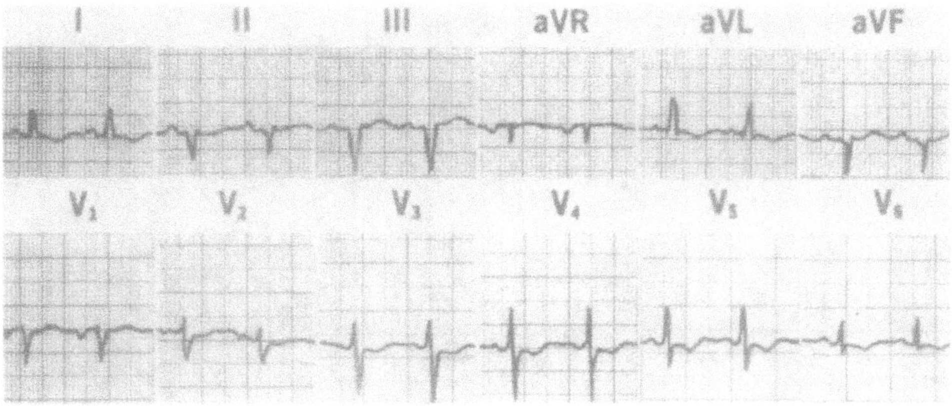

Fig. 1. ECG obtained 12 days before death. Pathologic Q waves are present in leads II, III, and aV_F and the ST segments and T waves in several leads are abnormal.

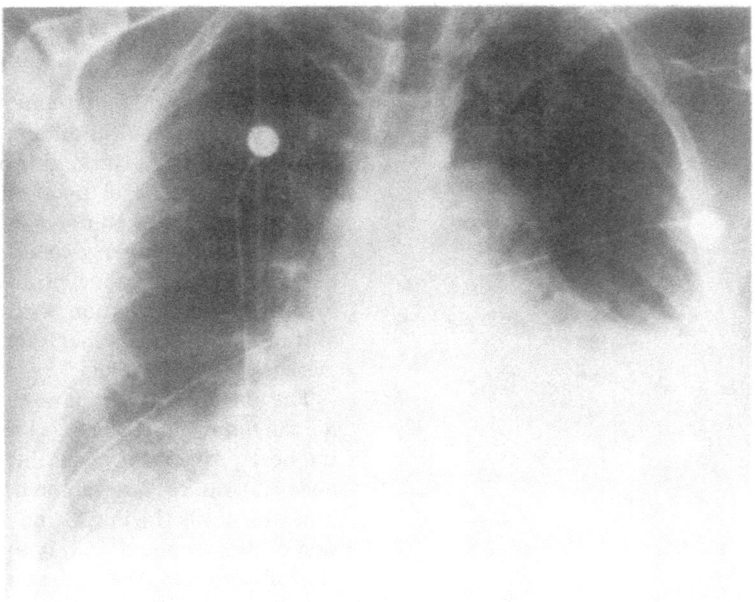

Fig. 2. Anteroposterior chest radiograph obtained 15 days before death. The cardiac silhouette is enlarged, pleural effusions are present, the pulmonary vessels are prominent, and the interstitial markings are abnormally prominent.

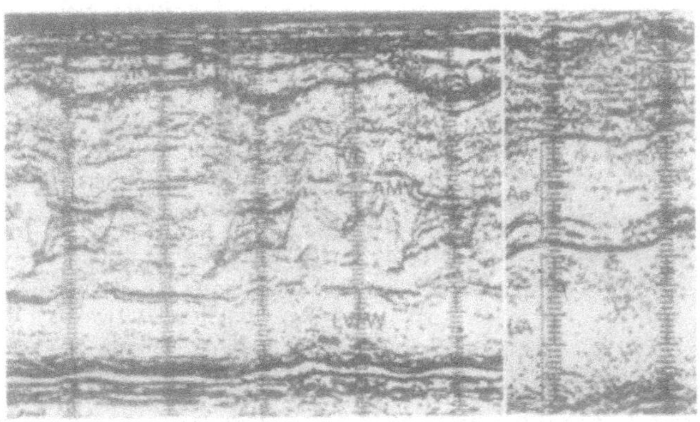

Fig. 3. M-mode echocardiograms obtained 18 days before death. The left ventricular free wall *(LVFW)* and ventricular septum *(VS)* are thickened. The LV cavity is of normal or less than normal size, the mitral leaflets move anteriorly during ventricular systole *(open arrow),* and the left atrium *(LA)* is dilated. *AMVL* = anterior mitral valve leaflet; *Ao* = aorta; *RVOT* = right ventricular outlfow tract.

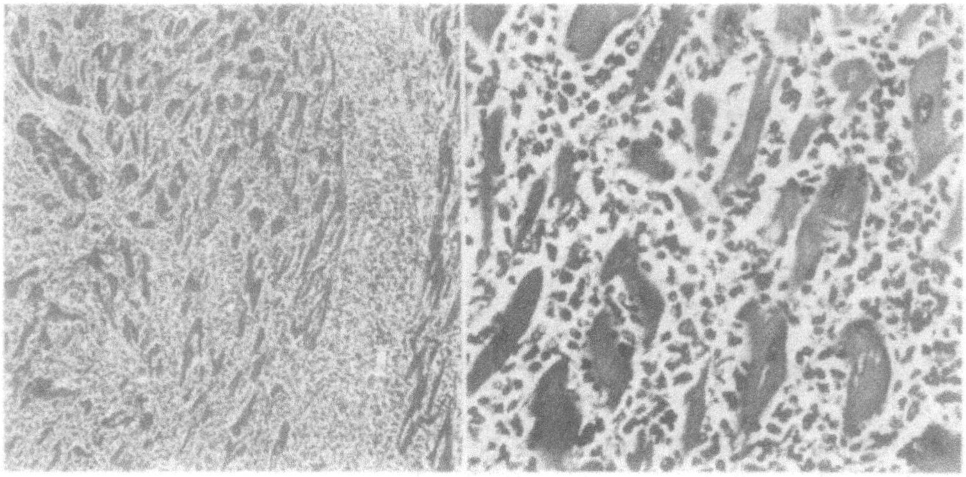

Fig. 4. Photomicrographs of lymphoma in the left ventricular wall. (Hematoxylin and eosin stains; original magnifications ×80 [*left*], ×330 [*right*].

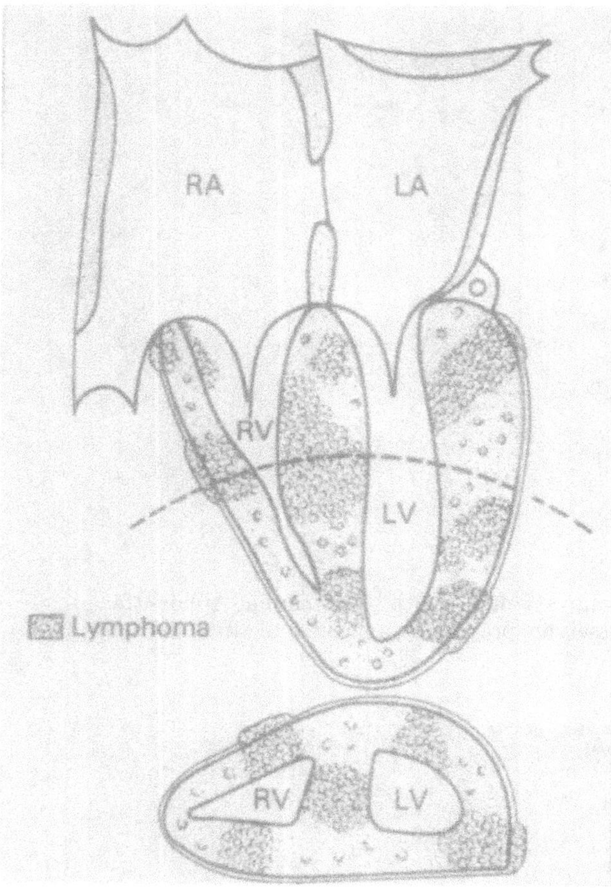

Fig. 5. Diagram showing locations of grossly visible lymphomatous nodules in the heart. *LA* = left atrium; *LV* = left ventricle; *RA* = right atrium; *RV* = right ventricle.

atrial cavity was dilated. With discontinuation of digoxin and furosemide and with institution of propranolol, CHF and intensity of the precordial murmur lessened. Three days later, however, cardiac arrest occurred. Although successfully resuscitated, he became comatose the next day and died 12 days later.

Necropsy disclosed diffuse fibrinous pericardial adhesions and extensive replacement of the cardiac ventricular walls by lymphoma (undifferentiated non-Burkitt's type) (Figs. 4 and 5). The thickening of the ventricular walls was entirely the result of neoplastic infiltration. The heart plus the infiltrating tumor weighed 910 gm. The lumina of the epicardial coronary arteries were free of significant narrowing and the four cardiac valves were normal. No myofiber disorganization was present in the ventricular septum. The only other site of lymphoma was in a mesenteric lymph node.

The above-described patient with lymphoma is unusual for the following reasons: (1) the neoplasm was limited to the heart, except for a small focus in a mesenteric lymph node; (2) the cardiac lymphoma caused cardiac dysfunction which was the initial and the only clinical manifestation of the lymphoma; (3) lymphoma was never suspected clinically; and (4) the cardiac involvement by the lymphoma mimicked hypertrophic cardiomyopathy (HC) (worsening of CHF and intensification of precordial systolic murmur by digitalis and diuretics and lessening of both by propranolol, and compatible echocardiographic findings). Although sarcoma primarily involving the ventricular septum has mimicked HC,[3] we have found no reports of other primary or secondary cardiac neoplasms simulating clinically HC.

We thank Dr. Elaine S. Jaffe, Chief, Hematopathology, Laboratory of Pathology, National Cancer Institute, National Institutes of Health, Bethesda, Maryland, for reviewing the histologic sections of the lymphoma and for classifying it for us.

REFERENCES

1. Roberts WC, Glancy DL, DeVita VT Jr: Heart in malignant lymphoma (Hodgkin's disease, lymphosarcoma, reticulum cell sarcoma and mycosis fungoides). A study of 196 autopsy cases. Am J Cardiol **22**:85, 1968.
2. Levitt LJ, Ault KA, Pinkus GS, Sloss LJ, McManus BM: Pericarditis and early cardiac tamponade as a primary manifestation of lymphosarcoma cell leukemia. Am J Med **67**:719, 1979.
3. Isner JI, Falcone MW, Virmani R, Roberts WC: Cardiac sarcoma causing "ASH" and simulating coronary heart disease. Am J Med **66**:1025, 1979.

Hypertrophic cardiomyopathy mimicking pericardial constriction or myocardial restriction

Bruce F. Waller, M.D., Barry J. Maron, M.D., Andrew G. Morrow, M.D., and William C. Roberts, M.D.
Bethesda, Md.

The occurrence of identical or nearly identical mean right atrial (RA), mean pulmonary arterial (PA) wedge, right (RV) and left ventricular (LV) and PA end-diastolic pressures is generally interpreted as indicative of pericardial constriction or myocardial restriction. Although the cardiac ventricles may restrict their filling in hypertrophic cardiomyopathy (HC),[1-2] the occurrence of similar pressures in the above-indicated pressure tracings in HC is rare. None such occurrence was observed in the first 64 patients with this condition reported by Braunwald et al.[3] or subsequently by others.

Recently, however, we studied a 53-year-old woman with HC who had typical hemodynamic features of pericardial constriction or myocardial restriction (Fig. 1). She had been well until age 48 when episodes of dizziness appeared, followed the next year by exertional dyspnea and chest pain. Cardiac catheterization (Table I) and echocardiogram (Fig. 2) disclosed features typical of HC and propranolol was started. Paroxysmal atrial fibrillation appeared at age 51 and at age 53 (February, 1981) she had repeat catheterization (Table I) which now disclosed the mean pressures in the RA and PA wedge position and the end-diastolic pressures in the PA, RV, and LV to be similar (approximately 25 mm Hg) and the RV and LV pressure tracings to have a square-root configuration (Fig. 1). The peak systolic pressure gradient at rest between LV

From the Pathology, Cardiology, and Surgery Branches, National Heart, Lung and Blood Institute, National Institutes of Health.

Received for publication May 22, 1981; accepted June 2, 1981.

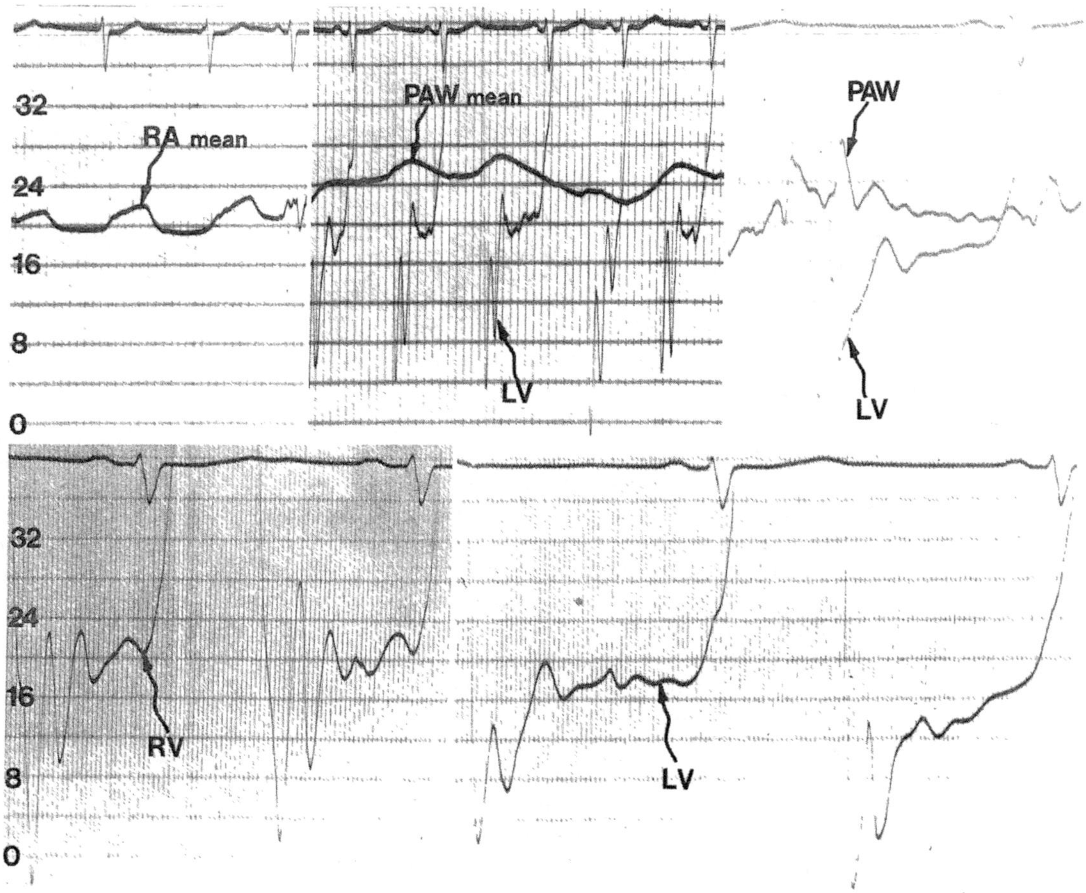

Fig. 1. Pressure tracings showing the mean pressures in the right atrium *(RA)* and pulmonary arterial wedge *(PAW)* position to be similar to the end-diastolic pressures in right *(RV)* and left *(LV)* ventricles.

Table I. Cardiac catheterization data (pressures in mm Hg)

	Ages (years) at catheterization	
	49	*53*
Pulmonary artery (systolic/diastolic, mean)	60/8(35)	70/25(35)
Right ventricular (s/d)	60/8	70/25
Right atrium (a:v:mean)	-:-:3	24:20:20
Pulmonary arterial wedge (a:v:mean)	20/28/18	-:-:25
Left ventricle (s/d)(LV)	244/30	180/25
Aorta (s/d)	110/70	160/80
LV-aorta peak systolic gradient		
rest	124	20
Valsalva	–	20
amyl nitrite	–	75
isoproterenol	–	35
Cardiac index (L/min/m^2)	2.4	1.3

and aorta was now only 20 mm Hg, whereas 4 years earlier it had been 124 mm Hg. Because of the unresponsiveness of the symptoms of cardiac dysfunction to beta blockade therapy, partial septectomy and septotomy were performed. At operation, the parietal and visceral pericardia were normal. Two days postoperatively, she developed fatal ventricular tachycardia.

At necropsy, the heart weighed 580 gm, the ventricular walls were hypertrophied, and the cavities were small (Fig. 3). Histologic study of the ventricular septum disclosed extensive myofiber disorganization and some intramural coronary arteries had thickened walls and narrowed lumina, findings typical of HC.[4] Although the above-described patient had hemodynamic evidence of cardiac

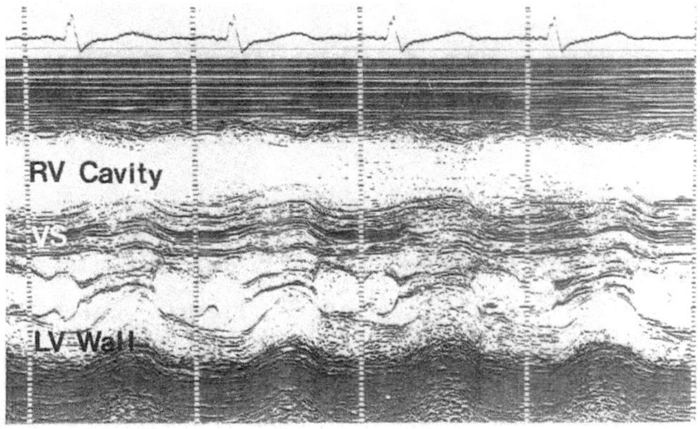

Fig. 2. Preoperative M-mode echocardiogram showing asymmetrically thickened ventricular septum *(VS)* with respect to left ventricular *(LV)* free wall and a small LV cavity. *RV* = right ventricular.

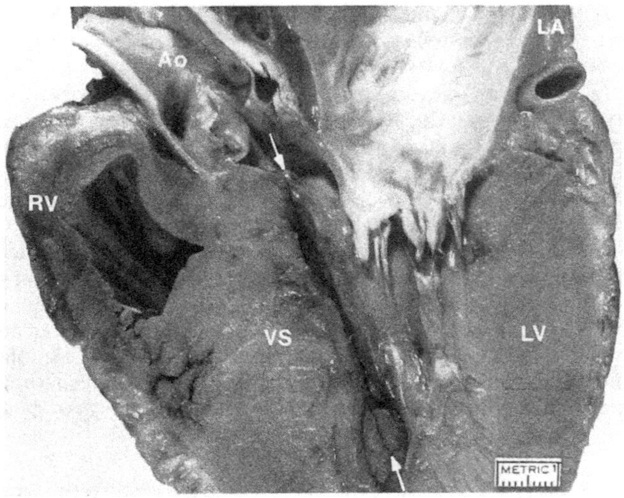

Fig. 3. Heart cut in a "long-axis" fashion showing the walls of the right *(RV)* and left *(LV)* ventricles and ventricular septum *(VS)* to be very thick and the LV cavity to be small. The two *white arrows* indicate the line of the operative vs incision and excision.

constriction or restriction, the mechanism by which the HC caused these hemodynamic alterations is uncertain but probably related to decreased LV diastolic compliance.

REFERENCES

1. Cohn J, Effat H, Goodwin JF, Oakley CM, Steiner RE: Hypertrophic obstructive cardiomyopathy. Br Heart J **26**:16, 1964.
2. Goodwin JE: Congestive and hypertrophic cardiomyopathies: A decade of study. Lancet **1**:731, 1970.
3. Braunwald E, Lambrew CT, Rockoff SD, Ross J, Morrow AG: Idiopathic hypertrophic subaortic stenosis. I. A description of the disease based upon an analysis of 64 patients. Circulation **29** (suppl IV):I, 1, 1964.
4. McReynolds, RA, Roberts WC: The intramural coronary arteries in hypertrophic cardiomyopathy. Am J Cardiol **35**:154, 1975.

Hypertrophic Cardiomyopathy in Infants: Clinical Features and Natural History

Barry J. Maron, M.D., Abdul J. Tajik, M.D., Herbert D. Ruttenberg, M.D., Thomas P. Graham, M.D., Gerald F. Atwood, M.D., Benjamin E. Victorica, M.D., J. T. Lie, M.D., and William C. Roberts, M.D.

SUMMARY **The clinical and morphologic features of hypertrophic cardiomyopathy in 20 patients recognized as having cardiac disease in the first year of life are described. Fourteen of these 20 infants were initially suspected of having heart disease solely because a heart murmur was identified. However, the infants showed a variety of clinical findings, including signs of marked congestive heart failure (in the presence of nondilated ventricular cavities and normal or increased left ventricular contractility) and substantial cardiac enlargement on chest radiograph. Other findings were markedly different from those usually present in older children and adults with hypertrophic cardiomyopathy (e.g., right ventricular hypertrophy on the ECG and cyanosis). Consequently, in 14 infants, the initial clinical diagnosis was congenital cardiac malformation other than hypertrophic cardiomyopathy.**

Twelve of the 14 infants who underwent left-heart catheterization showed substantial obstruction to left ventricular outflow (peak systolic pressure gradient ≥ 35 mm Hg). However, unlike older patients with hypertrophic cardiomyopathy, infants with this condition commonly had marked obstruction to right ventricular outflow (35–106 mm Hg) (nine patients); in six patients, the magnitude of obstruction to right ventricular outflow was at least as great as that to left ventricular outflow.

Asymmetric hypertrophy of the ventricular septum relative to the left ventricular free wall was present in the 16 patients who had echocardiographic or necropsy examination. Ventricular septal thickening was substantial in patients studied both before and after 6 months of age (mean 16 mm), indicating that in patients with hypertrophic cardiomyopathy, marked left ventricular hypertrophy may be present early in life and is probably congenital.

The clinical course was variable in these patients, but the onset of marked congestive heart failure in the first year of life appeared to be an unfavorable prognostic sign; nine of the 11 infants with congestive heart failure died within the first year of life. In infants with hypertrophic cardiomyopathy, unlike older children and adults with this condition, sudden death was less common (two patients) than death due to progressive congestive heart failure.

HYPERTROPHIC CARDIOMYOPATHY is a primary disease of cardiac muscle that usually is not recognized clinically until adulthood.[1-3] Therefore, most of the clinical and pathologic information regarding this disease is from older children and adults.[4-11] Hypertrophic cardiomyopathy does occur in infants, but only single cases or relatively small groups of patients have been reported.[7, 12-15] Hence, we assembled the clinical, hemodynamic and morphologic features of a large series of patients with hypertrophic cardiomyopathy in whom cardiac disease was identified in the first year of life.

Patients and Methods

The study includes 20 infants with hypertrophic cardiomyopathy evaluated at five institutions: eight patients from the National Heart, Lung, and Blood Institute, five from the Mayo Clinic, three from Vanderbilt University Hospital, three from the University of Utah Primary Children's Medical Center, and one patient from the University of Florida Shands Teaching Hospital and Clinics. Each patient met the following criteria: clinical identification of heart disease in the first year of life; echocardiographic, angiocardiographic or necropsy demonstration of a markedly hypertrophied but nondilated left ventricle in the absence of another cardiac or systemic disease capable of producing left ventricular hypertrophy;[16] and absence of maternal diabetes requiring insulin (to avoid confusion with the transient, nonfamilial form of hypertrophic cardiomyopathy that occurs in infants of diabetic mothers[17, 18]).

M-mode Echocardiography

M-mode echocardiography was performed using a 2.25-MHz, 1.25-cm-diameter unfocused Aerotech transducer and a Hoffrel 201 ultrasound receiver interfaced with a Honeywell 1856 strip-chart recorder. The methods of imaging the ventricular septum and posterior left ventricular free wall have been described.[19] Left ventricular internal dimensions at end-diastole and end-systole and aortic root and left atrial dimensions were measured echocardiographically in accord with published methods and criteria.[20, 21]

From the Cardiology and Pathology Branches, NHLBI, NIH, Bethesda, Maryland; The Mayo Clinic and Mayo Foundation, Rochester, Minnesota; the Department of Pediatrics, Vanderbilt University School of Medicine, Nashville, Tennessee; the Department of Pediatrics, University of Utah College of Medicine, Salt Lake City, Utah; and the Department of Pediatrics, University of Florida College of Medicine, Gainesville, Florida.

Address for correspondence: Dr. Barry J. Maron, Cardiology Branch, Building 10, Room 7B-15, National Heart, Lung, and Blood Institute, National Institutes of Health, Bethesda, Maryland 20205.

Received October 15, 1980; revision accepted March 27, 1981.

Circulation 65, No. 1, 1982.

Necropsy Analyses

Ventricular wall thicknesses were measured in the ventricular septum at the point of maximal thickness, usually halfway between the aortic valve and the apex of left ventricle, and in the left ventricular free wall behind the midpoint of the posterior mitral leaflet at a level corresponding to the tips of the mitral leaflets. Trabeculae, papillary muscles and the crista supraventricularis were not included in the measurements of ventricular wall thicknesses. The extent of cardiac muscle cell disorganization in tissue sections of ventricular septum was assessed quantitatively.[22, 23]

Results

Clinical Identification

Each of the 20 infants was a product of a term pregnancy; gestation was complicated by hydramnios in three. Birth weights ranged from 2.4–4.6 kg. Nineteen patients had no significant medical problems during the neonatal period; one patient had seizures associated with hypocalcemia and hypoglycemia of unknown cause. Eleven infants were male and nine were female. Heart disease was identified in each infant during the first year of life (from 1 day to 10 months of age; mean 3 months).

In 14 patients, the initial suspicion of heart disease arose solely because a systolic murmur was detected; the murmurs were usually judged to be ejection murmurs, were grade 2–4/6 and were heard loudest at the fourth left intercostal space or apex. Heart disease was initially identified because of the onset of congestive heart failure in three patients, bradycardia in one patient, and central cyanosis at rest or with crying associated with arterial oxygen desaturation in two patients.

In six infants, hypertrophic cardiomyopathy was correctly diagnosed during the initial clinical evaluation. In the other 14 patients, a cardiac disease other than hypertrophic cardiomyopathy was considered first: pulmonic valve stenosis in three patients, ventricular septal defect in three, cyanotic congenital heart disease in two, congenital mitral valve disease in two,

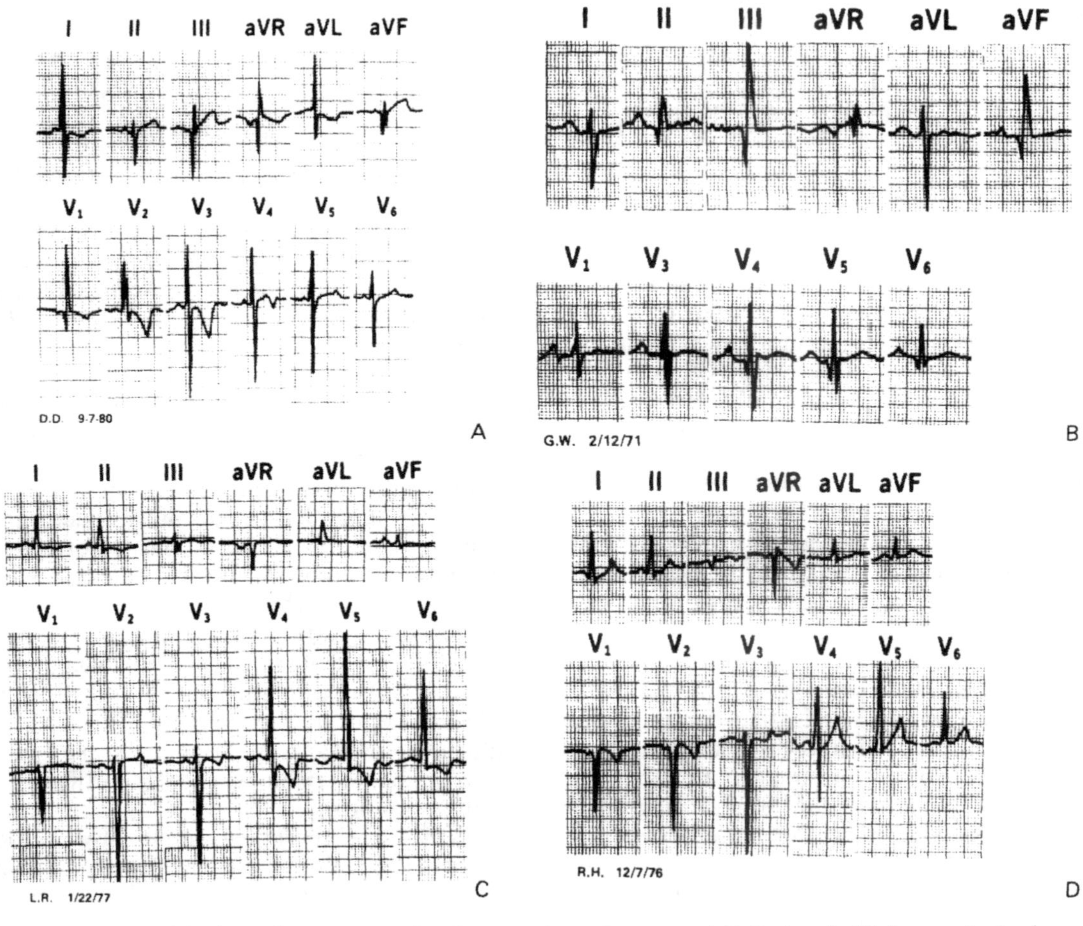

FIGURE 1. *ECGs from four patients showing a variety of patterns. (A) Patient 1. Right ventricular hypertrophy with predominant R waves in leads V_1 and V_2; deep but relatively narrow Q waves are evident in leads III, aV_F and V_1; left-axis deviation and left atrial enlargement are also present. (B) Patient 16. Probable right ventricular hypertrophy and wide Q waves in leads II, III, aV_F and V_4–V_6 and intraventricular conduction defect. (C) Patient 9. Left ventricular hypertrophy with ST-segment and T-wave abnormalities ("strain" pattern) and small R waves and deep S waves in right precordial leads. (D) Patient 4. Suggestive of left ventricular hypertrophy with deep S waves and absent or small R waves in leads V_1–V_3.*

aortic valve stenosis in one patient, left ventricular tumor in one, myocarditis in one, and congenital complete atrioventricular block in one. In seven of these 14 patients hypertrophic cardiomyopathy was correctly diagnosed at ages 10 days to 3 years (median 9 months).

An associated congenital noncardiac anomaly was also identified in four patients: lentiginosis with deafness,[24] Noonan syndrome,[25] tuberous sclerosis with pyloric stenosis and Pierre-Robin syndrome. Clinical and necropsy data for the 20 patients are summarized in table 1.

Electrocardiograms

The ECGs were abnormal in each infant. A wide variety of abnormalities was identified (fig. 1), but no ECG pattern was characteristic of the overall study group (table 1). Right ventricular hypertrophy, present in 11 patients, was the most common abnormality. Seven patients had left ventricular hypertrophy and five had diffuse ST-segment and T-wave abnormalities. Four patients had abnormal Q or QS waves. The ECG pattern showed no consistent relation to the hemodynamic state, although five of six patients with left ventricular hypertrophy on the ECG had marked and predominant obstruction to left ventricular outflow.

Chest Radiographic Findings

Heart size on the chest radiograph was larger than normal (cardiothoracic ratio > 0.55) in 19 of the 20 infants, including six of the seven who were asymptomatic. Cardiothoracic ratios ranged from 0.50–0.76 (mean 0.65). Of the eight infants in whom serial radiographs were obtained over a period of 10 months to 6.5 years, heart size was significantly decreased in three, increased in one and unchanged in four.

Hemodynamic, Angiographic and Functional Findings

Cardiac catheterization was performed in 16 infants, 2 weeks to 3.5 years of age. Of the 14 patients who underwent left-heart catheterization, 12 had a left ventricular outflow tract pressure gradient at rest (range 35–120 mm Hg; average 75 mm Hg) (fig. 2, table 1). The two other patients had no left ventricular outflow gradient. One other patient (no. 14), who did not undergo cardiac catheterization, was judged to have no left ventricular outflow tract obstruction based on the absence of systolic anterior motion of the anterior mitral leaflet on the echocardiogram.[26] Twelve patients had right ventricular outflow tract pressure gradients of 10 mm Hg or greater (range 10–106 mm Hg; average 46 mm Hg). In nine of these infants, the right ventricular outflow peak systolic gradient was substantial (35–106 mm Hg). In six infants, the magnitude of obstruction to right ventricular outflow equaled or exceeded that to left ventricular outflow (including patient 1, who had right ventricular outflow tract obstruction only). Left ventricular end-diastolic pressure was elevated in seven infants (range 12–25 mm Hg) and was normal in

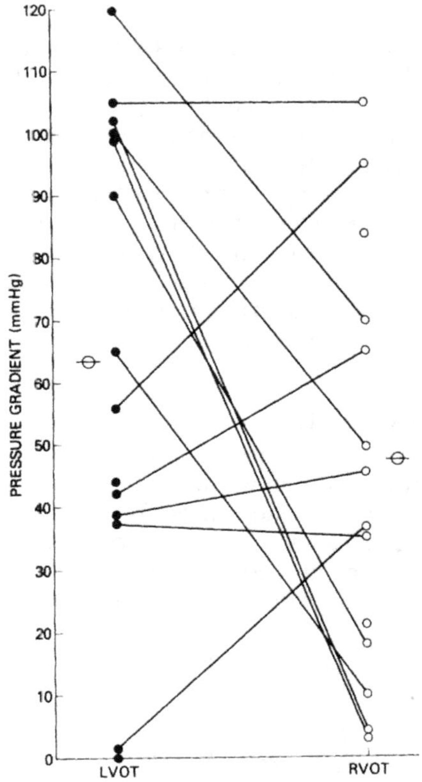

FIGURE 2. *Left ventricular outflow tract (LVOT) and right ventricular outflow tract (RVOT) peak systolic pressure gradients in 16 infants with hypertrophic cardiomyopathy. Data for each of the patients in whom both left and right ventricular outflow gradients were measured are connected by a line. Mean values are indicated by the symbol* ⊖.

seven. Right ventricular end-diastolic pressure was elevated (6–20 mm Hg) in 10 infants and normal (< 6 mm Hg) in four.

Left ventricular angiocardiograms were obtained in 13 infants and were abnormal in each (fig. 3). The angiocardiograms showed a variety of configurations in diastole, although no left ventricular appearance was particularly characteristic of the patient group. Mitral regurgitation was judged to be moderate or severe in three infants, mild in two, and absent in eight. In the eight patients who underwent right ventricular angiocardiography, right ventricular outflow tract narrowing was present during systole, and obstruction to right ventricular outflow was shown hemodynamically.

Each of the 16 patients studied by angiography or echocardiography showed evidence of normal or increased left ventricular contractility (ejection fraction 0.60–0.92 by angiography or 0.75–0.90 by echocardiography) (figs. 3C and 3E), including nine who had overt signs of congestive heart failure. However, no patient had evidence of left ventricular dilatation; the left ventricular cavity was assessed to be normal or small by angiography or at necropsy in 11 infants and left ventricular internal diastolic dimension by echocardiography was normal or decreased (15–33 mm)

TABLE 1. *Clinical and Necropsy Data in 20 Patients*

Pt	Age now or at death	Sex	Age heart disease identified	Reason heart disease suspected	Initial clinical diagnosis	Signs/symptoms	ECG* RVH	ECG* LVH	ECG* Q waves	Echo† VS Thickness (mm)	Echo† PW Thickness (mm)	Echo† VS/PW	Echo† SAM††	Echo† LVID$_d$ (mm)
Survivors														
1	1 yr 4 mo	M	2 mo	Murmur	HCM	None	+	0	+	13	6	2.2	0	21
2	2 yr 9 mo	F	2 wks	Murmur	HCM	None	+	0	0	12	6	2.0	1+	24
3	2 yr 9 mo	M	1 day	Murmur	HCM	None	+	0	+	22	7	3.1	4+	24
4	3 yr 4 mo	M	7 mo	Murmur	HCM	None	0	+	0	12	7	1.7	4+	29
5	4 yr	F	10 mo	Murmur	VSD	None	0	+‡	0	20	10	2.0	4+	31
6	4 yr 9 mo	M	3 wks	Murmur, cyanosis	Cyanotic CHD	None	+	+	0	14	6	2.3	2+	27
7	5 yr 8 mo	F	5 mo	Murmur	HCM	Fatigue, lightheadedness, syncope	0	+	+	—	—	—	—	—
8	9 yr 4 mo	F	10 days	Murmur	LV tumor	CHF, dyspnea, angina	0	+	0	24	11	2.1	4+	33
9	11 yr 7 mo	F	6 wks	Murmur	VSD	CHF	0	+	0	—	—	—	—	—
10	12 yr 5 mo	M	9 mo	Murmur	PS	Syncope (one episode only)	+‡	0	0	—	—	—	—	—
Nonsurvivors														
11	1 mo	M	4 days	CHF	PS	CHF→sudden death	+	0	0	—	—	—	—	—
12	1 mo	M	1 mo	CHF	Congenital MS	CHF	+	0	0	—	—	—	—	—
13	2 mo	F	1 day	Bradycardia	Congenital CAVB	CHF	0	0	0	—	—	—	—	—
14	2 mo	F	1 day	Murmur	HCM	CHF→sudden death	+	0	0	—	—	—	0	15
15	5 mo	M	6 wks	Murmur	Congenital MR	CHF	+	0	0	—	—	—	—	—
16	5 mo	M	3 wks	Murmur	VSD (& ASD)	CHF	0	0	+	—	—	—	—	—
17	8 mo	F	3 days	Murmur	Valvular PS	CHF→postop death	+‡	0	0	—	—	—	—	—
18	11 mo	M	1 wk	Murmur, cyanosis	TGV	CHF→postop death	+	0	0	13	7	1.9	3+	27
19	11 mo	M	10 mo	CHF	Myocarditis	CHF	0	0	0	—	—	—	—	—
20	9 yr 2 mo	M	9 mo	Murmur	Valvular AS	None→died of enterocolitis	0	+‡	0	—	—	—	—	—

*Data were obtained from the ECG recorded closest to 1 month of age.

†Data were obtained from the technically best echocardiographic study recorded closest to 2 years of age.

‡Left or right ventricular hypertrophy with "strain" pattern (i.e., with associated ST-segment and T-wave abnormalities).

§Postoperative left ventricular outflow tract gradient recorded in the operating room was zero.

¶Left and right ventricular outflow tract gradients recorded at cardiac catheterization 5 weeks after operation were each 20 mm Hg.

**The infant's father died suddenly at age 30 years, presumably of hypertrophic cardiomyopathy.

††Grading system for magnitude of systolic anterior motion of the anterior mitral leaflet (SAM): from 1+ (slight anterior motion) to 4+ (prolonged contact between anterior mitral leaflet and ventricular septal endocardium, consistent with the presence of marked obstruction to left ventricular outflow[26]).

‡‡Performed through aortotomy at age 21 months (body weight 10.5 kg).

§§Performed through left and right ventriculotomies, at age 16 months (body weight 8.1 kg).

¶¶Treated with digitalis briefly, before the diagnosis of hypertrophic cardiomyopathy was made; each patient showed clinical deterioration or lack of improvement while taking digitalis.

Abbreviations: AS = aortic stenosis; ASD = atrial septal defect; CAVB = complete atrioventricular block; CHD = congenital heart disease; CHF = congestive heart failure; EDP = end-diastolic pressure; EF = ejection fraction; TGV = transposition of the great vessels; HCM = hypertrophic cardiomyopathy; LV = left ventricular; LVID$_d$ = left ventricular internal dimension at end-diastole; LVOT = left ventricular outflow tract; LVH = left ventricular hypertrophy; M-M = ventricular septal myotomy and myectomy; MR = mitral regurgitation; MS = mitral stenosis; PS = pulmonary stenosis; PW = posterior left ventricular free wall; RV = right ventricular; RVH = right ventricular hypertrophy; SAM = systolic anterior motion of the anterior mitral leaflet; VS = ventricular septum; VS/PW = ventricular septal-to-posterior left ventricular free wall thickness

TABLE 1. (*Continued*)

Hemodynamics (mm Hg)									Necropsy			
Outflow gradients		EDP		Medications		Operation	Genetic transmission HCM	Thickness (mm)			% VS disorganization[22, 23]
LVOT	RVOT	LV	RV	Propranolol	Digitalis			VS	PW	VS/PW	
0	37	7	4	+	0	None	0	—	—	—	—
37	35	8	4	+	+¶¶	None	0	—	—	—	—
65	10	9	7	+	0	None	+	—	—	—	—
90	18	15	7	0	0	None	+	—	—	—	—
100	2	14	8	+	0	None	+	—	—	—	—
35	45	11	5	+	0	None	+**	—	—	—	—
104§	4	25	4	0	+	M-M‡‡	—	—	—	—	—
100	50	14	12	+	+¶¶	None	—	—	—	—	—
120	70	8	6	+	+¶¶	None	—	—	—	—	—
107¶	106¶	9	8	0	0	M-M; RV muscle resection§§	—	—	—	—	—
—	—	—	—	0	+	None	+	18	7	2.6	18
—	—	—	—	0	+	None	—	17	12	1.4	29
0	—	12	—	0	+	None	+	8	3	2.7	17
—	—	—	—	+	0	None	0	12	7	1.7	3
—	21	—	13	0	+	None	0	30	13	2.3	34
46	—	15	—	0	+	None	—	13	9	1.4	31
—	85	—	20	0	+	RV muscle resection	—	23	15	1.5	12
55	95	15	12	+	0	RV muscle resection	0	—	—	—	—
—	—	—	—	0	+	None	0	10	7	1.4	6
42	64	6	8	0	0	None	—	—	—	—	—

relative to body surface area in the other nine patients.

Structural Cardiac Features Identified by Echocardiography and at Necropsy

Asymmetric hypertrophy of the ventricular septum relative to the posterior left ventricular free wall[19, 27] (septal-to-free wall thickness ratio $\geq$ 1.3) was identified in all 16 patients studied by echocardiography or at necropsy (figs. 4 and 5, table 1). The septal–free wall ratio was 1.5 or greater in 13 of these 16 infants (fig. 6). Each of the 16 infants also had a marked increase in absolute ventricular septal thickness. The mean septal thickness was 16 mm (range 8–30 mm) and clearly exceeded the upper limit of normal relative to body surface area, based on normal diastolic or systolic echocardiographic values,[20] in each infant (fig. 7). There was no direct relation between septal thickness and body surface area. In seven infants who underwent echocardiographic or necropsy examination before 6 months of age, the mean ventricular septal thickness was also 16 mm. However, in the six patients with serial echocardiographic measurements (only one of whom showed clinical deterioration), neither ventricular septal thickness nor septal–free wall thickness ratio changed substantially with age during a follow-up of 9 months to 3 years (fig. 8).

Left atrial dimension measured echocardiographically was mildly increased relative to body surface area in two patients (27 mm and 28 mm) and was normal in seven. Five patients had marked systolic anterior motion of the anterior mitral leaflet (fig. 4), each of whom had left ventricular outflow gradients of 55–100 mm Hg at catheterization. Systolic anterior

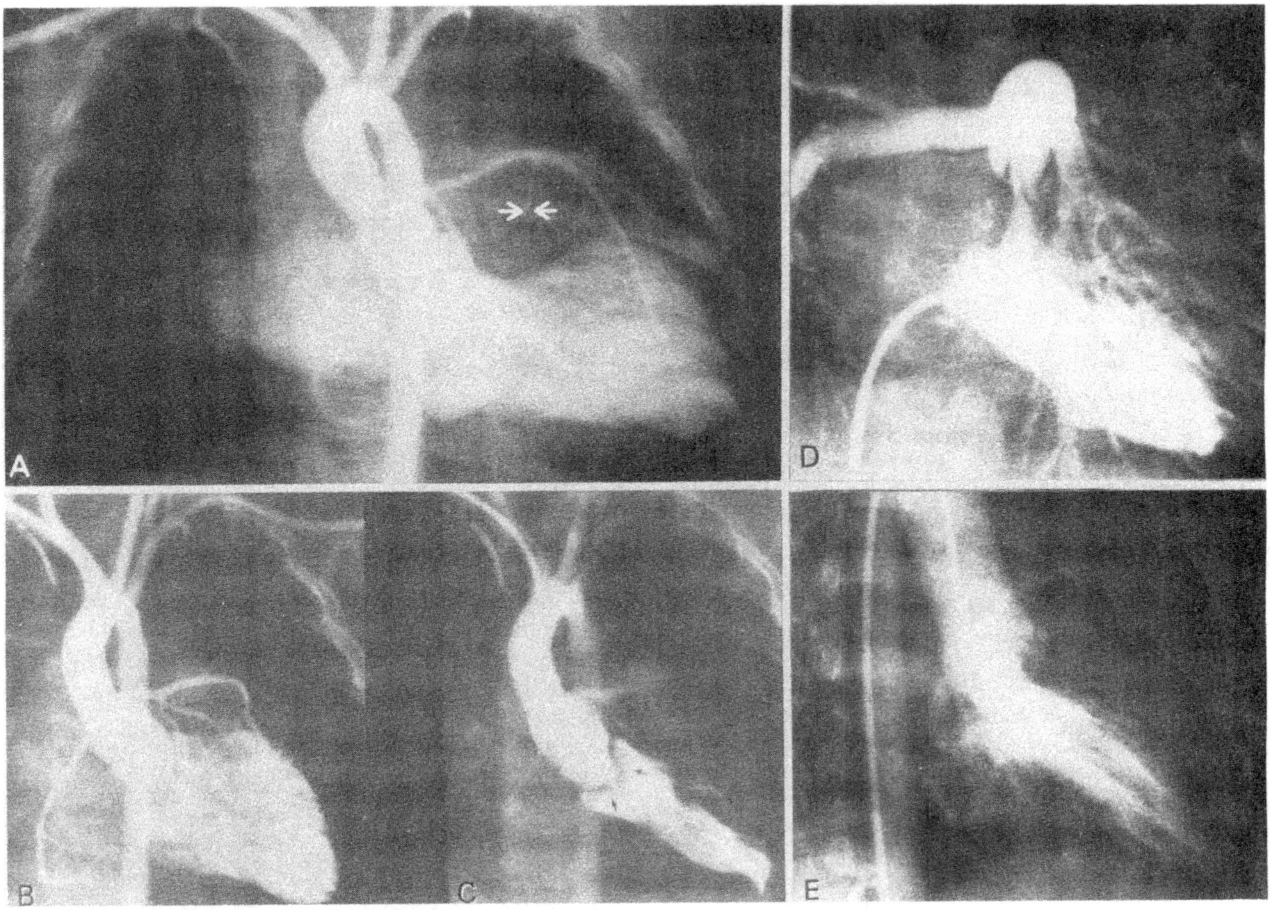

FIGURE 3. *Angiocardiograms obtained in the posteroanterior projection in four infants with hypertrophic cardiomyopathy showing a variety of diastolic and systolic abnormalities. (A) Abnormal diastolic left ventricular contour in which a superior indentation of the cavity is produced by marked hypertrophy of the ventricular septum. Septal coronary artery (arrows) arises from the left anterior descending coronary artery. Opacification of the left atrium indicates mitral regurgitation. (B) Diastolic and (C) systolic frames from the same patient, showing a hypercontractile left ventricle and marked systolic anterior motion of the anterior mitral leaflet (arrows). (D) Right ventricular angiocardiogram during systole from an infant with a right ventricular outflow tract gradient of 95 mm Hg, showing narrowing of the outflow tract. (E) Angiocardiogram in the lateral projection at end-systole showing marked emptying of the left ventricle, obliteration of the apex and a "ballerina slipper" configuration.*

motion was absent or mild in four other patients.

The extent of cardiac muscle cell disorganization in the ventricular septum was assessed quantitatively at necropsy in eight infants. Seven of these patients (five younger than 6 months of age) had marked septal disorganization that occupied more than 5% of the tissue section, consistent with the histologic diagnosis of hypertrophic cardiomyopathy;[22, 23] in the remaining patient, 3% of the section was involved (table 1).

Clinical Course and Treatment

Survivors

Ten patients survived during the observation period (mean follow-up of 5.5 years) (fig. 9, table 1). Seven of these 10 patients were asymptomatic when their heart disease was identified and have remained virtually asymptomatic throughout the period of follow-up (mean 3.5 years), although one, patient 10, had a single episode of syncope. Five of the seven asymptomatic patients received propranolol (3 mg/kg/day in each) and one underwent combined ventricular septal myotomy-myectomy[28] and resection of right ventricular outflow tract muscle, which resulted in substantial reduction of left and right ventricular outflow obstruction. Three other patients (nos. 7, 8 and 9) were symptomatic at the initial evaluation but improved substantially during the follow-up period, including two who had shown evidence of congestive heart failure; two of these three improved infants became asymptomatic. This improvement was evident after septal myotomy-myectomy in one (patient 7) and after treatment with propranolol (3 and 6 mg/kg/day) in the other two (patients 8 and 9).

Nonsurvivors

Ten patients died during the observation period, including one who died of noncardiac disease (enterocolitis with paralytic ileus) (fig. 9, table 1). The nine patients who died of heart disease had the onset of symptoms and died during the first year of life (age range 1–11 months; median 2 months). Five of these nine patients died of progressive congestive heart

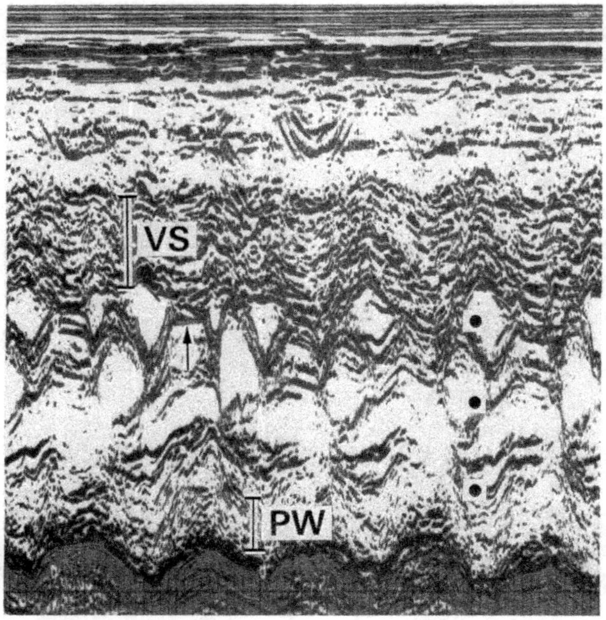

FIGURE 4. *M-mode echocardiogram from a 2-year-old patient with hypertrophic cardiomyopathy and marked left ventricular outflow tract obstruction (90-mm Hg peak systolic gradient at rest). The ventricular septum (VS) is thickened (12 mm) disproportionately with respect to the posterior left ventricular free wall (PW) and there is substantial systolic anterior motion of the anterior mitral leaflet (arrow). The calibration dots are 10 mm apart.*

failure, for which they had received digitalis; two other patients with severe heart failure died shortly after operation (resection of right ventricular outflow tract muscle). The remaining two patients (nos. 11 and 14) died suddenly, although each had evidence of congestive heart failure. Patient 11 was under treatment with digitalis for marked heart failure and died unexpectedly at 1 month of age; patient 14, who had relatively mild manifestations of congestive heart failure, died suddenly at 2 months of age despite propranolol therapy (5 mg/kg/day).

The patients who survived and those who died of heart disease did not differ substantially with regard to ventricular septal thickness, outflow tract gradient, end-diastolic pressure, or ECG pattern. For the overall study group, the follow-up period ranged from 3 days to 11.5 years (mean 3.3 years).

Family Studies

Genetic transmission of hypertrophic cardiomyopathy[1, 6, 8, 29, 30] was documented in the families of six infants (table 1). In five of these six families, echocardiographic studies[29] demonstrated genetic transmission of asymmetric septal hypertrophy in one first-degree relative of the index case. In the sixth family, the father of the infant died suddenly and unexpectedly at age 30 years; an autopsy was not performed.

Echocardiographic studies of first-degree relatives (i.e., both parents and two to five siblings) of six additional infants did not show evidence of hypertrophic cardiomyopathy. We could not perform comprehensive echocardiographic studies in relatives of the remaining eight infants; hence, genetic transmission of hypertrophic cardiomyopathy could not be determined definitively in these families.

Discussion

The clinical features and course of infants with hypertrophic cardiomyopathy may be quite variable. For example, although these infants were usually first suspected of having heart disease on the basis of a murmur, they also presented with signs of marked congestive heart failure, or even cyanosis (probably due to right-to-left shunting through a patent foramen ovale in the presence of right ventricular systolic hypertension). Hence, hypertrophic cardiomyopathy in infants may mimic other congenital heart diseases, and its clinical presentation often differs from that usually observed in children and adults with hypertrophic cardiomyopathy.[1-3, 10, 11] Indeed, in most of our patients, cardiac diseases other than hypertrophic cardiomyopathy were initially considered (most commonly, pulmonic valve stenosis, cyanotic congenital heart disease, ventricular septal defect, or congenital mitral or aortic valve disease).

Unlike older children and adults with hypertrophic cardiomyopathy,[1-3, 10, 11, 31] about one-fourth of our

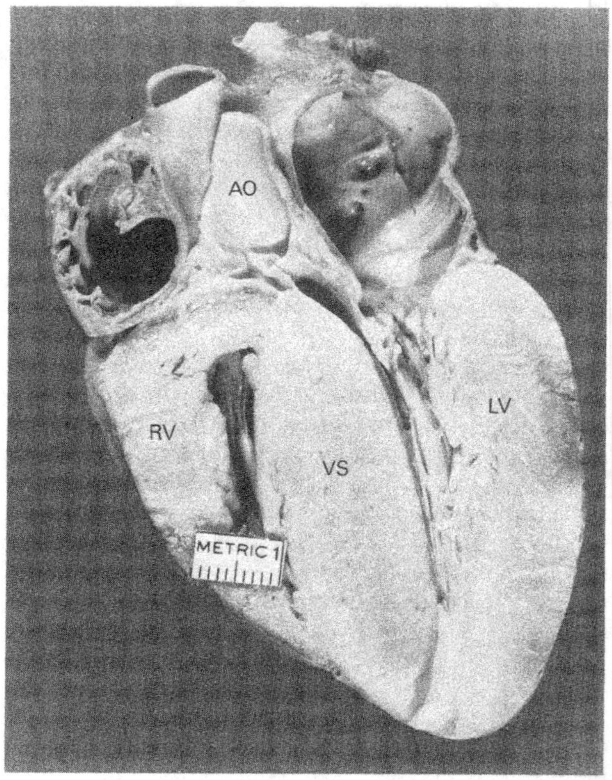

FIGURE 5. *Heart of a 1-month-old boy with hypertrophic cardiomyopathy. The ventricular septum (VS) is disproportionately thickened with respect to the left ventricular free wall (LV). The ventricular septal thickness is 17 mm, the free wall thickness is 12 mm, and the septal–free wall ratio is 1.4. Ao = aorta, RV = right ventricular cavity.*

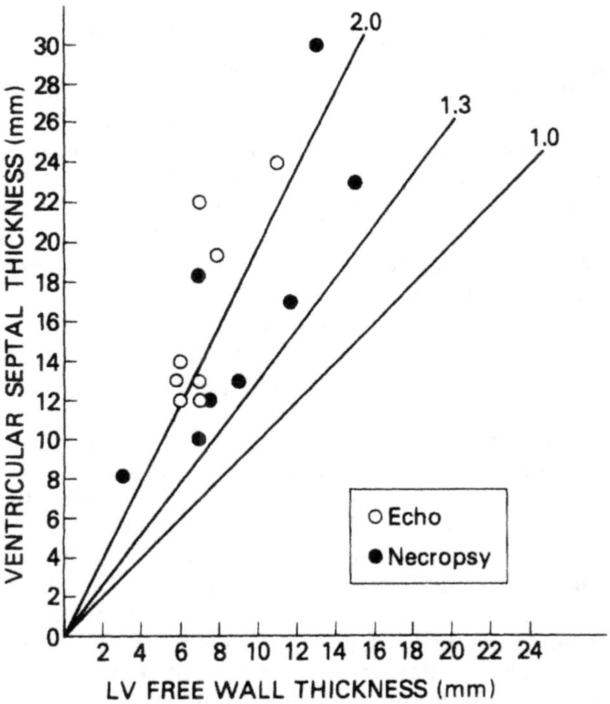

FIGURE 6. *Assessment by echocardiography (in diastole) or at necropsy of ventricular septal thickness, posterior left ventricular (LV) free wall thickness and septal–free wall thickness ratio in 16 infants. Identity lines define septal–free wall ratios of 1.0, 1.3, 1.5 and 2.0. The echocardiographic data were taken from the technically best study recorded closest to 2 years of age.*

patients became severely symptomatic (and died) with progressive congestive heart failure in the first year of life; only two died suddenly and unexpectedly. However, potential biases in our patient selection preclude definitive conclusions regarding the natural history of hypertrophic cardiomyopathy in infancy. For example, 70% of the patients in this study were identified as having heart disease in infancy solely because of the recognition of a loud heart murmur, indicative of outflow tract obstruction. Hence, patients with the nonobstructive form of hypertrophic cardiomyopathy (the most common hemodynamic variety of this disease in adults[29]) would be less likely to be identified in infancy because no murmur or only a soft murmur would be present.

Nevertheless, the onset of marked congestive heart failure during the first year of life appeared to be a poor prognostic sign; nine of the 11 patients with this clinical course died, either suddenly, of heart failure or after operation, before 1 year of age. Digitalis was administered to seven of the nine infants who died, including three with obstruction to ventricular outflow, and was ineffective in treating their marked congestive heart failure. The clinical profile of heart failure in these patients occurred in the presence of a nondilated heart with normal or increased systolic function. Hence, administration of digitalis would seem inappropriate, particularly if obstruction to ventricular outflow is present, and we do not recommend its use in such patients.

The two infants in this study group who had heart failure and survived had received propranolol. Although β blockers such as propranolol theoretically reduce left ventricular outflow obstruction, their negative inotropic effect on ventricular contractility may compromise their therapeutic value in infants with hypertrophic cardiomyopathy and heart failure. Thus, the safest course for infants with hypertrophic cardiomyopathy and severe congestive heart failure may be to administer diuretic agents alone. If this approach is ineffective, cautious use of a β-blocking agent might be warranted.

Infants with hypertrophic cardiomyopathy probably suffer importantly from impairment to ventricular filling.[32] Calcium-channel blockers such as verapamil improve diastolic filling[32] and functional capacity[33] in adults with hypertrophic cardiomyopathy. Therefore, verapamil may be beneficial for treating infants with hypertrophic cardiomyopathy. However, calcium-channel blockers have recognized side effects[34] and should be administered judiciously in such infants.

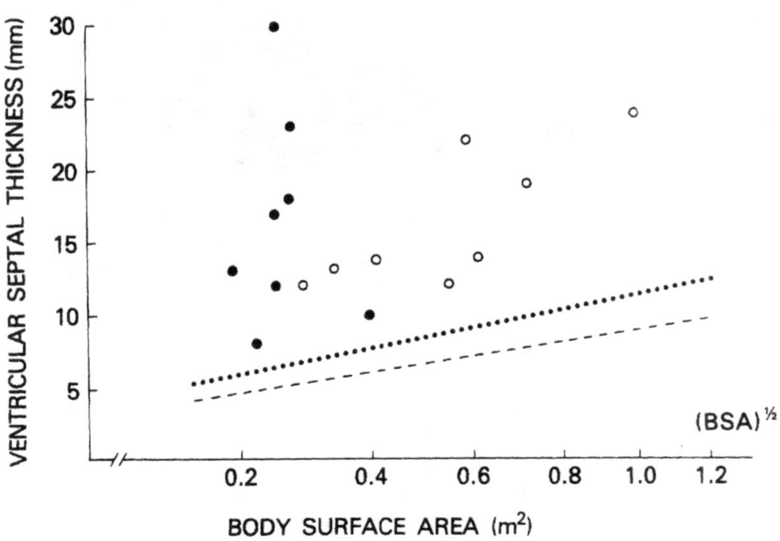

FIGURE 7. *Relation of ventricular septal thickness obtained by echocardiography in diastole (open symbols) or at necropsy (solid symbols) and body surface area (BSA) in 16 infants. Upper limits of normal (shown by the broken and dotted lines) were derived from analysis of echocardiograms from infants without heart disease.[20] The dotted line represents the 95% prediction interval for systolic measurements, with which the septal thicknesses obtained at necropsy are compared.[40] The broken line represents the 95% prediction interval for diastolic measurements, with which septal thicknesses obtained by echocardiography are compared.[40]*

Marked obstruction to right ventricular outflow under basal conditions was common in our infants with hypertrophic cardiomyopathy. What causes subpulmonic obstruction in patients with hypertrophic cardiomyopathy is not definitively known; it may be produced by the marked bulging of the hypertrophied ventricular septum[35] into the relatively small right ventricular outflow tract. Systolic anterior motion of the anterior tricuspid valve leaflet could be another mechanism by which right ventricular outflow tract obstruction occurs in such patients.[36]

The fact that subpulmonic obstruction is relatively common in infants and young children with hypertrophic cardiomyopathy,[1, 5, 7, 12, 15] but appears to be uncommon in patients who reach adulthood[1], can be explained in two ways. First, the right ventricular outflow obstruction present in some infants may resolve spontaneously with growth and aging, as a result of conformational changes in cardiac structure that increase the size of the right ventricular outflow tract. Second, the combined subaortic and subpulmonic obstruction may represent a particularly lethal hemodynamic alteration in infants with hypertrophic cardiomyopathy, predisposing them to premature death, which accounts for the rarity of marked obstruction to right ventricular outflow in adult patients with this disease.

Substantial evidence indicates that hypertrophic cardiomyopathy in children and adults is often genetically transmitted.[1, 6, 8, 29, 30, 37] Echocardiographic or historical evidence for genetic transmission of hypertrophic cardiomyopathy was found in only six of our 20 infants (30%); the rest either had no evidence for genetic transmission or insufficient data were available to make this assessment. Therefore, although our data clearly show that genetic transmission may occur in relatives of infants with hypertrophic cardiomyopathy, the true prevalence of genetically transmitted disease in our study population is uncertain. Nevertheless, our findings suggest that in addition to genetically transmitted hypertrophic cardiomyopathy, other etiologically distinct and nongenetic forms of this disease probably occur in infants.

The cardiac structural alterations characteristic of patients with hypertrophic cardiomyopathy can be evident quite early in life and are probably present at birth. Each of the seven patients studied by echocardiography or at necropsy before 6 months of age had substantial ventricular septal hypertrophy. Four of these seven patients, as well as a previously reported stillborn infant,[13] had an absolute septal thickness of 13 mm or more (range 13–30 mm). However, the fact that the average septal thickness in our infants younger than 6 months of age was 16 mm (compared

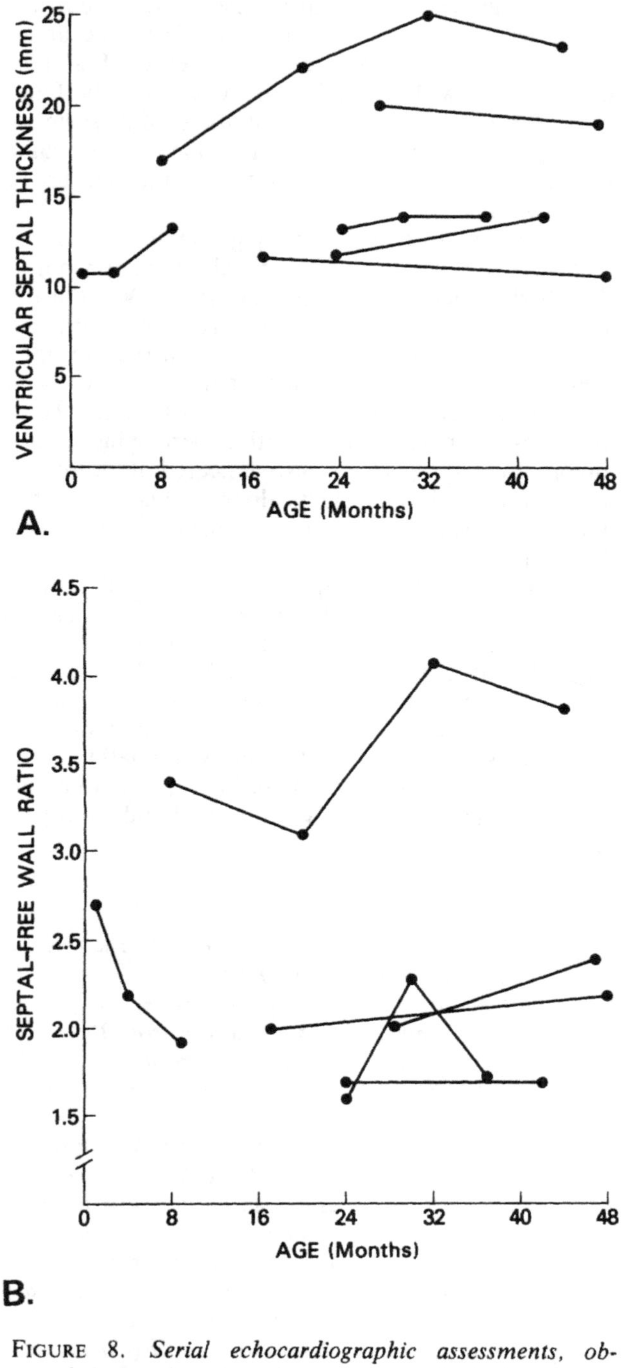

FIGURE 8. *Serial echocardiographic assessments, obtained during diastole, of ventricular wall thicknesses (A) and septal-free wall thickness ratios (B) in six infants.*

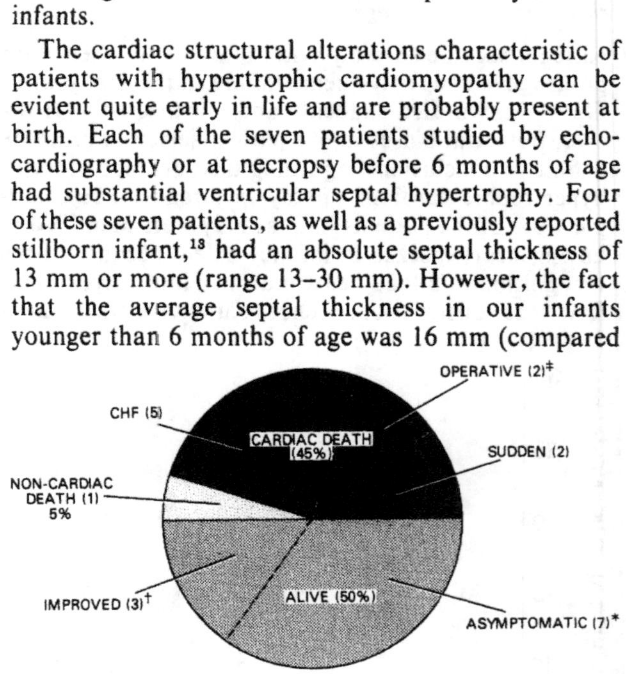

FIGURE 9. *Clinical course of 20 infants with hypertrophic cardiomyopathy. CHF = congestive heart failure. *Includes one patient who underwent combined septal myotomy-myectomy and resection of right ventricular outflow tract muscle. †Includes one patient who underwent septal myotomy-myectomy. ‡Includes two patients who underwent resection of right ventricular outflow tract muscle.*

with an average of 21 mm or 26 mm for populations of adult patients with hypertrophic cardiomyopathy studied by echocardiography[37] or at necropsy,[22] respectively) suggests that further thickening of the septum occurs with aging and growth. In addition, five of six patients studied at necropsy before 6 months of age showed marked disorganization of ventricular septal architecture, similar in appearance and extent to that present in older children and adults with hypertrophic cardiomyopathy.[4, 10, 22, 23]

A septal-free wall thickness ratio $\geq$ 1.3 has been shown at necropsy[38] and by echocardiography[39] to be relatively common in normal neonates and infants with congenital heart malformations other than hypertrophic cardiomyopathy. However, the asymmetry in ventricular wall thicknesses that occurs in such infants should not be confused with the asymmetric left ventricular hypertrophy present in our infants with hypertrophic cardiomyopathy. Infants with "true" hypertrophic cardiomyopathy can be distinguished from other infants with abnormal septal-free wall ratios by three criteria: absence of an associated cardiac lesion capable of producing disproportionate thickening of the ventricular septum;[27, 38] presence of marked absolute ventricular septal thickening; and no substantial decrease in the septal-free wall thickness ratio with increasing age and the persistence of an abnormal septal-free wall ratio (i.e., $\geq$ 1.3) after 2 years of age.

References

1. Frank S, Braunwald E: Idiopathic hypertrophic subaortic stenosis. Clinical analysis of 126 patients with emphasis on the natural history. Circulation **37:** 759, 1968
2. Adelman AG, Wigle ED, Ranganathan N, Webb GD, Kidd BSL, Bigelow WG, Silver MD: The clinical course in muscular subaortic stenosis. A retrospective and prospective study of 60 hemodynamically proved cases. Ann Intern Med **77:** 515, 1972
3. Hardarson T, De la Calzada CS, Curiel R, Goodwin JF: Prognosis and mortality of hypertrophic obstructive cardiomyopathy. Lancet **2:** 1462, 1973
4. Teare D: Asymmetrical hypertrophy of the heart in young patients. Br Heart J **20:** 1, 1958
5. Daoud G, Gallagher ME, Kaplan S: Muscular subaortic stenosis. Am J Cardiol **7:** 860, 1961
6. Wood RS, Taylor WJ, Wheat MW, Schiebler GL: Muscular subaortic stenosis in childhood. Report of occurrence in three siblings. Pediatrics **30:** 749, 1962
7. Rudhe U, Zetterquist P, Wallgren G: Angiocardiography of hypertrophic obstructive cardiomyopathy in infancy and childhood. Ann Radiol **9:** 185, 1966
8. Nasser WK, Williams JF, Mishkin ME, Childress RH, Helmen C, Merritt AD, Genovese PD: Familial myocardial disease with and without obstruction to left ventricular outflow. Clinical, hemodynamic, and angiographic findings. Circulation **35:** 638, 1967
9. Williams RG, Ellison RC, Nadas AS: Development of left ventricular outflow obstruction in idiopathic hypertrophic subaortic stenosis. N Engl J Med **288:** 868, 1973
10. Maron BJ, Henry WL, Clark CE, Redwood DR, Roberts WC, Epstein SE: Asymmetric septal hypertrophy in childhood. Circulation **53:** 9, 1976
11. Fiddler GL, Tajik AJ, Weidman WH, McGoon DC, Ritter DG, Giuliani ER: Idiopathic hypertrophic subaortic stenosis in the young. Am J Cardiol **42:** 793, 1978
12. Barr PA, Celermajer JM, Bowdler JD, Cartmill TB: Idiopathic hypertrophic obstructive cardiomyopathy causing severe right ventricular outflow tract obstruction in infancy. Br Heart J **35:** 1109, 1973
13. Maron BJ, Edwards JE, Henry WL, Clark CE, Bingle GJ, Epstein SE: Asymmetric septal hypertrophy (ASH) in infancy. Circulation **50:** 809, 1974
14. Lundquist CB, Amplatz K, Palma SP, Raghib G: Angiocardiographic findings in idiopathic myocardial hypertrophy with right and left ventricular outflow tract obstruction. AJR **93:** 315, 1965
15. Shand DG, Sell CG, Oates JA: Hypertrophic obstructive cardiomyopathy in an infant — propranolol therapy for three years. N Engl J Med **285:** 843, 1971
16. Maron BJ, Epstein SE: Hypertrophic cardiomyopathy: a discussion of nomenclature. Am J Cardiol **43:** 1242, 1979
17. Way GL, Wolfe RR, Eshaghpour E, Bender RL, Jaffe RB, Ruttenberg HD: The natural history of hypertrophic cardiomyopathy in infants of diabetic mothers. J Pediatr **95:** 1020, 1979
18. Gutgesell HP, Speer M, Rosenberg HS: Further characterization of the hypertrophic cardiomyopathy of infants of diabetic mothers. Circulation **61:** 441, 1980
19. Henry WL, Clark CE, Epstein SE: Asymmetric septal hypertrophy (ASH): echocardiographic identification of the pathognomonic anatomic abnormality of IHSS. Circulation **47:** 225, 1973
20. Henry WL, Ware J, Gardin JM, Hepner SI, McKay J, Weiner M: Echocardiographic measurements in normal subjects. Growth-related changes that occur between infancy and early adulthood. Circulation **57:** 278, 1978
21. Sahn DJ, DeMaria A, Kisslo J, Weyman A: Recommendations regarding quantitation in M-mode echocardiography: results of a survey of echocardiographic measurements. Circulation **58:** 1072, 1978
22. Maron BJ, Roberts WC: Quantitative analysis of cardiac muscle cell disorganization in the ventricular septum of patients with hypertrophic cardiomyopathy. Circulation **59:** 689, 1979
23. Maron BJ, Sato N, Roberts WC, Edwards JE, Chandra RS: Quantitative analysis of cardiac muscle cell disorganization in the ventricular septum: comparison of fetuses and infants with and without congenital heart disease and patients with hypertrophic cardiomyopathy. Circulation **60:** 685, 1979
24. Polani PE, Moynahan EJ: Progressive cardiomyopathic lentiginosis. Q J Med **41:** 205, 1972
25. Ehlers KH, Engle MA, Levin AR, Deely WJ: Eccentric ventricular hypertrophy in familial and sporadic instances of 46 XX, XY Turner phenotype. Circulation **45:** 639, 1972
26. Henry WL, Clark CE, Glancy DL, Epstein SE: Echocardiographic measurement of the left ventricular outflow gradient in idiopathic hypertrophic subaortic stenosis. N Engl J Med **288:** 989, 1973
27. Maron BJ, Clark CE, Henry WL, Fukuda T, Edwards JE, Mathews EC, Redwood DR, Epstein SE: Prevalence and characteristics of disproportionate ventricular septal thickening in patients with acquired or congenital heart disease: echocardiographic and morphologic findings. Circulation **55:** 489, 1977
28. Morrow AG: Hypertrophic subaortic stenosis: operative methods utilized to relieve left ventricular outflow obstruction. J Thorac Cardiovasc Surg **76:** 423, 1978
29. Clark CE, Henry WL, Epstein SE: Familial prevalence and genetic transmission of idiopathic hypertrophic subaortic stenosis. N Engl J Med **289:** 709, 1973
30. Pare JAP, Fraser RG, Pirozynski WJ, Shanks JA, Stubington D: Hereditary cardiovascular dysplasia. A form of familial cardiomyopathy. Am J Med **31:** 37, 1961
31. Maron BJ, Roberts WC, Edwards JE, McAllister HA, Foley DD, Epstein SE: Sudden death in patients with hypertrophic cardiomyopathy: characterization of 26 patients without functional limitation. Am J Cardiol **41:** 803, 1978
32. Hanrath P, Mathey DG, Kremer P, Sonntag F, Bleifeld W: Effect of verapamil on left ventricular isovolumic relaxation time and regional left ventricular filling in hypertrophic cardiomyopathy. Am J Cardiol **45:** 1258, 1980
33. Rosing DR, Kent KM, Maron BJ, Epstein SE: Verapamil therapy: a new approach to the pharmacologic treatment of hypertrophic cardiomyopathy. II. Effects on exercise capacity and symptomatic status. Circulation **60:** 1208, 1979
34. Epstein SE, Rosing DR: Verapamil: its potential for causing

serious complications in patients with hypertrophic cardiomyopathy. Circulation **64:** 437, 1981
35. Goodwin JP, Shah PM, Oakley CM, Cohen J, Yipinstoi T, Pocock W: The clinical pharmacology of hypertrophic obstructive cardiomyopathy. *In* Cardiomyopathies. A Ciba Foundation Symposium, edited by Wolstenholme GEW, O'Connor M. London, J & A Churchill, 1964, p 189
36. Brik H, Meller J, Bahler AS, Herman MV, Teichholz LE: Systolic anterior motion of the tricuspid valve in idiopathic hypertrophic subaortic stenosis. J Clin Ultrasound **6:** 121, 1978
37. Epstein SE, Henry WL, Clark CE, Roberts WC, Maron BJ, Ferrans VJ, Redwood DR, Morrow AG: Asymmetric septal hypertrophy. Ann Intern Med **81:** 650, 1974
38. Maron BJ, Edwards JE, Moller J, Epstein SE: Prevalence and characteristics of disproportionate ventricular septal thickening in infants with congenital heart disease. Circulation **59:** 126, 1979
39. Larter WE, Allen HD, Sahn DJ, Goldberg SJ: The asymmetrically hypertrophied septum. Further differentiation of its causes. Circulation **53:** 19, 1976
40. Maron BJ, Henry WL, Roberts WC, Epstein SE: Comparison of echocardiographic and necropsy measurements of ventricular wall thicknesses in patients with and without disproportionate septal thickening. Circulation **55:** 341, 1977

Left Atrial-to-Right Atrial Shunt without Atrial Septal Defect or Precordial Murmur*

Pulmonary Varix and Hypertrophic Cardiomyopathy

Frank C. Brosius, III, M.D.; David E. Schwartz, M.D.; William L. Gleason, M.D.; Barry Maron, M.D.; Michael Jones, M.D.; and William C. Roberts, M.D., F.C.C.P.

Pulmonary varix is infrequent, and when present, is usually clinically silent and found only as an incidental finding on chest roentgenogram. Hypertrophic cardiomyopathy, in contrast, is fairly frequent, and when present, is frequently clinically apparent. When the two occur together in the same patient, however, the pulmonary varix (with anomalous systemic venous connection) may become clinically apparent, the second (hypertrophy cardiomyopathy), the real culprit, may remain clinically silent and the combination may present challenging diagnostic and therapeutic difficulties which are described below.

A 49-year-old man who died on February 7, 1980, was found to have left ventricular hypertrophy on electrocardiogram during a routine examination at age 32 years (1963) (Fig 1). Cardiac catheterization disclosed a 19 mm Hg peak systolic pressure gradient between the left ventricle and aorta and a 2.8:1 left-to-right shunt via a large vein in the upper lobe of the left lung which connected to a vertical vein which in turn connected to the innominate vein. He was asymptomatic until age 43 when exertional dyspnea and excessive fatigue appeared. Intermittent atrial flutter and fibrillation appeared the following year, and congestive cardiac failure became overt and progressively worsened thereafter. Angiography at age 48 disclosed a dilated and diffusely hypocontractile left ventricle and a year later, the electrocardiogram showed marked diminution of amplitude of QRS complexes and loss or severe diminution of R waves in the precordial leads. At age 48, bilateral pleural effusions appeared and persisted thereafter.

When hospitalized on January 23, 1980, he was cachectic, dyspneic and dehydrated. He had never had chest pain. The neck veins were greatly distended; the liver, large, and the legs, non-edematous. The heart was large (Fig 2). A third heart sound was present but there was no precordial murmur. Electrocardiogram (Fig 1) now disclosed left

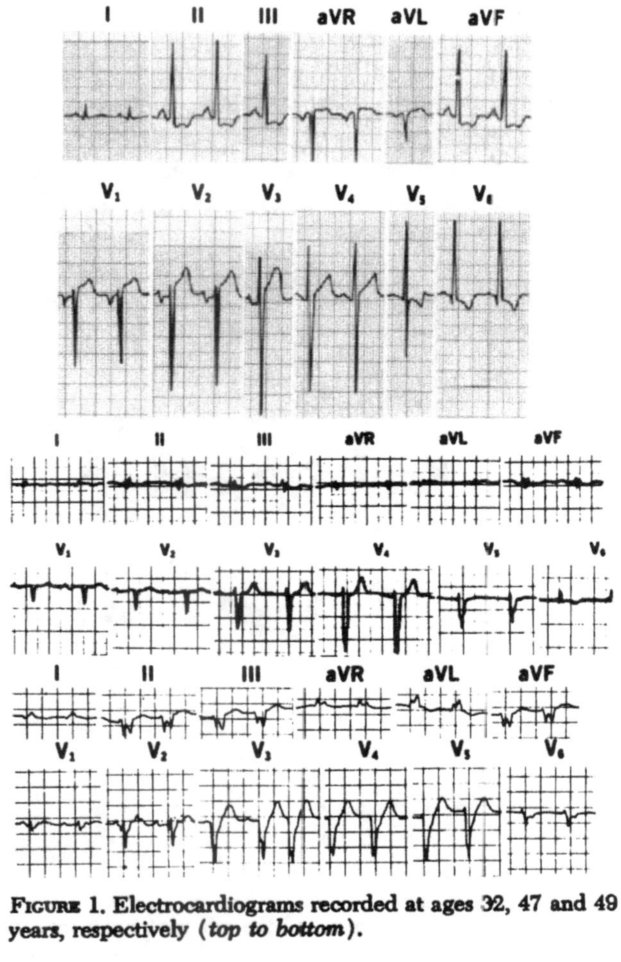

FIGURE 1. Electrocardiograms recorded at ages 32, 47 and 49 years, respectively (*top to bottom*).

*From the Pathology, Cardiology and Surgery Branches, National Heart, Lung and Blood Institute, National Institutes of Health, Bethesda, and the Department of Medicine, Watson Clinic, Lakeland, Florida.
Reprint requests: Dr. Roberts, Bldg 10A, Rm 3E30, National Institutes of Health, Bethesda 20205

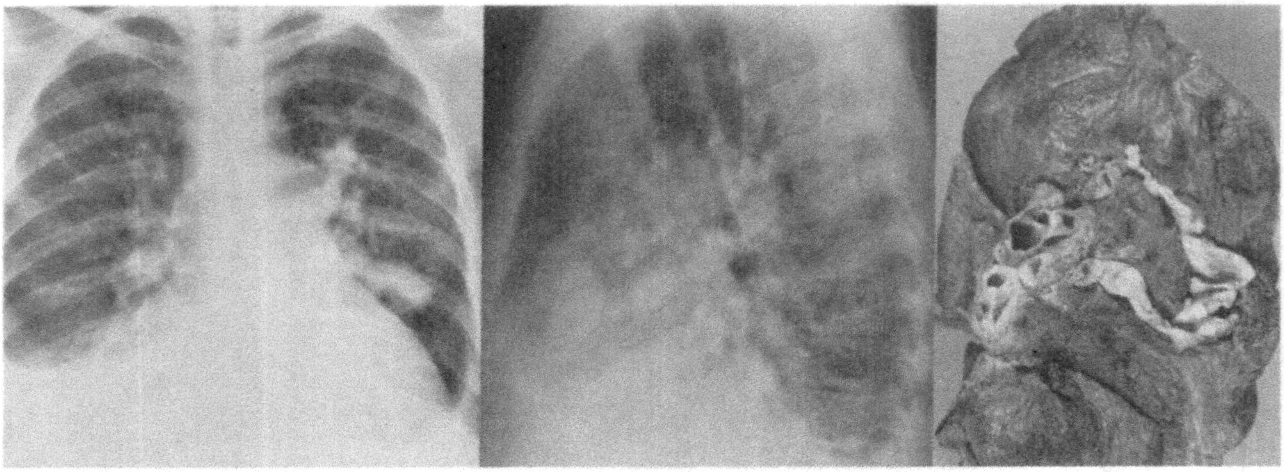

FIGURE 2. Posteroanterior (*left*) and lateral roentgenograms (*middle*) taken two weeks before death, and the left lung (*right*) at necropsy with the pulmonary varix dissected free. The pulmonary varix is seen well in both radiographs.

anterior hemiblock. On echocardiogram (Fig 3), both ventricular cavities were dilated and the ventricular septum and the left ventricular free wall were of similar thickness. Cardiac catheterization was repeated (Table 1). To exclude pericardial constriction, median sternotomy was performed: large pleural effusions were found but the pericardia were normal and the pericardial space was free of adhesions and excess fluid. The left vertical vein (Fig 4) measured up to 2.2 cm in diameter and the innominate vein, to 3.0 cm. Postoperation, he was hypotensive despite therapy with vasopressors and aortic balloon counterpulsation, the right-sided intracardiac pressures remained elevated, and the left-to-right shunt increased progressively from 3:1 to 11:1. Reoperation was done four hours after the first: the vertical vein was divided and anastomosed to the left atrium, but the patient could not be separated from cardiopulmonary bypass.

At necropsy, the heart weighed 540 gm. All four cardiac chambers were mildly dilated. The ventricular septum and left ventricular free wall were of similar thickness (1.7 cm). Both the ventricular septum and anterior portion of left ventricular free wall were extensively replaced by dense fibrous tissue (Fig 5). The cardiac valves and mural endocardium were normal. Of the 39 5-mm long segments of the left main, left anterior descending, left circumflex and right coronary arteries, none was narrowed 51-100 percent; 27 (69 percent) were narrowed 26-50 percent, and 12 (31 percent), 0-25 percent, in cross-sectional area by atherosclerotic plaques. Most of the intramural coronary arteries in the ventricular septum had thickened walls and a few, narrowed lumens. On quantitative analysis of transversely-cut sections of ventricular septum by a method described previously,[1] 40 percent of the myocardium was disorganized (normal = <5 per-

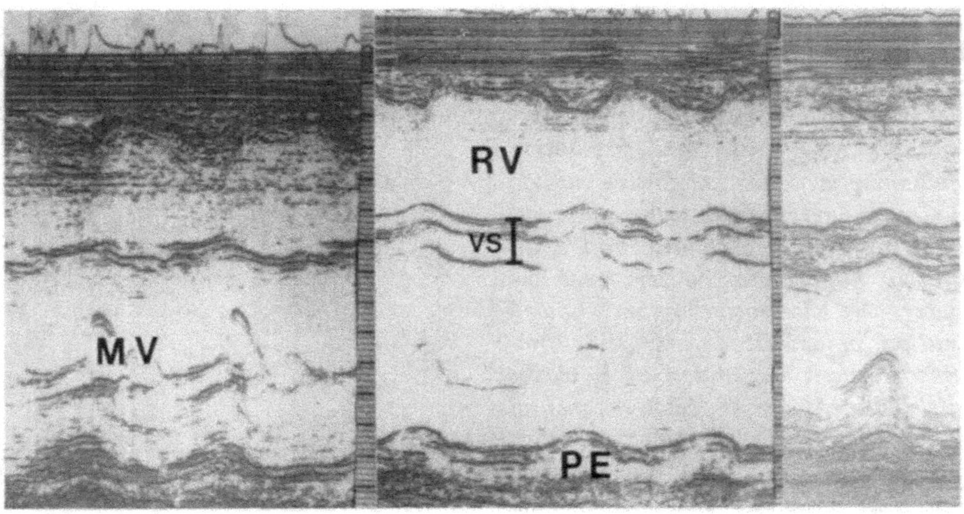

FIGURE 3. Echocardiogram recorded a week before death. The ventricular septum (VS) measures 15 mm and the left ventricular free wall, 14 mm in thickness. Both right (RV) and left ventricular cavities are dilated. A pericardial effusion (PE) is present. MV = mitral valve.

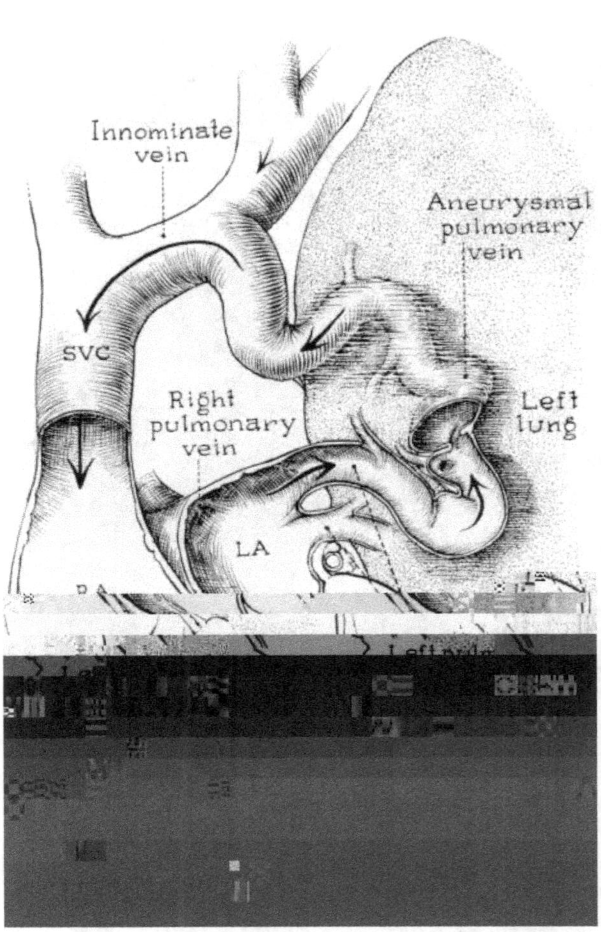

FIGURE 4. Diagram of the pulmonary varix and its connection to left atrium and to an anomalous systemic vein. The flow of blood in the varix is reverse of that which might have been expected had the heart been normal. IVC = inferior vena cava; LA = left atrium; LV = left ventricle; RA = right atrium; RV = right ventricle and SVC = superior vena cava.

cent); of similarly cut sections of anterior and posterior left ventricular free wall, 7 percent and 3 percent, respectively, were disorganized (normal < 10 percent). The varix was located in the lingular portions of the left upper lobe of the lung (Fig 2 and 4). Its maximal diameter was 2.5 cm and its wall was thin. The pulmonary parenchyma and pulmonary arteries were normal.

DISCUSSION

Although it was appreciated that the left-to-right shunt could hardly explain all the clinical, electrocardiographic, hemodynamic and radiographic findings, the presence of hypertrophic cardiomyopathy in the above described patient was never appreciated clinically. The diagnosis of hypertrophic cardiomyopathy at necropsy, however, was clear. He had left ventricular hypertrophy without (at least initially) left ventricular dilatation, systemic hypertension, supravalvular, valvular or discrete subvalvular aortic stenosis, and (at least initially) with a normal or supranormal cardiac output. He developed a large anteroseptal myocardial infarct which also was clinically silent, but which also is a well-recognized complication of hypertrophic cardiomyopathy.[2] Nearly one-half of the ventricular septum consisted of disorganized myocardial fibers and many intramural coronary arteries were thickened, both findings being typical of hypertrophic cardiomyopathy.[1,3]

The pulmonary varix which connected to an anomalous systemic vein and to the left atrium would probably have caused little to no symptoms of cardiac dysfunction had not hypertrophic cardiomyopathy also been present. With a normal left ventricle, its filling would have been unimpeded, thereby minimizing the left-to-right shunt through the pulmonary varix. The considerable left ventricular hypertrophy and scarring caused by the hypertrophic cardiomyopathy undoubtedly diminished left ventricular compliance, favoring drainage of oxygenated blood retrogradely through the pulmonary varix, with subsequent drainage into the anomalous systemic vein which in turn connected to the innominate vein, allowing for a left-atrial-to-right-atrial shunt without an atrial septal defect. A similar pathway, incidentally, has been described in several patients with mitral valve atresia and partial anomalous pulmonary venous connection.[4] Physiologically, the circumstance in our patient is similar to that in patients with mitral stenosis associated with atrial septal defect (Lutembacher's syndrome).[5] As in patients with Lutembacher's syndrome, the anomalous venous connection in our patient presumably relieved the left-sided congestive cardiac failure which might have been expected from the associated hypertrophic cardiomyopathy and augmented signs and symptoms of right-sided cardiac failure. Certainly, the presence of severe jugular venous distension and hepatomegaly without pulmonary edema, orthopnea or nocturnal dyspnea is atypical for hypertrophic cardiomyopathy and favors this hypothesis. The equal and elevated end-diastolic pressures in all four cardiac chambers also might be explained from the elevated left-sided pressures (due to the cardiomyopathy) which were transmitted to the right side of the heart through the anomalous venous connection.

The pulmonary varix in our patient was unusual not only in occurring in association with hypertrophic cardiomyopathy, but also in connecting to an anomalous systemic vein, an occurrence not hitherto reported. The varix was located in the left upper lobe which is the second most common site for varices.[6] The varix presented typical radiographic features (vascular shadow) with delayed filling in the levophase on angiogram.[7] At necropsy, the

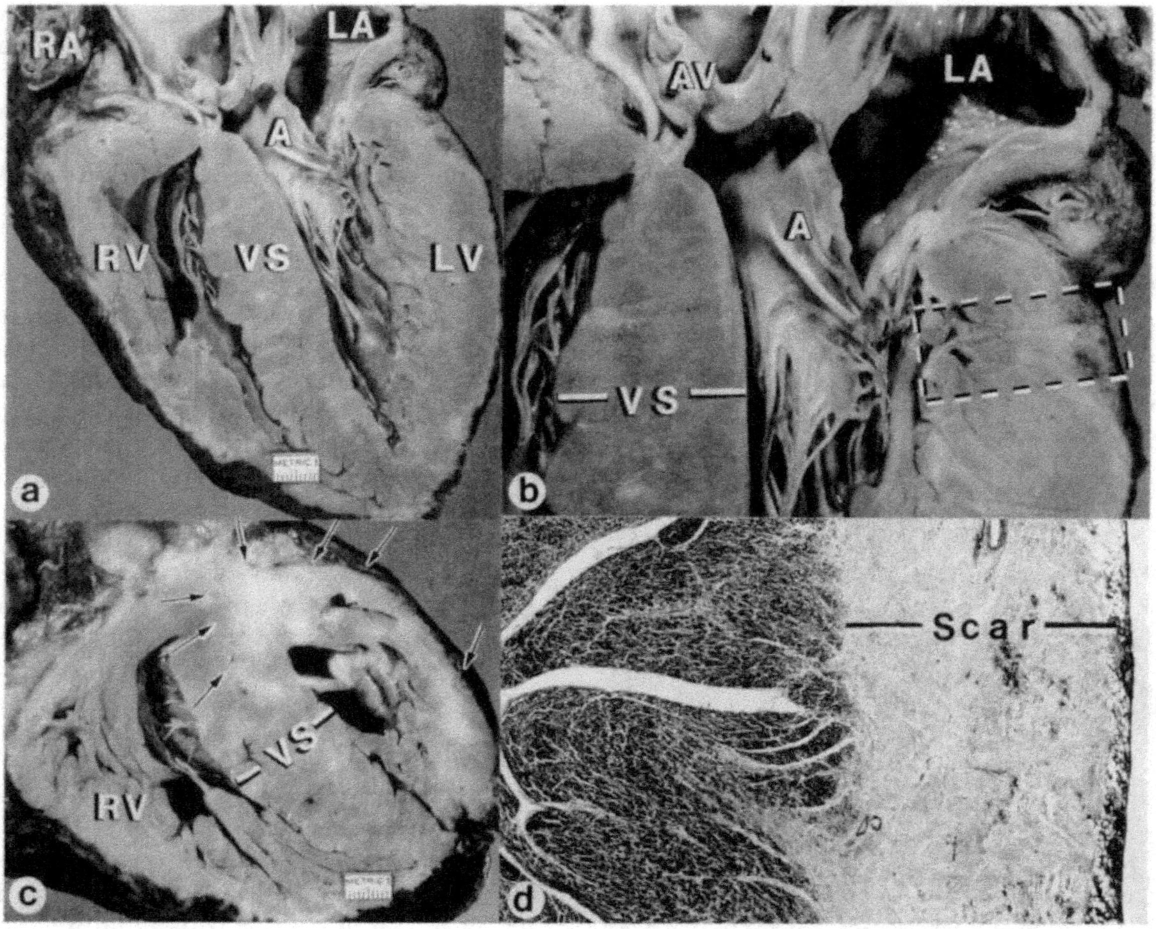

FIGURE 5. The heart. *a* anteroposterior cut (similar to that of the M-mode echo beam) showing the relative thickness of the right ventricular (RV), ventricular septal (VS) and left ventricular (LV) walls and the sizes of the ventricular cavities. A = anterior leaflet of the mitral valve; LA = left atrium; RA = right atrium. *b* close-up of mitral valve area. The most basal portion of left ventricular free wall is thinner than that in the mid-portion, the reverse of normal. A subepicardial scar, a fairly frequent occurrence in hypertrophic cardiomyopathy, is partially enclosed by brackets and a close-up photomicrograph (X16) of the area in brackets is shown in d. *c* A more anterior cut of the ventricles showing many transmural ventricular scars (*arrows*).

varix was tortuous, thin-walled and obviously aneurysmal compared to other pulmonary veins. Although usually benign, pulmonary varix may rupture, as described in at least three patients.[8,9] The relatively frequent association of pulmonary varices with other cardiac and pulmonary abnormalities,[10] however, indicates that patients with pulmonary varices should be examined for associated or additional cardiopulmonary abnormalities.

REFERENCES

1 Maron BJ, Roberts WC. Quantitative analysis of cardiac muscle cell disorganization in the ventricular septum of patients with hypertrophic cardiomyopathy. Circulation 1979; 59:689-706

2 Maron BJ, Epstein SE, Roberts WC. Hypertrophic cardiomyopathy and transmural myocardial infarction without significant atherosclerosis of the extramural coronary arteries. Am J Cardiol 1979; 43:1086-1102

3 McReynolds RA, Roberts WC. The intramural coronary arteries in hypertrophic cardiomyopathy (abstract). Am J Cardiol 1975; 35:154

4 Shone JD, Edwards JE. Mitral atresia associated with pulmonary venous anomalies. Br Heart J 1964; 26:241-49

5 Steinbrunn W, Cohn KE, Selzer A. Atrial septal defect associated with mitral stenosis: the Lutembacher syndrome revisited. Am J Med 1970; 48:295-302

6 Romanoff H, Manny J, Aviad I. Pulmonary varices. Report of two cases and review of the literature. Chest 1976; 70:395-97

7 Poller S, Wholey MH: Pulmonary varix: evaluation by selective pulmonary angiography. Radiology 1966; 86: 1078-81

8 Klinch GH Jr, Hunt HD. Pulmonary varix with spontaneous rupture and death. Arch Pathol 1933; 15:227-37

9 Perret L, Fortelius P. Ruptured aneurysm of a pulmonary vein. Acta Tuberc Scand 1962; 41:53-55

10 Moro C, Marin E, Sanchez A, Solozabal J. Pulmonary varix: report of a case with additional anomalies of the vascular pulmonary tree. Am Heart J 1978; 95:243-46

Sudden Death in Hypertrophic Cardiomyopathy: A Profile of 78 Patients

Barry J. Maron, M.D., William C. Roberts, M.D., and Stephen E. Epstein, M.D.

SUMMARY **The clinical profile of 78 patients with hypertrophic cardiomyopathy who died suddenly (or experienced cardiac arrest and survived) was analyzed. At the time of cardiac catastrophe, 71% of the patients were younger than 30 years of age, 54% were without functional limitation and 61% were performing sedentary or minimal physical activity. Nineteen of the 78 patients (24%) were taking propranolol in apparently adequate dosages, indicating that this drug does not provide absolute protection against sudden death.**

No clinical or morphologic variable was particularly reliable in identifying patients at risk for sudden death. Forty-eight of 62 patients (77%) who died suddenly had a markedly increased ventricular septal thickness of 20 mm or more; however, mean septal thickness was similar in patients who died suddenly (25.2 ± 0.9 mm) and in age- and sex-matched control patients with hypertrophic cardiomyopathy who have survived (23.6 ± 0.8 mm). An abnormal ECG was present as often in patients who died suddenly as in control patients who have survived, (51 of 53, 96%). In addition, no particular cardiac symptom or hemodynamic variable (such as the magnitude of left ventricular outflow tract obstruction under basal conditions or left ventricular end-diastolic pressure) was characteristic of the patients with hypertrophic cardiomyopathy who died suddenly.

PREMATURE SUDDEN DEATH is not uncommon in patients with hypertrophic cardiomyopathy.[1-10] Groups of patients with hypertrophic cardiomyopathy who died suddenly have been described,[6-9] but a detailed clinical and morphologic analysis of a large series of such patients is not available. It is not known whether certain clinical measurements can predict which patients with hypertrophic cardiomyopathy are at increased risk of sudden death. Thus, the present clinical profile of 78 patients with hypertrophic cardiomyopathy who died suddenly was assembled and is the subject of this report.

Patients

Autopsy records of the Pathology Branch and the patient records of the Cardiology Branch, 1960–1980, were reviewed. Sixty-six nonoperated patients with hypertrophic cardiomyopathy who died suddenly and unexpectedly were identified. Sudden death was defined as instantaneous collapse with subsequent death or documentation of ventricular fibrillation within minutes. Five of the 66 patients had survived a previous cardiac arrest with documented ventricular fibrillation 3 weeks to 26 months (median 20 months) before death.

Twelve other patients who experienced a cardiac arrest (with documented ventricular fibrillation), but who were successfully resuscitated and have survived to date were included in the study group and were considered to represent sudden deaths. These 12 patients have survived for 7 months to 15 years (mean 3.8 years) after their arrest, although one has had two subsequent occurrences of ventricular fibrillation; 10 of these 12 patients have also undergone ventricular septal myotomy-myectomy since the cardiac arrest.[11]

From the Cardiology and Pathology Branches, National Heart, Lung, and Blood Institute, National Institutes of Health, Bethesda, Maryland.

Address for correspondence: Barry J. Maron, M.D., National Heart, Lung, and Blood Institute, National Institutes of Health, Building 10, Room 7B-15, Bethesda, Maryland 20205.

Received March 2, 1981; revision accepted October 9, 1981.

Circulation 65, No. 7, 1982.

Of the 78 study patients, 29 had been evaluated at the National Heart, Lung, and Blood Institute before their death or cardiac arrest; the other 49 were either evaluated at institutions other than the National Heart, Lung, and Blood Institute or were never evaluated clinically. Fifteen patients had been chronically conditioned competitive athletes; seven of these 15 were initially identified because they were athletes who had died suddenly and were found to have hypertrophic cardiomyopathy only after examination of the heart at necropsy.[12]

The diagnosis of hypertrophic cardiomyopathy was based on the presence of a hypertrophied, nondilated left ventricle in the absence of another cardiac or systemic disease capable of producing left ventricular hypertrophy.[13] The presence of a hypertrophied, nondilated left ventricle was documented at necropsy in 45 patients, by echocardiography in 17 patients, by echocardiography and at necropsy in eight patients, and by left ventricular angiography in eight patients. Three patients in the study group had associated systemic hypertension, but are included because they demonstrated clinical or hemodynamic features consistent with hypertrophic cardiomyopathy[14] or because the extent of left ventricular hypertrophy clearly exceeded that which would have been expected to result from hypertension alone.[15, 16]

Sixteen other patients with hypertrophic cardiomyopathy who died suddenly were excluded from the present study group: Five had associated, hemodynamically significant coronary artery disease documented at necropsy (i.e., atherosclerotic luminal narrowing greater than 75% of the cross-sectional area of at least one major extramural coronary artery). In six, death was clearly related to a cerebrovascular accident or other embolic phenomena, including one with a pulmonary embolus. In five, the presence of coronary heart disease could not be definitively excluded; each of these patients was older than 40 years of age and did not undergo coronary arteriography during life or have a necropsy examination.

Fifteen of the 78 study patients did not undergo coronary arteriography or necropsy examination to definitively exclude coronary heart disease. However, based on patient age and clinical history, we believe that it is highly unlikely that any of these 15 patients with hypertrophic cardiomyopathy had associated hemodynamically significant coronary arterial narrowing, and therefore they have been included in the study group. Seven of the 15 patients were younger than 18 years of age; five others (three men and two women) were 21–37 years old, and had never experienced chest pain. The other three (two men and one woman) had experienced episodes of chest pain but were 29, 38 and 37 years of age.

Methods

Echocardiography

The echocardiographic technique used in this study has been described.[17] Echocardiograms were obtained with a 2.25-MHz, 1.2-cm-diameter Aerotech transducer connected to either a modified Ekoline 20A or a Hoffrel 201 ultrasound unit. The ultrasonic signal was connected by means of a custom-built video amplifier to a Honeywell 1856 Visicorder and recorded continuously on light-sensitive paper. The thickness of the ventricular septum was measured below the tips of the mitral valve leaflets just before atrial systole; the posterior left ventricular wall thickness was measured at the level of the tips of the mitral valve leaflets during the same phase of the cardiac cycle. The left ventricular outflow gradient (in mm Hg) was estimated from the M-mode echocardiogram based on the magnitude and duration of systolic anterior motion of the anterior mitral leaflet.[18]

Necropsy

Measurements of ventricular wall thicknesses were made at necropsy in the ventricular septum, just below the tips of the mitral leaflets, usually about one-half the distance between the base of the aortic valve and the apex of left ventricle; and in the posterior left ventricular wall, behind the midpoint of the posterior mitral leaflet, at a level corresponding to the tips of the mitral leaflets. In measuring ventricular wall thicknesses, we avoided including trabeculae, papillary muscles or crista supraventricularis. Two patients in whom transmural scarring of the ventricular septum and left ventricular free wall[19] was identified at necropsy (although significant atherosclerosis of the extramural coronary arteries was absent) were excluded from the analysis of left ventricular wall thicknesses.

Electrocardiograms

Electrocardiograms were obtained in 53 patients. The ECG analyzed for each patient was that obtained closest to the time of death or cardiac arrest (range 1 week to 6 years, median 10 months, and during the last year of life in 32). Criteria used for the electrocardiographic diagnosis of left ventricular hypertrophy were those of Cassel and Ziegler[20] for patients younger than 18 years of age and those of Romhilt and Estes[21] for patients 18 years and older; a score of five or more points by the Romhilt-Estes system was considered evidence for left ventricular hypertrophy. QT intervals (measured in standard lead II) were corrected for heart rate and compared with normal standards.[22, 23] Criteria used for identification of other electrocardiographic abnormalities have been summarized.[24]

Control Patients

Certain clinical, hemodynamic and morphologic findings in the study patients with sudden cardiac death (or cardiac arrest) were compared with a control group of surviving patients with hypertrophic cardiomyopathy. The control patients represented a consecutive series evaluated at the National Heart, Lung, and Blood Institute from February 1979 to April 1981, in whom a technically satisfactory one- or two-dimensional echocardiogram identified or confirmed the diagnosis of hypertrophic cardiomyopathy.

The presence and frequency of cardiac symptoms in 76 study patients who had died suddenly (exclusive of two infants) were compared with those in 76 surviving control patients with hypertrophic cardiomyopathy, matched for age and sex. Of the 76 surviving controls, 22 had no functional limitation, 27 had mild symptoms (New York Heart Association functional class II) and 27 had substantial functional limitation (class III). Fifty-four of the 76 controls had been taking propranolol for at least 1 year, within 5 years of the time of this study; 43 of these 54 were taking a daily dosage of propranolol that was considered clinically appropriate (120 mg/day or more in adults or 2 mg/kg/day or more in children). In addition, nine patients were taking quinidine, two Pronestyl, 17 verapamil, and seven digitalis.

Left ventricular wall thicknesses in the 62 patients who died suddenly were compared with those in the first 62 patients of the control group who could be matched for age and sex. Similarly, electrocardiographic patterns in 53 patients and hemodynamic data (left ventricular outflow gradient under basal conditions and left ventricular end-diastolic pressure) in 46 patients who died suddenly were compared with age- and sex-matched surviving control patients.

Statistical Analysis

Where appropriate, the *t* test, chi-square test or the Fisher exact test were used to assess statistical significance.

Results

Age at Death

The age at death (or cardiac arrest) ranged from 2 months to 58 years (median 19 years) (fig. 1). Sixty-seven of these 78 patients (89%) were younger than 40 years of age and 55 (71%) were younger than 30 years. Forty-nine (63%) of the patients were male and 29 were female. The 12 patients who experienced a cardiac arrest but survived were significantly older at the time of their arrest (mean age 32 ± 4 years [± SEM]) than the 66 patients who died (23 ± 8 years) ($p < 0.05$).

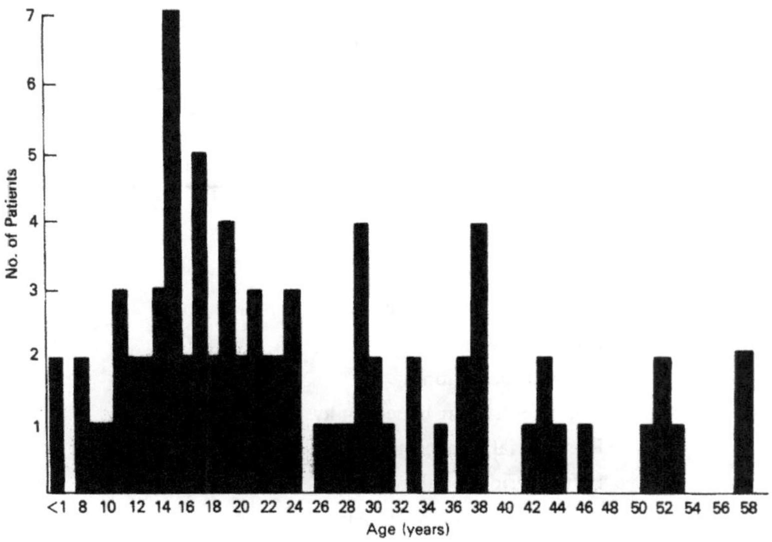

FIGURE 1. *Age distribution for 78 patients with hypertrophic cardiomyopathy who died suddenly or experienced cardiac arrest.*

Functional State Before Death

The functional state before death or cardiac arrest was assessed in 71 patients. Seven patients who were initially referred to us because they were athletes who had died suddenly and unexpectedly were excluded from this analysis because they could not have performed as competitive athletes unless they had been asymptomatic.

Thirty-eight of 71 patients (54%) had experienced no functional limitation (fig. 2). Of these 38 patients, 22 had been completely asymptomatic and 11 had experienced rare, transient symptoms that could have been due to hypertrophic cardiomyopathy (e.g., lightheadedness, palpitations and nonspecific chest pain). Hence, in 33 patients, sudden death was the first definitive manifestation of underlying cardiac disease. The remaining five patients without functional limitation, however, had demonstrated probable evidence of cardiac disease; i.e., they had experienced one or two episodes of syncope, supraventricular tachycardia, or both.

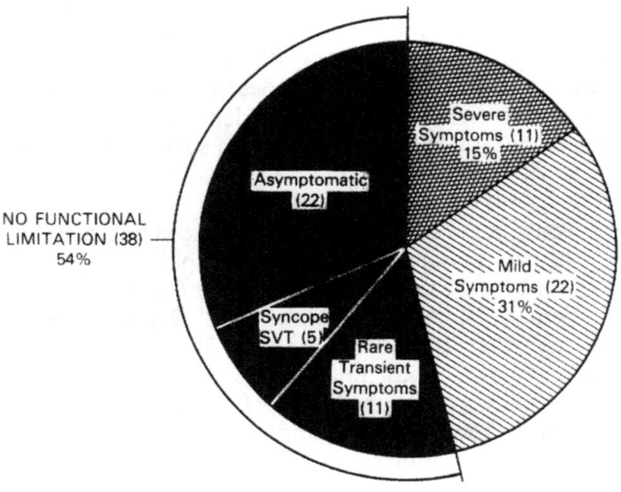

FIGURE 2. *Functional state before sudden death or cardiac arrest in 71 patients with hypertrophic cardiomyopathy. SVT = supraventricular tachycardia.*

Thirty-three of the 71 patients (46%) had functional limitation, including 22 who were considered to be in New York Heart Association functional class II and 11 who had substantial limitation and were in class III (fig. 2); three of these latter 11 patients had had overt clinical manifestations of pulmonary congestion in the presence of a nondilated left ventricle and normal ejection fraction. Eight of the 33 patients with functional limitation had also had supraventricular tachycardia, including five with atrial fibrillation.

The symptoms manifested by the study patients are summarized in table 1. No symptom was significantly more common among patients who died suddenly (or experienced cardiac arrest) than in surviving controls.

Circumstances of Death

Activity at the time of sudden death or cardiac arrest was assessed in 75 patients (fig. 3). Excluded from this analysis were one patient in whom the precise circumstances of death could not be determined and the two patients who died in infancy.

In 58 of the 63 patients who died suddenly (exclusive of the 12 patients who survived cardiac arrest), death was virtually instantaneous. Five other patients lived for 1 hour to 6 weeks after resuscitative measures were instituted. After the initial collapse, two of these five patients had hypotension, low cardiac output and pulmonary edema and died within 24 hours; two others had recurrent ventricular tachycardia followed by a terminal arrest; and one lived for 6 weeks in coma with evidence of cerebral anoxia before dying.

At the time of the cardiac catastrophe, 46 of 75 patients (61%) were engaged in sedentary activities (e.g., lying, sitting or standing, usually in the home but while in the hospital in three patients), or participating in activities that required mild exertion (e.g., walking, shopping, throwing or performing mild calisthenics); four of these 46 patients were known to be asleep. The other 29 patients were performing moderate-to-severe exertion (e.g., running, jogging, hiking, lifting, riding a horse or diving) at the time of death, including

TABLE 1. *Cardiac Symptoms in 76* Patients with Hypertrophic Cardiomyopathy and Sudden Death (or Cardiac Arrest) and in 76 Surviving Control Patients*

Symptoms	No. of patients: Sudden death	Survivors
Lightheadedness	36	39
Chest pain	24	42
Exertional dyspnea or fatigue	24	50
Syncope	20	16
Palpitations	14	28
Paroxysmal nocturnal dyspnea	4	3
Orthopnea	3	8
Pulmonary edema	1	0
Supraventricular tachyarrhythmia producing symptoms	8†	10‡

*Two infants were excluded from this analysis.
†Includes five patients with paroxysmal atrial fibrillation.
‡Includes eight patients with paroxysmal atrial fibrillation and two with chronic atrial fibrillation; three of these 10 also had other supraventricular arrhythmias.

four who died during or just after a competitive athletic contest. Sixty-eight of the 75 patients with sudden death or cardiac arrest had had no premonitory symptoms just before death; however, apparent "warning" symptoms occurred in six patients (fatigue in two and chest pain, syncope, presyncope, and combined chest pain and syncope in one each) from seconds to 2 hours before death.

Electrocardiograms

Electrocardiograms were obtained in 53 patients 1 week to 6 years (median 10 months) before death or

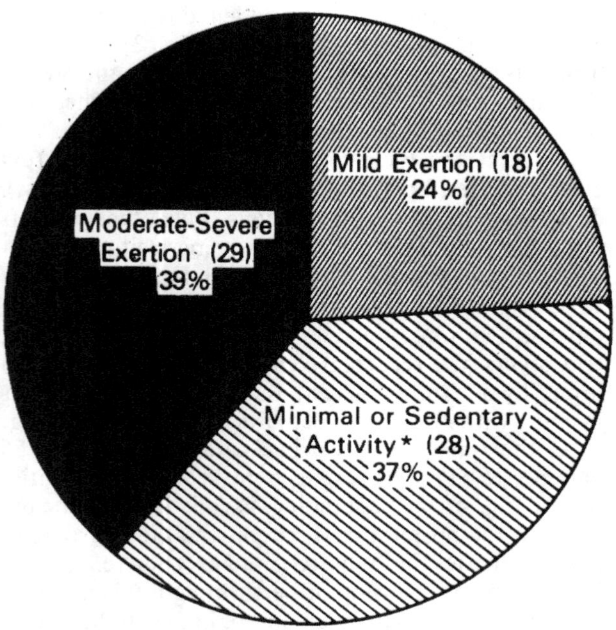

FIGURE 3. *Activity at the time of sudden death or cardiac arrest in 75 patients with hypertrophic cardiomyopathy. *Includes four patients who died during sleep.*

TABLE 2. *Electrocardiographic Findings in 53 Patients with Hypertrophic Cardiomyopathy and Sudden Death (or Cardiac Arrest) and in 53 Surviving Control Patients*

Abnormality	Sudden death (No. of patients)	Survivors (No. of patients)
ST-T abnormalities*	42†	43
Left ventricular hypertrophy	40‡	32
Q or QS waves*	21	12
Left atrial enlargement	16	13
QT prolongation§	16	31
Left-axis deviation	8	3
Right ventricular hypertrophy	6	1
Right atrial enlargement	4	4
Left anterior hemiblock	3	3
Wolff-Parkinson-White pattern	3	0
Intraventricular conduction defect	2	2
Right bundle branch block	1	1
First-degree AV block	1	1
Normal	2	2

Abbreviation: AV = atrioventricular.
*Present in two or more leads.
†Includes four patients with "giant T-wave inversion" (i.e., ≥ 10 mm deep in at least one lead).
‡Includes 17 patients with "strain" pattern (i.e., associated ST-segment and T-wave abnormalities) and seven patients who met Romhilt-Estes criterion for left ventricular hypertrophy without abnormal voltage magnitude.[21]
§Based on observations made in only 47 patients because QT interval could not be reliably measured in six patients who died suddenly.

cardiac arrest. They were abnormal in 51 patients and normal in two (table 2). No electrocardiographic pattern was characteristic of the study group. ST-segment and T-wave alterations were present in 42 patients, left ventricular hypertrophy in 40 and abnormal Q or QS waves in 21.

The prevalence of abnormal ECGs in the 53 patients who died suddenly (51 of 53, 96%) was the same as that in an age- and sex-matched control population of 53 surviving patients with hypertrophic cardiomyopathy (table 2). Electrocardiographic patterns among patients who died suddenly or had cardiac arrest did not differ from those in surviving controls.

Left Ventricular Wall Thicknesses

Ventricular septal thicknesses, assessed at necropsy in 45 patients and by echocardiography in 17, ranged from 12 to 44 mm (mean 25 mm) (fig. 4). In 48 of the 62 patients (77%), septal thickness was 20 mm or greater; in the other 14, it was less than 20 mm. Six of the patients with septal thickness less than 20 mm were chronically conditioned competitive athletes (including two who were also younger than 15 years old) and one was a member of a family with "malignant" hypertrophic cardiomyopathy.[7] However, ventricular septal thicknesses in the 62 patients with hypertrophic cardiomyopathy who died suddenly (mean 25.2 ± 0.9 mm) did not differ significantly from those in control

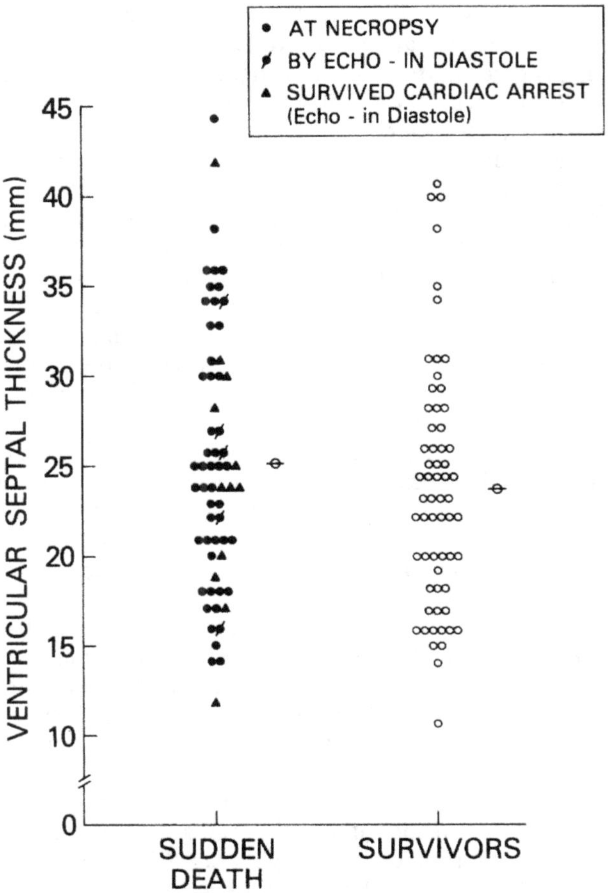

FIGURE 4. *Ventricular septal thickness in 62 patients with hypertrophic cardiomyopathy who died suddenly or had cardiac arrest, compared with a control group of 62 age- and sex-matched surviving patients with hypertrophic cardiomyopathy. Mean values are indicated.*

patients with hypertrophic cardiomyopathy who have survived (mean 23.6 ± 0.8 mm) (fig. 4).

Posterior left ventricular free wall thicknesses (mean 14.5 ± 0.6 mm, range 7–26 mm) were significantly greater than in controls (mean 11.8 ± 0.4 mm) ($p < 0.001$). Ventricular septal-to-posterior free wall thickness ratios ranged from 1.0 to 3.5 (mean 1.8 ± 0.1); in 58 of the 62 patients (94%), the septal-free wall ratio was 1.3 or greater and therefore met our criteria for asymmetric septal hypertrophy;[17] septal–free wall ratios in the controls (2.0 ± 0.1) were significantly greater ($p < 0.01$) than those in the patients with sudden death or cardiac arrest. The differences between control patients and patients who died suddenly with regard to posterior free wall thickness and septal–free wall ratio are probably due primarily to discrepancies inherent in comparing ventricular wall thickness measurements made at necropsy and those obtained by echocardiography during diastole.[25]

Hemodynamic Findings

The magnitude of the left ventricular outflow gradient was measured at cardiac catheterization in 46 patients and was estimated from the M-mode echocardiogram in three others who did not undergo catheterization. These 49 studies were performed 1 week to 10 years (median 15 months) before death and during the last year of life in 23 patients.

Left ventricular outflow tract gradients were present under basal conditions in 37 patients, and ranged from 5–120 mm Hg; in 12 other patients, no outflow gradient was present at rest (fig. 5). Eight of the patients who had no outflow obstruction or only a small gradient (less than 30 mm Hg) under basal conditions, had a gradient of more than 30 mm Hg with provocative interventions (Valsalva maneuver, isoproterenol infusion or amyl nitrite inhalation). Seven patients had no obstruction or a small gradient both under basal conditions and with provocative maneuvers. Patients who died suddenly and surviving control patients did not differ significantly with regard to the magnitude of the left ventricular outflow gradient measured at cardiac catheterization at rest (41 ± 5 mm Hg vs 39 ± 5 mm Hg). Only three patients had right ventricular outflow gradients of greater than 10 mm Hg (15, 47 and 55 mm Hg).

Left ventricular end-diastolic pressures ranged from 5 to 40 mm Hg (average 21 mm Hg) and were abnormal (more than 12 mm Hg) in 36 of the 46 patients. Patients who died suddenly and controls did not differ significantly with regard to the magnitude of left ventricular end-diastolic pressure (21 ± 1.2 mm Hg vs 18 ± 0.9 mm Hg) (fig. 5).

Cardiac Medications

Twenty-nine of the 78 patients had been taking propranolol in the period just before death. Nineteen of the 29 patients were reliably taking a daily dose that was considered clinically appropriate (120 mg/day or more in adults or 2 mg/kg/day or more in children) and the other 10 patients were taking less-than-ade-

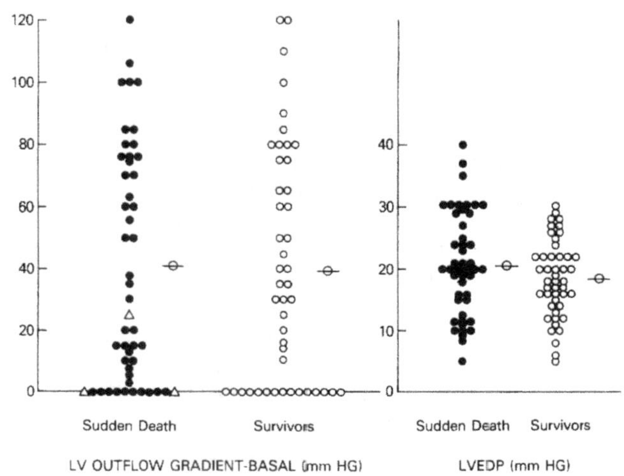

FIGURE 5. *Left ventricular (LV) outflow tract gradients under basal conditions and LV end-diastolic pressures (LVEDP) measured at cardiac catheterization in patients with sudden death (or cardiac arrest) compared with age- and sex-matched surviving controls. The triangle indicates that the basal left ventricular outflow gradient was estimated from the echocardiogram (three patients).*

quate dosages. Two of the patients taking appropriate dosages of propranolol also received either quinidine (1200 mg/day) or Norpace (400 mg/day). Nine patients were receiving digitalis, including three with clinical evidence of elevated pulmonary venous pressure and two with atrial fibrillation.

No cardiac medication regimen was characteristic of the 12 study patients who experienced ventricular fibrillation but were successfully resuscitated. Five of the 12 patients were taking no cardioactive medications before cardiac arrest. Of the remaining seven patients, five were taking propranolol (one in less-than-adequate dosages), one was taking a combination of propranolol and Norpace and one was taking digitalis.

Discussion

This study describes the clinical profile of patients with hypertrophic cardiomyopathy who experienced premature sudden death or cardiac arrest. Most of these patients were young, had experienced no or mild cardiac symptoms before death and were usually participating in sedentary or mild activity at the time of death.

The data show a particular predilection of sudden death for patients younger than 30 years of age and suggest that patients older than 40 years may be at low risk for sudden death. However, certain factors related to the selection of our patients could have influenced these data. For example, older patients who die suddenly outside the hospital are commonly assumed to have had coronary heart disease; often, a necropsy examination is not performed, and hence, the diagnosis of hypertrophic cardiomyopathy is unlikely to be made. In addition, older patients with hypertrophic cardiomyopathy who die suddenly often have associated coronary heart disease,[26] making it difficult to be certain which of the cardiac diseases was primarily responsible for death. In fact, our data suggest that the combination of hypertrophic cardiomyopathy and coronary heart disease may be particularly lethal; five of the 16 patients (30%) we evaluated with hypertrophic cardiomyopathy older than age 40 years who died suddenly had associated significant coronary arterial narrowing from atherosclerosis.

The fact that death usually occurred during sedentary or mild activity suggests that severe exertion may not per se be a substantial risk factor for sudden death in patients with hypertrophic cardiomyopathy. Nevertheless, since the proportion of the day during which most persons perform moderate-to-severe exertion is relatively small, the fact that about 40% of our patients died during or just after vigorous activity is impressive. Therefore, we continue to recommend that patients with hypertrophic cardiomyopathy not engage in competitive athletics or particularly strenuous physical exertion.

However, the patient with hypertrophic cardiomyopathy who died suddenly was not identified by the clinical, hemodynamic or morphologic measurements analyzed in this study, i.e., occurrence of a particular cardiac symptom, magnitude of left ventricular outflow tract obstruction under basal conditions or left ventricular end-diastolic pressure, electrocardiographic pattern or prevalence of an abnormal ECG, or degree of ventricular septal thickening. In particular, we found no significant increase in the incidence of syncope in patients with sudden death (or cardiac arrest) compared with surviving controls with hypertrophic cardiomyopathy. This finding is different from that of McKenna et al.,[10] who reported that syncope was more common among patients with hypertrophic cardiomyopathy who died suddenly. The present data also confirm our impression that the risk of sudden death in patients with hypertrophic cardiomyopathy is not related to severity of left ventricular outflow obstruction.[5, 7, 8]

Ventricular septal thickness also did not differ substantially between patients who died suddenly and the surviving controls. Therefore, absolute ventricular septal thickness cannot be used to predict sudden death in a population of patients with hypertrophic cardiomyopathy. However, in seven of our 14 patients who had a relatively thin ventricular septum (less than 20 mm), other factors were present that could have contributed to the occurrence of a premature cardiac catastrophe: a family history of "malignant" hypertrophic cardiomyopathy[7] or a competitive athletic lifestyle.

While the variables investigated in this study were not reliable in identifying that subgroup of patients with hypertrophic cardiomyopathy who are at increased risk for sudden death, two other clinical variables may be of more value. First, a familial predilection for sudden premature death may constitute a risk factor in certain families with unusually virulent expressions of hypertrophic cardiomyopathy.[7] Therefore, the occurrence of premature (younger than 50 years of age) sudden death in more than one first-degree relative of a person with known hypertrophic cardiomyopathy probably places that patient at an increased risk of sudden death. Second, preliminary data suggest that 24-hour ambulatory electrocardiographic monitoring may be useful in identifying certain patients with hypertrophic cardiomyopathy who are at increased risk for sudden death. Two prospective investigations[27, 28] of patients with hypertrophic cardiomyopathy, studied by 24- or 48-hour ambulatory ECGs, have shown a significant relationship between the presence of asymptomatic ventricular tachycardia on the ambulatory ECG and the subsequent occurrence of sudden cardiac death. In our study,[28] sudden cardiac catastrophe was significantly more common in patients with ventricular tachycardia on 24-hour ECG (four of 17, 25%) than in patients without ventricular tachycardia (two of 66, 3%) ($p < 0.02$). However, the fact that 13 of the 17 patients with ventricular tachycardia did *not* experience a catastrophic cardiac event suggests that other variables must coexist in patients with hypertrophic cardiomyopathy for ventricular instability to evolve into a terminal arrhythmia.

Patients with hypertrophic cardiomyopathy may die suddenly even while taking usual clinical dosages of propranolol. About one-fourth of the patients in this study were receiving apparently adequate amounts of propranolol during the period just before death. Thus, although propranolol does not eliminate the possibility of sudden death, well-controlled prospective studies have not, as yet, been performed to determine definitively whether patients with hypertrophic cardiomyopathy who are at high risk for sudden death and are receiving propranolol therapy have a lower mortality than untreated patients.

In the present study, surviving patients with hypertrophic cardiomyopathy had more often taken clinically appropriate dosages of propranolol than did the patients who died suddenly (43 of 78, 55%, vs 19 of 78, 24%). However, based on these data, we are hesitant to attribute to propranolol a role in enhancing survival of our patients with hypertrophic cardiomyopathy. The present study was not designed to critically determine whether propranolol reduced mortality rate. For example, patients with hypertrophic cardiomyopathy frequently may undergo alterations in their drug regimen. For the present investigation, we considered a patient in the control group to be treated with propranolol if the drug had been taken in clinically appropriate dosages for at least 1 year in the preceding 5 years, but the period these patients had actually been taking propranolol varied considerably, as did the drug dosage.

References

1. Frank S, Braunwald E: Idiopathic hypertrophic subaortic stenosis. Clinical analysis of 126 patients with emphasis on the natural history. Circulation **37:** 759, 1968
2. Adelman AG, Wigle ED, Ranganathan N, Webb GD, Kidd BSL, Bigelow WG, Silver MD: The clinical course in muscular subaortic stenosis. A retrospective and prospective study of 60 hemodynamically proved cases. Ann Intern Med **77:** 515, 1972
3. Hardarson T, De la Calzada CS, Curiel R, Goodwin JF: Prognosis and mortality of hypertrophic obstructive cardiomyopathy. Lancet **2:** 1462, 1973
4. Shah PM, Adelman AG, Wigle ED, Gobel FL, Burchell HB, Hardarson T, Curiel R, De la Calzada C, Oakley CM, Goodwin JF: The natural (and unnatural) course of hypertrophic obstructive cardiomyopathy. A multicenter study. Circ Res **35** (suppl II): II-179, 1973
5. Maron BJ, Henry WL, Clark CE, Redwood DR, Roberts WC, Epstein SE: Asymmetric septal hypertrophy in childhood. Circulation **53:** 9, 1976
6. Fiddler GL, Tajik AJ, Weidman WH, McGoon DC, Ritter DG, Giuliani ER: Idiopathic hypertrophic subaortic stenosis in the young. Am J Cardiol **42:** 793, 1978
7. Maron BJ, Lipson LC, Roberts WC, Savage DD, Epstein SE: "Malignant" hypertrophic cardiomyopathy: identification of a subgroup of families with unusually frequent premature deaths. Am J Cardiol **41:** 1133, 1978
8. Maron BJ, Roberts WC, Edwards JE, McAllister HA, Foley DD, Epstein SE: Sudden death in patients with hypertrophic cardiomyopathy: characterization of 26 patients without functional limitation. Am J Cardiol **41:** 803, 1978
9. Krelhaus W, Kuhn H, Loogen F: Analysis of deaths in the course of hypertrophic obstructive cardiomyopathy. *In* Cardiomyopathy and Myocardial Biopsy, edited by Kaltenbach M, Loogen F, Olsen EGJ. Berlin, Springer-Verlag, 1978, p 300
10. McKenna W, Deanfield J, Faruqui A, England D, Oakley C, Goodwin J: Prognosis in hypertrophic cardiomyopathy: role of age and clinical, electrocardiographic and hemodynamic features. Am J Cardiol **47:** 532, 1981
11. Morrow AG, Koch JP, Maron BJ, Kent KM, Epstein SE: Left ventricular myotomy and myectomy in patients with obstructive hypertrophic cardiomyopathy and previous cardiac arrest. Am J Cardiol **46:** 313, 1980
12. Maron BJ, Roberts WC, McAllister HA, Rosing DR, Epstein SE: Sudden death in young athletes. Circulation **62:** 218, 1980
13. Maron BJ, Epstein SE: Hypertrophic cardiomyopathy: a discussion of nomenclature. Am J Cardiol **43:** 1242, 1979
14. Epstein SE, Henry WL, Clark CE, Roberts WC, Maron BJ, Ferrans VJ, Redwood DR, Morrow AG: Asymmetric septal hypertrophy. Ann Intern Med **81:** 650, 1974
15. Maron BJ, Edwards JE, Epstein SE: Prevalence and characteristics of disproportionate ventricular septal thickening in patients with systemic hypertension. Chest **73:** 466, 1978
16. Savage DD, Drayer JIM, Henry WL, Mathews EC, Ware JH, Gardin JM, Cohen ER, Epstein SE, Laragh JH: Echocardiographic assessment of cardiac anatomy and function in hypertensive subjects. Circulation **59:** 623, 1979
17. Henry WL, Clark CE, Epstein SE: Asymmetric septal hypertrophy (ASH): echocardiographic identification of the pathognomonic anatomic abnormality of IHSS. Circulation **47:** 225, 1973
18. Henry WL, Clark CE, Glancy DL, Epstein SE Echocardiographic measurement of the left ventricular outflow gradient in idiopathic hypertrophic subaortic stenosis. N Engl J Med **288:** 989, 1973
19. Maron BJ, Epstein SE, Roberts WC: Hypertrophic cardiomyopathy and transmural myocardial infarction without significant atherosclerosis of the extramural coronary arteries. Am J Cardiol **43:** 1086, 1979
20. Cassel DE, Ziegler RF: Electrocardiography in Infants and Children. New York, Grune & Stratton, 1966, p 355
21. Romhilt DW, Estes EH: A point score system for the ECG diagnosis of left ventricular hypertrophy. Am Heart J **75:** 752, 1968
22. McCammon RW: A Longitudinal Study of Electrocardiographic Intervals in Healthy Children. Acta Paediatr Scand (Uppsala) **50** (suppl 126): 1961
23. Simonson E, Cady LD Jr, Woodbury M: The normal Q-T interval. Am Heart J **63:** 747, 1962
24. Savage DD, Seides SF, Clark CE, Henry WL, Maron BJ, Robinson FC, Epstein SE: Electrocardiographic findings in patients with obstructive and nonobstructive hypertrophic cardiomyopathy. Circulation **58:** 402, 1978
25. Maron BJ, Henry WL, Roberts WC, Epstein SE: Comparison of echocardiographic and necropsy measurements of ventricular wall thicknesses in patients with and without disproportionate septal thickening. Circulation **55:** 341, 1977
26. Lardani H, Serrano JA, Villamil RJ: Hemodynamics and coronary angiography in idiopathic hypertrophic subaortic stenosis. Am J Cardiol **41:** 476, 1978
27. McKenna WJ, England D, Oakley CM, Goodwin JF: Detection of arrhythmia in hypertrophic cardiomyopathy: prospective study. (abstr) Circulation **62** (suppl III): III-187, 1980
28. Maron BJ, Savage DD, Wolfson J, Epstein SE: Prognostic significance of 24-hour ambulatory electrocardiographic monitoring in patients with hypertrophic cardiomyopathy: a prospective study. Am J Cardiol **48:** 252, 1981

Hypertrophic Cardiomyopathy With Ventricular Septal Hypertrophy Localized to the Apical Region of the Left Ventricle (Apical Hypertrophic Cardiomyopathy)

BARRY J. MARON, MD, FACC
ROBERT O. BONOW, MD, FACC
TIPPUR N. R. SESHAGIRI, MD, FACC
WILLIAM C. ROBERTS, MD, FACC
STEPHEN E. EPSTEIN, MD, FACC

Bethesda, Maryland

Clinical and morphologic features are described in a unique subgroup of seven patients with hypertrophic cardiomyopathy. Five patients either died suddenly or are alive but severely symptomatic. In each patient ventricular septal hypertrophy was demonstrated on two dimensional echocardiography or at necropsy to be virtually confined to its apical one-half. However, conventional M mode echocardiography was unreliable in identifying this site of hypertrophy because it was often inaccessible to the path of the M mode beam. Apical distribution of septal hypertrophy does not constitute a separate disease entity, but rather appears to be part of the morphologic spectrum of hypertrophic cardiomyopathy, as judged from two findings: (1) genetic transmission of hypertrophic cardiomyopathy in relatives of each study patient; and (2) marked disorganization of cardiac muscle cells in the left ventricular wall of the two patients studied at necropsy.

Apical distribution of septal hypertrophy in these patients was associated with relatively mild T wave inversion in the electrocardiogram and characteristic angiographic appearance of the left ventricle with mid ventricular constriction and a small, often poorly contractile apical segment. These electrocardiographic and angiographic features differ from those previously described in Japanese patients with "apical hypertrophic cardiomyopathy" in whom "giant" T wave inversion and a "spade-like" appearance of the left ventricle were characteristic.

Hypertrophic cardiomyopathy is a primary disease of cardiac muscle that may manifest a variety of clinical and morphologic features.[1–7] Marked variation in the distribution of left ventricular hypertrophy among patients within this disease spectrum has been shown by wide angle two dimensional echocardiography.[8–10] In this regard, investigators in Japan[11,12] recently described a form of nonobstructive hypertrophic cardiomyopathy in which hypertrophy was localized to the apical region of the left ventricle, producing a distinctive angiographic appearance and electrocardiographic pattern. The purpose of this communication is to describe the clinical and morphologic features in a subgroup of patients with hypertrophic cardiomyopathy evaluated at our institution in whom hypertrophy was confined primarily to the region of the left ventricular apex.

Methods

Selection of patients: The case records of the Pathology Branch as well as the two dimensional echocardiograms of those patients with hypertrophic cardiomyopathy studied in the Cardiology Branch from 1979 to 1981 were reviewed. On the basis of two dimensional echocardiographic and necropsy observations, seven patients met the morphologic criterion for inclusion into the study group: ventricular septal hypertrophy virtually confined to its apical one-half in the absence of an associated cardiac or systemic disease. Each of the seven patients had normal systemic blood pressure. Significant narrowing of the extramural

From the Cardiology and Pathology Branches, National Heart, Lung, and Blood Institute, National Institutes of Health, Bethesda, Maryland. Manuscript received June 27, 1981; revised manuscript received November 10, 1981, accepted December 4, 1981.

Address for reprints: Barry J. Maron, MD, Cardiology Branch, Building 10, Room 7B-15, National Heart, Lung, and Blood Institute, National Institutes of Health, Bethesda, Maryland 20205.

coronary arteries was excluded by coronary arteriography or necropsy examination in five of the seven patients; in the other two patients the presence of coronary heart disease was considered unlikely because of their youthful age (15 and 21 years).

M mode echocardiography: M mode echocardiograms were obtained using a 2.25 megahertz, 1.25 cm in diameter unfocused Aerotech transducer and a Hoffrel 201 ultrasonic receiver interfaced with a Honeywell 1856 strip chart recorder. Echocardiograms were recorded using "standard" transducer placement (that is, where the anterior mitral leaflet is imaged with the transducer held perpendicular to the chest wall, in the third or fourth intercostal space near the left sternal border, with the patient rotated 30° into the left lateral decubitus position.[13]

The methods used for imaging the ventricular septum and posterior left ventricular free wall have been described previously.[14] The thickness of the ventricular septum was measured just before atrial systole with the ultrasonic beam directed slightly below the distal margins of the mitral leaflets. Thickness of the posterior left ventricular free wall was measured during the same phase of the cardiac cycle, with the ultrasonic beam passing through the distal portions of the mitral leaflets. A switch-gain circuit was utilized to simplify identification of the epicardium of the posterior left ventricular free wall.

Two dimensional echocardiography: A Varian (V-3000 or V-3400) real time, phased array, ultrasonic sector scanner with a hand-held 2.25 megahertz transducer was used to perform the two dimensional echocardiographic studies. The field of view was 80° in an azimuthal direction and 15 or 21 cm deep. Images were produced at 32 frames/s and recorded on 1 inch (2.54 cm) (Sony) reel to reel videotape or an Ampex DR-10 rhodium-plated chromium disc for subsequent review in real time, slow motion or stop action modes. Single still frame photographs were made from a television monitor using a 35 mm camera.

The two dimensional echocardiographic examination included the imaging of several cross-sectional planes through the heart. Serial *short axis views* of the left ventricle were obtained by initially orienting the sector plane perpendicular to the long axis of the left ventricle from a standard transducer placement. The "short axis sweep" was performed by maintaining the transducer in a fixed location and slowly angling the image plane from the aorta (cephalad) to the apex (caudad).[15] Care was taken to assure proper transducer angulation so that the left ventricle appeared circular rather than oval or elliptical.

The long axis view was obtained by orienting the sector plane parallel to the longitudinal axis of the left ventricle, taking care to avoid improper angulation of the scan plane tangentially through the ventricle. The *apical four chamber view* was obtained with the transducer placed at the cardiac apex and the tomographic plane directed perpendicular to the ventricular and atrial septa and through the plane of the mitral and tricuspid valve orifices.[16]

TABLE I

Clinical and Morphologic Findings in Seven Study Patients

	Patients						
	1	2	3	4	5	6	7
Age and sex	15M	21M	26F	34F	38M	48F	59M
Functional class (NYHA)	II	I	II (and SD)	III	III (and SD)	III	III
Electrocardiogram							
T wave inversion (maximal depth in mm)	+(1)	+(4)	+(1)	+(4)	+(2)	+(1)	+(6)
LVH	+	0	+[ϕ]	+[*]	+[ϕ]	+	+[*]
RVH	0	0	0	0	+	0	0
LAE	+	0	+	0	+	+	+
Abnormal Q waves	0	0	0	0	0	+	0
Echocardiogram							
$LVID_d$ (mm)	46	43	–	48	51	43	49
EF (%)[†]	0.66	0.83	–	0.82	0.80	0.66	0.87
% systolic thickening of septum	50	23	–	43	33	8	50
MV position[‡]	0.53	0.52	–	0.61	0.86	0.61	0.53
Ventricular wall thickness (mm)							
Maximal VS[#]	23	21	23[Δ]	32	25[Δ]	14[a]	27
PBLV	10	10	14	9	15[Δ̸]	10	11
VS:PBLV	2.3	2.1	1.6	3.5	1.7	1 4	2.5
LV outflow gradient (mm Hg)							
Basal	—	—	63	0	0	0	0
Provoked	—	—	—	0	0	10	—
LVEDP (mm Hg)	—	—	40	10	30	28	12

* With "strain" pattern. ϕ Met Romhilt and Eştes criterion[17] for left ventricular hypertrophy *without* abnormally tall voltage. † Measured at the caudal margins of mitral valve leaflets and, hence, not in the area of cavity obliteration. ‡ Measure of the relative position of the mitral valve in the left ventricular cavity at the onset of systole. The mitral valve position index was computed by dividing the ventricular septal-mitral valve distance into the mitral valve-posterior free wall distance[22]; an index of greater than 0.3 indicates that the mitral valve is displaced anteriorly in the left ventricular cavity—that is, closer to the ventricular septum.[22] # Approximate measurements made from two dimensional echocardiogram utilizing primarily parasternal long axis or apical views or at necropsy (Patients 3 and 5), in areas of the ventricular septum not accessible to the conventional M mode beam. Δ Heart weights exceeded normal values [20]; 500 g in Patient 3 and 560 g in Patient 5. Δ̸ Transmural scarring of the posterior and anterolateral left ventricular free wall was present from base to apex. This finding has been previously observed in patients with hypertrophic cardiomyopathy (and absence of significant coronary atherosclerosis) who showed ventricular dilatation and progressive congestive heart failure.[21] a Contiguous region of left ventricular apex showed more substantial hypertrophy. + = present. 0 = absent. – = data not available.

LAE = left atrial enlargement; LV = left ventricle; LVEDP = left ventricular end-diastolic pressure; LVH = left ventricular hypertrophy; $LVID_d$ = left ventricular internal dimension at end-diastole; MV = mitral valve; NYHA = New York Heart Association; PBLV = posterobasal left ventricular free wall; SD = sudden death; VS = ventricular septum; VS:PBLV = ventricular septal to posterobasal left ventricular free wall thickness ratio.

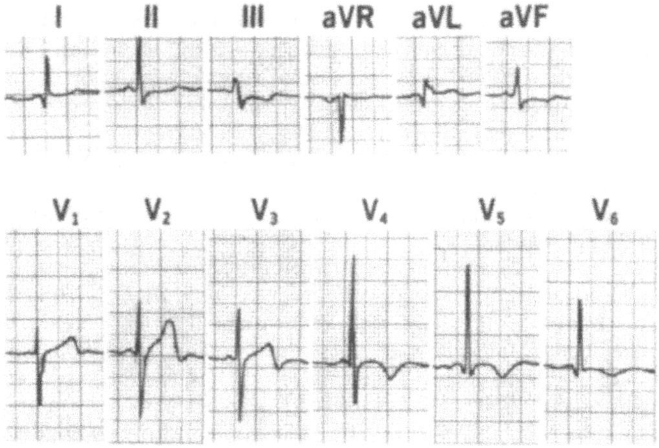

FIGURE 1. Case 2. Electrocardiogram showing relatively mild symmetric T wave inversion in leads I, aVL and $V_2 - V_6$.

The location of left ventricular hypertrophy was described in two cross-sectional planes.[8,9] In the *anteroposterior plane*, hypertrophy involved either the ventricular septum or the left ventricular free wall. The septum was divided into two equal segments (anterior and posterior). The free wall was divided into three segments (anterior, lateral and posterior). In the *cephalad-caudad plane*, hypertrophy involved either the basal or apical segments; the basal portion extended from cardiac base to just below the caudal margins of the mitral leaflets and the apical portion included the remainder of the ventricle visualized caudal to the mitral leaflets.

Electrocardiography: Criteria employed for the electrocardiographic diagnosis of left ventricular hypertrophy were those of Romhilt and Estes[17]; five or more points by the Romhilt and Estes system were considered evidence for left ventricular hypertrophy. Criteria used for identification of other electrocardiographic abnormalities were those which have been previously summarized.[18]

Necropsy: Necropsy studies were performed in both study patients who died (Cases 3 and 5). Ventricular wall thickness measurements were made at four equally spaced transverse planes from the cardiac base to the apex. Trabeculations, papillary muscles and the crista supraventricularis were not included in the measurement of ventricular wall thickness. Sites of hypertrophy were described by the same convention used for the two-dimensional echocardiograms.[8,9]

With use of a previously described method,[19] the disorganized arrangement of cardiac muscle cells was assessed quantitatively in each of the four transverse planes for the ventricular septum and in the most basal transverse plane for the left ventricular free wall.

Results

Clinical features and course: The seven patients ranged in age from 15 to 59 years (median 34); four were male and three female (Table I). Six patients were white and one was black. One patient was asymptomatic, but the other six had experienced functional limitation. Four of these six patients had moderate to severe symptoms (New York Heart Association functional class III) and the other two had only mild symptoms (class II).

Two of the seven patients (Cases 3 and 5) died suddenly at ages 26 and 38 years, respectively. Patient 3 had been only mildly symptomatic before death. Patient 5 had been severely symptomatic with evidence of congestive heart failure; both patients had been taking propranolol and digitalis.

Each study patient had a systolic ejection murmur that was loudest at the lower left sternal border or apex. The intensity of the murmur was grade 1 or 2/6 in four patients and grade 3/6 in the other three. In only two patients did the intensity of the murmur increase with the Valsalva maneuver.

Electrocardiograms: Electrocardiograms were abnormal in each patient (Table I), and the most consistent alteration was inversion of the T waves. T wave inversion involved all or virtually all leads in two patients, or was limited to the standard leads (two patients), leads I, aVL and the left precordial leads (two patients, Fig. 1), or only lead V_6 (one patient). T wave inversion was relatively mild in amplitude (1 to 6 mm) in each patient. Six patients showed a pattern of left ventricular hypertrophy (including two with "strain"); only one patient had abnormal Q waves.

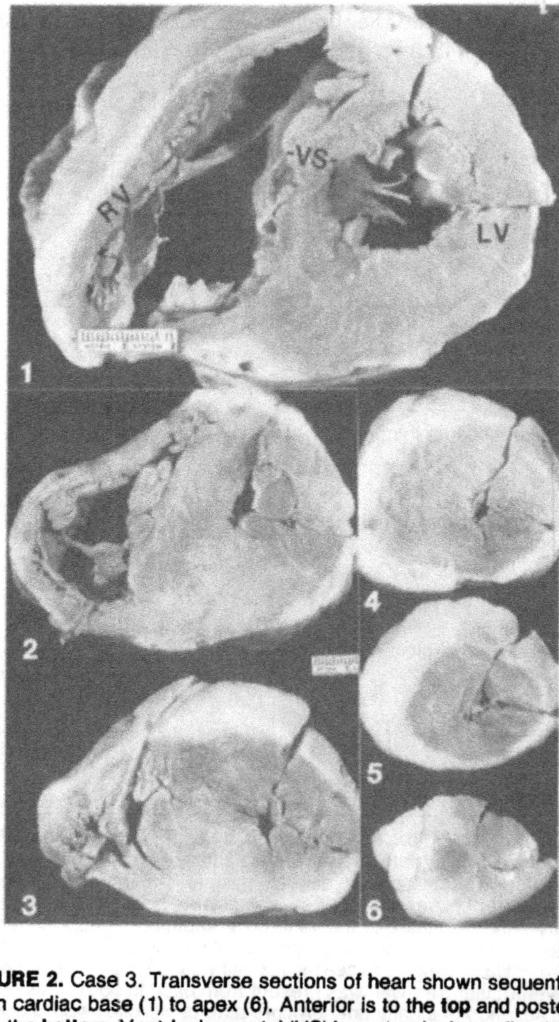

FIGURE 2. Case 3. Transverse sections of heart shown sequentially from cardiac base (1) to apex (6). Anterior is to the **top** and posterior is to the **bottom.** Ventricular septal (VS) hypertrophy is confined to its apical one-half. The portion of the posterior left ventricular (LV) free wall contiguous with the posterior aspect of the ventricular septum also is thickened (in sections 1, 2 and 3). RV = right ventricle.

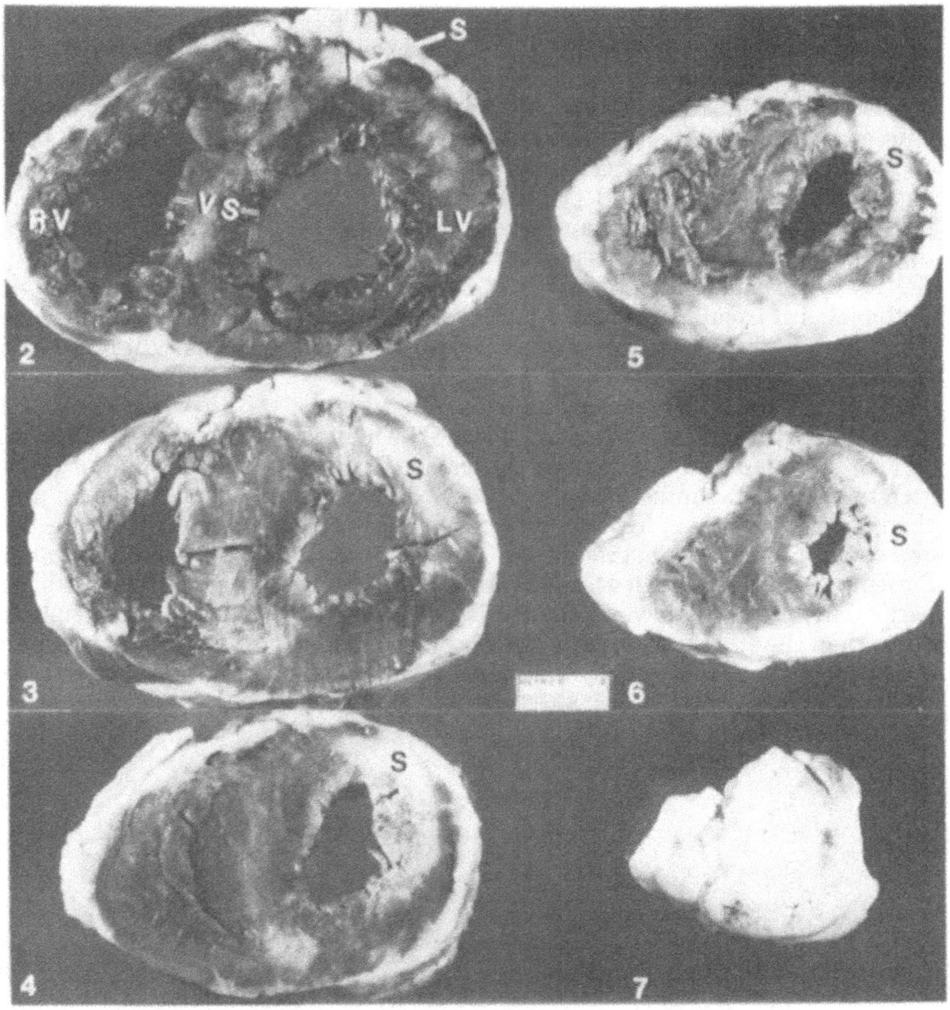

FIGURE 3. Case 5. Transverse sections of heart shown sequentially from near cardiac base (2) to apex (7). Same orientation as in Figure 1; the section at a level equivalent to section 1 in Figure 1 is not shown. Ventricular septal (VS) hypertrophy is virtually confined to its apical one-half. Anterolateral left ventricular (LV) free wall in section 2 and posterior free wall in sections 3 and 5 are also thickened. Note transmural scarring (S) in the anterolateral free wall. RV = right ventricle.

Gross anatomic findings (echocardiography or necropsy): Two dimensional echocardiographic studies or examination of the heart at necropsy showed each of the seven patients to have a nondilated, hypertrophied left ventricle (Table I; Fig. 2 and 3). In the six patients studied with M mode echocardiography the mitral valve was shown to be positioned anteriorly within the left ventricular cavity (Fig. 4), to a degree similar to that in patients with nonobstructive hypertrophic cardiomyopathy.[22]

In each patient the basal half of the ventricular septum was of normal thickness, but the anterior and posterior segments of the septum were hypertrophied in its apical half (Fig. 2, 3 and 5). The transition from normal to increased septal thickness was often abrupt and resembled a "shelf" (Fig. 6B). Maximal ventricular septal thickness ranged from 14 to 32 mm (mean 24). Septal-free wall ratio, calculated as the ratio of maximal ventricular septal thickness to posterobasal free wall thickness, ranged from 1.4 to 3.5 (mean 2.2) (Table I).

Portions of the left ventricular free wall also were thickened in six of the seven patients (Fig. 2, 3 and 5). Most commonly, free wall hypertrophy was located predominantly in the anterolateral free wall contiguous with the thickened ventricular septum near the apex (four patients); in one patient free wall hypertrophy involved only the posterior segment, and in another, both the basal anterolateral free wall and apical posterior free wall were hypertrophied (Fig. 3). In addition, Patient 5 (who died suddenly) showed marked transmural scarring of the anterolateral and posterior left ventricular free wall from base to apex (Fig. 3).

M mode echocardiograms obtained in five patients (in whom wall thicknesses could be measured) were not definitively diagnostic of hypertrophic cardiomyopathy. This occurred because neither the ventricular septum nor the posterior free wall was substantially thickened in the basal portion of the left ventricle (areas through which the conventional M mode beam passes). Ventricular wall thicknesses were normal in four of these five patients, and showed mild asymmetry in the other patient (septal thickness of 13 mm and posterior free wall thickness of 10 mm). In two of these patients, a second M mode echocardiogram was performed after two dimensional echocardiography demonstrated substantial ventricular septal hypertrophy near the apex. By angulating the M mode ultrasonic beam in a particularly acute angle toward the apex in both these patients it was possible to image areas of marked ventricular septal thickening (Fig. 4B).

Histologic findings (Table II): In both patients studied at necropsy (Cases 3 and 5) the overall extent of ventricular septal disorganization was marked (43 and 46 percent, respectively). Cell disorganization was particularly extensive in the apical regions of the septum and less marked in the basal portion of the septum (Fig. 7). In both patients, the extent of disorganization in the left ventricular free wall was marked (6 and 15 percent), although much less extensive than in the ventricular septum.

Findings in family members: The seven patients came from five families; Patients 3, 4 and 5 are related (Fig. 8). In four of the five families at least one first degree relative of the index case died prematurely (less than 55 years of age) of hypertrophic cardiomyopathy or was symptomatic from that disease. In the family of Patients 3, 4 and 5, sudden death (or cardiac arrest) was particularly prevalent, having occurred in eight relatives other than the study patients; in addition, three other members of that family are symptomatic from hypertrophic cardiomyopathy (Fig. 8).

Echocardiography or cardiac catheterization (or both) was performed in 20 relatives from four of the five families (no relatives of Patient 7 were studied). Evidence of hypertrophic cardiomyopathy was present in 11 of these 20 persons. Two dimensional echocardiograms were obtained in 8 of the 11 affected relatives and showed a variety of patterns of left ventricular hypertrophy. In seven of the eight patients both the basal and apical regions of ventricular septum were hypertrophied; the remaining patient showed hypertrophy of the anterolateral free wall but not of the septum. In four of the eight relatives studied with two dimensional echocardiography the anterior basal ventricular septum, through which the M mode beam passes,[8] was not thickened (Fig. 9A); however, the four other relatives showed more typical hypertrophy of the anterior basal septum, which produced asymmetric septal hypertrophy on M mode echocardiography (Fig. 9B).

Hemodynamic findings: A left ventricular outflow tract gradient between the left ventricular cavity and the aorta was absent under basal conditions in four of the five patients who underwent cardiac catheterization. Patient 3 had a 63 mm Hg peak systolic pressure difference recorded across the area of mid ventricular

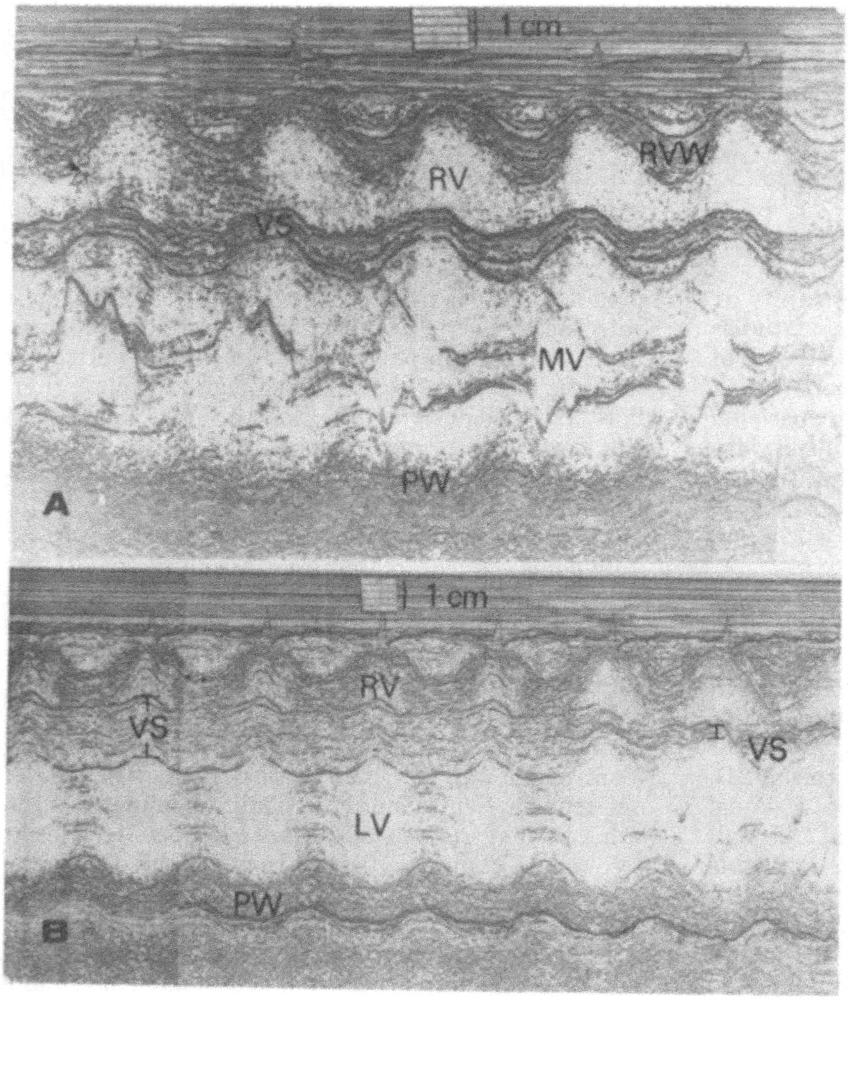

FIGURE 4. Case 4. M mode echocardiograms. **A,** at level of mitral valve (MV), which is displaced anteriorly in the normal-sized left ventricular cavity. Both the ventricular septum (VS) and posterior free wall (PW) are of normal thickness. **B,** continuous scan from body of left ventricle (LV) toward left ventricular outflow tract. Note that the ventricular septum (VS) is of normal thickness at the mitral valve level (seen to the **right**) but increases abruptly and markedly in thickness as the ultrasonic beam is directed far below the mitral valve (seen to the **left**); compare with biventricular angiocardiogram from the same patient (Fig. 6B). RV = right ventricle; RVW = right ventricular wall.

constriction, which did not appear to be artifactually created by entrapment of the left ventricular catheter during systole[23–25] (Table I). Six of the seven patients had no systolic anterior motion of the anterior mitral leaflet on echocardiography, suggesting that obstruction at the level of the left ventricular outflow tract also was absent[26]; in Patient 5 systolic anterior motion of the anterior mitral leaflet was mild and insufficient to produce outflow obstruction. Left ventricular end-diastolic pressure was markedly elevated in three patients, and normal in two (Table I).

Angiographic findings: Four of the five patients in whom angiocardiograms were obtained showed hypercontractility of the left ventricle (Fig. 10); Patient 6 had a normally contractile ventricle without apical cavity obliteration. The appearance of the left ventricular cavity (in the right anterior oblique projection) was similar in the four patients with a hypercontractile left ventricle. These four patients showed a marked narrowing or constriction at the mid ventricular level (Fig. 6A and 10B). The proximal portion of the cavity was of normal size in each; however, the distal part of the left ventricle was substantially smaller and often contracted poorly. This configuration of the left ventricle was most prominent in systole in three patients (Fig. 10B), but was evident in diastole in one patient (Case 4) (Fig. 6A) who showed extreme left ventricular cavity obliteration in systole. Mitral regurgitation was mild in three patients and absent in two.

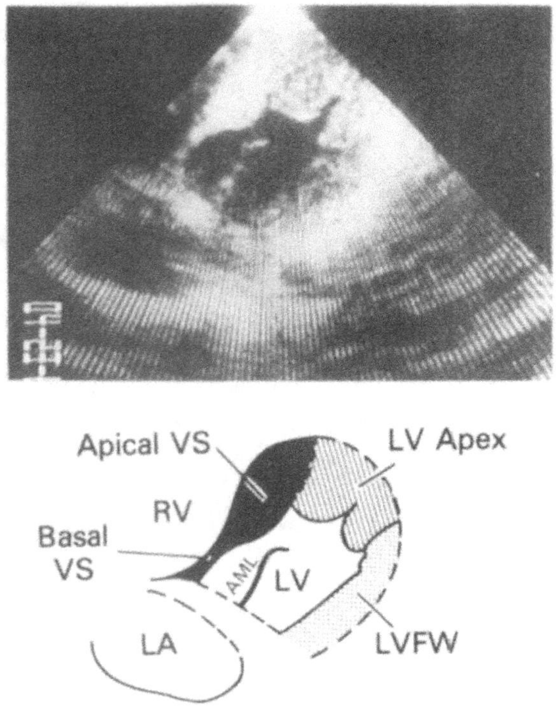

FIGURE 5. Case 1. Stop-frame of apical two chamber view of two dimensional echocardiogram (obtained during diastole) **(above)** and schematic illustration **(below)**. The basal septum (Basal VS) is of normal thickness, but the apical portion (Apical VS) is thickened. There is also marked hypertrophy of the left ventricular (LV) apex and the contiguous portion of left ventricular free wall (LVFW). Other similar views of the left ventricle from the apex involving slightly different transducer angulation also showed this pattern and magnitude of wall thickening. Orientation is such that the cardiac apex is to the **top,** the base is to the **bottom** and the left ventricle is to the **right.** AML = anterior mitral leaflet; Ao = aorta; LA = left atrium; RV = right ventricle.

Discussion

Distribution of left ventricular hypertrophy: Two dimensional echocardiographic studies[8,9] have demonstrated that marked variation in the distribution of left ventricular hypertrophy occurs in patients with hypertrophic cardiomyopathy. In the majority of such patients, hypertrophy involves both the ventricular septum and left ventricular free wall, although either may be selectively involved. In addition, hypertrophy usually involves to some extent both the basal and apical regions of the left ventricle.[6,9,10,27] However, this paper describes the clinical and morphologic features of a unique subgroup of patients with hypertrophic cardiomyopathy, that is, those in whom ventricular septal hypertrophy is *virtually confined to the apical region of the left ventricle.*

Despite the unusual location of left ventricular hypertrophy, the findings in these patients appear to represent part of the spectrum of hypertrophic cardiomyopathy, rather than a separate and etiologically distinct disease entity. This conclusion is based on two lines of evidence. First, genetic transmission of hypertrophic cardiomyopathy was identified in each of four families studied. The pattern of inheritance in these families was compatible with the autosomal dominant transmission that is typical of hypertrophic cardiomyopathy.[28] Although affected relatives in these families occasionally showed an apical distribution of left ventricular hypertrophy (as in the family of Patients 3, 4 and 5), such persons more commonly demonstrated a variety of other morphologic patterns usually observed in patients with hypertrophic cardiomyopathy.[9] Second, histologic examination of myocardium at necropsy in the two study patients who died demonstrated extensive disorganization of cardiac muscle cells that was particularly marked in the ventricular septum and was similar in extent and distribution to that observed in more typical morphologic forms of hypertrophic cardiomyopathy.[19,29]

Comparison with Japanese studies: Our findings in the seven patients presented here are relevant to those of investigators in Japan,[11,12] who have described a similar disease entity that they termed "apical hypertrophic cardiomyopathy" and that commonly occurs in their population of patients with cardiac disease. An apparently unique feature of the Japanese form of the disease is the presence of particularly deep ("giant") T wave inversion (defined as greater than 10 mm in depth) in the lateral precordial leads of the scalar electrocardiogram. Although T wave inversion was present in each of our seven patients, it was mild in amplitude (6 mm or less). In fact, in a review of electrocardiograms of 200 patients with hypertrophic cardiomyopathy at our institution in whom the hypertrophy was *not* predomi-

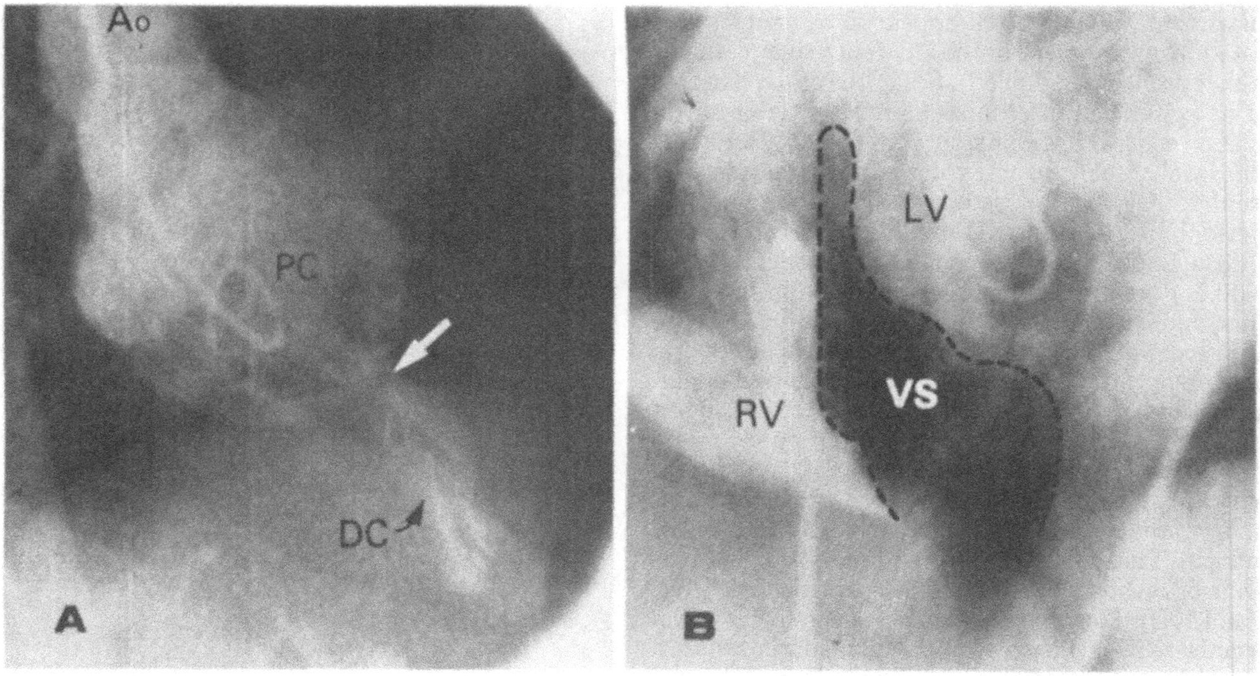

FIGURE 6. Case 4. Ventricular angiograms. **A,** left ventricular angiogram in the right anterior oblique projection during diastole. Note small distal cavity (DC), normal-sized proximal cavity (PC) and marked mid ventricular constriction (**arrow**). **B,** biventricular angiogram in the left anterior oblique projection during diastole. Contrast material fills the left ventricular (LV) and right ventricular (RV) cavities simultaneously, delineating the ventricular septum (VS) which is outlined by the **broken line.** The cephalad portion of septum (toward the **top**) is of normal thickness and the left and right endocardial surfaces are parallel. Toward the apex the septum increases abruptly in thickness, producing a "shelf-like" appearance (compare with Fig. 5). Ao = aorta.

nantly apical in distribution, only 6 (3 percent) showed T wave inversion greater than 10 mm in depth. Hence, in our experience, hypertrophic cardiomyopathy is rarely associated with "giant" T wave inversion; furthermore, when this electrocardiographic pattern is present in a patient with hypertrophic cardiomyopathy it is not indicative of left ventricular hypertrophy localized to the apex.

In addition, the angiographic appearance of the left ventricle in our patients and that reported from Japan are not identical, although both reflect the apical distribution of left ventricular hypertrophy. In Japanese patients, the distal aspect of the left ventricle (as seen in the right anterior oblique projection during diastole) was described as "spade-like" with the edge of the spade directed toward the apex. In contrast, most of our pa-

TABLE II

Gross Anatomic and Histologic Findings in Two Patients Studied at Necropsy

	Patient 3			Patient 5		
	Disorganization			Disorganization		
Tissue Location	%*	Type†	Wall Thickness (mm)	%*	Type†	Wall Thickness (mm)
Ventricular septum						
Basal	13	IA	8	4	IA	12
Mid ventricular	65	IB	12	17	IB	14
Proximal apex	47	IA	23	69	IA	25
Distal apex	36	IB	18	65	IB	22
Total	46			43		
LV free wall (basal)						
Anterolateral	17	IA	14	9	IA	20
Posterior	9	IA	24	0	IA	15
Total	15			6		

* Percent area of the relevant portions of the tissue section occupied by disorganized cardiac muscle cells.[19] † We have previously classified cardiac muscle cell disorganization into four major types[19] of which two are represented in two patients presented here. Type IA disorganization consists of areas of myocardium in which adjacent cardiac muscle cells are aligned perpendicularly and obliquely to each other, usually forming tangled masses or "pinwheel" configurations; type IB disorganization consists of relatively broad bundles of muscle cells oriented at oblique and perpendicular angles to each other; cells within these bundles are, however, normally arranged.
LV = left ventricular.

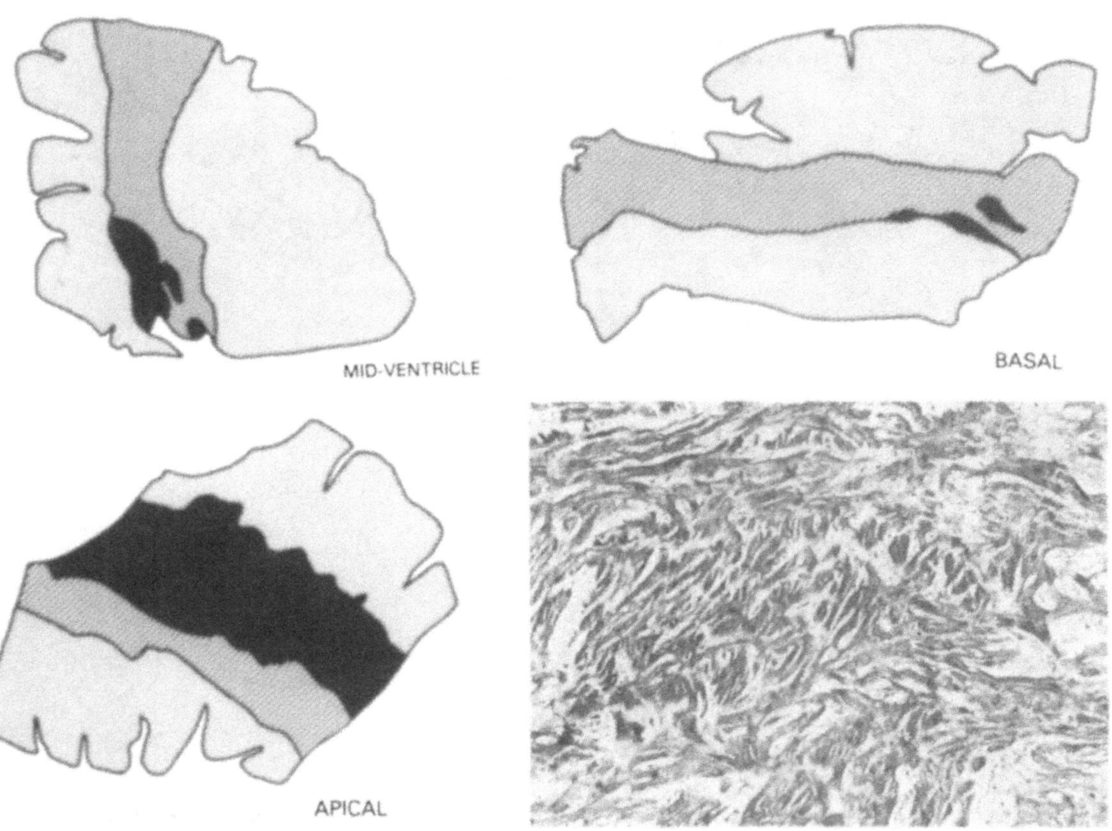

FIGURE 7. Case 5. Histologic findings including "maps" of histologic sections showing distribution of cardiac muscle cell disorganization in the basal, mid ventricular and apical regions of ventricular septum, respectively. **Solid areas** contain cellular disorganization, which constitutes 4 percent of the relevant parts of the basal tissue section, 17 percent of the mid ventricle section and 65 percent of the apical section. **Striped areas** represent normally arranged cardiac muscle cells that have been cut longitudinally. **Shaded areas** at the periphery of the section contain cells cut transversely. **Lower right,** photomicrograph of myocardium showing cellular disorganization typical of that present in the apical portion of ventricular septum. Bundles of cardiac muscle cells are oriented at oblique and perpendicular angles to each other (Type IB).

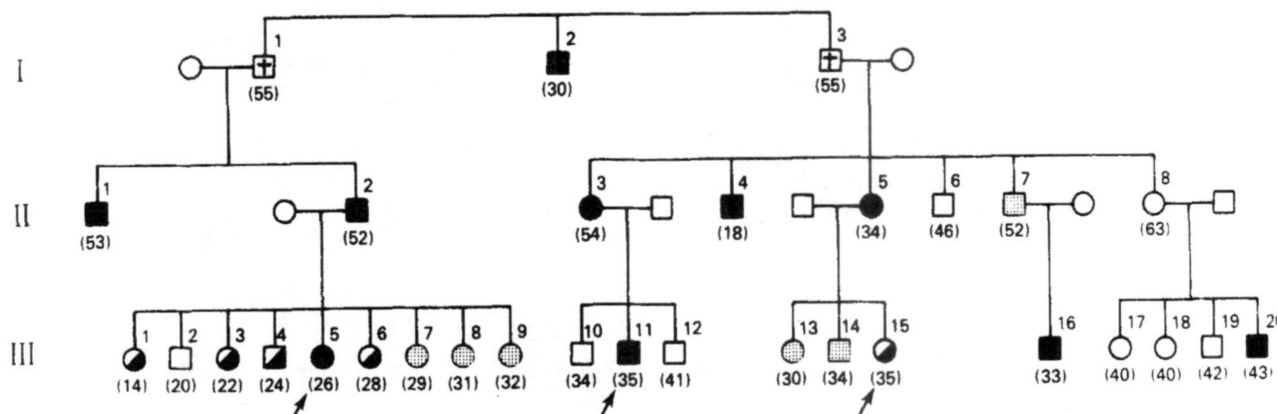

FIGURE 8. Pedigree of family in which study Patients 3, 4 and 5 (**arrows**) are members (Patients III. 5, III.11 and III.15, respectively, in the diagram). Patients' ages (yr) are shown in **parentheses** below the symbols; patient identification numbers are to the **upper right** of the symbols. Patients I. 1 and I. 3 both died of heart disease but not suddenly; a precise diagnosis was not made. In Patient II. 2, the left ventricular angiocardiogram suggested apical distribution of hypertrophy but no echocardiogram was obtained. Patient II. 3 with hypertrophic cardiomyopathy and severe mitral regurgitation died after mitral valve replacement. Patient III.16 survived a cardiac arrest (with documented ventricular fibrillation) at age 18 and has survived for 15 years. **Solid symbols,** sudden death probably or definitely due to hypertrophic cardiomyopathy; **half-filled symbols,** alive with hypertrophic cardiomyopathy that was identified by echocardiography or cardiac catheterization, or both; **dotted symbols,** hypertrophic cardiomyopathy absent on echocardiographic studies; **clear symbols,** not studied. **circles,** female subjects; **squares,** male subjects.

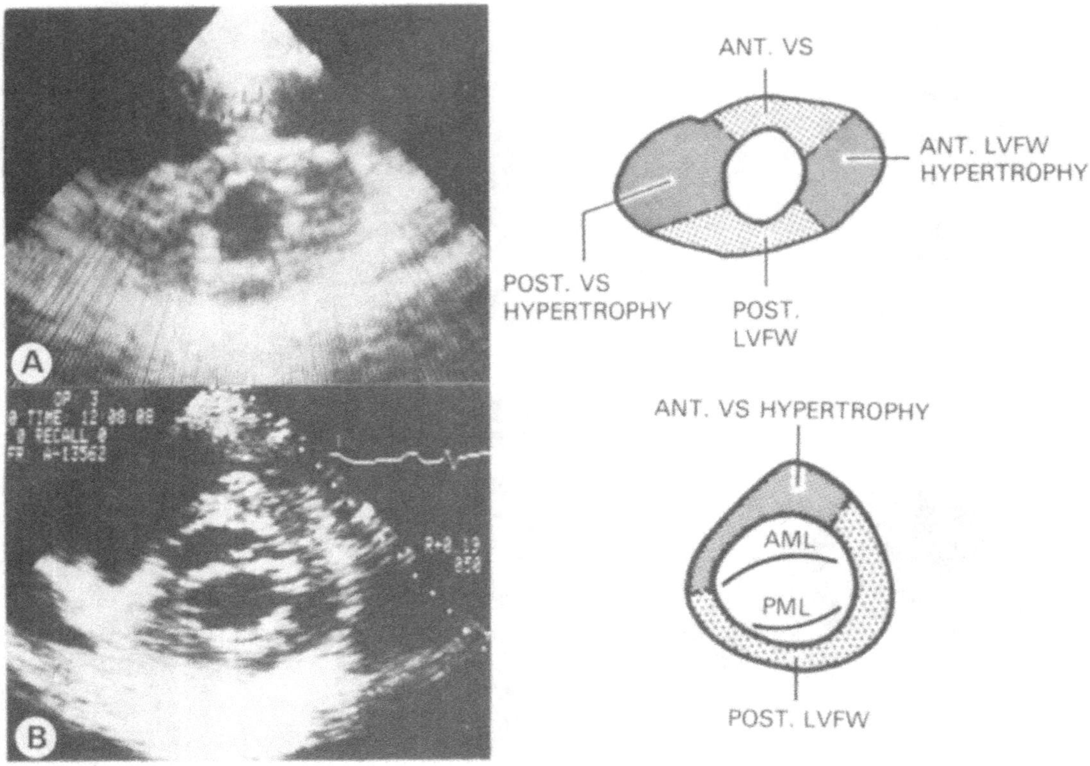

FIGURE 9. Stop-frames of two dimensional echocardiograms (obtained during diastole in the short axis view) from two relatives of Patients 3, 4 and 5 with apical distribution of hypertrophy. Each stop-frame (**left**) is accompanied by a schematic illustration (**right**). Heart sections are viewed from area of cardiac apex with anterior to the **top,** posterior to the **bottom** and patient's left to the **right. A,** from relative III.1 (in Figure 8), a 14 year old girl, showing hypertrophy at the level of the mitral leaflets involving the posterior ventricular septum (POST. VS) and anterolateral left ventricular free wall (ANT. LVFW). The anterior portion of septum is not thickened in this or any other cross-sectional plane and, hence, the M mode echocardiogram was normal and not diagnostic of hypertrophic cardiomyopathy. **B,** from relative III.16, a 33 year old man who survived a cardiac arrest at age 18 showing an anterior basal ventricular septum (ANT. VS) which is asymmetrically thickened relative to the posterior left ventricular free wall (POST. LVFW) (at the level of the mitral valve leaflets). AML and PML = anterior and posterior mitral leaflet, respectively.

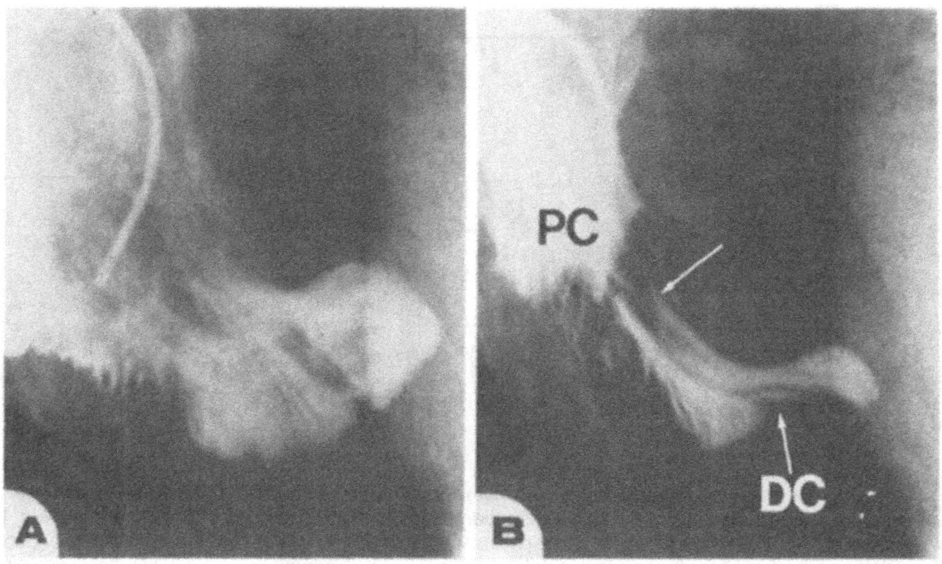

FIGURE 10. Case 3. Left ventricular angiogram obtained in right anterior oblique projection. **A,** during diastole the cavity is normal-sized with a bizarre "cauliflower" appearance; **B,** during systole mid ventricular constriction is apparent (**arrow**); the distal cavity (DC) is relatively small compared with the proximal cavity (PC).

tients showed a small, poorly contractile apical segment of left ventricle that communicated with the normal-sized proximal cavity through a markedly narrowed mid ventricular channel. These observations suggest that genetic and racial differences may account for the variation in clinical and morphologic features of hypertrophic cardiomyopathy in the United States and Japan.

Diagnosis: The diagnosis of hypertrophic cardiomyopathy could not always be made definitively from the conventional M mode echocardiogram in our study patients. In each patient, ventricular septal hypertrophy was virtually confined to regions of the ventricular wall not ordinarily traversed by the M mode ultrasonic beam. Only wide angle two dimensional echocardiography permitted definitive identification of the unusually located regions of hypertrophy near the left ventricular apex and confirmation of the diagnosis of hypertrophic cardiomyopathy.

We[8] have also previously described patients with hypertrophic cardiomyopathy and other patterns of left ventricular hypertrophy, in whom the M mode echocardiogram did not show hypertrophy and two dimensional echocardiography was necessary to make the correct diagnosis. Such patients, who also had an abnormal scalar electrocardiogram and family history of hypertrophic cardiomyopathy, usually showed hypertrophy that was limited to the posterior segment of ventricular septum, anterolateral left ventricular free wall, or both.

One of our patients (Case 3) had an intraventricular systolic pressure difference measured. This gradient appeared to be present across the area of severe midcavity narrowing identified by left ventricular angiography (the absence of systolic anterior motion of the anterior mitral leaflet in the echocardiogram also suggested that obstruction at the level of the left ventricular outflow tract was not present). The occurrence of mid ventricular obstruction has rarely been reported in patients with hypertrophic cardiomyopathy.[30] However, the clinical and physiologic significance of an intraventricular pressure difference, in which the highest left ventricular pressure is obtained from a diminutive distal segment of cavity, is unknown.

References

1. **Braunwald E, Lambrew CT, Rockoff SD, Ross J Jr, Morrow AG.** Idiopathic hypertrophic subaortic stenosis. I. A description of the disease based upon an analysis of 64 patients. Circulation 1964;30:(Suppl IV):IV-3–217.
2. **Goodwin JF, Hollman A, Cleland WP, Teare RD.** Obstructive cardiomyopathy simulating aortic stenosis. Br Heart J 1960;22: 403–4.
3. **Wigle ED, Heimbecker RO, Gunton RW.** Idiopathic ventricular septal hypertrophy causing muscular subaortic stenosis. Circulation 1962;26:325–40.
4. **Epstein SE, Henry WL, Clark CE, et al.** Asymmetric septal hypertrophy. Ann Intern Med 1974;81:650–80.
5. **Maron BJ, Epstein SE.** Hypertrophic cardiomyopathy. Recent observations regarding the specificity of three hallmarks of the disease: asymmetric septal hypertrophy, septal disorganization, and systolic anterior motion of the anterior mitral leaflet. Am J Cardiol 1980;45:141–54.
6. **Roberts WC, Ferrans VJ.** Pathologic anatomy of the cardiomyopathies. Idiopathic types, infiltrative types, and endomyocardial disease with and without eosinophilia. Hum Pathol 1975;6:288–342.
7. **Abbasi AS, MacAlpin RN, Eber LM, Pearce ML.** Echocardiographic diagnosis of idiopathic hypertrophic cardiomyopathy without outflow obstruction. Circulation 1972;46:897–904.
8. **Maron BJ, Gottdiener JS, Bonow RO, Epstein SE.** Hypertrophic cardiomyopathy with unusual locations of left ventricular hypertrophy undetectable by M-mode echocardiography: identification by wide-angle, two-dimensional echocardiography. Circulation 1981;63:409–18.
9. **Maron BJ, Gottdiener JS, Epstein SE.** Patterns and significance of the distribution of left ventricular hypertrophy in hypertrophic cardiomyopathy: a wide angle, two dimensional echocardiographic study of 125 patients. Am J Cardiol 1981;48:418–28.
10. **Tajik AJ, Seward JB, Hagler DJ.** Detailed analysis of hypertrophic obstructive cardiomyopathy by wide-angle two-dimensional sector echocardiography (abstr). Am J Cardiol 1979;43:348.
11. **Sakamoto T, Tei C, Murayama M, et al.** Giant negative T wave inversion as a manifestation of asymmetric apical hypertrophy (AAH) of the left ventricle. Echocardiographic and ultrasonocardiotomographic study. Jpn Heart J 1976;17:611–29.
12. **Yamaguchi H, Ishimura T, Nishiyama S, et al.** Hypertrophic nonobstructive cardiomyopathy with giant negative T waves (apical hypertrophy): ventriculographic and echocardiographic features in 30 patients. Am J Cardiol 1979;44:401–12.
13. **Popp RL, Filly K, Brown OR, Harrison DC.** Effect of transducer placement on echocardiographic measurement of left ventricular dimensions. Am J Cardiol 1975;35:537–40.
14. **Henry WL, Clark CE, Epstein SE.** Asymmetric septal hypertrophy (ASH): echocardiographic identification of the pathognomonic anatomic abnormality of IHSS. Circulation 1973;47:225–33.
15. **Kisslo J, von Ramm OT, Thurstone FL.** Cardiac imaging using phased array ultrasound system. II. Clinical technique and application. Circulation 1976;53:262–7.
16. **Silverman NH, Schiller NB.** Apex echocardiography. A two-dimensional technique for evaluating congenital heart disease. Circulation 1978;57:503–11.
17. **Romhilt DW, Estes EH.** A point score system for the ECG diagnosis of left ventricular hypertrophy. Am Heart J 1968;75:752–8.
18. **Savage DD, Seides SF, Clark CE, et al.** Electrocardiographic findings in patients with obstructive and nonobstructive hypertrophic cardiomyopathy. Circulation 1978;58:402–7.
19. **Maron BJ, Roberts WC.** Quantitative analysis of cardiac muscle cell disorganization in the ventricular septum of patients with hypertrophic cardiomyopathy. Circulation 1979;59:689–706.
20. **Gould SE.** Pathology of the Heart and Blood Vessels. 3rd ed. Springfield IL: Charles C Thomas, 1968:1139.
21. **Maron BJ, Epstein SE, Roberts WC.** Hypertrophic cardiomyopathy and transmural myocardial infarction without significant atherosclerosis of the extramural coronary arteries. Am J Cardiol 1979;43:1086–1102.
22. **Henry WL, Clark CE, Griffith JM, Epstein SE.** Mechanism of left ventricular outflow obstruction in patients with obstructive asymmetric septal hypertrophy (idiopathic hypertrophic subaortic stenosis). Am J Cardiol 1975;35:337–45.
23. **Criley JM, Lewis KB, White RI Jr, Ross RS.** Pressure gradients without obstruction. A new concept of "hypertrophic subaortic stenosis." Circulation 1965;32:881–7.
24. **Ross J, Braunwald E, Gault JH, Mason DT, Morrow AG.** The mechanism of the intraventricular pressure gradient in idiopathic hypertrophic subaortic stenosis. Circulation 1966;34:558–78.

25. **Adelman AG, Wigle ED.** Two types of intraventricular pressure difference in the same patient. Left ventricular catheter entrapment and right ventricular outflow tract obstruction. Circulation 1968; 38:649–55.
26. **Henry WL, Clark CE, Glancy DL, Epstein SE.** Echocardiographic measurement of the left ventricular outflow gradient in idiopathic hypertrophic subaortic stenosis. N Engl J Med 1973;288:989–93.
27. **Redwood DR, Scherer JL, Epstein SE.** Biventricular cineangiography in the evaluation of patients with asymmetric septal hypertrophy. Circulation 1974;49:1116–21.
28. **Clark CE, Henry WL, Epstein SE.** Familial prevalence and genetic transmission of idiopathic hypertrophic subaortic stenosis. N Engl J Med 1973;289:709–15.
29. **Maron BJ, Anan TJ, Roberts WC.** Quantitative analysis of the distribution of cardiac muscle cell disorganization in the left ventricular wall of patients with hypertrophic cardiomyopathy. Circulation 1981;63:882–94.
30. **Falicov RE, Resnekov L, Bharati S, Lev M.** Mid-ventricular obstruction: a variant of obstructive cardiomyopathy. Am J Cardiol 1976;37:432–7.

Coexistence of asymmetric and symmetric left ventricular hypertrophy in a family with hypertrophic cardiomyopathy

Elisabetta Ciró, M.D., Barry J. Maron, M.D., and William C. Roberts, M.D. *Bethesda, Md.*

A characteristic feature of the pattern of hypertrophy in patients with hypertrophic cardiomyopathy (HC) is its asymmetric distribution[1-4] and in the vast majority of instances the ventricular septum is disproportionately thickened with respect to the left ventricular (LV) free wall.[1-6] However, an occasional patient with the clinical features of HC may show concentric (symmetric) LV hypertrophy.[7-11] It is often unclear whether the cardiac disease manifested by such patients should be regarded as part of the disease spectrum of HC.[11] Hence, it is of value to describe a family with genetically transmitted HC in whom there is the unusual coexistence of closely related individuals who manifest either the asymmetric or symmetric morphologic forms of this disease.

From the Cardiology and Pathology Branches, National Heart, Lung and Blood Institute, National Institutes of Health.

Received for publication May 13, 1982; accepted May 21, 1982.

Reprint requests: Elisabetta Ciró, M.D., NHLBI-NIH, Bldg. 10, Room 7B-15, Bethesda, MD 20205.

Seven members of the family have been demonstrated to have HC (patients No. II.3, II.7, II.8, III.1. III.3, III.6, and IV.1) (Fig. 1). The index case (No. II.7) was a 56-year-old woman who died 1 day following LV myotomy-myectomy of complications emanating from ventricular septal infarction and rupture. This patient demonstrated clinical findings consistent with obstructive HC. She had marked functional limitation (New York Heart Association functional class III) with symptoms of dyspnea, fatigue, syncope, lightheadedness, angina pectoris, and palpitations. A 3/6 systolic ejection murmur was present at the lower left sternal border; alterations in the intensity of the murmur that occurred with various maneuvers were typical of patients with obstructive cardiomyopathy (i.e., increased with the Valsalva maneuver or with the administration of amyl nitrite and diminished with squatting). Blood pressure was slightly elevated (140/100 mm Hg); the patient had a history of labile systemic hypertension since childhood, although normalization of blood pressure had been achieved with diuretic therapy during the last 9 years of her life.

A 12-lead ECG showed the pattern of LV hypertrophy with "strain." M-mode echocardiogram showed a concentrically thickened LV wall; ventricular septal thickness was 18 mm, posterior free wall thickness was 17 mm, and septal–free wall ratio was 1.1. Ventricular septal excursion and thickening were markedly reduced (percent systolic thickening = 0). LV transverse dimension in diastole was normal (i.e., 36 mm). Marked systolic anterior motion of the mitral valve was present, resulting in prolonged contact of the anterior mitral leaflet with the ventricular septum. At left heart catheterization a LV outflow tract gradient of 40 mm Hg was present under basal conditions and it increased to 80 mm Hg with infusion of isoproterenol. LV end-diastolic pressure was within normal limits (12 mm Hg). Angiography showed a hypercontractile LV (ejection fraction = 90%) with cavity obliteration and characteristic "ballerina slipper" appearance in end-systole.

Necropsy confirmed the echocardiographic findings by demonstrating that the entire LV wall was symmetrically (concentrically) thickened; ventricular septum and LV free wall measured 18 mm and 17 mm, respectively (Fig. 2, *A*). The heart weighed 310 gm. The LV cavity was reduced in size, and both atria were dilated. An endocardial contact plaque was present on the ventricular septum in the LV outflow tract in apposition to the thickened anterior mitral leaflet. Histologic examination of ventricular septal myocardium revealed a markedly disordered arrangement of numerous cardiac muscle cells in which adjacent cells were aligned perpendicularly and obliquely to each other (Fig. 3, *A*, and *C*). Abnormally arranged cardiac muscle cells occupied 27% of the ventricular septal tissue section analyzed (Fig. 3, *A*).[12] The extramural coronary arteries were free of significant narrowing by atherosclerotic plaques.

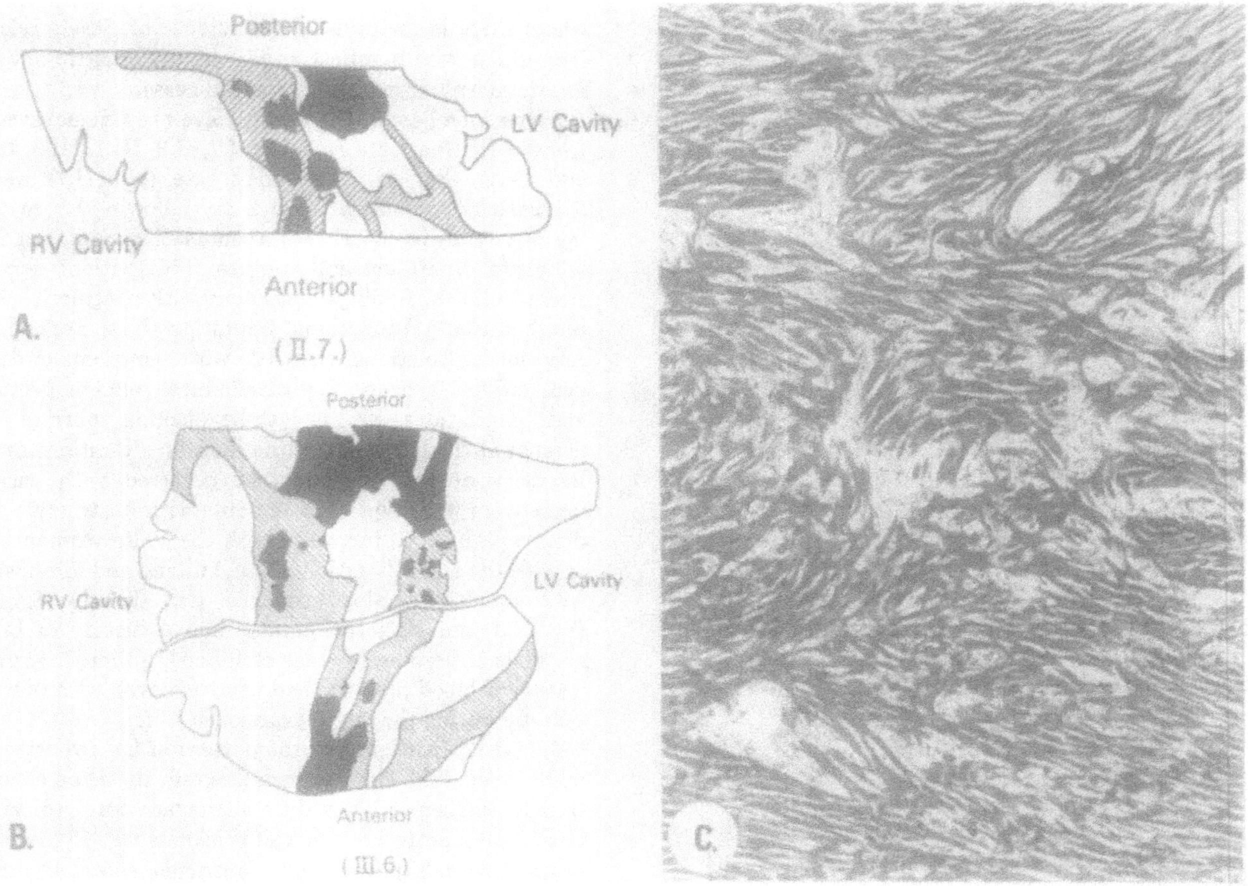

Fig. 3. *A* and *B*, "Maps" of ventricular septal tissue sections analyzed in the index case, II.7 *(A)*, and in her niece, III.6 *(B)*. Sections were obtained in the transverse plane—i.e., perpendicular to the long axis of the left ventricle. *Striped areas* represent normally arranged cardiac muscle cells cut longitudinally. *Solid areas* represent foci of disorganized cardiac muscle cells. In the index case *(A)*, disorganized cardiac muscle cells occupy about 25% of the striped area; in the niece *(B)*, the disorganized areas are more extensive, involving about 50% of the striped area. Clear areas adjacent to the left ventricular *(LV)* and right ventricular *(RV)* cavities contain cells cut transversely in which assessment of cellular arrangement can not be made. *C*, Photomicrograph of a representative tissue section of ventricular septum from the index case (patient No. II.7) showing cellular disorganization. Adjacent cardiac muscle cells are aligned perpendicularly and obliquely to each other. This pattern of myocardial architecture is similar to that found in the patient's niece (No. III.6). (Hematoxylin and eosin stain; original magnification ×55.)

index case. Histologic examination of myocardium showed marked septal disorganization involving 54% of the tissue section (Fig. 3, *B*); disorganization was of the type in which relatively broad bundles of cardiac muscle cells were oriented at oblique or perpendicular angles to each other, although cells within the bundles were normally arranged.[12]

Three affected relatives (No. II.8, III.3, and IV.1) are alive and asymptomatic. In each, two-dimensional echocardiography (2DE) showed thickening which was located predominantly in the posterior portion of the ventricular septum and anterolateral LV free wall. Because hypertrophy only involved portions of the LV wall not traversed by the M-mode echo beam, the conventional M-mode echocardiogram was normal in each of these three affected relatives.[13] Hence, while the distribution of hypertrophy was asymmetric in these three patients, it nevertheless differed from the particular pattern of asymmetric hypertrophy observed in the niece of the index case (patient III.6). The remaining two family members known definitely to have HC (No. II.3 and III.1) died of progressive congestive heart failure. However, the precise distribution of LV hypertrophy was not defined by 2DE or at necropsy in these two patients.

The family described in this report demonstrates that within the wide disease spectrum of genetically transmitted HC a variety of morphologic expressions may be observed, including symmetric (concentric) as well as asymmetric LV hypertrophy, and that these forms may coexist in the same family. The index case, a severely symptomatic 56-year-old woman with marked subaortic obstruction, showed concentric LV hypertrophy. Six other relatives showed a variety of patterns of asymmetric hypertrophy, including a niece of the index case who died suddenly at 15 years of age without having previously experienced cardiac symptoms. Of note, substantial disorganization of ventricular septal architecture was present in both the index patient with relatively mild concentric hypertrophy and in her niece with particularly marked asymmetric hypertrophy. Septal disorganization in each of these two relatives was extensive and similar to that found in other patients with HC, and far exceeded the degree of disorganization reported in patients with cardiac diseases other than HC.[12] Therefore, disordered septal architecture represented a morphologic link between these two patients with HC who had markedly different patterns and magnitude of LV hypertrophy.

Of note, the index case of this family with concentric LV hypertrophy had experienced systemic hypertension for several years. Nevertheless, the vast amount of clinical and pathologic information in this patient suggests it is appropriate to consider her cardiac disease to be within the clinicopathologic spectrum of HC and not primarily related to systemic hypertension. First, she experienced severe functional limitation with typical symptoms of HC such as exertional dyspnea, lightheadedness, chest pain, and palpitations. Also typical of this disease was the presence of marked obstruction to LV outflow associated with systolic anterior motion of the mitral valve and the angiographic appearance of a hypercontractile LV. Finally, the widespread distribution of cardiac muscle cell disorganization involving over 25% of the ventricular septal myocardium analyzed is typical of patients with HC and far exceeds the usual extent of involvement observed in patients with systemic hypertension.[12] It is also conceivable that this patient with concentric LV hypertrophy may have demonstrated asymmetric LV hypertrophy at an earlier stage in the natural history of her disease but, as a consequence of systemic hypertension, thickening of the posterior wall occurred and resulted in the morphologic appearance of symmetric LV hypertrophy.

"True" concentric LV hypertrophy, as demonstrated by the index case, is probably a particularly uncommon occurrence in patients with HC.[4] A number of patients with HC and normal septal-to-free wall thickness ratios of < 1.3 have been identified with M-mode echocardiography[8-11]; however, in such patients 2DE usually shows asymmetric hypertrophy in regions of the LV wall inaccessible to the M-mode echo beam.[4] Hence, the appearance of concentric LV on the M-mode echocardiogram of patients with HC usually results when those relatively small regions of LV wall sampled by this technique (portions of anterior ventricular septum and posterobasal free wall) are of similar thickness, although other regions of the LV may show more substantial wall thickening.

REFERENCES

1. Teare D: Asymmetrical hypertrophy of the heart in young patients. Br Heart J **20**:1, 1958.
2. Roberts WC: Valvular, subvalvular and supravalvular aortic stenosis: Morphologic features. Cardiovasc Clin **5**:104, 1973.
3. Menges H, Brandenburg RO, Brown AL: The clinical, hemodynamic and pathologic diagnosis of muscular subvalvular aortic stenosis. Circulation **24**:1126, 1961.
4. Maron BJ, Gottdiener JS, Epstein SE: Patterns and significance of distribution of left ventricular hypertrophy in hypertrophic cardiomyopathy. A wide-angle, two-dimensional echocardiographic study of 125 patients. Am J Cardiol **48**:418, 1981.
5. Henry WL, Clark CE, Epstein SE: Asymmetric septal hypertrophy (ASH); echocardiographic identification of the pathognomonic anatomic abnormality of IHSS. Circulation **47**:225, 1973.
6. Abbasi AS, MacAlpin RN, Eber LM, Pearce ML: Left ventricular hypertrophy diagnosed by echocardiography. N Engl J Med **289**:118, 1973.
7. Bercu BA, Diettert GA, Danforth WH, Pund EE, Ahlvin RC, Belliveau RR: Pseudoaortic stenosis produced by ventricular hypertrophy. Am J Med **25**:814, 1958.
8. Chahine RA, Raizner AE, Ishimori T, Montero AC: Echocardiographic, hemodynamic and angiographic correlations in hypertrophic cardiomyopathy. Br Heart J **39**:945, 1977.
9. Come PC, Bulkley BH, Goodman ZD, Hutchins GM, Pitt B, Fortuin NJ: Hypercontractile cardiac states simulating hypertrophic cardiomyopathy. Circulation **55**:901, 1977.
10. Rossen RM, Goodman DJ, Ingham RE, Popp RL: Echocardiographic criteria in the diagnosis of idiopathic hypertrophic subaortic stenosis. Circulation **50**:747, 1974.
11. Maron BJ, Gottdiener JS, Roberts WC, Henry WL, Savage DD, Epstein SE: Left ventricular outflow tract obstruction due to systolic anterior motion of the anterior mitral leaflet in patients with concentric left ventricular hypertrophy. Circulation **57**:527, 1978.
12. Maron BJ, Roberts WC: Quantitative analysis of cardiac muscle cell disorganization in the ventricular septum of patients with hypertrophic cardiomyopathy. Circulation **59**:689, 1977.
13. Maron BJ, Gottdiener JS, Bonow RO, Epstein SE: Hypertrophic cardiomyopathy with unusual locations of left ventricular hypertrophy undetectable by M-mode echocardiography: Identification by wide-angle, two-dimensional echocardiography. Circulation **63**:409, 1981.

Systolic anterior motion of the posterior mitral leaflet: a previously unrecognized cause of dynamic subaortic obstruction in patients with hypertrophic cardiomyopathy

BARRY J. MARON, M.D., ANTHONY M. HARDING, PAOLO SPIRITO, M.D., WILLIAM C. ROBERTS, M.D., AND BRUCE F. WALLER, M.D.

ABSTRACT Dynamic obstruction to left ventricular outflow in patients with hypertrophic cardiomyopathy usually occurs when the anterior mitral leaflet moves forward in systole and approaches or contacts the ventricular septum. However, we have recently identified, by M mode and two-dimensional echocardiography, 21 patients with hypertrophic cardiomyopathy who had a unique pattern of mitral valve motion characterized by abnormal mitral valve coaptation and systolic anterior motion of the posterior mitral leaflet. This abnormality of mitral valve motion was most reliably identified with two-dimensional echocardiography in views of the left ventricle obtained from the apex. At end-diastole the anterior and posterior mitral leaflets did not appear to coapt at their distal free margins. Rather, at mitral valve closure, the anterior mitral leaflet contacted the basal portion of posterior mitral leaflet. Subsequently, during systole the "residual" distal portion of posterior mitral leaflet approached or contacted the ventricular septum. Morphologic observations in nine other patients with hypertrophic cardiomyopathy suggested that systolic anterior motion of the posterior mitral leaflet is due to elongation of the middle scallop of the posterior leaflet, which probably comes into apposition with the ventricular septum during systole by passing through the space created by the normal pattern of chordal attachments onto the anterior mitral leaflet. Of the 16 patients who underwent cardiac catheterization, nine had basal subaortic gradients of 20 to 85 mm Hg, which were apparently due to moderate or marked systolic anterior motion of the posterior mitral leaflet. Ventricular septal myotomy-myectomies were performed in two patients and resulted in markedly diminished systolic anterior motion of the posterior mitral leaflet in each and abolition of subaortic gradient in the one patient who underwent postoperative cardiac catheterization. Hence, in patients with hypertrophic cardiomyopathy, systolic anterior motion of the posterior mitral leaflet (1) is not uncommon (identifiable in about 10% of a consecutively studied series of patients), (2) constitutes a previously undescribed mechanism for dynamic subaortic obstruction, and (3) is due to a malformation of the posterior mitral leaflet.
Circulation 68, No. 2, 282–293, 1983.

A SUBSTANTIAL PROPORTION of patients with hypertrophic cardiomyopathy demonstrate obstruction to left ventricular outflow.[1-5] Most available angiographic[6, 7] and echocardiographic[8-25] data appear to indicate that this dynamic subaortic obstruction occurs when the anterior mitral leaflet (AML) (with or without its attached chordae tendineae) approaches or comes into contact with the ventricular septal endocardium. Others have suggested that the chordae tendineae or papillary muscles may primarily produce left ventricular outflow obstruction.[26-28] However, the role played by the posterior mitral leaflet (PML) in this obstructive process has not been defined. In this regard, we have identified a subgroup of patients with hypertrophic cardiomyopathy in whom the PML showed systolic anterior motion (SAM) that appeared to be responsible for subaortic obstruction.

Methods

Selection of patients. Between July 1979 and April 1980, 150 consecutively studied patients with a technically satisfactory two-dimensional echocardiogram were diagnosed at the National Heart, Lung and Blood Institute as having hypertrophic cardiomyopathy. In each patient, the diagnosis of hypertrophic cardiomyopathy was established by the characteristic clinical findings[1-5] and the echocardiographic demonstration of a hypertrophied and nondilated left ventricle in the absence of

From the Echocardiography Laboratory and Cardiology and Pathology Branches of the National Heart, Lung and Blood Institute, National Institutes of Health, Bethesda.

Address for correspondence: Barry J. Maron, M.D., Cardiology Branch, National Heart, Lung and Blood Institute, National Institutes of Health, Bldg. 10, Room 7B-15, Bethesda, MD 20205.

Received Jan. 4, 1983; revision accepted April 7, 1983.

another cardiac or systemic disease that could produce left ventricular hypertrophy.[29–31]

Of the 150 patients with hypertrophic cardiomyopathy, 77 had SAM of the mitral valve that was evident on their M mode echocardiograms. In nine (12%) of these 77 patients, two-dimensional echocardiography demonstrated that this SAM was produced by the PML.

In addition, between May 1980 and May 1982, another 12 patients with hypertrophic cardiomyopathy were identified as having SAM of the PML by two-dimensional echocardiography and were added to the patient group. Therefore, the overall study group comprised 21 patients with hypertrophic cardiomyopathy and SAM of the PML.

Patient characteristics. The 21 study patients ranged in age from 9 to 50 years (mean 28); 13 (62%) were male patients. Nine patients were asymptomatic, the activities of five were mildly limited by their symptoms (New York Heart Association class II), and the activities of seven were moderately to severely limited (classes III and IV). The symptoms most commonly experienced were dyspnea on exertion and fatigue (seven patients), lightheadedness (six patients), and palpitations (five patients). Fifteen patients were taking cardiac medications at the time of the echocardiographic studies (propranolol in nine and verapamil in six).

The two other groups of patients were studied by echocardiography and compared with the patients with hypertrophic cardiomyopathy and SAM of the PML. One control group consisted of 48 subjects in whom there was no evidence of heart disease; their ages ranged from 20 to 50 years (mean 24) and 15 (60%) were male patients. The second group consisted of 137 patients with cardiac diseases other than hypertrophic cardiomyopathy, including coronary heart disease (51 patients), aortic valve disease (48 patients), congenital heart malformations (18 patients), mitral valve disease other than prolapse (13 patients), and dilated cardiomyopathy (seven patients). Ages ranged from 2 to 73 years (mean 45); 102 (75%) were male patients.

Hemodynamic studies. Cardiac catheterization was performed in 16 of the 21 patients with hypertrophic cardiomyopathy and SAM of the PML after cardioactive medications were discontinued. Left ventricular outflow tract gradients of 20 to 85 mm Hg were present under basal conditions in nine patients, including five with gradients of 40 mm Hg or more. In six of the nine patients with basal subaortic obstruction, higher gradients of 40 to 110 mm Hg were produced by provocative intervention (i.e., isoproterenol infusion, Valsalva maneuver, or amyl nitrite inhalation).

Seven other patients had small (5 mm Hg) or no left ventricular outflow gradient under basal conditions. Five of these seven patients had provoked gradients of 30 to 60 mm Hg, one had no gradient with provocation, and the remaining patient underwent no provocative maneuvers.

M mode echocardiography. M mode echocardiograms were performed with an IREX System II Ultrasound unit with a 2.25 MHz unfocused transducer 1.3 cm in diameter. Maximal thickness of the ventricular septum was measured just before atrial systole, with the ultrasound beam directed either through or slightly below the mitral leaflets.[29, 31] Thickness of the posterior left ventricular free wall was measured during the same phase of the cardiac cycle, with the ultrasound beam passing through the mitral leaflets.

Position of the mitral valve in the left ventricular cavity was assessed at the point of closure of the valve leaflets. Mitral valve position index was calculated by dividing the distance between mitral valve and posterior free wall endocardium by the distance between mitral valve and ventricular septal endocardium.[18]

Other M mode echocardiographic parameters were measured in accordance with the recommendations of the American Society of Echocardiography.[32] When appropriate, echocardiographic dimensions were adjusted for body surface area and compared with normal standards.[33]

SAM of the mitral valve was evaluated in a semiquantitative fashion. SAM was defined as mild if the minimal mitral-septal distance was greater than 10 mm; moderate, if this distance was 10 mm or less but there was no mitral-septal contact; and marked if there was either brief or prolonged (greater than 30% of echocardiographic systole[24]) mitral-septal contact.

Two-dimensional echocardiography. A Varian (V-3400) real-time, phased-array, ultrasonic sector scanner with a hand-held 2.25 MHz transducer was used to perform the two-dimensional echocardiographic studies. The field of view is 80 degrees in an azimuthal direction and 15 or 21 cm deep. Azimuthal resolution is 2 to 5 mm within the field of view and range resolution is 1.5 to 2 mm. Images were produced at 32 frames/sec and recorded on 1 inch (Sony) reel-to-reel videotape or an Ampex DR-10 rhodium-plated chromium disc for subsequent review in real-time, slow-motion, or stop-action modes. Single still-frame photographs were made from a television monitor with the use of a 35 mm camera.

Two-dimensional echocardiographic examination included the imaging of a number of cross-sectional planes through the heart.[34] Serial short-axis views of the left ventricle were obtained by initially orienting the sector plane perpendicular to the long axis of the left ventricle from a standard parasternal transducer location and slowly angling the image plane from aorta (cephalad) to apex (caudad).[35] The long-axis view was obtained from the same transducer placement by orienting the sector plane parallel to the longitudinal axis of the left ventricle, with care being taken to avoid improper angulation of the scan plane tangentially through the ventricle.

The apical four-chamber view was obtained with the transducer at the cardiac apex and the tomographic plane directed perpendicular to the ventricular and atrial septa and through the plane of the mitral and tricuspid valve orifices. This permitted simultaneous display of atria and ventricles and atrioventricular valves and cardiac septae.[36] The right anterior oblique equivalent (two-chamber) view of the left ventricle was obtained by rotating the transducer clockwise 60 to 90 degrees so that the ultrasound beam was in a plane approximately parallel to the ventricular septum, permitting simultaneous visualization of the aorta (and aortic valve), left ventricular outflow tract, and mitral valve leaflets.[34]

Valvular motion is best appreciated by analysis of real-time (motion) video recordings. The freeze-frame photographs we use for illustration do not permit the visual integration that is possible with the real-time movie, and the quality of such static images is therefore unavoidably degraded optically compared with the dynamic real-time display. We also recognize the difficulty in reliably establishing the precise point of demarcation between the distal portions of mitral valve leaflet and the attached chordae tendineae. To aid in making this distinction (as well as that between the anterior and posterior leaflets), M mode recordings were made while the cardiac anatomy was being directly observed with two-dimensional echocardiography in the long-axis view. In addition, imaging the left ventricle in the right anterior oblique view from the apex was often helpful in discerning the proximal extent of the chordae from the distal portion of the mitral leaflets. Nevertheless, for the purposes of simplicity and clarity, we have referred to the adjacent portions of mitral valve leaflet and attached chordae tendineae as either the AML or PML.

The cross-sectional orifice area of the left ventricular outflow tract was assessed by a method described in detail elsewhere.[37] In brief, the outflow tract was outlined in the short-axis plane at the level of the mitral valve during diastole, and the cross-

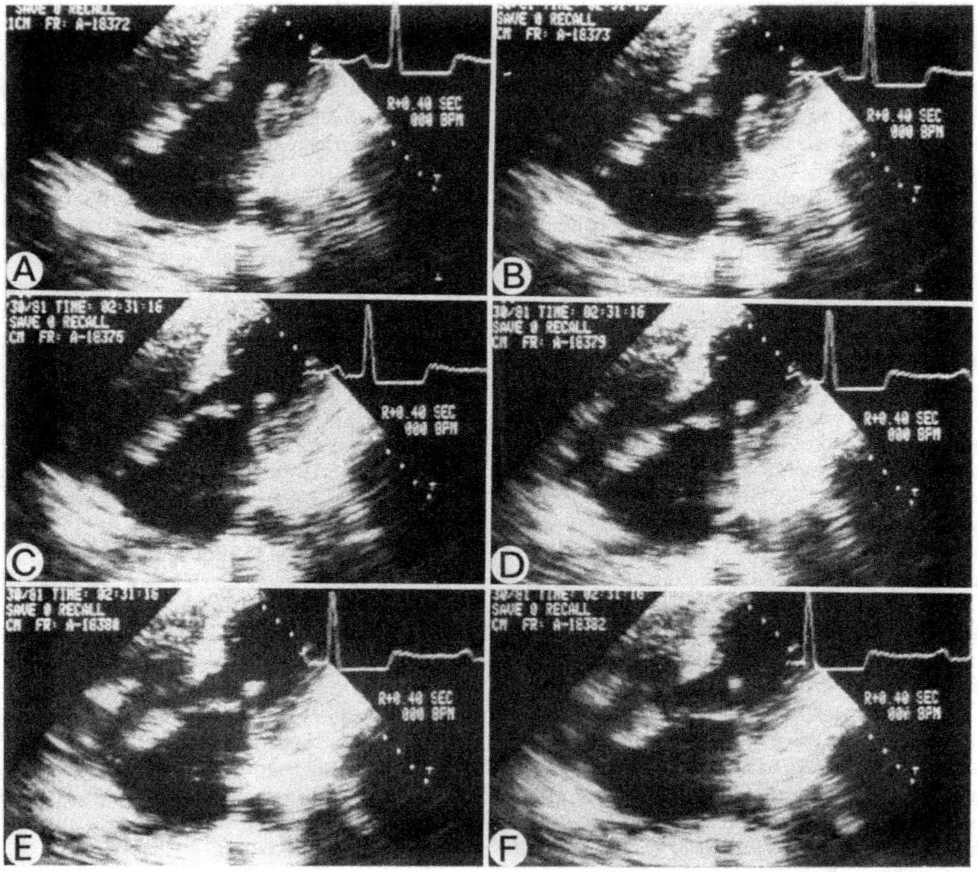

FIGURE 1. Sequential two-dimensional echocardiographic stop-frame images obtained during the same cardiac cycle in the apical four-chamber view, in a 45-year-old woman with hypertrophic cardiomyopathy and a 50 mm Hg subaortic gradient under basal conditions. Frames *A* through *E* were obtained during diastole; *F* was obtained during the early portion of the subsequent systole. Each stop-frame is accompanied by a schematic illustration shown separately in figure 2. During diastole the AML and PML approach each other, although the PML shows relatively little motion. In frame *C* it is apparent that the leaflets have failed to meet (i.e., not coapted) at their distal margins, and in *E* the AML tip comes into apposition with the base of the posterior leaflet. In frame *F*, at the onset of systole, the residual portion of the PML shows marked anterior motion and approaches the ventricular septum (VS). In subsequent systolic frames (not shown here) the posterior leaflet contacted the septum. FW = free wall of left ventricle; LA = left atrium; LV = left ventricle; RV = right ventricle. In this and other illustrative echocardiograms, calibration dots are 1 cm apart.

sectional area was quantitated with a video planimetry system.

Four basic patterns of distribution of left ventricular hypertrophy were identified by two-dimensional echocardiography in the study patients. This classification has been reported in detail previously.[31]

Morphologic studies. The case records of the Pathology Branch and those of the Echocardiography Laboratory were reviewed and nine patients were identified in whom (1) the gross heart specimen (seven patients) or operatively excised mitral valve (two patients) were in suitable condition to permit examination and measurement of the mitral valve leaflets[38] and (2) a technically adequate two-dimensional echocardiogram had been obtained while they were alive. None of these patients are included among the 21 patients who comprise the primary study group.

Results

Mitral valve motion

Two-dimensional echocardiography. An abnormality of mitral valve motion and coaptation was identified in each of the 21 study patients by two-dimensional echocardiography (figures 1 through 6).

In the apical view of the left ventricle (figures 1 through 3) it was evident that the distal margins of the AML and PML did not come into apposition at end-diastole in the normal fashion. Rather, the distal portion of the PML passed caudal to the anterior leaflet while the anterior leaflet coapted at or near the base of the posterior leaflet (figures 1 through 3). Hence, the distal portion of the PML did not participate in mitral valve coaptation. This "residual" posterior leaflet distal to the site of coaptation varied in length depending on precisely where the anterior leaflet made contact with the posterior leaflet. For example, when the AML coapted at the base of the posterior leaflet the residual portion of posterior leaflet was relatively long (figures 1 through 3). If the point of coaptation was closer to the

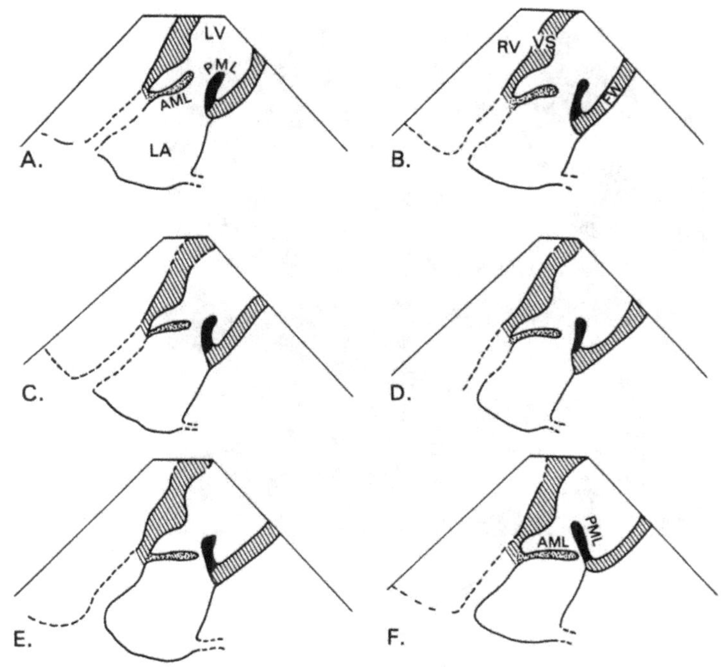

FIGURE 2. Schematic illustrations of stop-frame images shown in figure 1. Abbreviations are as in figure 1.

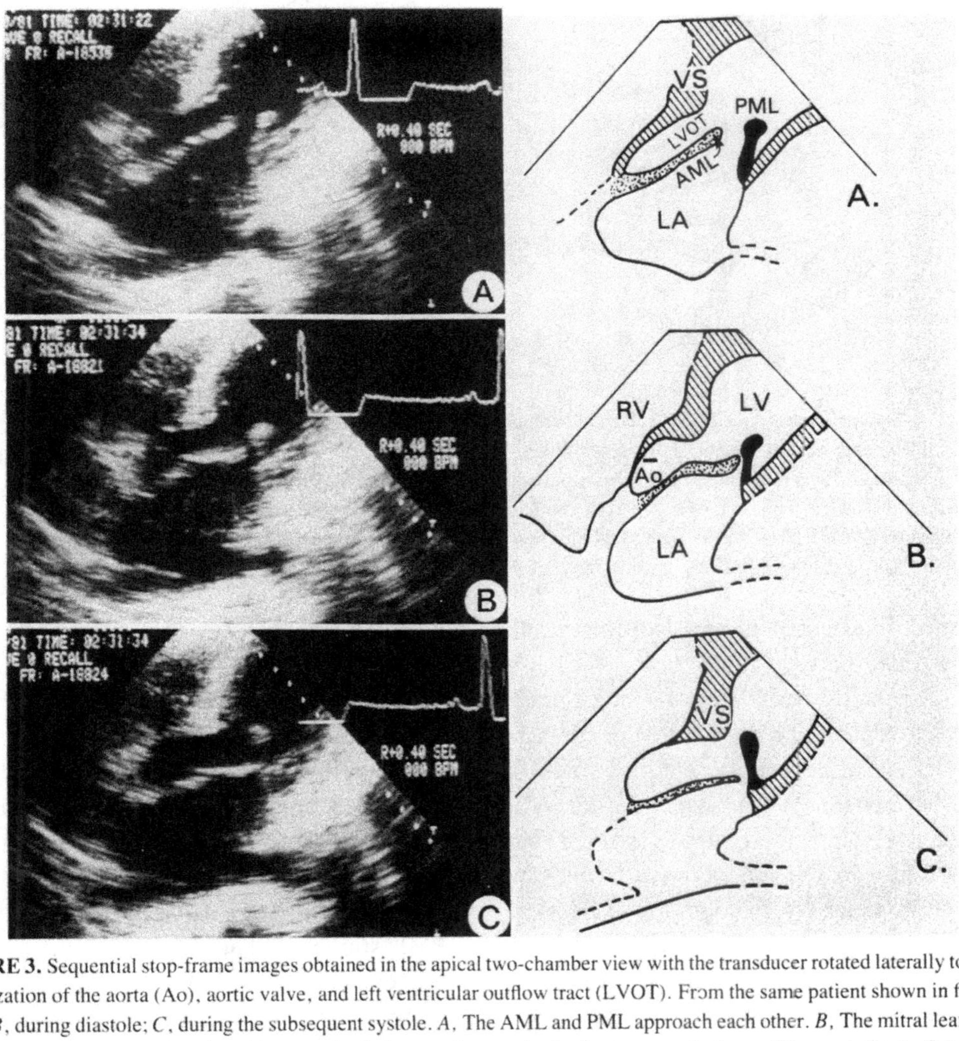

FIGURE 3. Sequential stop-frame images obtained in the apical two-chamber view with the transducer rotated laterally to permit visualization of the aorta (Ao), aortic valve, and left ventricular outflow tract (LVOT). From the same patient shown in figure 1. *A* and *B*, during diastole; *C*, during the subsequent systole. *A*, The AML and PML approach each other. *B*, The mitral leaflets fail to coapt normally at their distal margins; at mitral closure, the anterior leaflet contacts the base of the posterior leaflet. *C*, The portion of posterior leaflet distal to the site of coaptation protrudes into the left ventricular outflow tract and approaches the ventricular septum (VS). LA = left atrium; LV = left ventricle; RV = right ventricle.

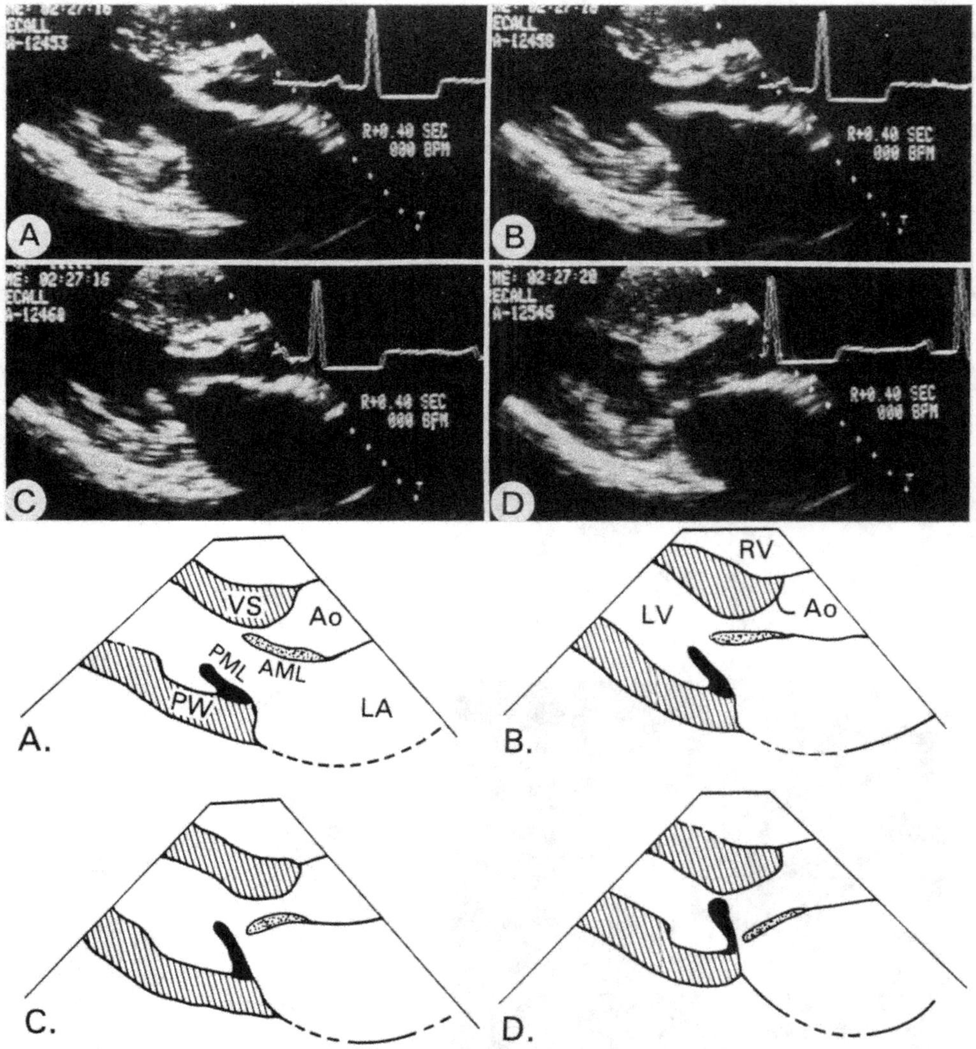

FIGURE 4. Sequential two-dimensional echocardiographic stop-frame images obtained during the same cardiac cycle in the parasternal long-axis view. *A* through *C*, during diastole; *D*, during the subsequent systole. Mitral valve motion corresponds to that shown in the apical views in figure 1. *A*, Mitral valve is wide open; the AML is in apposition to ventricular septum (VS) and the PML apposes the posterior free wall. *B* and *C*, The mitral leaflets approach each other. *D*, The anterior leaflet coapts at the base of the posterior leaflet and the free residual portion of the posterior leaflet comes into apposition with the ventricular septum. Ao = aorta; LV = left ventricle; RV = right ventricle; PW = posterior free wall.

tip of the posterior leaflet, the residual portion of that leaflet was relatively short.

In early systole, the residual posterior leaflet continued its anterior movement and approached or contacted the ventricular septal endocardium during midsystole (figures 1 through 3). When imaged in the right anterior oblique equivalent view, it was evident that the PML projected into the left ventricular outflow tract during systole (figure 3). Recognition of SAM of the PML could usually be achieved in the conventional four-chamber view; however, it was often necessary to tilt or rotate the transducer slightly clockwise or counterclockwise in order to identify that segment of the PML that showed SAM.

In each study patient, the PML appeared to be elongated (in the base to apex plane); the length of the posterior leaflet was approximately equal to or greater than that of the anterior leaflet in each patient. In five of the 21 patients, the site of attachment of the PML to the posterobasal free wall appeared to be displaced toward the apex relative to the AML; in the other 16 patients the mitral leaflets were normally positioned with respect to each other.

Abnormal mitral valve coaptation and SAM of the PML similar to that observed in the apical views was also evident in the parasternal long-axis view (figures 4 and 6). The distal margins of posterior leaflet appeared to pass caudal to the tip of anterior leaflet and approach the ventricular septum in systole.

Analysis of the short-axis views confirmed and sup-

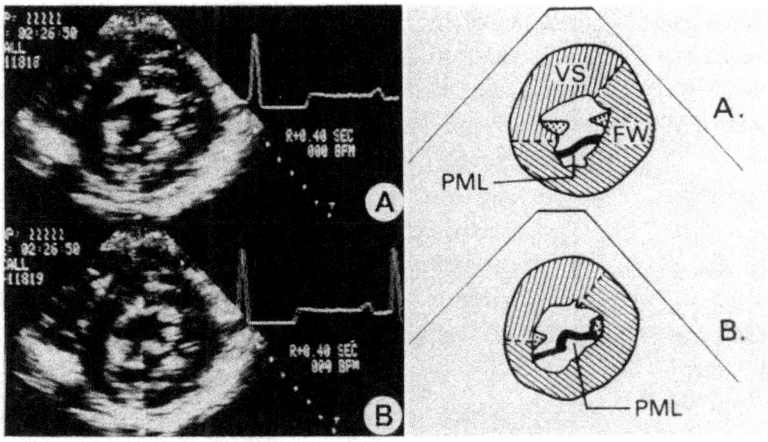

FIGURE 5. Two-dimensional echocardiographic stop-frame images obtained during late diastole *(A)* and systole *(B)* in the parasternal short-axis view. From the same patient shown in figure 4. *A*, At this cross-sectional level, the PML is imaged alone since the entire anterior leaflet is positioned more cephalad. *B*, At the onset of systole, the middle one-third of the posterior leaflet has moved anteriorly and appears to pass between bundles of chordae tendineae (dotted structures on schematic drawings). In subsequent systolic frames (not shown here) the posterior leaflet came into contact with the ventricular septum (VS). FW = free wall of left ventricle.

plemented findings obtained in the other tomographic planes. In the short-axis planes through the most basal portions of the left ventricle, both mitral leaflets could be imaged together and showed normal anatomic relationships and valvular motion. However, when the echocardiographic beam was directed more distally (to a level where the chordae tendineae were visualized) it was often possible to image the PML alone (figure 5). At this level, the posterior leaflet was observed to move anteriorly during systole between the chordal bundles; the middle one-third of the leaflet appeared to most closely approach or contact the septum (figure 5).

SAM involving the PML (or AML) was absent in 177 of the 185 control subjects studied by echocardiography. The remaining eight subjects (two normal subjects and six with other cardiac diseases) showed SAM of the PML that was particularly trivial in magnitude — i.e., did not come within 18 mm of the ventricular septum during systole.

M mode echocardiography. It was also possible to identify SAM of the PML by M mode echocardiography in each study patient (figures 7 through 9). In diastole, the PML occupied a relatively posterior position in the left ventricular cavity and showed the normal peaks of anterior and posterior motion (i.e., E′, F′, and A′) at appropriate times in the cardiac cycle. Diastolic excursion of the posterior leaflet was, however, often exaggerated.

At the onset of ventricular systole (just after the peak of the R wave on electrocardiogram) the PML moved abruptly anteriorly toward the ventricular septum, reaching its maximum forward excursion in midsystole, and then moved sharply posteriorly, returning to baseline position just before the end of systole (figure 8). Usually one or two notches, produced by rapid anterior and posterior systolic leaflet motion, were evident in the upstroke of the PML contour (figure 8).

The contour of the posterior leaflet on the echograms varied among the study patients. In nine patients the leaflet showed a rapid, relatively smooth upstroke and descent (figure 8); in the other 12 patients the initial rapid ascent was directly anterior, but as the

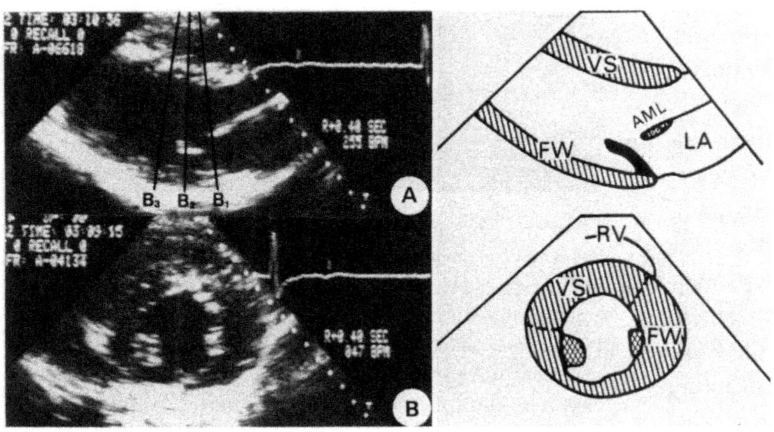

FIGURE 6. Two-dimensional echocardiographic stop-frame images from a 41-year-old man with hypertrophic cardiomyopathy in whom hypertrophy was primarily confined to the apical one-half of the left ventricle. *A*, In the long-axis view, mitral valve motion is shown during early systole *(A)*. Magnitude of SAM of the PML is mild and left ventricular outflow tract dimension is normal; hence, the PML does not closely approach the ventricular septum (VS), accounting for the absence of subaortic obstruction under basal conditions. Solid lines B_1, B_2, and B_3 denote sampling sites for the M mode echocardiograms shown in figure 7. *B*, Short-axis view at papillary muscle level shows hypertrophy of anterolateral free wall and posterior portion of septum, which can not be identified by M mode echocardiography or seen in the long-axis view. FW = free wall of left ventricle; LA = left atrium; RV = right ventricle.

leaflet approached the septum its velocity diminished and it assumed a "squared-off" appearance (figure 7). The magnitude and duration of SAM of the PML also varied greatly among individual patients and was mild in three (figure 7), moderate in seven, and severe in 11 (figure 8). Since the PML occupies a posterior position in the cavity during diastole, moderate-to-marked SAM of the PML represents an example of particularly exaggerated leaflet excursion.

In six study patients the residual portion of PML was particularly long and extended far caudal to the anterior leaflet. Therefore, it was possible to pass the M mode beam preferentially through the posterior leaflet and record its motion without imaging the anterior leaflet (figures 6 through 8). Verification that this isolated valve structure represented the posterior leaflet was obtained by scanning the M mode beam (either conventional or derived from the two-dimensional echocardiogram) until it was possible to identify continuity between the distal portion of posterior leaflet that was imaged alone and its more proximal segment (visualized with the anterior leaflet).

In 15 other patients the residual portion of the posterior leaflet was shorter and the distal margins of the two mitral leaflets were relatively close together. Hence, the posterior leaflet could not be selectively imaged without the anterior leaflet by M mode echocardiography. In such patients, the images of the mitral leaflets were superimposed and appeared to criss-cross each other at onset of systole (figure 9).

In seven patients M mode and two-dimensional echocardiograms were obtained during provocative maneuvers (i.e., Valsalva maneuver or amyl nitrite inhalation). A distinct increase in the magnitude and duration of SAM of the PML was evident with provocation in four of these seven patients, including two in whom the subaortic gradient had been shown at catheterization to be greater with provocation than under basal conditions. In the other three patients little or no change in SAM of the PML was observed with provocation.

Correlation of echocardiographic and hemodynamic findings. A relationship was apparent between the severity of the basal left ventricular outflow tract gradient and the magnitude and duration of SAM of the PML under basal conditions.[14] In eight of nine patients with a gradient of 20 mm Hg or more at catheterization, SAM of the PML was marked — i.e., the PML came into contact with the ventricular septum during systole; in three of these patients mitral-septal contact was particularly prolonged. The other patient (with a basal subaortic gradient of 20 mm Hg) showed moderate SAM of the PML in which the posterior leaflet approached but did not contact the septum.

In seven other patients the basal subaortic gradient was 0 or 5 mm Hg. SAM of the PML was mild in four of these seven patients, moderate in two, and marked in one.

Postoperative echocardiographic findings. Two patients underwent ventricular septal myotomy-myectomy.[39] Before surgery these patients had obstruction to left ventricular outflow (gradients of 40 and 50 mm Hg)

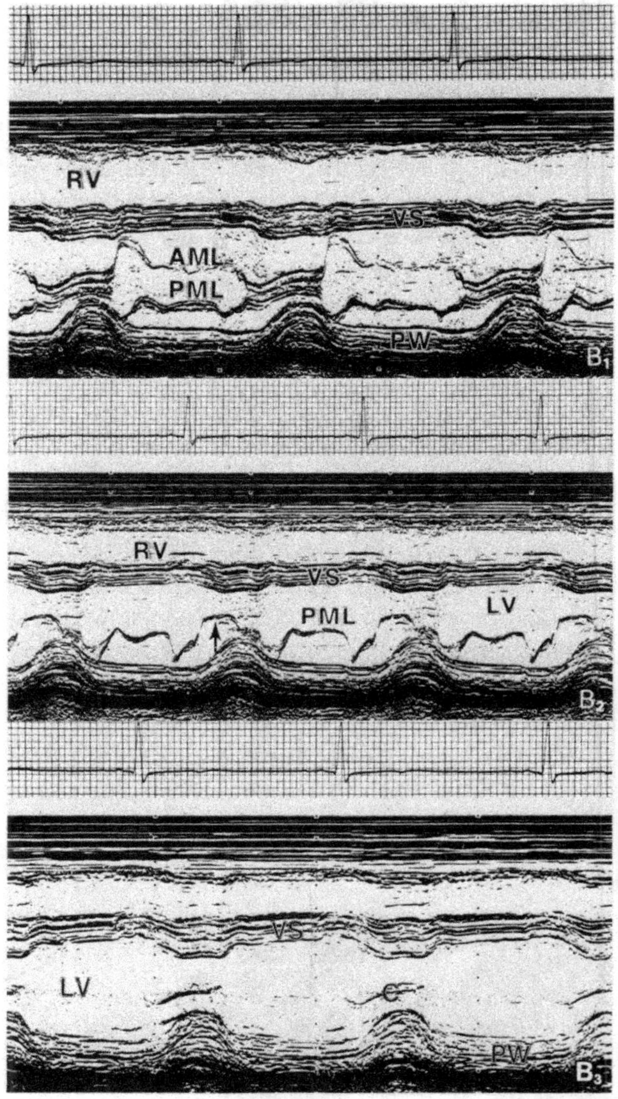

FIGURE 7. M mode echocardiograms obtained at three levels in the left ventricular cavity (along solid lines B_1, B_2, and B_3, shown in figure 6). *B_1*, From cephalad portion of outflow tract in which AML and PML are imaged together. SAM is absent at this level. *B_2*, from a slightly more distal location in the left ventricular cavity, where it is possible to preferentially image the PML; SAM of the PML is evident (arrow). *B_3*, even more distal location in the cavity below level of mitral valve. Ventricular septum (VS) and posterior free wall (PW) are of normal thickness at each of the three levels. C = chordae tendineae; LV = left ventricular cavity; RV = right ventricle.

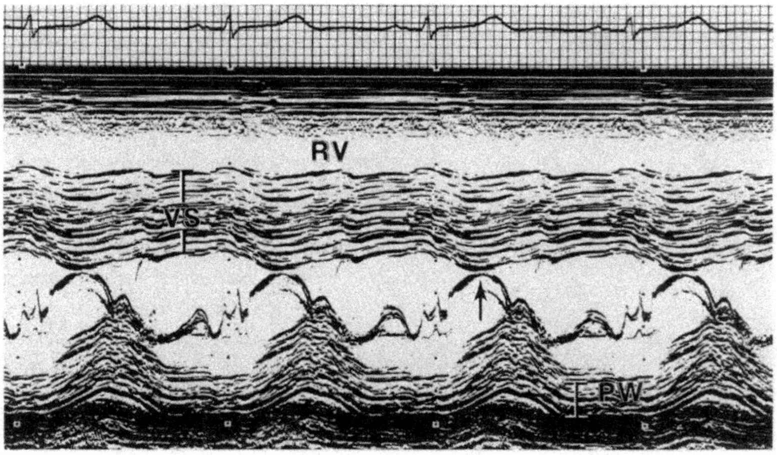

FIGURE 8. M mode echocardiogram obtained from a 25-year-old woman with obstructive hypertrophic cardiomyopathy. Mitral valve anatomy permitted selective imaging of the residual portion of the PML. Note that the posterior leaflet moves abruptly anteriorly at the onset of ventricular systole, makes prolonged contact with the septum in midsystole (arrow), and then moves sharply posteriorly, returning to baseline position before the end of systole. Marked asymmetric hypertrophy of the ventricular septum (VS) relative to the posterior free wall (PW) is also evident. RV = right ventricle.

and their echocardiograms showed that they had marked SAM of the PML (figure 4). After surgery only a trivial degree of SAM of the PML was evident in each patient (figure 10). Cardiac catheterization performed 6 months after surgery in one of these patients showed no subaortic gradient under basal conditions and only a 5 mm Hg gradient with provocation; the other patient refused to undergo a postoperative catheterization.

Ventricular wall thicknesses and distribution of left ventricular hypertrophy. On M mode echocardiograms ventricular septal thicknesses ranged from 9 to 32 mm (mean 22) and posterior free wall thicknesses ranged from 9 to 21 mm (mean 13). Ventricular septal to free wall thickness ratios were 0.9 to 2.7 (mean 1.7).

Two-dimensional echocardiography demonstrated a wide variety of patterns of left ventricular hypertrophy. Most patients had hypertrophy of both the anterior and posterior portions of ventricular septum, but not of the left ventricular free wall (eight patients), or of both the septum and anterolateral free wall (seven patients). Three other patients had hypertrophy confined to only the anterior segment of septum and the remaining three patients showed involvement of portions of the left ventricle other than the basal anterior ventricular septum[40]; of the latter three patients, two had hypertrophy of the posterior septum and/or anterolateral free wall and one had septal and free wall hypertrophy confined to the apical one-half of the left ventricle (i.e., apical hypertrophic cardiomyopathy)[41, 42] (figure 6, *B*).

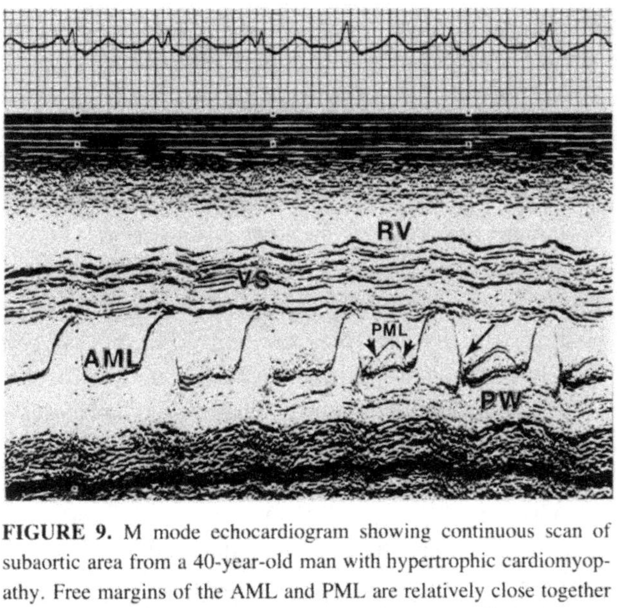

FIGURE 9. M mode echocardiogram showing continuous scan of subaortic area from a 40-year-old man with hypertrophic cardiomyopathy. Free margins of the AML and PML are relatively close together and appear superimposed in this one-dimensional view. To the left, at a location just below the aortic valve, the AML is imaged alone and its contour can be followed continuously from left to right until the PML (arrows) is seen. The posterior leaflet appears to "cross" the anterior leaflet at the onset of systole and then moves anteriorly and closely approaches the ventricular septum (VS) in midsystole. PW = posterior wall; RV = right ventricle.

Other echocardiographic findings. In each of the 21 patients, the left ventricular internal dimension at end-diastole was either normal or reduced (range 30 to 49 mm, mean 38). Left atrial dimension was increased in 12 patients (45 to 60 mm) and normal in nine (30 to 38 mm). Premature systolic closure of the aortic valve was identified in 11 patients, absent in five, and could not be reliably assessed in five. No consistent relationship was evident between the magnitude and degree of SAM of the PML (or basal subaortic gradient) and either left atrial dimension or the presence of premature aortic valve closure.

Left ventricular outflow tract cross-sectional areas ranged from 1.7 to 8.8 cm^2 (mean 4.3) and each was reduced compared with normal. The small outflow tract area appeared to be largely due to the abnormal anterior position of the mitral valve in the left ventricular cavity (mitral valve position index of 0.3 to 1.1, mean 0.8; normal < 0.3).

Angiographic findings. Left ventricular angiocardiograms were available for analysis in five patients, in-

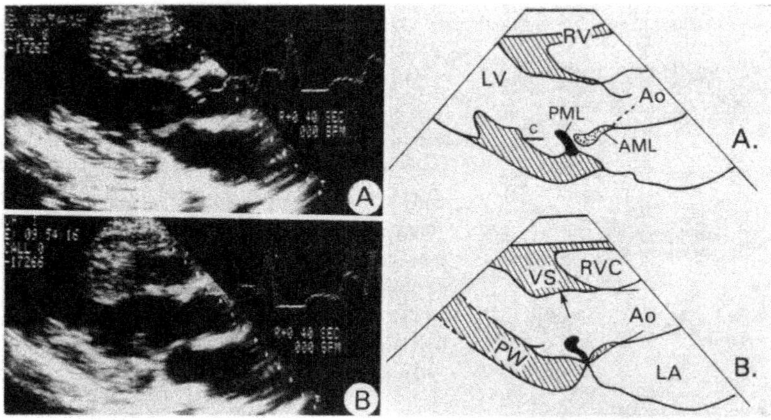

FIGURE 10. Two-dimensional echocardiographic stop-frame images obtained during late diastole *(A)* and early systole *(B)* in the parasternal long-axis view. From the same patient shown in figure 4, but 6 months after ventricular septal myotomy-myectomy. Site of operative excision of muscle from the anterior basal septum is evident (arrow) and the transverse dimension of the left ventricular outflow tract has been greatly increased by the operation. Magnitude of SAM of the PML shown here is trivial and much reduced when compared with the preoperative echocardiogram (compare with figure 4). Ao = aorta; C = chordae tendineae; LA = left atrium; LV = left ventricle; PW = posterior wall; RV = right ventricular wall; RVC = right ventricular cavity.

cluding four with marked and one with moderate SAM of the PML on the two-dimensional echocardiogram. SAM of the mitral valve was identified in each of the three patients in whom an angiogram was obtained in the left anterior oblique projection. Mitral regurgitation (of a mild degree) was present in only one patient.

Morphologic observations. Of the nine patients studied morphologically, three had SAM of the PML that was evident on their two-dimensional echocardiograms. In each of these three patients the middle segment of the PML appeared elongated (in the cephalad-caudad axis) compared with the anterolateral and posteromedial segments[38] (figure 11). The elongated segment measured 19, 21, and 24 mm from anulus attachment to leaflet tip (mean for normal valves, 13 mm[38]), was approximately the same length or slightly longer than the anterior leaflet, and comprised about one-third the total width of the posterior leaflet (figure 11, *a* and *b*). In addition, when the mitral valve leaflets were positioned in their correct anatomic relationships, the elongated segment of the posterior leaflet extended distal to the caudal margins of the anterior leaflet and also was capable of passing through the V-shaped gap created by the normal pattern of chordal insertions onto the anterior leaflet (figure 11, *c* and *d*.)[43]

In each of the three patients, the elongated middle segment was thickened and had an indentation located parallel to the mitral anulus about two-thirds the distance from the anulus to the leaflet tip (figure 11, *b*); this groove appeared to correspond to the point of impact of the anterior leaflet tip on the posterior leaflet body during systole. Each of the remaining six patients had neither SAM of the PML nor an elongated segment of PML extending distal to the anterior leaflet.

Discussion

In this study we describe a newly recognized echocardiographic pattern of mitral valve motion in patients with hypertrophic cardiomyopathy in which the PML shows SAM. Furthermore, this SAM of the PML appears to occur not infrequently in patients with hypertrophic cardiomyopathy. In our consecutively studied series of patients with this disease and mitral SAM, about 10% showed SAM that was due to the posterior leaflet alone. The magnitude and duration of SAM of the PML varied considerably among our patients; in the majority, however, SAM was marked and was associated with left ventricular outflow tract systolic pressure gradients.

Some divergence of opinion exists among investigators regarding the precise mechanism by which subaortic gradients are produced in patients with obstructive hypertrophic cardiomyopathy. Most observers have concluded that the free edges of the mitral leaflets are primarily involved in this process and that obstruction to left ventricular outflow occurs at the site at which the AML contacts the ventricular septal endocardium.[8-25] The PML also may appear to move anteriorly in synchrony with the AML, but does not itself contact the septum because of its posterior position.

In contrast, the type of mitral valve SAM described in this report differs distinctly from that previously described in hypertrophic cardiomyopathy[8-25] (figure 12). In our patients, it was the PML that moved anteriorly in systole. Furthermore, each patient had a reduction in the cross-sectional area of the left ventricular outflow tract.[37] Hence, it appears that the mechanism by which SAM of the PML occurs may be similar to that previously postulated[44] for other patterns of mitral SAM. For example, the residual portion of the posterior leaflet may be pulled anteriorly toward the ventricular septum by the high-velocity jet of blood ejected through an anatomically narrow left ventricular outflow tract (i.e., a Venturi effect).[44]

In our experience, SAM of the PML is most reliably demonstrated with two-dimensional echocardiogra-

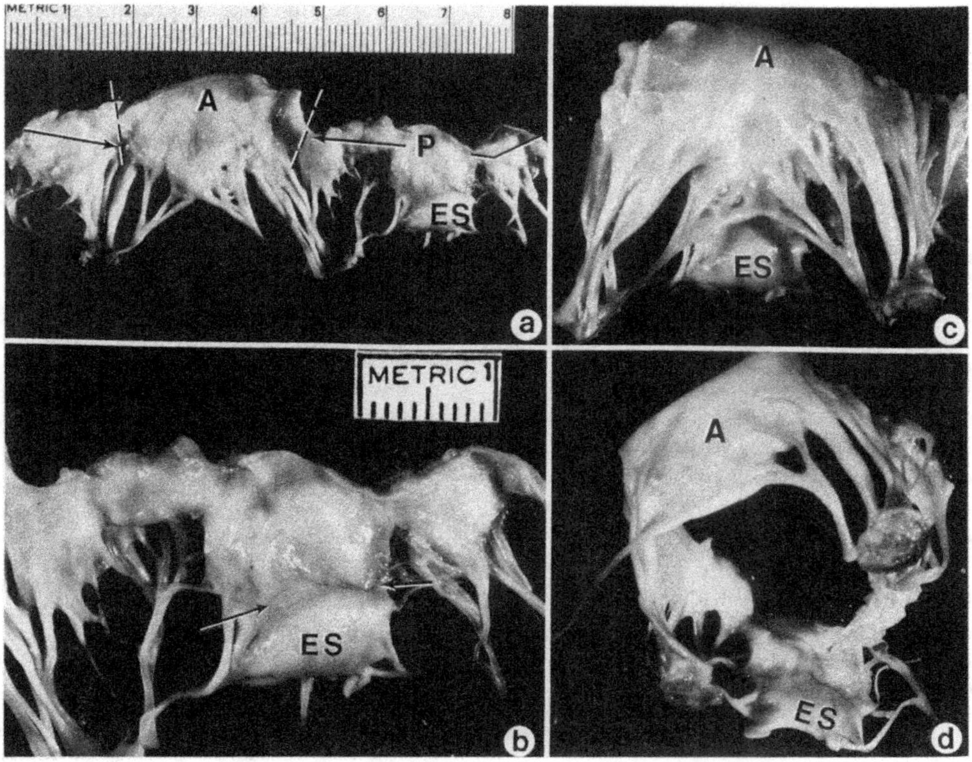

FIGURE 11. Mitral valve removed at operation from a 60-year-old woman with hypertrophic cardiomyopathy and mitral regurgitation. SAM of the PML was evident on two-dimensional echocardiogram. *a*, Valve is displayed so that AML (A) is between the broken lines and portions of PML (P) are seen to either side of the anterior leaflet. Elongated middle scallop (ES) of the PML is situated to the right of the anterior leaflet and between the two other normally appearing segments of posterior leaflet. *b*, Higher magnification view of the elongated middle scallop (ES) of posterior leaflet. The indentation or groove (arrows) located two-thirds of the distance from mitral anulus attachment to leaflet tip and parallel to the plane of the anulus was probably produced by impact of the distal margins of anterior leaflet on the middle scallop during systole. Four nonthickened chordae tendineae insert onto the elongated scallop of posterior leaflet. *c*, Intact valve demonstrating anatomic relationships that permit the elongated scallop of the posterior leaflet to contact the septum during systole; the posterior leaflet is able to pass distal to the anterior leaflet through the V-shaped space created by the normal pattern and location of chordal insertions onto the anterior leaflet. *d*, Intact valve viewed from below, showing relation of elongated scallop of posterior leaflet (ES) to the anterior leaflet.

phy, particularly in the tomographic planes obtained from the left ventricular apex. However, it was also possible to identify SAM of the PML with M mode echocardiography. This was accomplished most convincingly in those patients in whom the posterior leaflet appeared displaced toward the apex relative to the anterior leaflet. In such patients this abnormality in mitral valve anatomy permitted the M mode beam to be directed preferentially through the posterior leaflet. SAM of the PML in such patients may be missed by conventional M mode echocardiography if care is not taken to scan the entire cephalad-caudad extent of the mitral valve apparatus. In other patients the distal margins of the two mitral leaflets were closer together, and an M mode echocardiographic image was created in which the posterior leaflet (showing SAM) and the anterior leaflet (showing no SAM) appeared to be superimposed (figures 9 and 12).

Our gross anatomic data, obtained in a separate group of patients with hypertrophic cardiomyopathy in whom the mitral valve could be studied morphologically, offer a probable structural basis for the occurrence of SAM of the PML. Each of these patients, who had SAM of the PML on their two-dimensional echocardiograms, showed a marked segmental elongation that was confined to the middle scallop of the PML; in addition, the free caudal margins of this abnormal portion of the posterior leaflet appeared to extend distal to the caudal margins of the AML. These findings have led us to postulate that it is the elongated scallop of the posterior leaflet that contacts the septum during systole by passing beyond the free edge of the anterior leaflet into the space created by the divergent sites of attachment of the chordae tendineae onto the anterior leaflet.[43] Hence, our patients with SAM of the PML probably represent a subset of the overall population with hypertrophic cardiomyopathy in whom this particular malformation of the mitral valve occurs.

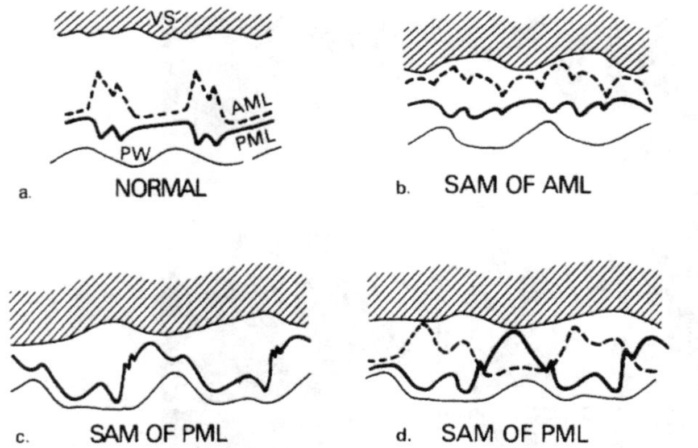

FIGURE 12. Schematic drawings of M mode echocardiograms showing normal pattern of mitral valve motion, compared with patterns of SAM identified in patients with hypertrophic cardiomyopathy. In each panel, the AML is depicted as a broken line and PML as a solid line. *a,* Normal subject without SAM. *b,* SAM of the type commonly observed in patients with hypertrophic cardiomyopathy. Both mitral leaflets move anteriorly in systole, but the anterior leaflet actually contacts the septum. *c,* SAM of the PML in a patient with hypertrophic cardiomyopathy, with the ultrasound beam directed preferentially through the posterior leaflet. *d,* SAM of PML in a patient with cardiomyopathy with ultrasound beam directed through both the AML (showing no SAM) and PML (showing SAM).

Segmental posterior leaflet elongation similar to that observed in our patients with hypertrophic cardiomyopathy appears to be uncommon in normal subjects or in patients with other heart diseases. In each of the 50 mitral valves examined by Ranganathan et al.,[38] the length of the AML exceeded that of all three scallops of the posterior leaflet. Furthermore, a gross anatomic analysis of PML morphology in 29 patients with coronary heart disease and mitral regurgitation identified no instance of a mitral leaflet abnormality similar to that which occurred in our patients with hypertrophic cardiomyopathy.[45] In 60 patients with mitral valve prolapse who also demonstrated mitral regurgitation and one or more elongated scallops of the PML, either the AML was also elongated or an elongated middle scallop of the PML was present but buckled cephalad, which produced a relatively short mitral anulus-to-leaflet tip distance.[45] Furthermore, the transverse groove in the middle scallop of the PML produced by the impact of the anterior leaflet that we observed in some study patients with hypertrophic cardiomyopathy was not present in patients with mitral valve prolapse.

Recognition of SAM of the PML may alter the operative approach in selected patients with hypertrophic cardiomyopathy and subaortic obstruction. This is a particularly pertinent consideration for those patients in whom the caudal margins of the posterior leaflet contact the ventricular septum at a point far distal to the anterior leaflet. In such patients, the longitudinal extent of the myotomy-myectomy[39] should incorporate that region of septal muscle adjacent to the caudal margins of PML in order to include the site of subaortic obstruction.

We thank Ms. Bonnie Wesley and Mr. Robert Fatula for their expert technical assistance, and M. M. Moore for her photography of the gross anatomy.

References

1. Wigle ED, Heimbecker RO, Gunton RW: Idiopathic ventricular septal hypertrophy causing muscular subaortic stenosis. Circulation **26:** 325, 1962
2. Braunwald E, Lambrew CT, Rockoff SD, Ross J, Morrow AG: Idiopathic hypertrophic subaortic stenosis. I. A description of the disease based upon an analysis of 64 patients. Circulation **30** (suppl IV): IV-3, 1964
3. Cohen J, Effat H, Goodwin JF, Oakley CM, Steiner RE: Hypertrophic obstructive cardiomyopathy. Br Heart J **26:** 16, 1964
4. Goodwin JF, Oakley CM: The cardiomyopathies. Br Heart J **34:** 545, 1972
5. Epstein SE, Henry WL, Clark CE, Roberts WC, Maron BJ, Ferrans VJ, Redwood DR, Morrow AG: Asymmetric septal hypertrophy. Ann Intern Med **81:** 650, 1974
6. Dinsmore RE, Sanders CA, Harthorne JW: Mitral regurgitation in idiopathic hypertrophic subaortic stenosis. N Engl J Med **275:** 1225, 1966
7. Simon AL, Ross J, Gault JH: Angiographic anatomy of the left ventricle and mitral valve in idiopathic hypertrophic subaortic stenosis. Circulation **36:** 852, 1967
8. Popp RL, Harrison DC: Ultrasound in the diagnosis and evaluation of therapy in idiopathic hypertrophic subaortic stenosis. Circulation **40:** 905, 1969
9. Shah PM, Gramiak R, Kramer DH: Ultrasound location of left ventricular outflow obstruction in hypertrophic obstructive cardiomyopathy. Circulation **40:** 3, 1969
10. Pridie RB, Oakley CM: Mechanism of mitral regurgitation in hypertrophic obstructive cardiomyopathy. Br Heart J **32:** 203, 1970
11. Shah PM, Gramiak R, Adelman AG, Wigle ED: Role of echocardiography in diagnostic and hemodynamic assessment of hypertrophic subaortic stenosis. Circulation **44:** 891, 1971
12. Shah PM, Gramiak R, Adelman AG, Wigle ED: Echocardiographic assessment of the effects of surgery and propranolol on the dynamics of outflow obstruction in hypertrophic subaortic stenosis. Circulation **45:** 516, 1972
13. King JF, DeMaria AN, Reis RL, Bolton MR, Dunn MI, Mason DT: Echocardiographic assessment of idiopathic hypertrophic subaortic stenosis. Chest **6:** 723, 1973
14. Henry WL, Clark CE, Glancy DL, Epstein SE: Echocardiographic measurement of the left ventricular outflow gradient in idiopathic hypertrophic subaortic stenosis. N Engl J Med **288:** 989, 1973
15. Bolton MR, King JF, Polumbo RA, Mason D, Pugh DM, Reis RL, Dunn MI: The effects of operation on the echocardiographic features of idiopathic hypertrophic subaortic stenosis. Circulation **50:** 897, 1974
16. Reis RL, Bolton MR, King JF, Pugh DM, Dunn MI, Mason DT: Anterior-posterior displacement of papillary muscles producing obstruction and mitral regurgitation in idiopathic hypertrophic subaortic stenosis: Operative relief by posterior-superior realignment of papillary muscles following ventricular-septal myectomy. Circulation **50** (suppl II): II-181, 1974
17. Feizi O, Emanuel R: Echocardiographic spectrum of hypertrophic cardiomyopathy. Br Heart J **37:** 1286, 1975
18. Henry WL, Clark CE, Griffith JM, Epstein SE: Mechanism of left ventricular outflow obstruction in patients with obstructive asymmetric septal hypertrophy (idiopathic hypertrophic subaortic stenosis). Am J Cardiol **35:** 337, 1975
19. Maron BJ, Gottdiener JS, Roberts WC, Henry WL, Savage DD, Epstein SE: Left ventricular outflow tract obstruction due to systolic anterior motion of the anterior mitral leaflet in patients with concentric left ventricular hypertrophy. Circulation **57:** 527, 1978
20. Martin RP, Rakowski H, French J, Popp RL: Idiopathic hypertro-

phic subaortic stenosis viewed by wide-angle, phased-array echocardiography. Circulation **59:** 1206, 1979

21. Tajik AJ, Seward JB, Hagler DJ: Detailed analysis of hypertrophic obstructive cardiomyopathy by wide-angle two-dimensional sector echocardiography. Am J Cardiol **43:** 348, 1979 (abst)
22. Maron BJ, Epstein SE: Hypertrophic cardiomyopathy: Recent observations regarding the specificity of three hallmarks of the disease: asymmetric septal hypertrophy, septal disorganization and systolic anterior motion of the anterior mitral leaflet. Am J Cardiol **45:** 141, 1980
23. Shah PM, Taylor RD, Wong M: Abnormal mitral valve coaptation in hypertrophic obstructive cardiomyopathy: Proposed role in systolic anterior motion of mitral valve. Am J Cardiol **48:** 258, 1981
24. Gilbert BW, Pollick C, Adelman AG, Wigle ED: Hypertrophic cardiomyopathy: Subclassification by M-mode echocardiography. Am J Cardiol **45:** 861, 1980
25. Pollick C, Morgan CD, Gilbert BW, Rakowski H, Wigle ED: Muscular subaortic stenosis: The temporal relationship between systolic anterior motion of the anterior mitral leaflet and the pressure gradient. Circulation **66:** 1087, 1982
26. Ballester M, Donaldson R, Richards A, McDonald L: Systolic anterior motion of mitral valve: Chordal or valve participation and its relevance to presence and degree of obstruction in patients with hypertrophic cardiomyopathy. Br Heart J **47:** 196, 1982 (abst)
27. Rodger JC: Motion of mitral apparatus in hypertrophic cardiomyopathy with obstruction. Br Heart J **38:** 732, 1976
28. Gehrke J, Goodwin JF: The significance of systolic anterior motion (SAM) on the mitral echo pattern in hypertrophic cardiomyopathy. Clin Cardiol **1:** 152, 1978
29. Henry WL, Clark CE, Epstein SE: Asymmetric septal hypertrophy (ASH): echocardiographic identification of the pathognomonic anatomic abnormality of IHSS. Circulation **47:** 225, 1973
30. Maron BJ, Epstein SE: Hypertrophic cardiomyopathy: a discussion of nomenclature. Am J Cardiol **43:** 1241, 1979
31. Maron BJ, Gottdiener JS, Epstein SE: Patterns and significance of distribution of left ventricular hypertrophy in hypertrophic cardiomyopathy. A wide-angle two-dimensional echocardiographic study of 125 patients. Am J Cardiol **48:** 418, 1981
32. Sahn DJ, DeMaria A, Kisslo J, Weyman A: Recommendations regarding quantitation in M-mode echocardiography: Results of a survey of echocardiographic measurements. Circulation **58:** 1072, 1978
33. Henry WL, Gardin JM, Ware JH: Echocardiographic measurements in normal subjects from infancy to old age. Circulation **62:** 1054, 1980
34. Tajik AJ, Seward JB, Hagler DJ, Mair DD, Lie JT: Two-dimensional real-time ultrasonic imaging of the heart and great vessels. Mayo Clin Proc **53:** 271, 1978
35. Kisslo J, Von Ramm OT, Thurstone FL: Cardiac imaging using phased array ultrasound system. II. Clinical technique and application. Circulation **53:** 262, 1976
36. Silverman NH, Schiller NB: Apex echocardiography. A two-dimensional technique for evaluating congenital heart disease. Circulation **57:** 503, 1978
37. Spirito P, Maron BJ: Significance of left ventricular outflow tract cross-sectional area in hypertrophic cardiomyopathy: a two-dimensional echocardiographic assessment. Circulation (in press)
38. Ranganathan N, Lam JHC, Wigle ED, Silver MD: Morphology of the human mitral valve: II. The valve leaflets. Circulation **41:** 459, 1970
39. Morrow AG: Hypertrophic subaortic stenosis: operative methods utilized to relieve left ventricular outflow obstruction. J Thorac Cardiovasc Surg **76:** 423, 1978
40. Maron BJ, Gottdiener JS, Bonow RO, Epstein SE: Hypertrophic cardiomyopathy with unusual locations of left ventricular hypertrophy undetectable by M-mode echocardiography: Identification by wide-angle, two-dimensional echocardiography. Circulation **63:** 409, 1981
41. Maron BJ, Bonow RO, Seshagiri TN, Roberts WC, Epstein SE: Hypertrophic cardiomyopathy with ventricular septal hypertrophy localized to the apical region of the left ventricle (apical hypertrophic cardiomyopathy). Am J Cardiol **49:** 1838, 1982
42. Yamaguchi H, Ishimura T, Nishiyama S, Nagasaki F, Nakanishi S, Takatsu F, Nishijo T, Umeda T, Machii K: Hypertrophic nonobstructive cardiomyopathy with giant negative T waves (apical hypertrophy): Ventriculographic and echocardiographic features in 30 patients. Am J Cardiol **44:** 401, 1979
43. Lam JHC, Ranganathan N, Wigle ED, Silver MD: Morphology of the human mitral valve: I. Chordae tendineae: A new classification. Circulation **41:** 449, 1970
44. Wigle ED, Adelman AG, Silver MD: Pathophysiological considerations in muscular subaortic stenosis. *In* Wolstenholme GEW, O'Connor M, editors: Hypertrophic obstructive cardiomyopathy. 1971, London, J and A Churchill, p 63
45. Waller BF, Morrow AG, McIntosh CL, Maron BJ, Del Negro AA, Kent KM, Wallace RB, Roberts WC: Etiology of clinically isolated, severe, chronic, pure mitral regurgitation: analysis of 97 patients over 30 years of age with mitral valve replacement. Am Heart J **104:** 276, 1982

Hypertrophic cardiomyopathy: a common cause of sudden death in the young competitive athlete

B. J. MARON, S. E. EPSTEIN AND W. C. ROBERTS

Cardiology and Pathology Branches, National Heart, Lung and Blood Institute, National Institutes of Health, Bethesda, Maryland, USA

KEY WORDS: Sudden death, hypertrophic cardiomyopathy, athletes.

The causes of sudden, unexpected death in highly-conditioned competitive athletes are summarized. In the vast majority of young athletes (less than 35 years of age) sudden death is due to underlying structural cardiovascular disease. Hypertrophic cardiomyopathy appears to be the most common cause of such deaths and may account for about one-half of the sudden deaths in a youthful athletic population. Cardiovascular abnormalities that appear to be less frequent important causes of sudden death include anomalous origin of the left coronary artery from the anterior sinus of Valsalva, ruptured aorta (due to cystic medial necrosis), idiopathic concentric left ventricular hypertrophy and coronary artery atherosclerosis. Other diseases which are probably particularly uncommon causes of sudden death in the young athlete include mitral valve prolapse, aortic valvular stenosis, acute myocarditis, QT interval prolongation syndromes, hypoplasia of the coronary arteries or sarcoidosis. Cardiovascular disease in young athletes is usually unsuspected during life. In only about 25% of those competitive athletes who die suddenly is underlying disease identified prior to participation and rarely is the correct clinical diagnosis made. In contrast, when sudden death occurs in older competitive or recreational athletes (over 35 years of age) it is usually due to coronary artery disease.

Introduction

Highly conditioned competitive athletes epitomize the most healthy segment of our society. For this reason, the occurrence of sudden death in an athlete is particularly shocking and tragic (Fig. 1). For many years our ignorance of the causes of such catastrophes was clothed in esoteric sounding phrases, such as 'sudden death syndrome', which merely masked the fact that the precise causes were unknown. Recently, careful morphologic studies performed after death have revealed that a variety of congenital or acquired structural malformations of the heart and great vessels are responsible for the vast majority of sudden deaths that occur in athletes[1-5].

Sudden death in young competitive athletes

Considering the large numbers of participants in competitive and recreational athletic programs, sudden death must be considered an uncommon event. Nonetheless, an occasional young athlete, apparently in excellent health, will die suddenly and unexpectedly. Such individuals participate in a variety of sports and most commonly are high school athletes at the time of death[1]; however, some young athletes reach the collegiate or even professional level[6] of competition before dying suddenly. Usually such catastrophes occur during or just following exertion on the athletic field and death is thereby often attributed to intense physical activity. However, while extreme effort may be the precipitating cause of death in some instances, the underlying cause of death in the vast majority of young athletes (less than 35 years of age) is a congenital cardiovascular malformation[1]. Despite the fact that these malformations are present at birth, individuals so afflicted can compete for many years without either being aware of their cardiovascular disease or experiencing significant symptoms.

In our series of 29 young competitive athletes who died suddenly, 28 had a structural cardiovascular disease identified at necropsy that represented an unequivocal or probable cause of death[1] (Fig. 2).

Address correspondence to: Dr Barry J. Maron, Senior Investigator, National Heart, Lung, and Blood Institute, Building 10, Room 7B-15, Bethesda, Maryland 20205, USA.

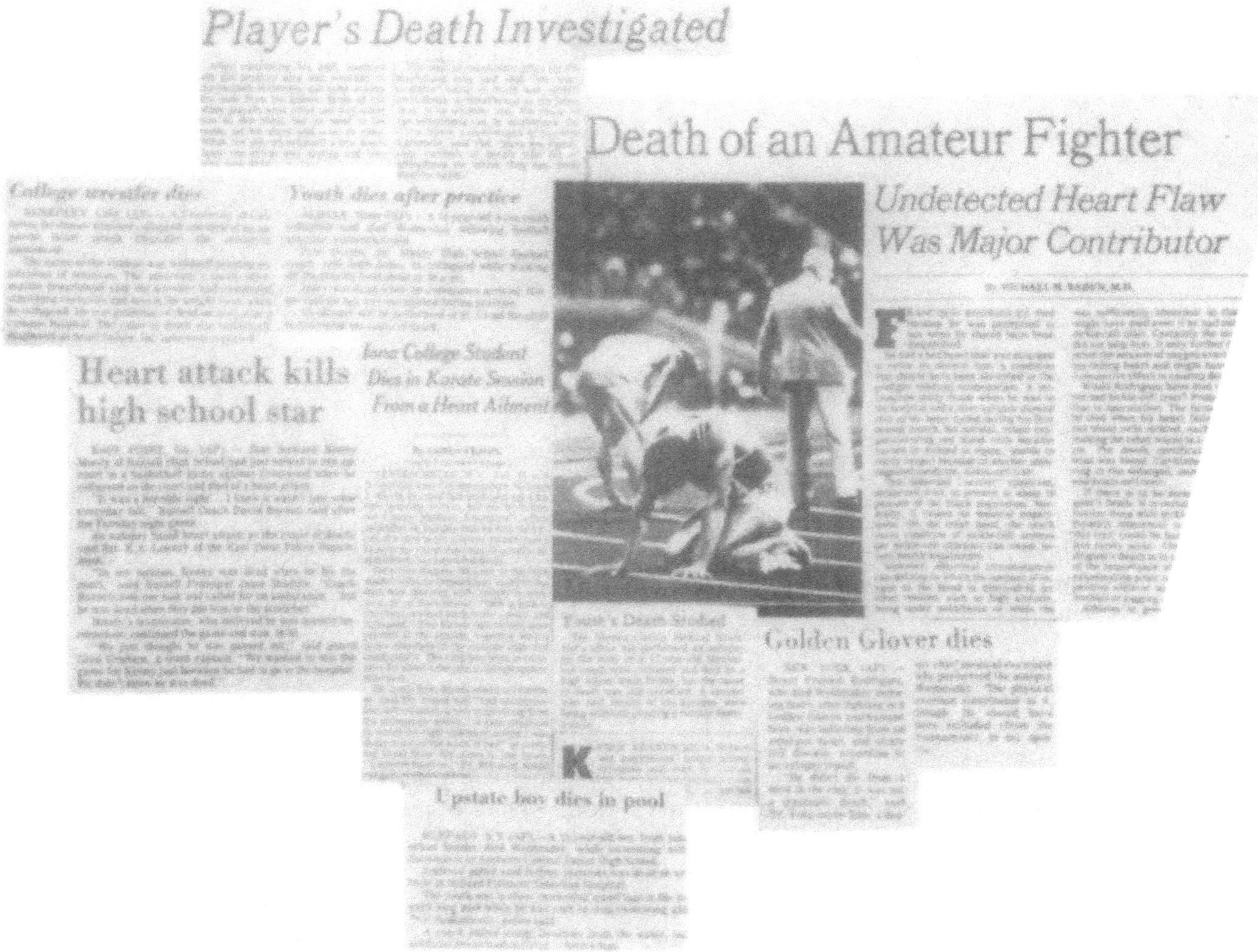

Player's Death Investigated
Death of an Amateur Fighter
Undetected Heart Flaw Was Major Contributor
College wrestler dies
Youth dies after practice
Heart attack kills high school star
Iona College Student Dies in Karate Session From a Heart Ailment
Youth's Death Studied
Golden Glover dies
Upstate boy dies in pool

Figure 1 Media reports of sudden unexpected deaths in young athletes.

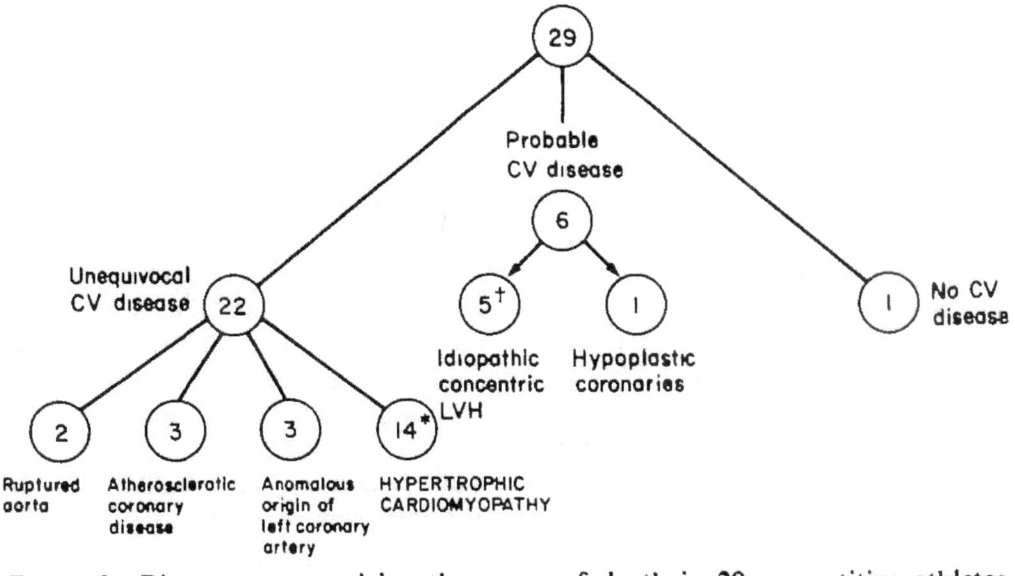

Figure 2 Diagram summarizing the cause of death in 29 competitive athletes. CV = cardiovascular; LVH = left ventricular hypertrophy. The asterisk indicates that this group includes one patient who also had anomalous origin of the left coronary artery from the anterior sinus of Valsalva. The daggar indicates that this group includes one patient who had gross and histologic findings at necropsy consistent with mitral valve prolapse, as well as a family history of that condition.

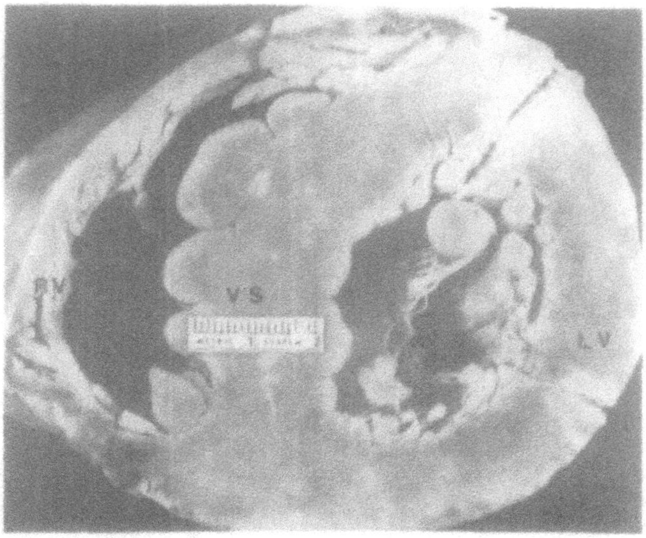

Figure 3 Heart of a 13 year old male (gridiron) football player showing disproportionate thickening of the ventricular septum (VS) with respect to the posterior left ventricular free wall (LV). RV = right ventricular wall.

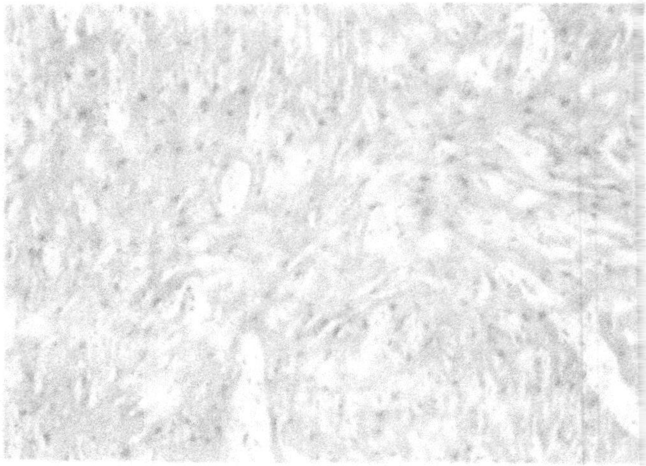

Figure 4 Histologic section of ventricular septal myocardium from a 14 year old competitive athlete showing marked cellular disorganization in which adjacent cardiac muscle cells are oriented at oblique and perpendicular angles to each other.

HYPERTROPHIC CARDIOMYOPATHY

The most common cause of such deaths appears to be ***hypertrophic cardiomyopathy***, which occurred in almost one-half (i.e. 14) of the athletes. Each of these individuals had a hypertrophied, nondilated left ventricle in the absence of another cardiac or systemic disease that could produce left ventricular hypertrophy (such as valvular, hypertensive or coronary heart disease or infiltrative cardiomyopathy)[7]. The heart weights in these 14 patients were all increased over normal[8] and ranged from 360 to 630 g (mean 475 g). None of the 12 patients with blood pressure recordings during life had systemic hypertension. Mild to moderate right ventricular dilatation also was present in five patients.

For the diagnosis of hypertrophic cardiomyopathy to be made, each of these patients also had to have at least one of the following characteristic features of the disease: (1) asymmetric septal hypertrophy (ventricular septal-to-left ventricular free wall thickness ratio $\geqslant 1 \cdot 3$; range $1 \cdot 3$ to $2 \cdot 2$)[9–11] Fig. 3); (2) marked disorganization of cardiac muscle cells in the ventricular septum[12] involving at least 5% of the relevant areas of the tissue section[13] (Fig. 4); (3) clinical or echocardiographic evidence of hypertrophic cardiomyopathy in one or more closely related family members[14]. Seven of the 14 athletes with hypertrophic cardiomyopathy had both asymmetric septal hypertrophy and marked ventricular septal cellular disorganization and three had asymmetric septal hypertrophy without disorganization. The other four athletes had concentric (symmetric) left ventricular hypertrophy (septal – free wall ratio $<1 \cdot 3$), including two with marked septal disorganization and two without disorganization; each of these four athletes had at least one first degree relative with echocardiographic evidence of hypertrophic cardiomyopathy.

Abnormal intramural coronary arteries (two or more per tissue section) were identified in the ventricular septal myocardium of four athletes with hypertrophic cardiomyopathy. The abnormal arteries had thickened walls (due to intimal proliferation or medial hypertrophy or both) and narrowed lumens. One other athlete with hypertrophic cardiomyopathy showed marked narrowing (due to fibromuscular hyperplasia) of only the arteries to the sinoatrial and atrioventricular nodes. The conduction system was otherwise normal, as were the other intramural coronary arteries.

In athletes with hypertrophic cardiomyopathy the scalar electrocardiogram may show a wide variety of alterations (Figs 5 and 6). It should also be emphasized that electrocardiographic abnormalities in patients with hypertrophic cardiomyopathy may be similar to those in some athletes *without* underlying heart disease. However, in such athletes without cardiac disease the inversion of T waves may normalize with exercise or isoproterenol infusions[15] or spontaneously after deconditioning (Fig. 7).

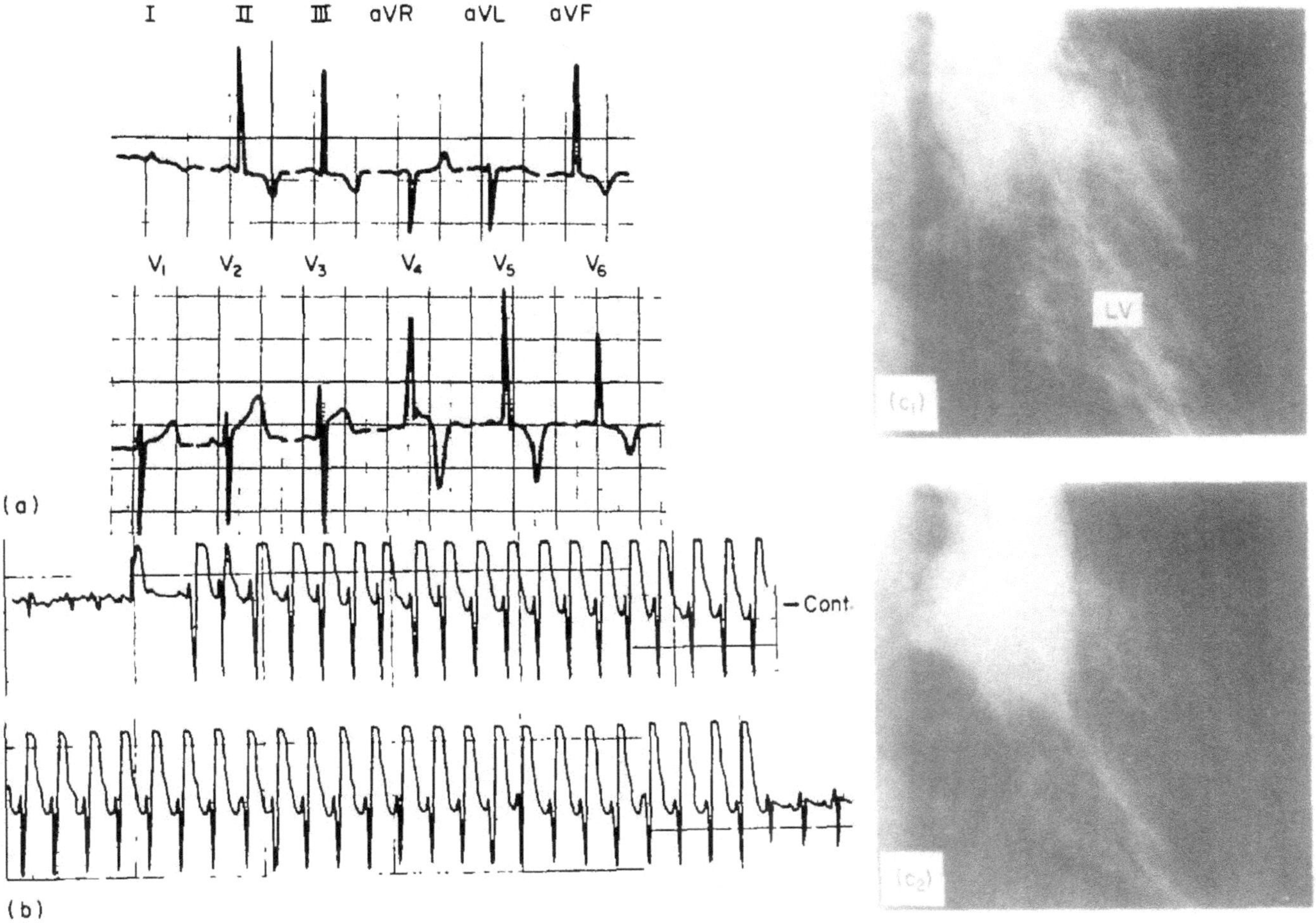

Figure 5 Electrocardiographic and angiographic findings in a 23 year old collegiate basketball player in whom the diagnosis of hypertrophic cardiomyopathy was made at necropsy. (a) Standard 12-lead ECG obtained under basal conditions showing marked symmetric T-wave inversion (as much as 15 mm in depth), as well as left ventricular hypertrophy. (b) Four-second period of ventricular tachycardia that occurred in the second minute of recovery and terminated spontaneously, after a routine treadmill exercise test. (c) Left ventricular angiocardiogram in diastole (c_1) and end-systole (c_2) showing marked cavity obliteration (ejection fraction of 95%). LV = left ventricular cavity. Electrocardiograms have been retraced for clarity.

IDIOPATHIC CONCENTRIC LEFT VENTRICULAR HYPERTROPHY

Five other athletes had a hypertrophied, nondilated left ventricle unassociated with a cardiac lesion that could produce left ventricular hypertrophy; heart weights were increased[8] and ranged from 420 to 530 g. However, each of these five hearts differed from the other hearts in this study considered to represent hypertrophic cardiomyopathy by virtue of *the absence of* (1) asymmetric septal hypertrophy (septal – free wall thickness ratios ranged from 1·0 to 1·2). (2) disorganization of cardiac muscle cells in the ventricular septum; and (3) clinical or echocardiographic evidence of hypertrophic cardiomyopathy in closely related family members.

The five patients with idiopathic concentric left ventricular hypertrophy ranged in age from 16 to 28 years. Two were normotensive, but blood pressure recordings had not been obtained during life in the other three. In three of these five patients the degree of left ventricular wall thickening was particularly marked (i.e. 20 to 23 mm) (Fig. 8); in the other two patients, left ventricular wall thickening was only moderate (thicknesses of 16 and 18 mm). The magnitude of ventricular wall thickening that these athletes with idiopathic concentric left ventricular hypertrophy exhibited at necropsy greatly exceeded that which could be considered to be 'physiologic' ventricular hypertrophy produced by athletic conditioning[16,17].

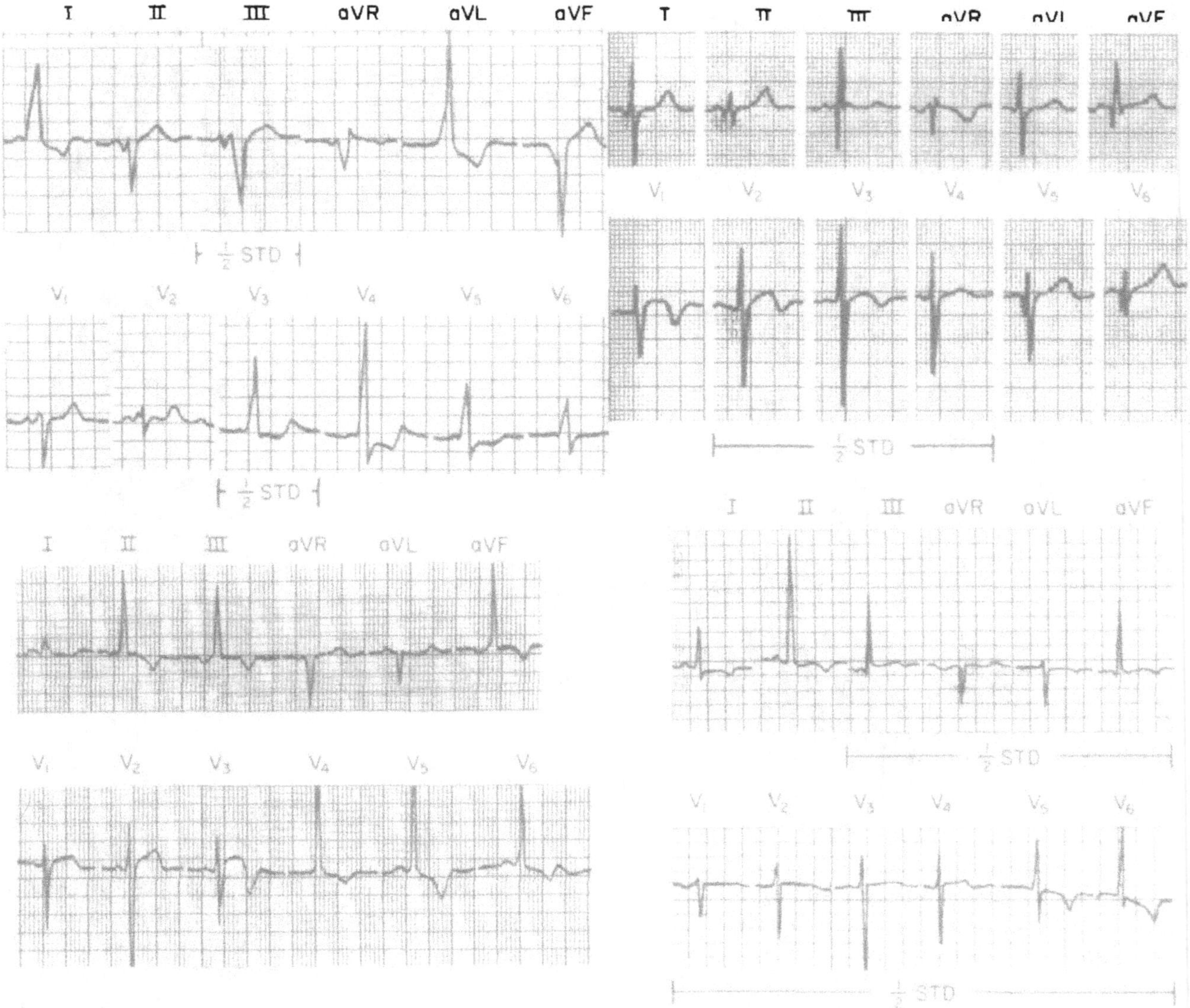

Figure 6 Electocardiograms showing the spectrum of abnormalities in four athletes with hypertrophic cardiomyopathy. Although cardiovascular disease was suspected in each athlete during life, a clinical diagnosis other than hypertrophic cardiomyopathy had been made in each. *Top left:* From a 14 year old wrestler showing Wolff–Parkinson–White pattern, left axis deviation, diffuse T-wave inversion in leads I, AVL and V_4 to V_6 and probable left ventricular hypertrophy. *Top right:* From a 17 year old (gridiron) football player showing deep Q waves in leads III, AVF, V_5 and V_6 and probable left ventricular hypertrophy. *Bottom left:* From a 20 year old basketball player showing deep symmetric T-wave inversion in leads II, III, AVF and V_5 to V_6 and left ventricular hypertrophy. Compare with a similar ECG from another athlete shown in Fig 5(a). *Bottom right:* From a 30 year old tennis player showing left ventricular hypertrophy with 'strain' and diffuse T-wave flattening and inversion. Electrocardiograms have been retraced for clarity.

Two of the five athletes with idiopathic concentric left ventricular hypertrophy had an associated cardiac malformation. In one, a 17 year old football (soccer) player with a 530 g heart, the anterior and posterior mitral leflets had an appearance consistent with relatively mild mitral valve prolapse; the leaflets were thickened, gelatinous and mildly scalloped with excessive mucoid material observed histologically. This patient's mother and two siblings had clinical or echocardiographic evidence of mitral valve prolapse.

In addition, this athlete (and one other with concentric ventricular wall thickening) had an anatomic alteration of the artery to the atrioventricular node, consisting of severe fibromuscular hyperplasia of the vessel wall and marked narrowing of the lumen (Fig. 9). One additional athlete with concentric ventricular wall thickening had a similar alteration in the artery to the atrioventricular node.

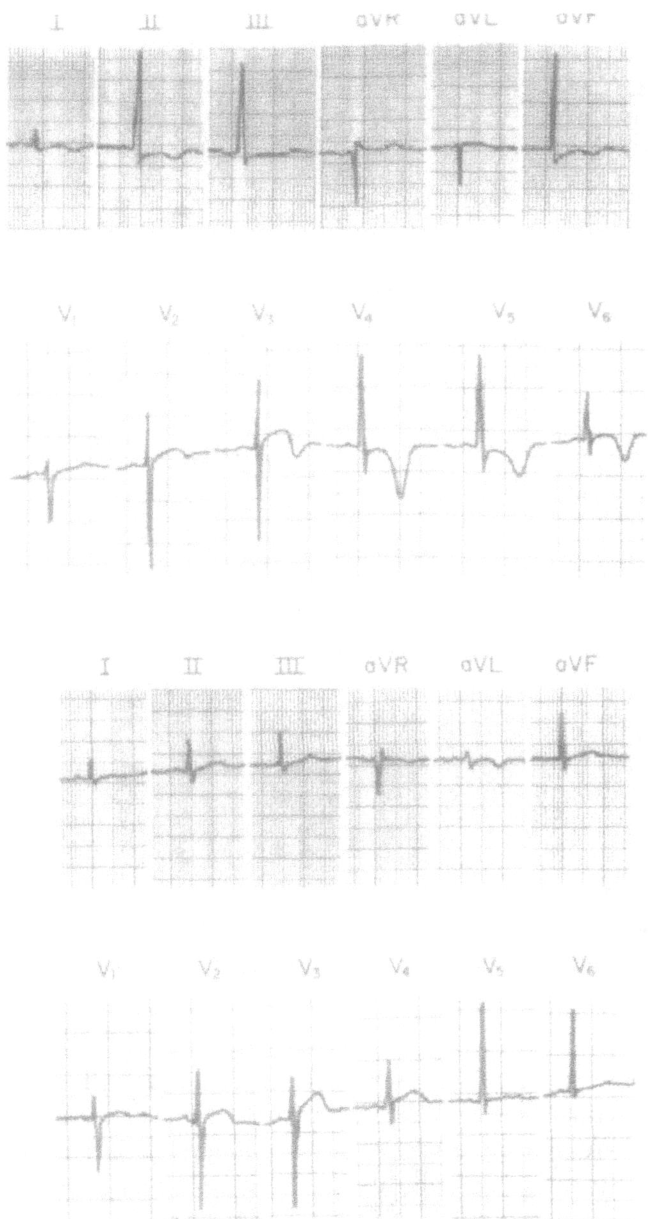

Figure 7 Serial 12-lead ECGs obtained under basal conditions from a professional basketball player *without* underlying structural cardiac disease. *Top:* Recorded during a period of time when the athlete was highly conditioned and competing actively in his sport, showing diffuse T-wave inversion that is particularly deep and symmetric in leads V_4 to V_6. *Bottom:* Three years later at a time when the athlete was no longer training and was deconditioned; the deep T-wave inversions have virtually normalized, although T-waves in V_5 and V_6 still appear flattened.

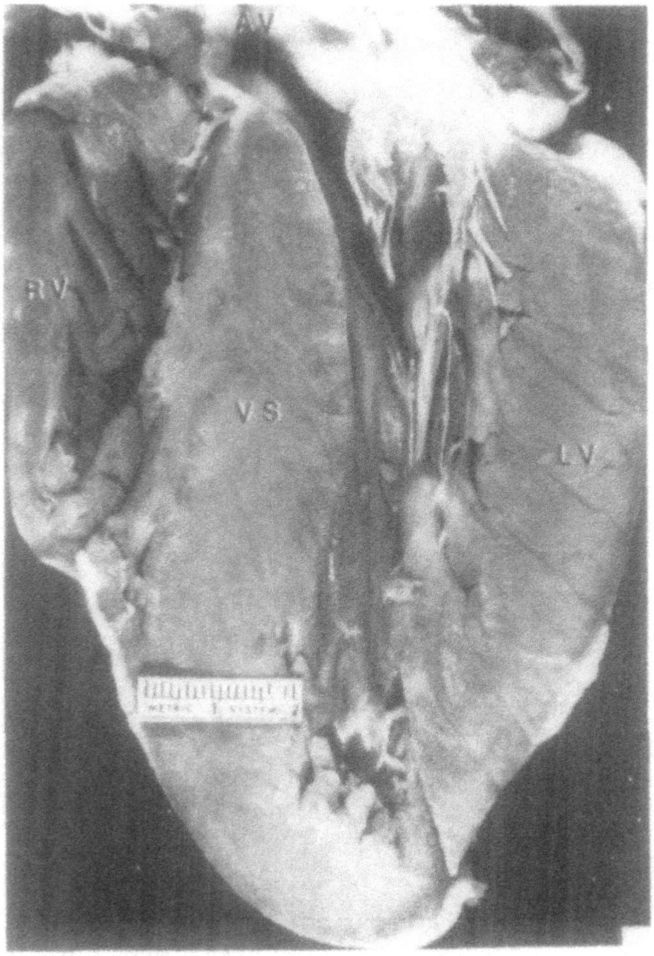

Figure 8 Heart of a 17 year old soccer player showing marked idiopathic concentric (symmetric) thickening of the ventricular septum (VS) and left ventricular free wall (LV). RV = right ventricular wall; AV = aortic valve.

The conducting tissue was otherwise normal in these latter two athletes. None of the athletes who had idiopathic concentric left ventricular hypertrophy, with or without alterations in the artery to the atrioventricular node, had abnormal intramural coronary arteries in other areas of ventricular myocardium.

CONGENITAL CORONARY ARTERY ANOMALY

In addition to hypertrophic cardiomyopathy and idiopathic concentric left ventricular hypertrophy, a number of other malformations of the heart and blood vessels may be responsible for sudden death in young athletes. In three of our 29 patients, the left main coronary artery had an anomalous origin from the right (anterior) sinus of Valsalva and followed a course through the narrow area between aorta and main pulmonary artery[18]. Because the left coronary artery followed this unusual course, it necessarily assumed a very acute angle at its origin from the aorta (Fig. 10). It is believed that this acute bend is potentially hazardous. During severe exertion (when the great vessels expand), the left main coronary artery probably becomes severely kinked and

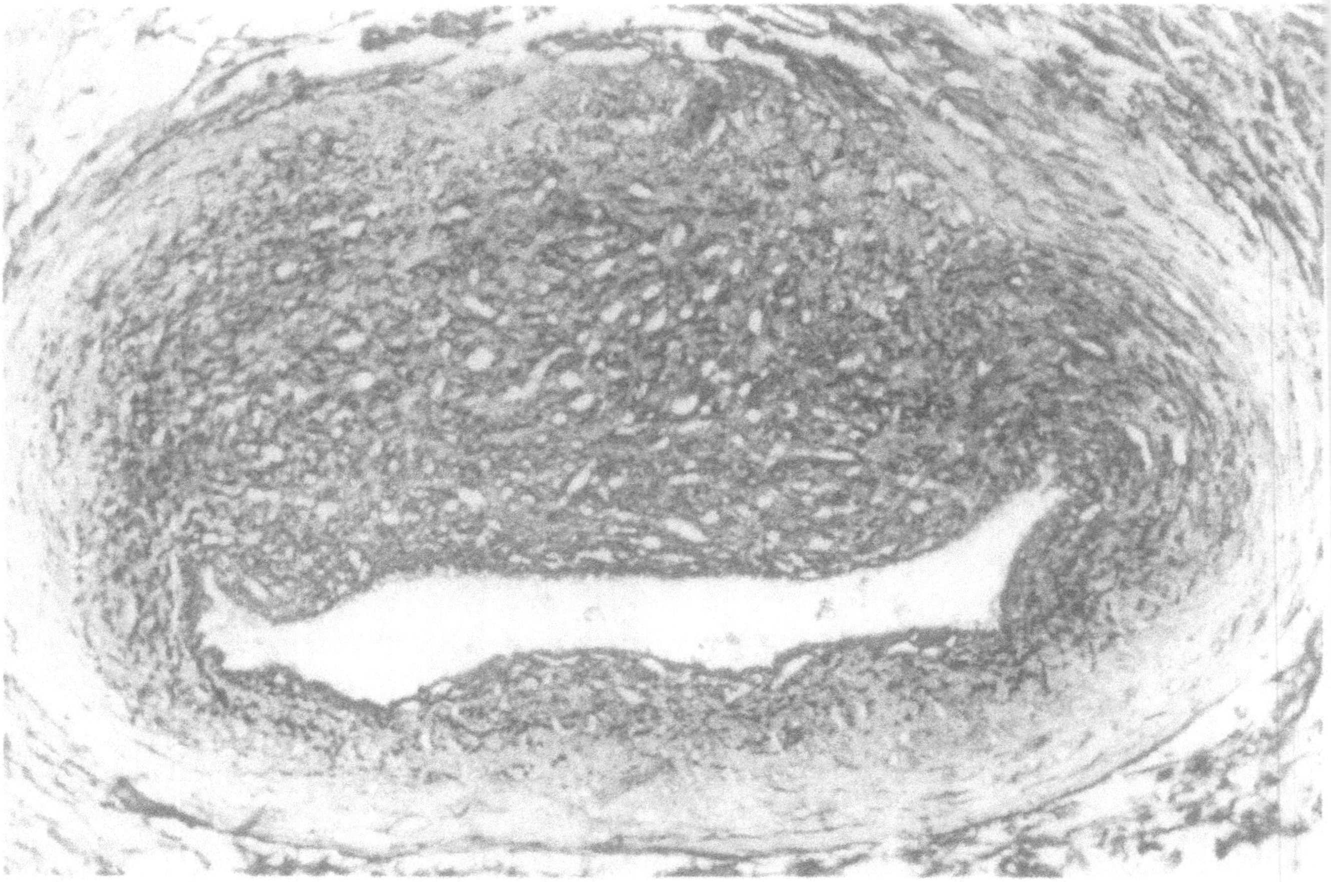

Figure 9 Small artery to atrioventricular node of a 17 year old basketball player with idiopathic concentric left ventricular hypertrophy. The lumen is markedly narrowed due to extreme thickening of the arterial wall.

narrowed, thereby critically diminishing the myocardial oxygen supply.

AORTIC RUPTURE

Two athletes died suddenly from rupture of the aorta. These individuals showed decreased numbers of elastic fibers in their aortic media that produced intrinsic weakening of the wall ('cystic medial necrosis'). Eventually, when such a malformed aorta is unable to maintain the normal blood pressure to which it is exposed, aortic rupture occurs. It is of interest that individuals with cystic medial necrosis may successfully participate in competitive athletics for many years without experiencing a catastrophic event. Many such individuals also have the systemic manifestations of the Marfan syndrome, potentially facilitating their clinical recognition (such as one of our two patients).

CORONARY HEART DISEASE

Three athletes had acquired abnormalities of the coronary arteries. These patients were 24, 26 and 28 years of age. Two of the three athletes showed severe atherosclerosis in each of the three major extramural coronary arteries (>75% cross-sectional area luminal narrowing by atherosclerotic plaque), including one with total occlusion of the right coronary artery by an antemortem thrombus and hemorrhage into atherosclerotic plaque. This athlete, a 28 year old professional (gridiron) football player had a large myocardial infarct that was about 2 months old in the posterior left ventricular wall at necropsy[6]. The remaining patient had 50% cross-sectional area luminal narrowing of the left anterior descending coronary artery by atherosclerotic plaque and no, or only minimal, atherosclerosis in each of the other two major extramural coronary arteries. However, the left anterior descending artery was completely occluded by an antemortem thrombus 2 cm from the bifurcation of the left main coronary artery.

OTHER CAUSES OF SUDDEN DEATH

Certain other cardiovascular diseases such as isolated mitral valve prolapse, QT interval prolongation syndromes, acute myocarditis and

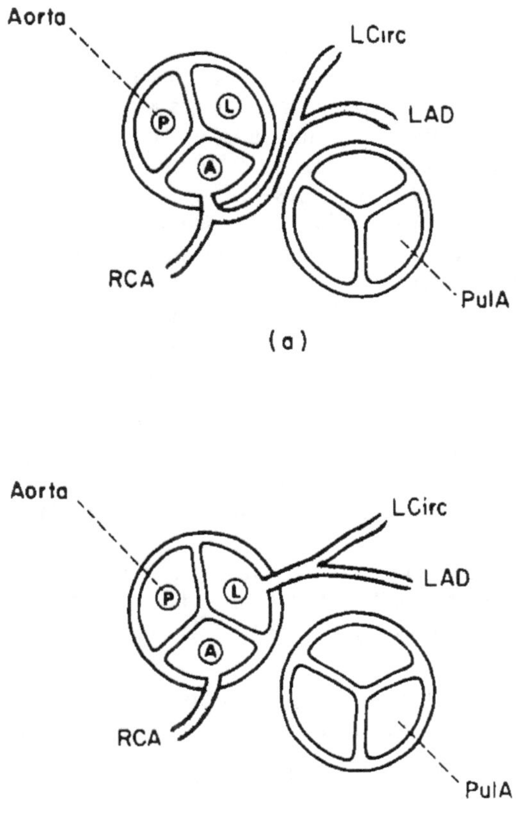

Figure 10 (a) A diagrammatic representation of anomalous origin of the left coronary artery from the right (anterior) sinus of Valsalva. Note the acute leftward and posterior course of the left coronary artery between the aorta and pulmonary artery. (b) Normal origins of the left coronary artery from the left sinus of Valsalva and of the right coronary artery from the right sinus of Valsalva are shown for comparison. A = anterior (right) coronary sinus; L = left coronary sinus; P = posterior (noncoronary) sinus; LAD = left anterior descending coronary artery; LCirc = left circumflex coronary artery; PulA = pulmonary artery; RCA = right coronary artery.

sarcoidosis did not appear in our study group and are probably less common causes of sudden death in athletes. Also, lesions such as aortic valvular stenosis would likely have been identified early in life because of a loud heart murmur or some other obvious physical finding, thereby leading to eventual disqualification from competitive athletics. Infrequently, sudden death may occur in young athletes who have no demonstrable organic heart disease. In such individuals (one of the 29 athletes in our series) death was probably due to a primary arrhythmia that arose independently of any structural abnormality of the heart that could be demonstrated at autopsy.

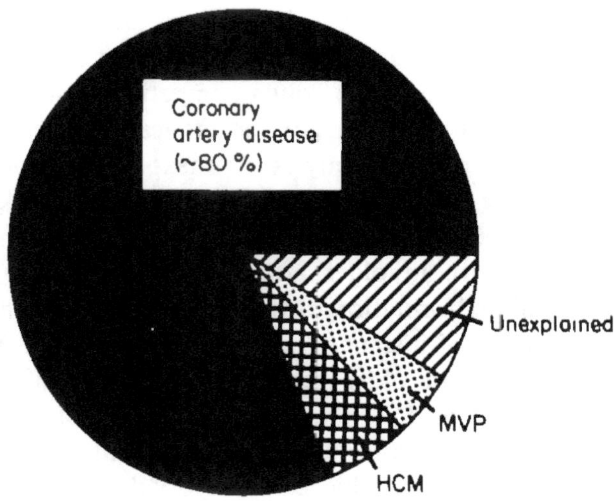

Figure 11 Causes of sudden death in older athletes (>35 years of age). Approximate prevalence figures have been summarized from the literature[2–4]. MVP = mitral valve prolapse; HCM = hypertrophic cardiomyopathy.

CLINICAL FEATURES

Cardiovascular disease had been suspected by an examining physician during life in only seven of our 29 athletes (two with transient symptoms and five who were asymptomatic). In the latter five asymptomatic athletes, the suspicion of cardiovascular disease initially arose because of a heart murmur in two, a family history of heart disease in one, identification of ventricular tachycardia on an exercise electrocardiogram (Fig. 5(b)) performed as a routine part of a preparticipation athletic examination in one, and during evaluation for the Marfan syndrome in one.

In six of the seven athletes in whom cardiovascular disease was suspected during life, hypertrophic cardiomyopathy was confirmed at necropsy. However, in only one of those six athletes was the correct diagnosis of hypertrophic cardiomyopathy made clinically. In the other five athletes, the diagnosis during life was 'normal athletic heart' in three, ventricular septal defect in one and Wolff–Parkinson–White syndrome in one. Each of these five athletes with hypertrophic cardiomyopathy had a distinctly abnormal electrocardiogram, and one also had an abnormal left ventricular angiocardiogram (Fig. 5(c)).

SUDDEN DEATH IN OLDER ATHLETES

Increasing numbers of middle-aged or older individuals (over the age of 35) are now participating in competitive and recreational sports, as well as in physical conditioning programs (such as jogging and swimming). Superior physical fitness at any age, however, does not assure protection against exercise-related death. Similar to young competitive athletes, older athletes may harbor occult cardiovascular disease and die suddenly and unexpectedy while participating in athletic activities. However, unlike the more youthful athletes previously discussed, the cause of death in older athletes is usually not a congenital malformation of the heart. Rather, in the vast majority of instances (about 80%) the cause of sudden death in older athletes is coronary heart disease[2-4] (Fig. 11). The remaining 20% of such deaths are due to other diseases such as mitral valve prolapse or hypertrophic cardiomyopathy[19] or, in some instances, no cause of death is established at necropsy.

References

(1) Maron BJ, Roberts WC, McAllister HA, Rosing DR, Epstein SE. Sudden death in young athletes. Circulation 1980; 62: 218–29.

(2) Thompson PD, Stern MP, Williams P, Duncan K, Haskell WL, Wood PD. Death during jogging or running. A study of 18 cases. JAMA 1979: 242: 1265–7.

(3) Waller BF, Roberts WC. Sudden death while running in conditioned runners aged 40 years or over. Am J Cardiol 1980; 45: 1292–300.

(4) Virmani R, Rabinowitz M, McAllister HA. Non-traumatic death in joggers: a series of 30 autopsy patients. Am J Med 1982: 72: 874–82.

(5) James TN, Froggatt P, Marshall TK. Sudden death in young athletes. Ann Int Med 1967: 67: 1013–21.

(6) Roberts WC, Maron BJ. Sudden death while playing professional football. Am Heart J 1981: 102: 1061–3.

(7) Maron BJ, Epstein SE. Hypertrophic cardiomyopathy: a discussion of nomenclature. Am J Cardiol 1979: 43: 1242–4.

(8) Gould SE. Pathology of the heart and blood vessels, 3rd edn. Springfield, Illinois: Charles C. Thomas, 1968: 1139.

(9) Henry WL, Clark CE, Epstein SE. Asymmetric septal hypertrophy (ASH): echocardiographic identification of the pathognomonic anatomic abnormality of IHSS. Circulation 1973: 47: 225–33.

(10) Menges H, Brandenburg RO, Brown AL. The clinical, hemodynamic, and pathologic diagnosis of muscular subvalvular aortic stenosis. Circulation 1961: 24: 1126–36.

(11) Roberts WC. Valvular, subvalvular and supravalvular aortic stenosis: Morphologic features. Cardiovasc Clin 1973: 5: 104–26.

(12) Teare D. Asymmetrical hypertrophy of the heart in young patients. Br Heart J 1958: 20: 1–8.

(13) Maron BJ, Roberts WC. Quantitative analysis of cardiac muscle cell disorganization in the ventricular septum of patients with hypertrophic cardiomyopathy. Circulation 1979; 59: 689–706.

(14) Maron BJ, Nichols PF, Pickle LW, Muvihill JJ. Patterns of inheritance in hypertrophic cardiomyopathy. Circulation (submitted for publication).

(15) Zeppilli P, Pirrami MM, Sassara M, Fenici R. T wave abnormalities in top-ranking athletes: effects of isoproterenol, atropine and physical exercise. Am Heart J 1980: 100: 213–22.

(16) Morganroth J, Maron BJ, Henry WL, Epstein SE. Comparative left ventricular dimensions in trained athletes. Ann Int Med 1975: 82: 521–4.

(17) Roeske WR, O'Rourke RA, Klein A, Leopold G, Karliner JS. Noninvasive evaluation of ventricular hypertrophy in professional athletes. Circulation 1976: 53: 286–292.

(18) Cheitlin MD, De Castro CM, McAllister HA. Sudden death as a complication of anomalous left coronary origin from the anterior sinus of Valsalva. A not-so-minor congenital anomaly. Circulation 1974: 50 780–7.

(19) Noakes TD, Rose AG, Opie LH. Hypertrophic cardiomyopathy associated with sudden death during marathon racing. Br Heart J 1979: 41: 624–7.

Loogen If I understood you correctly, you say this giant T inversion is sometimes found in men or in athletes without any other signs of heart disease. What is your policy in such cases? Do you allow them to go on in sports or do you recommend thorough investigation – that means invasive methods, determination of lactate production, and all the other steps that are necessary to exclude a cardiac disease?

Maron I think, certainly, an ECG like that demands a careful non-evasive workup to exclude particularly hypertrophic cardiomyopathy and mitral valve prolapse. But having not found those conditions, I think that I would construe the ECG to be innocent, even though it is dramatic in appearance. This is particularly true since we know that such ECGs may be dynamic, in the sense that they may revert to normal (often with deconditioning). I have been to Italy to speak to a group of sport medicine physicians who had followed athletes in Italy for the 20 years or so since the last Olympiad was in Rome. They have accumulated, over the years, hundreds of ECGs in athletes. These ECGs looked just like the one I showed and they are not indicative of organic heart disease. For the most part such athletes continue to compete and lead active lives.

Kuhn We have observed four people who were not champions, but very active athletes. In three of them we found pronounced asymmetric septal hypertrophy with giant negatives T-waves. In three athletes left ventricular angiography was performed. There was the complete picture of hypertrophic non-obstructive cardiomyopathy. We are not quite sure how to interpret this. I should like to speculate that there is a latent hypertrophic process in these patients and that physical activity during sports would lead to the manifestation of the disease.

Secondly, I should like to comment on the case you showed with an abnormally thickened septum of more than 20 mm. There is an echocardiographic study performed by Dr Ross of Cologne. He found that septal thickness of more than 15 mm hardly ever occurs in athletes. So from this evidence I would suggest that this is really a hypertrophy in the sense of hypertrophic cardiomyopathy. I have now tried to review the literature on autopsy findings in athletes, mainly in Germany, and what I found several times was a diagnosis of myocarditis or chronic myocarditis. However, at autopsy the hearts were described as having a weight of more than 700 or even 800 g, and a septal thickness of more than 20 mm. So I have no doubt that these patients did not have myocarditis, because there were only a few or no inflammatory cells present.

Maron Certainly, in the United States, medical examiners who are responsible for providing a diagnosis after death have a tendency to over-diagnose myocarditis. The awareness of a condition such as hypertrophic cardiomyopathy has not been great, and a few round cells in the myocardium has often been enough to ensure the diagnosis of myocarditis. Myocarditis certainly can be a cause of sudden death in young people, but I think that much of the older literature is a little misleading.

Das I think Dr Maron has addressed the question I had in mind, particularly concerning the four patients, for whom no ideology was discerned. I wonder whether detailed investigation for active myocarditis was carried out in the four patients that you mentioned.

Maron You mean the four patients with idiopathic left ventricular hypertrophy? Certainly, these are not instances of myocarditis. The amount of hypertrophy seen in those four patients would have to be considered pathologic from what we know about a living population of athletes studied echocardiographically. It's pathologic because the athlete is dead and because it represents an obvious increase in left ventricular mass.

Frank Mine is more of a comment rather than a question. I'd like to congratulate Dr Maron on his restraint with the four patients with symmetrical hypertrophy. I remember discussing this with him at an evening meeting and we came to the conclusion that the only way we're going to understand hypertrophic cardiomyopathy as an entity – if indeed it is an entity – was by exclusion of cases that missed one more of the important characteristics of the condition. So, in the absence of myocardial fibre disarray and in the absence of first-degree relatives demonstrating a positive echo, I think that it is quite proper that we continue to call this group idiopathic left ventricular hypertrophy.

Harmjanz In rather young patients having giant T-waves and left ventricular hypertrophy we observed, on a number of occasions, a slowly arising delay in left ventricular exitation up to left ventricular bundle branch block while the patient underwent cardiac catheterization; this declined in a stepwise manner within about 10 beats. I want to ask whether you had the same experience in your cases?

Maron We don't really have much experience catheterizing this type of patient. This is a retrospective study and most of the limited catheterization data is from other institutions. I really couldn't give you an answer to that.

Massive Cardiac Ventricular Scarring in First-Degree Relatives with Hypertrophic Cardiomyopathy

CAROLE A. WARNES, MB, BS, MRCP
BARRY J. MARON, MD
WILLIAM C. ROBERTS, MD

Although most adults with hypertrophic cardiomyopathy (HC) have at necropsy small scars in the left ventricular (LV) free walls or ventricular septum (VS) or both, extensive scarring of these structures is uncommon.[1] We recently studied at necropsy a father and daughter with HC and both had massively scarred cardiac ventricular walls, a finding not described previously in more than 1 family member.

Pertinent clinical and morphologic features of the father and daughter are summarized in Table I. Symptoms of cardiac dysfunction were present in the father for 8 years and in the daughter for 9 years, but each had a different clinical course: The father had progressive and eventually fatal congestive heart failure; the daughter had mild dyspnea, occasional dizziness and chest pain, and died suddenly. No peak systolic gradient at rest between left ventricle and aorta was present in either father or daughter. The LV cavity was always of normal size in the daughter; in the father it was dilated during his final 2 years. On electrocardiogram (Fig. 1), both father and daughter had absent or small R waves in the precordial leads, QRS duration of ≥0.12 second and T-wave abnormalities. M-mode echocardiograms of both

From the Pathology and Cardiology Branches, National Heart, Lung, and Blood Institute, National Institutes of Health, Bethesda, Maryland 20205.
Manuscript received and accepted August 13, 1984.

TABLE I Clinical and Morphologic Features of Father and Daughter

	Father	Daughter
Clinical symptoms		
Age (yr) at death	33	21
Age (yr) precordial murmur noted	11	3
Age (yr) symptoms began	25	12
Chest pain	+	+
Syncope or dizziness	+	+
Paroxysmal atrial tachycardia	+	0
Congestive heart failure	+	0
Cerebrovascular accident	+	0
Systolic precordial murmur	+	+
Electrocardiogram		
QRS duration (second)	0.13	0.12
Absent or small R waves in precordial leads	+	+
T-wave abnormalities	+	+
Cardiac catheterization		
Pulmonary artery wedge mean (mm Hg)	9*	24†
Pulmonary artery (s/d) (mm Hg)	28/10*	50/25†
Right ventricle (s/d) (mm Hg)	40/6*	50/12†
Left ventricle (s/d) (mm Hg)	115/16*	90/25†
Systemic artery (s/d) (mm Hg)	115/70*	90/60†
LV-SA peak systolic gradient (mm Hg) at rest (provocation)	0 (0)	0 (17)
Necropsy		
Heart weight (g)	580	615
Asymmetric septal hypertrophy	0‡	+
Dilated RV and LV cavities	+	0
Scarred LV and RV walls and ventricular septum	+	+
Endocardial plaque, LV outflow tract	0	—
Thickened mitral valve	0	+
Intracardiac thrombus	+	0
Myocardial fiber disarray	+	+
Abnormal intramural coronary arteries	+	+

* Performed at 27 years. † Performed at age 12 years. ‡ An echocardiogram recorded 14 months earlier showed the ventricular septum to be 18 mm and the LV free wall 13 mm thick.

LV = left ventricular; SA = systemic arterial; RV = right ventricular; s/d = systolic/diastolic; + = present; 0 = absent; — = no information available.

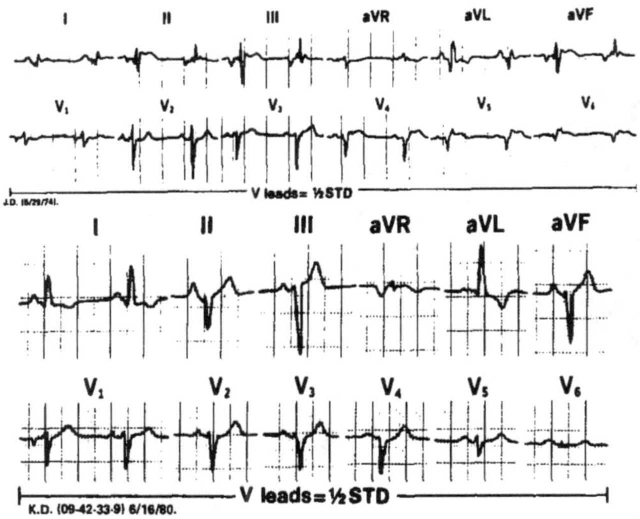

FIGURE 1. Electrocardiogram of the father (**top**) and daughter (**bottom**).

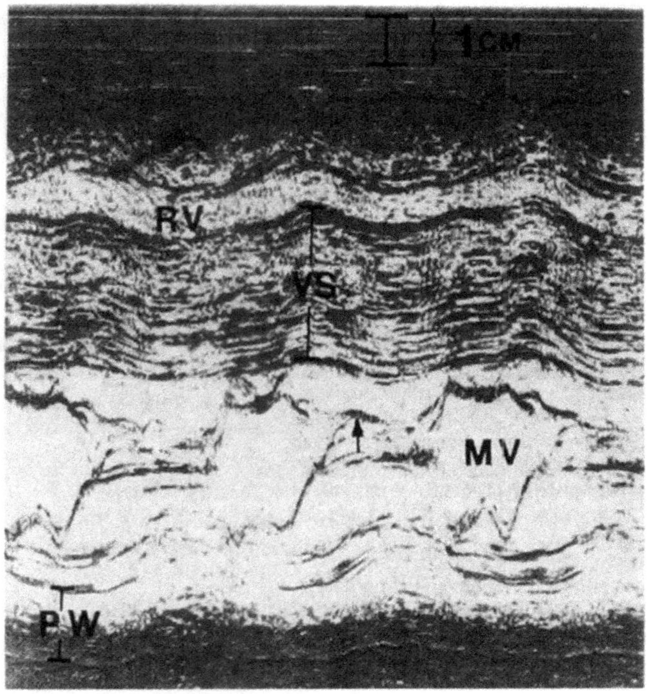

FIGURE 2. Daughter. M-mode echocardiogram recorded when she was 12 years old. The ventricular septum (VS) is much thicker than the posterior left ventricular free wall (PW). The **arrow** points to the anterior mitral leaflet, which has moved slightly toward the septum during systole. MV = mitral valve orifice during diastole; RV = right ventricular cavity.

father and daughter showed asymmetric septal hypertrophy; in the father, 14 months before death, the VS measured up to 18 mm in thickness, and the LV free wall up to 13 mm. Serial echocardiograms in the daughter showed that the septal disproportion lessened; at age 12 years the VS was up to 28 mm thick, and the LV free wall was 11 mm thick (Fig. 2); at age 20 years the VS was 20 mm and the LV free wall was 14 mm.

At necropsy in each, the ventricular walls were massively scarred, the myocardial fibers were disarrayed, the intramural coronary arteries were strikingly abnormal (Fig. 3 and 4) and the extramural coronary arteries were insignificantly narrowed or normal. The scarring in both patients involved the walls of both ventricles and the VS. Within each wall the scarring was both "interstitial" (increased fibrous tissue between most myocardial cells) and "replacement" (collections of myocardial cells were completely replaced with scar) in type.

At least 3 factors need consideration as a cause of the "massive" ventricular wall scarring in the 2 patients: coronary arterial narrowing; excessive myocardial mass in relation to coronary arterial size; and genetic etiology.

Abnormality of the *epicardial* coronary arteries clearly was not the cause of the scarring because these

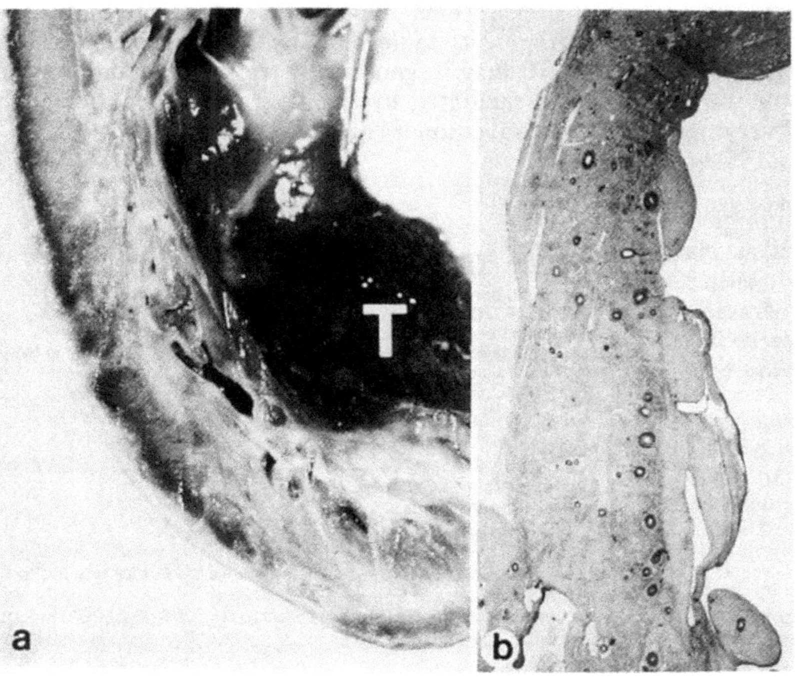

FIGURE 3. Father. **a**, portion of scarred left ventricular free wall with a superimposed mural thrombus (T). **b**, photomicrograph of a section of ventricular septum showing extensive scarring and numerous intramural coronary arteries with thickened walls and narrowed lumens. Elastic van Gieson stain; magnification × 4, reduced 22%.

FIGURE 4. Daughter. a, transverse section of the left ventricle showing a normal-sized cavity and a thickened and extensively scarred wall. b, photomicrograph of ventricular septum showing extensive scarring and numerous thickened and narrowed intramural coronary arteries. Movat stain; magnification × 12. c, photomicrograph of ventricular septum showing extensive scarring and disarray of the myocardial fibers. Hematoxylin-eosin stain; magnification × 20. d, high-power photomicrograph of intramural coronary arteries in the ventricular septum. Both the media and intima of each artery is thickened and the lumens are narrowed. Movat stain; magnification × 68. All panels reduced 38%.

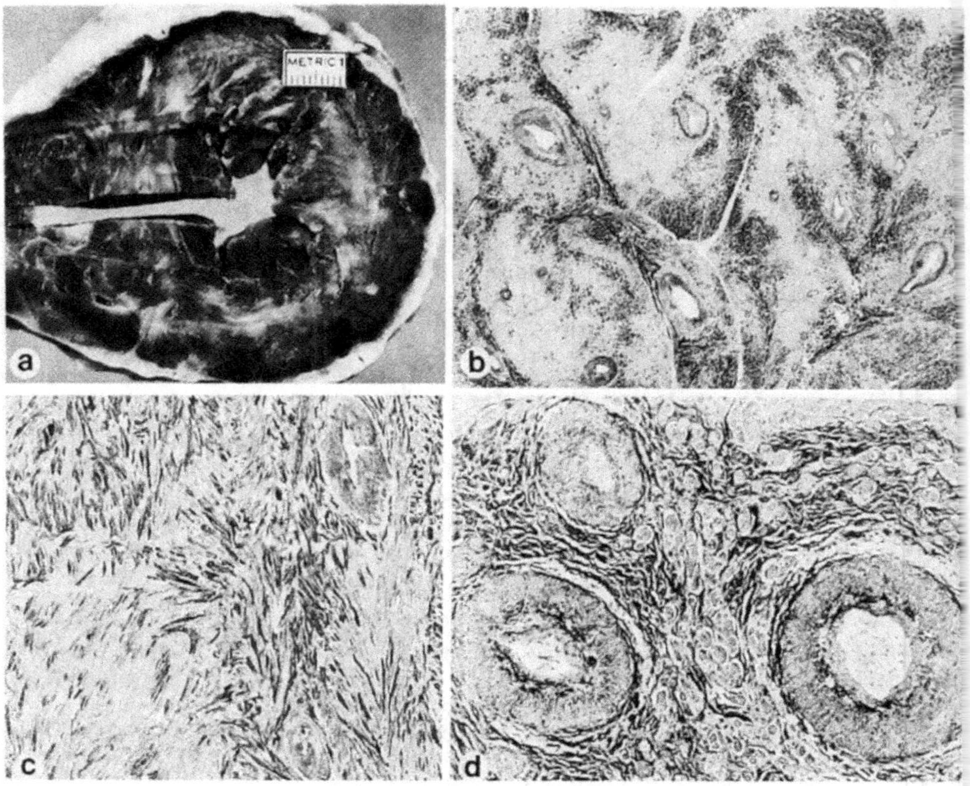

vessels were normal, or nearly so, in both patients. Furthermore, the distribution of the ventricular scarring was different from that seen in patients with atherosclerotic coronary heart disease. There was nothing in the epicardial coronary arteries to suggest the presence of an embolus or in situ thrombus at any time.[2] Coronary spasm has not been demonstrated in patients with HC, and moreover there is no evidence that spasm of these arteries produces ventricular wall fibrosis. Abnormality of the *intramural* coronary arteries, however, may be the explanation for the scarring. In both patients the changes in these arteries were severe; hardly any were normal. The intramural coronary arteries in both patients appeared increased in number, they were clearly increased in size, and their lumens often were severely narrowed. Similar abnormalities of varying degrees of severity have been observed in about 50% of necropsy patients with HC.[3]

Ventricular wall fibrosis resulting from too large a myocardial mass in relation to coronary arterial size is not a reasonable cause for the cardiac scarring in either patient. The heart weight was less than 100% increased in both patients, and it is likely that the myocardial mass must increase nearly 4 times normal for this mechanism to be applicable. We have studied at necropsy a 23-year-old woman with HC, and her heart weighed 1,250 g, the coronary arteries were normal, and yet a large transmural infarct was present; she weighed 46 kg. We believe that the myocardial mass exceeded the ability of the coronary bed in her, but not in the 2 patients described herein. Their hearts weighed 580 and 615 g.

Finally, the occurrence of the ventricular scarring in both father and daughter suggests a genetic etiology. Could the scarring have been present at birth? This occurrence seems unlikely. It seems most tenable that the propensity to develop massive scarring associated with HC may be genetically transmitted and perhaps may be mediated by the severe abnormalities of the intramural coronary arteries.

References

1. **Maron BJ, Epstein SE, Roberts WC.** Hypertrophic cardiomyopathy and transmural myocardial infarction without significant atherosclerosis of the extramural coronary arteries. Am J Cardiol 1979;43:1086–1102.
2. **Roberts WC.** Coronary embolism: a review of causes, consequences, and diagnostic considerations. Cardiovasc Med 1978;3:699–710.
3. **McReynolds RA, Roberts WC.** The intramural coronary arteries in hypertrophic cardiomyopathy (abstr). Am J Cardiol 1975;35:154.

Causes of Sudden Death in Competitive Athletes

BARRY J. MARON, MD, FACC, STEPHEN E. EPSTEIN, MD, FACC,
WILLIAM C. ROBERTS, MD, FACC

Bethesda, Maryland

Cardiovascular diseases responsible for sudden unexpected death in highly conditioned athletes are largely related to the age of the patient. In most young competitive athletes (<35 years of age) sudden death is due to congenital cardiovascular disease. Hypertrophic cardiomyopathy appears to be the most common cause of such deaths, accounting for about half of the sudden deaths in young athletes. Other cardiovascular abnormalities that appear to be less frequent but important causes of sudden death in young athletes include congenital coronary artery anomalies, ruptured aorta (due to cystic medial necrosis), idiopathic left ventricular hypertrophy and coronary artery atherosclerosis. Diseases that appear to be very uncommon causes of sudden death include myocarditis, mitral valve prolapse, aortic valve stenosis and sarcoidosis. Cardiovascular disease in young athletes is usually unsuspected during life, and most athletes who die suddenly have experienced no cardiac symptoms. In only about 25% of those competitive athletes who die suddenly is underlying cardiovascular disease detected or suspected before participation and rarely is the correct clinical diagnosis made. In contrast, in older athletes (≥35 years of age) sudden death is usually due to coronary artery disease, and rarely results from congenital heart disease.

(J Am Coll Cardiol 1986;7:204–14)

The highly conditioned competitive athlete epitomizes the most healthy segment of our society. Nevertheless, both youthful and older competitive athletes may occasionally die suddenly and unexpectedly, and such events take on a particularly shocking and tragic tone. For many years, our ignorance of the causes of such catastrophes was clothed in esoteric sounding descriptions, such as "sudden death syndrome," which merely masked the fact that the precise causes were unknown. Over the past several years, the cardiovascular diseases responsible for sudden death in highly trained athletes have been the subject of several reports (1–5). This communication reviews these published findings and updates our own observations on the causes of sudden death in young competitive athletes (1).

Definitions

In our modern society, a substantial proportion of the population may consider themselves to be "athletes." However, for the purposes of this discussion, a *competitive* athlete is considered to be an individual who participates in an organized team or individual sport in which regular competition is a component, a high priority is placed on excellence and achievement and vigorous training in a systematic fashion is required (6). Such competitive participation may occur at any age and encompass sports at either the youth, interscholastic, intercollegiate, professional or master's (>40 years old) level.

Sudden death is defined as a witnessed or unwitnessed natural death resulting from sudden cardiac arrest occurring unexpectedly within 6 hours of a previously witnessed usual normal state of health.

Causes of Sudden Death in Young Athletes (<35 years of age)

Considering the large number of youthful participants in competitive athletic programs in the United States, sudden death in such individuals must be considered a relatively uncommon event. The causes of such catastrophes differ considerably, but age has proved to be the most useful variable in predicting the cause of an unexpected catastrophe in an athlete (and, hence, in determining which cardiovascular lesions should be most vigorously pursued in the diagnostic evaluation of an athlete during life) (Fig. 1).

Young athletes who die suddenly are usually male, have

From the Cardiology and Pathology Branches, National Heart, Lung, and Blood Institute, National Institutes of Health, Bethesda, Maryland.

Manuscript received January 22, 1985; revised manuscript received March 26, 1985, accepted May 7, 1985.

Address for reprints: Barry J. Maron, MD, National Heart, Lung, and Blood Institute, Building 10, Room 7B-15, National Institutes of Health, Bethesda, Maryland 20892

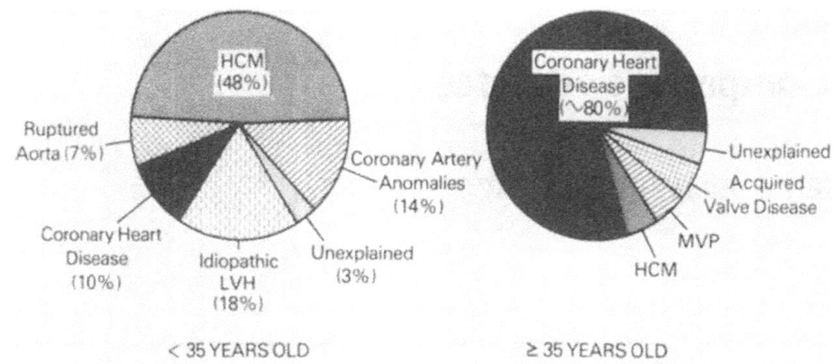

Figure 1. Causes of sudden death in competitive athletes. Estimated prevalences of diseases responsible for death are compared in young (<35 years old) and older (≥35 years old) athletes. Data shown are taken from Maron et al. (1) for young athletes and by collating several studies (2,3,5,65–67,70,71) for older athletes. HCM = hypertrophic cardiomyopathy; LVH = left ventricular hypertrophy; MVP = mitral valve prolapse.

participated in a variety of sports (most frequently basketball and football) and most commonly are junior high school or high school athletes at death (1). Some sudden deaths, however, occur in young athletes who reach the collegiate or even professional level of competition. Usually such catastrophes occur during or just after exertion on the athletic field, and as a result death is often attributed to intense physical activity.

At necropsy, most youthful, highly trained athletes who die suddenly show structural congenital cardiovascular lesions that probably or unequivocably could be ascertained to be the cause of death. In a series (1) of 29 young competitive athletes who had died suddenly and prematurely, we found evidence of structural cardiovascular disease in 28; in only 1 athlete was the heart structurally normal (Fig. 2). We inferred that this individual may have died of a primary ventricular arrhythmia.

A variety of cardiovascular diseases were responsible for sudden death in the 29 trained athletes (Fig. 2). The most common cause was hypertrophic cardiomyopathy, which occurred in about half of the patients. It should be emphasized, however, that the precise prevalence of cardiovascular diseases in a group of athletes dying suddenly probably cannot be derived from our series because of unavoidable limitations in patient selection. We did not study a consecutive series of sudden deaths in athletes occurring in a well defined geographic area. Instead, such deaths were identified from several locations in the United States in several ways: 1) through news media reports describing sudden death in athletes, or 2) referral through hospital-based pathology registries or medical examiner offices. Furthermore, we also required that the athlete's heart be available for examination, a stipulation that excluded many instances of sudden death from our series. In this report, we will describe each cardiovascular lesion that is a proved cause of sudden death in the young competitive athlete on the basis of data in our original study group (1) and in additional cases that were identified subsequently.

Hypertrophic Cardiomyopathy

Hypertrophic cardiomyopathy is a primary disease of cardiac muscle that is usually genetically transmitted (7) and is characterized by a hypertrophied but nondilated left ventricle, in the absence of another cardiac or systemic disease that may produce left ventricular hypertrophy (8). This increase in left ventricular mass usually results in impaired ventricular filling and compliance (9–12).

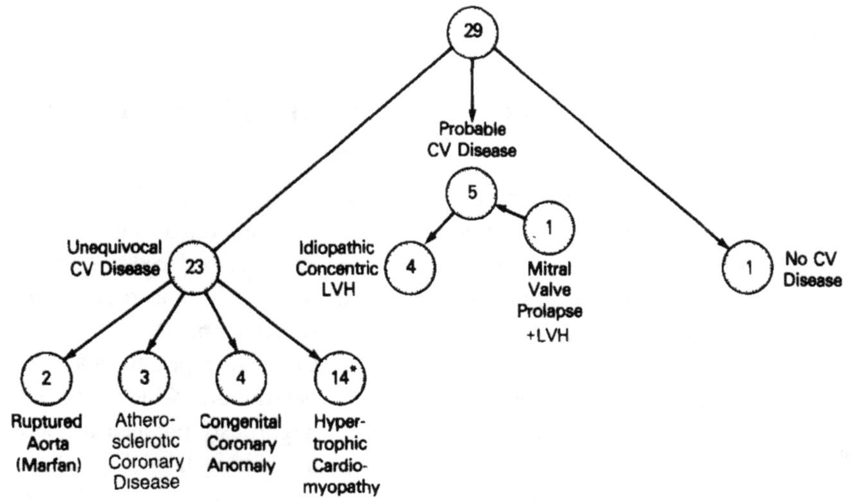

Figure 2. Diagram summarizing the cause of death in 29 competitive athletes. CV = cardiovascular; LVH = left ventricular hypertrophy. *Includes one patient who also had anomalous origin of the left coronary artery from the anterior sinus of Valsalva.

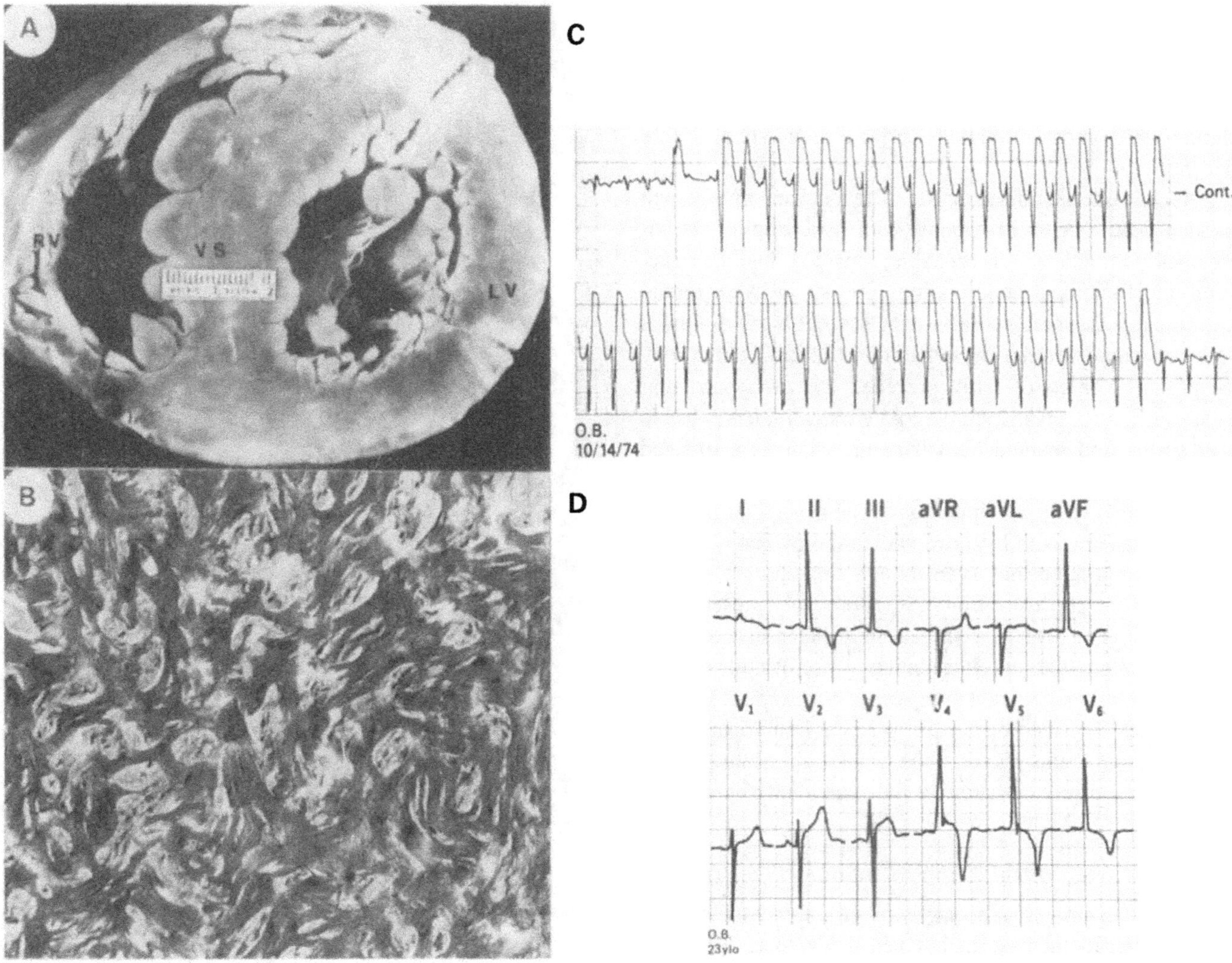

Figure 3. Clinical and morphologic features of athletes with hypertrophic cardiomyopathy. **A**, Heart of a 13 year old male football and baseball player, showing disproportionate thickening of the ventricular septum (VS) with respect to the posterior left ventricular (LV) free wall. RV = right ventricular wall. **B**, Marked disorganization of cardiac muscle cells in the disproportionately thickened ventricular septum. Adjacent hypertrophied cardiac muscle cells are oriented at oblique and perpendicular angles. **C**, Four second period of ventricular tachycardia, which occurred in the second minute of recovery after a routine treadmill exercise test and terminated spontaneously, in a 23 year old collegiate basketball player with hypertrophic cardiomyopathy who died suddenly. **D**, Standard 12 lead electrocardiogram obtained under basal conditions, showing marked symmetric T wave inversion (as much as 15 mm in depth) as well as left ventricular hypertrophy from the same athlete shown in **C**.

Anatomic features. Competitive athletes in our series (1) who died suddenly of hypertrophic cardiomyopathy ranged in age from 13 to 30 years (mean 19). Heart weight was 360 to 630 g, and ventricular septal thickness ranged from 15 to 30 mm (mean 20). Ventricular wall thickening was usually asymmetric (13), with the septum disproportionately thicker than most of the left ventricular free wall (Fig. 3); the ratio of septal thickness to that of the posterior free wall was usually 1.3 or greater (mean 1.5) (14). In addition, the thickened left ventricular wall (particularly the ventricular septum) characteristically showed two other morphologic features that are of potential pathophysiologic significance: 1) bizarre cellular architecture in which there is a markedly disordered arrangement of cardiac muscle cells (Fig. 3B) (15), and 2) an increased number of abnormal intramural coronary arteries with thickened walls and narrowed lumen (16).

Clinical profile. Hypertrophic cardiomyopathy is known to be an important cause of sudden death in the young (17–20), usually occurring in individuals without significant prior symptoms, including many in whom sudden death was the first manifestation of their disease (21). A clinical profile of 78 patients with hypertrophic cardiomyopathy who died suddenly (19) showed that 70% died before 30 years of age, 55% experienced no functional limitation before death and about 40% were actively engaged in moderate to severe physical activity just before death. That many patients with hypertrophic cardiomyopathy died during or just after vigorous activity is particularly impressive, especially when one considers the relatively small proportion of the day during which most individuals perform moderate to severe exertion.

Mechanism of sudden death. The mechanism by which sudden death occurs in patients with hypertrophic cardiomyopathy is unclear. It is probable, however, that the structural and functional abnormalities present in hypertrophic cardiomyopathy predispose certain susceptible individuals to a malignant ventricular arrhythmia (22,23) (which may be primary, or conceivably preceded by supraventricular tachycardia or bradyarrhythmia). Alternatively, it is possible that abrupt and marked hemodynamic changes associated with a reduction in left ventricular volume (in the absence of arrhythmia) may precipitate syncope or sudden death in selected patients with hypertrophic cardiomyopathy (24).

It is remarkable that even though this cardiac malformation (or the predisposition to it) is probably present at or near the time of birth, individuals so afflicted can compete for many years without either being aware of their disease or experiencing significant symptoms. For example, one of our athletes who died of hypertrophic cardiomyopathy was a professional tennis player at the time of her death, having competed intensely in that sport for more than 15 years (1).

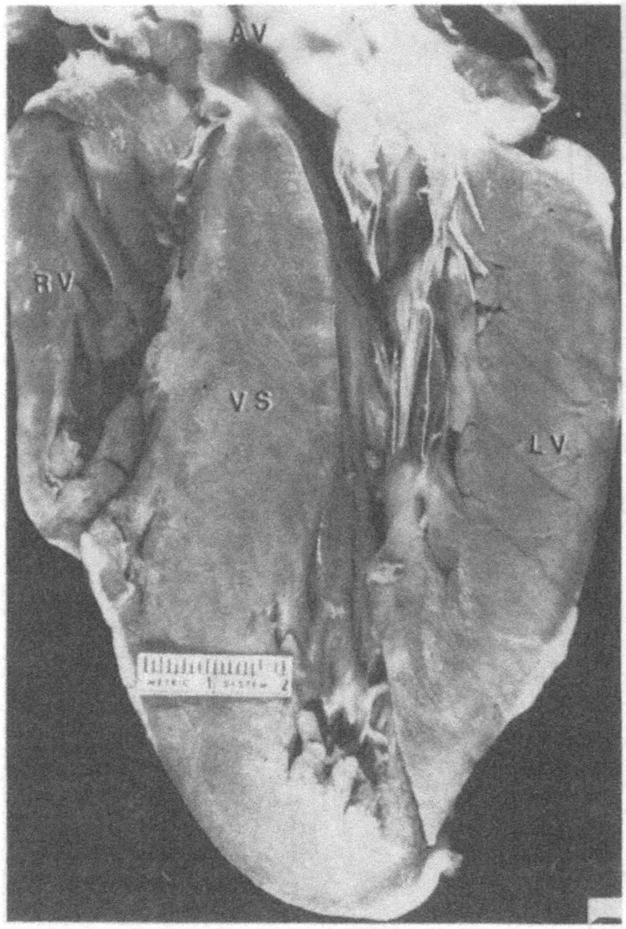

Figure 4. Heart of 17 year old soccer player showing marked concentric (symmetric) thickening of the ventricular septum (VS) and left ventricular (LV) free wall. The heart weighed 465 g. The ventricular septum is 23 mm thick and the left ventricular free wall is 20 mm. Histologic examination of the left ventricular myocardium and echocardiographic studies in first degree relatives failed to show evidence supportive of the diagnosis of hypertrophic cardiomyopathy. AV = aortic valve; RV = right ventricle.

Idiopathic Concentric Left Ventricular Hypertrophy

We also examined at necropsy other young athletes with an unexplained increase in left ventricular mass (Fig. 4). Although each of these athletes had a hypertrophied, nondilated left ventricle (heart weight 420 to 530 g; maximal wall thickness 16 to 23 mm), we considered these athletes to have "idiopathic concentric left ventricular hypertrophy" rather than hypertrophic cardiomyopathy since they differed from the usual patient with hypertrophic cardiomyopathy in several important respects: 1) the pattern of left ventricular hypertrophy was symmetric (concentric); 2) disorganization of cardiac muscle cells was not present in left ventricular myocardium (15); and 3) there was no clinical or echocardiographic evidence of genetic transmission of hypertrophic cardiomyopathy in first degree relatives (7). Some athletes with idiopathic concentric left ventricular hypertrophy (as well as hypertrophic cardiomyopathy) may show distinctive abnormalities of the intramural arteries to the sinoatrial or atrioventricular nodes, consisting of fibromuscular hyperplasia with thickening of the vessel wall and marked narrowing of the lumen (Fig. 5). Of note, the magnitude of ventricular wall thickening that athletes with idiopathic left ventricular hypertrophy exhibited at necropsy greatly exceeded that which could be considered "physiologic" left ventricular hypertrophy induced by athletic conditioning (25–32). It is also possible that idiopathic left ventricular hypertrophy (as described in our athletes) represents a variant of hypertrophic cardiomyopathy, which is not characterized by genetic transmission or asymmetric left ventricular hypertrophy. Alternatively, it is conceivable that some of these athletes may have had undetected severe systemic hypertension as the cause of their left ventricular hypertrophy.

Congenital Anomalies of Coronary Arteries

Left coronary artery arising from right sinus of Valsalva. Congenital malformations of coronary artery anatomy and distribution have been incriminated as the cause of sudden death in several young athletes (4,33–40). These potentially lethal malformations are usually of two types. The most common is anomalous origin of the *left* main coronary artery from the *right (anterior)* sinus of Valsalva. Cheitlin et al. (33) were the first to point out that the origin

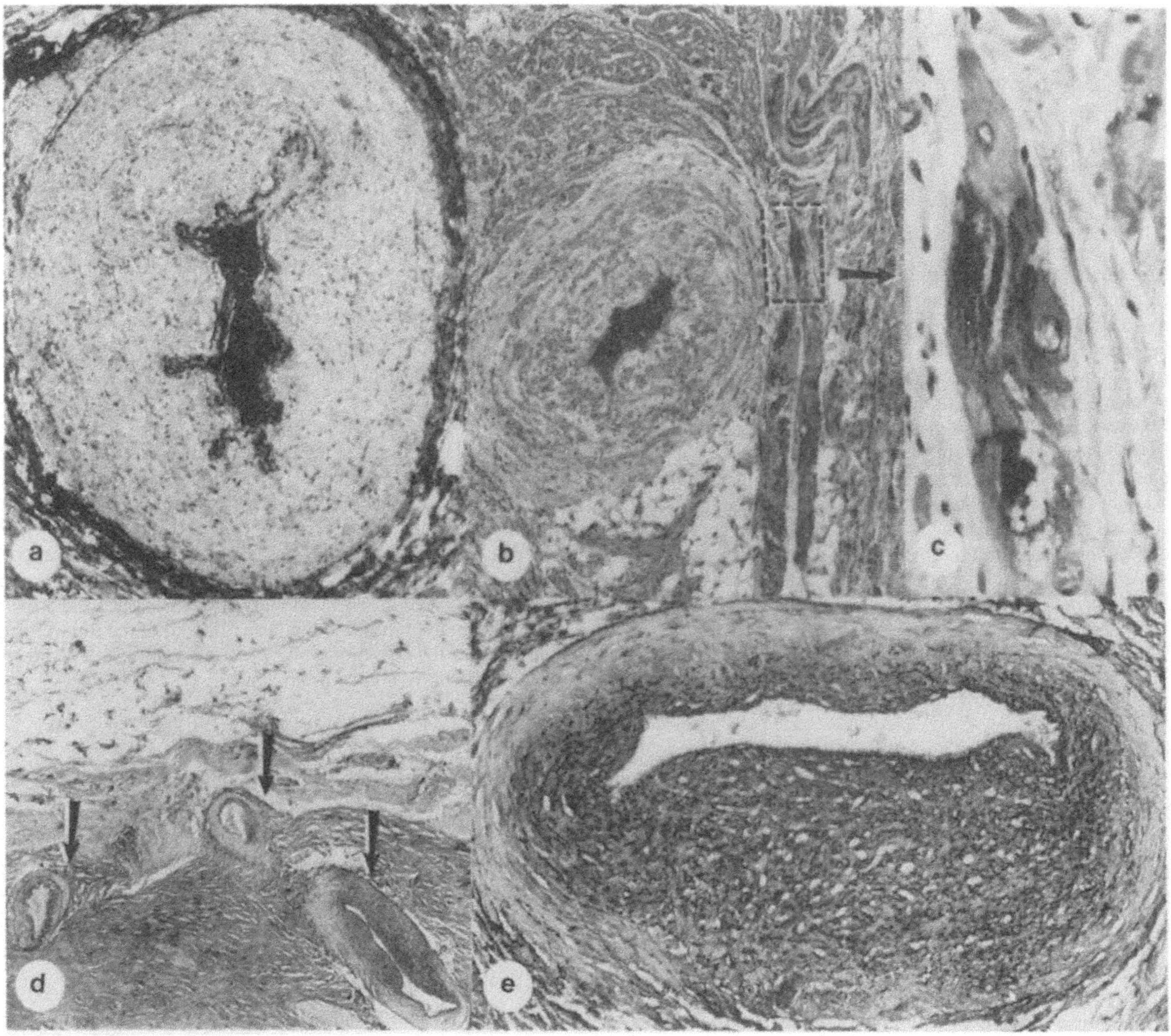

Figure 5. Small arteries in the conduction system of two athletes who died suddenly. **a**, **b**, and **c**, The artery to the sinoatrial node of a 24 year old basketball player with hypertrophic cardiomyopathy (hematoxylin- eosin stain). **d** and **e**, Arteries to the atrioventricular node of a 17 year old basketball player with idiopathic concentric left ventricular hypertrophy (elastic van Gieson stain). **a**, Artery to the sinoatrial node has a markedly narrowed lumen as a result of extreme thickening of the arterial wall. **b**, Same artery as in **a**, but at a different level and at a lower magnification, showing calcium deposits in adjacent myocardial fibers (outlined by **broken line**). **c**, Higher magnification view of the calcium-containing fiber shown in **b**. **d**, Low magnification view of the portion of atrioventricular node tissue that penetrates the central fibrous body. Three distinctly abnormal small arteries are evident (**arrows**). **e**, Higher magnification of one of the vessels shown in **d**, but at a different level. The lumen is markedly narrowed because of thickening of the arterial wall. Original magnification: **a**, ×95; **b**, ×50; **c**, ×400; **d**, ×40; **e**, ×130; all reduced by 25%.

of both the left main and the right coronary arteries from the right sinus (emanating from either a common ostium or two separate ostia), with passage of the left main coronary between the aorta and pulmonary trunk, was a clinically significant malformation (Fig. 6).

The exact mechanism by which this coronary anomaly may produce sudden death is not definitively known. However, it has been postulated (33,35) that the important anatomic feature is the acute takeoff angle of the left main coronary artery from the right sinus, which results in a narrowing of the coronary ostium. The increased stroke volume caused by physical activity probably causes dilation of the ascending aorta; this, in turn, leads to an even greater acute takeoff angle with the coronary ostium assuming an even more narrowed "slit-like" configuration, presumably resulting in diminished coronary blood flow and myocardial ischemia. It is also possible that dilation of the aorta and pulmonary trunk during exercise "squeezes" the left main

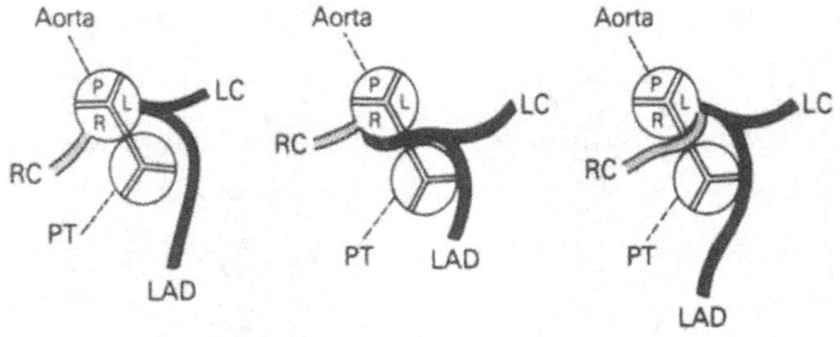

Figure 6. Diagrammatic representation of congenital coronary artery anomalies capable of causing sudden death in the young athlete. **Left**, Normal anatomy is shown for comparison. **Center**, Anomalous origin of the left coronary artery from the right (anterior) sinus of Valsalva. The left coronary artery may have a common (or separate) ostium with the right coronary artery, which also arises from the right (R) sinus of Valsalva. Note the acute leftward bend at its origin and the posterior course of the left coronary artery between the aorta and pulmonary trunk (PT). **Right**, The right coronary (RC) artery may arise from the left (L) coronary sinus and show a similar acute bend at its origin before it courses between the great arteries. LAD = left anterior descending coronary artery; LC = left circumflex coronary artery; P = posterior (noncoronary) cusp.

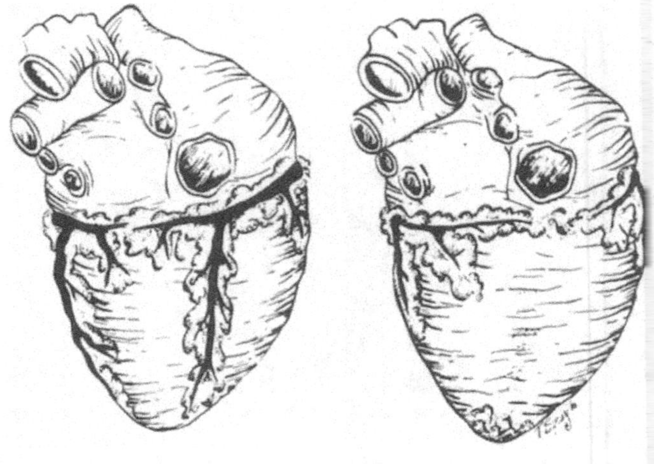

Figure 7. Diagrammatic representation of a rare congenital coronary artery abnormality in a 17 year old female distance runner who died suddenly at the end of a race (**right**). Coronary artery distribution to the posterior surface of the heart is greatly diminished because only two small posterior descending branches to the posterior left ventricular wall arose from the left circumflex coronary artery. Also, the right coronary artery was short and provided only two small branches to the posterior wall of the right ventricle and none to the posterior wall of the left ventricle. The drawing on the **left** shows normal arterial supply.

coronary artery as it passes between these two great arteries (38).

Right coronary artery arising from left sinus of Valsalva. Recently, Roberts et al. (34) emphasized that the "mirror image" coronary anomaly in which the *right* coronary artery arises from the *left* sinus of Valsalva (and courses between the aorta and the pulmonary trunk) may also convey a risk for sudden death in young conditioned individuals (Fig. 6). In this lesion, an anatomic and pathophysiologic situation exists at the right coronary ostium, which is analogous to that previously described for the left main coronary artery ostium (when that vessel originated from the right sinus). With origin of the right coronary artery from the aortic wall behind the left sinus, there is an acute rightward takeoff of the right coronary artery, which may become obstructed with exercise as the acute angle increases further as a result of increased stroke volume and aortic dilation.

Other variants. Other unusual variants of coronary artery anatomy may be occasional causes of exercise-related sudden deaths in young conditioned individuals (35). These include single coronary artery (in which the left coronary artery is absent), hypoplasia of the right and left circumflex coronary arteries (Fig. 7) or origin of the left main, left anterior descending or right coronary artery from the pulmonary trunk. Also, one of us (W.C.R.) examined the heart of a 19 year old collegiate football player who died unexpectedly and showed at necropsy an intussusception of a large ramus intermedius coronary artery branch off the left main coronary artery; this intussusception occluded the arterial lumen for 1 cm of its length. Atherosclerosis was absent from any portion of the coronary tree, and myocardial fibrosis was not evident.

Myocardial bridging. It has been suggested that "tunneled" major coronary arteries (myocardial "bridges") constitute a potential lethal anatomic variant and may cause sudden unexpected death in otherwise healthy young individuals (41). Such tunneled major coronary arteries (usually the left anterior descending artery) are completely surrounded by myocardium for at least a portion of their course, and it has been postulated that in certain susceptible individuals the artery may be critically constricted during systole and produce myocardial ischemia. Necropsy studies, however, have shown that tunneling of the left anterior descending coronary artery occurs in at least 20% of all hearts. We, therefore, believe that there is no convincing evidence that a tunneled coronary artery may be responsible for such sudden catastrophes in young athletes.

Aortic Rupture

Young athletes may die suddenly because of rupture of the aorta (Fig. 8). At necropsy, such individuals have a decreased number of elastic fibers in the aortic media, an abnormality that is presumably responsible for intrinsic weakening of the wall (commonly known as "cystic medial necrosis") (Fig. 8B). Certain individuals with cystic medical necrosis may participate successfully in strenuous competitive sports for many years without experiencing a catastrophic event. Some of these athletes also manifest aortic regurgitation or features of Marfan's syndrome (including mitral valve prolapse) that may facilitate their clinical recognition.

Figure 8. **a**, Posteroanterior chest radiograph obtained from an 18 year old male collegiate swimmer with Marfan's syndrome who died 2 months later of a ruptured aorta during a practice session. Note the prominent dilation of the ascending aorta. In this patient, the correct diagnosis was made during life and the athlete was apprised of the risks of continued competition. **b**, Histologic section of the ascending aorta from another athlete who died of a ruptured aorta. Note the markedly diminished number of elastic fibers (which stain darkly) in the media. The intima is toward the **top** and the adventitia is toward the **bottom**. Elastic van Gieson stain; magnification ×80.

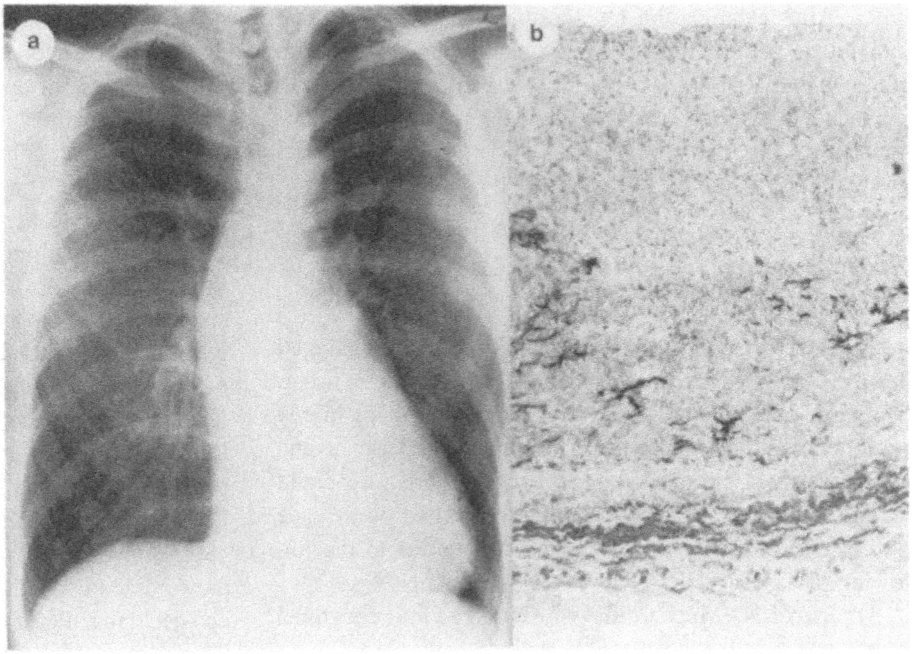

Coronary Heart Disease

Coronary heart disease is infrequently responsible for sudden death in young athletes (1,42). We studied three such athletes (24, 26, and 28 years of age, respectively) who had coronary artery atherosclerosis when they died. Two of these athletes had severe (>75%) cross-sectional area luminal narrowing by atherosclerotic plaque of each of the three major extramural coronary arteries. One of these two had total occlusion of the right coronary artery by an antemortem thrombus and hemorrhage into an atherosclerotic plaque. He was a 28 year old professional football player with type II hyperlipoproteinemia who, at necropsy, had a large healed posterior wall myocardial infarct (42). On retrospective analysis of his medical history, it was apparent that he had experienced symptoms compatible with myocardial infarction about 45 days before death, and also had had frequent episodes of chest pain with exertion thereafter. During life, however, these symptoms had not been considered to be due to heart disease, but rather as manifestations of a traumatic injury.

One other patient had approximately 50% cross-sectional area luminal narrowing of the left anterior descending coronary artery by atherosclerotic plaque and no, or only minimal, atherosclerosis in each of the other two major extramural coronary arteries. However, the left anterior descending coronary artery was completely occluded by an antemortem thrombus 2 cm from the bifurcation of the left main coronary artery.

Idiopathic causes of death. Occasionally young athletes die unexpectedly and, even after careful gross and histologic examination of the heart at necropsy (often including microscopic analysis of the conduction system), no structural abnormalities that could possibly have been the cause of death can be identified (1,4,43). Some of these patients may, however, show patchy areas of fibrosis in the left and right ventricular walls. Obviously, one can only speculate on the potential etiology of such deaths. It is possible, however, that some of these catastrophes resulted from a primary arrhythmia (1,44) or exercise-induced coronary spasm (45).

Clinical Features

Sudden death in young athletes is rarely preceded by symptoms. On retrospective questioning of surviving relatives, we found that only 8 of our 29 young athletes who died suddenly had experienced transient symptoms (for example, lightheadedness, syncope or chest discomfort) that could conceivably have been cardiovascular in origin (1). Only 2 of the 29 athletes had the correct diagnosis established during life; 1 with obvious clinical stigmata of Marfan syndrome and the other with hypertrophic cardiomyopathy, in whom there was a family history of sudden death due to that disease.

Five other athletes were suspected clinically of having cardiac disease, and all died of hypertrophic cardiomyopathy. Each of these five individuals had a distinctly abnormal electrocardiogram and one had an abnormal left ventricular angiocardiogram, but the correct diagnosis was not made clinically in any of the five. During life, three of the five athletes were mistakenly considered to have "athlete's heart syndrome" (46,47), one was thought to have a small ventricular septal defect and one was given the diagnosis of Wolff-Parkinson-White syndrome because his electrocardiographic pattern was characteristic of that disorder. After examination for possible heart disease, these individuals were permitted by the examining physician to continue participating in competitive athletics and each subsequently died on the practice field or during an athletic contest.

Other Less Common or Potential Causes of Sudden Death

The cardiac conditions described in this section have all been documented to cause sudden death in patients and, therefore, are potential causes of sudden death in highly conditioned athletes. However, in our own experience and after review of the available published reports, we could identify either no instances or only an isolated occurrence of sudden death in a highly trained athlete due to the following diseases.

Myocarditis. Myocarditis (with either a viral, undefined or other origin) has been traditionally considered to be an important cause of otherwise unexplained death in young individuals (20,48). Although myocarditis may occur in this context (with either no or relatively innocent prodromal symptoms), its prevalence and importance as a cause of sudden death in the young have probably been exaggerated owing to "overinterpretation" at necropsy of relatively small numbers of interstitial round cells. Jokl (49) reported a 25 year old runner who died after a 12 mile road race and proved to have unsuspected myocarditis. We also identified one exercise-related sudden death due to myocarditis in a 25 year old soldier who was not, however, a competitive athlete.

Mitral valve prolapse. Despite its high prevalence (probably about 5%) in the general population (50), mitral valve prolapse is not a frequent cause of sudden death in competitive athletes. Only approximately 40 subjects (average age about 35 years) with mitral valve prolapse and sudden death have been reported (51–53); death was rarely related to exercise and no subject was a trained athlete. In our series of 29 athletes studied at necropsy (1), one showed mitral valve morphology consistent with "floppy" mitral valve prolapse syndrome (that is, thickened, gelatinous and mildly scalloped leaflets with excessive mucoid material histologically) and a family history of mitral valve prolapse. However, this patient also had a marked increase in left ventricular mass, a finding that cannot be explained by the mitral valve prolapse syndrome; hence, this particular athlete may have had more than one cardiac abnormality that contributed to his unexpected death on the athletic field.

Aortic valve stenosis. Aortic stenosis is another disease that has traditionally been considered to be a common cause of sudden death in children and young adults (20). It is perhaps surprising, however, that on the basis of available information, aortic stenosis does not appear to be a frequent cause of sudden death in young athletes. This is probably due to the likelihood that this lesion will be identified early in life because of a loud heart murmur, thereby leading to prompt disqualification from competitive athletics.

Sarcoidosis. Sarcoid heart disease may cause sudden unexpected death in previously asymptomatic individuals. In a review by Roberts et al. (54) of 26 patients with cardiac dysfunction resulting from sarcoid granulomatous infiltration of the heart, 17 patients were reported to have died suddenly, including 6 in whom death occurred during exertion and was the initial manifestation of sarcoidosis. We evaluated a 25 year old professional basketball player who had recurrent ventricular tachyarrhythmias (including symptomatic ventricular tachycardia) before dying suddenly, and proved to have sarcoid infiltration of the heart at necropsy.

Abnormalities in the cardiac conduction system. Some investigators have suggested that abnormalities in the cardiac conduction system may be responsible for sudden death in athletes without other structural cardiac disease. Thiene et al. (55) reported a 26 year old cyclist whose only cardiac abnormality was a fascicle of right atrial myocardium that bypassed the atrioventricular node and connected with the His bundle. James et al. (56) described abnormalities of the small intramural artery to the sinus node in which the vessel wall was thickened and the lumen narrowed. We (1) also identified similar abnormal intramural arteries to either the sinoatrial or atrioventricular nodes in some of the young athletes dying with hypertrophic cardiomyopathy, idiopathic left ventricular hypertrophy or a mitral valve morphologically compatible with mitral valve prolapse syndrome.

Other conditions. Extremely uncommon diseases, such as QT interval prolongation syndrome (57,58) and arrhythmogenic right ventricular dysplasia (59,60), are potential casues of sudden death because of their intrinsic propensity to produce serious arrhythmias or sudden death. Although there are no reports of competitive athletes dying with these conditions, this may be due largely to the infrequency with which these lesions occur. In addition, Green et al. (61) reported on a 44 year old marathon runner who collapsed after completing 24 miles of a race, and at necropsy proved to have transmural myocardial infarction in the absence of extramural coronary artery disease. Exercise-related sudden death also has been described in individuals with such rare conditions as isolated thinning of right ventricular myocardium (62) and lipomatous infiltration of the heart (63).

Sudden Death in Older Athletes (≥35 years of age)

Increasing numbers of middle-aged or older individuals (≥35 years of age) are now participating in organized competitive sports and in extremely vigorous physical conditioning programs (for example, jogging and swimming). Superior physical fitness in this age group (or at any other age), however, does not guarantee protection against exercise-related death. As is the case with the young competitive athlete, older athletes also may harbor occult cardiovascular disease and die suddenly and unexpectedly while participating in athletic activities (2,3,5,35,64–71). Nevertheless, the prevalence of such catastrophes is probably quite low considering the large number of individuals in the older age groups participating in sports (66).

Causes of sudden death. Unlike the more youthful athletes previously discussed, the cause of death in older conditioned athletes is usually not a congenital malformation of the heart. On the basis of the available data from several published studies (2,3,5,64–71), the cause of sudden death in the vast majority of older athletes is coronary heart disease. At necropsy, such individuals usually have severe (>75%) narrowing of the cross-sectional area by atherosclerotic plaque of one, two or three major extramural coronary arteries (left anterior descending, left circumflex or right) (Fig. 9), but rarely of the left main coronary artery. The remaining deaths in older athletes appear to be due to a variety of noncoronary causes such as hypertrophic cardiomyopathy (or idiopathic left ventricular hypertrophy), mitral valve prolapse or acquired mitral or aortic valve heart disease (3,5,70); in a few athletes, the cause of death could not be established definitively at necropsy (3,5).

Coronary heart disease. To date, about 100 older athletes who died suddenly of coronary heart disease have been reported in eight separate necropsy investigations (2,3,5,65–67,70,71). These individuals comprise a heterogeneous group of athletes, including runners (some in training for competitive long distance races) and joggers, and others participating in sports such as rugby and squash. Unlike the young competitive athletes who died of congenital heart disease, approximately half of the older athletes with coronary heart disease had experienced prodromal cardiovascular symptoms before death or had a known medical history of coronary artery disease. In addition, these athletes are usually described as having "severe" coronary artery narrowing at necropsy, although only a few studies provide

Figure 9. Sections of coronary arteries from a 49 year old man who ran an average of about 170 km/week and successfully completed six marathons and seven 80 km races, but died suddenly of coronary heart disease. The right (R), left anterior descending (LAD) and left circumflex (LC) coronary arteries are shown at the sites of maximal narrowing by atherosclerosis, both in the proximal (**upper panels**) and distal (**lower panels**) halves of the respective arteries.

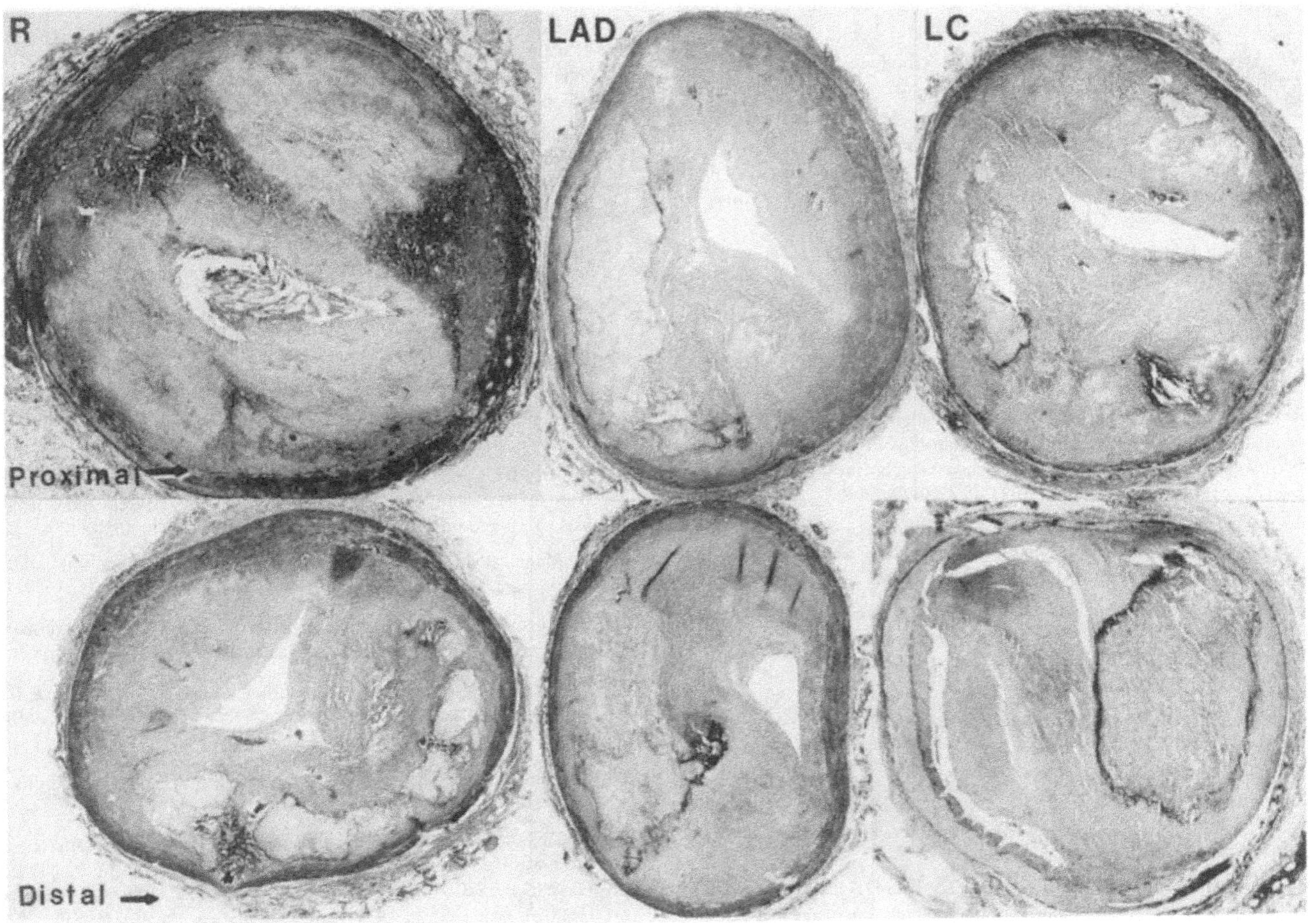

detailed or quantitative morphologic descriptions of the severity and distribution of arterial narrowing.

Sudden death due to coronary heart disease may also occur in highly conditioned older athletes who have trained for and completed particularly long competitive races, including the marathon distance (26 miles) (Fig.9) (2,69,71). Hence, marathon running itself does not provide "immunity to atherosclerosis," as previously suggested (72).

References

1. Maron BJ, Roberts WC, McAllister HA, Rosing DR, Epstein SE Sudden death in young athletes. Circulation 1980:62:218–29
2. Waller BF, Roberts WC. Sudden death while running in conditioned runners aged 40 years or over. Am J Cardiol 1980:45:1292–300
3 Virmani R, Robinowitz M, McAllister HA. Nontraumatic death in joggers A series of 30 patients at autopsy. Am J Med 1982:72·874–81
4. Tsung SH, Huang TY, Chang MH. Sudden death in young athletes Arch Pathol Lab Med 1982;106:168–70.
5 Northcote RJ, Evans ADB, Ballantyne D. Sudden death in squash players. Lancet 1984;1·148–51.
6. Maron BJ, Epstein SE, Mitchell JH The competitive athlete with cardiovascular disease: definitions, guidelines, and considerations. Introduction to Bethesda Conference #16 J Am Coll Cardiol, 1986;6:1189–90
7 Maron BJ, Nichols PF, Pickle LW, Wesley YE, Mulvihill JJ Patterns of inheritance in hypertrophic cardiomyopathy: assessment by M-mode and two-dimensional echocardiography. Am J Cardiol 1984;53.1087–94
8. Maron BJ, Epstein SE. Hypertrophic cardiomyopathy. a discussion of nomenclature Am J Cardiol 1979;43.1242–4.
9. Sanderson JE, Gibson DG, Brown DJ, Goodwin JF Left ventricular filling in hypertrophic cardiomyopathy An angiographic study Br Heart J 1977;39:661–70
10. St. John Sutton MG, Tajik AJ, Gibson DG, Brown DJ, Seward JB, Giuliani ER Echocardiographic assessment of left ventricular filling and septal and posterior wall dynamics in idiopathic hypertrophic subaortic stenosis Circulation 1978;57.512–20.
11 Hanrath P, Mathey DB, Siegert R, Bleifeld W Left ventricular relaxation and filling in different forms of left ventricular hypertrophy· an echocardiographic study Am J Cardiol 1980,45·15–23
12 Bonow RO, Rosing DR, Bacharach SL, et al. Effects of verapamil on left ventricular systolic function and diastolic filling in patients with hypertrophic cardiomyopathy Circulation 1981,64:787–96
13. Maron BJ, Gottdiener JS, Epstein SE Patterns and significance of the distribution of left ventricular hypertrophy in hypertrophic cardiomyopathy. a wide-angle, two-dimensional echocardiographic study of 125 patients Am J Cardiol 1981,48·418–28.
14. Henry WL, Clark CE, Epstein SE Asymmetric septal hypertrophy (ASH): echocardiographic identification of the pathognomonic anatomic abnormality of IHSS. Circulation 1973,47:225–33
15. Maron BJ, Anan TJ, Roberts WC Quantitative analysis of the distribution of cardiac muscle cell disorganization in the left ventricular wall of patients with hypertrophic cardiomyopathy Circulation 1981;63:882–94
16. Maron BJ, Wolfson JK, Epstein SE, Roberts WC Intramural "small vessel" coronary artery disease in hypertrophic cardiomyopathy. Prevalence and potential significance (abstr). J Am Coll Cardiol 1985;5:395.
17 Maron BJ, Henry WL, Clark CE, Redwood DR, Roberts WC, Epstein SE. Asymmetric septal hypertrophy in childhood Circulation 1976,53:9–18
18. McKenna W, Deanfield J, Faruqui A, England D, Oakley C, Goodwin JF Prognosis in hypertrophic cardiomyopathy: role of age and clinical, electrocardiographic and hemodynamic features. Am J Cardiol 1981;47.532–8
19. Maron BJ, Roberts WC, Epstein SE Sudden death in hypertrophic cardiomyopathy. a profile of 78 patients. Circulation 1982:65:1188–94.
20. Lambert EC, Menon VA, Wagner HR, Vlad P. Sudden unexpected death from cardiovascular diseases in children. A cooperative international study Am J Cardiol 1974;34:89–96.
21. Maron BJ, Roberts WC, Edwards JE, McAllister HA Jr, Foley DD, Epstein SE Sudden death in patients with hypertrophic cardiomyopathy· characterization of 26 patients without functional limitation. Am J Cardiol 1978,41:803–10.
22 Maron BJ, Savage DD, Wolfson JK, Epstein SE. Prognostic significance of 24-hour ambulatory electrocardiographic monitoring in patients with hypertrophic cardiomyopathy. a prospective study Am J Cardiol 1981;48:252–7
23 McKenna WJ, England D, Doi YL, Deanfield JE, Oakley CM, Goodwin JF Arrhythmia in hypertrophic cardiomyopathy: I Influence on prognosis. Br Heart J 1981;46:168–72.
24. McKenna W, Harris L, Deanfield J. Syncope in hypertrophic cardiomyopathy. Br Heart J 1982;47·177–9
25 Morganroth J, Maron BJ, Henry WL, Epstein SE. Comparative left ventricular dimensions in trained athletes Ann Intern Med 1975;82:521–4
26. Roeske WR, O'Rourke RA, Klein A, Leopold G, Karliner JS Noninvasive evaluation of ventricular hypertrophy in professional athletes. Circulation 1976;53:286–92.
27 Gilbert CA, Nutter DO, Felner JM, Perkins JV, Heymsfield SB, Schlant RC. Echocardiographic study of cardiac dimensions and function in the endurance-trained athlete. Am J Cardiol 1977,40:528–33
28 Ehsani AA, Hagberg JM, Hickman RC Rapid change in left ventricular dimensions and mass in response to physical conditioning and deconditioning Am J Cardiol 1978;42.52–6.
29 Ikaheimo MJ, Palatsi IJ, Takkunen JT. Noninvasive evaluation of the athletic heart sprinters versus endurance runners. Am J Cardiol 1979,44:24–30.
30 Longhurst JC, Kelly AR, Gonyea WJ, Mitchell JH. Echocardiographic left ventricular masses in distance runners and weight lifters. J Appl Physiol 1980;48:154–62.
31. Nishimura T, Yamada Y, Kawai C. Echocardiographic evaluation of long-term effects of exercise on left ventricular hypertrophy and function in professional bicyclists. Circulation 1980;61:832–40.
32. Fagard R, Aubert A, Lysens R, Staessen J, Vanhees L, Amery A. Noninvasive assessment of seasonal variations in cardiac structure and function in cyclists. Circulation 1983,67:896–901
33 Cheitlin MD, DeCastro CM, McAllister HA. Sudden death as a complication of anomalous left coronary origin from the anterior sinus of Valsalva. Circulation 1974;50:780–7
34 Roberts WC, Siegel RJ, Zipes DP. Origin of the right coronary artery from the left sinus of Valsalva and its functional consequences. analysis of 10 necropsy patients Am J Cardiol 1982;49:863–8
35 McManus BM, Waller BE, Graboys TB, et al. Exercise and sudden death, part I Curr Prob Cardiol 1981;6:17–78
36. Liberthson RR, Dinsmore RE, Bharati A, et al. Aberrant coronary artery origin from the aorta Circulation 1974;50.774–9.
37 Cohen LS, Shaw LD Fatal myocardial infarction in an 11 year old boy associated with a unique coronary artery anomaly. Am J Cardiol 1967;19.420–3
38. Benson PA, Lack AR Anomalous aortic origin of the left coronary artery Arch Pathol Lab Med 1968,86:214–6
39 McClellan JT, Jokl E Congenital anomalies of coronary arteries as cause of sudden death associated with physical exertion. In. McClellan JT, Jokl E , eds. Medicine and Sport, Vol. 5: Exercise and Cardiac Death. Basel· Karger, 1971.91–8

40. Jokl E, McClellan JT, Ross GD. Congenital anomaly of left coronary artery in a young athlete JAMA 1962.182:572–3

41. Morales AR, Romanelli R, Boucek RJ. The mural left anterior descending coronary artery, strenuous exercise and sudden death. Circulation 1980;62:230–7.

42. Roberts WC, Maron BJ. Sudden death while playing professional football. Am Heart J 1981;102:1061–3.

43. Benson DW Jr, Benditt DG, Anderson RW, et al. Cardiac arrest in young, ostensibly healthy patients: clinical, hemodynamic, and electrophysiologic findings. Am J Cardiol 1983;52.65–9.

44. Pedersen DH, Zipes DP, Foster PR, Troup PJ Ventricular tachycardia and ventricular fibrillation in a young population. Circulation 1979;60.988–97.

45. Yasue H, Omote S, Takizawa A, Nagao M, Miwa K, Tanaka S. Circadian variation of exercise capacity in patients with Prinzemetal's variant angina: role of exercise-induced coronary arterial spasm. Circulation 1979;59:938–48.

46. Rost R. The athlete's heart. Eur Heart J 1982;3(suppl A):193–8.

47. Maron BJ. Structural features of the athlete's heart as defined by echocardiography. J Am Coll Cardiol 1986;7:190–203.

48. Noren GJ, Staley NA, Brandt CM, Kaplan EL Occurrence of myocarditis in sudden death in children. J Forensic Sci 1977;22.188–96.

49. Jokl E Sudden death after exercise due to myocarditis. In Ref 39: 99–101.

50. Jeresaty RM. Mitral Valve Prolapse. New York: Raven, 1979.

51 Chesler E, King RA, Edwards JE. The myxomatous mitral valve and sudden death. Circulation 1983;67:632–9.

52. Jeresaty RM. Sudden death in the mitral valve prolapse-click syndrome. Am J Cardiol 1976;37:317–9.

53 Pocock WA, Bosman CK, Chesler E, Barlow JB, Edwards JE. Sudden death in primary mitral valve prolapse. Am Heart J 1984;107.378–82.

54. Roberts WC, McAllister HA, Ferrans VJ Sarcoidosis of the heart. A clinicopathologic study of 35 necropsy patients (group I) and review of 78 previously described necropsy patients (group II). Am J Med 1977;63:86–108.

55. Thiene G, Pennelli N, Rossi L Cardiac conduction system abnormalities as a possible cause of sudden death in young athletes Hum Pathol 1983;14:706–9.

56. James TN, Froggart P, Marshall TK. Sudden death in young athletes. Ann Intern Med 1967;67.1013–21.

57. Schwartz PJ, Periti M, Malliani A. The long Q-T syndrome. Am Heart J 1975;89:378–90

58. James TN, Frogatt P, Atkinson WJ, et al. De subitaneis mortibus. XXX. Observations on the pathophysiology of the long QT syndromes with special reference to the neuropathology of the heart. Circulation 1978;57:1221–31.

59. Marcus FI, Fontaine GH, Guiraudon G, et al. Right ventricular dysplasia: a report of 24 adult cases. Circulation 1982;65:384–98.

60. Olsson SB, Edvardsson N, Emanuelsson H, Eneström S. A case of arrhythmogenic right ventricular dysplasia with ventricular fibrillation. Clin Cardiol 1982;5:591–6.

61. Green LH, Cohen SI, Kurland G. Fatal myocardial infarction in marathon racing. Ann Intern Med 1976;84.704–6.

62. Virmani R, Robinowitz M, Clark MA, McAllister HA. Sudden death and partial absence of the right ventricular myocardium. Arch Pathol Lab Med 1982;106:163–7.

63. Voigt J, Agdal N. Lipomatous infiltration of the heart. An uncommon cause of sudden, unexpected death in a young man. Arch Pathol Lab Med 1982;106:497–8.

64. Noakes TD, Rose AG, Opie LH. Hypertrophic cardiomyopathy associated with sudden death during marathon racing. Br Heart J 1979;41:624–7.

65. Jackson RT, Beaglehole R, Sharpe N. Sudden death in runners. NZ Med J 1983;96:289–92.

66. Thompson PD, Funk EJ, Carleton RA, Sturner WQ. Incidence of death during jogging in Rhode Island from 1975 through 1980. JAMA 1982;247.2535–8.

67. Opie LH, Sudden death and sport. Lancet 1975;1:263–6.

68. Waller BA, Csere RS, Baker WP, Roberts WC. Structure-function correlations in cardiovascular and pulmonary diseases (CPC). Running to death. Chest 1981;79:346–9.

69. Ludmerer KM, Kissane JM. Clinicopathologic conference: sudden death in 47-year-old marathon runner Am J Med 1984;76:517–26.

70. Thompson PD, Stern MP, Williams P, Duncan K, Haskell WL, Wood PD Death during jogging or running A study of 18 cases. JAMA 1979;242.1265–7.

71. Noakes TD, Opie LH, Rose AG, Kleynhans PHT. Autopsy-proved coronary atherosclerosis in marathon runners. N Engl J Med 1979;301:86–9

72. Bassler TJ. Marathon running and immunity to atherosclerosis. Ann NY Acad Sci 1977;301.579–92.

Impaired Left Ventricular Systolic and Diastolic Function Without Left Ventricular Dilatation Associated With Papillary Muscle Calcification in Hypertrophic Cardiomyopathy

ELIZABETH M. ROSS, MD
DOUGLAS R. ROSING, MD
JAMES C. LAIDLAW, MD
LOCKHART B. McGUIRE, MD
BARRY M. MARON, MD
WILLIAM C. ROBERTS, MD

Impairment of left ventricular (LV) systolic function in hypertrophic cardiomyopathy (HC) is unusual, and when it occurs the LV cavity often dilates.[1] This report describes a patient with chronic severe impairment in LV contractility associated with congestive heart failure (CHF) but without LV dilatation.

From the Pathology and Cardiology Branches, National Heart, Lung, and Blood Institute, National Institutes of Health, Bethesda, Maryland 20205, the Department of Medicine, Winchester Memorial Hospital, Winchester, Virginia, and the Division of Cardiology, Department of Medicine, University of Virginia School of Medicine, Charlottesville, Virginia. Manuscript received October 4, 1985, accepted October 7, 1985.

A 52-year-old man (CC#15-66-24-6) had been well until age 42, when chest pain, palpitations and dizziness developed associated with rapid atrial fibrillation. These findings prompted cardiac catheterization (Table I). Thoracotomy shortly thereafter excluded pericardial constriction. During the next 10 years he was hospitalized on more than 60 occasions. At age 44 he had 2 nonfatal cardiac arrests and a pacemaker was inserted. Evidence of CHF appeared shortly thereafter, and it progressively worsened and became intractable during the next 8 years. Five months before death the patient was referred to the National Heart, Lung, and Blood Institute, and a second cardiac catheterization was performed (Table I). At that time, his activities were limited to sitting or reclining. Ejection fraction at rest by radionuclide angiography was 32%. Chest radiograph (Fig. 1) disclosed a calcific deposit in the area of the mitral valve and the posteromedial papillary muscle. Although 2-dimensional echocardiography showed that the maximal thickness of the ventricular septum was 20 mm, the anterior portion of the ventricular septum in the path of the M-mode beam was 13 mm (Fig. 2); LV cavity (transverse dimension) was 45 mm in ventricular diastole and 40 mm in systole; left atrial dimension was 65 mm and

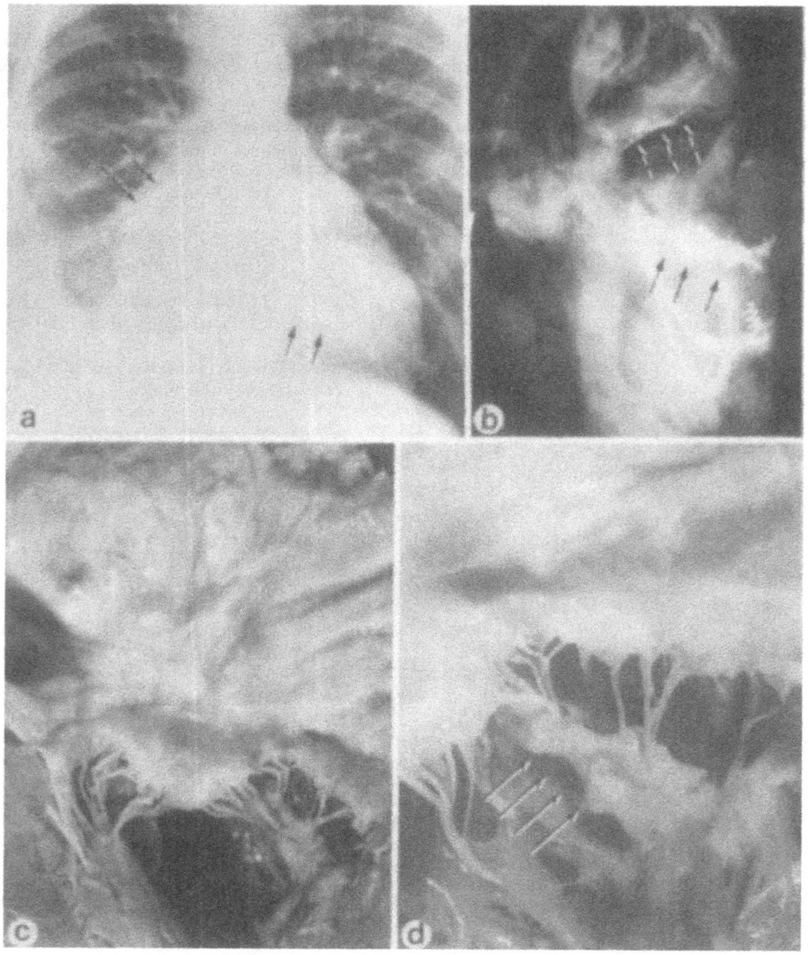

FIGURE 1. Chest radiograph taken 5 months before death (*A*); radiograph of heart specimen at necropsy (*B*); opened left atrium, mitral valve and left ventricle (*C*), and close-up of left ventricular posteromedial papillary muscle (*D*). The papillary muscle calcific deposit is designated by *solid arrows* and the left atrial calcific deposits by *dashed arrows.*

TABLE I Hemodynamic Findings

	May 1972 (age 42)	July 1982 (age 53)
Pulmonary artery wedge (m:a:v)	29:28:41	30:–:45
Pulmonary artery (s/d)	49/22	55/30
Right ventricle (s/d)	49/14	55/19
Right atrium (m:a:v)	14:17:23	19:–:22
Left ventricle (s/d)	96/35	90/26
Systemic artery (s/d)	96/70	90/60
Cardiac index (liters/min/m^2)	1.8	2.1
LV cineangiogram		
Mitral regurgitation	0	0
Calcium, papillary muscle	+	+
LV cavity size	Normal	Normal

a = a wave; d = diastole; LV = left ventricular; m = mean; s = systole; v = v wave; + = present; 0 = absent.

right ventricular transverse dimension was 30 mm. Systolic anterior motion of the mitral valve was absent. Prominent, bright echo densities were present in the posteromedial papillary muscle (Fig. 2 and 3). The patient died of progressive CHF 5 months later. The patient's 13-year-old son had characteristic echocardiographic features of HC.

At necropsy, the heart weighed 500 g. The epicardial surfaces were focally fibrotic, presumably the result of previous thoracotomy. The epicardial coronary arteries were free of significant luminal narrowing. Both ventricular cavities were of normal size. The LV free wall measured up to 12 mm and the ventricular septum up to 20 mm in thickness. Heavy calcific deposits almost totally replaced the posteromedial LV papillary muscle (Fig. 1 and 4). Focal calcific deposits also were present on the mural endocardium of the body of the left atrium but not in the appendage and not in the mitral anulus (Fig. 1). The cardiac valve leaflets and chordae tendineae were normal. Small focal scars were present in the ventricular septum but no grossly visible foci of fibrosis or necrosis were present in the LV free wall. Histologic examination dis-

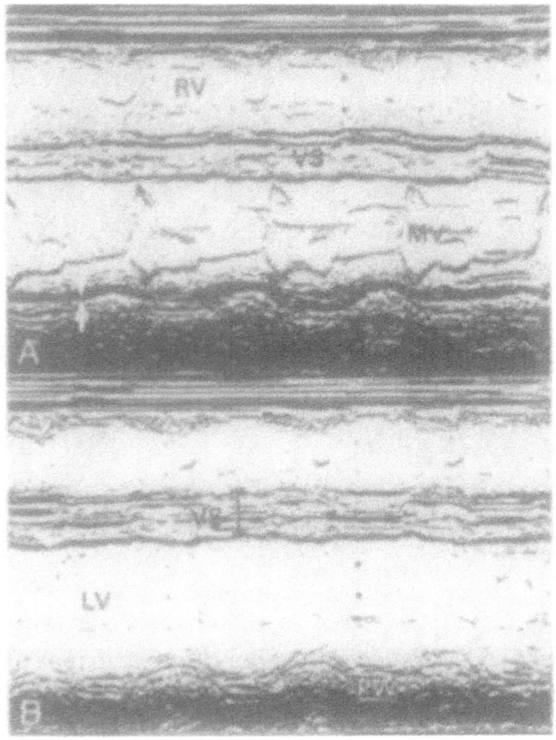

FIGURE 2. M-mode echocardiogram shown at the level of the mitral valve (*A*) and below mitral valve (*B*) showing a 13-mm thick ventricular septum (VS), a nondilated left ventricular (LV) cavity and a bright echo-dense band, presumed to be calcium behind the mitral valve (MV) (*arrows in A*). PW = posterior wall; RV = right ventricular cavity.

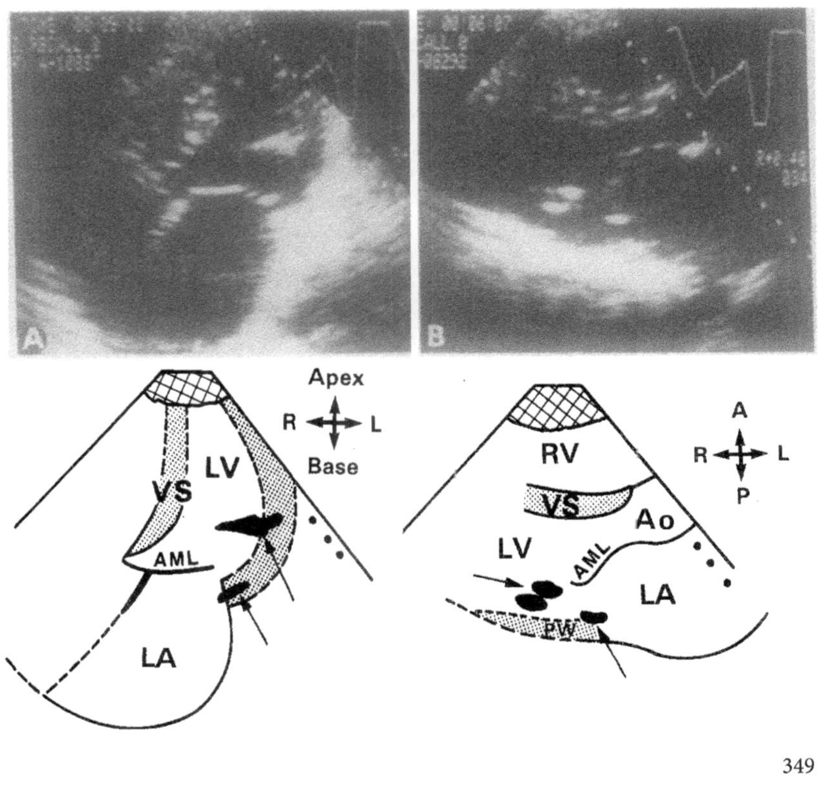

FIGURE 3. Two-dimensional echocardiograms obtained in the apical 4-chamber (*A*) and parasternal long axis (*B*) views. Each image is accompanied by a schematic illustration. Both echocardiograms show a mildly hypertrophied and nondilated left ventricle, and bright echo-dense structures in the region of the posteromedial papillary muscle and also at the junction of left atrial (LA) and left ventricular (LV) free walls (*arrows*), which represent calcific deposits. *Calibration dots* are 1-cm apart. A = anterior; AML = anterior mitral leaflet; Ao = aorta; L = left; P = posterior; PW = posterior left ventricular free wall; R = right; RV = right ventricle; VS = ventricular septum.

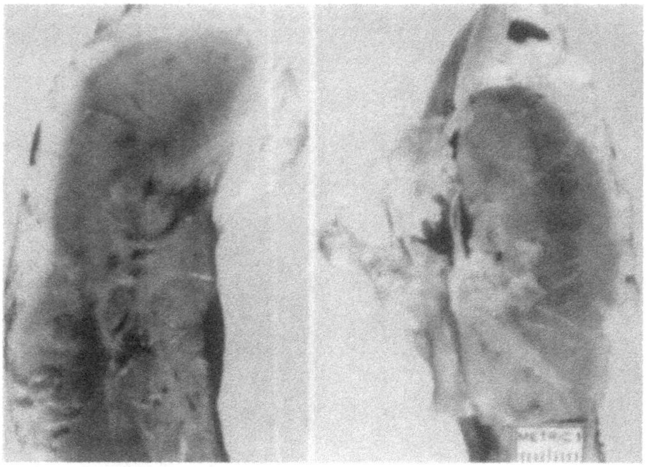

FIGURE 4. Longitudinal section of the normal anterolateral (*left*) and calcified posteromedial (*right*) left ventricular papillary muscles.

closed severe myocardial fiber disarray in the ventricular septum and virtually normal intramural coronary arteries.

This patient demonstrates that poor systolic function and chronic CHF can occur in patients with HC without associated LV dilatation and without significant coronary arterial narrowing or LV fibrosis or necrosis. Chronic, severe LV failure without LV dilatation has not been emphasized previously in patients with HC.

During the past 25 years, the hearts of 174 patients with HC have been studied in the Pathology Branch of the National Heart, Lung, and Blood Institute. Of these hearts, the only one with calcific deposits in one or more ventricular papillary muscles or in the left atrial wall was from the patient described herein. Additionally, we have not found any published report describing calcific deposits in a cardiac papillary muscle or in the left atrial wall in a patient with HC. The cause of the almost total replacement by calcific deposits of the posteromedial papillary muscle in the patient described herein is unclear. Older patients frequently have small calcific deposits in the apices of 1 or both LV papillary muscles, but almost total replacement of them by a presumed aging mechanism has not been described, and our patient was only 52 years old. Another possible mechanism for gross myocardial calcification is ischemia from fixed coronary arterial narrowing, but this mechanism is not applicable in this patient because his major epicardial coronary arteries were only insignificantly narrowed. Furthermore, his intramural coronary arteries were normal.

The cause of the left atrial calcific deposits also is unclear. Calcific deposits have been observed in the left atrial wall in patients with mitral stenosis (never in patients with pure mitral regurgitation) and in patients with large left-to-right shunts from patent ductus arteriosus.[2] Our patient, however, had no diastolic gradient between pulmonary artery wedge position and left ventricular or a left-to-right shunt.

References

1. Maron BJ, Epstein SE, Roberts WC. *Hypertrophic cardiomyopathy and transmural myocardial infarction without significant atherosclerosis of the extramural coronary arteries. Am J Cardiol 1979;43:1086–1102.*

2. Roberts WC. *Morphologic features of the normal and abnormal mitral valve. Am J Cardiol 1983;51:1005–1028.*

Intramural ("Small Vessel") Coronary Artery Disease in Hypertrophic Cardiomyopathy

BARRY J. MARON, MD, FACC, JAMES K. WOLFSON, MS, STEPHEN E. EPSTEIN, MD, FACC, WILLIAM C. ROBERTS, MD, FACC

Bethesda, Maryland

Many patients with hypertrophic cardiomyopathy have signs and symptoms of myocardial ischemia and dysfunction. Although hypertrophy and increased left ventricular pressure can account for such abnormalities, altered small intramural coronary arteries have also been described in such patients. To determine the prevalence and extent as well as the clinical relevance of abnormal intramural coronary arteries, a histologic analysis of left ventricular myocardium obtained at necropsy was performed in 48 patients with hypertrophic cardiomyopathy (but without atherosclerosis of the extramural coronary arteries) and in 68 control patients with either a normal heart or acquired heart disease.

In hypertrophic cardiomyopathy, abnormal intramural coronary arteries were characterized by thickening of the vessel wall and a decrease in luminal size. The wall thickening was due to proliferation of medial or intimal components, or both, particularly smooth muscle cells and collagen. Of the 48 patients with hypertrophic cardiomyopathy, 40 (83%) had abnormalities of intramural coronary arteries located in the ventricular septum (33 patients), anterior left ventricular free wall (20 patients) or posterior free wall (9 patients); an average of 3.0 ± 0.7 abnormal arteries were identified per tissue section. Altered intramural coronary arteries were also significantly more common in tissue sections having considerable myocardial fibrosis (31 [74%] of 42) than in those with no or mild fibrosis (31 [30%] of 102; $p < 0.001$). Abnormal intramural coronary arteries were also identified in three of eight infants who died of hypertrophic cardiomyopathy before 1 year of age.

In contrast, only rare altered intramural coronary arteries were identified in 6 (9%) of the 68 control patients (0.1 ± 0.05 abnormal arteries per section; $p < 0.001$) and those arteries showed only mild thickening of the wall and minimal luminal narrowing. Moreover, of those patients with abnormal intramural coronary arteries, such vessels were about 20 times more frequent in patients with hypertrophic cardiomyopathy (0.9 ± 0.2/cm^2 myocardium) than in control patients (0.04 ± 0.02/cm^2 myocardium).

Hence, abnormal intramural coronary arteries with markedly thickened walls and narrowed lumens are present in increased numbers in most patients with hypertrophic cardiomyopathy studied at necropsy and may represent a congenital component of the underlying cardiomyopathic process. Although the clinical significance of "small vessel coronary artery disease" in hypertrophic cardiomyopathy is unclear, the occurrence of structurally altered intramural coronary arteries in areas of substantial myocardial fibrosis suggests a causal role for these arteries in producing ischemia.

(J Am Coll Cardiol 1986;8:545–57)

Hypertrophic cardiomyopathy is a cardiac disease with a variety of clinical and morphologic features (1–11). Many patients with hypertrophic cardiomyopathy manifest evidence of myocardial ischemia or damage, including angina pectoris or atypical chest pain (4,6,12), certain electrocardiographic abnormalities (13–16), myocardial fibrosis (10,17) and abnormalities in coronary blood flow and lactate production during stress (18,19). In this investigation, we considered the possibility that structural alterations in the intramural coronary arteries (20–22) could contribute to myocardial ischemia in patients with hypertrophic cardiomyopathy. We examined histologic sections of ventricular myocardium from 48 patients with hypertrophic cardiomyopathy and from 68 patients with acquired cardiac disease or a normal heart to determine the prevalence and severity of abnormal intramural coronary arteries and their relation to areas of fibrosis.

From the Cardiology and Pathology Branches of the National Heart, Lung, and Blood Institute, National Institutes of Health, Bethesda, Maryland.

Manuscript received November 22, 1985; revised manuscript received February 24, 1986, accepted April 24, 1986.

Address for reprints: Barry J. Maron, MD, National Institutes of Health, National Heart, Lung, and Blood Institute, Building 10, Room 7B-15, Bethesda, Maryland 20892.

Methods

Selection of patients. The cardiovascular registry of the Pathology Branch of the National Heart, Lung, and Blood Institute was reviewed and 154 hearts of children and adults with hypertrophic cardiomyopathy were identified and considered for inclusion in the study. Of this number, 106 were excluded for one or more of the following reasons: 1) there was associated cardiac disease such as systemic hypertension, aortic valve stenosis, mitral valve prolapse or coronary heart disease (>50% narrowing of the cross-sectional lumen of one or more extramural [epicardial] coronary arteries) (37 patients) or systemic disease including insulin-dependent diabetes mellitus (7 patients); 2) the patient had had a previous operation (ventricular septal myotomy-myectomy) and had survived more than 1 month postoperatively (19 patients); 3) the specimen was in poor condition and tissue suitable for histologic analysis could not be obtained from the standard three sites in the septum and left ventricular free wall described below (18 patients); or 4) the heart was considered to be a particularly good example of hypertrophic cardiomyopathy that we wished to preserve intact (25 patients). The remaining 48 patients constitute the study group. Each patient met our definition of hypertrophic cardiomyopathy by virtue of having a hypertrophied, nondilated left ventricle in the absence of another cardiac or systemic disease that could produce left ventricular hypertrophy (23). In addition to these 48 patients, 8 infants who died of hypertrophic cardiomyopathy (24,25) (7 live-born and 1 stillborn) were examined separately as part of this investigation.

Control patients. In addition, 68 patients without hypertrophic cardiomyopathy were selected as controls, including 14 without evidence of cardiac disease and 54 with a variety of relatively common acquired cardiac diseases characterized by an increase in left ventricular mass (Table 1). Because our control group was defined in this fashion, it did not include several congenital cardiac or systemic diseases in which intramural coronary artery abnormalities had already been described (21,26,27). Each of the 54 patients with cardiac disease had clinically or hemodynamically significant lesions and died suddenly, or of complications of surgery or cardiac catheterization, or of congestive heart failure. Certain demographic, clinical and morphologic data in patients with hypertrophic cardiomyopathy and control patients are summarized in Tables 2 and 3.

Table 1. Cardiac Disease in 68 Control Patients

	No. of Patients	No. With Abnormal IMCAs
Disease		
Coronary heart disease*	18	1
Aortic valvular disease	15†	2‡
Systemic hypertension	13	1
Dilated cardiomyopathy	8	0
Normal	14	2
Total	68	6

*Heart weight > 400 g. †Includes 11 patients with predominant or pure aortic stenosis as well as 2 with combined aortic stenosis and regurgitation, 1 with associated coronary heart disease and 1 with an associated atrial septal defect. ‡Includes one patient with combined aortic stenosis and atrial septal defect and one patient with aortic stenosis and associated coronary heart disease. IMCAs = intramural coronary arteries.

Preparation of tissue. Each of the 124 hearts utilized in this study (from 48 children or adults with hypertrophic cardiomyopathy, 8 infants with hypertrophic cardiomyopathy and 68 control subjects) was fixed in formalin. Tissue blocks were taken from the full thickness of the ventricular wall in a plane perpendicular to the long axis of the left ventricle (that is, a transverse plane), about half the distance between the aortic valve and left ventricular apex. Tissue sections were obtained from three locations: ventricular septum, anterior left ventricular free wall (about 2 cm lateral to the left anterior descending coronary artery) and posterior left ventricular free wall (between the papillary muscles) (Fig. 1) (28). Each tissue block was embedded in paraffin, sectioned at 6 μ and stained with Movat's pentachrome stain (29).

Analysis of intramural coronary arteries. Assessment of intramural coronary artery anatomy was confined to those arteries (<1,500 μ in diameter) that were viewed in cross section (transverse cut) without obvious obliquity and that did not appear to be branches of another intramural vessel, or portions of a "tunneled" epicardial vessel. Small coronary arteries in trabeculae or papillary muscles were excluded from analysis.

The extent to which abnormal intramural coronary arteries occurred in each tissue section was graded semiquantitatively based on the number of abnormal arteries and on an estimation of the degree of wall thickening and luminal narrowing. The grading system used to express the magnitude of these abnormalities was as follows. First, the *frequency* of altered arteries in a tissue section was assessed and numeric values of 0.5 to 9.5 were assigned to reflect the number of abnormal intramural coronary arteries identified. Sections with only a single altered intramural coronary artery were not considered abnormal. Second, for each intramural coronary artery judged to be abnormal the *severity* of wall thickening and apparent luminal narrowing was graded qualitatively as mild (1+), moderate (2+) or severe (3+). Grades for frequency and severity were then averaged to yield an overall assessment of abnormal intramural coronary artery morphology for each section. These values were then summed for all three tissue sections taken from each patient, giving an overall "abnormal intramural coronary artery tissue section grade."

Prior knowledge of whether or not tissue sections studied were from patients with hypertrophic cardiomyopathy or control patients was usually unavoidable because particularly large tissue section size or the presence of marked cardiac muscle cell disorganization suggested the presence of hypertrophic cardiomyopathy.

Analysis of myocardial fibrosis. The extent of fibrous tissue formation was assessed qualitatively in each tissue section: 0 (none), 1+ (mild), 2+ (moderate) and 3+ (severe). Mild fibrosis was judged to be present when an isolated small scar or interstitial fibrous tissue formation, or both, was identified; severe fibrosis was characterized by extensive replacement scarring occupying substantial portions of the section. Moderate fibrosis consisted of degrees of replacement scarring intermediate in extent between that observed with the mild and severe grades. Transmural infarction was defined as involving at least the inner two-thirds of the ventricular wall.

Measurement of tissue section area. The area of each of the 348 tissue sections analyzed in this study was calculated using a previously described method (30). The boundaries of each section (exclusive of trabeculae and papillary muscles) were traced on ordinary tablet paper with a fine point marking pen and the area was then measured (in square centimeters) utilizing a video planimeter.

Clinical features. Of the 48 patients with hypertrophic cardiomyopathy, 26 died suddenly and unexpectedly; 9 died from progressive congestive heart failure, 10 died at operation and 1 each died from cerebrovascular accident, complications of cardiac catheterization and suicide. Sixteen patients (34%) had been asymptomatic or minimally symptomatic; the remaining 32 (66%) had experienced substantial functional limitation, including 10 with moderate symptoms (New York Heart Association functional class II) and 22 with marked symptoms (class III or IV). Nineteen (40%) of the 48 patients had chest pain.

Of 33 patients having cardiac catheterization, 18 had a subaortic gradient of 30 mm Hg or more under basal conditions (40 to 160 mm Hg; average 88), and the remaining 15 patients had zero basal gradient or a small gradient of 15 mm Hg or less. Of the latter 15 patients, 10 had provocative maneuvers performed in the cardiac catheterization laboratory (Valsalva maneuver, isoproterenol infusion or amyl nitrite inhalation), which induced a gradient of 20 mm Hg or less in 8 patients and 50 mm Hg or more in the other 2. Five other patients with no or a small gradient at rest did not have provocative maneuvers performed.

The eight infants with hypertrophic cardiomyopathy ranged in age at the time of death from stillborn to 11 months (mean 4 months); six were male and two were female. Of the seven live-born infants, four died of progressive congestive heart failure, one died suddenly and two died postoperatively.

Interobserver variation. To assess interobserver variability in the identification of abnormal intramural coronary arteries, 36 tissue sections (12 each of ventricular septum, anterior and posterior free wall) from 12 study patients (10 with hypertrophic cardiomyopathy and 2 with other cardiac diseases) were analyzed independently by two observers. Each investigator determined whether or not individual tissue sections showed two or more abnormal arteries.

Statistical methods. Data were expressed as the mean ± SEM. Differences between means were assessed with the Student's *t* test. Differences between proportions were evaluated with the chi-square test.

Results

Histologic features of abnormal intramural coronary arteries. Compared with normal intramural coronary arteries (Fig. 2), abnormal arteries were characterized by increased size and thickened walls (Fig. 3 to 6); usually the lumen was narrowed, although some of these arteries had a normal-sized or apparently dilated lumen. Thickening of the arterial wall was due to proliferation of medial or intimal components, particularly smooth muscle cells and collagen. Also, increased numbers of elastic fibers were often present in the intima, and mucoid deposits (acid mucopolysaccharide) were occasionally identified in the intima or media. In some arteries isolated intimal proliferation was localized to only a portion of the luminal circumference. The internal elastic membrane was frequently distorted or obscured, making it difficult or impossible to discern the relative contribution of the intima or media to thickening of the arterial wall.

Control patients. Of the 68 control patients with a normal heart or cardiac disease other than hypertrophic cardiomyopathy, 6 (9%) had abnormal intramural coronary arteries present in at least one tissue section, including ventricular septum (5 patients) or posterior free wall (1 patient) (Fig. 7 and 8). Therefore, abnormal arteries were present in only 6 (3%) of the 204 individual tissue sections analyzed, and were most common in the ventricular septum. The remaining 62 (91%) patients did not show altered intramural arteries in any of the tissue sections examined.

A total of 15 abnormal intramural coronary arteries were identified in the 204 sections, an average of 0.1 ± 0.05/section and 0.04 ± 0.02/cm^2 of myocardium analyzed (Table 4). The maximal number of abnormal arteries present in any single section was three.

Altered intramural coronary arteries ranged in external diameter from 90 to 390 μ (mean 215). Most abnormal arteries (13 [87%] of 15) were midly or moderately narrowed with localized or modest intimal or medial thickening; only 2 (13%) of 15 were considered to be markedly thickened and appeared narrowed. The overall abnormal intramural coronary artery tissue section grade, reflecting the frequency and severity of arterial abnormalities for combined ventricular septum and free wall, was 0.08 ± 0.03 (Fig. 9; Table 4).

Patients with hypertrophic cardiomyopathy. Of the 48 patients with hypertrophic cardiomyopathy, 40 (83%) had abnormal intramural coronary arteries in at least one

Table 2. Clinical and Morphologic Data in 48 Patients With Hypertrophic Cardiomyopathy

Case	Age (yr) & Sex	Mode of Death	CP	FC	LVOT PSG (mm Hg) Rest	LVOT PSG (mm Hg) Prov.	HW (g)	VS (mm)	PW (mm)	VS/PW
1	11F	SD	0	1	—	—	400	17	9	1.9
2	12M	SD	0	1	—	—	270	18	10	1.8
3	13M	CHF	0	3	15	50	520	23	17	1.3
4	13M	SD	0	1	—	—	450	21	14	1.5
5	14M	SD	0	1	15	—	360	18	12	1.5
6	15F	SD	0	1	55	115	400	38	16	2.6
7	15F	SD	0	1	—	—	320	22	11	2.0
8	15M	SD	0	1	—	—	650	35	18	1.9
9	17M	SD	0	1	—	—	370	27	13	2.1
10	17M	SD	0	1	—	—	530	21	12	1.8
11	19F	SD	+	2	40	—	320	24	15	1.6
12	19F	Op	+	3	160	—	730	28	25	1.1
13	20F	CHF	+	2	40	55	1,250	42	10	4.2
14	20M	SD	0	1	—	—	630	33	20	1.7
15	21F	Op	+	3	80	100	390	29	15	1.9
16	21F	SD	0	1	—	—	400	24	9	2.7
17	22M	SD	0	1	—	—	500	21	13	1.6
18	23M	SD	0	1	0	—	500	20	15	1.3
19	23M	SD	0	1	—	—	750	30	15	2.0
20	24F	SD	0	2	—	—	720	44	26	1.7
21	24F	CVA	0	2	0	—	385	24	11	2.2
22	25F	Op	+	3	0	0	400	25	15	1.7
23	26F	SD	+	2	65	—	500	23	14	1.6
24	26F	CHF	0	3	10	—	390	22	16	1.4
25	27F	SD	+	3	100	—	640	33	20	1.6
26	27M	Op	+	3	70	—	950	34	27	1.3
27	27F	Cath	+	2	130	—	490	30	19	1.6
28	28F	Op	+	3	80	—	580	28	17	1.6
29	29M	SD	0	4#	0	0	450	25	12	2.1
30	30F	SD	0	1	—	—	445	17	15	1.1
31	30F	CHF	+	2	0	20	525	17	21	0.8
32	33M	SD	+	2	0	15	1,020	34	25	1.4
33	33F	CHF	+	4	0	10	430	27	13	2.1
34	33M	CHF	+	3	0	0	580	15	15	1.0
35	33F	SD	0	2	120	—	550	35	19	1.8
36	35F	SD	+	3	100	—	620	36	25	1.4
37	37M	Op	+	3	65	160	680	27	18	1.5
38	38M	SD	+	3	0	0	560	25	15	1.7
39	38M	SD	0	2	85	130	600	26	21	1.2
40	41F	Op	0	4	0	—	530	25	16	1.6
41	41M	Op	0	3	15	100	700	27	17	1.6
42	43F	SD	0	1	—	—	300	18	11	1.6
43	43F	CHF	0	4	55	75	310	18	16	1.1
44	50F	Su	+	3	130	—	450	20	19	1.1
45	50F	CHF	0	3	0	5	550	15	10	1.5
46	53M	Op	0	3	110	140	800	32	18	1.8
47	59F	Op	+	3	100	—	610	23	23	1.0
48	60M	CHF	0	4	—	—	530	16	12	1.3

*Denotes number of abnormal intramural coronary arteries per tissue section. †Qualitative assessment (1+ to 3+) of the degree of wall thickening and luminal narrowing in all abnormal intramural coronary arteries in the tissue section (with 1+ the most mild and 3+ the most severe). ‡Mean external diameter of all abnormal intramural coronary arteries in the tissue section. §Qualitative assessment (1+ to 3+) of the degree and extent of fibrosis observed in the tissue section; mild (1+) fibrosis was judged to be present when an isolated small scar or interstitial fibrous tissue formation, or both, was identified; severe (3+) fibrosis was characterized by extensive replacement scarring occupying substantial portions of the section; moderate (2+) fibrosis consisted of degrees of replacement scarring intermediate in extent between that observed with the mild or severe grades. ‖"Tissue section grade" (TSG) is a numeric expression of the frequency and severity of abnormal intramural coronary arteries in combined ventricular septal and free wall tissue

Table 2. *(continued)*

Abnormal Intramural Coronary Arteries																
Ventricular Septum				Anterior LVFW				Posterior LVFW				Overall
No.*	S†(0 to 3+)	D‡(μ)	Fi§	No.*	S†(0 to 3+)	D‡(μ)	F§	No.*	S†(0 to 3+)	D‡(μ)	Fi§	TSG‖
2	2+	315	1+	2	2+	355	1+	0	0	0	0	2.35
12	2+	370	2+	4	1+	215	1+	0	0	0	1+	3.35
4	2+	335	3+	0	0	0	1+	0	0	0	0	1.40
2	2+	700	1+	0	0	0	0	0	0	0	0	1.30
4	2+	410	2+	0	0	0	1+	0	0	0	0	1.30
0	0	240	1+	3	3+	355	1+	0	0	0	1+	1.60
0	0	0	1+	0	0	0	0	0	0	0	0	0
7	1+	300	3+	4	3+	580	2+	0	0	0	1+	3.35
5	2+	350	2+	2	1+	150	1+	0	0	0	1+	2.25
0	0	0	1+	0	0	0	1+	0	0	0	0	0
2	1+	305	1+	0	0	0	0	2	1+	185	1+	1.60
2	3+	370	1+	2	1+	270	1+	0	0	0	2+	2.15
5	1+	155	3+**	3	1+	175	3+	6	1+	225	3+	3.75
15	2+	455	1+	0	0	0	0	0	0	0	1+	2.75
0	0	0	1+	0	0	0	1+	0	0	0	0	0
10	2+	395	2+	2	2+	400	1+	2	1+	140	1+	4.10
0	0	0	1+	0	0	0	1+	2	2+	240	0	1.30
0	0	0	0	0	0	0	0	2	1+	295	0	0.80
0	0	0	1+	0	0	0	1+	0	0	0	2+	0
0	0	0	1+	2	2+	205	1+	0	0	0	1+	1.05
18	2+	250	3+	3	2+	205	2+	4	2+	360	2+	5.90
6	2+	360	2+	5	2+	205	2+	3	1+	225	1+	4.25
4	1+	290	1+	0	0	0	0	0	0	0	0	1.05
2	1+	305	2+	0	0	0	0	0	0	0	1+	0.80
50	3+	290	3+**	0	0	0	2+	0	0	0	1+	6.50
3	2+	295	0	4	2+	195	3+	0	0	0	2+	2.70
0	0	0	1+	0	0	0	2+	0	0	0	1+	0
0	0	0	2+	0	0	0	1+	0	0	0	0	0
3	1+	205	1+	0	0	0	0	0	0	0	0	0.95
0	0	0	0	5	1+	200	1+	0	0	0	0	1.40
4	2+	230	3+**	2	2+	230	3+	0	0	0	1+	1.75
3	2+	355	2+	2	2+	475	3+	0	0	0	1+	2.50
16	2+	360	3+	0	0	0	3+	0	0	0	1+	2.00
76	3+	345	3+**	0	0	0	2+	0	0	0	1+	9.25
0	0	0	2+	0	0	0	1+	0	0	0	1+	0
4	2+	295	1+	0	0	0	1+	0	0	0	1+	1.30
0	0	0	0	8	1+	100	0	0	0	0	1+	1.50
4	2+	145	1+	7	2+	160	3+**	0	0	0	1+	3.10
7	1+	255	1+	0	0	0	1+	0	0	0	1+	1.55
7	2+	215	3+**	0	0	0	2+	0	0	0	1+	1.76
0	0	0	0	3	2+	360	0	0	0	0	1+	1.30
8	2+	325	1+	0	0	0	1+	0	0	0	0	1.95
3	1+	315	2+	3	1+	270	2+	0	0	0	1−	2.05
3	2+	190	1+	0	0	0	0	0	0	0	1−	1.30
22	2+	370	3+**	0	0	0	2+	5	2+	355	2+	4.90
4	1+	360	1+	7	1+	180	0	2	1+	180	0	3.55
0	0	0	0	0	0	0	0	0	0	0	1+	0
15	2+	245	3+**	0	0	0	1+	0	0	0	1+	2.80

sections for each patient (see text for details). #Assigned to functional class IV by virtue of experiencing and surviving an episode of cardiovascular collapse (associated with documented ventricular fibrillation) 8 months before his sudden death. **Replacement fibrosis is transmural. Cath = cardiac catheterization; CHF = congestive heart failure; CP = chest pain; CVA = cerebrovascular accident; D = (external) diameter; F = female; FC = functional class; Fi = fibrosis; HW = heart weight; IMCA = intramural coronary artery; LVFW = left ventricular free wall; LVOT = left ventricular outflow tract; M = male; Op = operation; Prov. = provokable; PSG = peak systolic gradient; PW = posterior left ventricular free wall thickness; S = severity; SD = sudden death; Su = suicide; TSG = tissue section grade; VS = ventricular septal thickness; + = present; 0 = absent.

Table 3. Demographic, Clinical and Morphologic Data in 48 Patients with Hypertrophic Cardiomyopathy and 68 Control Patients*

	No. Patients	Age at Death (yr)	Sex (% male)	VS† (mm)	PW† (mm)	VS/PW	No. (%) With Abnormal IMCAs	Heart weight (g)
Hypertrophic cardiomyopathy	48‡	29 (11 to 60)	44	26 (15 to 44)	16 (9 to 26)	1.7 (0.8 to 4.2)	40/48 (83%)	542 (270 to 1,250)
Controls	68	48 (13 to 80)	69	16 (10 to 34)	15 (9 to 23)	1.1 (0.8 to 2.0)	6/68 (9%)	526 (250 to 900)
p Value		<0.001		<0.001	NS	<0.001	<0.001	NS

*Data presented as mean and range, where applicable. †Ventricular septal measurements were made at the point of maximal thickness, usually about half the distance between the aortic valve and left ventricular apex. Left ventricular posterior wall measurements were taken behind the midpoint of the posterior mitral leaflet, at a level corresponding to the tips of the mitral leaflets; trabeculae, papillary muscles and crista supraventricularis muscle were, by convention, excluded from these measurements. ‡Does not include eight infants with hypertrophic cardiomyopathy who were analyzed separately; ventricular septal thicknesses were 8 to 30 mm (mean 16), posterior free wall thicknesses were 3 to 15 mm (mean 9) and septal-free wall ratios were 1.4 to 2.7 (mean 1.9). IMCAs = intramural coronary arteries; NS = nonsignificant; PW = posterior left ventricular free wall; VS = ventricular septum; VS/PW = ventricular septal to free wall thickness ratio.

tissue section; hence, the prevalence of abnormal sections was significantly greater in the patients with hypertrophic cardiomyopathy than in control patients (83 versus 9%; $p < 0.001$) (Fig. 7). In patients with hypertrophic cardiomyopathy, altered intramural coronary arteries were identified in the ventricular septum (33 patients), anterior free wall (20 patients) or posterior free wall (9 patients) (Table 2; Fig. 8). Therefore, abnormal arteries were present in 62 (43%) of the 144 individual tissue sections analyzed and most commonly appeared in ventricular septum. Of the 40 patients with abnormal intramural coronary arteries, such vessels were identified in one of the three tissue sections in 23 patients, in two sections in 12 patients and in all three sections in only 5 patients.

A total of 433 abnormal intramural coronary arteries were identified in the 144 tissue sections, an average of 3.0 $\pm$ 0.7/section and 0.9 $\pm$ 0.2/cm^2 of myocardium analyzed; their frequency was significantly greater in patients with hypertrophic cardiomyopathy than in control patients, ($p < 0.001$) (Table 4). The maximal number of altered arteries present in any single section was 76.

Occasionally, numerous abnormal intramural coronary arteries appeared in clusters, but the distribution of abnormal arteries throughout the tissue section showed no particular predilection for the subendocardial or subepicardial regions. There was no significant relation between the frequency of abnormal arteries and thickness of either ventricular septum ($r = 0.18$) or posterior free wall ($r = 0.43$).

Abnormal intramural coronary arteries in patients with hypertrophic cardiomyopathy were also larger (range 50 to 1,330 μ in external diameter; mean 300) (Table 2) than those in controls (90 to 390 μ; mean 215). Most altered arteries (288 [64%] of 452) were markedly thickened and usually narrowed, whereas the remainder (164 or 36%) were judged only mildly or moderately narrowed with mild or localized intimal or medial thickening.

The overall "abnormal intramural coronary artery tissue section grade" (for septum and free wall combined) was substantially greater in patients with hypertrophic cardio-

Figure 1. Section of left ventricle (LV) in the anteroposterior (transverse) plane about half the distance between base and apex, showing the location of the three tissue sections that were analyzed quantitatively in each study patient. LVFW = left ventricular free wall; RV = right ventricle.

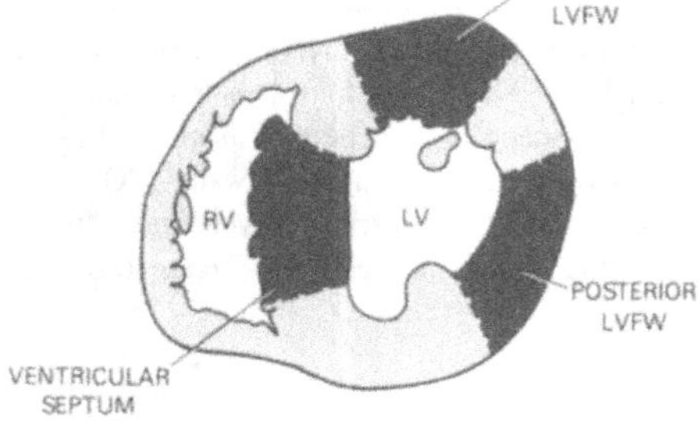

Figure 2. Normal intramural coronary artery in the ventricular septum. The internal elastic membrane (IEM) is well visualized adjacent to the sizeable lumen. Original magnification ×220, reduced by 26%.

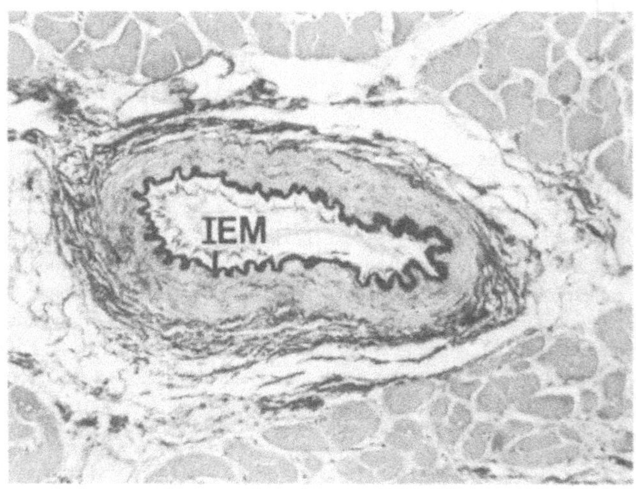

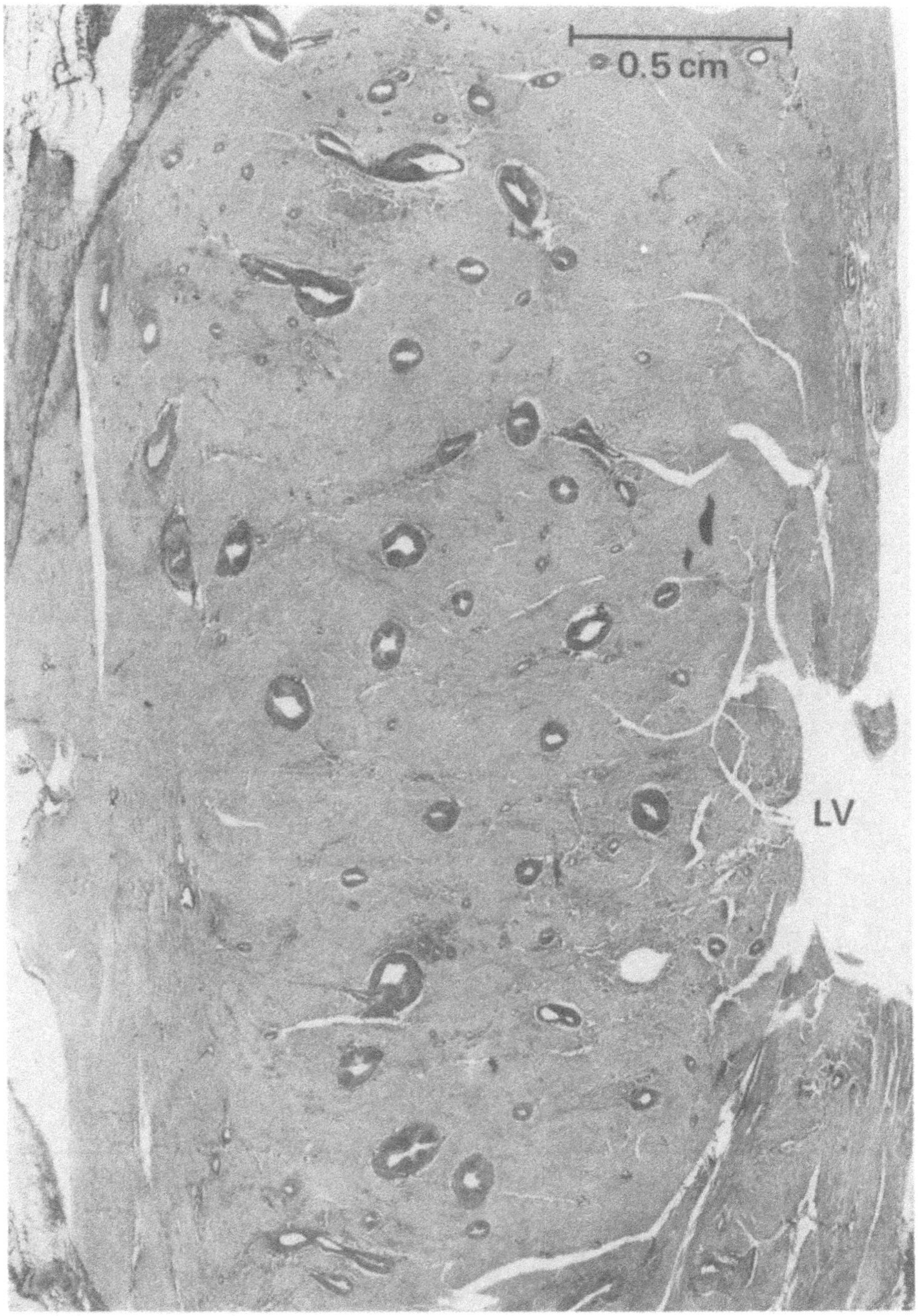

Figure 3. Portion of ventricular septum from a patient with hypertrophic cardiomyopathy. Numerous abnormal intramural coronary arteries are present; most are larger than normal and have a thicker wall than normal and a small lumen. This patient is not included in the present study group because she died more than 1 month after the septal myotomy-myectomy operation. Original magnification ×5, reduced by 26%. LV = left ventricular cavity.

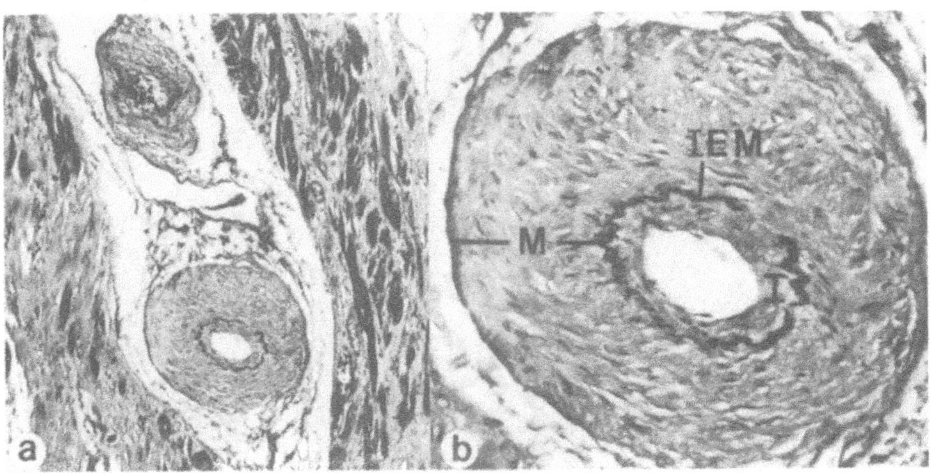

Figure 4. a, A single large abnormal intramural coronary artery is seen in an interstitial space of the left ventricular free wall. Original magnification ×100. **b**, The same vessel at higher magnification (×350). The wall thickening is due primarily to proliferation of medial (M) components, although the intima (I) is also mildly thickened. The internal elastic membrane (IEM) is well defined. Both panels reduced by 26%.

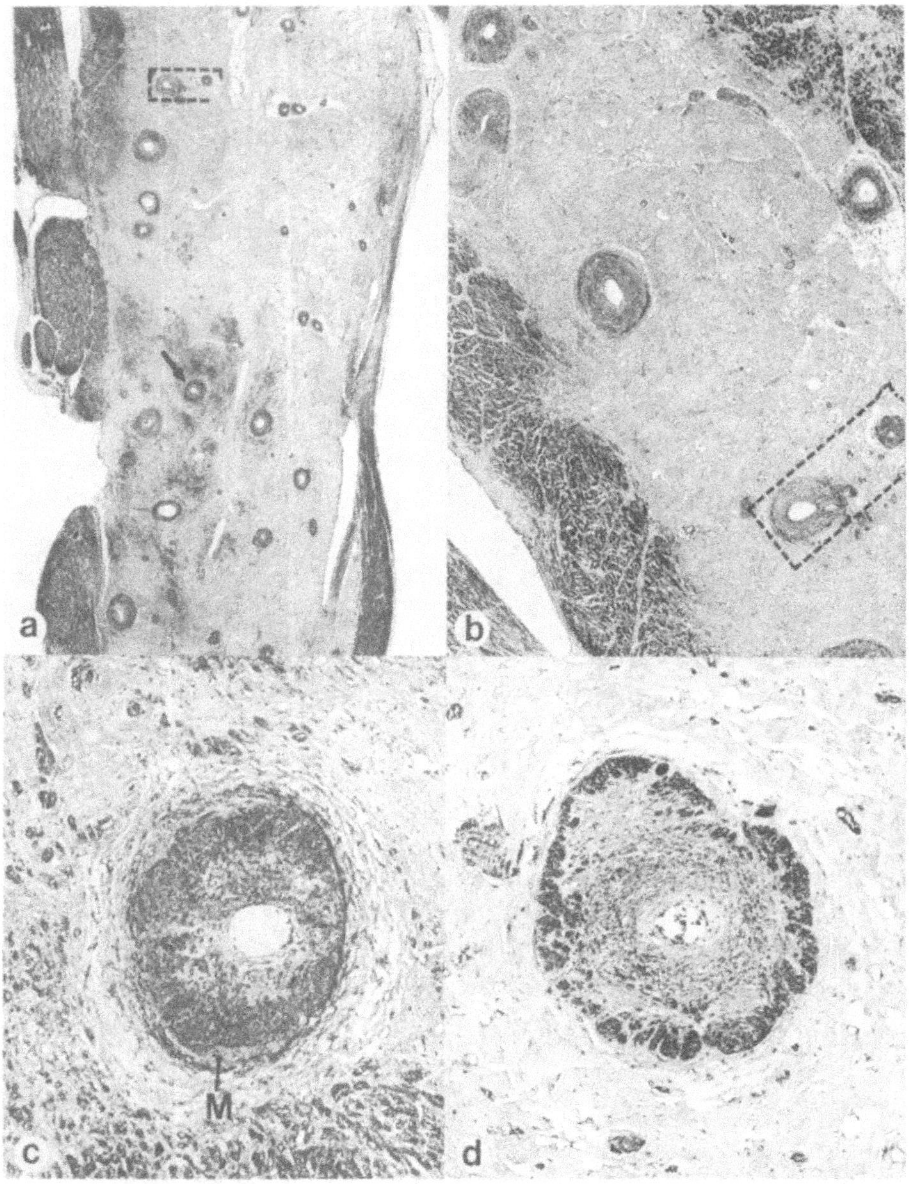

Figure 5. Four photomicrographs (**a** to **d**) showing substantial replacement scarring of the ventricular septum and abnormal intramural coronary arteries. **a**, Low power view showing transmural scarring of the septum and numerous altered intramural coronary arteries; some intramural coronary arteries have a thickened wall and narrowed lumen. Original magnification ×8. **b**, Higher power view of the septum shown in **a**; the two intramural coronary arteries within the **box** are indicated in a similar fashion in **a**. Original magnification ×20. **c**, High power micrograph of an abnormal intramural coronary artery surrounded by fibrous tissue that is designated by the **arrow** in **a**; luminal narrowing is due primarily to proliferation of intimal smooth muscle; the small medial (M) layer is evident at the periphery. Original magnification ×100. **d**, Abnormal intramural coronary artery in which luminal narrowing is due primarily to medial fibrous tissue proliferation. Original magnification ×100. All reduced by 26%.

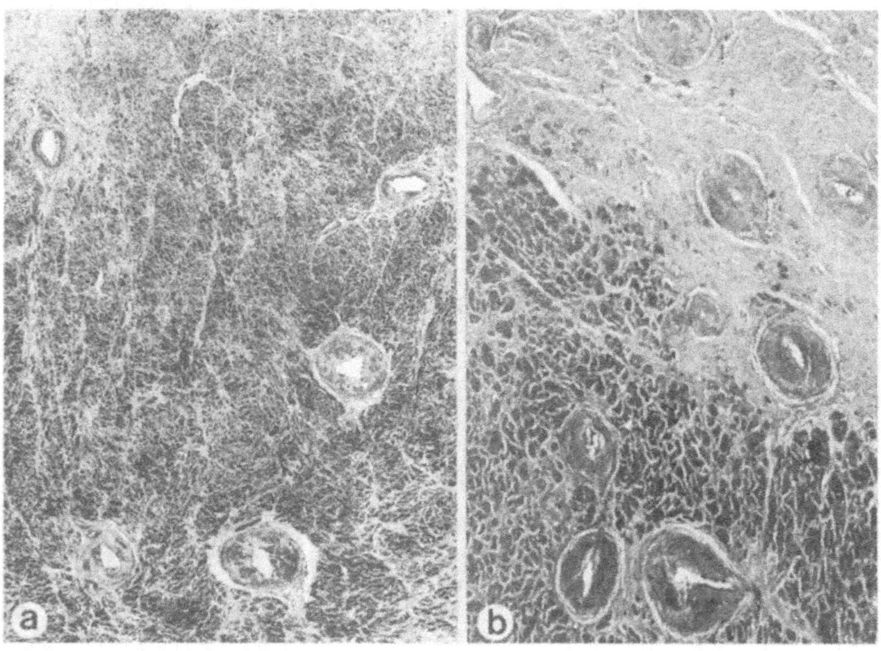

Figure 6. **a**, A portion of ventricular septum with only small patchy areas of fibrosis. Abnormal intramural coronary arteries are present in or near both scarred and nonscarred areas. Original magnification ×20. **b**, Area of left ventricular free wall in which numerous abnormal intramural coronary arteries are present in a region of scarring, as well as in an adjacent area of myocardium that is not scarred. Original magnification ×55. Both reduced by 26%.

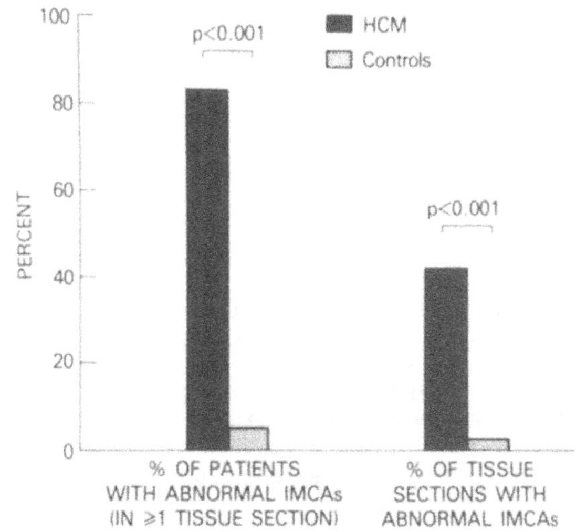

Figure 7. Prevalence of abnormal intramural coronary arteries (IMCAs) in patients with hypertrophic cardiomyopathy (HCM) and control subjects, and in tissue sections from these two groups of patients.

myopathy (2.1 ± 0.1) than in control patients (0.08 ± 0.03; $p < 0.001$) (Fig. 9; Table 3). Furthermore, in patients with hypertrophic cardiomyopathy, the magnitude of intramural coronary artery abnormalities was significantly greater in the ventricular septum than in the anterior free wall and greater in the anterior free wall than in the posterior free wall (Fig. 9).

Abnormal intramural coronary arteries were identified in the ventricular septum from three of the eight infants with hypertrophic cardiomyopathy. In two of these three infants numerous altered arteries had moderate to marked thickening of the vessel wall and luminal narrowing; in the remaining infant, milder arterial abnormalities were identified. Fibrosis was not associated with the abnormal arteries in the three infants.

Relation between abnormal intramural coronary arteries and myocardial fibrosis. In the 48 patients with hypertrophic cardiomyopathy, myocardial scarring was absent or mild in 102 tissue sections and moderate to severe in 42 sections. Abnormal intramural coronary arteries were significantly more common in those tissue sections with moderate or severe fibrosis (31 [74%] of 42) than in sections with no or mild fibrosis (31 [30%] of 102; $p < 0.001$) (Fig. 10). The association between altered intramural arteries and fibrosis was most significant in ventricular septal sections; abnormal arteries were present in 19 (90%) of 21 septal sections with moderate to marked fibrosis, but in only 14 (52%) of 27 septal sections with no or mild fibrosis ($p < 0.025$). In 24 of the 31 sections in which abnormal intramural coronary arteries and substantial fibrosis were present, a particularly close association between the two was apparent, with abnormal arteries located either within or at the margins of areas of replacement fibrosis (Fig. 5 and 6).

Transmural scarring was present in tissue sections from eight patients, including ventricular septum in seven and anterior free wall in one. In each of these sections, clusters of large numbers of abnormal intramural coronary arteries were present either within or adjacent to the scar (Fig. 5 and 6). Most of these arteries had a small, narrowed lumen, although in occasional vessels the arterial lumen appeared normal or even dilated. The relation between abnormal intramural arteries and myocardial fibrosis was not influenced by the age or sex of the patient. Of the six tissue sections with abnormal intramural coronary arteries in the control group, only one showed moderate fibrosis, while the remainder had either no or mild fibrosis.

Correlation of abnormal intramural coronary arteries with other clinical or morphologic findings. Various clinical, hemodynamic and morphologic findings in the 48 patients with hypertrophic cardiomyopathy were correlated with the prevalence and severity of abnormal intramural coronary arteries. There was no correlation between the occurrence or magnitude of intramural coronary artery abnormalities and age of the patient, sex distribution, presence or absence or severity of symptoms, mode of death (sudden versus chronic decompensation), left ventricular end-diastolic pressure, heart weight, ventricular septal thickness or septal to free wall thickness ratio. Although there was no statistically significant relation between the presence, absence or magnitude of left ventricular outflow obstruction and small artery abnormalities (in the 32 patients who underwent cardiac catheterization), the abnormal intramural coronary artery tissue section grade in patients with nonobstructive hypertrophic cardiomyopathy (2.8 ± 0.6) tended to exceed that of patients with obstructive hypertrophic cardiomyopathy (1.6 ± 0.4; $p < 0.2$). Altered arteries were present in each of the 15 patients with nonobstructive hy-

Figure 8. Distribution of abnormal intramural coronary arteries (IMCAs) in the left ventricle (LV) of patients with hypertrophic cardiomyopathy (HCM) and control subjects. ANT. FW = anterior free wall; POST. FW = posterior free wall; VS = ventricular septum.

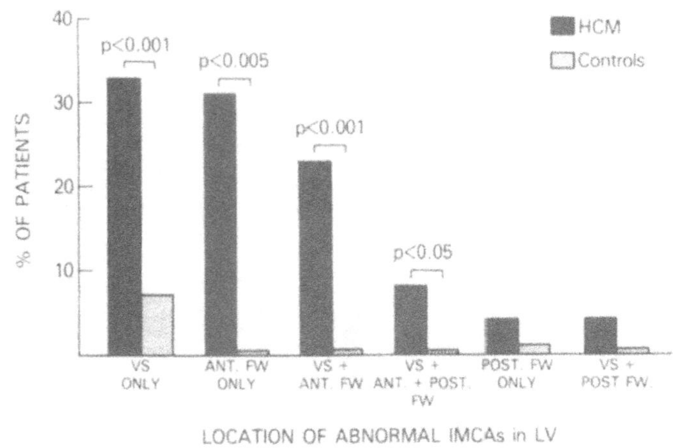

Table 4. Frequency of Abnormal Intramural Coronary Arteries in Patients With Hypertrophic Cardiomyopathy and Control Subjects

	Hypertrophic Cardiomyopathy	Control Group
No. of patients	48	68
Total no. of abnormal IMCAs	433	15
Avg. no. of abnormal IMCAs/tissue section	3.0 ± 0.7*	0.1 ± 0.05*
Maximal no. of abnormal IMCAs/tissue section	76	3
Avg. tissue section area (cm^2)†	3.5 ± 0.2*	2.3 ± 0.1*
Avg. no. of abnormal IMCAs/cm^2 of myocardium‡	0.9 ± 0.2*	0.04 ± 0.02*
IMCA tissue section grade§	2.1 ± 0.1*	0.08 ± 0.03*

*Comparison of these variables in patients with hypertrophic cardiomyopathy and control patients achieved statistical significance, $p < 0.001$. †Expressed here for ventricular septum, anterior free wall and posterior free wall combined. ‡Analysis of only those tissue sections with abnormal intramural coronary arteries. §Reflects the frequency as well as the severity of abnormal intramural coronary arteries; data presented here combine ventricular septal and both free wall tissue sections in each patient (see text for details). Avg. = average; IMCAs = intramural coronary arteries.

pertrophic cardiomyopathy and in 12 of 17 patients with obstructive hypertrophic cardiomyopathy.

Of the 48 patients with hypertrophic cardiomyopathy, 19 had experienced clinically significant and recurrent episodes of chest pain. Of these 19 patients, 15 (79%) had abnormal intramural coronary arteries in at least one tissue section; however, these altered arteries were also commonly identified in patients without chest pain (25 [86%] of 29). Furthermore, there was no relation between the occurrence of chest pain and the extent of myocardial fibrosis; chest pain was present in 12 (63%) of 19 patients with moderate to marked fibrosis and in 14 (48%) of 29 patients with no or mild fibrosis.

Interobserver variation. There was agreement between two observers with regard to the presence or absence of abnormal intramural arteries in 88% of observations (32 of 36 tissue sections analyzed).

Discussion

Occurrence and pathogenesis of abnormal intramural coronary arteries in hypertrophic cardiomyopathy. The findings of this study demonstrate that many patients (over 80%) with hypertrophic cardiomyopathy have structural abnormalities of the intramural coronary arteries. There was great variation in the magnitude of these abnormalities, which were striking in some patients and relatively mild in others. Altered intramural coronary arteries were most common in the ventricular septum, but were also frequently identified in the anterior or posterior left ventricular free wall. These

Figure 9. Semiquantitative expression of magnitude of intramural coronary artery (IMCAs) abnormalities in the 48 patients with hypertrophic cardiomyopathy (HCM) and 68 control patients. Tissue section grade utilized here takes into account both the *frequency* of abnormal intramural coronary arteries and the apparent *severity* of wall thickening and luminal narrowing (see text for details).

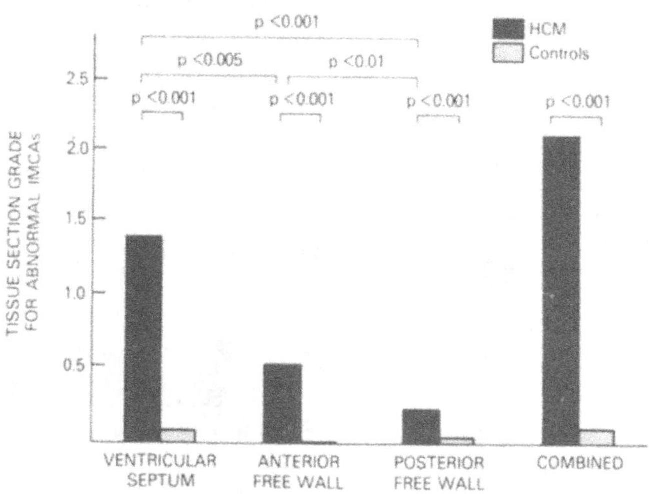

Figure 10. Relation between occurrence of abnormal intramural coronary arteries (IMCAs) and myocardial fibrosis in 144 tissue sections obtained from the ventricular septum and anterior and posterior left ventricular free walls in 48 patients with hypertrophic cardiomyopathy. Marked fibrosis includes those tissue sections graded as moderate or severe.

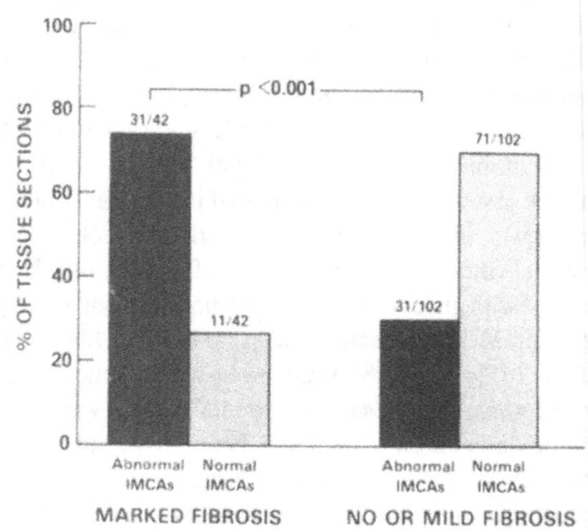

findings of abnormal intramural coronary arteries in hypertrophic cardiomyopathy are similar to those described in several patients by James and Marshall (22). The present study extends their observations, however, because our results allow a quantitative assessment of the prevalence, distribution and severity of these abnormal intramural coronary arteries in patients who died of hypertrophic cardiomyopathy, as well as in control patients with a variety of other cardiac diseases.

Our findings indicate that the presence of abnormal intramural coronary arteries is not unique for hypertrophic cardiomyopathy; such vessels were also present in a few control patients with a variety of cardiac diseases characterized by left ventricular hypertrophy. However, the altered intramural coronary arteries identified in our control patients were much less frequent and less severe than those observed in patients with hypertrophic cardiomyopathy. In particular, their prevalence was much lower in patients with systemic hypertension and in patients with valvular aortic stenosis. Because these latter diseases lead to a pressure load on the left ventricular myocardium, this finding indicates that myocardial wall stress alone is not sufficient to produce these abnormal intramural arteries in the frequency with which they are found in hypertrophic cardiomyopathy. In addition, our observations that intramural coronary artery abnormalities were equally severe in patients with and without left ventricular outflow obstruction and the lack of relation between left ventricular wall thickness and frequency or location of abnormal intramural coronary arteries, further substantiate the conclusion that these abnormal arteries are not solely related to elevated intramyocardial wall tension. Although we have no definitive data that define the pathogenesis of the abnormal intramural coronary arteries present in most patients with hypertrophic cardiomyopathy, the fact that these altered arteries cannot be ascribed to high ventricular pressures suggests that they may constitute an independent marker of hypertrophic cardiomyopathy and a component of the cardiomyopathic process, which may be present at birth (three of the eight infants with hypertrophic cardiomyopathy we studied had abnormal intramural coronary arteries). On the other hand, it is possible that in some patients these abnormal intramural arteries arise secondary to substantial or transmural fibrous tissue formation, as a form of neovascularization.

Abnormal intramural coronary arteries in other diseases. Previous investigators (26,27,31–37) have reported alterations in small left ventricular intramural coronary arteries (as well as in small arteries in the sinoatrial and atrioventricular nodes) similar to those described in this report. These observations, made primarily in patients with diseases *other than hypertrophic cardiomyopathy,* included systemic or metabolic diseases in which hypertrophy was absent or mild, such as diabetes mellitus (26), progressive muscular dystrophy (27), Friedreich's ataxia (27,31), scleroderma (32), homocystinuria (33) and the Marfan syndrome (27). Abnormal intramural coronary arteries have also been described in a diverse group of primary cardiovascular diseases with or without left ventricular hypertrophy such as tunnel subaortic stenosis (34), primary pulmonary hypertension (27), Newfoundland dogs (35,36) with discrete fibrous subaortic stenosis, newborns with aortic or pulmonic atresia (37) and the syndrome of congenital deafness, syncope and sudden death associated with QT interval prolongation (27). In addition, small arteries with similar morphologic features have been observed to be limited to the specialized sinoatrial or atrioventricular conduction tissue of apparently healthy young individuals (including competitive athletes) who died suddenly and either had left ventricular hypertrophy (38) or had no gross evidence of structural heart disease (39,40). Although none of these studies attempted to quantitate the frequency and severity of altered intramural coronary arteries, it is our impression (based on a review of the published papers) that these arteries occurred in relatively small numbers, and therefore did not constitute the widespread and potentially significant lesion that we observed in most patients with hypertrophic cardiomyopathy.

Considerations regarding control subjects. The control group assembled for this study was comprised of patients with a normal heart, dilated cardiomyopathy and acquired heart disease associated with increased left ventricular pressure, mass, or both (for example, systemic hypertension, aortic valve disease and coronary heart disease). Therefore, this particular control group was designed to reflect a population of adult patients with heart diseases that are relatively common in cardiologic practice. As a result, many of the congenital cardiac or systemic diseases in which abnormal intramural coronary arteries have occasionally been reported (as described earlier) are not represented. However, it was not our intention in this investigation to suggest that abnormal intramural coronary arteries are more common in hypertrophic cardiomyopathy than in *any* other cardiac or systemic disease. Our study design permits only an assessment of the relative frequency of these altered arteries in hypertrophic cardiomyopathy as compared with other common cardiac diseases associated with left ventricular hypertrophy.

Relation between abnormal intramural coronary arteries and myocardial fibrosis. In our study there was no clear relation between the presence of abnormal intramural coronary arteries and the clinical history of chest pain in patients with hypertrophic cardiomyopathy. Whereas about 80% of patients who had chest pain had altered intramural coronary arteries, about 85% of patients who had no chest pain also showed abnormal intramural coronary arteries. It is conceivable that this lack of specificity of abnormal intramural arteries for patients with chest pain may be due in part to the fact that clinical assessment of chest pain in a retrospective analysis such as ours is a difficult and subjective judgment. In addition, "silent" ischemia has now been well documented in patients with coronary artery disease (41), and there is no reason to assume that this phenomenon would be less common in hypertrophic cardiomyopathy. Most importantly, however, our study identified an important association between abnormal intramural coronary arteries and objectively determined evidence of severe prolonged ischemia, that is, myocardial fibrosis. Altered intramural coronary arteries were more commonly present near or within areas of substantial fibrosis, and clusters of increased numbers of these arteries were often identified in transmural scars. In our view, this finding suggests that the intramural coronary artery abnormalities identified in hypertrophic cardiomyopathy are of pathophysiologic significance. We hypothesize that abnormal narrowed small arteries compromise coronary blood flow, resulting in myocardial ischemia which, if prolonged and severe, produces myocardial necrosis and fibrous tissue formation.

Conclusions. The "small vessel" intramural coronary artery disease identified in this study (in patients with and without left ventricular outflow obstruction) constitutes a common morphologic component of the disease process in patients with hypertrophic cardiomyopathy. The presence of abnormal intramural coronary arteries in some infants who died of hypertrophic cardiomyopathy implies that these abnormal arteries may be present from birth as part of the developmental abnormality in hypertrophic cardiomyopathy. The association of altered intramural arteries with myocardial fibrosis suggests that these vessels may contribute to the formation of myocardial fibrosis.

References

1. Braunwald E, Morrow AG, Cornell WP, Aygen MM, Hilbish TF. Idiopathic hypertrophic subaortic stenosis. Am J Med 1960;29:924–45.
2. Goodwin JF, Hollman A, Cleland WP, Teare D. Obstructive cardiomyopathy simulating aortic stenosis. Br Heart J 1960;22:404–14.
3. Wigle ED, Heimbecker RO, Gunton RW. Idiopathic ventricular septal hypertrophy causing muscular subaortic stenosis. Circulation 1962;26:325–40.
4. Braunwald E, Lambrew CT, Rockoff SD, Ross J Jr, Morrow AG. Idiopathic hypertrophic subaortic stenosis. I. A description of the disease based upon an analysis of 64 patients. Circulation 1964;30(suppl IV):IV-217.
5. Henry WL, Clark CE, Epstein SE. Asymmetric septal hypertrophy (ASH): echocardiographic identification of the pathognomonic abnormality of IHSS. Circulation 1973;47:225–33.
6. Epstein SE, Henry WL, Clark CE, et al. Asymmetric septal hypertrophy. Ann Intern Med 1974;81:650–80.
7. Shah PM, Sylvester LJ. Echocardiography in the diagnosis of hypertrophic obstructive cardiomyopathy. Am J Med 1977;62:830–5.
8. Abbasi AS, MacAlpin RN, Eber LM, Pearce ML. Echocardiographic diagnosis of idiopathic hypertrophic cardiomyopathy without outflow obstruction. Circulation 1972;46:897–904.
9. Gilbert BW, Pollick C, Adelman AG, Wigle ED. Hypertrophic cardiomyopathy: subclassification by M-mode echocardiography. Am J Cardiol 1980;45:861–72.
10. Roberts WC, Ferrans VJ. Pathologic anatomy of the cardiomyopathies. Idiopathic dilated and hypertrophic types, infiltrative types and endomyocardial disease with and without eosinophilia. Human Pathol 1975;6:287–342.
11. Maron RJ, Gottdiener JS, Epstein SE. Patterns and significance of distribution of left ventricular hypertrophy in hypertrophic cardiomyopathy. A wide-angle, two-dimensional echocardiographic study of 125 patients. Am J Cardiol 1981;48:418–28.
12. St. John Sutton MG, Tajik AJ, Smith HC, Ritman EL. Angina in idiopathic hypertrophic suboartic stenosis. A clinical correlate of regional left ventricular dysfunction: a videometric and echocardiographic study. Circulation 1980;61:561–8.
13. Estes EH Jr, Whalen RE, Roberts SR Jr, McIntosh HD. The electrocardiographic and vectorcardiographic findings in idiopathic hypertrophic subaortic stenosis. Am Heart J 1963;65:155–61.
14. Braudo M, Wigle ED, Keith JD. Distinctive electrocardiogram in muscular subaortic stenosis due to ventricular septal hypertrophy. Am J Cardiol 1964;14:599–607.
15. Prescott R, Quinn JS, Littmann D. Electrocardiographic changes in hypertrophic subaortic stenosis which simulate myocardial infarction. Am Heart J 1963;66:43–8.
16. Maron BJ, Wolfson JK, Ciró E, Spirito P. Relation of electrocardiographic abnormalities and patterns of left ventricular hypertrophy identified by two-dimensional echocardiography in patients with hypertrophic cardiomyopathy. Am J Cardiol 1983;51:189–94.
17. Maron BJ, Epstein SE, Roberts WC. Hypertrophic cardiomyopathy and transmural myocardial infarction without significant atherosclerosis of the extramural coronary arteries. Am J Cardiol 1979;43:1086–102.
18. Pasternac A, Noble J, Streulens Y, Elie R, Henschke C, Bourassa MG. Pathophysiology of chest pain in patients with cardiomyopathies and normal coronary arteries. Circulation 1982;65:778–89.
19. Cannon RO, Rosing DR, Maron BJ, et al. Myocardial ischemia in hypertrophic cardiomyopathy: contribution of inadequate vasodilator reserve and elevated left ventricular filling pressures. Circulation 1985;71:234–43.
20. McReynolds RA, Roberts WC. The intramural coronary arteries in hypertrophic cardiomyopathy (abstr). Am J Cardiol 1975;35:154.
21. Roberts WC. Congenital cardiovascular abnormalities usually "silent" until adulthood: morphologic features of the floppy mitral valve, valvular aortic stenosis, hypertrophic cardiomyopathy, sinus of Valsalva aneurysm and the Marfan syndrome. Cardiovasc Clin 1979;10:407–53.
22. James TN, Marshall TK. De Subitaneis Mortibus. XII. Asymmetrical hypertrophy of the heart. Circulation 1975;51:1149–66.
23. Maron BJ, Epstein SE. Hypertrophic cardiomyopathy: a discussion of nomenclature. Am J Cardiol 1979;43:1242–4.
24. Maron BJ, Edwards JE, Henry WL, Clark CE, Bingle GJ, Epstein SE. Asymmetric septal hypertrophy (ASH) in infancy. Circulation 1974;50:809–20.
25. Maron BJ, Tajik AJ, Ruttenberg HD, et al. Hypertrophic cardiomyopathy in infants: clinical features and natural history. Circulation 1982;65:7–17.
26. James TN. Small arteries of the heart. Circulation 1977;56:2–14.
27. James TN. An etiologic concept concerning the obscure myocardiopathies. Prog Cardiovasc Dis 1964;7:43–64.
28. Maron BJ, Anan TJ, Roberts WC. Quantitative analysis of the distribution of cardiac muscle cell disorganization in the left ventricular wall of patients with hypertrophic cardiomyopathy. Circulation 1981;63:882–94.
29. Movat HZ. Demonstration of all connective tissue elements in a single section. Arch Pathol 1955;60:289–95.
30. Maron BJ, Roberts WC. Quantitative analysis of cardiac muscle cell disorganization in the ventricular septum of patients with hypertrophic cardiomyopathy. Circulation 1979;59:689–706.

31. James TN, Fisch C. Observations on the cardiovascular involvement in Friedreich's ataxia. Am Heart J 1963;66:164–75.

32. James TN. De Subitaneis Mortibus. VIII. Coronary arteries and conduction system in scleroderma heart disease. Circulation 1974;50:844–56.

33. James TN, Carson NAJ, Froggatt P. De Subitaneis Mortibus. IV. Coronary vessels and conduction system in homocystinuria. Circulation 1974;49:367–74.

34. Maron BJ, Redwood DR, Roberts WC, Henry WL, Morrow AG, Epstein SE. Tunnel subaortic stenosis. Left ventricular outflow tract obstruction produced by fibromuscular tubular narrowing. Circulation 1976;54:404–16.

35. Flickinger GL, Patterson DF. Coronary lesions associated with congenital subaortic stenosis in the dog. J Pathol Bacteriol 1967;93:133–40.

36. Muna WFT, Ferrans VJ, Pierce JE, Roberts WC. Discrete subaortic stenosis in Newfoundland dogs: association of infective endocarditis. Am J Cardiol 1978;41:746–54.

37. Bulkley BH, Weisfeldt ML, Hutchins GM. Isometric cardiac contraction. A possible cause of the disorganized myocardial pattern of idiopathic hypertrophic subaortic stenosis. N Engl J Med 1977; 296:135–9.

38. Maron BJ, Roberts WC, McAllister HA, Rosing DR. Epstein SE. Sudden death in young athletes. Circulation 1980;62:218–29.

39. James TN, Froggatt P, Marshall TK. Sudden death of young athletes. Ann Intern Med 1967;67:1013–21.

40. James TN, Marshall TK. De Subitaneis Mortibus. XVII. Multiple stenoses due to fibromuscular dysplasia of the sinus node artery. Circulation 1976;53:736–42.

41. Cohn PF. Silent myocardial ischemia in patients with a defective anginal warning system. Am J Cardiol 1980;45:697–702.

Regional Myocyte Hypertrophy and Increased Interstitial Myocardial Fibrosis in Hypertrophic Cardiomyopathy

DONALD V. UNVERFERTH, MD, PETER B. BAKER, MD, LEESA I. PEARCE, BS, JEFFREY LAUTMAN, BA, and WILLIAM C. ROBERTS, MD

The purpose of this study was to determine if the thickened cardiac walls of patients with hypertrophic cardiomyopathy (HC) are due to increased size or number of myocytes or increased amounts of fibrous tissue. Eight patients, aged 18 to 42 years, who died from complications of HC and 8 age-matched control subjects without heart disease were studied. A 1.5-cm³ block of tissue was removed from the left ventricular free wall, right ventricular free wall and ventricular septum (VS). Each region of each wall was evaluated for fibrous tissue by point counting; cell diameter was measured using an ocular micrometer disc. Cell layers were counted across the walls. The results revealed that increased cell size, cell layers and fibrous tissue are characteristic of HC, but only in the VS are all 3 significantly increased. The fibrous tissue was most extensive in the VS (19 ± 9%), but it was more extensive than in the control subjects in all 3 walls. Cell diameters were largest in the layers closest to the left ventricular cavity.

(Am J Cardiol 1987;59:932–936)

In patients with hypertrophic cardiomyopathy (HC), the right and left ventricular (RV and LV) free walls and the ventricular septum (VS) are thickened,[1-3] the amount of fibrous tissue between myocardial cells usually is increased and most cardiac myocytes are enlarged.[4-6] The amount of ventricular wall thickening produced by the increased amounts of fibrous tissue and by enlargement of the myocytes has not been determined. The present study attempts to determine how much of the wall thickening is due to fibrous tissue increase and how much to myocyte enlargement, and also if differences exist in the cardiac ventricular walls compared to the ventricular septum.

From the Division of Cardiology, Department of Medicine, and the Department of Pathology, Ohio State University College of Medicine, Columbus, Ohio, and the Pathology Branch, National Heart, Lung, and Blood Institute, National Institutes of Health, Bethesda, Maryland. This study supported in part by the Samuel J. Roessler Research Foundation, the Central Ohio Heart Chapter of the American Heart Association, and by the James D. Casto Research Fund, Columbus, Ohio. Manuscript received June 9, 1986; revised manuscript received October 27, 1986, accepted October 30, 1986.

Address for reprints: Donald V. Unverferth, MD, Ohio State University College of Medicine, 657 Means Hall, 1655 Upham Drive, Columbus, Ohio 43210.

Methods

Patient selection: Eight necropsy patients (3 women 5 men), aged 18 to 43 years (mean 30), were studied. Seven were studied clinically and all 8 at necropsy at the National Heart, Lung, and Blood Institute (Fig. 1 through 5). Six had 1 to 5 other family members who had HC. Seven of the 8 patients had died suddenly and unexpectedly outside the hospital; patient 8 died from an intracerebral hemorrhage secondary to warfarin therapy for atrial fibrillation. Sudden death was the first and only symptom of HC in patient 1. The other 7 patients had symptoms of cardiac dysfunction for 2 to 20 years. Of the 5 patients who had undergone cardiac catheterization, only 1 (patient 5) had LV outflow obstruction at rest or with provocation. Echocardiograms in 7 patients disclosed small or normal-sized LV cavities in all 7, ventricular septums thicker than LV free walls in 5 and absence of systolic anterior motion of the anterior mitral leaflet in all 7. All 8 patients had normal systemic arterial pressures. Only patient 5 had a thickened mitral valve or thickened mural endocardium in the LV outflow tract in apposition to the anterior mitral leaflet, and this was the only patient with documented LV outflow obstruction; absence of mural endocardial plaque in the LV outflow tract and absence of fibrous thickening of either mitral leaflet in the other 7 patients is anatomic evidence for the lack of

LV outflow obstruction in them. The heart at necropsy in the 3 women weighed 616, 460 and 490 g (mean 522) and in the 5 men from 540 to 610 g (mean 568). The VS was thicker than the LV free wall in 6 patients and thicknesses were similar in 2 patients. Four patients had grossly visible scars in the VS or LV free wall or both. None of the 8 patients had significant narrowing of any of the major epicardial coronary arteries. Histologic sections, however, showed abnormalities of many intramural coronary arteries in the VS in 5 patients and myofiber disorganization in the VS in 7. Eight age-matched control subjects died of head trauma. No control subject had a history of heart disease and none had gross or histologic morphologic cardiac abnormalities; all had normal coronary arteries.

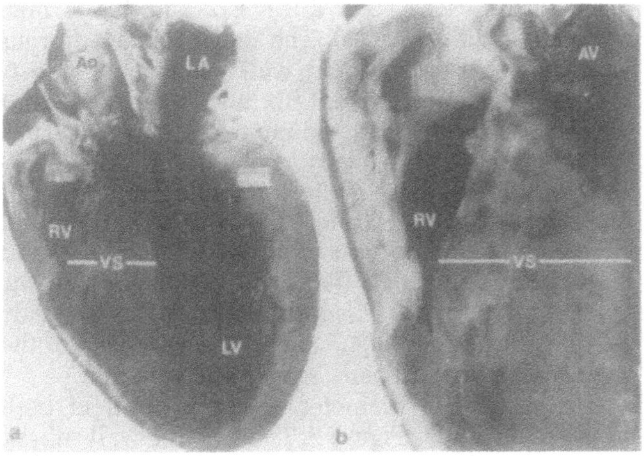

FIGURE 1. Patient 1. Heart from an 18-year-old boy (WBH #A84-8) who had cardiac arrest while jogging. He had had no previous symptoms of cardiac dysfunction. *a*, longitudinal view of heart showing the ventricular septum (VS) to be thicker than the left ventricular free wall. *b*, close-up of the thickened VS. Ao = aorta; AV = aortic valve; LA = left atrium; LV = left ventricle; RV = right ventricle.

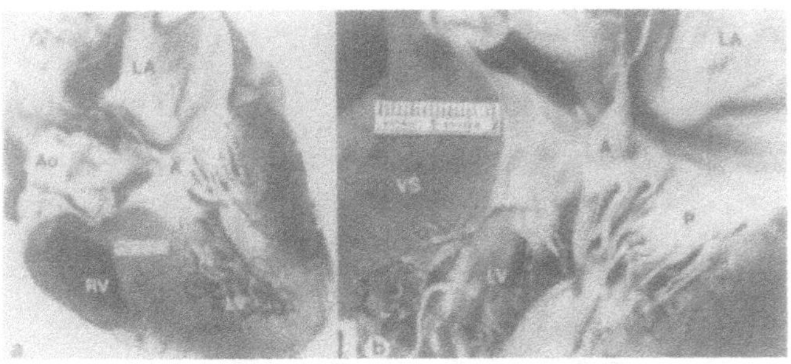

FIGURE 2. Patient 5. Heart from a 38-year-old man (MMH #A78-89) who had an 85-mm Hg peak systolic pressure gradient between the left ventricle and aorta (Ao) at rest. This was the only patient of the 8 to have documented left ventricular outflow obstruction. He had symptoms of cardiac dysfunction for 12 years and, periodically, runs of atrial tachycardia. He was found dead in his bed at home. *a*, longitudinal view of heart showing severe thickening of both ventricular septum (VS) and left ventricular free wall (LV). An endocardial mural plaque is present in apposition to the thickened anterior mitral leaflet (A). This mural plaque is the anatomic equivalent of systolic anterior motion of the anterior mitral leaflet and is indicative of a left ventricular output pressure gradient at some time. *b*, close-up of left ventricular outflow tract. This patient was the only one of the 8 with a left ventricular outflow mural plaque. LA = left atrium; P = posterior mitral leaflet; RV = right ventricle.

Tissue handling: Transmural blocks of tissue approximately 1.5 cm^2 at the wall surfaces were obtained from the LV free wall, RV free wall and VS (halfway between the aortic valve and the apex) and fixed in 10% formalin. Four transmural planes were sectioned from the block at orientations that allowed each layer of myocardial fibers to be examined in both cross and longitudinal sections. Routine light microscopic slides 3 to 5 μ thick were prepared from each of the paraffin-

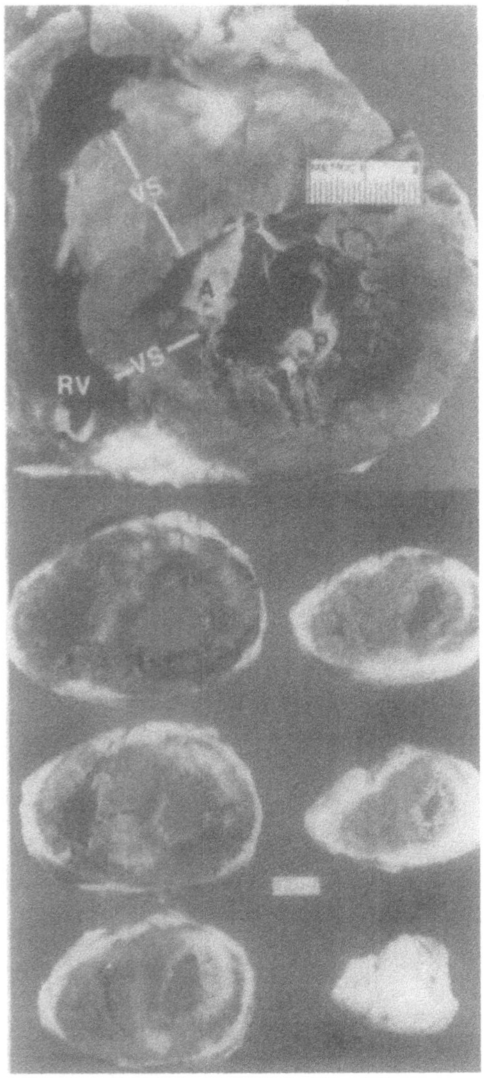

FIGURE 3. Patient 6. Heart from a 38-year-old man (YH #79-223-5) who had severe congestive heart failure for years and died suddenly while walking upstairs at home. At necropsy, the left ventricular free wall and ventricular septum (VS) were severely scarred. *a*, transverse view of the most basal portion of the left ventricle. The anterior portion of the VS is much thicker than the posterior half of the VS. *b*, transverse slices of the cardiac ventricles. The VS in the apical half of the slices is thicker than the VS in the more basal half of the slices. A = anterior mitral leaftlet; P = posterior mitral leaflet; RV = right ventricular cavity.

embedded sections. The slides were stained by hematoxylin-eosin and Masson's trichrome stains by the methods of Sheehan and Hrapchak.[7] Under a stereoscope the mounted sections of the LV free wall and VS were separated into fifths and the RV free wall was separated into thirds. Fibrous tissue was quantified in each area of each ventricular wall by the stereologic techniques of Weibel.[8] The amount of fibrous tissue in each area was quantified on the trichrome-stained slides by means of a grid of 243 cross-points laid on each area at a magnification of 400×. The number of cross-points lying on fibrosed areas was divided by the total number of cross-points evaluated to determine the percent of fibrous tissue per area. More than 2,000 points were evaluated for each area; 13 areas (5 from the LV free wall, 5 from the VS and 3 from the RV free wall) were evaluated for each patient.

Each area from each section was examined by a 43× objective lens and a 10× eyepiece with an ocular micrometer disc. The diameter of at least 100 cells from each area was determined by measuring the distance across the cell at its narrowest plane across the nucleus. The mean of these measurements was calculated. The measurements for each region inscribed a normal distribution. The techniques of determining cell diameter and extent of fibrosis have been previously described by our laboratory.[9]

In addition to myocyte diameter and percent fibrous tissue, cell layers were counted across each ventricular wall. Two lines perpendicular to the endocardial and epicardial surface were drawn across each of the tissue sections (8 lines per wall). The number of cells touching the line were counted and mean and standard deviations were recorded. The length of the lines was also measured.

Statistical analysis: The cell diameter data were compared between the heart failure and control subjects by the analysis of variance for nested data.[10] Fibrous tissue analysis required an arcsine transformation for the dependent variable. Wall level data were analyzed by repeated measures and Tukey's pairwise comparison procedure.[10]

Results

The mean widths (± SD) of the LV free wall, VS and RV free wall in the HC group were 13 ± 2, 22 ± 4 and 5 ± 1 mm, respectively. The mean widths in the normal group was 12 ± 2, 12 ± 2 and 4 ± 1 mm, respectively (all $p < 0.05$). The mean percent fibrous tissue for each region of each wall is shown in **Figure 6**. In every region the percent fibrous tissue was greater for the HC group than the control group ($p < 0.05$). Within the HC group, every region of the VS had significantly greater percent fibrous tissue than the RV or LV free walls (all $p < 0.05$). The LV free wall did not have greater fibrous tissue than the RV free wall and no 1 region in the VS had greater fibrosis than the other septal regions. The normal group had a steady percent fibrous tissue (4.7 to 5.9%) across each of the walls with no statistically significant variation.

The mean cell diameter of each region of both groups is shown in Figure 7. The RV free wall subendocardial region as well as the mid-subendocardial and endocardial regions about the LV cavity had a significantly larger cell size in the HC subjects than the normal control subjects (Fig. 7). A pattern of cellular hypertrophy was also noted in the HC group. In the RV free wall, the endocardial region had significantly larger cells than the RV epicardial region. Each of the RV free wall regions had smaller myocyte diameters

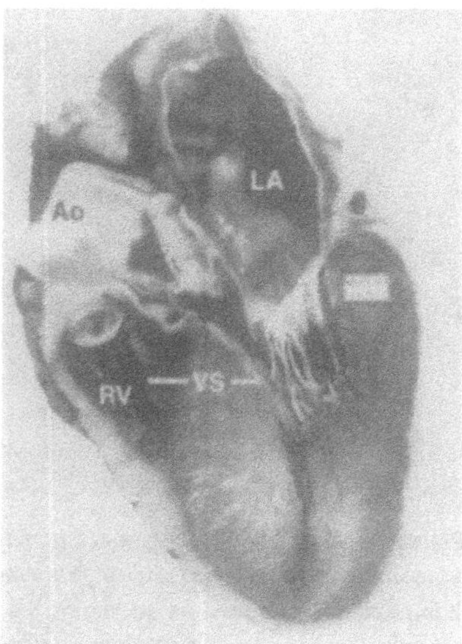

FIGURE 4. Patient 7. Heart from a 38-year-old woman (LCH #A83-717) who died suddenly at home. She had had periodic runs of documented ventricular tachycardia. A longitudinal view of the ventricular septum (VS) is shown. The VS is much thicker than the left ventricular free wall. The left atrium is dilated. Ao = aorta; LA = left atrium; RV = right ventricle.

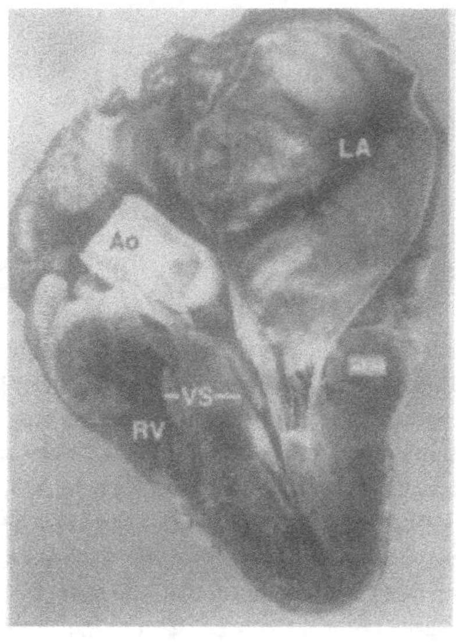

FIGURE 5. Patient 8. Heart in a 43-year-old woman (NH #A82-73) who had an enormously dilated left atrium (LA) (84 mm by echocardiogram) and atrial fibrillation for many years. She had been receiving warfarin sodium in her last several years. She had equally thickened ventricular septum (VS) and left ventricular free wall. Ao = aorta; RV = right ventricle.

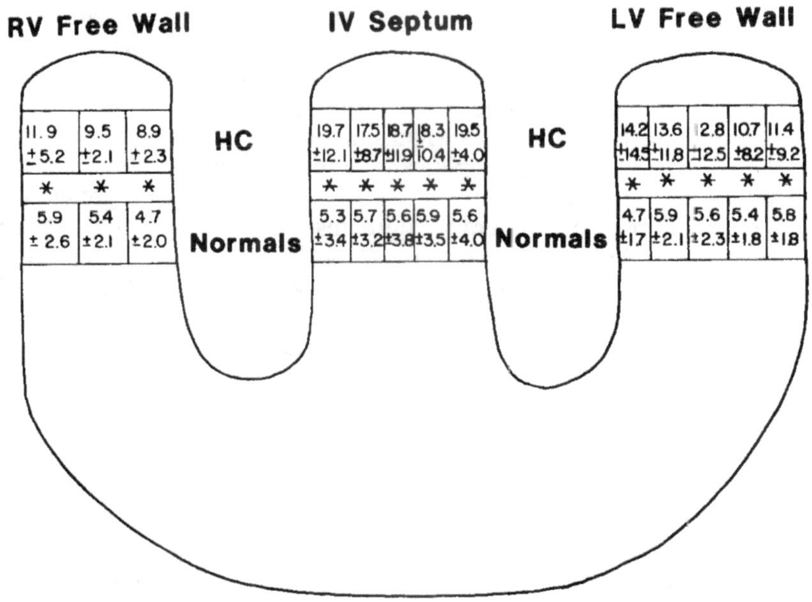

FIGURE 6. Mean percent fibrous tissue for each region of each wall for patients with hypertrophic cardiomyopathy (HC) and normal control patients. *p <0.05 between the 2 groups for that region. IV Septum = ventricular septum; LV = left ventricular; RV = right ventricular.

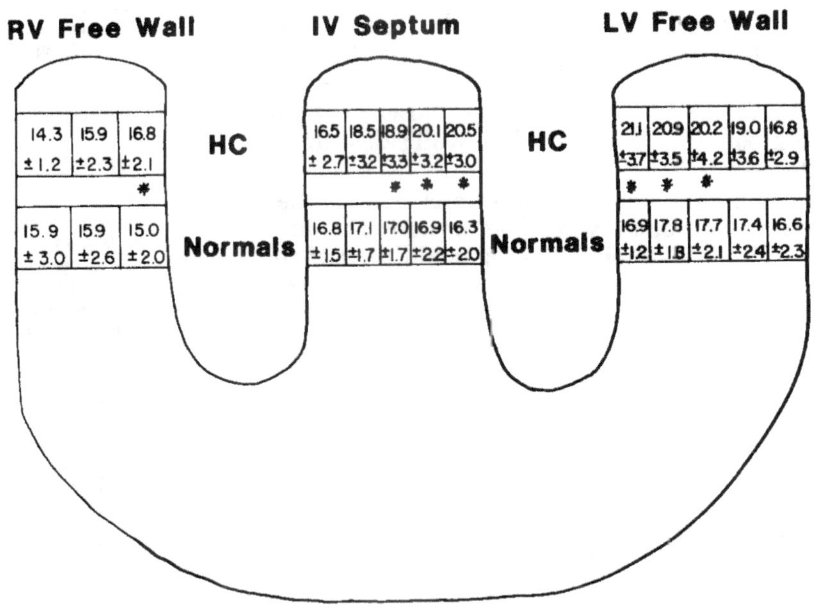

FIGURE 7. Mean cell diameter for each region of each wall for the group of patients with hypertrophic cardiomyopathy (HC) and normal control groups. *p <0.05 between the 2 groups for that region. Abbreviations as in Figure 6.

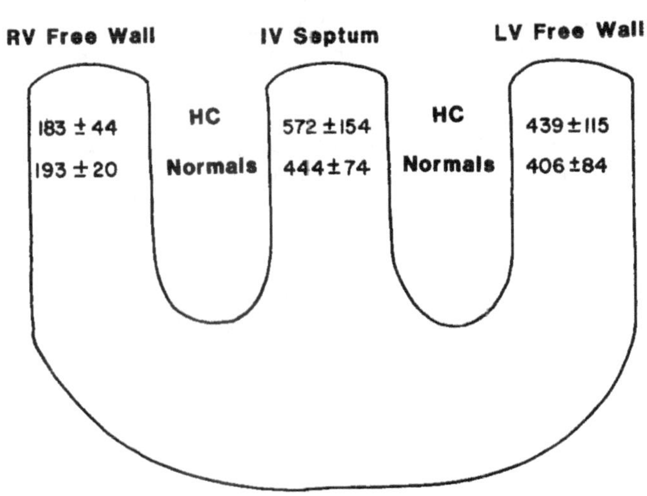

FIGURE 8. Mean number of cell layers counted across each wall for both groups. The number across the ventricular septum (IV Septum) approached statistical significance (p <0.1). Abbreviations as in Figure 6.

than the middle regions of the VS and the LV free walls ($p < 0.05$). The endocardial and subendocardial regions on the left side of the VS and LV free wall had cells with the greatest diameters. These regions were significantly different from the right side of the VS, all of the RV free wall and the epicardial and subepicardial regions of the LV free wall.

The number of cell layers was greatest across the VS in patients in the HC group ($p < 0.1$) (Fig. 8). Although the number of cell layers across the VS was not significantly greater than in the LV free wall, it was greater than that of any of the walls of the control group.

Discussion

This study has addressed the questions of what increases the ventricular wall thicknesses in patients with HC and whether regional wall differences exist. Fibrous tissue was the most important factor; it was significantly greater in hearts of HC patients than in control subjects in all regions. Increased numbers of cell layers and increased cell diameters also contributed to wall thickness in some regions (Fig. 6 to 8). Regional differences existed in HC hearts. The VS contained the most fibrous tissue ($p < 0.005$) and cell layers ($p < 0.1$). The cell layers closest to the LV cavity (on both the VS and LV free wall sides) contained the largest cells.

Increased myocardial fibrous tissue in the HC cardiac ventricular walls has been found in previous studies,[11,12] although the regional distribution has not. The cause of the increased fibrous tissue (especially in the VS) is not known. Several factors—cellular hypertrophy,[13] myofibril disarray,[12,14] myocyte loss[12] and ischemia—may play a role.[15,16] Myocardial ischemia, especially in the VS, has been reported in patients with HC[15]; myocardial infarction has occurred in the absence of significant narrowing of the epicardial coronary arteries.[16] A recent positron-emission tomography report, however, has questioned the presence of myocardial ischemia at rest or exercise in patients with HC.[17]

The increased number of cell layers across the VS in patients with HC relative to the VS of normal patients and the LV free wall of the HC patients has been shown.[5] Because neither the study of Fujiwara et al[5] nor our study is 3-dimensional, it is not possible to determine if this finding represents cellular hyperplasia or a rearrangement of myocytes. It may be that the HC myocytes are extremely long and that cells from other areas have forced their way into the regions of each heart we examined. This possibility, however, is counter to observations that HC myocytes are increased in diameter yet short.[18,19] Thus, the VS in HC may actually be a region with increased numbers of myocytes. The normal control mechanisms that limit or prevent cardiomyocyte cell division may be lacking in HC.

Several studies have described the increased cardiac cell diameter in HC.[2,3,5,6,11] Hoshino et al[6] quantitated the increase and compared HC subjects to normal and hypertensive subjects. Although they found that the largest cells were in the midportion of the VS,[6] we found that the greatest cellular hypertrophy was in the layers closest to the cavity. The most likely cause for this distribution is that the greatest stress is in the LV endocardium and subendocardium.[20-22] The endocardial third of the RV free wall also had larger cells than the control subjects.

Acknowledgment: We thank Carl V. Leier, MD, for review of the manuscript and Tami Smith for preparation of the manuscript.

References

1. Oakley C. *Ventricular hypertrophy in cardiomyopathy. Br Heart J* 1971;33:179–186.
2. Roberts WC, Ferrans VJ, Buja LM. *Pathologic aspects of the idiopathic cardiomyopathies. Adv Cardiol* 1974;13:349–367.
3. Olsen EGJ. *The pathology of cardiomyopathies. A critical analysis. Am Heart J* 1979;98:385–392.
4. Moore GW, Hutchins GM, Bulkley BH, Tseng JS, Ki PF. *Constituents of the human ventricular myocardium: connective tissue hyperplasia accompanying muscular hypertrophy. Am Heart J* 1980;100:610–616.
5. Fujiwara H, Hoshino T, Yamana K, Fujiwara T, Furuta M, Hamashima Y, Kawai C. *Number and size of myocytes and amount of interstitial space in the ventricular septum and in the left ventricular free wall in hypertrophic cardiomyopathy. Am J Cardiol* 1983;52:818–823.
6. Hoshino T, Fujiwara H, Kawai C, Hamashima Y. *Myocardial fiber diameter and regional distribution in the ventricular wall of normal adult hearts, hypertensive hearts and hearts with hypertrophic cardiomyopathy. Circulation* 1983;67:1109–1116.
7. Sheehan DC, Hrapchak BB. *Connective tissue and muscle fiber stains. In: Theory and Practice of Histotechnology. St. Louis: C.V. Mosby,* 1973.
8. Weibel ER. *Stereological principles for morphometry in electron microscopic cytology. Int Rev Cytol* 1969;26:235–271.
9. Dick MR, Unverferth DV, Baba N. *The pattern of myocardial degeneration in nonischemic congestive cardiomyopathy. Hum Pathol* 1982;13:740–744.
10. Winer BJ. Statistical Principles in Experimental Design. 2nd Ed. New York: McGraw-Hill, 1971.
11. Noda S. *Histopathology of endomyocardial biopsies from patients with idiopathic cardiomyopathy; quantitative evaluation based on multivariate statistical analysis. Jpn Circ J* 1980;44:95–116.
12. Anderson KR, St John Sutton MG, Lie JT. *Histopathological types of cardiac fibrosis in myocardial disease. J Pathol* 1979;128:79–85.
13. Montfort I, Perez-Tamayo R. *The muscle-collagen ratio in normal and hypertrophic human hearts. Lab Invest* 1962;7:463–469.
14. St John Sutton MG, Lie JT, Anderson KR, O'Brien PC, Frye RL. Histopathological specificity of hypertrophic obstructive cardiomyopathy. *Br Heart J* 1980;44:433–443.
15. Cannon RO III, Rosing DR, Maron BJ, Leon MB, Bonow RO, Watson RM, Epstein SE. *Myocardial ischemia in patients with hypertrophic cardiomyopathy: contribution of inadequate vasodilator reserve and elevated left ventricular filling pressures. Circulation* 1985;71:234–243.
16. Maron BJ, Epstein SE, Roberts WC. *Hypertrophic cardiomyopathy and transmural myocardial infarction without significant atherosclerosis of the extramural coronary arteries. Am J Cardiol* 1979;43:1086–1091.
17. Grover-McKay M, Schwaiger M, Krivokapich J, Phelps ME, Schelbert HR. *Relative reduction of exogenous glucose utilization in the septum of patients with hypertrophic cardiomyopathy (abstr). JACC* 1986;7:202A.
18. Ferrans VJ, Morrow AG, Roberts WC. *Myocardial ultra-structure in idiopathic hypertrophic subaortic stenosis. A study of operatively excised left ventricular outflow tract muscle in 14 patients. Circulation* 1972;45:769–792.
19. Davies MJ. *The current status of myocardial disarray in hypertrophic cardiomyopathy. Br Heart J* 1984;51:361–363.
20. Wong AYK, Rautaharja PM. *Stress distribution within the left ventricular wall approximated as a thick ellipsoidal shell. Am Heart J* 1968;75:649–657.
21. Mirsky I. *Left ventricular stresses in the intact human heart.* Biophys J 1969;9:189–198, 1969.
22. Gould P, Ghista D, Brombolich L, Mirsky I. *In vivo stresses in the human left ventricular wall: analysis accounting for irregular three dimensional geometry and comparison with idealized geometry analyses. J Biomech* 1972;5:521–531.

Frequency and Significance of Mitral Anular Calcium in Hypertrophic Cardiomyopathy: Analysis of 200 Necropsy Patients

HAMID E. MOTAMED, MD, and WILLIAM C. ROBERTS, MD

To determine the frequency and significance of mitral anular calcium (MAC) in hypertrophic cardiomyopathy (HC), 43 clinical and morphologic variables in 200 necropsy cases of HC were examined. Of 100 patients <40 years of age, none had MAC. Of the 100 necropsy patients >40 years, 30 (30%) had MAC, 21 (70%) of whom were women. The mean age of the 30 MAC patients was older than that of the 70 non-MAC patients >40 years of age (66 years vs 53 years). The frequency of MAC increased with age. MAC was present in 3 of 31 patients (10%) aged 41 to 50 years; in 6 of 34 patients (18%) aged 51 to 60 years; in 11 of 21 patients (52%) aged 61 to 70 years; and in 10 of 14 patients (71%) aged 71 to 90 years. Compared with the 70 patients >40 years of age without MAC, the 30 patients >40 years of age with MAC had higher average systemic arterial peak systolic pressure (133 mm Hg vs 113 mm Hg); a larger percentage of the MAC patients had calcific deposits in the epicardial coronary arteries (93% vs 41%) and in the aortic valve cusps (33% vs 6%); and a larger percentage of the MAC patients had severe narrowing by atherosclerotic plaques of 1 or more of the 4 major epicardial coronary arteries (47% vs 24%). The frequency of a history of systemic hypertension, diabetes mellitus and total serum cholesterol levels >200 mg/dl in the patients with and without MAC was similar. In no patient with MAC by hemodynamic studies was there evidence of obstruction to left ventricular inflow. The frequency of mitral regurgitation by left ventricular angiography was similar in the patients with and without MAC. (Am J Cardiol 1987;60:877–884)

Hypertrophic cardiomyopathy (HC) is a relatively uncommon disease. In the Western world, calcific deposits in the mitral anular region (mitral anular calcium [MAC]) are common, particularly in persons older than 65 years.[1-4] During the last 27 years, we and others have observed patients with HC who also had MAC.[5-7] This report describes the frequency of MAC in 200 necropsy patients with HC, and compares 43 variables in patients >40 years of age with and without MAC to determine the clinical significance of MAC in HC.

Patients

Sources of patients: In the files of the Pathology Branch, National Heart, Lung, and Blood Institute, National Institutes of Health, 220 necropsied cases are coded as having HC. On examination of our records of these 220 cases, the heart itself was never examined in 9 cases—only histologic sections of heart—and these cases were therefore eliminated from this study. Eleven other cases originally coded as HC also were eliminated because of an associated noncoronary cardiovascular disease (cardiovascular syphilis in 1, Marfan syndrome in 1, carcinoid syndrome in 1) or because these cases did not fulfill our present definition of HC (see below). In 10 of these latter 11 cases the diagnosis of HC was not made during life. A total of 200 cases of HC remained and form the basis of this study. The hearts in all 200 cases were examined initially by WCR. Of the 30 hearts with MAC, 21 were reexamined by WCR and also examined by HEM. In addition to reviewing the records in the Pathology Branch in all 200 patients, the medical records in the 100 patients >40 years of age were reviewed. Of the 100 cases >40 years of age, 67 had been studied clinically at the National Institutes of Health, and the diagnosis of HC in each was established clinically; in the other 33 patients

From the Pathology Branch, National Heart, Lung, and Blood Institute, National Institutes of Health, Bethesda, Maryland. Manuscript received June 4, 1987, accepted June 15, 1987.

Address for reprints: William C. Roberts, MD, Pathology Branch, National Heart, Lung, and Blood Institute, Building 10, Room 2N-258, National Institutes of Health, Bethesda, Maryland 20892.

aged >40 years, the clinical records from the submitting hospital were examined.

Definition of hypertrophic cardiomyopathy: All 200 cases had hearts of increased weight for their body size, all at necropsy had nondilated right or left ventricular cavities or the few who did have dilated ventricles at necropsy were found earlier in life by angiogram or echocardiogram or both to have nondilated ventricular cavities; all had a normally functioning aortic valve (neither stenosis nor regurgitation); all had dilated right and left atria; and none had a condition other than HC that could explain the following cardiac features of HC present in most cases: (1) a ventricular septum thicker at some point than the left ventricular free wall; (2) a mural endocardial fibrous plaque in the left ventricular outflow tract in apposition to anterior mitral leaflet; (3) focally thickened mitral leaflets and chordae tendineae; (4) abnormal intramural coronary arteries in the ventricular septum—about half the patients; and (5) characteristic myofiber disorganization in the ventricular septum—about 90% of the patients. Of the 200 necropsy patients, 154 were >20 years of age; of them, 83 were women and of them the heart weighed >350 g in 78 (94%); of the 154 patients >20 years of age, 71 were men and 70 (98%) of them had hearts weighing >400 g. Of the 6 men and women with smaller sized hearts, all 6 had the other characteristic anatomic features of HC, and all of them had small body weights.

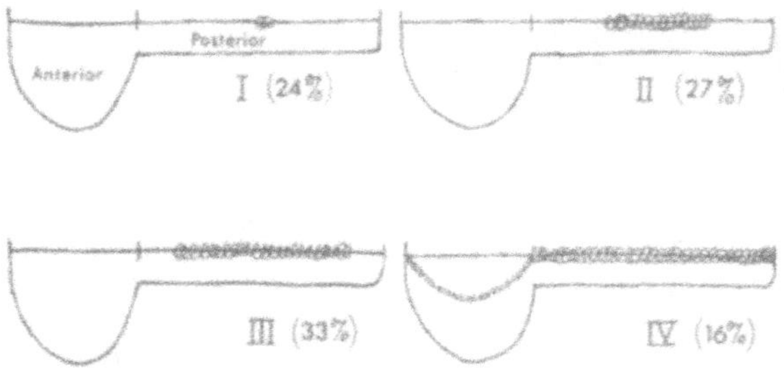

FIGURE 1. Method of grading mitral anular calcium. Grade I indicates only a single small deposit: grade II, a large single or more than one small deposit. Grade III and IV represents extensive deposits. The entire anulus behind the posterior leaflet is involved in grade IV, and, on rare occasion, calcific deposits also may extend across the anterior leaflet. Reproduced with permission from Roberts WC and Perloff JK. Mitral valvular disease. A clinicopathologic survey of the conditions causing the mitral valve to function abnormally. Ann Intern Med 1972;77:939–975.

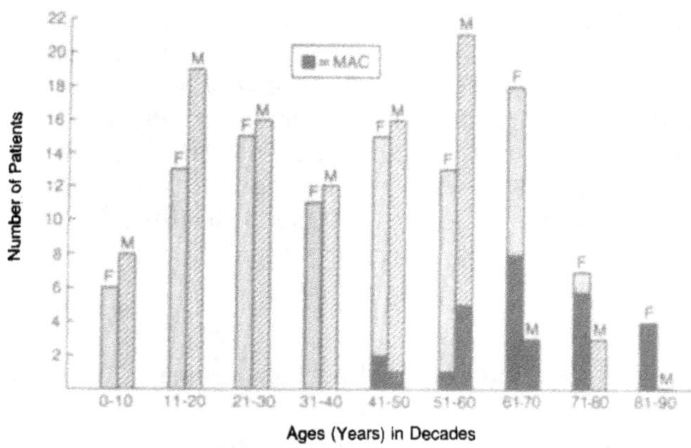

FIGURE 2. Bar graph subdividing the 200 necropsy patients with hypertrophic cardiomyopathy by age decade and by sex and indicating those patients with associated mitral anular calcium (MAC).

Quantitation of mitral anular calcium: MAC was quantitated on a scale of 1+ to 4+ (Fig. 1): 1+ = small deposits involving <50% of the circumference of the posterior leaflet or a single large deposit involving <25% of the posterior leaflet; 2+ = large deposits involving less than half of the posterior mitral leaflet or smaller deposits involving up to 75% of the circumference of the posterior mitral leaflet; 3+ = smaller deposits involving the entire posterior mitral leaflets or huge deposits involving less than the entire mitral leaflet; and 4+ = huge deposits beneath the entire posterior mitral leaflet with or without involvement of anterior mitral leaflet.

Statistical methods: Statistical analysis between groups was done by chi-square analysis and Student t tests when appropriate. A p value <0.05 was considered significant.

Results

Frequency of mitral anular calcium: Of the 200 HC patients, 30 (15%) had MAC. Of the 100 patients ≤40 years of age with HC, none had MAC (Fig. 2). Of the

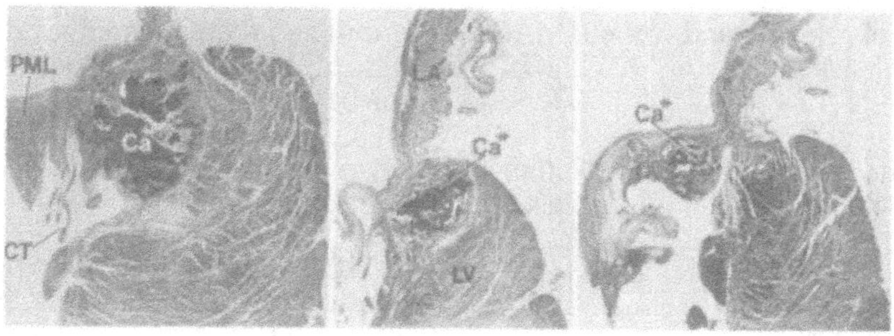

FIGURE 3. Patient 18 (Table I). Photomicrographs from 3 areas of posterior mitral leaflet (PML) showing calcific deposits of differing sizes beneath posterior mitral leaflet (*left*), within the most basal portion of left ventricular free wall and unattached to posterior mitral leaflet (*middle*) and within the posterior mitral leaflet only (*right*) in a 70-year-old woman. When calcific deposits are heavy, they are never limited to the anulus, which is the site where left atrial mural endocardium, left ventricular wall (LV) and posterior mitral leaflet meet. CT = chordae tendineae; LA = left atrial wall. Hematoxylin-eosin stains; original magnification × 4.5 (*left*), × 4.0 (*middle* and *right*).

TABLE I Clinical and Morphologic Observations in Each of 30 Necropsy Patients with Hypertrophic Cardiomyopathy and Mitral Anular Calcium

Case	Age (yr) at Death	Sex	SH by H	DM	TC (mg/dl)	AF	Interval (days) CC to Death	RV (s/d) mm Hg	LV (s/d) mm Hg	SA (s/d) mm Hg	LV-SA psg (R) mm Hg	LV-SA psg (P) mm Hg	PAW (mean) mm Hg
							1+ Mitral Anular Calcium						
1	57	M	+	0	300	+	2,520	56/14	192/25	105/68	87	175	26
2	61	F	+	+	201	0	8	80/10	200/26	110/60	90	—	40
3	65	F	+	0	118	+	5	85/24	240/25	120/80	140	—	24
4	68	M	0	0	269	0	14	32/9	115/12	115/60	0	120	12
5	76	F	0	0	—	+	—	—	—	—	—	—	—
							2+ Mitral Anular Calcium						
6	42	M	0	0	231	0	53	32/5	180/20	125/70	55	80	16
7	45	F	0	0	155	0	6,120	35/13	190/18	95/48	94	—	—
8	51	M	+	0	177	0	2,280	45/	200/28	130/70	70	82	13
9	59	F	+	0	194	+	450	/14	135/19	75/58	60	84	27
10	63	M	+	0	176	+	180	49/9	189/20	163/69	25	100	—
11	65	F	+	0	—	0	—	—	—	—	—	—	—
12	65	F	+	0	239	+	210	—	190/08	195/90	0	100	—
13	69	F	+	+	—	0	—	—	—	—	—	—	—
14	81	F	+	0	268	0	2,220	24/4	140/15	160/70	80	130	10
15	82	F	+	0	199	0	—	—	—	—	—	—	—
							3+ Mitral Anular Calcium						
16	59	M	0	+	168	+	6,120	96/11	224/26	90/56	134	—	—
17	69	M	0	0	196	0	22	28/10	135/15	130/70	5	100	10
18	70	F	0	0	—	+	2	—	160/20	95/70	65	—	34
19	71	F	+	0	268	+	4,170	32/5	230/10	95/60	155	159	8
20	72	F	0	0	174	+	1,170	30/6	250/14	170/75	80	125	10
							4+ Mitral Anular Calcium						
21	45	F	—	+	—	0	—	—	—	—	—	—	—
22	60	M	+	0	—	+	—	—	—	—	—	—	—
23	60	M	0	+	255	+	2,520	—	213/10	117/68	95	—	—
24	64	F	0	0	240	0	1	42/6	230/12	160/70	60	—	13
25	70	F	+	0	126	0	4	115/20	245/20	120/65	125	—	20
26	72	F	+	0	272	+	1,890	24/7	165/10	100/50	65	—	7
27	74	F	+	+	—	0	—	—	—	—	—	—	—
28	79	F	0	0	—	0	—	—	—	—	—	135	—
29	81	F	0	0	120	+	—	—	—	—	—	—	—
30	87	F	0	0	—	+	—	—	—	—	—	—	—

*Operative myotomy and myectomy (Morrow procedure) performed.

†The catheterization data in the patients having ventricular septotomy-septectomy (myotomy and myectomy) are that obtained preoperatively. In the unoperated patients, the data are from the last catheterization.

AF = atrial fibrillation; AV = aortic valve; CA^{++} = calcium; CAs = coronary arteries; CC = cardiac catheterization; CHF = congestive heart failure; CI = cardiac index; CSA = cross-sectional-area; DM = diabetes mellitus; F = fibrosis; H = history; HW = heart weight; IE = infective endocarditis; LAD = left anterior descending; LC = left circumflex; LV = left ventricle; M&M = myotomy and myectomy; MR = mitral regurgitation; P = with provocation; PAW = pulmonary artery wedge; psg = peak systolic gradient; R = rest; RV = right ventricle; SA = systemic arterial; s/d = peak systole/end diastole; SH = systemic hypertension; TC = serum total cholesterol; VS = ventricular septum.

100 necropsy patients >40 years of age with HC, 30 (30%) had MAC (Fig. 2) (Table I). Of the 57 women >40 years of age with HC, 21 (37%) had MAC; of the 43 men >40 years of age with HC, 9 (21%) had MAC. The frequency of MAC increased with age. MAC was present in 3 of 31 patients (10%) aged 41 to 50 years; in 6 of 34 patients (18%) aged 51 to 60 years; in 11 of 21 patients (52%) aged 61 to 70 years, and in 10 of 14 patients (71%) aged 71 to 90 years.

Clinical and morphologic features in the patients with mitral anular calcium: These data in each patient are presented in Table I. Morphologic features of MAC in patients with heavy calcific deposits are illustrated in Figures 3 to 9.

Similar and different variables between patients with and without mitral anular calcium: Table II compares 43 variables between the 30 necropsy patients >40 years of age with HC and MAC vs the 70 necropsy patients >40 years of age with HC and without MAC. Of the 43 variables analyzed, 8 (17%) were significantly different between the 2 groups. Compared to the 70 patients >40 years of age without MAC, the 30 patients >40 years of age with MAC had a higher mean age (66 years vs 53 years); a larger per-

TABLE I (continued)

Case	CI (l/min/m²)	MR by LV cine (0–3+)	M&M	Interval (days) M&M → Death	Mode of Death	HW (g)	Ca^{++} CAs	No. Right, LAD & LC CAs >75% ↓ in CSA	AV Ca^{++}	VS (mm)	LV (mm)	LV F
					1+ Mitral Anular Calcium							
1	2.6	1+	0	—	Cancer	490	+	0	+	25	19	0
2	1.7	3+	+	0	M&M	665	+	3	0	—*	—*	0
3	1.5	0	+	0	M&M	615	+	0	0	—*	—*	0
4	2.2	—	+	1	M&M	540	+	3	+	—*	—*	+
5	—	—	0	—	Sudden	510	+	1	+	18	16	0
					2+ Mitral Anular Calcium							
6	2.9	2+	+	0	M&M	650	+	1	0	—*	—*	+
7	2.8	0	+	6,120	CHF	590	0	0	0	—*	—*	+
8	3.0	—	0	—	Sudden	885	+	0	+	25	20	0
9	1.8	3+	+	0	M&M	460	+	0	0	—*	—*	0
10	2.6	0	+	0	M&M	735	+	0	0	—*	—*	+
11	—	—	0	—	Alcoholism	450	0	0	0	23	22	0
12	1.4	—	+	215	Reoperation	475	+	3	0	—*	—*	0
13	—	—	0	—	Sudden	530	+	3	0	19	19	+
14	2.1	—	+	2,190	Sudden	550	+	2	0	—*	—*	+
15	—	—	0	—	Sudden	310	+	0	+	20	15	0
					3+ Mitral Anular Calcium							
16	2.8	2+	+	6,120	CHF	670	+	0	+	—*	—*	+
17	3.3	0	+	1	M&M	550	+	2	0	—*	—*	+
18	1.9	3+	0	—	CHF	450	+	0	0	31	29	0
19	2.5	1+	+	4,170	CHF	720	+	0	+	—*	—*	+
20	2.0	2+	+	1,170	Sudden	550	+	0	0	—*	—*	0
					4+ Mitral Anular Calcium							
21	—	—	+	4,320	CHF	1,150	+	0	0	—*	—*	+
22	—	—	0	—	Suicide	645	+	0	0	21	19	0
23	—	0	0	—	CHF	745	+	0	0	25	23	0
24	—	1+	0	—	Sudden	355	+	2	0	30	25	0
25	1.2	1+	0	—	Sudden	664	+	2	0	29	24	0
26	2.7	2+	+	1,860	CHF	815	+	0	+	—*	—*	+
27	—	—	0	—	CHF	650	+	0	0	37	25	+
28	—	—	0	—	Sudden	430	+	2	+	25	18	0
29	—	—	0	—	IE	550	+	0	+	—	—	0
30	—	—	0	—	Leukemia	460	+	1	0	26	20	+

centage of women with MAC compared to the women without MAC were >65 years of age (62% vs 5%); the MAC patients had higher average systemic artery peak systolic pressure (133 mm Hg vs 113 mm Hg); a larger percentage of the MAC patients had calcific deposits in the epicardial coronary arteries (93% vs 41%) and the aortic valve cusps (33% vs 6%), and a larger percentage of the MAC patients had severe (>75% decrease in cross-sectional area) narrowing by atherosclerotic plaques of 1 or more of the 4 major epicardial coronary arteries (47% vs 24%).

Discussion

Frequency of mitral anular calcium: Examination of the hearts and medical records of the 200 necropsy patients with HC disclosed that 30 (15%) had MAC: of the 100 patients ≤40 years of age, none had MAC and of the 100 patients >40 years of age, 30 (30%) had MAC. Of the 100 patients >40 years of age, 57 (57%) were women and of them, 21 (37%) had MAC. Of the 43 men >40 years of age with HC, 9 (21%) had MAC.

Functional significance of mitral anular calcium: An attempt was made to determine differences in HC patients >40 years of age with MAC and in HC patients >40 years of age without MAC. Analysis of 43 variables (Table II) indicated that the 30 patients >40 years of age with MAC compared to the 70 patients >40 years of age without MAC, as a group, were older by a mean of 13 years and a larger percentage of them were >65 years of age. The MAC patients compared to the non-MAC patients >40 years of age also had higher systemic arterial peak systolic pressures. In no patient with MAC was there evidence of obstruction by hemodynamic studies to left ventricular inflow. The frequency of mitral regurgitation by left ventricular

TABLE II Comparison of Hypertrophic Cardiomyopathy Patients >40 Years of Age With and Without Mitral Anular Calcium (MAC)

	With MAC (n = 30)	Without MAC (n = 70)	p Values
Number of men	9 (30%)	34 (49%)	NS
Number of women	21 (70%)	36 (51%)	NS
Age (yr): range (mean)	42–87 (66)	41–78 (53)	<0.01
Ages (yr): Men: Range (mean)	42–69 (59)	41–78 (52)	<0.05
Number >65 years	2/9 (22%)	3/34 (9%)	NS
Ages (yr): Women: Range (mean)	45–87 (69)	41–71 (54)	<0.01
Number >65 years	13/21 (62%)	2/36 (5%)	<0.001
Number with history of systemic hypertension	16/29 (55%)	25/68 (37%)	NS
Number having diabetes mellitus	6 (20%)	5/58 (9%)	NS
Number having left-sided cardiac catheterization*	10 (20%)	24 (34%)	
Average LV peak systolic pressure (mm Hg)	188	175	NS
Number of LV peak systolic pressure >140 mm Hg	7 (70%)	12/20 (60%)	NS
Average SA peak systolic pressure (mm Hg)	133	113	<0.05
Number with LV-SA psg @ rest >20 mm Hg	7 (70%)	14 (53%)	NS
Range (mean) LV-SA psg @ rest	25–140 (79)	30–175 (95)	NS
Number without LV-SA psg @ rest	3 (15%)	10 (42%)	NS
Range (mean) LV-SA psg @ rest	0–5 (2)	0–20 (8)	NS
Number with serum TC measured	21	45	
TC (mg/dl): range (mean)	118–300 (207)	125–476 (220)	NS
Number TC >200 mg/dl	10 (48%)	27 (60%)	NS
Number TC >240 mg/dl	6 (29%)	12 (27%)	NS
Number with chronic atrial fibrillation	15 (50%)	27/63 (43%)	NS
Number with cardiac operation	15 (50%)	36 (51%)	NS
Ventricular myotomy and myectomy	15† (50%)	33‡ (47%)	NS
Mitral valve replacement	0	2	
Number having LV angiogram	8	21	
MR by LV angiogram (severe)	5 (2) (62%)	17 (4) (81%)	NS
Number with PA wedge mean pressure	8	22	
Number ≤12 mm Hg	2 (25%)	12 (54%)	NS
Number 13–20 mm Hg	3 (37%)	2 (9%)	NS
Number >20 mm Hg	3 (37%)	8 (36%)	NS
Number with RV peak systolic pressure	8	18	
Number ≤35 mm Hg	3 (37%)	7 (39%)	NS
Number 36–60 mm Hg	2 (25%)	6 (33%)	NS
Number >60 mm Hg	3 (37%)	5 (28%)	NS
Mode of death			
Noncardiac	4 (13%)	5 (7%)	NS
Cardiac	26 (87%)	65 (93%)	NS
Sudden	8 (31%)	34 (52%)	NS
Chronic CHF	8 (31%)	11 (17%)	NS
Operation	8 (31%)	15 (23%)	NS
Infective endocarditis	1 (3%)	1 (1%)	NS
Catheterization	1 (3%)	1 (1%)	NS
Stroke	0	3 (5%)	NS
Heart weight (g) (mean)	595	600	NS
Men: range (mean)	490–885 (656)	350–1,030 (693)	NS
Women: range (mean)	340–1,150 (568)	290–900 (513)	NS
Number with ≥1 major coronary arteries >75%↓ in CSA	14 (47%)	17 (24%)	<0.05
Number with calcific deposits			
Epicardial coronary arteries	28 (93%)	29 (41%)	<0.001
Aortic valve cusps	10 (33%)	4 (6%)	<0.001

*The catheterization data in the patients having ventricular septotomy (myotomy and myectomy) and septectomy are that obtained preoperatively. In the unoperated patients, the data are from the last catheterization. The catheterization data used in this table in patients with and without MAC was that obtained in the last 1 year of the patient's life.

†Three patients also had CABG.

‡Two patients also had CABG. One other patient also had CABG without either myotomy and myectomy or mitral valve replacement.

CABG = coronary artery bypass grafting; CHF = congestive heart failure; CSA = cross-sectional area; LV = left ventricular; MR = mitral regurgitation; NS = not significant; PA = pulmonary artery; psg = peak systolic gradient; RV = right ventricular; SA = systemic artery; TC = total cholesterol.

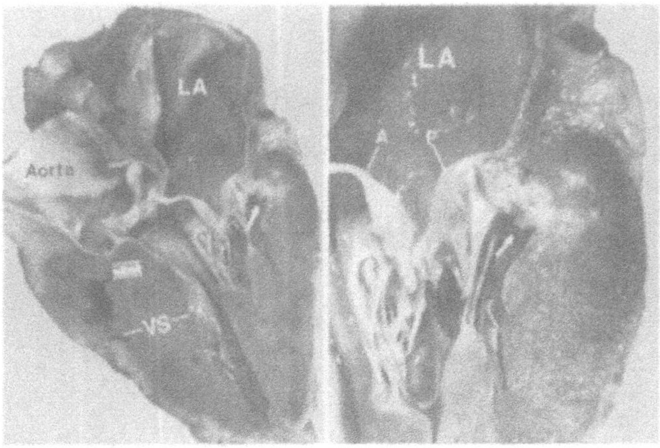

FIGURE 4. Patient 20 (Table I). Long-axis view of the left side of the heart in 72-year-old woman who died suddenly 39 months after partial ventricular septotomy and septectomy ("myotomy and myectomy"). *Left, arrow* designates the location of calcium behind posterior mitral leaflet. LA = left atrium; VS = ventricular septum. *Right*, close-up view of anterior (A) and posterior (P) mitral leaflets again showing the calcific deposit (*arrow*), which had burrowed into the left ventricular wall behind the posterior mitral leaflet.

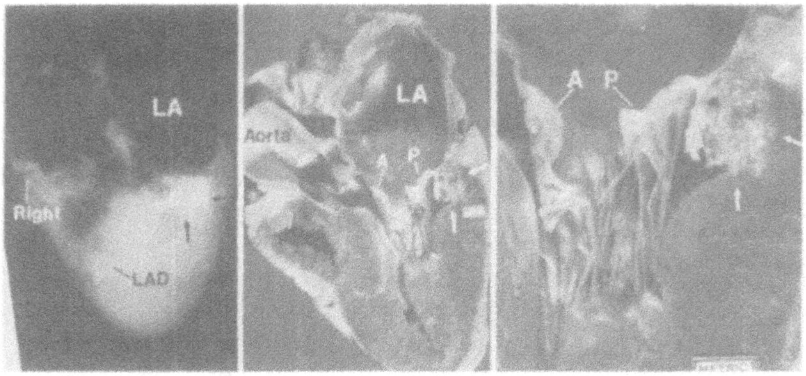

FIGURE 5. Patient 22 (Table I). Heart in a 60-year-old man who died from a noncardiac cause. *Left*, radiograph of heart at necropsy showing a large calcific deposit (*arrows*) in the mitral valve area and also calcific deposits in the right and left anterior descending (LAD) coronary arteries. LA = left atrial cavity. *Center*, long-axis view of left side of heart showing the heavy calcific deposit (*arrows*) behind posterior (P) mitral leaflet. A = anterior mitral leaflet. *Right*, close-up view of the calcific deposit (*arrows*) behind posterior mitral leaflet. The calcific deposit has burrowed into the left ventricular wall.

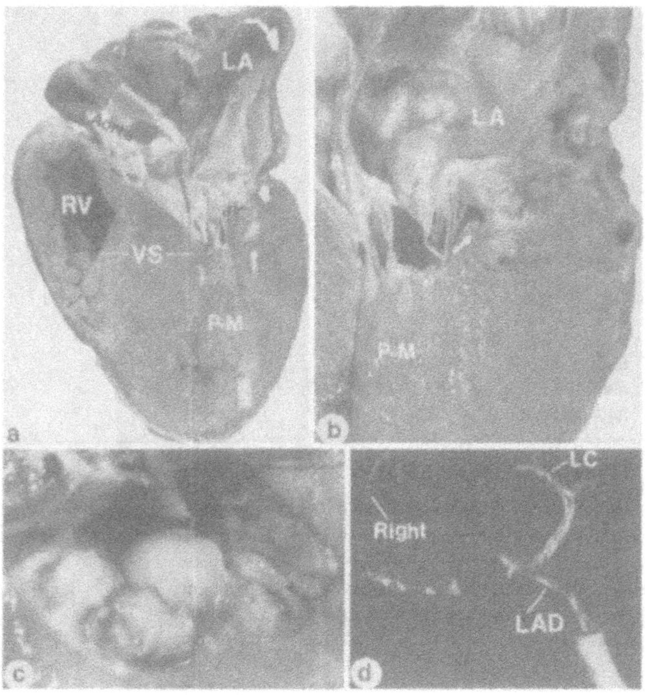

FIGURE 6. Patient 25 (Table I). Heart in a 70-year-old woman who died suddenly. *a*, long-axis view of heart showing calcific deposit (*arrow*) behind the posterior mitral leaflet and in the basal portion of left ventricular wall. LA = left atrium; P-M = posteromedial papillary muscle; RV = right ventricular cavity; VS = ventricular septum. *b*, close-up view of anterior (A) and posterior (P) mitral leaflets again showing the calcific deposit (*arrow*). *c*, mitral valve viewed from the left atrium showing the posterior mitral leaflet bulging toward the left atrium and the calcific deposit behind it. *d*, radiograph of the excised epicardial coronary arteries showing calcific deposits in the right, left circumflex (LC) and left anterior descending (LAD) arteries.

angiography was similar in the patients with and without MAC.

Relation of mitral anular calcium to atherosclerosis: There is considerable evidence that MAC is a form of atherosclerosis and therefore it is not surprising to see that the MAC patients had more coronary atherosclerosis than did the non-MAC patients.[4] The MAC patients had considerably more atherosclerotic plaquing in the major epicardial coronary arteries and also a higher frequency of calcific deposits in the epicardial coronary arteries and aortic valve cusps than did the non-MAC patients >40 years of age. Deposits of calcium on the aortic aspects of the aortic valve cusps in persons >60 years of age is common and this deposition also may be considered a form of atherosclerosis in this older population.[4] Thus, it also is not surprising to find that the MAC patients had a higher frequency of associated aortic valve calcific deposits than did the non-MAC patients.

Relation of mitral anular calcium and diabetes mellitus: Diabetes mellitus also has been considered a factor predisposing to MAC.[1,8] The frequency of this condition in our patients with and without MAC, however, was not significantly different.

Previous studies of mitral anular calcium in hypertrophic cardiomyopathy: Previous studies have shown that MAC occurs only in populations where the total serum cholesterol is >150 mg/dl.[8] Of the 21 patients with MAC and cholesterol levels available, 3 (14%) were <150 mg/dl and of the 45 patients without MAC and cholesterol levels available, 2 (4%) were <150 mg/dl. These numbers represent single determinations on all 66 patients, and therefore their significance is uncertain. The mean total cholesterol values for the group of patients with MAC was similar to that of the group of patients without MAC.

No previous publication has focused on the frequency or significance of MAC in necropsy patients with HC. Two echocardiographic and/or fluoroscopic studies, however, have provided data. Kronzon and Glassman[6] studied 46 patients with HC by cardiac fluoroscopy and found MAC in 16 (35%). The ages of the 16 patients with MAC ranged from 51 to 78 years (mean 65), whereas the 30 patients without MAC were 17 to 50 years (mean 48). MAC was found in 12 of 18 patients (66%) >55 years of age and in 4 of 28 patients (14%) <55 years of age. No hemodynamic or angiographic differences were observed by these authors between the 16 patients with MAC and the 30 patients without MAC. Kronzon and Glassman[6] also studied 22 patients with HC by echocardiography without cardiac catheterization. Of them, 7 (32%) had MAC. Of their 46 patients studied by M-mode echocardiography, 16 (35%) had thick dense echoes consistent with MAC. Nair and associates[7] studied 42 patients with HC by both M-mode and cross-sectional echocardiography and found MAC in 12 (29%) of them. The ages of the 12 patients with MAC ranged from 60 to 88 years (mean 75 ± 8) and of the 30 patients without MAC, 39 to 96 years (mean 65 ± 13). These authors found the "systolic excursion of the left ventricular posterior wall" to be less in the patients with MAC than in those without MAC.

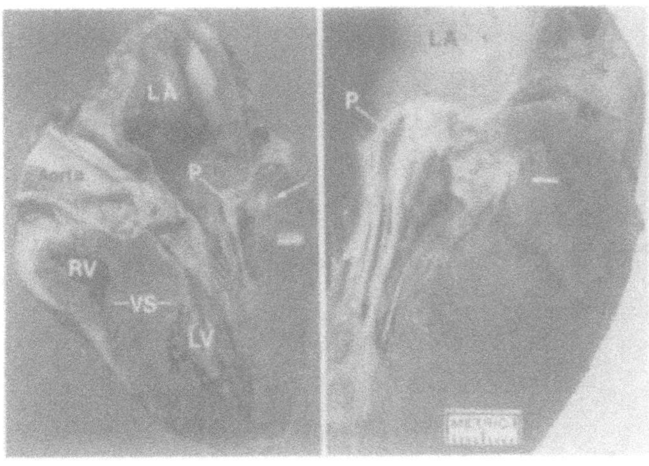

FIGURE 7. Patient 26 (Table I). Long-axis view of the left side of the heart in a 72-year-old woman who died of congestive heart failure 62 months after partial ventricular septotomy and septectomy ("myotomy and myectomy"). *Left,* the *arrow* designates the location of calcium behind the posterior (P) mitral leaflet. LA = left atrium; LV = left ventricle; RV = right ventricle; VS = ventricular septum. *Right,* close-up view of the calcific deposit (*arrow*) behind the posterior mitral leaflet.

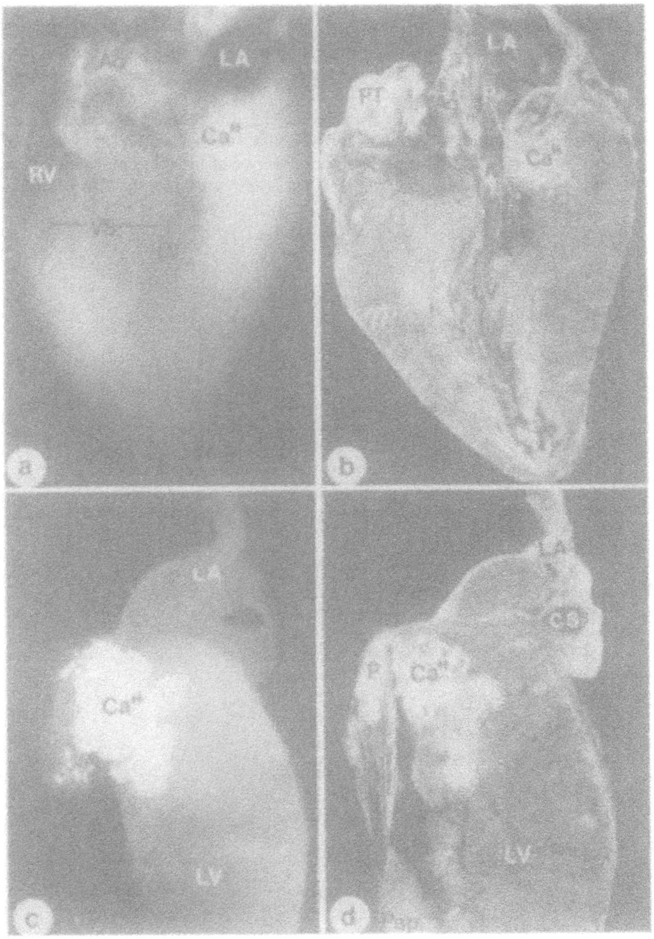

FIGURE 8. Patient 27 (Table I). Heart in a 74-year-old woman who died of congestive heart failure. *a,* radiograph of heart at necropsy showing a large calcific deposit (Ca^{++}) in the mitral valve area. Ao = aorta; LA = left atrium; RV = right ventricle; VS = ventricular septum. *b,* long-axis view of the left side of the heart showing the heavy calcific deposit behind posterior (P) mitral leaflet. A = anterior mitral leaflet; PT = pulmonary trunk. *c* and *d,* longitudinal section and radiograph of the left atrial (LA) and left ventricular (LV) walls and the posterior mitral leaflet (P) showing a large calcific deposit behind the posterior mitral leaflet. The calcific deposit has burrowed into the left ventricular wall. CS = coronary sinus; Pap = papillary muscle. The photographs shown in *a* and *b* are reproduced with permission from Ewy GA, Marcus FI, Bohajalian O, Burke HL, Roberts WC. Muscular subaortic stenosis. Clinical and pathologic observations in an elderly patient. Am J Cardiol 1968;22:126–132.

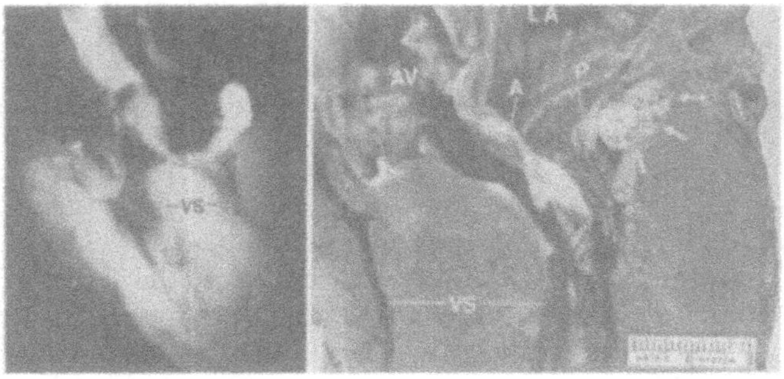

FIGURE 9. Patient 30 (Table I). Heart in a 87-year-old woman who died from a noncardiac cause. *Left,* radiograph of heart at necropsy showing a large J-shaped calcific deposit in the mitral valve area. VS = ventricular septum. *Right,* close-up view of the left ventricular inflow and outflow tracts showing the heavy calcific deposit (*arrows*) behind posterior (P) mitral leaflet. A = anterior mitral leaflet; AV = aortic valve; LA = left atrium.

References

1. Roberts WC. *Morphologic features of the normal and abnormal mitral valve.* Am J Cardiol 1983;51:1005–1028.
2. Nair CK, Sudhakaran C, Aronow WS, Thomson W, Woodruff MP, Sketch MH. *Clinical characteristics of patients younger than 60 years with mitral anular calcium: comparison with age- and sex-matched control subjects.* Am J Cardiol 1984;54:1286–1287.
3. Aronow WS, Schwartz KS, Koenigsberg M. *Correlation of serum lipids, calcium and phosphous, diabetes mellitus, aortic valve stenosis and history of systemic hypertension with presence or absence of mitral anular calcium in persons older than 62 years in a long-term health care facility.* Am J Cardiol 1987;59:381–382.
4. Roberts WC. *The senile cardiac calcification syndrome.* Am J Cardiol 1986;58:572–574.
5. Ewy GA, Marcus FI, Bohjalian O, Burke HL, Roberts WC. *Muscular subaortic stenosis. Clinical and pathologic observations in an elderly patient.* Am J Cardiol 1968;22:126–132.
6. Kronzon I, Glassman E. *Mitral ring calcification in idiopathic hypertrophic subaortic stenosis.* Am J Cardiol 1978;42:60–66.
7. Nair CK, Kudesia V, Hansen D, Thomson W, Panago T, Ryschon K, Sketch MH. *Echocardiographic and electrocardiographic characteristics of patients with hypertrophic cardiomyopathy with and without mitral anular calcium.* Am J Cardiol 1987;59:1428–1430.
8. Savage DD, Garrison RJ, Castelli WP, McNamara PM, Anderson SJ, Kannel WB, Feinleib M. *Prevalence of submitral (anular) calcium and its correlates in a general population-based sample (the Framingham study).* Am J Cardiol 1983;51:1375–1378.

MORPHOLOGIC FEATURES

Charles Stewart Roberts
William Clifford Roberts

Since 1958, numerous publications have described various morphologic cardiac findings in patients with hypertrophic cardiomyopathy (HCM).[1-39] Although it was Teare in 1958 who first described certain characteristic features of the heart in HCM,[40] earlier descriptions were suggestive of this condition.

In 1869, Liouville and Hallopeau each reported a patient probably having HCM.[41,42] Both authors noted striking hypertrophy of the ventricular septum, and each considered the left ventricular outflow tract to be obstructed by the hypertrophied septal muscle; Hallopeau also noted thickening of the anterior mitral leaflet in his 69-year-old patient.

In 1907, Schmincke described severe hypertrophy of the ventricular septum in the hearts of 2 women, aged 50 and 56 years.[43] In addition to the thickening of the septum, the left ventricular free wall in each patient was severely hypertrophied. Schmincke considered the ventricular septal hypertrophy to be primary and of congenital origin, leading to obstruction to left ventricular ejection and to secondary hypertrophy of the left ventricular free wall. He further speculated that the latter, in turn, aggravated the degree of obstruction, thereby initiating a vicious cycle.

In 1910, Bernheim described a syndrome of right-sided congestive cardiac failure in 10 patients with left ventricular hypertrophy of various causes.[44] Proper function of the right ventricle was thought to be impeded by severe hypertrophy of the ventricular septum, which protruded into the right ventricular outflow tract. It has been suggested that some of Bernheim's cases were examples of HCM.[45] Because of the marked left ventricular dilatation in 9 of the 10 hearts described, a finding rarely seen in adults with HCM, it seems unlikely that the cases described by Bernheim were examples of this disease.

After Schmincke's report in 1907,[43] a period of nearly 50 years elapsed before another report of the structural abnormalities of the disease appeared. In 1952, Davies described a family in whom many members had heart disease, a history of sudden death, and systolic precordial murmurs.[46] At necropsy, the heart in one patient showed "diffuse subaortic stenosis" associated with left ventricular hypertrophy. He described an area of fibrosis 4 cm^2 in the left ventricular outflow tract opposite the anterior mitral leaflet, a lesion suggestive of HCM.

In 1957, Brock operated on a 63-year-old woman thought to have valvular aortic stenosis and systemic hypertension.[47] At operation, however, the aortic valve was normal, and no obstruction to left ventricular outflow was encountered by dilating instruments, despite direct pressure tracings showing subvalvular obstruction. The patient died shortly after operation, and necropsy showed a hypertrophied, nondilated left ventricle and no subaortic fibrous stricture.

Although the cases reported by Liouville,[41] Hallopeau,[42] Schmincke,[43] Davies,[46] and Brock[47] are probably examples of HCM, the comparative thicknesses of the ventricular septum and left ventricular free wall and other features of HCM were not described in any of them. Thus, it can only be presumed that these patients had HCM. The first unequivocal description of HCM was by Teare from London, and the report appeared in the *British Heart Journal* in January of 1958.[40] Although Brock's clinical report was published in *Guy's Hospital Reports* in the final quarterly issue of 1957,[47] Teare's article had been received by the journal office in January of 1957, that is, *before* Brock had operated on his patient. Therefore, it seems fair to credit Teare with the first detailed anatomic description and to credit Brock with the first description of the functional nature of this entity.

Teare described gross and histologic cardiac findings in 9 patients, aged 14 to 45 years (mean 26), 2 women and 7 men, 8 of whom died suddenly. Although Teare did not give measurements of the thicknesses of the ventricular septum and left ventricular free wall, he clearly indicated that the septum was thicker than the left ventricular free wall and, indeed, called the condition "asymmetrical hypertrophy of the heart." He considered the localized septal hypertrophy to be a "benign tumor" or "hamartoma." He observed on histologic examination a "bizarre arrangement of muscle bundles" and "considerable variation in size" of the myocardial fibers in the ventricular septum. Teare also noted similar disordered arrangement of muscle bundles in the adjacent anterior free wall of the left ventricle. In one patient, the posterior left ventricular free wall "appeared thinner than normal," and histologic examination showed normal arrangement and uniform size of the myocardial fibers. Although one of Teare's 9 patients underwent valvulotomy for suspected mitral stenosis (this was the only patient in his study who did not die suddenly), there were no descriptions of the mitral valve, no mention of mural endocardial thickening in the left ventricular outflow tract, and no comments regarding the sizes of the various cardiac chambers. This report, however, established HCM as a distinct entity and described the peculiar arrangement of and variation in size of the fibers in the ventricular septum.

DEFINITION

Probably no cardiovascular disease in recent years has engendered as much controversy or "professional" emotional display as has HCM. Since Teare applied the term "asymmetrical hypertrophy of the heart" to HCM, at least 57 other terms, including "functional subaortic stenosis," "diffuse muscular subaortic stenosis," "idiopathic hypertrophic subaortic stenosis," "hypertrophic obstructive cardiomyopathy," and "asymmetric septal hypertrophy" have been applied.[48] Terms that include the word "stenosis" or "obstruction" are inappropriate because obstruction is more often absent than present. Terms that emphasize asymmetry of the walls bordering the left ventricular cavity have served a useful purpose in emphasizing a frequent morphologic feature of this condition, but the ventricular septum may be thicker than the left ventricular free wall in some conditions other than HCM, and some patients with HCM do not have asymmetric septal hypertrophy (i.e., septum thicker than free wall), and the free wall in HCM is not always thickened.

A major obstacle to understanding and discussing HCM is the lack of agreement among its students as to what it is. It is readily apparent that evidence of left ventricular outflow obstruction is not necessary for a diagnosis of HCM. The presence of asymmetric septal hypertrophy is not required for diagnosis because other conditions can cause the ventricular septum to be thicker than the left ventricular free wall, and in many patients with HCM the septum and free wall are of similar thicknesses. Rapid upstroke of the arterial pulse, cardiomegaly, a systolic precordial murmur, and an abnormal electrocardiogram are usually present, but none of these are diagnostic or specific. Systolic anterior motion of the anterior mitral leaflet also is often present by echocardiogram, but any condition in which the left ventricular cavity is relatively small and the percentage of left ventricular volume ejected each beat is relatively high can also cause systolic anterior motion. Thus, what is HCM? It appears most reasonable simply to consider HCM a condition characterized by: (1) hypertrophy of all or a portion of the walls of left ventricle, that is, ventricular septum or free wall or both; (2) dilated right and left atria; (3) nondilatation of the cavities of both cardiac ventricles, except in the presence of transmural ventricular wall necrosis or fibrosis or complete heart block; (4) absence of another cardiac condition that could produce left ventricular hypertrophy (focal or diffuse) without ventricular cavity dilatation, such as systemic hypertension or valvular heart disease; (5) presence of a normal or "supernormal" cardiac output and stroke volume; and (6) absence of other states such as hyperthyroidism or pheochromocytoma that independently might increase cardiac output abnormally. Atherosclerotic coronary artery disease can coexist with HCM.

Personal study of 220 patients with HCM at necropsy has disclosed certain predictable, grossly visible, characteristic, although not absolutely specific, features of HCM (Table 1): (1) dilated atria (100%); (2) increased heart weight (95%); (3) nondilated left ventricle (79%); (4) thickened mitral valve (75%); (5) mural endocardial plaque in the left ventricular outflow tract in apposition to the anterior mitral leaflet (72%); (6) greater maximal thickness of the ventricular septum than that of the left ventricular free wall (69%); and (7) grossly visible left ventricular scarring (42%), usually in the absence of significant narrowing of the epicardial coronary arteries. The hearts in

TABLE 1. CARDIAC MORPHOLOGIC FEATURES OF HYPERTROPHIC CARDIOMYOPATHY: FINDINGS IN 220 NECROPSY CASES

Characteristics	Cardiac Operation 0 (n = 145)	Cardiac Operation + (n = 75)	Total (n = 220)
1. Dilated atria	145 (100%)	75 (100%)	220 (100%)
2. Increased heart weight*	138 (95%)	72 (96%)	210 (95%)
3. Nondilated left ventricle	118 (81%)	56 (76%)	174 (79%)
4. Thickened mitral valve	90/137 (66%)	64/68 (94%)	154/205 (75%)
5. Fibrous plaque, left ventricular outflow	83/137 (61%)	66/71 (93%)	149/208 (72%)
6. Ventricular septum > left ventricle	102/142 (72%)	46/73 (63%)	148/215 (69%)
7. Gross left ventricular fibrosis	60/145 (41%)	32/73 (44%)	92/218 (42%)

* Adult women > 350 g; adult men > 400 g.

no 2 patients with HCM are alike. Almost invariably, the atria are dilated and the heart weight is increased, but the remaining 5 gross characteristics are variable.

MORPHOLOGIC FEATURES

A chief morphologic abnormality in HCM resides in the ventricular septum. As pointed out by Teare in his initial description of this condition in 1958, the ventricular septum usually is thicker than the left ventricular free wall. Among our adult necropsy patients, the maximal thickness of ventricular septum was usually about 3.0 cm and that of the left ventricular free wall, about 2.0 cm. The thickest portion of the septum is that part located about midway between aortic valve and left ventricular apex. This level corresponds approximately to the apex of right ventricle. Although in nearly all our necropsy patients the ventricular septum was thicker than normal, the left ventricular free wall was usually, but not always, thicker than normal.

Although ventricular asymmetry, that is, a significant difference in maximal thickness of ventricular septum and left ventricular free wall, is a characteristic morphologic feature of HCM, about 30% of our patients at necropsy had ventricular symmetry, that is, equal maximal thicknesses of the ventricular septum and left ventricular free wall. Thus, although asymmetric septal hypertrophy is a sensitive marker for HCM, it is not specific for this condition. Ventricular septa thicker than left ventricular free walls may occur in conditions causing thinning of the left ventricular free wall relative to the septum and in conditions causing thickening of the septum relative to the free wall. The most common cause of preferential free wall thinning is myocardial infarction, and the most common cause of preferential septal thickening is right ventricular systolic hypertension of any cause.

Among patients with HCM, the thickness of the ventricular septum is not dependent on the presence of left ventricular outflow tract obstruction at rest, and indeed, the thickness of the septum is similar in patients with and without outflow obstruction at rest. Although examination of the septum in patients with HCM is not helpful in separating patients *with* from those *without* left ventricular outflow obstruction at rest, examination of the basal portion of the left ventricular free wall (posterior or posterolateral portion) does permit delineation between these two groups of patients. In patients with the nonobstructive type of HCM, this posterobasal portion is thinner than normal and is often pointed like a bird's bill. In patients without obstruction at rest, the thickest portion of the left ventricular free wall is about midway between the base of posterior mitral leaflet and apex of the left ventricle.[14]

Another abnormality in the ventricular septum in patients with HCM is focal myocardial fiber disarray or disorganization. This abnormality, described initially by Teare, occurs in about 95% of these patients, depending on how "septal disorganization" is defined. Small foci of groups of myocardial fibers not parallel to one another in the ventricular septum are common in normal developing and adult hearts. When, however, the definition of "septal disorganization" is rigid and quantitation of the amount of disorganization is introduced, about 90% of the patients with HCM can be clearly delineated from persons with normal hearts or from patients with cardiac conditions other than HCM. Studies by Maron and associates have shown that, among patients with HCM, nearly 90% had >5% of the area of the ventricular septum showing myofiber disorganization.[15,20,22,26] In contrast, among persons with normal hearts or heart conditions other than HCM, <5% and usually <1% of the area of the ventricular septum showed myofiber disorganization.

Although "septal disorganization" of >5% of the area of the ventricular septum occurs in about 90% of the patients with HCM, about 10% of these patients have <5% of the area of the septum showing disarray, and of them a few patients have no disarray at all. Thus, like ventricular asymmetry, "septal disorganization" of >5% of the area of the septum occurs in most patients with HCM, but this abnormality may involve a smaller area of septum or, rarely, may be entirely absent.

Not only does disorganization of myocardial fibers occur, but in addition, ultrastructural studies have shown disarray of myofibrils and myofilaments within individual cells.[4] Again, the abnormalities of myofibrils and myofilaments are not specific for HCM, but when disorganization of these subcellular components is found in other cardiac conditions, the abnormal cells are found in small numbers. The individual septal myocardial cells in HCM also appear to have increased amounts of Z-band material and nonspecific changes of cellular hypertrophy and degeneration.

Myofiber disarray also occurs in the left and right ventricular free walls, but not to the extent observed in the ventricular septum. Ultrastructural examination of the left and right ventricular free walls, however, has disclosed many bizarrely shaped, disorganized cells in the ventricular free walls of patients *without* obstruction, whereas the bizarrely shaped and disorganized myocardial fibers are less numerous in the ventricular free walls in the patient *with* obstruction.[4] Thus, the disorientation of groups of myocardial cells and the disarray of myofibrils and myofilaments within individual myocardial cells are not the result of left ventricular outflow obstruction or high intraventricular systolic pressures.

The functional or clinical significance of "septal disorganization" among patients with HCM is not clear. Among patients studied at necropsy, those with high percentages of area of septum with disorganization were younger, had a higher frequency of premature death involving >1 member of the same family, and had thicker ventricular septa than those with low percentages of area of involved septum.[20] The presence or degree of left ventricular outflow obstruction, length of symptoms of cardiac dysfunction, mode of death, arrhythmias, and so forth were not significantly different in patients with high than in those with low percentages of septal area involved by disorganization.

Another abnormality of ventricular septum in patients with HCM is the presence of abnormal intramural coronary arteries in >50% of the patients.[12,34] The abnormalities observed in the intramural coronary arteries in these patients are striking and consist of increased number and size of arteries with thickened walls and narrowed lumens. The thickening results from increased numbers of smooth-muscle cells and increased amounts of fibrous tissue in both the media and the intima. Moreover, mucoid deposits (acid mucopolysaccharide material) are increased. Like asymmetric ventricular septal thickening and septal disorganization, however, abnormality of the intramural coronary arteries is not specific for HCM, but it is certainly more striking in HCM than in other conditions. Similar abnormality of the intramural coronary arteries may be observed in patients and in Newfoundland dogs with discrete subaortic stenosis,[49] in patients with tunnel subaortic stenosis,[50] in normal human fetuses,[22] and in newborns with aortic valve atresia.[51]

The significance of the changes in the intramural coronary arteries in patients with HCM is unknown. Their presence or absence does not correlate with any analyzed clinical parameter, including presence or degree of left ventricular outflow tract obstruction, age, sex, presence of cardiac dysfunction or ischemia including chest pain, or length of symptoms of cardiac dysfunction. The cause of the striking abnormalities of the intramural coronary arteries also is uncertain. In each of the four conditions in which this degree of abnormality has been observed, namely, HCM, discrete and tunnel subaortic stenosis, and aortic valve atresia, the septum is extremely thick, and movement of the septum during life is limited, as shown by echocardiogram. It is possible that the severe septal thickening prevents adequate expansion of these arteries during ventricular diastole, so flow through them during this phase of the cardiac cycle is greatly reduced. The fibrous-smooth muscle cell response, in turn, may obliterate the unused lumen. This hypothesis, however, does not explain the large size of these arteries. It is possible that the proliferation of the smooth-muscle cells in the walls of these arteries represents a response to the same stimulus that causes severe hypertrophy and abnormal configuration of many striated myocardial cells.

Another abnormality of the ventricular septum in adults with HCM is the occurrence of a fibrous plaque on the mural endocardium of left ventricle in apposition to the anterior mitral leaflet (Figs. 1 to 4). This fibrous thickening is the result of contact between the valvular and mural endocardium. The mural plaque, in other words, is the anatomic equivalent of "systolic anterior motion" of the anterior mitral leaflet observed on echocardiogram in HCM and occasionally in other conditions. The obstruction in HCM, when present, almost certainly begins at a level corresponding to the distal margin of the anterior mitral leaflet and with the caudal margin of the septal endocardial plaque. The mural endocardial septal plaque is present more frequently and is thicker in patients with obstruction at rest than in those without obstruc-

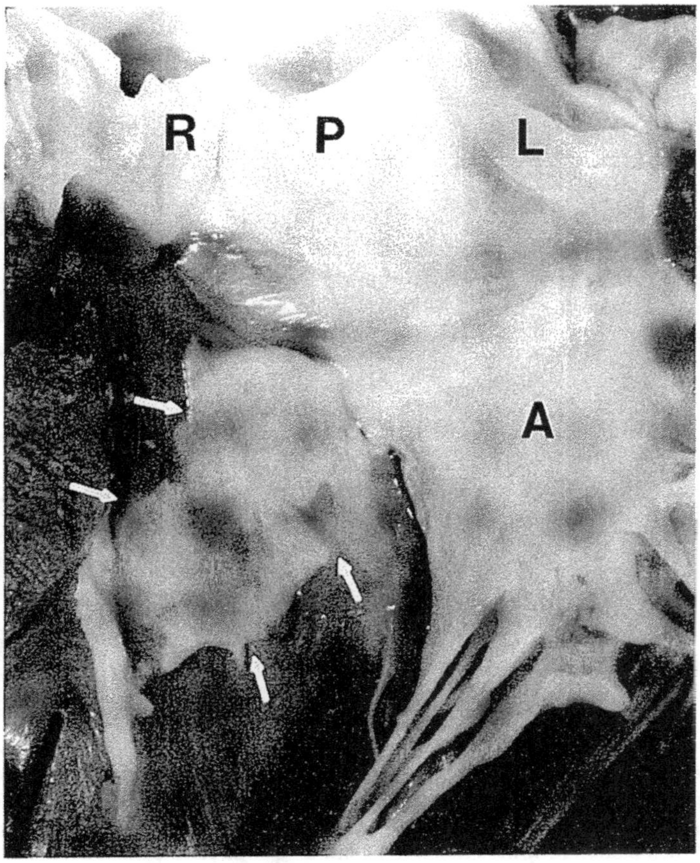

Fig. 1. Opened left ventricular outflow tract and aortic valve of a 14-year-old adopted boy who died suddenly during a basketball game. Sudden death was his first symptom of hypertrophic cardiomyopathy. He was known, however, to have had a precordial murmur, and an echocardiogram had shown systolic anterior motion of the anterior mitral leaflet. At necropsy, the heart weighed 410 g. Neither ventricular cavity was dilated, and both atria were dilated. A mural endocardial fibrous plaque (arrows) was present in the left ventricular outflow tract in apposition to the anterior mitral leaflet (A). The anterior mitral leaflet was mildly thickened by fibrous tissue. R, Right; P, posterior; L, left aortic valve cusp.

tion at rest. The mural outflow plaque, however, is often absent (Figs. 5 to 11).

It appears that HCM is primarily a disease of the ventricular septum, and the morphologic abnormalities in it are apparent at the gross, microscopic, and ultrastructural levels. Other portions of the heart, however, are affected in HCM, but it seems likely that these other abnormalities are secondary, at least in part, to the abnormalities of the ventricular septum. These other abnormalities include decreased ventricular cavity size or at least lack of ventricular cavity dilatation, increased atrial cavity size, varying degrees of interstitial and replacement myocardial fibrosis (Fig. 12), particularly in the ventricular septum, thickening of the posterior as well as the anterior mitral leaflet, and in elderly patients, calcification of the mitral anulus.

The cause of the relatively small sizes

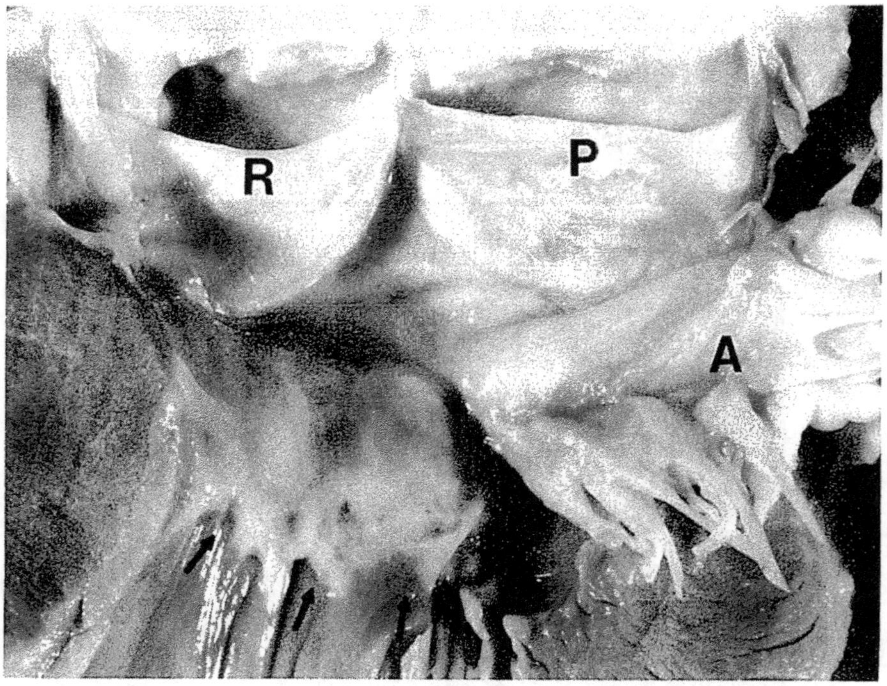

Fig. 2. Opened left ventricular outflow tract and aortic valve of a 56-year-old man who died suddenly in bed shortly after awaking. Sudden death was his first and only symptom of hypertrophic cardiomyopathy. On routine physical examination to obtain a commercial pilot's license, he was found to have a precordial murmur. Echocardiogram had disclosed the maximal thickness of the ventricular septum to be greater than that of the left ventricular free wall, and the ventricles were not dilated. At necropsy, the heart weighed 670 g, and a mural fibrous plaque (arrows) was present in the left ventricular outflow tract in apposition to the anterior mitral leaflet (A), which was thickened by fibrous tissue. R, Right and P, posterior aortic valve cusp.

of the ventricular cavities in HCM is unclear. The septum, being on average about twice normal thickness, surely occupies space normally represented by cavity. Furthermore, the ventricular free walls, on average about one third thicker than normal, also probably compromise the intracavitary space slightly. Additionally, the greater thickness of the septum makes this structure relatively noncompliant, as shown by its absent or minimal movement on echocardiogram. Although the left ventricular free wall in HCM (by echocardiogram) usually contracts vigorously, in contrast to the septum, it appears to have little capacity to distend outwardly. Whatever the explanation, ventricular cavity size is infrequently enlarged in these patients. Those with dilated ventricular cavities have either unscarred left or right ventricular free walls of normal thickness or scarred ventricular free walls of less than normal thickness. Left ventricular dilatation also may occur after operative septotomy-septectomy in HCM.

The impression of ventricular cavity size, as observed at necropsy in patients with HCM, may be misleading because the cavity at necropsy in patients with

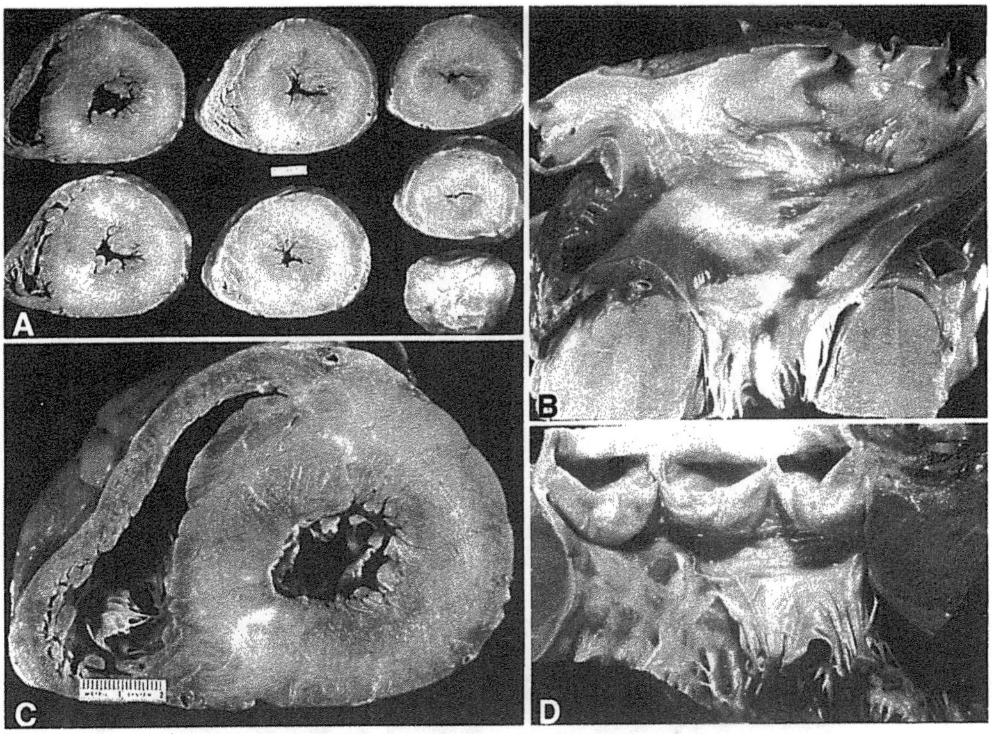

Fig. 3. Heart of a 53-year-old man who died suddenly at home. At age 33, he was found to have labile systemic hypertension. At age 45, although still asymptomatic, cardiac catheterization disclosed an 8-mm Hg peak systolic pressure difference between left ventricle (150/10 mm Hg) and radial artery (142/73 mm Hg) and a 69-mm Hg gradient with provocation. Symptoms of cardiac dysfunction (dyspnea) began at age 47, when his indirect systemic arterial pressure was 170/110 mm Hg. Episodes of dizziness and angina occurred in his fifties. Atrial fibrillation appeared 6 weeks before his sudden death. At necropsy, the heart weighed 750 g. *A,* Transverse sections of the cardiac ventricles disclosed no cavity dilatation, and the septum and left ventricular free wall were of similar thickness. *B,* View of the opened and dilated left atrium and of the atrial aspect of the anterior mitral leaflet, which is thickened. *C,* View of the cardiac base at the level of the distal margins of the mitral leaflets; a small scar is present in the septum posteriorly. *D,* Opened left ventricular outflow tract showing a mural endocardial fibrous plaque in apposition to the thickened anterior mitral leaflet.

HCM represents the size at the end of ventricular systole. This information was derived by comparing the left ventricular free wall thickness at necropsy to that measured by echocardiogram during life. The thickness at necropsy corresponds to the thickness during ventricular systole, not diastole, as observed by echocardiogram.[14]

In contrast to the ventricular cavities, the atrial cavities in HCM, at least in adults, are always dilated. The dilatation appears to be a response to difficulty in filling the relatively small ventricular cavities.

Not only is the anterior mitral leaflet thickened, but often, more frequently in patients with outflow obstruction, the posterior mitral leaflet is also. The thickening of both mitral leaflets is probably

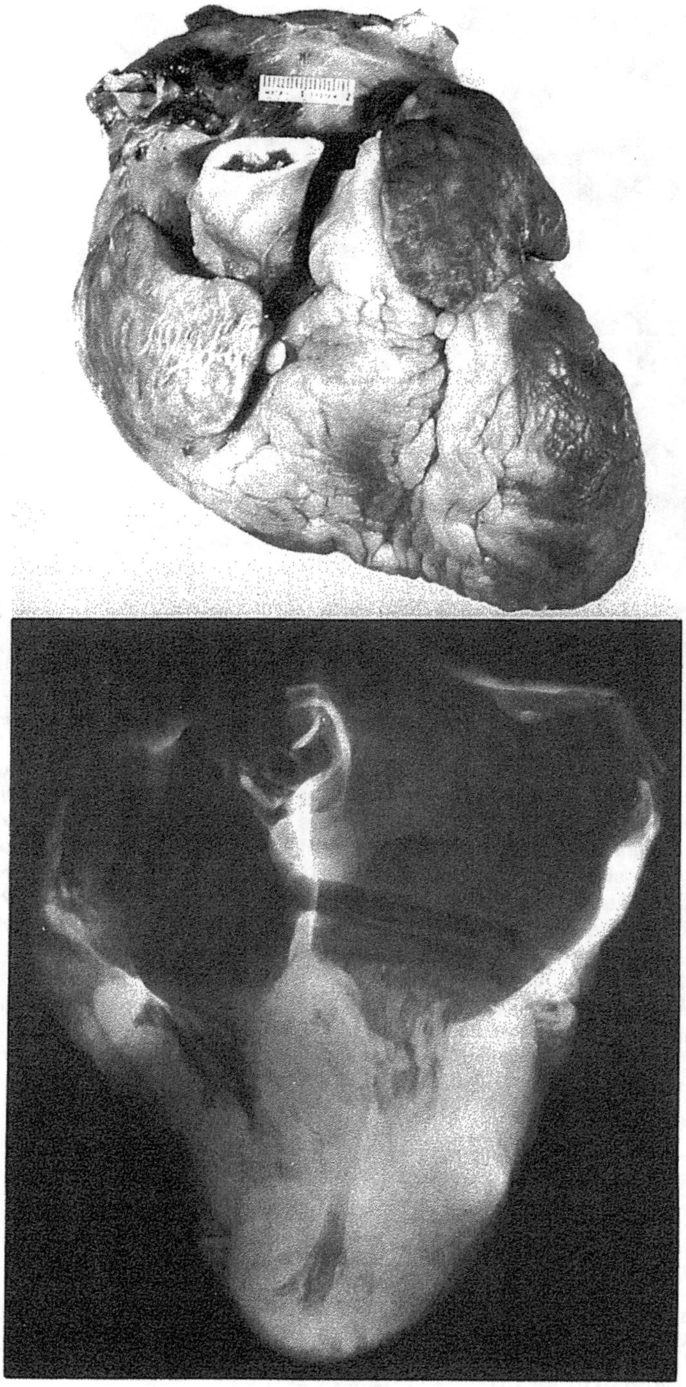

A

B

Fig. 4. Photograph of heart anteriorly (*A*) and radiograph of the heart specimen (*B*) of a 43-year-old woman who died of progressive congestive heart failure. At cardiac catheterization when 33 years old, she had a 54-mm Hg peak systolic pressure gradient at rest between the left ventricle (146/18 mm Hg) and a systemic artery (92/56 mm Hg). Both her mother and 2 siblings died of hypertrophic cardiomyopathy. She had had evidence of congestive heart failure for many years and atrial fibrillation for at least 6 years. At necropsy, the heart weighed only 310 g, but the patient weighed only 40 kg. Both atria were huge, and neither ventricular cavity was dilated. A mural endocardial plaque was present in the left ventricular outflow tract in apposition to the thickened anterior mitral leaflet. The maximal thickness of both ventricular septum and left ventricular free wall was similar.

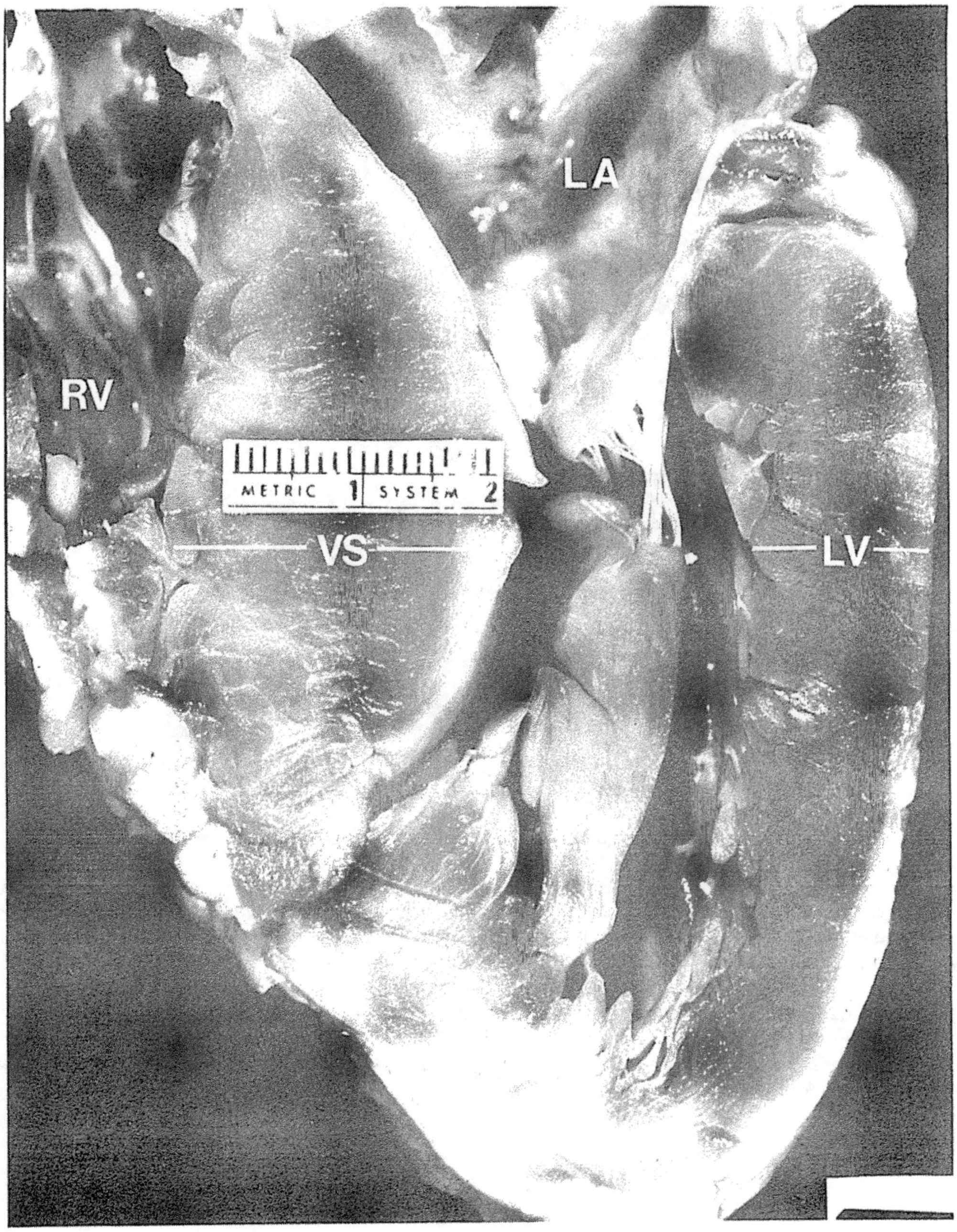

Fig. 5. Longitudinal view of the heart of a 12-year-old girl who died suddenly. Sudden death was her first and last symptom of hypertrophic cardiomyopathy, which was not known to have been present clinically. At necropsy, the heart weighed 275 g. Both atria were dilated; both ventricles were slightly dilated. The maximal thickness of the ventricular septum (VS) was 26 mm and that of the left ventricular (LV) free wall 14 mm. The mitral valve was normal, and no mural endocardial plaque was present in the left ventricular outflow tract. LA, Left atrium; RV, right ventricle.

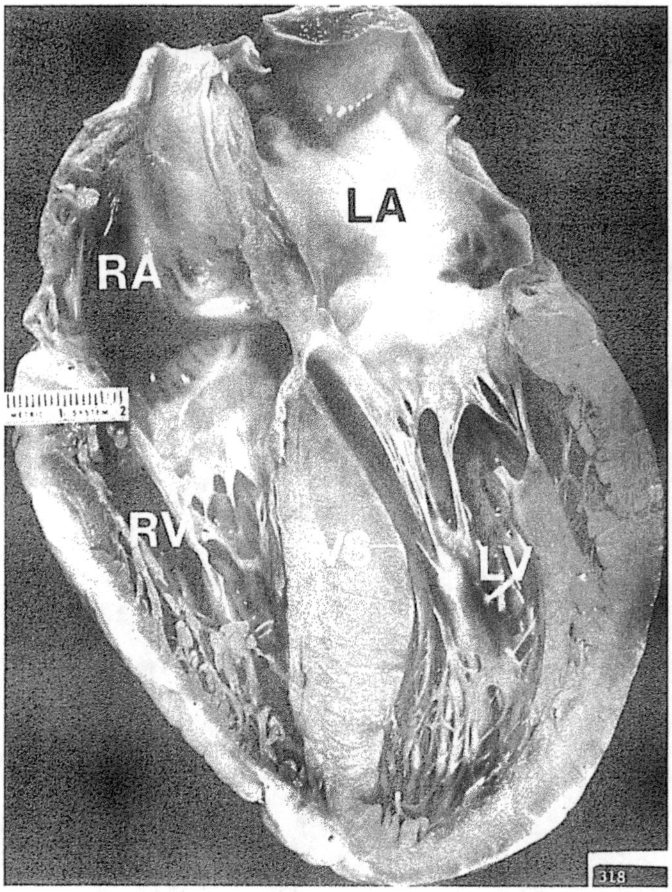

Fig. 6. Longitudinal cut of the heart of a 16-year-old girl who died suddenly while jogging. Her mother had symptomatic (angina) hypertrophic cardiomyopathy, nonobstructive, and she was 45 years old. A maternal aunt had died at 3 months of age; 3 siblings had died at 4, 10, and 13 years of age, and all had documented hypertrophic cardiomyopathy. The child whose heart is shown here had been asymptomatic, but by echocardiogram, the ventricular septum was 14 mm thick, and the left ventricular free wall was 8 mm thick. Systolic anterior motion of the anterior mitral leaflet had been present. The photograph shows that all 4 cavities are dilated, the ventricular septum (VS) is much thicker than the left ventricular (LV) free wall, and the mitral valve is normal. No endocardial mural plaque was present in the left ventricular outflow tract. LA, Left atrium; RA, right atrium; RV, right ventricle.

the consequence of the small left ventricular cavity. The mitral valve resides in the left ventricle, which, being small, causes abnormal contact of the leaflets with themselves and also causes the anterior leaflet to contact the septum. In the patients without obstruction, the basal portion of the left ventricular cavity is larger than in the patients with obstruction because of the thinning of the basal portion of free wall posteriorly and laterally. The focal fibrous thickening of the posterior mitral leaflet probably results from abnormal contact during ventricular systole because there is not enough room in the ventricular cavity to accom-

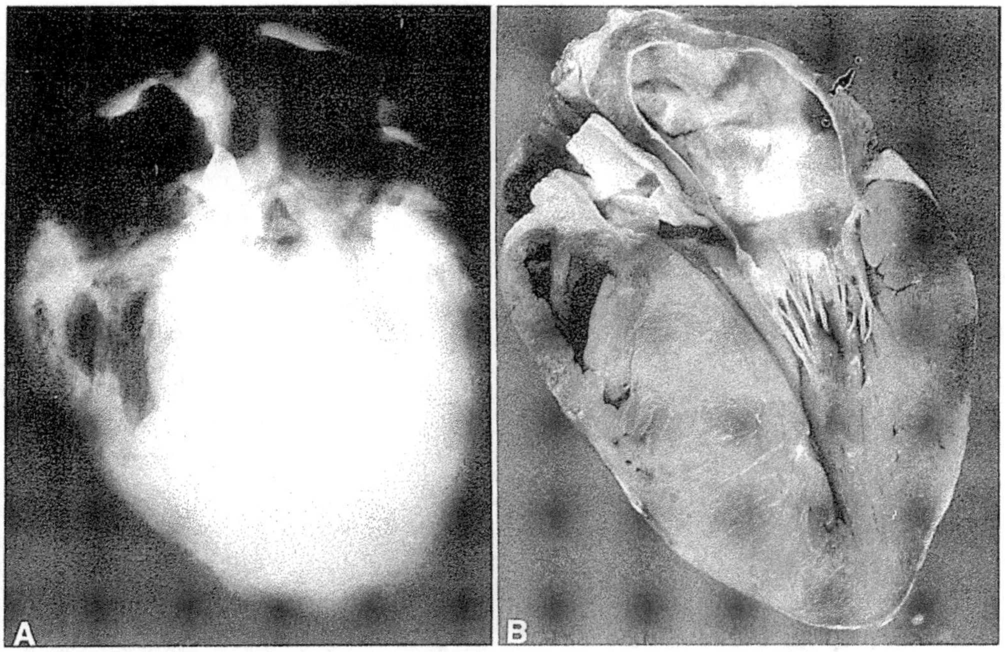

Fig. 7. Radiograph of heart specimen (*A*) and longitudinal cut of heart (*B*) of a previously asymptomatic 18-year-old woman who died suddenly at home shortly after running up some stairs. Her father, a paternal uncle, and a sister had hypertrophic cardiomyopathy. On echocardiogram, the ventricular septum was 35 mm thick, and the left ventricular free wall, 8 mm thick. Systolic anterior motion of the anterior mitral leaflet was absent. The heart weighed 490 g. The radiograph shows the small ventricular cavities and the massiveness of the ventricular myocardium. The right view shows the septum (35 mm) to be much thicker than the left ventricular free wall (10 mm), the mitral leaflets to be normal, and the absence of a left ventricular mural endocardial plaque in apposition to the anterior mitral leaflet.

modate the leaflets and chordae easily. The ventricle and mitral leaflets in this respect may be regarded as similar to an accordion. The mitral leaflet thickening in HCM is analogous to that which occurs normally as a consequence of aging. With aging, the left ventricular cavity becomes smaller, presumably in response to increased work required to fill the small left ventricle. Similar mechanisms appear to be accelerated in HCM.

Most patients with HCM have some degree of mitral regurgitation. It is not related to annular dilatation because the mitral anulus in this condition is not dilated. Furthermore, the leaflet thickening, in and of itself, is not extensive enough to cause valvular regurgitation. The most likely explanation appears to be abnormal bending of the papillary muscles, particularly the anterolateral one. These structures may be bent abnormally by the bulging ventricular septum, with resulting excessive tension on the chordae tendineae preventing closure of the mitral orifice. Although they are usually present in the papillary muscles in HCM, focal scars cannot account for the regurgitation. Although it is usually mild in HCM, mitral regurgitation may be the dominant clinical feature of this condition. Despite its advocacy by some in-

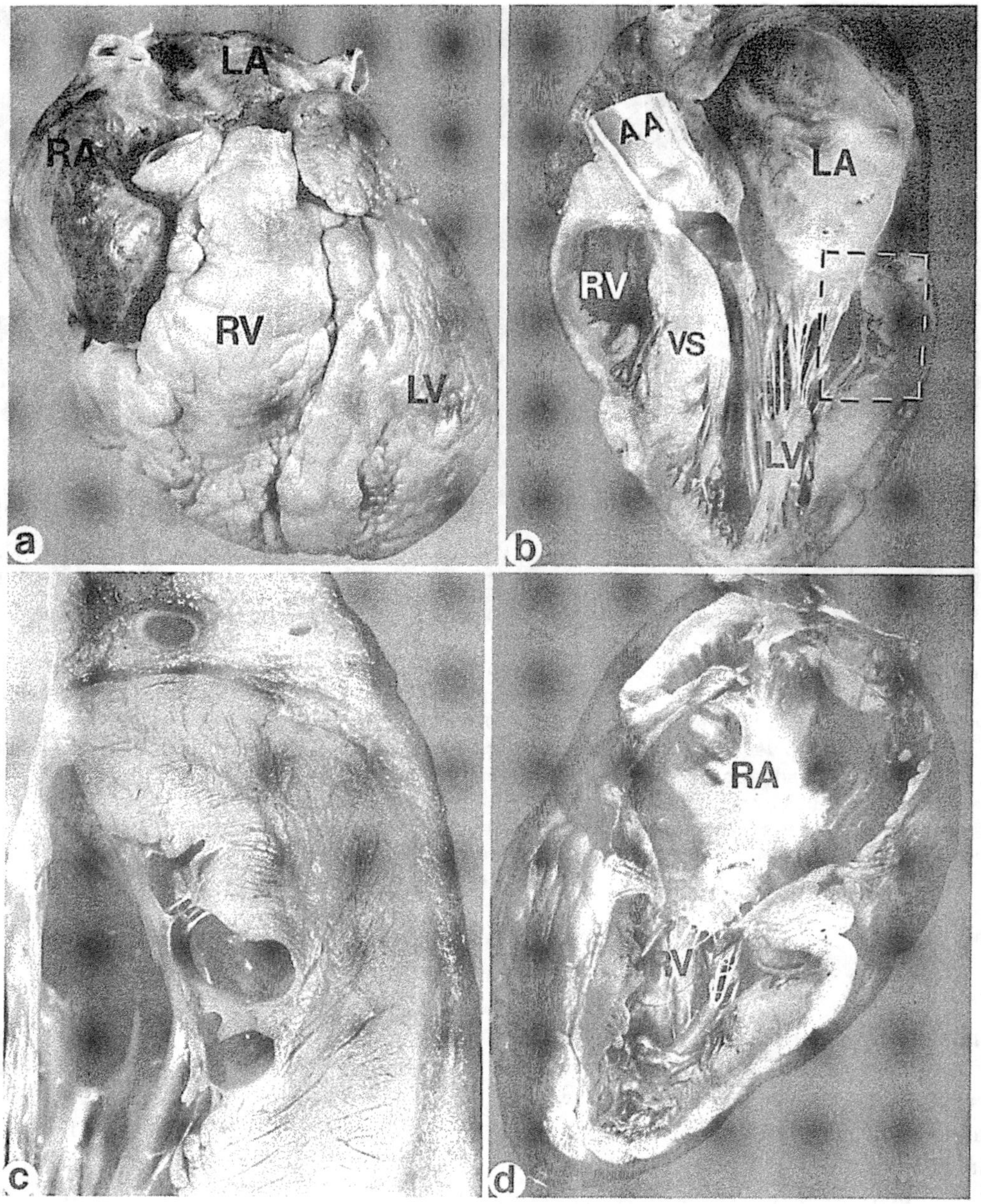

Fig. 8. Heart of a 21-year-old woman who died of massive congestive heart failure. She had been well until age 17, when the heart was found to be enlarged and the electrocardiogram to be abnormal. Echocardiogram showed the ventricular septum (26 mm) to be thicker than the left ventricular free wall (11 mm) and the ventricular cavities to be of normal size. Systolic anterior motion of the anterior mitral leaflet was present, and the left atrial diameter was 48 mm. At 2 cardiac catheterizations, no peak systolic outflow pressure gradient was present either at rest or on provocation. Atrial fibrillation appeared about a year before death. No other family members had hypertrophic cardiomyopathy. At necropsy, the heart weighed 410 g. *a,* Exterior view; both the right (RA) and the left atrium (LA) are dilated; extensive adipose tissue covers the right (RV) and the left ventricle (LV). *b,* Longitudinal view of the heart; the ventricular septum (VS) is thicker than the left ventricular free wall; the left atrium is dilated, and the ascending aorta (AA) is of normal size. *c,* A close-up of the rectangular, dotted area in *b;* when the free wall behind the posterior mitral leaflet is thinner (0.8 cm) than the free wall more caudally, left ventricular outflow obstruction is nearly always absent. *d,* Longitudinal view of the dilated right atrium and the right ventricle.

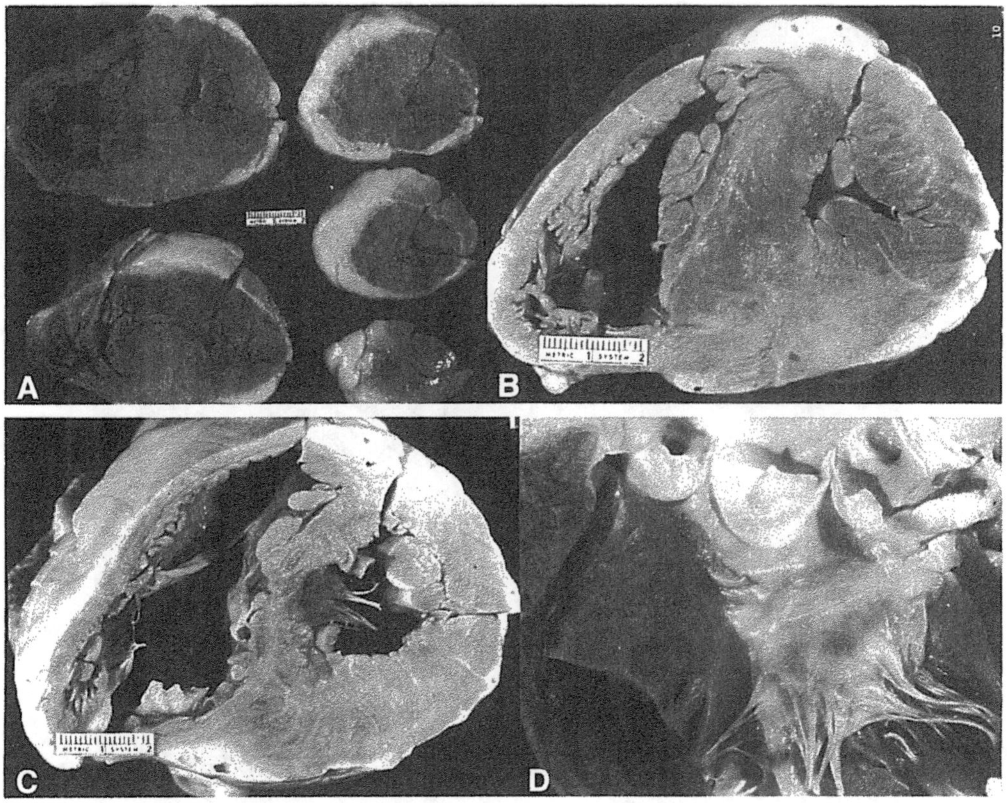

Fig. 9. Heart of a 26-year-old woman who died suddenly outside the hospital. Several family members also had hypertrophic cardiomyopathy. At necropsy, the heart weighed approximately 500 g. *A,* Transverse sections of the ventricles showing the cavities to be of normal size and the septum to be thicker than the left ventricular free wall. *B,* Close-up of a section not shown in *A. C,* Basal section showing the septum at this level to be thinner than the left ventricular free wall. *D,* Opened left ventricular outflow tract and aortic valve showing the mitral valve to be normal and the absence of a mural endocardial outflow plaque. The ventricular septum in this patient was thicker in the apical half than in the basal half.

vestigators,[52-55] mitral valve replacement in HCM is potentially hazardous and rarely warranted.[6] The exception is the patient with severe mitral regurgitation from superimposed infective endocarditis, a condition not rare in patients with HCM. The small left ventricular cavity makes mitral valve replacement difficult, and the small cavity may prevent a prosthesis or bioprosthesis in the mitral position from functioning properly. Furthermore, the mitral regurgitation in patients with HCM, except when due to valvular damage from infective endocarditis, nearly always either disappears or is strikingly lessened by adequate partial septectomy and septotomy.

GROSS MORPHOLOGIC DIFFERENCES BY AGE AND SEX

Patients with HCM can die in any decade of life. Figure 13 presents the ages of

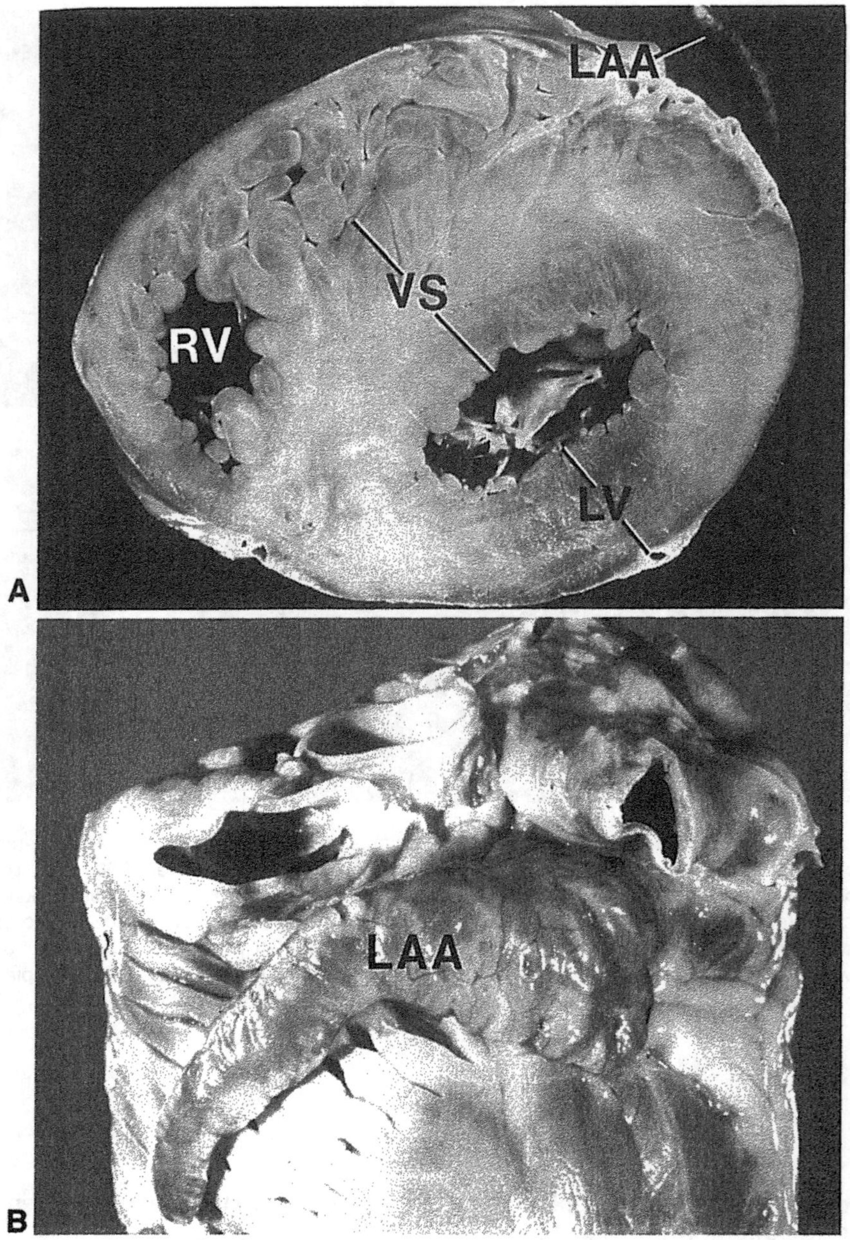

Fig. 10. Heart of a 28-year-old man in whom sudden death was the first and only manifestation of hypertrophic cardiomyopathy, which was not diagnosed clinically. At necropsy, the heart weighed 970 g. *A,* Transverse section of the ventricles at the level of the margins of the mitral leaflets; the septum is 35 mm, and the left ventricular free wall is 20 mm thick; the mitral valve is normal, and the mural endocardium of the left ventricular outflow tract is normal. LAA, Left atrial appendage; LV, left ventricular wall; VS, ventricular septum; RV, right ventricular cavity. *B,* View of the dilated left atrial appendage, which has a tail-like appearance.

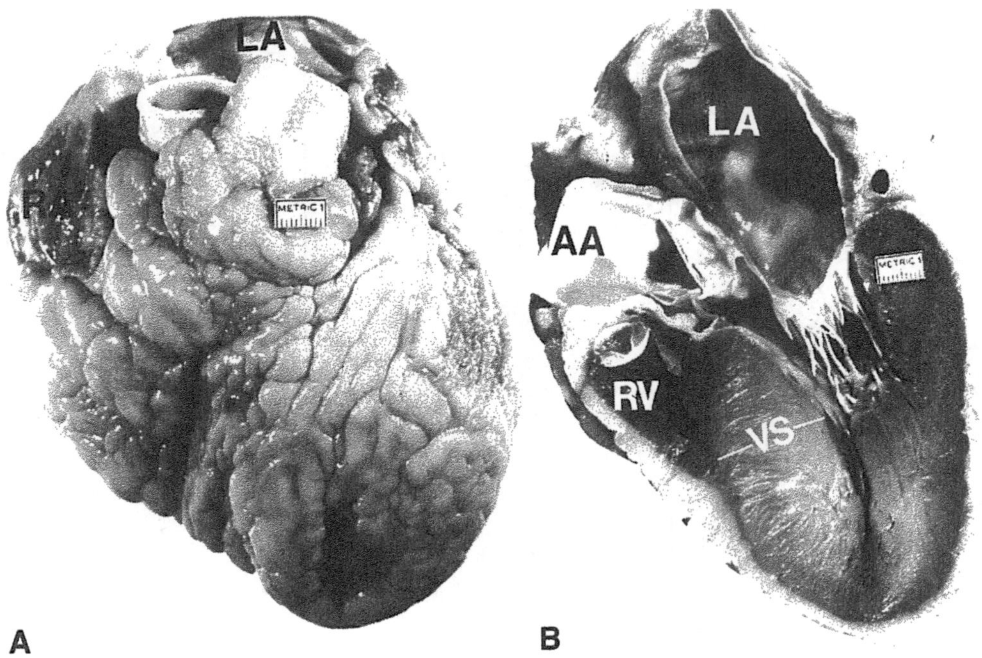

Fig. 11. Heart of a 38-year-old woman who died suddenly at home. At least 6 other members of her family also had hypertrophic cardiomyopathy. She had had episodic chest pain since age 18; by age 36, she was having 20 to 30 episodes of chest pain daily. At catheterization on 3 occasions, no left ventricular outflow obstruction was present. By echocardiogram, systolic anterior motion of the anterior mitral leaflet was absent. At necropsy, the heart weighed 460 g. *A,* Exterior of the heart showing considerable subepicardial fat. RA, Right atrium; LA, left atrium. *B,* Longitudinal view of the heart. The septum measures about 25 mm, and the left ventricular free wall is about 19 mm in maximal thickness. Neither ventricular cavity is dilated, but right and left atria are dilated. The mitral valve is normal, and there is no thickening of mural endocardium in the left ventricular outflow tract. AA, Ascending aorta; RV, right ventricle; VS, ventricular septum.

death by decade of the 220 patients studied in the Pathology Branch of the National Heart, Lung, and Blood Institute. In the first 2 decades of life, a higher percentage of the necropsied patients were male, whereas most necropsy patients over 60 years of age were women. Between 20 and 60 years of age, the percentage of males and females among necropsied patients was similar.

Among the 220 patients studied at necropsy, 145 had not had a cardiac operation, and 75 had undergone such a procedure. The 145 patients with unoperated HCM were separated into 3 groups according to the age of death (Table 2). In the 118 patients who died from ages 11 to 70 years, the diagnosis of HCM at necropsy was not difficult. In the 13 extremely young (age ≤10 years) and in the 14 oldest patients (age >70 years), however, diagnosis of HCM both clinically and at necropsy was usually difficult. Tables 3 and 4 present clinical and morphologic findings in the 13 patients ≤10 years of age and the 14 patients >70 years of age at death, respectively.

In all 13 patients who died at <10 years of age (see Table 3; Figs. 14 to 16), the heart at necropsy was increased in

TABLE 2. CLINICAL AND CARDIAC MORPHOLOGIC CHARACTERISTICS IN 3 DIFFERENT AGE GROUPS OF 145 NECROPSY PATIENTS WITH UNOPERATED HYPERTROPHIC CARDIOMYOPATHY

Group	Age (yr)	Number of Patients	Age (yr) Range (mean)	Males/ females	Heart weight (g) Range (mean)	VS > LV	Fibrous Plaque, LVOT	Thickened MV	Dilated LV Cavity	Gross Fibrosis LV/VS	Epicardial CAD
I	≤10	13	0.2–9	8/5	28–670 (190) (male = 256) (female = 57)	9/13 (69%)	2/13 (15%)	3/13 (23%)	4/13 (31%)	0/13 (0)	0/13 (0)
II	11–70	118	11–70 (35)	63/55	250–1250 (559) (male = 606) (female = 506)	82/115 (71%)	69/110 (63%)	73/110 (66%)	22/118 (19%)	53/118 (45%)	9/114 (8%)
III	>70	14	71–87 (79)	3/11	265–710 (468) (men = 558) (women = 443)	11/14 (79%)	12/14 (86%)	14/14 (100%)	1/14 (7%)	7/14 (50%)	7/14 (50%)
	TOTALS or MEAN	145	(36)	74/71	(526) (men = 574) (women = 476)	102/142 (72%)	83/137 (61%)	90/137 (66%)	27/145 (19%)	60/145 (41%)	16/141 (11%)

CAD, Significant coronary artery disease; LV, left ventricular or left ventricle; OT, outflow tract; MV, mitral valve; VS, ventricular septum.

TABLE 3. CLINICAL AND CARDIAC MORPHOLOGIC CHARACTERISTICS OF 13 PATIENTS AGED ≤10 YEARS WITH HYPERTROPHIC CARDIOMYOPATHY

Case	Age	Sex	LV-SA PSG at rest (mm Hg)	HCM Diagnosed During Life	FH of HCM	Mode of Death	Heart Weight (g)	VS > LV	Fibrous Plaque, LVOT	Thickened MV	Dilated LV Cavity	Gross Fibrosis LV/VS	MFD in VS
1	1 mo	M	—	0*	0	Operation†	—	+	0	0	0	0	—
2	1 mo	M	—	0*	0	CHF	80	0	+	+	0	0	+
3	2 mo	M	—	0*	—	Unknown	50	+	0	+	0	0	+
4‡	2 mo	F	0	0*	0	CHF	62	+	0	0	+§	0	+
5	2 mo	F	—	+	0	Sudden	28	+	0	0	0	0	—
6	6 mo	F	—	0*	0	Sudden	80	0	0	0	0	0	+
7	7 mo	F	100	+	0	Procedure‖	—	+	+	+	0	0	—
8	9 mo	F	—	+	0	Pneumonia	—	+	0	0	0	0	+
9	12 mo	M	—	0*	0	CHF	270	+	0	0	0	0	+
10	18 mo	M	0	0*	0	Unknown	—	+	0	0	+	0	—
11	7 yr	M	0	0*	0	Sudden	227	+	0	0	+	0	+
12	9 yr	M	0	0*	0	Sudden	240	0	0	0	+#	0	+
13	9 yr	M	0	+	0	Sudden	670	0	0	0	0	0	—

* Heart disease diagnosed, but not hypertrophic cardiomyopathy.

† This patient underwent operative ligation of the left main coronary artery for presumed anomalous origin from the pulmonary trunk; no coronary anomaly was found at necropsy.

‡Case reported by Maron, B. J., et al.: Am. Heart J., *101*:857, 1981.

§ This patient had complete heart block from birth and the cavity dilatation may have resulted from the conduction disturbance.

‖ Right ventricular wall perforated during endomyocardial biopsy producing hemopericardium.

\# Left ventricular cavity normal in size at angiogram several months before death.

CHF, Congestive heart failure; F, female; FH, family history; HCM, hypertrophic cardiomyopathy; LV, left ventricle or left ventricular; LVOT, left ventricular outflow tract; M, male; MFD, myocardial fiber disorganization; MV, mitral valve; PSG, peak systolic gradient; SA, systemic artery; VS, ventricular septum; +, present or positive; 0, absent or negative; —, no information available.

TABLE 4. CLINICAL AND CARDIAC MORPHOLOGIC CHARACTERISTICS OF PATIENTS >70 YEARS OF AGE WITH HYPERTROPHIC CARDIOMYOPATHY WITHOUT A CARDIAC OPERATION

Case	Age (yr)	Sex	HCM diagnosed in Life	SH	FH of HCM	Mode of Death	Heart Weight (g)	VS > LV	Thickness VS	Thickness LV	Fibrous Plaque, LVOT	Thickened MV	MAC (0–4)	Dilated LV Cavity	Gross Fibrosis, LV/VS	No. 4 CAs >75% in CSA
1	71	M	0	+	0	NC (C)	710	+	3.5	2.5	0	+	0	0	+	1
2	71	F	+(e)	+	0	CHF	475	+	2.5	1.4	+	+	0	0	0	1
3	73	F	+	—	+	NC (C)	430	0	0.6	1.1	0	+	0	+	+*	0
4	74	F	0	—	0	NC (C)	360	+	2.1	1.5	+	+	1	0	0	0
5	74	F	+	+	0	CHF	650	+	3.7	2.5	+	+	4	0	+	0
6	76	F	+(e)	0	0	Sudden	510	+	1.8	1.4	+	+	2	0	0	1
7	78	M	0	+	0	NC	450	+	—	—	+	+	0	0	+	0
8	79	F	0	0	0	Sudden	430	+	2.5	1.8	+	+	4	0	+	2
9	81	F	0	0	0	NC	265	0	1.2	1.2	+	+	0	0	0	0
10	82	F	+(e)	—	0	Sudden	310	+	2.0	1.5	+	+	2	0	0	1
11	83	F	+(e)	—	0	CHF†	450	+	3.0	2.0	+	+	0	0	0	0
12	84	M	0	0	0	Operation‡	515	0	2.0	2.0	+	+	1	0	+	3
13	86	F	0	+	0	Sudden	520	+	3.0	2.0	+	+	0	0	+	0
14	87	F	+(e)	—	0	NC (C)	470	+	2.5	2.0	+	+	4	0	0	1

* Involves nearly all the ventricular septum.

† Patient also had active infective endocarditis involving the mitral valve.

‡ Patient died shortly after thoracotomy for planned pericardiectomy for suspected pericardial constriction.

NC, Noncardiac; C, cancer; CHF, congestive heart failure; CAs, major epicardial coronary arteries; CSA, cross-sectional area; e, echocardiogram; F, female; FH, family history; HCM, hypertrophic cardiomyopathy; LV, left ventricle; LVOT, left ventricular outflow tract; M, male; MAC, mitral annular calcium; MV, mitral valve; SH, systemic hypertension by history; VS, ventricular septum; +, present or positive; 0, absent or negative; —, no information available.

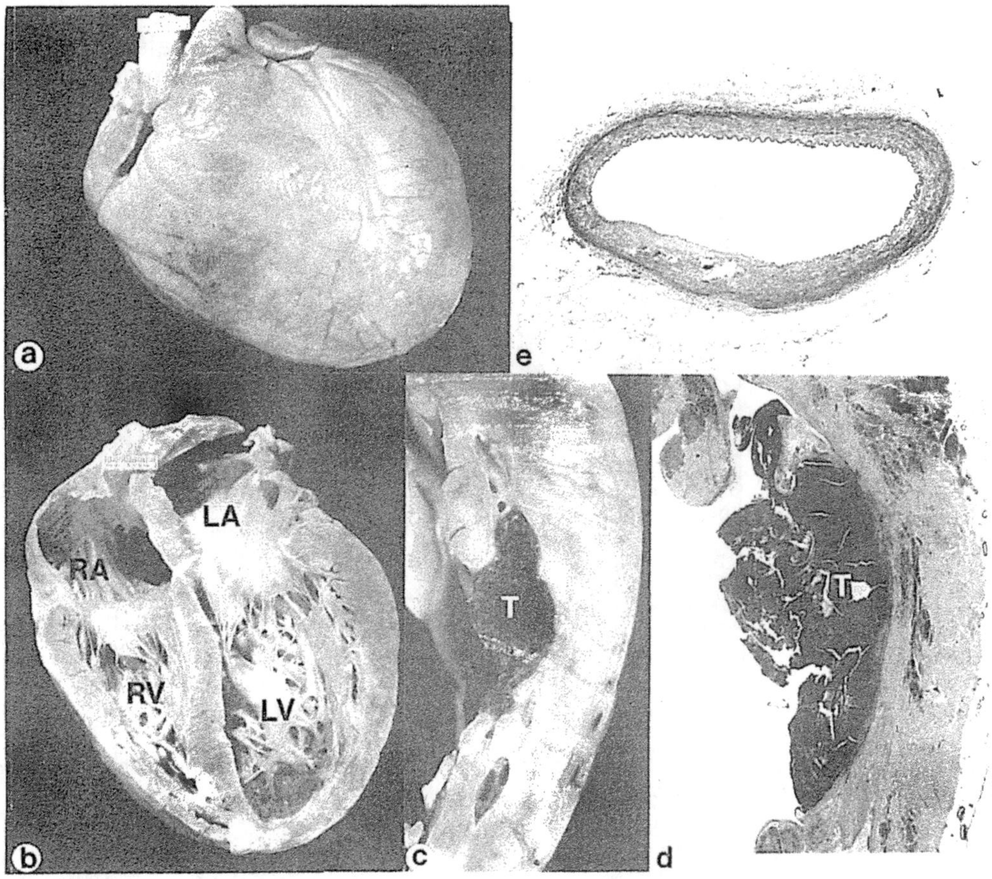

Fig. 12. Heart of a 19-year-old woman who died of progressive congestive heart failure. Her mother and a brother had evidence of hypertrophic cardiomyopathy. At cardiac catheterization when asymptomatic at age 11, the left ventricular cavity was normal in size by angiogram, and a small (<30 mm Hg) pressure gradient was present on provocation, but not at rest. Exertional dyspnea began at age 12 and slowly progressed thereafter. Two months before death, she had acute pulmonary edema. A month before death, echocardiogram disclosed the left ventricular cavity to be 57 mm in transverse diameter in end-diastole and 50 mm in end-systole; the left atrium was 42 mm, and the ejection fraction was 30%. The maximal thickness of the ventricular septum and left ventricular free wall were similar. *a,* Heart from the anterior view. *b,* Four-chamber view showing a dilated right (RV) and left (LV) ventricle and a lesser dilated right (RA) and left (LA) atrium. *c,* Longitudinal view of severely scarred left ventricular free wall with a superimposed thrombus (T). *d,* Photomicrograph of a portion of the wall shown in *c;* only a few islands of myocardial cells remain. *e,* Left main coronary artery; all major epicardial coronary arteries were normal.

weight. The thickness of the septum was greater than that of the left ventricular free wall in 9 patients (69%), a percentage similar to that in the other age groups. A fibrous plaque in the left ventricular outflow tract, however, was present in only 2 patients (15%), and the mitral valve was thickened in only 3 patients (23%). Furthermore, the left ventricle at necropsy was dilated in 4 patients (31%). No patient had a grossly visible left ventricular or septal scar. In

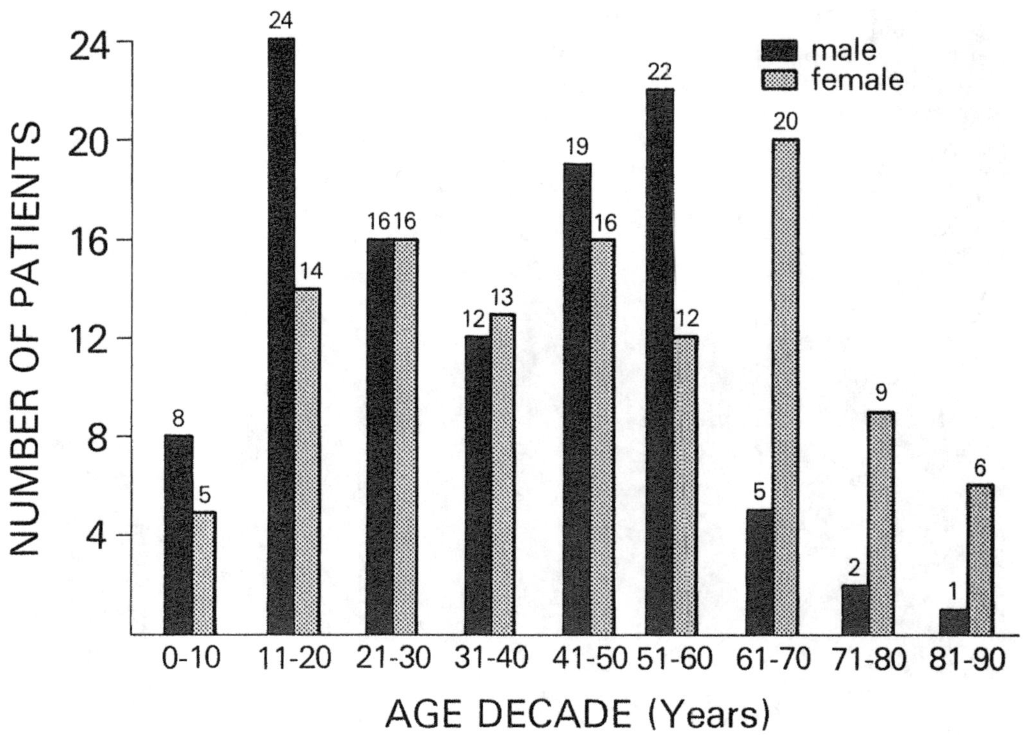

Fig. 13. Ages by decade and sex of the 220 patients with hypertrophic cardiomyopathy studied at necropsy in the Pathology Branch of the National Heart, Lung, and Blood Institute.

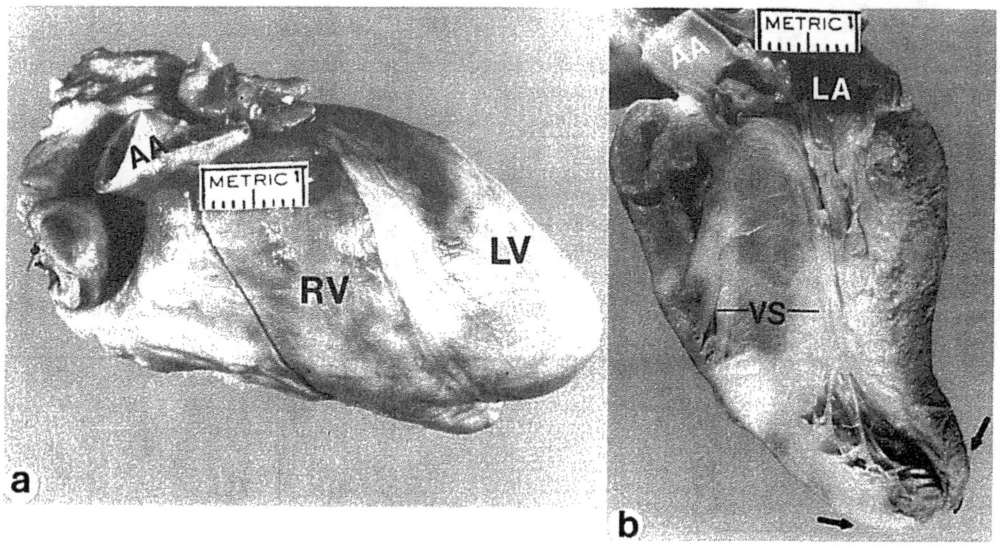

Fig. 14. Heart of a 2-month-old boy who died suddenly. Echocardiogram shortly before death disclosed the ventricular septum to be thicker than the left ventricular free wall, possible systolic anterior motion of the anterior mitral leaflet, hyperdynamic ventricles, and a dilated left atrium. *a,* Exterior of the heart; AA, ascending aorta; LV, left ventricle; RV, right ventricle. *b,* Longitudinal view of the heart showing the ventricular septum (VS) to be thicker than the left ventricular free wall, a thickened mitral valve, but no mural endocardial plaque in the left ventricular outflow tract; LA, left atrium.

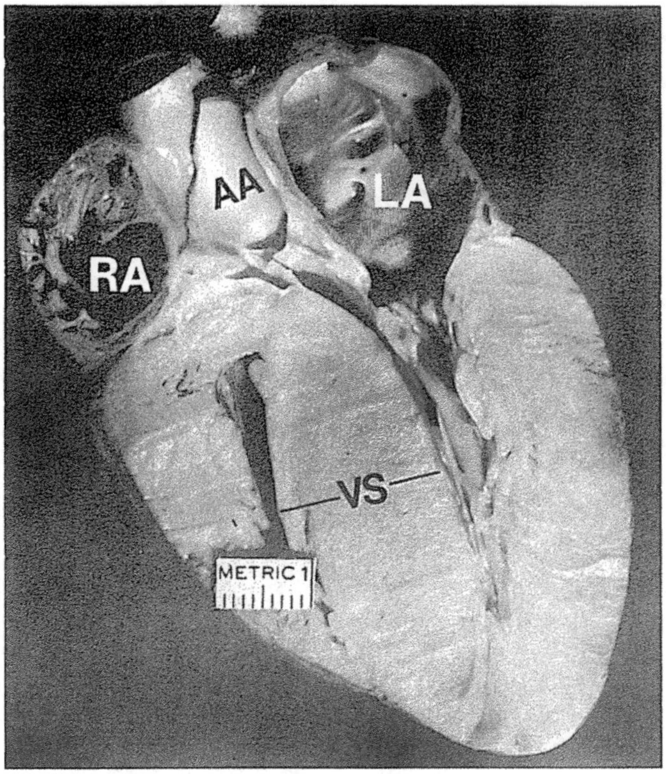

Fig. 15. Longitudinal view of heart of a 7.5-year-old boy who began having grand mal seizures at the age of 4 months and was found to have an enlarged heart with poor ventricular contractions and an abnormal electrocardiogram. A grade 3/6 systolic precordial murmur was recorded. He was found dead in bed. At necropsy, the heart weighed 230 g. Shown here is a longitudinal cut showing the ventricular septum (VS) to be thicker than the left ventricular wall and a dilated right (RA) and left atrium (LA). The mitral valve is normal, and the mural endocardial in apposition to the anterior leaflet is normal. AA, Ascending aorta.

only 4 patients was the diagnosis of HCM made during life, although all 13 were considered clinically to have heart disease.

Of the 14 patients >70 years of age at death, only 3 (21%) were men (Table 4). Diagnosis of HCM was made in 7 of these 14 patients during life. Only 1 patient had a family history of HCM, and 5 had had systemic hypertension. All but 2 patients had a heart of increased weight; the mean increase, however, was not as great as that in the patients aged 11 to 70 years. The maximal thickness of the ventricular septum was greater than that of the left ventricular free wall in 11 patients (79%). The mitral valve was thickened in all 14 patients. A fibrous plaque was present in the left ventricular outflow tract in 12 patients (86%), and the left ventricular cavity was of normal or smaller-than-normal size in 13 patients (93%). Gross left ventricular fibrosis was present in 7 of the 14 elderly patients, and 7 had significant narrowing of 1 or more major epicardial coronary arteries.

In the necropsied patients with HCM aged 11 to 70 years, the numbers of males and females were similar. Heart weight was increased in 113 patients (96%); 71%

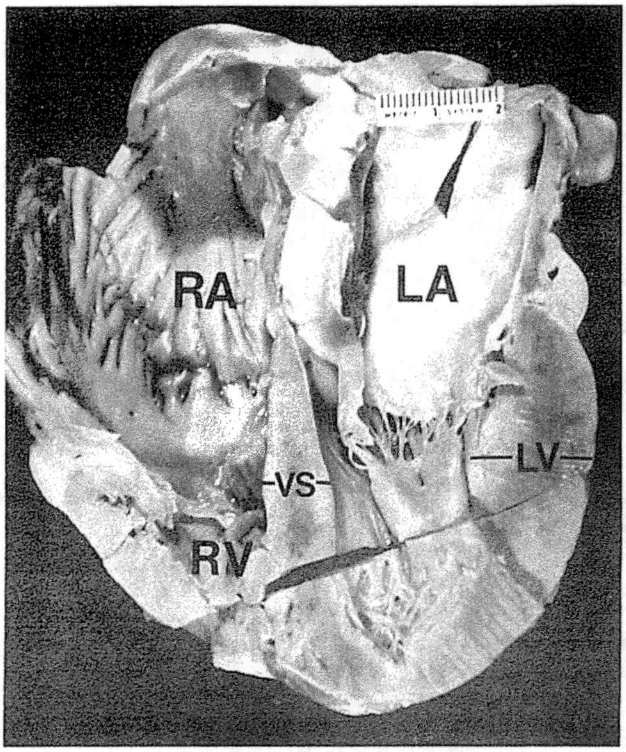

Fig. 16. Four-chamber view of the heart of a 9-year-old boy. He was well until about 1 year before death, when evidence of congestive heart failure appeared, and it rapidly progressed. At catheterization, the following pressures in mm Hg were recorded: right ventricle, 90/27; pulmonary artery 90/60; left ventricle, 90/34, and femoral artery, 105/60. At angiogram, the left ventricular cavity was of normal size, but it contracted poorly. He died suddenly. At necropsy, the heart weighed 240 g. Both the right (RA) and left (LA) atrium are enormously dilated. The ventricular septum (VS) is thinner than the left ventricular (LV) free wall. Neither right (RV) nor left ventricle (LV) is dilated. The 4 valves are normal, and no endocardial mural plaque is present in the left ventricular outflow tract. The cause of the severe pulmonary hypertension is unclear, but it may have been the result of the extremely depressed left ventricular function.

had a septum thicker than the left ventricular free wall; 66% had a thickened mitral valve, and 63% had a fibrous endocardial plaque in the left ventricular outflow tract. The left ventricular cavity was of normal or smaller-than-normal size in 96 patients (81%), and gross left ventricular fibrosis was present in 53 patients (45%). Only 8% of these 113 patients had 1 or more major epicardial coronary arteries severely (> 75% decrease in cross-sectional area lumen) narrowed.

OBSTRUCTIVE VERSUS NONOBSTRUCTIVE TYPES

The 145 patients with unoperated HCM were separated into 3 groups (Table 5): those in whom a left ventricular outflow tract gradient was present at rest (group I), absent (group II), and unknown (group III) (cardiac catheterization not performed). Certain morphologic features of the obstructive type (group I) were different from those of the nonob-

TABLE 5. COMPARISON OF CLINICAL AND CARDIAC MORPHOLOGIC CHARACTERISTICS IN 145 UNOPERATED NECROPSY PATIENTS WITH HYPERTROPHIC CARDIOMYOPATHY IN WHOM A LEFT VENTRICULAR OUTFLOW TRACT PRESSURE GRADIENT WAS PRESENT, ABSENT, OR UNKNOWN

Group	LVOT Gradient	Number of Patients	Ages (yr) Range (mean)	M/F	Heart weight (g) Range (mean)	VS > LV	Fibrous Plaque, LVOT	Thickened MV	Dilated LV Cavity	Gross Fibrosis LV/VS	Epicardial CAD
I	Present	32	0.2–70 (43)	11/21	310–1250 (613) (male = 736) (female = 546)	25/32 (78%)	31/32 (97%)	31/32 (97%)	2/32 (6%)	15/32 (47%)	7/32 (22%)
II	Absent	33	0.2–54 (31)	18/15	62–1065 (507) (male = 560) (female = 446)	21/33 (64%)	15/32 (47%)	15/32 (47%)	13/33 (39%)	15/33 (45%)	2/33 (6%)
III	Unknown	80	0.1–87 (35)	45/35	28–1200 (499) (male = 539) (female = 450)	56/77 (73%)	37/73 (51%)	44/73 (60%)	12/80 (15%)	30/80 (38%)	7/76 (9%)
TOTALS or MEAN		145	(36)	74/71	28–1250 (526) (male = 574) (female = 476)	102/142	83/137	90/137	27/145	60/145 (41%)	16/141 (11%)

LVOT, Left ventricular outflow tract; M, male; F, female; VS, ventricular septum; LV, left ventricular or left ventricle; MV, mitral valve; CAD, coronary artery disease.

structive type (group II). The mean heart weights of male and female patients with left ventricular outflow tract gradients were greater than in patients without a gradient, and disproportionately thickened septa also were more common (78% versus 64%). A thickened mitral valve and a fibrous plaque in the left ventricular outflow tract were present in 31 (97%) of 32 patients with a gradient and in 15 (47%) of 32 patients without a gradient. A dilated left ventricular cavity was found more frequently in patients without a gradient (39% versus 6%). The frequency of gross left ventricular fibrosis was similar in both groups, but epicardial coronary artery disease occurred in a higher percentage of patients with the obstructive type.

Cardiac catheterization was not done in 80 of the 145 patients with unoperated HCM. This group presumably included both obstructive and nonobstructive types, and as expected, the frequency of disproportionately thickened septa, fibrous plaque in the outflow tract, thickened mitral valve, and nondilated left ventricular cavity were between those of groups I and II.

CARDIAC MORPHOLOGIC FEATURES AFTER OPERATIVE TREATMENT

Of the 220 necropsy patients with HCM, 75 underwent operative treatment: partial septal myectomy in 66 (Fig. 17); septal myotomy alone in 4; and mitral valve replacement in 7. The patients were separated into 3 groups according to length of survival after operation (Table 6). Thirty-seven patients survived ≤60 days; 15 patients, 61 days to 42 months; and 23 patients, >42 months. The average age of death for all 75 patients was 47 years. In the patients who died ≤60 days after operation, a disproportionately high number were women, and the mean left ventricular outflow tract gradient preoperatively was higher than in those who survived longer periods. A fibrous plaque in the left ventricular outflow tract and a thickened mitral valve were present in >90% of patients who underwent operation. An impressive morphologic change after operation was dilation of the left ventricular cavity. Only 2 of 52 patients who died ≤42 months after operation had dilated left ventricular cavities, whereas 16 (73%) of 22 patients who survived >42 months after operation had dilated left ventricular cavities.

SUMMARY

The morphologic features of 220 patients with HCM are described. The major gross morphologic features of HCM, in order of decreasing frequency, are as follows: (1) dilated atria (100%); (2) increased heart weight (95%); (3) nondilated left ventricle (79%); (4) thickened mitral valve (75%); (5) fibrous endocardial mural plaque, left ventricular outflow tract (72%); and (6) a ventricular septum thicker than the left ventricular free wall (69%). Gross left ventricular fibrosis occurred in 42% of the patients and rarely was a consequence of associated narrowing of an epicardial coronary artery disease. HCM may cause death in any decade of life. The diagnosis of HCM in the extremely young (age ≤10 years) and the extremely old (age >70) is more difficult clinically and at necropsy than in the intermediate age group. Patients with the obstructive type of HCM usually have larger hearts, a higher frequency of a fibrous plaque in the left ventricular outflow tract, and a higher frequency of a thickened mitral valve than those without obstruction. Left ventricular cavity dilation is present in about 20% of patients with HCM and is a result of either operation (with survival >42 months) or extensive left ventricular wall scarring.

TABLE 6. CLINICAL AND CARDIAC MORPHOLOGIC CHARACTERISTICS OF 75 NECROPSY PATIENTS WITH HYPERTROPHIC CARDIOMYOPATHY WHO HAD CARDIAC OPERATIVE TREATMENT

Group	Survival After Operation	Number of Patients	Age (yr) Range (mean)	Males/ females	LV–SA PSG at Rest (mm Hg) Range (mean)	Cardiac Operation		
						Septal Myotomy	Septal Myectomy	MVR
I	≤60 days	37	18–69 (48)	13/24	0–162 (70)	0	32	5
II	61 days–42 mo	15	22–72 (47)	8/7	0–130 (50)	2	13	0
III	>42 mo	23	21–81 (47)	13/10	0–130 (48)	2	21	2
TOTAL		75	18–81 (47)	34/41	0–162 (61)	4	66	7

Interval 0 to Death Range (mean)	Heart weight (g) Range (mean)	VS > LV	Fibrous Plaque, LVOT	Thickened MV	Dilated LV Cavity	Gross Fibrosis LV/VS	Epicardial CAD
0–57 days (6)	290–1070 (582) (men = 733) (women = 500)	23/37 (62%)	31/35 (89%)	32/35 (91%)	2/37 (5%)	12/37 (32%)	10/37 (27%)
2–39 months (20)	450–870 (603) (men = 678) (women = 517)	10/15 (67%)	15/15 (100%)	15/15 (100%)	0/15 (0)	6/15 (40%)	4/15 (27%)
47–204 months (111)	550–1150 (718) (men = 717) (women = 718)	13/21 (62%)	20/21 (95%)	17/18 (94%)	16/22 (73%)	14/21 (67%)	4/22 (18%)
0–204 months (38)	290–1150 (628)	46/73 (63%)	66/71 (93%)	64/68 (94%)	18/74 (24%)	32/73 (44%)	18/74 (24%)

MVR, Mitral valve replacement; 0, cardiac operation; PSG, peak systolic gradient; SA, systemic artery; LV, left ventricular or left ventricle; VS, ventricular septum; LVOT, left ventricular outflow tract; CAD, coronary artery disease.

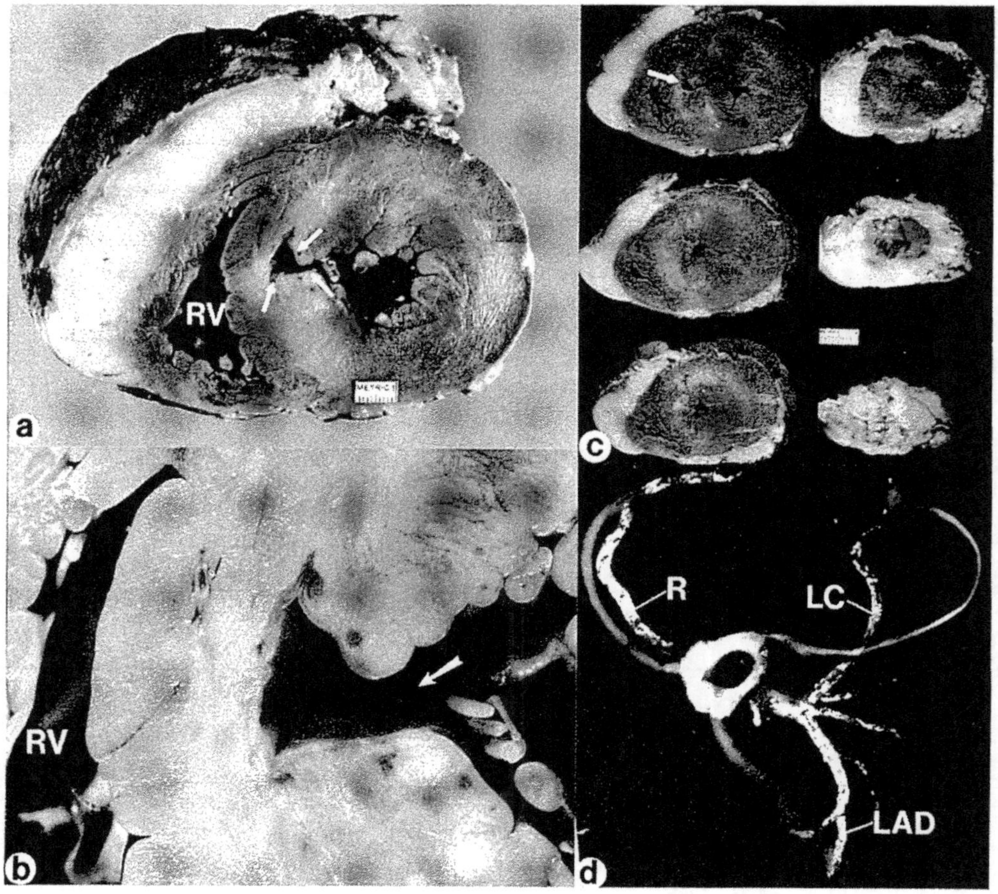

Fig. 17. Operative partial ventricular septectomy and septotomy in a 51-year-old man who died 35 days after this procedure and simultaneous coronary artery bypass grafting. *a,* Transverse section of basal portion of the heart showing a wedge-shaped space (arrows) designating the site of septectomy; RV, right ventricle. *b,* A close-up view of the septum where the myoectomy (arrow) had been done. *c,* Transverse slices of the ventricles showing the minute left and right ventricular cavities; the arrow points to the myectomy site. *d,* Radiograph of the native calcified coronary arteries and the saphenous vein grafts; R, right; LAD, left anterior descending artery; LC, left circumflex artery.

REFERENCES

1. Menges, H., Jr., Brandenburg, R.O., and Brown, A.L., Jr.: The clinical, hemodynamic, and pathologic diagnosis of muscular subvalvular aortic stenosis. Circulation, *24:*1126, 1961.
2. Ewy, G.A., et al.: Muscular subaortic stenosis: clinical and pathologic observations in an elderly patient. Am. J. Cardiol., *22:*126, 1968.
3. Buja, L.M., and Roberts, W.C.: Pulmonary parenchymal ossific nodules in idiopathic hypertrophic subaortic stenosis. Am. J. Cardiol., *25:*710, 1970.
4. Ferrans, V.J., Morrow, A.G., and Roberts, W.C.: Myocardial ultrastructure in idiopathic hypertrophic subaortic stenosis: a study of operatively excised left ventricular outflow tract muscle in 14 patients. Circulation, *45:*769, 1972.
5. Roberts, W.C.: Valvular, subvalvular and supravalvular aortic stenosis: morphologic features. Cardiovasc. Clin., *5:*104, 1973.
6. Roberts, W.C.: Operative treatment of hypertrophic obstructive cardiomyopathy. Am. J. Cardiol., *32:*377, 1973.

7. Roberts, W.C., and Ferrans, V.J.: Morphologic observations in the cardiomyopathies. *In* Myocardial Disease. Edited by N.O. Fowler. New York, Grune & Stratton, 1973, p. 59.
8. Roberts, W.C., and Ferrans, V.J.: Pathological aspects of certain cardiomyopathies. Circulation, *34/35* (Suppl. 2): 128, 1974.
9. Maron, B.J., et al.: Differences in distribution of myocardial abnormalities in patients with obstructive and nonobstructive asymmetric septal hypertrophy (ASH): light and electron microscopic findings. Circulation, *50*:436, 1974.
10. Roberts, W.C., and Ferrans, V.J.: Pathologic anatomy of the cardiomyopathies: idiopathic dilated and hypertrophic types, infiltrates types, and endomyocardial disease with and without eosinophilia. Hum. Pathol. *6*:287, 1975.
11. Epstein, S.E., et al.: Asymmetric septal hypertrophy. Ann. Intern. Med., *81*:650, 1974.
12. McReynolds, R.A., and Roberts, W.C.: The intramural coronary arteries in hypertrophic cardiomyopathy. (Abstract.) Am. J. Cardiol., *35*:154, 1975.
13. Maron, B.J., et al.: Asymmetric septal hypertrophy in childhood. Circulation, *53*:9, 1976.
14. Maron, B.J., Henry, W.L., Roberts, W.C., and Epstein, S.E.: Comparison of echocardiographic and necropsy measurements of ventricular wall thicknesses in patients with and without disproportionate septal thickening. Circulation, *55*:341, 1977.
15. Maron, B.J., et al.: Prevalence and characteristics of disproportionate ventricular septal thickening in patients with acquired or congenital heart diseases. Circulation, *55*:489, 1977.
16. Maron, B.J., et al.: Left ventricular outflow tract obstruction due to systolic anterior motion of the anterior mitral leaflet in patients with concentric left ventricular hypertrophy. Circulation, *57*:528, 1978.
17. Spray, T.L., et al.: A discussion of hypertrophic cardiomyopathy. Am. Heart J., *95*:511, 1978.
18. Maron, B.J., et al.: Sudden death in patients with hypertrophic cardiomyopathy: characterization of 26 patients without functional limitation. Am. J. Cardiol., *41*:803, 1978.
19. Maron, B.J., et al.: "Malignant" hypertrophic cardiomyopathy: identification of a subgroup of families with unusually frequent premature death. Am. J. Cardiol., *41*:1133, 1978.
20. Maron, B.J., and Roberts, W.C.: Quantitative analysis of cardiac muscle cell disorganization in ventricular septum of patients with hypertrophic cardiomyopathy. Circulation, *59*:689, 1979.
21. Maron, B.J., Epstein, S.E., and Roberts, W.C.: Hypertrophic cardiomyopathy and transmural myocardial infarction without significant atherosclerosis of the extramural coronary arteries. Am. J. Cardiol., *43*:1086, 1979.
22. Maron, B.J., et al.: Quantitative analysis of cardiac muscle cell disorganization in the ventricular septum: comparison of fetuses and infants with and without congenital heart disease and patients with hypertrophic cardiomyopathy. Circulation, *60*:685, 1979.
23. Isner, J.M., Maron, B.J., and Roberts, W.C.: Comparison of amount of myocardial cell disorganization in operatively excised septectomy specimens with amount observed at necropsy in 18 patients with hypertrophic cardiomyopathy. Am. J. Cardiol., *46*:42, 1980.
24. Waller, B.F., Maron, B.J., Epstein, S.E., and Roberts, W.C.: Transmural myocardial infarction in hypertrophic cardiomyopathy. Chest, *79*:461, 1981.
25. Maron, B.J., Connor, T.M., and Roberts, W.C.: Hypertrophic cardiomyopathy and complete heart block in infancy. Am. Heart J., *101*:857, 1981.
26. Maron, B.J., and Roberts, W.C.: Hypertrophic cardiomyopathy and cardiac muscle cell disorganization revisited: relation between the two and significance. Am. Heart J., *102*:95, 1981.
27. Waller, B.F., Maron, B.J., Morrow, A.G., and Roberts, W.C.: Hypertrophic cardiomyopathy mimicking pericardial constriction or myocardial restriction. Am. Heart J., *102*:790, 1981.
28. Maron, B.J., et al.: Hypertrophic cardiomyopathy in infants: clinical features and natural history. Circulation, *65*:7, 1982.
29. Maron, B.J., Roberts, W.C., and Epstein, S.E.: Sudden death in hypertrophic cardiomyopathy: a profile of 78 patients. Circulation, *65*:1388, 1982.
30. Ciro, E., Maron, B.J., and Roberts, W.C.: Coexistence of asymmetric and symmetric left ventricular hypertrophy in a family with hypertrophic cardiomyopathy. Am. Heart J., *104*:643, 1982.
31. Maron, B.J., et al.: Systolic anterior motion of the posterior mitral leaflet: a previously unrecognized cause of dynamic subaortic obstruction in patients with hypertrophic cardiomyopathy. Circulation, *68*:282, 1983.
32. Warnes, C.A., Maron, B.J., and Roberts, W.C.: Massive cardiac ventricular scarring in first-degree relatives with hypertrophic cardiomyopathy. Am. J. Cardiol., *54*:1377, 1984.
33. Wigle, E.D., et al.: Hypertrophic cardiomyopathy. The importance of the site and the extent of hypertrophy: a review. Prog. Cardiovasc. Dis., *28*:1, 1985.
34. Maron, B.J., Wolfson, J.K., Epstein, S.E., and Roberts, W.C.: Intramural ("small vessel") cor-

onary artery disease in hypertrophic cardiomyopathy. J. Am. Coll. Cardiol., *8*:545, 1986.

35. Ross, E.M., et al.: Impaired left ventricular systolic and diastolic function without left ventricular dilatation associated with papillary muscle calcification in hypertrophic cardiomyopathy. Am. J. Cardiol., *57*:488, 1986.
36. Roberts, W.C.: Congenital cardiovascular abnormalities usually "silent" until adulthood: morphologic features of the floppy mitral valve, valvular aortic stenosis, discrete subvalvular aortic stenosis, hypertrophic cardiomyopathy, sinus of Valsalva aneurysm, and the Marfan syndrome. *In* Adult Congenital Heart Disease. Edited by W.C. Roberts. Philadelphia, F.A. Davis, 1987, p. 407.
37. Maron, B.J., et al.: Hypertrophic cardiomyopathy: interrelations of clinical manifestations, pathophysiology, and therapy. N. Engl. J. Med., *316*:780, 1987.
38. Unverferth, D.V., et al.: Regional myocyte hypertrophy and increased interstitial myocardial fibrosis in hypertrophic cardiomyopathy. Am. J. Cardiol. *59*:932, 1987.
39. Motamed, H.E., and Roberts, W.C.: Frequency and significance of mitral anular calcium in hypertrophic cardiomyopathy: analysis of 200 necropsy patients. Am. J. Cardiol., *60*:877, 1987.
40. Teare, D.: A symmetrical hypertrophy of the heart in young adults. Br. Heart J., *20*:1, 1958.
41. Liouville, H.: Rétrécissement cardiaque sous aortique. Gazette Med. Paris, *24*:161, 1869.
42. Hallopeau, M.: Rétrécissement ventriculo-aortique. Gazette Med. Paris, *24*:683, 1869.
43. Schmincke, A.: Ueber linkseitige muskulose Conusstenosen. Dtsch. Med. Wochenschr., *33*:2082, 1907.
44. Bernheim, P.I.: De L'asystolie veineuse dans l'hypertrophie du coeur gauche par sténose concomitante du ventricle droit. Rev. Med., *30*:785, 1910.
45. Braunwald, E., et al.: Idiopathic hypertrophic subaortic, stenosis. American Heart Association Monograph No. 10. New York, American Heart Association, 1984, p. 1.
46. Davies, L.G.: Familial heart disease. Br. Heart J., *14*:206, 1952.
47. Brock, R.: Functional obstruction of the left ventricle (acquired aortic subvalvular stenosis). Guy's Hosp. Rep., *106*:221, 1957.
48. Maron, B.J., and Epstein, S.E.: Hypertrophic cardiomyopathy: a discussion of nomenclature. Am. J. Cardiol., *43*:1242, 1979.
49. Muna, W.F.T., Ferrans, V.J., Pierce, J.E., and Roberts, W.C.: Discrete subaortic stenosis in Newfoundland dogs: association of infective endocarditis. Am. J. Cardiol., *41*:746, 1978.
50. Maron, B.J., et al.: Tunnel subaortic stenosis: left ventricular outflow tract obstruction produced by fibromuscular tubular narrowing. Circulation, *54*:406, 1976.
51. Roberts, W.C., et al.: Aortic valve atresia: a new classification based on necropsy study of 73 cases. Am. J. Cardiol., *37*:753, 1976.
52. Ellis, J.G., Terneny, O.J., Winters, W.L., and Leachman, R.D.: Critical role of the mitral valve leaflet in hypertrophic subaortic stenosis and amelioration of the disease by mitral valve replacement. Chest, *59*:378, 1971.
53. Cooley, D.A., Leachman, R.D., and Wukasch, D.C.: Diffuse muscular subaortic stenosis: surgical treatment. Am. J. Cardiol., *31*:1, 1973.
54. Cooley, D.A., Grace, R.R., Wukasch, D.C., and Leachman, R.D.: Replacement and/or repair of the mitral valve as treatment of idiopathic hypertrophic subaortic stenosis. Cardiovasc. Dis., *3*:381, 1976.
55. McIntosh, C.L., and Maron, B.J.: Current operative treatment of obstructive hypertrophic cardiomyopathy. Circulation, *78*:487, 1988.

Usefulness of Total 12-Lead QRS Voltage Compared with Other Criteria for Determining Left Ventricular Hypertrophy in Hypertrophic Cardiomyopathy: Analysis of 57 Patients Studied at Necropsy

ALLEN L. DOLLAR, M.D., WILLIAM C. ROBERTS, M.D. *Bethesda, Maryland*

PURPOSE: The sensitivity of electrocardiographic indicators of left ventricular (LV) hypertrophy is known to be rather poor. To date, no study has undertaken a comparison of the various electrocardiographic criteria for LV hypertrophy among patients with hypertrophic cardiomyopathy (HC). In this study, we compared the sensitivity of the total 12-lead QRS amplitude with the sensitivity of certain standard electrocardiographic criteria for LV hypertrophy in necropsy patients with HC.

MATERIALS AND METHODS: A total of 57 hearts were studied. The last technically satisfactory electrocardiogram available from each necropsy patient was used. Electrocardiographic criteria employed to diagnose LV hypertrophy included the Sokolow and Lyon index, the Romhilt-Estes voltage criteria, the Romhilt-Estes point score, the ratio of RV6:RV5 greater than 1 proposed by Holt and Spodick, and a method utilizing the sum of the amplitudes of the QRS complexes of all 12 leads.

RESULTS: The total 12-lead QRS amplitude ranged from 66 to 339 mm (mean: 197 mm) (10 mm = 1 mV). Using 175 mm as the upper limit of normal, this technique yielded a sensitivity of 53%, which was the highest sensitivity of any criteria tested. The Sokolow-Lyon index had a sensitivity of 39%; the Romhilt-Estes voltage criteria, 37%; the Romhilt-Estes point score system, 49%; and the criterion of RV6 more than RV5, 39%. No correlation was found between total 12-lead QRS voltage and heart weight, LV free wall thickness, LV peak systolic and end-diastolic pressures, or LV outflow tract peak systolic pressure gradient. The 10 patients (18%) with transmural LV scars had significantly lower total 12-lead QRS voltage than did the 48 patients (78%) without such scars (155 mm versus 205 mm, p = 0.02).

CONCLUSION: Total 12-lead QRS amplitude more than 175 mm is a useful indicator of LV hypertrophy and, among patients with HC, it is more sensitive than other more commonly employed criteria.

From the Pathology Branch, National Heart, Lung, and Blood Institute, National Institutes of Health, Bethesda, Maryland. Requests for reprints should be addressed to Pathology Branch, Building 10, Room 2N258, National Institutes of Health, Bethesda, Maryland 20892. Manuscript submitted March 9, 1989, and accepted in revised form July 10, 1989.

Electrocardiographic indicators of left ventricular (LV) hypertrophy are known to be relatively nonspecific and insensitive. The sensitivity of these criteria also varies with the various etiologies of LV hypertrophy [1]. Although many studies have described electrocardiographic abnormalities in hypertrophic cardiomyopathy (HC) [2–12], none have compared the various electrocardiographic criteria for LV hypertrophy among patients with HC. In this investigation, we describe electrocardiographic findings in 57 patients with HC studied both clinically and at necropsy and determine which electrocardiographic criteria are most sensitive for LV hypertrophy in these patients.

MATERIALS AND METHODS

From July 1959 to July 1988, the hearts of 210 patients with HC were studied in the Pathology Branch, National Heart, Lung, and Blood Institutes (NHLBI), Bethesda, Maryland. Of this number, 179 were 12 years of age or older and, of these, electrocardiograms obtained during the last year of life were available in 57. Most of the other 122 patients had not been seen at the National Institutes of Health (NIH) during their last year of life or they had never been studied at NIH and only their hearts had been submitted to the Pathology Branch (NHLBI). Various clinical, electrocardiographic, and morphologic observations in these 57 patients are summarized in **Table I**. Of the 57 patients, 31 died shortly after a cardiac operation, and the other 26 never had a cardiac operation. Of these 26, 13 died suddenly outside the hospital, six of progressive congestive heart failure, two of consequences of strokes, and five of noncardiac causes. The last technically satisfactory electrocardiogram available from each patient was analyzed. The interval from the studied electrocardiogram until death ranged from 0 to 327 days (average, 37 days). In the 31 patients who died perioperatively, the immediate preoperative 12-lead electrocardiogram was analyzed.

The amplitudes of the QRS complexes were measured from the peak of the R wave to the nadir of either the Q wave or the S wave, whichever was deeper, according to the method of Siegel and Roberts [13] (**Figure 1**). The electrocardiographic criteria used to diagnose LV hypertrophy included the Sokolow and Lyon index [14] (sum of SV1 plus the larger of RV5 or RV6 greater than 35 mm), the Romhilt-Estes voltage criteria [15] (either tallest limb-lead R or deepest limb-lead S greater than 20 mm or tallest RV4-6 or deepest SV1-3 greater than 25 mm), the Romhilt-Estes point score [15] (a system utilizing ST-T segment changes, QRS axis, left atrial abnormality, QRS duration, and duration of the intrinsicoid deflection in addition to electrocardiographic voltage criteria), the ra-

TABLE I

Clinical, Electrocardiographic, and Morphologic Observations in 57 Patients with HC

Patient	Age (years)	Interval ECG-Death (days)	HR (beats/minute)	Rhythm	QRS Axis (o)	Interval(s) PR	Interval(s) QRS (BBB)	Interval(s) QTc	P Wave Abnormality	Romhilt-Estes Score	Sokolow-Lyon Index	Total QRS Voltage (mm)	HW (g)	Thickness (mm) VS	Thickness (mm) LV	Transmural LV Scar	Interval CC-Death (days)	Pressure (mm Hg) RV (s/d)	Pressure (mm Hg) LV (s/d)	Pressure (mm Hg) SA (s/d)	Pressure (mm Hg) LV-SA psg (rest)	Pressure (mm Hg) LV-SA psg (p)	CI
Women																							
1	36	1	80	S	−90	0.20	0.12 (R)	0.34	|	6	3	68	500	22	15	+	—	—	—	—	—	—	—
2	65	0	80	AF	−45	—	0.16 (L)	0.42	—	4	13	87	475	19	24	−	210	75/20	190/8	195/90	0	100	1.4
3	30	9	125	S	−60	0.24	0.14 (R)	0.46	|	6	3	111	510	15	18	+	—	—	—	—	—	—	—
4	45	7	50	S	70	0.16	0.08	0.40	|	3	24	131	290	15	15	−	26	20/4	110/12	105/60	5	115	2.9
5	46	10	100	S	−60	0.22	0.12 (L)	0.46	|	3	23	134	460	18	17	+	—	—	—	—	—	—	—
6	61	2	60	S	−30	0.20	0.12 (L)	0.46	—	3	32	136	580	28	17	−	192	30/6	110/30	100/70	10	125	2.4
7	21	120	78	S	90	0.20	0.12	0.55	|	4	7	144	390	27	18	−	270	30/6	170/18	90/—	80	105	—
8	54	10	72	S	−45	0.22	0.10	0.48	|	6	26	150	455	20	20	−	30	55/5	230/18	120/65	120	—	3.4
9	65	21	100	S	30	0.12	0.06	0.39	|	1	27	151	430	19	15	−	6	65/12	260/45	110/65	150	—	2
10	62	48	72	S	30	0.20	0.10	0.44	—	2	23	153	450	19	15	−	60	40/4	225/14	135/90	90	150	2.8
11	52	19	55	S	−30	0.20	0.12	0.48	|	6	27	158	470	22	20	−	21	65/8	140/28	120/70	20	80	—
12	19	5	85	S	−20	0.16	0.08	0.45	b	1	40	160	360	25	20	−	30	50/12	210/28	130/80	80	110	—
13	65	1	54	S	60	0.20	0.10	0.42	—	2	26	166	615	25	20	−	5	85/24	240/25	120/80	140	—	1.5
14	25	33	90	S	0	0.22	0.10	0.44	|	4	23	171	720	38	25	−	—	—	—	—	—	—	—
15	20	68	52	S	−90	0.16	0.12	0.48	—	4	14	173	1230	45	32	+	—	—	—	—	—	—	—
16	59	3	67	S	−30	0.20	0.16 (L)	0.55	|	6	31	182	610	23	23	+	6	98/10	275/30	100/60	160	—	1.5
17	87	8	85	S	−30	0.16	0.10	0.38	—	4	32	190	460	26	20	−	—	—	—	140/50	—	—	—
18	19	12	80	S	0	0.20	0.12	0.44	|	4	34	195	730	—	—	−	120	28/8	260/14	98/75	162	—	3.1
19	25	265	67	S	0	0.20	0.16 (R)	0.49	|	4	26	198	650	18	15	+	—	—	—	—	—	—	—
20	70	15	120	AF	0	—	0.08	0.40	—	4	51	205	450	31	29	−	2	—	160/20	95/70	65	—	1.9
21	56	2	65	S	45	0.18	0.10	0.42	—	8	37	206	310	18	19	−	7	—	165/14	115/70	40	90	—
22	61	1	65	S	0	0.20	0.08	0.46	|	3	39	207	500	19	16	−	90	26/11	188/10	108/80	80	115	2.5
23	58	327	82	S	0	0.22	0.12	0.47	|	7	31	214	900	—	—	−	—	—	—	—	—	—	—
24	65	18	70	S	20	0.18	0.10	0.43	|	8	45	219	410	26	22	−	5	32/—	210/20	110/60	100	140	—
25	35	41	78	S	60	0.16	0.08	0.43	—	1	42	232	600	35	20	−	—	—	—	—	—	—	—
26	40	2	82	S	45	0.20	0.10	0.51	|	7	48	240	475	18	18	−	5	24/9	208/12	104/—	104	115	—
27	70	5	70	S	120	0.20	0.12	0.48	—	4	25	263	664	29	24	−	4	115/20	245/20	120/65	125	—	1.2
28	58	23	90	S	90	0.18	0.12	0.39	|	8	44	265	490	22	15	−	300	—	205/5	108/53	100	—	2.5
29	64	2	130	S	45	0.12	0.08	0.41	—	4	44	266	355	30	25	−	1	42/6	230/12	160/70	60	—	—
30	81	1	60	S	0	0.12	0.20 (L)	0.44	|	7	55	272	550	25	13	−	—	—	—	—	—	—	—
31	59	115	95	S	30	0.20	0.12	0.45	|	8	58	277	460	20	15	−	450	—/14	135/19	75/58	60	84	1.8
32	62	3	68	S	−45	0.14	0.12	0.47	|	9	38	281	730	30	25	−	90	22/2	160/10	140/70	20	68	2.3
33	25	1	73	S	−30	0.20	0.12	0.42	|	3	38	286	400	22	22	−	270	—	130/38	130/80	0	0	—
34	64	4	70	S	−25	0.20	0.12 (L)	0.45	|	7	44	290	670	22	21	−	5	36/18	180/22	145/50	35	84	2
35	56	18	42	S	15	0.16	0.12	0.42	|	8	64	314	680	33	25	−	180	50/3	230/25	105/60	130	—	3
36	61	10	60	S	15	0.19	0.08	0.44	—	4	60	327	665	25	18	−	8	80/10	200/26	110/60	90	—	1.7
Mean	51	34	77		4	0.19	0.11	0.43		5	33	201	547	25	20	−	92	51/10	195/20	118/68	78	99	2.2

Men																						
1	59	1	57	J	130	—	0.18 (L)	0.47	—	1	13	107	670	20	16	—	720	55/—	—	—	0	0	—
2	33	13	74	S	−60	0.18	0.10	0.44	I	7	11	110	450	27	13	—	14	—	—	—	0	—	2
3	60	54	87	S	−90	0.18	0.16 (R)	0.46	I	6	12	112	475	16	12	+	—	—	—	100/65	—	—	—
4	45	122	87	AF	−60	—	0.20	0.55	—	3	21	120	760	20	15	+	515	—	120/25	120/75	0	0	—
5	56	99	150	S	−30	0.14	0.12 (L)	0.44	I	4	23	134	680	25	18	—	630	44/8	220/12	130/80	90	190	2
6	55	27	60	S	30	0.16	0.10	0.44	I	5	25	151	790	22	20	—	—	—	—	—	—	—	—
7	54	96	150	S	0	0.16	0.06	0.44	I	1	27	161	515	20	25	—	671	31/10	200/35	145/85	50	75	—
8	41	2	75	AF	30	—	0.10	0.45	—	2	25	162	700	25	21	—	4	40/—	—	—	80	—	—
9	57	219	90	AF	−30	—	0.12	0.44	—	4	21	163	580	20	18	—	—	—	—	—	—	—	—
10	50	2	95	S	20	0.22	0.12	0.38	I	5	43	168	655	25	16	—	—	—	—	—	—	—	—
11	51	18	110	S	30	0.12	0.16 (L)	0.49	—	5	32	170	890	20	20	—	90	41/8	150/15	136/85	40	100	—
12	68	2	85	S	−30	0.16	0.08	0.45	I	5	28	170	540	21	24	—	14	32/9	115/12	115/60	0	120	2.2
13	58	66	55	S	−45	0.22	0.16	0.46	I	10	12	183	585	20	15	+	—	—	—	—	—	—	—
14	63	15	85	S	0	0.24	0.12	0.48	—	2	36	207	735	25	20	—	180	49/9	189/4	163/69	26	100	2.6
15	29	2	70	S	0	0.22	0.10	0.43	I	8	46	228	995	21	21	—	30	52/13	180/40	110/80	70	110	—
16	24	4	56	S	−90	0.24	0.16 (R)	0.46	I	9	30	232	750	33	24	—	30	—	—/24	120/80	50	80	—
17	55	45	60	S	−45	0.20	0.16 (L)	0.50	I	10	56	237	735	30	25	—	90	28/7	160/13	125/65	30	130	1.9
18	41	6	50	S	20	0.18	0.10	0.38	I	5	38	266	750	28	19	+	396	40/5	188/8	110/60	76	110	2.8
19	29	17	72	S	−60	0.28	0.12	0.42	—	3	28	279	450	28	20	—	150	22/5	110/12	110/65	0	0	—
20	21	38	60	S	−45	0.28	0.12 (R)	0.44	I	10	30	281	1070	33	24	—	30	100/15	140/24	128/70	12	55	4.1
21	14	18	55	S	60	0.12	0.08	0.38	I	7	48	339	325	17	12	—	30	40/9	118/24	118/70	0	40	3
Mean	46	41	80		−13	0.19	0.12	0.45		5	29	190	671	33	19		225	44/9	158/19	124/72	33	79	2.6

+ = present; AF = atrial fibrillation; b = biatrial enlargement; BBB = bundle branch block; bpm = beats per minute; CC = cardiac catheterization; CI = cardiac index in L/minute/m²; HR = heart rate; HW = heart weight; I = intraventricular conduction delay; J = junctional; L = left; l = left atrial abnormality; p = peak; psg = peak systolic gradient; QTc = QT interval corrected for heart rate; R = right; S = sinus; s/d = peak systole/end diastole; SA = systemic artery; VS = ventricular septum.

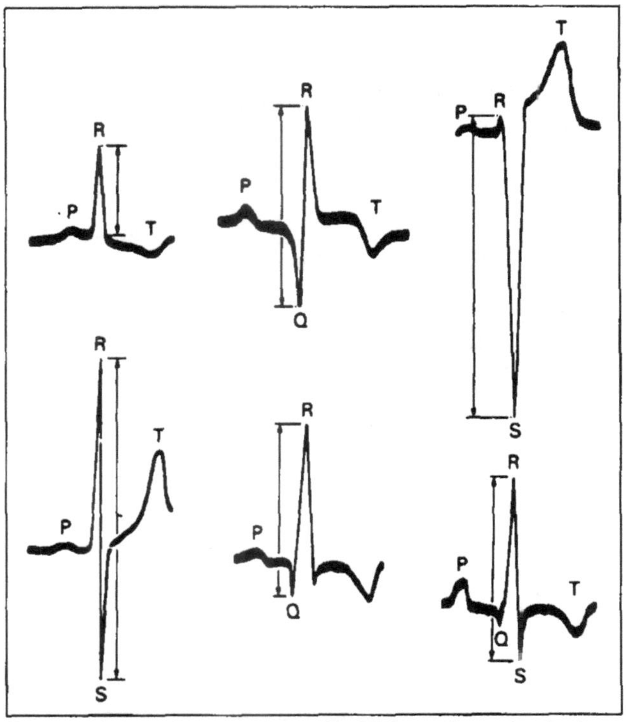

Figure 1. Various electrocardiographic QRS complexes showing how the voltage (in mm) was measured. Reproduced with permission from [13].

tio of RV6:RV5 greater than 1 as proposed by Holt and Spodick [16], and a method utilizing the sum of the amplitudes of the QRS complexes of all 12 leads. Patients with bundle branch block were included in all analyses. Amplitudes were standardized to 10 mm equaling 1 mV.

At necropsy, the heart weight used was that of the formalin-fixed heart. The fixation period before the heart was weighed varied from about two to 20 days, a period during which heart weight of the fresh specimen is the same as the fixed specimen.

Statistical methods included linear regression analysis, unpaired two-tailed Student's t-test, and chi-square analysis applied where appropriate. Significance was determined if the p value was <0.05.

RESULTS

The 57 patients ranged in age from 14 to 87 years (mean: 49 years). Of these, 21 (37%) were men and 36 (63%) were women; 53 (93%) were white and four (7%) were black. Heart weights ranged from 290 to 1,230 g (mean: 593 g). The LV free wall thicknesses ranged from 1.2 to 3.2 cm (mean: 2.0 cm), and the ventricular septa, from 1.5 to 4.5 cm (mean: 2.4 cm). Cardiac catheterization data within two years of death were available in 42 patients. Left ventricular to aortic (or another systemic artery) peak systolic pressure gradients greater than 10 mm Hg were present at rest in 32 (77%) patients and with provocation in 35 patients (85%). The resting peak systolic gradients ranged from 12 to 162 mm Hg (mean: 79 mm Hg), and the provoked gradients, from 40 to 190 mm Hg (mean: 104 mm Hg). There were no differences between patients with and without LV-to-systemic arterial peak systolic gradients at rest with regards to heart weight, ventricular

TABLE II

Sensitivity of Electrocardiographic Criteria for Diagnosing LV Hypertrophy in 57 Necropsy Patients with HC

Electrocardiographic Criteria	Number (%) of Patients Above Normal Limit
Total 12-lead QRS amplitude >175 mm	30 (53)
Romhilt-Estes Point Score ≥5	28 (49)
Sokolow-Lyon Index (SV1 + RV5 or RV6 [larger] > 35 mm)	22 (39)
RV6:RV5 > 1	22 (39)
Romhilt-Estes Voltage Criteria (either tallest limb-lead R or deepest limb-lead S > 20 mm or tallest RV1-3 or deepest SV1-3 > 25 mm)	21 (37)

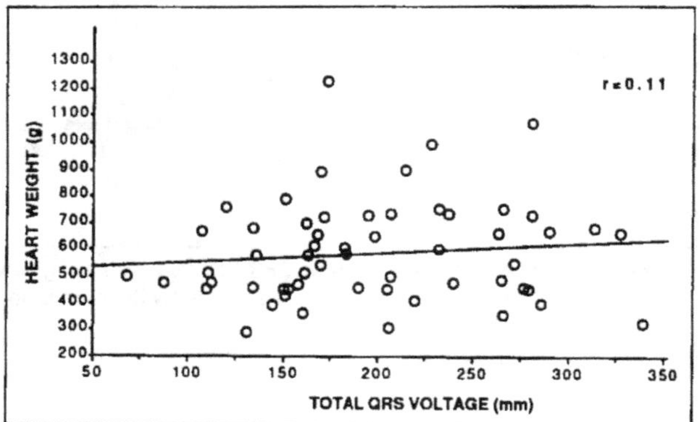

Figure 2. Relation between total QRS amplitude and heart weight at necropsy in 57 patients with HC who had an electrocardiogram recorded within one year of death.

TABLE III

Comparison of Previous Studies Determining the Sensitivity of Various Criteria for LV Hypertrophy in HC

References	Number of Patients Meeting Criteria for LV Hypertrophy/Number of Patients Studied (Sensitivity)
Sokolow-Lyon Index	
Braunwald *et al* [4]	47/64 (73%)
Harmjanz *et al* [5]	9/25 (36%)
McKenna *et al* [9]	45/100 (45%)
Dollar and Roberts (present study)	22/57 (39%)
Romhilt-Estes Point Score (≥5 points)	
Walston *et al* [6]	22/33 (67%)
Maron *et al* [10]	72/153 (47%)
Alcini *et al* [11]	8/20 (40%)
Dollar and Roberts (present study)	28/57 (49%)

septal thickness, total QRS amplitude, and Romhilt-Estes scores. The Sokolow-Lyon index was significantly different in the patients with and without obstruction: the mean index was 37 in the obstructive group and 28 in the non-obstructive group (p <0.02). Mean values for age, heart rate, axis, electrocardiographic intervals, total 12-lead QRS amplitude, ventricular wall thickness, LV outflow tract gradient, and heart weight were compared between men and women. Only mean heart weight was significantly different between the two groups: mean heart rate of men equal to 671 g and that of women equal to 547 g (p <0.02).

The cardiac rhythm was sinus in 51 patients (89%), atrial fibrillation in five (9%), and junctional in one (2%). A history of atrial fibrillation was present in 17 (30%) patients. Left atrial abnormality was present in 37 (73%) of the 51 patients in sinus rhythm and biatrial abnormality in one (2%). The QRS complex width was 0.12 seconds or greater in 33 patients (58%), with a left bundle branch block pattern in 10 (18%), a right bundle branch block pattern in six (11%), and a nonspecific conduction delay in 17 (30%).

The total 12-lead QRS amplitude in the 57 patients ranged from 66 to 339 mm (mean: 197 mm). (The upper limit of normal for total QRS amplitude of 175 mm was first suggested by Roberts and Day [17] and validated by Odom *et al* [18] who found that this upper limit yielded a specificity of 93% in a group of normal hearts.) Of the criteria examined, the total 12-lead QRS amplitude had the highest sensitivity (53%) (**Table II**). Although the total 12-lead QRS amplitude was the most sensitive criterion tested, there was no correlation of heart weight with the total 12-lead QRS amplitude (**Figure 2**). This observation was demonstrated both by linear regression analysis and by comparison of the mean heart weights for those patients with total 12-lead QRS amplitudes greater than 175 mm to those with amplitudes equal to or less than 175 mm, and there was no difference in mean heart weights (605 and 579 g, respectively, p = 0.6). Total QRS amplitude also was compared to ventricular wall thicknesses, LV peak systolic and end-diastolic pressures at rest, and provoked LV outflow tract gradients using linear regression analysis. No comparison was significant.

Transmural (involving all the inner one half and a portion of the outer one half of the LV free wall or ventricular septum) scars were present in 10 of the 57 patients (six women, four men). The mean heart weight of the group with transmural LV or septal scars was not significantly different from that of the group without scars. There was, however, a significantly lower total 12-lead QRS amplitude in the group with transmural scars (155 mm versus 205 mm, p = 0.02) and a lower mean Sokolow-Lyon index (11.6 versus 13.2, p = <0.001). The mean Romhilt-Estes score was not statistically different in the two groups.

COMMENTS

This study examined total 12-lead QRS voltage and other more standard electrocardiographic criteria for diagnosing LV hypertrophy in patients with HC studied at necropsy (Table II). The highest sensitivity among the criteria for LV hypertrophy in patients with HC was achieved by the total 12-lead QRS voltage (53%). In the patients with HC, the voltage criteria of Romhilt and Estes and the Sokolow-Lyon index were relatively insensitive (37% and 39%, respectively). The criterion of RV6 greater than RV5 proposed by Holt and Spodick [16] was 39% sensitive. Koito and Spodick [19] reported an overall 52% sensitivity of the criterion of RV6 greater than RV5 in a group of patients with LV hypertrophy of various etiologies but noted that there was a trend toward less sensitivity of this criterion in patients with HC. Several previous studies have evaluated the sensitivity of these criteria in patients with HC [4–6,9–11], and they are summarized in **Table III**.

Our study is the first to examine total 12-lead QRS

TABLE IV

Comparison of the Sensitivity of Total QRS Voltage in Identifying LV Hypertrophy of Various Etiologies

	Valvular Aortic Stenosis (n = 30)	Aortic Regurgitation (n = 12)	HC (n = 57)	Idiopathic Dilated Cardiomyopathy (n = 49)	Amyloid (n = 30)	Normal (n = 30)
Age (years)	52 ± 5	52 ± 6	49 ± 17	48 ± 15	58 ± 17	56 ± 10
Heart weight (g)	630 ± 14	745 ± 132	593 ± 189	614 ± 126	532 ± 139	393 ± 57
Total QRS voltage (mm)	245 ± 56	274 ± 87	197 ± 67	153 ± 48	104 ± 36	127 ± 29
Number > 175 mm (%)	43 (93)	27 (90)	30 (53)	16 (33)	2 (7)	2 (7)

voltage in patients with HC. Several studies, however, have evaluated the relation between the total 12-lead QRS voltage and heart weight at necropsy in other cardiac diseases (**Table IV**) [13,17,18,20,21]. Measurement of the total 12-lead QRS voltage provides a sensitive marker for LV hypertrophy among patients with aortic stenosis and aortic regurgitation (93% and 90%, respectively). Among patients with HC, this criterion is moderately sensitive (53%), albeit the most sensitive of the criteria examined. Total QRS amplitude in patients with idiopathic dilated cardiomyopathy identified 33% as having LV hypertrophy. As expected, a low total amplitude was observed in patients with cardiac amyloidosis severe enough to cause cardiac dysfunction.

REFERENCES

1. Murphy ML, Thenabadu PN, de Soyza N, Meade J, Doherty JE, Baker BJ: Sensitivity of electrocardiographic criteria for left ventricular hypertrophy according to type of cardiac disease. Am J Cardiol 1985; 55: 545–549.
2. Braunwald E, Morrow AG, Cornell WP, Aygen MM, Hilbish TF: Idiopathic hypertrophic subaortic stenosis. Clinical, hemodynamic and angiographic manifestations. Am J Med 1960; 29: 924–945.
3. Estes EH Jr, Whalen RE, Roberts SR Jr, McIntosh HD: The electrocardiographic and vectorcardiographic findings in idiopathic hypertrophic subaortic stenosis. Am Heart J 1963; 65: 155–161.
4. Braunwald E, Lambrew CT, Rockoff SD, Ross J Jr, Morrow AC: Idiopathic hypertrophic subaortic stenosis. I. A description of the disease based upon an analysis of 64 patients. Circulation 1964; 30 (suppl IV): IV-3–IV-119.
5. Harmjanz D, Bottcher D, Schertlein G: Correlations of electrocardiographic pattern, shape of ventricular septum and isovolumetric relaxation time in irregular hypertrophic cardiomyopathy (obstructive cardiomyopathy). Br Heart J 1971; 33: 928–937.
6. Walston A II, Behar VS, Wagner GS, Greenfield JC Jr: Electrocardiographic and hemodynamic correlations in patients with idiopathic hypertrophic subaortic stenosis. Am Heart J 1976; 91: 11–17.
7. Savage DD, Seides SF, Clark CE, *et al*: Electrocardiographic findings in patients with obstructive and nonobstructive hypertrophic cardiomyopathy. Circulation 1978; 58: 402–408.
8. McKenna W, Deanfield J, Faruqui A, England D, Oakley C, Goodwin J: Prognosis in hypertrophic cardiomyopathy: role of age and clinical, electrocardiographic and hemodynamic features. Am J Cardiol 1981; 47: 532–538.
9. McKenna WJ, Borggrefe M, England D, Deanfield J, Oakley CM, Goodwin JF: The natural history of left ventricular hypertrophy in hypertrophic cardiomyopathy: an electrocardiographic study. Circulation 1982; 66: 1233–1240.
10. Maron BJ, Wolfson JK, Ciro E, Spirito P: Relation of electrocardiographic abnormalities and patterns of left ventricular hypertrophy identified by 2-dimensional echocardiography in patients with hypertrophic cardiomyopathy. Am J Cardiol 1983; 51: 189–194.
11. Alcini E, Mottironi P, Martinelli MM, Ale E, Aratari D: Hypertrophic cardiomyopathy: electrocardiographic and 2-dimensional echocardiographic correlations. Panminerva Med 1984; 27: 165–173.
12. Nair CK, Kudesia V, Hansen D, *et al*: Echocardiographic and electrocardiographic characteristics of patients with hypertrophic cardiomyopathy with and without mitral annular calcium. Am J Cardiol 1987; 59: 1428–1430.
13. Siegel RJ, Roberts WC: Electrocardiographic observations in severe aortic valve stenosis: correlative necropsy study to clinical, hemodynamic, and ECG variables demonstrating relation of 12-lead QRS amplitude to peak systolic transaortic pressure gradient. Am Heart J 1982; 103: 210–221.
14. Sokolow M, Lyon TP: The ventricular complex in left ventricular hypertrophy as obtained by unipolar precordial and limb leads. Am Heart J 1949; 37: 161–186.
15. Romhilt DW, Estes EH Jr: A point-score system for the ECG diagnosis of left ventricular hypertrophy. Am Heart J 1968; 75: 752–758.
16. Holt DH, Spodick DH: The RV6:RV5 voltage ratio in left ventricular hypertrophy. Am Heart J 1962; 63: 65–66.
17. Roberts WC, Day PJ: Electrocardiographic observations in clinically isolated, pure, chronic, severe aortic regurgitation: analysis of 30 necropsy patients aged 19 to 65 years. Am J Cardiol 1985; 55: 432–438.
18. Odom H II, Davis JL, Dinh H, Baker BJ, Roberts WC, Murphy ML: QRS voltage measurements in autopsied men free of cardiopulmonary disease: a basis for evaluating total QRS voltage as an index of left ventricular hypertrophy. Am J Cardiol 1986; 58: 801–804.
19. Koito H, Spodick DH: Accuracy of the RV6:RV5 voltage ratio for increased left ventricular mass. Am J Cardiol 1988; 62: 985–987.
20. Roberts WC, Waller BF: Cardiac amyloidosis causing cardiac dysfunction: analysis of 54 necropsy patients. Am J Cardiol 1983; 52: 137–146.
21. Roberts WC, Siegel RJ, McManus BM: Idiopathic dilated cardiomyopathy: analysis of 152 necropsy patients. Am J Cardiol 1987; 60: 1340–1355.

Hypertrophic Cardiomyopathy as a Cause of Massive Cardiomegaly (>1,000 g)

Charles Stewart Roberts, MD, and William C. Roberts, MD

The normal adult human heart in women weighs ≤350 g and in men it weighs ≤400 g. The occurrence of heart weights in humans >1,000 g is exceedingly rare.

From the Surgery and Pathology Branches, National Heart, Lung, and Blood Institute, National Institutes of Health, Bethesda, Maryland 20892. Manuscript received and accepted August 1, 1989.

During the past 30 years, approximately 10,000 human adult hearts with various types of cardiovascular diseases have been examined in this laboratory. Of that number, 30 weighed >1,000 g.[1] The most common (15 patients) cause of the massive cardiomegaly was aortic regurgitation with or without other volume lesions, such as mitral regurgitation or ventricular septal defect. Pressure lesions

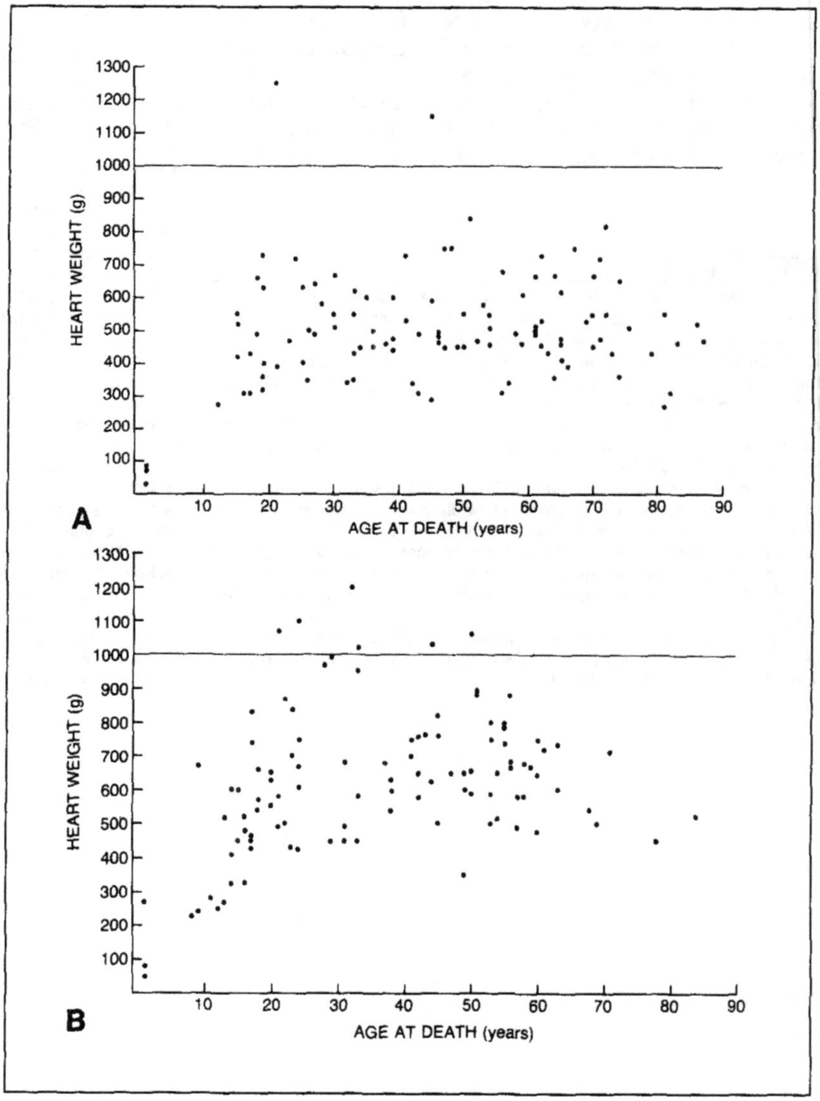

FIGURE 1. Relation of age at death and heart weight in 110 women (*A*) and in 105 men (*B*) with hypertrophic cardiomyopathy.

TABLE I Clinical and Cardiac Morphologic Characteristics of Eight Necropsy Patients with Hypertrophic Cardiomyopathy and Heart Weighing >1,000 g

Pt	Age at Death (yrs)	Sex	Age at CC (yrs)	BP (s/d) (mm Hg)	LV (s/d) (mm Hg)	LV-SA PSG at Rest (mm Hg)	S&S	Mode of Death	BH (cm)	BW (kg)	HW (g)	HW/BW	Thickness (cm) VS	Thickness (cm) LV	Fibrous Plaque LVOT	Thickened MV	Dilated LV Cavity	Gross Fibrosis LV/VS	Abnormal IMCAs	MFD VS
1	21	M	21	140/24	128/70	12*	+†	CHF	183	99	1070	1.1	3.3	2.4	+	+	0	0	+	+
2	21	F	14	158/10	108/57	50	0	AMI	161	47	1250	2.7	4.5	3.2	0	0	+	+	+	+
3	24	M	—	—	—	—	0	Sudden	—	—	1100	—	4.0	2.5	+	+	0	0	+	+
4	32	M	—	—	—	—	0	Sudden	—	—	1200	—	4.0	2.8	0	0	+	0	+	+
5	33	M	29	115/28	117/70	0	0	Sudden	179	82	1020	1.2	3.7	2.6	0	0	0	0	0	0
6	44	M	41	220/29	175/100ǁ	45	0	Sudden	182	87	1030	1.2	3.0	2.0	+	+	0	+§	0	+
7	45	F	—	—	—	—	+‡	CHF	178	103	1150	1.1	3.0	2.5	+	+	+	+	0	+
8	50	M	49	95/10	100/60	0	0	Sudden	174	83	1065	1.3	2.5	2.5	0	0	0	+	+	+

* At cardiac catheterization at age 1, the LV-SA PSG at rest was varied from 50 to 100 mm Hg.
† Partial ventricular septectomy and septotomy 2 days before death.
‡ Partial ventricular septectomy and septotomy 12 years before death.
§ Apical left ventricular aneurysm.
ǁ Systemic hypertension.
AMI = acute myocardial infarction; BH = body height; BP = blood pressure; BW = body weight; CC = cardiac catheterization; CHF = congestive heart failure; HW = heart weight; IMCA = intramural coronary artery; LV = left ventricular or left ventricle; MFD = myocardial fiber disarray; OT = outflow tract; MV = mitral valve; PSG = peak systolic gradient; s/d = systolic diastolic; SA = systemic artery; S&S = septectomy and septotomy; VS = ventricular septum; + = present; 0 = absent.

as the cause of massive cardiomegaly were far less common: 4 patients had aortic valve stenosis, but all also had associated aortic regurgitation or mitral regurgitation.

Cardiomyopathy is a rare cause of massive cardiomegaly. Of >200 patients with idiopathic dilated cardiomyopathy studied at necropsy in this laboratory, none had hearts weighing >1,000 g. Of 70 patients with cardiac amyloidosis extensive enough to cause cardiac dysfunction, none had massive cardiomegaly. During the past 30 years, we have studied at necropsy 220 patients with hypertrophic cardiomyopathy (HC) and 200 of them were >20 years of age. Of this latter number, 8 had hearts weighing >1,000 g. This report summarizes findings in these 8 patients and also describes the heart weights in 207 other patients with HC studied by us at necropsy.

Certain clinical and necropsy findings in the 8 patients are summarized in Table I, and the cardiac weights in the men and women with HC studied by us are summarized in Figure 1. Our definitions of HC are summarized in a previous publication.[2] The scale used to weigh the hearts was accurate to <1 g.

Thus, HC needs to be added to the list of causes of massive cardiomegaly. What led to the massive cardiomegaly in our 8 patients is unclear. These 8 patients did not appear to have larger bodies than did the patients with HC without massive cardiomegaly. It is extremely rare for massive cardiomegaly to occur in women. Yet, 2 of our 8 patients were women, and the largest heart among the 8 belonged to a 21-year-old woman who weighed only 103 pounds (47 kg). She had a large myocardial infarct in the absence of narrowed epicardial coronary arteries, suggesting that she simply had too much myocardium to be perfused even by normal—albeit dilated—epicardial coronary arteries.

Left ventricular outflow obstruction was not a prerequisite for massive cardiomegaly. Only 4 of the 8 patients had either a thickened anterior mitral leaflet or a mural endocardial fibrous plaque in the left ventricular outflow tract in apposition to the anterior mitral leaflet. The latter 2 lesions are considered the anatomic equivalents of systolic anterior motion of the anterior mitral leaflet, a finding usually associated with left ventricular outflow obstruction. Furthermore, of the 5 patients having cardiac catheterization, 2 had no outflow pressure gradients, and in the 3 who did, the peak systolic pressure gradients were ≤50 mm Hg. Thus, outflow obstruction is not the cause of the massive cardiomegaly.

1. Roberts WC, Podolak MJ. The king of hearts: analysis of 23 patients with hearts weighing 1,000 grams or more. *Am J Cardiol 1985;55:485–494.*

2. Roberts CS, Roberts WC. Morphologic aspects of hypertrophic cardiomyopathy. In: Zipes DP, ed. Progress in Cardiology 2/2. *Philadelphia: Lea & Febiger, 1989:3–32.*

Sudden death in hypertrophic cardiomyopathy with normal left ventricular mass

Barry J Maron, Amy H Kragel, William C Roberts

Abstract

An active, healthy, and symptom free 16 year old boy with a family history of hypertrophic cardiomyopathy died suddenly while walking home from school. Necropsy showed absence of left ventricular hypertrophy (that is, normal heart weight), though the characteristic histological abnormalities of hypertrophic cardiomyopathy, such as cardiac muscle cell disorganisation and abnormal intramural coronary arteries, were present. It is likely that this patient had hypertrophic cardiomyopathy and died before left ventricular hypertrophy developed.

Cardiology and Pathology Branches, National Heart, Lung, and Blood Institute, National Institutes of Health, Bethesda, Maryland, USA
B J Maron
A H Kragel
W C Roberts

Correspondence to Dr Barry J Maron, National Institutes of Health, National Heart, Lung, and Blood Institute, Building 10, Room 7B15, Bethesda, MD 20892, USA.

Hypertrophic cardiomyopathy is a primary myocardial disease, often inherited, in which the morphological and clinical features are diverse.[1–4] The most characteristic anatomical feature of the disease is left ventricular hypertrophy in the absence of ventricular dilatation, unassociated with another cardiac or systemic disease which itself could produce left ventricular hypertrophy.[5]

In patients with hypertrophic cardiomyopathy, however, left ventricular hypertrophy is not always fully expressed within the first two decades of life.[6] In children with this disease left ventricular hypertrophy is often progressive or develops for the first time when body growth and maturation accelerate.[1,6]

Sudden death and cardiac arrest are the most devastating consequences of hypertrophic cardiomyopathy and they are most common in youthful patients with few or no symptoms[2,7,8] and substantial left ventricular hypertrophy.[1,2,8,9] The boy with hypertrophic cardiomyopathy that we describe died suddenly before the typical gross morphological features of the disease developed.

Case report

A 16 year old boy complained of feeling unwell at the end of the school day. Shortly afterwards he collapsed while walking home. Onlookers promptly started cardiopulmonary resuscitation, but these measures were unsuccessful.

According to his mother, the boy had been active, healthy, and in generally good physical condition until the day he died. He had not been involved in competitive athletics, but had often participated in bowling and occasionally lifted weights. He used neither drugs nor alcohol. There was, however, a strong family history of cardiac disease[1] (fig 1). His mother, brother, maternal aunt, and two maternal uncles have clinically and echocardiographically confirmed hypertrophic cardiomyopathy. These relatives showed various patterns of asymmetrical left ventricular hypertrophy.[1–4] The maximum ventricular septal thickness in the relatives ranged from 17 mm to 28 mm; none had systolic anterior motion of the mitral valve. The patient's maternal grandmother died at age 42 with congestive heart failure of uncertain cause (heart weight at necropsy was 530 g).

A complete necropsy was performed. The patient was 1·70 m tall and weighed 66 kg. He

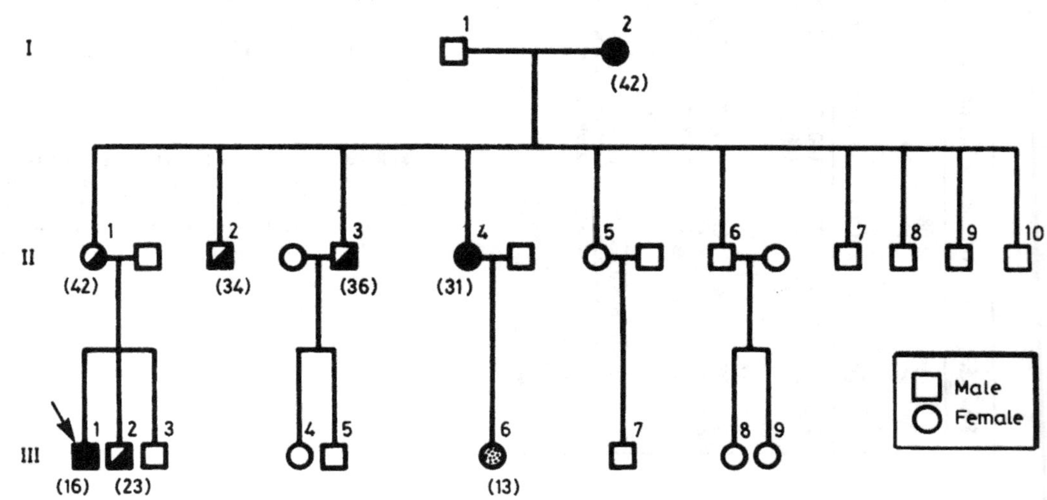

Figure 1 Pedigree of the patient (arrow) described in this report. Solid symbols indicate death from hypertrophic cardiomyopathy; those represented by half filled symbols are alive but affected by hypertrophic cardiomyopathy. Open symbols indicate that no clinical data are available. The stippled symbol represents a patient with symptoms suggestive of hypertrophic myopathy who was never investigated clinically. Ages are given in parentheses.

was well developed and well nourished. Mass spectrophotometric analysis for over 300 drugs (including volatile alcohols, narcotics, antihistamines, phenothiazines, barbiturates, synthetic narcotics, various sedatives, and cocaine) were performed on blood, urine, and lung tissue, and all were negative. All non-cardiac organs were normal.

The heart weighed 330 g and was judged to be within normal limits for sex and body size (that is ⩽345 g according to Ludwig,[10] <380 g by the standards of Reiner,[11] and <420 g according to Kitzman *et al*[12]). In addition, the absolute heart weight (and heart weight corrected for body weight) of the patient was the lowest among the 75 weighed specimens from male patients ⩾15 years old with hypertrophic cardiomyopathy who died of cardiac or non-cardiac causes and were studied in the Pathology Branch from 1960 to 1988 (fig 2D).

The epicardium was smooth and glistening and subepicardial adipose tissue was not increased. The ventricular and atrial chambers were non-dilated and the cardiac valves were normal (fig 2A). The thickness of the ventricular septum and left ventricular free wall did not exceed 15 mm (normal thickness ⩽15 mm) in nearly all segments of the left ventricular wall (fig 2A). Limited portions of the distal (caudal) left ventricular free wall were up to 17 or 18 mm in thickness. Thickening of these small regions of wall were believed to be postmortem changes[13] rather than segmental hypertrophy,[14] in view of the patient's overall normal heart weight. There was no grossly visible myocardial necrosis or fibrosis nor any mural endocardial plaques. The epicardial coronary arteries were widely patent without evidence of atherosclerotic plaques.

The sinoatrial and atrioventricular nodal areas were dissected, serially sectioned, and examined every 8 μm; no abnormalities of the conducting tissue or small arteries were identified. In addition, seven transverse blocks of left ventricular myocardium were obtained, including four from the proximal (cephalad), middle, and distal (caudal) regions of the ventricular septum and three from the left ventricular free wall at the same levels. Histological sections (6 μm thick) were stained with haematoxylin and eosin and by the Movat method and examined by light microscopy.

Numerous foci of disorganised cardiac muscle cells were identified in which adjacent cells or bundles of cells were arranged at oblique and perpendicular angles to one another (fig 2B).

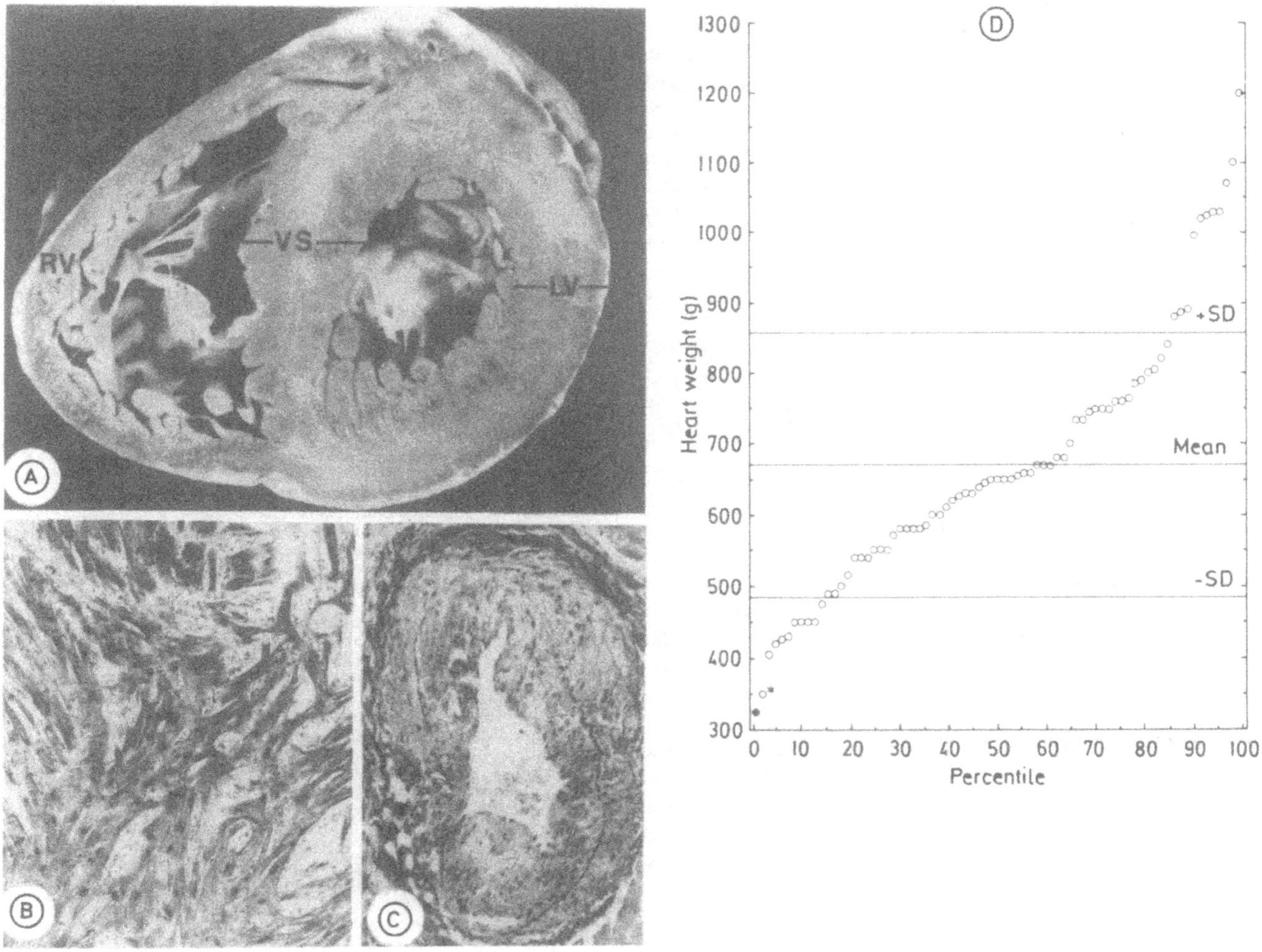

Figure 2 (A) Transverse section of the basal portion of the heart (which was of normal overall weight) showing non-dilated left ventricular cavity and normal ventricular septal (VS) and left ventricular free wall (LV) thicknesses; RV, right ventricular wall. (B) Region of cardiac muscle cell disorganisation in the left ventricular free wall, in which adjacent cells were oriented obliquely and perpendicularly. Haematoxylin and eosin stain, original magnification × 80. (C) Abnormal intramural coronary artery showing thickened wall and apparently narrowed lumen. Movat method; original magnification × 80. (D) Heart weights of 75 male patients with hypertrophic cardiomyopathy in the Pathology Branch registry. The solid symbol represents the patient reported here; the asterisk identifies the patient with the next lowest heart weight, a 49 year old man without a history of cardiac symptoms who died of renal cell carcinoma.

We measured the overall extent of cellular disorganisation from photographic enlargements of the histological sections.[14] Of the cardiac muscle cells analysed, 17% in the left ventricular free wall and 4% in the ventricular septum were judged to be disorganised. In addition, we identified eight abnormal intramural coronary arteries with thickened walls and apparently narrowed lumen[15] (five in the septum and three in the free wall) (fig 2C).

Discussion

All earlier studies of patients with hypertrophic cardiomyopathy who died suddenly (or survived a cardiac arrest) reported left ventricular hypertrophy and usually a considerable increase in left ventricular mass.[1 2 9 16] Our patient, however, did not show the gross morphological features that are typical of hypertrophic cardiomyopathy. The heart weight was within normal limits,[10–12] and there was no mitral valve thickening, mural endocardial plaque in the left ventricular outflow tract, or left atrial enlargement. Therefore, the anatomical diagnosis of hypertrophic cardiomyopathy in our patient depended on the histological findings. For example, disorganisation of cardiac muscle cells in the left ventricular myocardium was more extensive than that found in diseases other than hypertrophic cardiomyopathy or in normal controls.[14] Using a previously described morphometric mapping technique,[14] we calculated that cellular disorganisation constituted almost 20% of left ventricular free wall myocardium (while the ventricular septum was less severely affected). In addition, we identified several abnormal intramural coronary arteries with thickened walls and apparently narrowed lumens, typical of those commonly seen in hypertrophic cardiomyopathy.[15] These histological findings and the family predisposition to hypertrophic cardiomyopathy (five had the disease) strongly suggest that he died of hypertrophic cardiomyopathy before left ventricular hypertrophy developed.

At present, members of families with hypertrophic cardiomyopathy are advised that those relatives who seem to be unaffected by the disease (that is, do not show left ventricular hypertrophy on echocardiography) are not at that time at risk of sudden death or the development of symptoms. It is possible that the identification of other patients who die suddenly in the absence of hypertrophy will alter our perceptions about the course of hypertrophic cardiomyopathy and our approach to the genetic counselling of affected families. None the less cases of sudden death from hypertrophic cardiomyopathy before left ventricular hypertrophy appears are likely to be uncommon.

We cannot be certain that left ventricular hypertrophy and wall thickening would not have developed in our patient. Indeed, previous echocardiographic studies have shown that children with a genetic predisposition to hypertrophic cardiomyopathy can develop left ventricular hypertrophy for the first time during adolescence when body growth and development are accelerated.[6]

Our patient seems to be an unusual example of an individual who was genetically predisposed to develop hypertrophic cardiomyopathy and who died suddenly before left ventricular mass increased. The only structural evidence of hypertrophic cardiomyopathy at necropsy was cardiac muscle cell disorganisation and abnormal intramural coronary arteries.

1 Maron BJ, Bonow RO, Cannon RO, Leon MB, Epstein SE. Hypertrophic cardiomyopathy: interrelation of clinical manifestations, pathophysiology, and therapy. *N Engl J Med* 1987;**316**:780–9, 844–52.

2 Wigle ED, Sasson Z, Henderson MA, *et al.* Hypertrophic cardiomyopathy: the importance of the site and the extent of hypertrophy: a review. *Prog Cardiovasc Dis* 1985;**28**: 1–83.

3 Shapiro LM, McKenna WJ. Distribution of left ventricular hypertrophy in hypertrophic cardiomyopathy: a two-dimensional echocardiographic study. *J Am Coll Cardiol* 1983;2:437–44.

4 Maron BJ, Gottdiener JS, Epstein SE. Patterns and significance of the distribution of left ventricular hypertrophy in hypertrophic cardiomyopathy: a wide-angle, two-dimensional echocardiographic study of 125 patients. *Am J Cardiol* 1981;**48**:418–28.

5 Maron BJ, Epstein SE. Hypertrophic cardiomyopathy: a discussion of nomenclature. *Am J Cardiol* 1979;**43**: 1242–4.

6 Maron BJ, Spirito P, Wesley YE, Arce J. Development and progression of left ventricular hypertrophy in children with hypertrophic cardiomyopathy. *N Engl J Med* 1986; **315**:610–4.

7 McKenna W, Deanfield J, Faruqui A, England D, Oakley C, Goodwin JF. Prognosis in hypertrophic cardiomyopathy: role of age and clinical, electrocardiographic and hemodynamic features. *Am J Cardiol* 1981;**47**:532–8.

8 Maron BJ, Roberts WC, Epstein SE. Sudden death in hypertrophic cardiomyopathy: profile of 78 patients. *Circulation* 1982;**65**:1388–94.

9 Spirito P, Maron BJ. Relation between extent of left ventricular hypertrophy and occurrence of sudden cardiac death in hypertrophic cardiomyopathy. *J Am Coll Cardiol* (in press).

10 Ludwig J. *Current methods of autopsy practice.* 2nd ed. Philadelphia: WB Saunders, 1979:670–1.

11 Reiner L. Gross examination of the heart. In: Gould SE, ed. *Pathology of the heart and blood vessels.* 3rd ed. Springfield, Illinois: Charles C Thomas, 1968:1137.

12 Kitzman DW, Scholz DG, Hagen PT, Ilstrup DM, Edwards WD. Age-related changes in normal human hearts during the first 10 decades of life. Part II (maturity): a quantitative anatomic study of 765 specimens from subjects 20 to 99 years old. *Mayo Clin Proc* 1988;**63**: 137–46.

13 Maron BJ, Henry WL, Roberts WC, Epstein SE. Comparison of echocardiographic and necropsy measurements of ventricular wall thicknesses in patients with and without disproportionate septal thickening. *Circulation* 1977; 55:341–5.

14 Maron BJ, Anan TJ, Roberts WC. Quantitative analysis of the distribution of cardiac muscle cell disorganisation in the left ventricular wall of patients with hypertrophic cardiomyopathy. *Circulation* 1981;**63**:882–94.

15 Maron BJ, Wolfson JK, Epstein SE, Roberts WC. Intramural ("small vessel") coronary artery disease in hypertrophic cardiomyopathy. *J Am Coll Cardiol* 1986; **8**:545–57.

16 Olsen EG. Anatomic and light microscopic characterisation of hypertrophic obstructive and non-obstructive cardiomyopathy. *Eur Heart J* 1983;**4**(suppl F):1–8.

Combined Obstructive Hypertrophic Cardiomyopathy and Stenotic Congenitally Bicuspid Aortic Valve

Paul S. Brown, Jr., MD, Charles Stewart Roberts, MD, Charles L. McIntosh, MD, PhD, William C. Roberts, MD, and Richard E. Clark, MD

Hypertrophic cardiomyopathy (HC) is a congenital heart disease. Persons with 1 type of congenital heart disease are more prone to a second congenital heart condition than are persons without any congenital cardiac condition. The frequency of the congenitally bicuspid aortic valve in the general population is believed to be about 1%.[1] Therefore, it might be expected to be present in an occasional patient with a more uncommon condition, such as HC. The present report describes findings in 4 patients with coexisting HC and a congenitally bicuspid aortic valve.

The records of the Surgery Branch, National Heart, Lung, and Blood Institute, were searched for all patients who had a cardiac operation for HC and who had coexisting aortic valve disease. From 1960 to 1990 a total of 525 patients with HC underwent ventricular septotomy and partial septectomy (hereafter referred to as myotomy and myectomy) and 29 (5%) of them had coexisting aortic valve disease: pure aortic regurgitation in 20 patients and aortic valve stenosis with or without regurgitation in 9 patients. Of the latter 9 patients, 5 had tricuspid aortic valves, and 4 had bicuspid aortic valves. This report focuses on the 4 patients with combined HC and stenotic congenitally bicuspid aortic valves.

Pertinent findings in the 4 patients are summarized in Table I. All 4 patients were in New York Heart Association Functional class III or IV. Patients 1 and 2 had other family members with HC. Grade 3/6 systolic precordial murmurs, loudest along the left sternal border, were audible in all 4 patients, and the murmur was made louder by standing or by the Valsalva maneuver. Patients 1, 3 and 4 had a second systolic murmur that radiated to the neck, suggestive of valvular aortic stenosis. By echocardiogram the thickness of the ventricular septum was considerably greater (ratio >1.6) than that of the left ventricular free wall, and systolic anterior motion of the anterior mitral leaflet was present in all 4 patients. The peak systolic pressure gradient between the left ventricle and ascending aorta was >70 mm Hg in all 4 patients (Figure 1). At operation, all 4 patients had calcified, stenotic, congenitally bicuspid aortic valves (Figure 2). A typical mural endocardial plaque in apposition to the anterior mitral leaflet was present in all 4 patients. The ventricular septum by palpation was severely thickened and typical of that found in HC associated with a normal aortic valve. The portions of excised ventricular septum histologically had myofibril disorganization consistent with HC. All 4 patients had a lessening of their symptoms of cardiac dysfunction late postoperatively.

Coexisting HC and valvular aortic stenosis have been reported in at least 30 patients since 1960,[2-4] but usually the only evidence of HC was a ventricular septum thicker than the left ventricular free wall. Although asymmetric septal hypertrophy is usually present in HC, it also occurs in about 10% of patients with valvular aortic stenosis, and in about 10% of patients with systemic hypertension.[5,6] Thus, to diagnose HC in the presence of valvular aortic stenosis, findings other than a disproportionately thickened ventricular septum are necessary, and such was the case in the 4 patients described here.

The congenitally bicuspid aortic valve appears to occur with the same frequency in patients with obstructive HC as in the general population (each about 1%). At least 2 patients with HC and a congenitally bicuspid stenotic aortic valve have been reported by others. One,[3] a 52-year-old man, had a 73-mm Hg peak systolic left ventricular outflow pressure gradient, a ventricular septum con-

From the Surgery and Pathology Branches, National Heart, Lung, and Blood Institute, National Institutes of Health, Room 2N244, Building 10, Bethesda, Maryland 20892. Manuscript received June 7, 1990; revised manuscript received and accepted July 5, 1990.

TABLE I Findings in Four Patients with Combined Hypertrophic Cardiomyopathy and Congenitally Bicuspid Stenotic Aortic Valves

		Preoperative Catheterization								Echo Data				Morphologic Data				AV Prosthesis		Six Months Postoperative Catheterization					Follow-Up After MM+AVR		
				LVP	AAP	LV–AA															LVP	AAP	LV–AA psg[§]				
Pt. No.	Age (Yr)/ & Sex	FH of HC	FC (1–4)	s/d (mm Hg)		psg (mm Hg)	CI	AR (0–4)	+VPC Response	VS (mm)	LVFW (mm)	LA (mm)	SAM	Amount Excised (g)	VS LVOT Mural Plaque	AV Ca (0–4)	AV Weight (g)	Type	(Size)	FC (1–4)	s/d (mm Hg)		Rest (mm Hg)	Provoked (mm Hg)	CI	(yrs)	FC
1	57/F	+	4	235/12	93/56	142*	2.4	2+	+	22	12	45	+	4.7	+	4+	4.7	BS	(21)	1	150/5	140/72	10	50	2.2	16.5	1
2	57/M	+	3	238/10	123/62	115*	2.3	0	+	21	13	46	+	1.1	+	2+	1.4	BS‡	(19)	2	160/10	142/80	22	50	2.8	7.2	2
3	58/M	0	3	195/5	110/65	95*,†	2.6	1+	+	21	12	45	+	1.4	+	4+	7.2	SJM‡	(27)	1	150/10	125/80	25	30	2.5	2.6	1
4	64/M	0	4	220/9	145/60	75	1.8	2+	+	25	10	48	+	1.0	+	3+	—	H	(27)	2	—	130/80	—	—	—	7.3	2

* Left ventricle to ascending aorta pullback pressure measurements demonstrated <25 mm Hg aortic valvular component to the gradient; † provokable gradient to 125 mm Hg with isoproterenol; ‡ concomitant coronary artery bypass grafting; § highest provokable gradient measured during Valsalva maneuver, inhalation of amyl nitrite or infusion of isoproterenol; ǁ all patients were alive at 4/1/90.

AA = ascending aorta; AAP = ascending aortic pressure; AR = aortic regurgitation; AV = aortic valve; AVR = aortic valve replacement; BS = Bjork Shiley; Ca = calcification; CI = cardiac index (liters/min/m²); F = female; FC = functional class (New York Heart Association); FH = family history; H = Hancock bioprosthesis; HC = hypertrophic cardiomyopathy; LA = left atrium; LV = left ventricular; LVFW = left ventricular free wall; LVP = left ventricle pressure; M = male; MM = myotomy and myectomy; psg = peak systolic gradient; SAM = systolic anterior motion of the anterior mitral leaflet; s/d = peak systolic/end-diastolic pressure; SJM = St. Jude Medical; VPC = ventricular premature complex; VS = ventricular septum; + = present; 0 = absent; — = unknown.

siderably thicker than the left ventricular free wall, and systolic anterior motion of the anterior mitral leaflet; he underwent both aortic valve replacement and myotomy and myectomy. The second,[4] a 48-year-old woman with a family history of HC, had a 120-mm Hg peak systolic pressure gradient between the left ventricle and aorta, and a ventricular septum considerably thicker than the left ventricular free wall; she underwent aortic valve replacement only.

The operatively excised valves in our 4 patients actually appeared considerably more stenotic than was the degree of valvular stenosis found at preoperative cardiac catheterization. In our 4 patients, however, valvular aortic stenosis was anticipated because of the presence of an additional precordial murmur, calcific deposits in the aortic valve on chest x-ray, and aortic regurgitation.

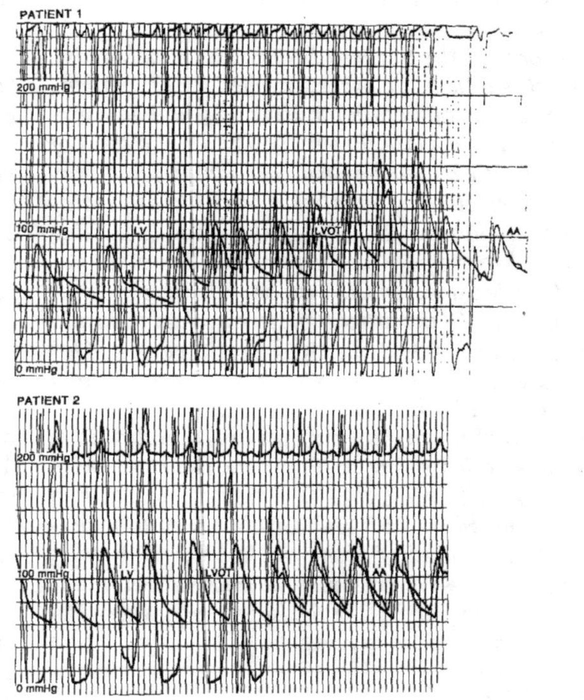

FIGURE 1. Left ventricle to ascending aorta pullback pressure tracings. The pressure gradient was primarily subvalvular with a <25 mm Hg valvular component in patients 1 to 3. AA = ascending aorta; LV = left ventricle; LVOT = left ventricular outflow tract.

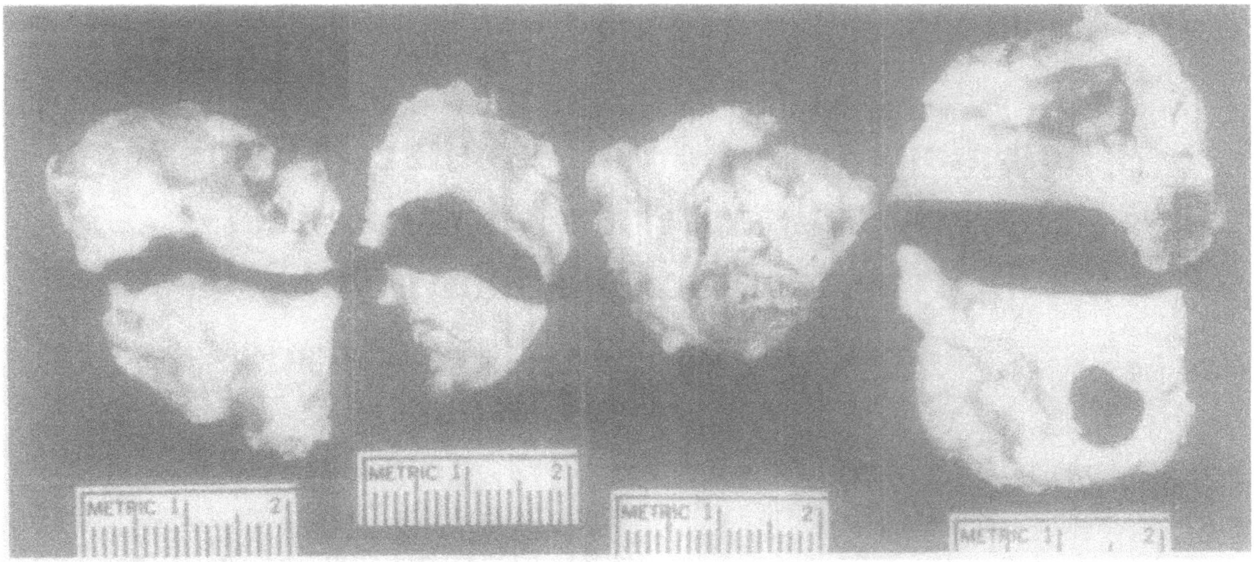

FIGURE 2. Excised stenotic bicuspid aortic valves from the 4 patients are shown from left to right. Valve no. 4 had a large perforation that was blocked by an area of calcium from the opposite leaflet.

1. Roberts WC. The congenitally bicuspid aortic valve. A study of 85 autopsy cases. *Am J Cardiol* 1970;26:72–83.

2. Nanda NC, Gramiak R, Shaw PM, Stewart S, DeWeese JA. Echocardiography in the diagnosis of idiopathic hypertrophic subaortic stenosis co-existing with aortic valve disease. *Circulation* 1974;50:752–757.

3. Stewart S, Nanda N, DeWeese J. Simultaneous operative correction of aortic valve stenosis and idiopathic hypertrophic subaortic stenosis. *Circulation* 1975; 51/52(suppl 1):I-34–I-39.

4. Feize O, Farrer-Brown G, Emanuel R. Familial study of hypertrophic cardiomyopathy and congenital aortic valve disease. *Am J Cardiol* 1978;41:956–964.

5. Parker D, Kaplan MA, Connolly JE. Coexistent aortic valvular and functional hypertrophic subaortic stenosis. *Am J Cardiol* 1969;24:307–317.

6. Panza JA, Maron BJ. Valvular aortic stenosis and asymmetric septal hypertrophy; diagnostic consideration and clinical and therapeutic implication. *Eur Heart J* 1988;9(suppl E):71–76.

Anomalous Insertion of Papillary Muscle Directly Into Anterior Mitral Leaflet in Hypertrophic Cardiomyopathy

Significance in Producing Left Ventricular Outflow Obstruction

Heinrich G. Klues, MD; William C. Roberts, MD; and Barry J. Maron, MD

Background. **Obstruction to left ventricular outflow in hypertrophic cardiomyopathy (HCM) is usually due to systolic anterior motion of the mitral valve. Occurrence of structural mitral valve abnormalities in HCM and their significance in producing outflow obstruction (even in the absence of typical systolic anterior motion) has not been fully appreciated.**

Methods and Results. **Analysis of 78 mitral valves excised from patients with obstructive HCM showed that 10 (13%) had anomalous insertion of one or both left ventricular papillary muscles directly into the anterior mitral leaflet. This malformation was identified by echocardiography, which demonstrated direct continuity between the hypertrophied papillary muscle and mitral leaflet, resulting in a long rigid area of midcavity narrowing that appeared to be solely or largely responsible for outflow obstruction. Basal subaortic pressure gradients were large (70–150 mm Hg). Mitral valve replacement reduced the outflow gradient substantially to 0–15 mm Hg in four patients with postoperative cardiac catheterization. However, two other patients who underwent septal myotomy/myectomy had persistent symptoms and incomplete relief of obstruction (gradients 60 and 70 mm Hg) because of continued midcavity apposition of papillary muscle and ventricular septum.**

Conclusions. **Anomalous papillary muscle insertion into anterior mitral leaflet represents a mechanism of obstruction to left ventricular outflow in patients with HCM and differs considerably from typical dynamic obstruction caused by mitral valve systolic anterior motion that occurs in many other patients with HCM. Recognition of this malformation emphasizes the diverse morphological expression of HCM and also has important clinical implications for patients requiring operation because the gradient is likely to persist even after adequate myotomy/myectomy; consequently, mitral valve replacement would appear to be the operation of choice in most such patients. (*Circulation* 1991;84:1188–1197)**

Obstruction to left ventricular outflow in patients with hypertrophic cardiomyopathy (HCM) usually results from systolic anterior motion of the mitral valve and midsystolic contact of mitral valve with ventricular septum.[1–9] The valve itself has often been described as free of intrinsic disease.[10–14] In the course of recent morphologic investigations of mitral valves in HCM, we observed a variety of structural mitral valve alterations including increased leaflet area and asymmetric or segmental leaflet elongation.[15] Also, a subset of patients was identified as having a congenital deformity of the mitral valve apparatus not fully appreciated as a cause of subaortic obstruction[16,17] in which one or both papillary muscles inserted directly into the ventricular surface of the anterior mitral leaflet. This study describes clinical recognition of this anomaly and focuses on its echocardiographic features and their diagnostic, hemodynamic, therapeutic, and prognostic implications.

From the Pathology (H.G.K., W.C.R.) and Cardiology (B.J.M.) Branches, National Heart, Lung, and Blood Institute, National Institutes of Health, Bethesda, Md.

Address for correspondence: Barry J. Maron, MD, National Institutes of Health, Building 10, Room 7B-15, Bethesda, MD 20892.

Received January 18, 1991; revision accepted May 21, 1991.

Methods

Selection of Study Patients

The cardiovascular registry of the Pathology Branch, 1982–1989, was reviewed and, of the 78 mitral valve specimens removed at operation or necropsy from patients with obstructive HCM in suitable morphological condition, 10 (13%) were identified as having a

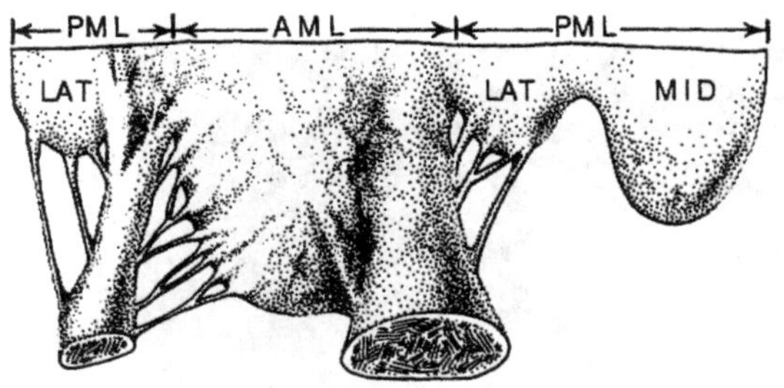

FIGURE 1. *Schematic drawing of an opened mitral valve with the ventricular aspect exposed. Orientation is with annular margin to the top and distal free edge of the valve to the bottom. Both the posteromedial and anterolateral papillary muscles insert directly (without interpositioned chordae tendineae) into the anterior mitral leaflet (AML). Note that the anomalous papillary muscle insertion largely involves the commissural regions between anterior leaflet and lateral portions of the posterior leaflet (PML). As drawn here for the purpose of illustration, the anomalous anterolateral papillary muscle is significantly larger and occupies greater portions of the anterior leaflet body (similar to that shown in Figure 4C). The anomalous posteromedial papillary muscle is smaller, does not extensively involve the anterior leaflet, and leaves the distal portion of the valve to be free and mobile (similar to that shown in Figure 2). LAT, lateral portion of posterior leaflet; MID, mid portion of posterior leaflet.*

distinctive morphological appearance in which one or both left ventricular papillary muscles inserted directly into the anterior mitral leaflet (Figure 1). The 10 study patients ranged in age from 24 to 62 years (mean, 41); six were men and four were women.

Control Patients

Mitral valves from 100 patients with normal hearts (45 patients) or aortic valve disease (55 patients) were selected as controls solely to determine the prevalence of anomalous papillary muscle insertion into anterior mitral leaflet. Patients ranged in age from 15 to 74 years (mean, 45); 59 were men and 41 were women.

Echocardiography

M-mode and two-dimensional echocardiograms were performed with commercially available ATL Mark 500 and Hewlett-Packard Sonos 500 instruments with 2.25 and 2.5 MHz transducers. Images were obtained in standard cross-sectional planes[18] as well as adaptations of these planes where judged appropriate. Intraoperative epicardial echocardiograms were also performed in eight of the 10 study patients just before and after the operative procedure.

Statistical Methods

Data are expressed as mean±SD. Differences between group means were analyzed by the unpaired Student's t test. Proportions were compared by the χ^2 test.

Results

Morphology of Mitral Valve Apparatus

Each of the 10 valves had direct insertion of the cephalad portion of one or both left ventricular papillary muscles into the ventricular surface of the anterior mitral leaflet (Figures 1–4). Anomalous papillary muscle insertion involved the commissural region in each valve but also extended to contiguous portions of the anterior and posterior mitral leaflets (Figures 1–4). Chordae tendineae were absent in the area of direct anomalous muscle insertion but otherwise were present in usual numbers with normal anatomic relation. In eight of the 10 patients, a single papillary muscle inserted into the mitral leaflet near either the anterolateral (six patients) (Figures 2, 3B, and 4C) or posteromedial commissure (two patients) (Figure 2). In the other two valves (patients 1 and 4 in Table 1), both papillary muscles inserted into the anterior mitral leaflet, each near its respective commissure. Mitral leaflet size was normal or only slightly increased in each patient (6.8–13.0 cm^2; mean, 10.2 cm^2).[15]

Only one (1%) of the 100 valves from control patients had direct insertion of a papillary muscle into the ventricular surface of the anterior mitral leaflet (a 36-year-old man with a normal heart).

Echocardiographic–Morphological Correlations

In nine of the 10 study patients, the morphology of the mitral valve apparatus (initially defined by visual inspection of the excised valve specimen) was subsequently identified by retrospective analysis of the echocardiographic studies. In the other patient (who was the last evaluated), anomalous papillary muscle insertion was identified prospectively before surgery by both transthoracic and intraoperative echocardiography (Figure 4).

In each of the 10 patients (as viewed in the parasternal and apical views), the anterior mitral leaflet appeared to be in continuity with one or both papillary muscles, creating the image of a large mass inserting directly into the ventricular surface of the anterior mitral leaflet (Figures 3–7); delicate thin echos characteristic of chordae tendineae were not evident. In addition, the aberrant papillary muscle showed an exaggerated anterior displacement within the left ventricular cavity (Figures 3–7). Consequently, the mitral apparatus was situated in particularly close proximity to (or in direct apposition with) the ventricular septum, producing extreme reduction in end-diastolic left ventricular outflow tract dimension. During systole, a long area of midseptal contact was produced by the anomalous papillary muscle with the most caudal extent located about 3–6 cm from the aortic valve (Figures 4–6).

In six of the 10 patients, the anomalous papillary muscle was very large and occupied substantial portions of the anterior mitral leaflet body beyond the commissural region (Figures 3B and 4C); there was complete absence of associated mitral systolic anterior motion on echocardiogram (Figures 4–7). The

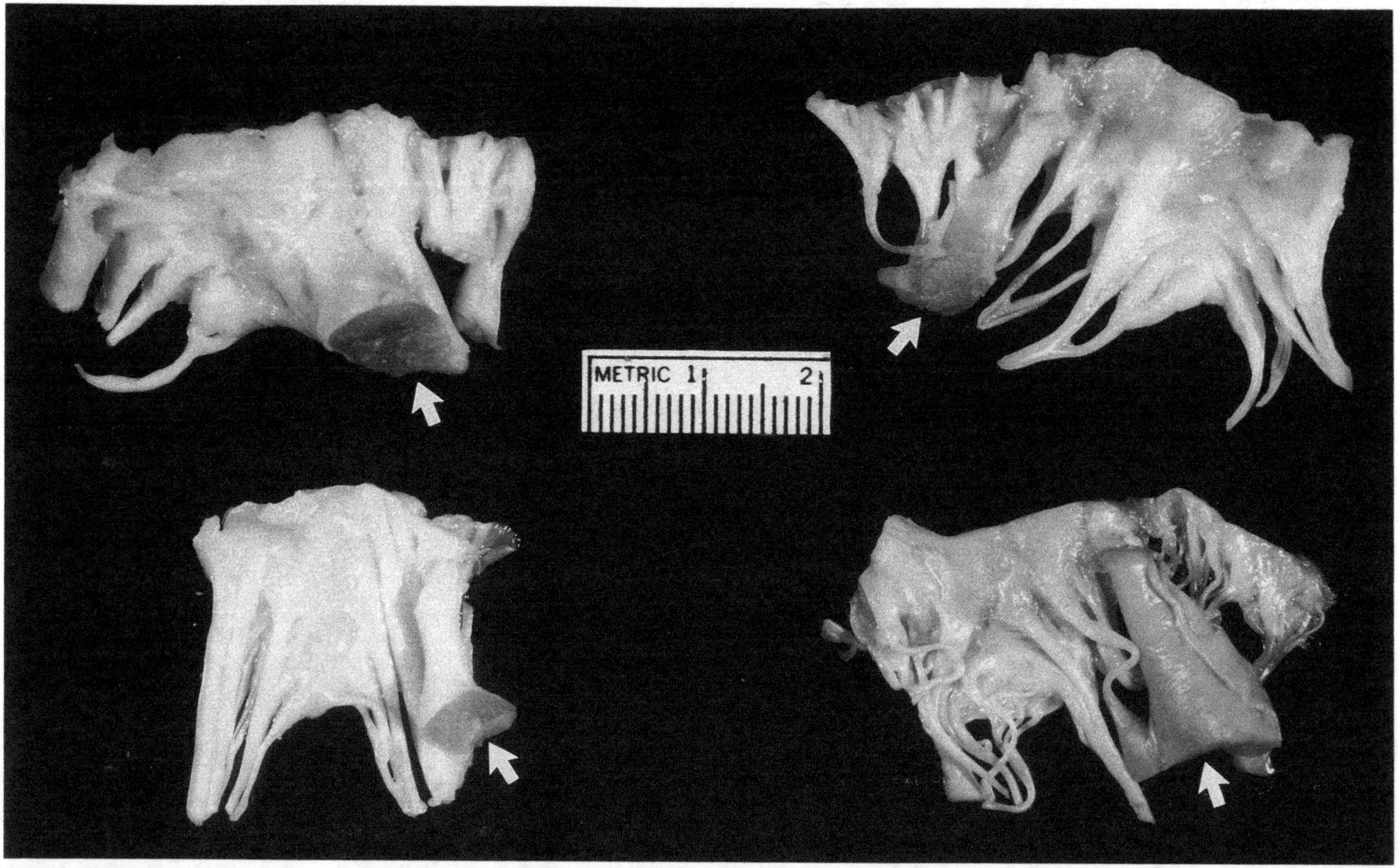

FIGURE 2. *Photograph of mitral valve specimens (with ventricular aspect exposed) excised at operation from four patients with obstructive hypertrophic cardiomyopathy showing anomalous papillary muscle insertion directly into anterior mitral leaflet (arrows). Papillary muscles are of various sizes and insert into the region of either the posteromedial (valve at upper right) or anterolateral commissure (the other three valves).*

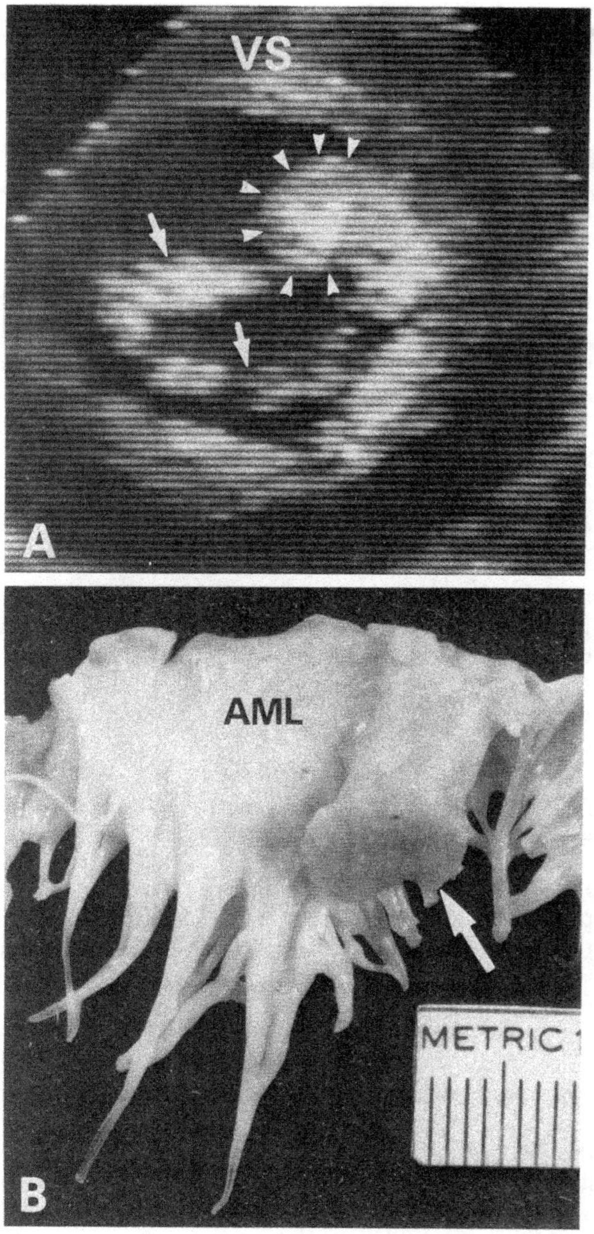

FIGURE 3. *Echocardiographic stop-frame image obtained intraoperatively (before mitral valve replacement) and mitral valve specimen from a 45-year-old man with obstructive hypertrophic cardiomyopathy and anomalous papillary muscle insertion.* Panel A: *Short-axis cross-sectional plane showing hypertrophied anomalous papillary muscle (arrowheads) in close proximity to the anterior ventricular septum (VS) during diastole. Large portions of the mitral valve (arrows) are also visualized and appear to be contiguous with the papillary muscle. Calibration marks are 1 cm apart.* Panel B: *Anterior mitral leaflet (AML) excised at operation to relieve obstruction to left ventricular outflow. Hypertrophied papillary muscle (arrow) inserts directly into region of the anterolateral commissure near the annular margin.*

other four patients had relatively small anomalous papillary muscles that were situated almost entirely in the commissural area, involving the anterior leaflet less extensively and sparing the distal margins (Figure 2); also, the distal portion of anterior leaflet appeared to make contact with the septum, usually in a passive fashion (with a relatively flat motion pattern) as the papillary muscle moved forward in systole.

The anatomic relation between papillary muscle and mitral valve was often not evident in the standard parasternal long-axis plane oriented through the center of the left ventricular cavity (Figure 5). Only when the cross-sectional plane was angulated slightly medially or laterally with respect to the center of the cavity (toward the posteromedial or anterolateral commissures) was the true anatomic continuity between papillary muscle and mitral leaflet visualized. Also, when the left ventricle was scanned slowly from base to apex in the short-axis plane, the anomalous papillary muscle could be visualized as directly contiguous with anterior mitral leaflet, without imaging interposed structures, which appeared to be chordae tendineae (Figure 3A).

Hemodynamic Findings

All 10 study patients had marked obstruction to left ventricular outflow under basal conditions measured at cardiac catheterization; subaortic pressure gradients were 70–150 mm Hg (average, 93). Left ventricular end-diastolic pressures ranged from 8 to 26 mm Hg (average, 17) and were greater than 15 mm Hg in five patients.

Clinical Findings

Each of the 10 patients had severe symptoms of cardiac dysfunction: exertional dyspnea in eight, angina in eight, and syncope in four. All 10 underwent operation to relieve symptoms and left ventricular outflow tract obstruction. Eight patients had mitral valve replacement as a primary operative procedure; four of these eight underwent postoperative cardiac catheterization studies and each showed abolition or marked reduction in basal outflow gradient to 0–15 mm Hg.

The other two patients had septal myotomy/myectomy (Patients 1 and 4 in Table 1); postoperative echocardiograms showed an apparently adequate resection of septal muscle (1.8–2.5 cm wide; 3.0–3.5 cm long), which extended caudal to the mitral leaflet tips in the long-axis plane. Nevertheless, large basal outflow gradients (60 and 70 mm Hg) remained after operation, a result of persistent muscular apposition between the anomalous papillary muscle and septum in the midcavity region beyond the caudal extent of the myotomy/myectomy. One of these two patients died 4 days after operation as a consequence of persistent congestive heart failure and outflow obstruction. The other patient had a second more extensive myotomy/myectomy performed 10 years later (because of persistent symptoms and obstruction), which also did not achieve a reduction in the outflow gradient.

Seven of the 10 patients showed evidence of genetic transmission of HCM in at least one first-degree relative based on echocardiographic and clinical

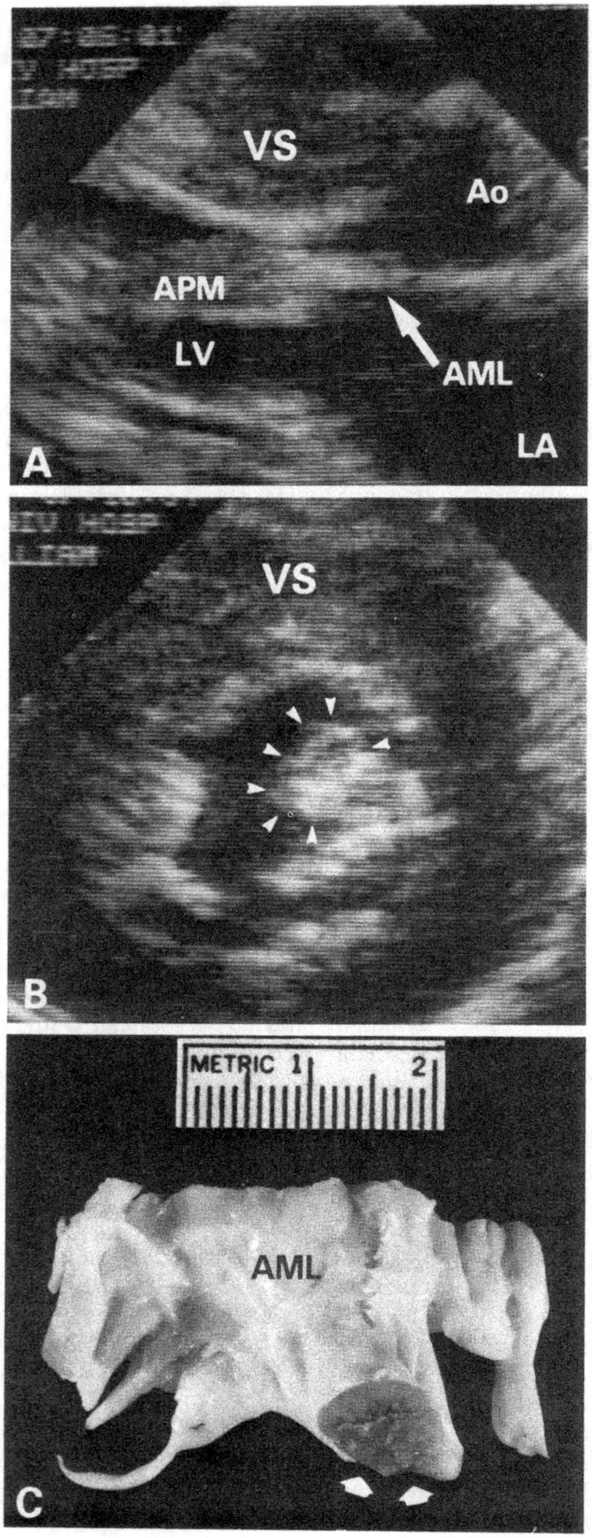

FIGURE 4. *Stop-frame images obtained intraoperatively (before mitral valve replacement) and mitral valve specimen from a 31-year-old man with obstructive hypertrophic cardiomyopathy and anomalous papillary muscle insertion.* Panel A: *Long-axis plane showing direct continuity between anomalous papillary muscle (APM) and anterior mitral leaflet (AML) creating a long area of midventricular outflow narrowing. Calibration marks are 1 cm apart.* Panel B: *Short-axis cross-sectional plane showing hypertrophied anomalous papillary muscle (arrowheads) in close proximity to the anterior ventricular septum (VS) during diastole.* Panel C: *Mitral valve excised at operation; a massively hypertrophied anterolateral anomalous papillary muscle (arrows) inserts directly into large portions of the anterior mitral leaflet (AML) body. This patient was prospectively identified by echocardiography as having aberrant papillary muscle insertion. Ao, aorta; LA, left atrium; LV, left ventricle.*

studies.[19] Systematic echocardiographic studies, however, were not performed in the other two pedigrees.

Discussion

In about 15% of mitral valves removed from patients with obstructive HCM, we identified anomalous insertion of one or both left ventricular papillary muscles directly into the anterior mitral leaflet. The findings of the present integrated morphological and echocardiographic investigation describe the clinical significance of this congenital mitral valve malformation responsible for obstruction to left ventricular outflow in some patients with HCM.

These patients had a distinctive left ventricular geometry with a strikingly narrowed outflow tract and greatly exaggerated anterior displacement of the papillary muscles beyond that usually present in HCM.[20,21] Consequently, subaortic obstruction appeared to occur largely by virtue of systolic apposition between the hypertrophied papillary muscle and septum in the midportion of the left ventricular cavity; typically the papillary muscle (as well as the contiguous distal mitral leaflets in some patients) came forward together as an intact single, rigid structure to make contact with the septum, creating a long area of midcavity apposition. It appeared that the absence of chordae tendineae between papillary muscle and mitral leaflet restricted leaflet motion and usually prohibited the distal leaflet from achieving the flexibility necessary to bend and produce the pattern of systolic anterior motion typical of patients with obstructive HCM. This finding was particularly true of those valves in which the anomalous papillary muscle was large and extensively involved the anterior leaflet.

In nine of our 10 study patients, the initial echocardiographic assessment failed to identify the morphological abnormality of the mitral apparatus. This was partly because anomalous papillary muscle insertion directly into mitral valve[16,17] had not been previously recognized as an established cause of subaortic obstruction in HCM. However, on retrospective analysis of the echocardiograms, we did identify this malformation. Critical to echocardiographic diagnosis was recognition that the aberrant papillary muscle inserts into the commissural regions of the mitral valve (and not into the central portion of the anterior leaflet). Therefore, standard parasternal long-axis

Table 1. Clinical, Hemodynamic, and Echocardiographic Data in 10 Patients With Hypertrophic Cardiomyopathy and Direct Insertion of Papillary Muscle Into Anterior Mitral Leaflet

				Functional class (NYHA)		LV–SA PSG (mm Hg)		LV (S/D) (mm Hg)		Preop echo measurements								
										Thickness (mm)		Cavity (mm)						
Patient No.	Age (yr)	Sex	Cardiac operation	Preop	Postop	Preop	Postop	Preop	Postop	VS	LVFW	S	D	Postop follow-up (months)	No. anomalous papillary muscles	Mitral leaflet area (cm^2)	SAM (preop)	Family history of HCM
1	7	F	M+M	3	2	150	120	240/8	200/14	...	...	...	...	168	...	9.9	−	−
	22		M+M	3	3	50*	70	190/10	210/10	22	16	30	44	34	...	...	−	
	24		MVR	3	3	75	0	215/21	120/26	14	16	33	48	6‡	1	...	−	
2	31	M	MVR	3	1	118	...	120/14	...	18	16	28	40	1	1	11.8	−	+
3	31	M	MVR	3	2	90	15	185/24	125/19	19	18	16	36	67	1	13.0	+	+
4	33	F	M+M	3	4	100	60†	218/26	...	28	20	21	37	0.06‡	2	7.9	−	+
5	39	F	MVR	3	2	70	0	200/23	115/14	18	14	17	32	43	1	12.2	+	+
6	39	F	MVR	3	2	70	0	160/16	140/7	21	13	23	40	68	2	6.8	−	+
7	45	M	MVR	3	1	100	...	190/10	...	19	18	21	38	41	1	12.0	+	+
8	49	M	MVR	3	2	85	...	170/21	...	16	...	14	32	18	1	11.0	−	−
9	54	M	MVR+CABG	3	2	70	...	170/10	...	18	20	29	42	6‡	1	11.5	...	...
10	62	F	MVR	3	3	90	5	170/24	140/24	18	15	28	43	13‡	1	7.6	−	+

NYHA, New York Heart Association; LV, left ventricle; SA, systemic artery; S, systolic; D, diastolic; VS, ventricular septum; LVFW, left ventricular free wall; SAM, systolic anterior motion; HCM, hypertrophic cardiomyopathy; M+M, ventricular septal myotomy/myectomy; MVR, mitral valve replacement; CABG, coronary artery bypass grafting; M, male; F, female; +, present; −, absent.

*Gradient measured at time patient was taking propranolol.

†Gradient estimated by continuous wave Doppler echocardiography; recorded 2 days after operation and probably represents an underestimation because patient was clinically in a state of low cardiac output and congestive heart failure.

‡Death (patients No. 1 and 4 due to congestive heart failure and No. 9 and 10 due to sudden cardiac death, patient No. 10 also had marked pulmonary hypertension present before as well as after operation: 85/30 mm Hg; mean, 59).

cross-sectional planes directed through the midportion of left ventricular cavity usually fail to image the abnormal anatomic relation between mitral leaflet and papillary muscle and the true geometric proximity of these structures to the ventricular septum. Accurate identification depends on sweeping the transducer medially or laterally from the center of the cavity to obtain nonstandard cross-sectional planes. Consequently, in a patient with HCM, the combination of left ventricular outflow tract obstruction and absence of mitral systolic anterior motion would strongly suggest the possibility of midcavity obstruction caused by anomalous papillary muscle insertion. Indeed, in the last (or 10th) patient in our series, anomalous papillary muscle insertion was diagnosed prospectively by both transthoracic and intraoperative echocardiography applying these anatomic and spatial principles derived from retrospective analysis of the other nine patients.

Direct insertion of papillary muscle into the anterior mitral leaflet represents a congenital malformation with selective failure of chordal development at about 12 weeks' gestation.[22,23] At this stage of normal cardiac development, the papillary muscles are contiguous with the mitral leaflets. Under normal circumstances, cephalad portions of the papillary muscles are first transformed into thick muscular chordae tendineae, which ultimately become delicate fibrous chordae positioned between the mitral leaflets and the papillary muscles. The arrest in normal embryological development demonstrated by our patients is not pathognomonic of HCM but may occur occasionally in otherwise normal hearts (as evidenced in our control group) or in patients with other types of heart disease.[24]

Each of our 10 patients had severe symptoms of congestive heart failure refractory to medical treatment as well as marked basal obstruction to left ventricular outflow. Recognition in such patients that outflow obstruction is due to a malformation of the mitral apparatus may have important implications with regard to planning operative strategy. Our data suggest that conventional septal myotomy/myectomy (Morrow procedure)[25] is not the optimal procedure for relieving obstruction in this subgroup of patients. Indeed, the two patients in this study who underwent myotomy/myectomy with an apparently adequate muscular resection nevertheless had only partial reduction in subaortic gradient and persistent marked outflow tract obstruction caused by continued systolic contact between anomalous papillary muscle and ventricular septum. In addition, these two patients continued to have substantial cardiac symptoms and ultimately died from heart failure. We have also evaluated two other patients with obstructive HCM (who are not formally part of this study) and the characteristic echocardiographic images of anomalous papillary muscle insertion; the malformation was described by the surgeon at operation but the mitral valve specimen was not available for examination because neither valve replacement nor necropsy was performed. After septal myotomy/myectomy, these patients had persistence of severe symptoms (or

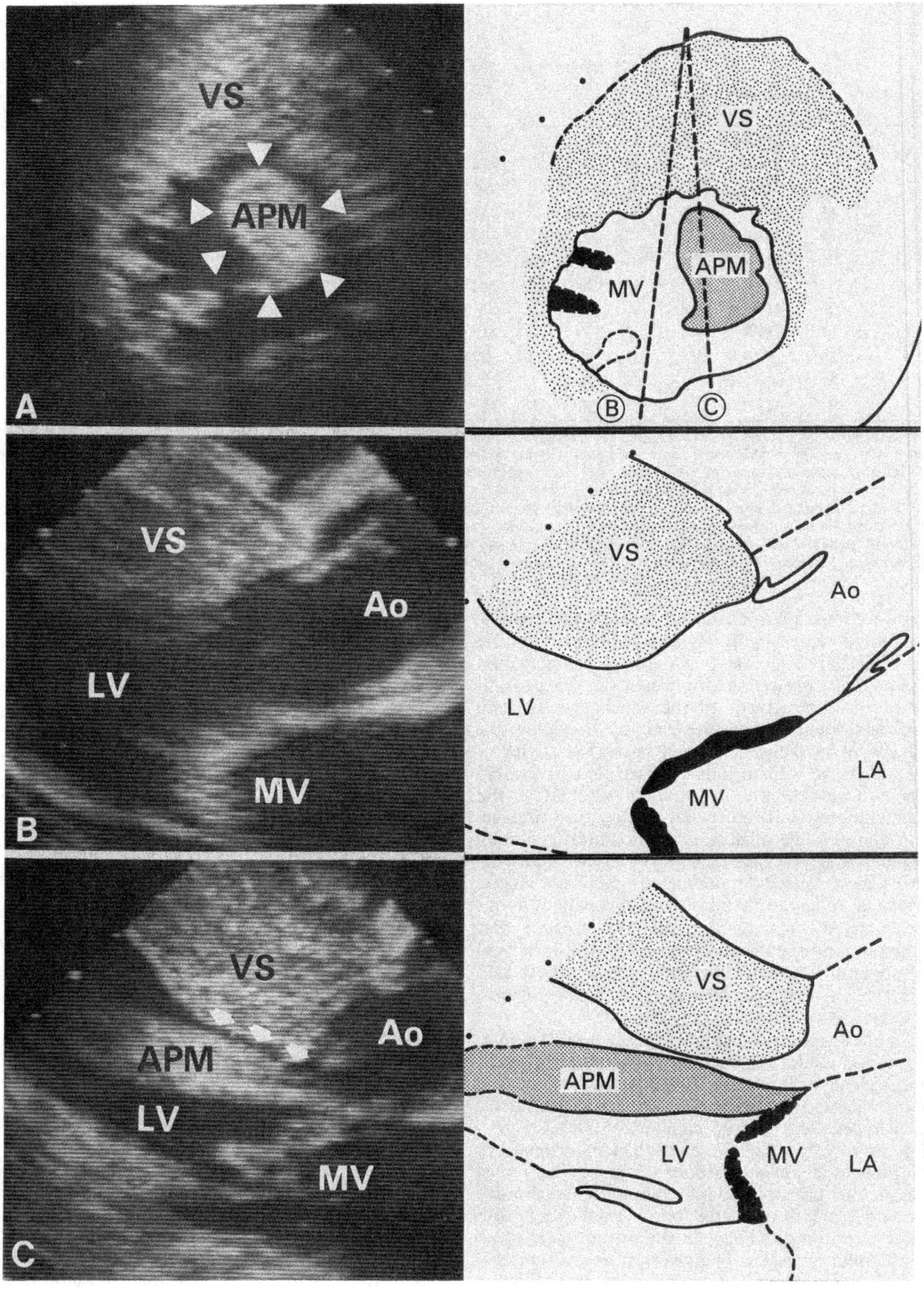
VS
APM
A
VS
MV
APM
B
C
VS
Ao
LV
MV
B
VS
Ao
LV
LA
MV
VS
Ao
APM
LV
MV
C
VS
Ao
APM
LV
MV
LA

FIGURE 5. *Composite of stop-frame images obtained intraoperatively (before myotomy/myectomy) during diastole in a 56-year-old man with obstructive hypertrophic cardiomyopathy and direct anterolateral papillary muscle insertion into anterior mitral leaflet.* Panel A: *Short-axis view in diastole shows massive anterolateral papillary muscle (arrowheads) in an exaggerated anterior position in close proximity to ventricular septum (VS). When the echo beam is passed perpendicular to the short-axis plane but without traversing the anomalous papillary muscle (broken line B), the long-axis view shows a wide-open left ventricular outflow tract without anatomic evidence of subaortic obstruction during systole (see* panel B*). In contrast, when the echo beam is swept laterally and passes through the anomalous papillary muscle (APM) (broken line C), the systolic image shown in* panel C *is obtained; the hypertrophied aberrant papillary muscle is in direct continuity with the anterior mitral leaflet without evidence of interposed chordae tendineae. Anomalous papillary muscle makes prolonged contact with the anterior ventricular septum in the midcavity region, producing left ventricular outflow obstruction. Calibration marks are 1 cm apart. Ao, aorta; LA, left atrium; LV, left ventricle; MV, mitral valve.*

postoperative death) and subaortic obstruction caused by papillary muscle–septal contact.

The standard septal myotomy/myectomy operation[11,25] probably fails to reduce the magnitude of the subaortic gradient adequately in patients with anomalous papillary muscle because it is fundamentally designed to relieve obstruction by enlarging outflow tract cross-sectional area and reducing dynamic systolic anterior motion of the mitral valve[26–29] (by virtue of minimizing the Venturi phenomenon).[16] Conversely, obstruction in our patients is not due to dynamic mitral leaflet motion,[1–9,16,26,28] but rather is a form of midcavity obstruction[30–32] that occurs by virtue of a different pathophysiological mechanism. This muscular obstruction occurs deep within the ventricle and is largely inaccessible to the standard myotomy/myectomy resection, which is commonly performed through an aortotomy.

Awareness that congenital papillary muscle insertion may occur in patients with obstructive HCM is critical to its identification either by echocardiography or at the time of operation. Inspection of mitral valve anatomy by the surgeon may confirm the presence of this anomaly and also aid in the assessment of whether a particularly extensive myotomy/myectomy or mitral valve replacement[33–36] would most likely afford relief of obstruction. Indeed, in the study patient most recently evaluated, the decision to perform mitral valve replacement was predicated on the prospective identification (before operation) of direct papillary muscle insertion.

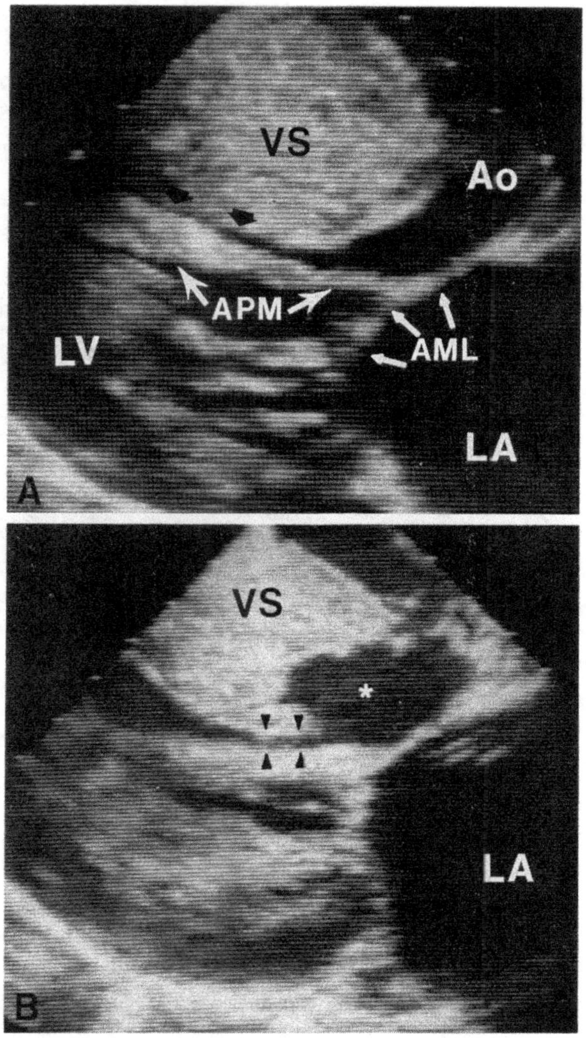

FIGURE 6. *Long-axis views obtained intraoperatively during systole from a 33-year-old woman with obstructive hypertrophic cardiomyopathy and anomalous papillary muscle insertion.* Panel A: *Before myotomy/myectomy. Anterior mitral leaflet (AML) is in direct continuity with the hypertrophied anomalous papillary muscle (APM), which is displaced anteriorly within the left ventricular cavity, producing a long area of midcavity contact with the anterior ventricular septum (VS) and outflow obstruction (arrowheads); note that tips of mitral leaflets coapt in the usual position and typical systolic anterior motion of the distal mitral leaflets is absent (small arrows).* Panel B: *After myotomy/myectomy. Extensive muscular resection (*) extends from base of septum beyond the distal margins of the anterior mitral leaflet; nevertheless, a large area of direct contact between papillary muscle and ventricular septum remains (arrowheads) that is responsible for persistent obstruction to left ventricular outflow. Ao, aorta; LA, left atrium; LV, left ventricle. Calibration marks are 1 cm apart.*

References

1. Shah PM, Gramiak R, Kramer DH: Ultrasound location of left ventricular outflow obstruction in hypertrophic obstructive cardiomyopathy. *Circulation* 1969;40:3–11
2. Pollick C, Rakowski H, Wigle ED: Muscular subaortic stenosis: The quantitative relationship between systolic anterior motion and the pressure gradient. *Circulation* 1984;69:43–49
3. Shah PM, Taylor RD, Wong M: Abnormal mitral valve coaptation in hypertrophic obstructive cardiomyopathy: Proposed role in systolic anterior motion of mitral valve. *Am J Cardiol* 1981;48:258–262

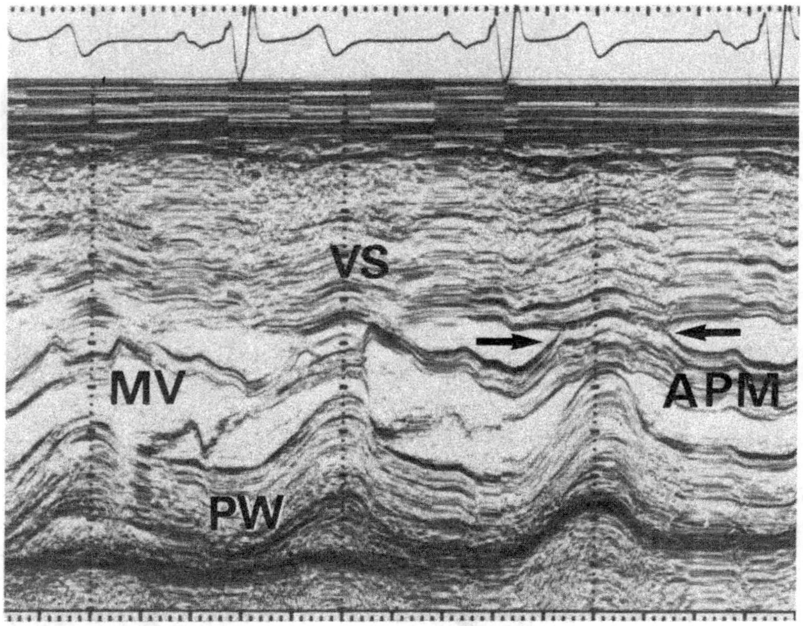

FIGURE 7. *Continuous M-mode echocardiographic sweep in a 62-year-old patient with obstructive hypertrophic cardiomyopathy and anomalous papillary muscle insertion. Toward the left, mitral valve (MV) motion is evident but typical systolic anterior motion is absent. Toward the right, the anterior mitral leaflet is contiguous with a thicker echo dense structure – anomalous papillary muscle (APM) characterized by a more restricted motion pattern and systolic contact with ventricular septum (VS) (arrows), even in the presence of paradoxic septal motion. PW, posterior free wall.*

4. Spirito P, Maron BJ: Patterns of systolic anterior motion of the mitral valve in hypertrophic cardiomyopathy: Assessment by two-dimensional echocardiography. *Am J Cardiol* 1984;54: 1039–1046
5. Maron BJ, Harding AM, Spirito P, Roberts WC, Waller BF: Systolic anterior motion of the posterior mitral leaflet: A previously unrecognized cause of dynamic subaortic obstruction in patients with hypertrophic cardiomyopathy. *Circulation* 1983;68:282–293
6. Henry WL, Clark CE, Glancy DL, Epstein SE: Echocardiographic measurement of the left ventricular outflow gradient in idiopathic hypertrophic subaortic stenosis. *N Engl J Med* 1973;288:989–993
7. Gilbert BW, Pollick C, Adelman AG, Wigle ED: Hypertrophic cardiomyopathy: Subclassification by M-mode echocardiography. *Am J Cardiol* 1980;45:861–872
8. Sasson Z, Yock PG, Hatle LK, Alderman EL, Popp RL: Doppler echocardiographic determination of the pressure gradient in hypertrophic cardiomyopathy. *J Am Coll Cardiol* 1988;11:752–756
9. Popp RL, Harrison DC: Ultrasound in the diagnosis and evaluation of therapy of idiopathic hypertrophic subaortic stenosis. *Circulation* 1969;40:905–914
10. Teare D: Asymmetrical hypertrophy of the heart in young adults. *Br Heart J* 1958;20:1–8
11. Morrow AG, Roberts WC, Ross J Jr, Fisher RD, Behrendt DM, Mason DT, Braunwald E: Obstruction to left ventricular outflow: Current concepts of management and operative treatment. *Ann Intern Med* 1968;69:1255–1286
12. Olsen EG: Anatomic and light microscopic characterization of hypertrophic obstructive and non-obstructive cardiomyopathy. *Eur Heart J* 1983;4(suppl F):1–8
13. Roberts WC: Operative treatment of hypertrophic obstructive cardiomyopathy: The case against mitral valve replacement. *Am J Cardiol* 1973;32:377–381
14. Roberts CS, Roberts WC: Morphologic features, in Zipes DP, Rowlands DJ (eds): *Progress in Cardiology 2/2.* Philadelphia, Lea & Febiger, 1989, pp 3–22
15. Klues HG, Dollar AL, Roberts WC, Maron BJ: Diversity of mitral valve structure in patients with hypertrophic cardiomyopathy: Evidence for a primary mitral valve abnormality (abstract). *Circulation* 1990;82(suppl III):III-293
16. Wigle ED, Sasson Z, Henderson MA, Ruddy TD, Fulop J, Rakowski H, Williams WG: Hypertrophic cardiomyopathy: The importance of the site and the extent of hypertrophy: A review. *Prog Cardiovasc Dis* 1985;28:1–83
17. Wigle ED, Adelman AG, Auger P, Marquis Y: Mitral regurgitation in muscular subaortic stenosis. *Am J Cardiol* 1969;24: 698–706
18. Tajik AJ, Seward JB, Hagler DJ, Mair DD, Lie JT: Two-dimensional real-time ultrasonic imaging of the heart and great vessels. *Mayo Clin Proc* 1978;53:271–303
19. Maron BJ, Nichols PF, Pickle LW, Wesley YE, Mulvihill JJ: Pattern of inheritance in hypertrophic cardiomyopathy: Assessment by M-mode and two-dimensional echocardiography. *Am J Cardiol* 1984;53:1087–1094
20. Reis RL, Bolton MR, King JF, Pugh DM, Dunn MI, Mason DT: Anterior-superior displacement of papillary muscles producing obstruction and mitral regurgitation in idiopathic hypertrophic subaortic stenosis: Operative relief by posterior-superior realignment of papillary muscles following ventricular septal myectomy. *Circulation* 1974;49 and 50(suppl II):II-181–II-187
21. Jiang L, Levine RA, King ME, Weyman AE: An integrated mechanism for systolic anterior motion of the mitral valve in hypertrophic cardiomyopathy based on echocardiographic observations. *Am Heart J* 1987;113:633–644
22. Wennick ACG, Gittenberger-de Groot AC, Brom AG: Developmental considerations of mitral valve anomalies. *Int J Cardiol* 1986;11:85–98
23. Teal SI, Moore GW, Hutchins GM: Development of aortic and mitral valve continuity in the human embryonic heart. *Am J Anat* 1986;176:447–460
24. Del Guzzo L, Sherrid MV: Anomalous papillary muscle insertion contributing to obstruction in discrete subaortic stenosis. *J Am Coll Cardiol* 1983;2:379–382
25. Morrow AG, Reitz BA, Epstein SE, Henry WL, Conkle DM, Itscoitz SB, Redwood DR: Operative treatment in hypertrophic subaortic stenosis: Techniques and the results of pre- and postoperative assessments in 83 patients. *Circulation* 1975;52:88–102
26. Schapira JN, Stemple DR, Martin RP, Rakowski H, Stinson EB, Popp RL: Single and two-dimensional echocardiographic visualization of the effects of septal myectomy in idiopathic hypertrophic subaortic stenosis. *Circulation* 1978;58:850–860
27. Spirito P, Maron BJ, Rosing DR: Morphologic determinants of hemodynamic state after ventricular septal myotomy in patients with obstructive hypertrophic cardiomyopathy: M-mode and two-dimensional echocardiographic assessment. *Circulation* 1984;70:984–994
28. Maron BJ, Bonow RO, Cannon RO III, Leon MB, Epstein SE: Hypertrophic cardiomyopathy: Interrelation of clinical

manifestations, pathophysiology, and therapy. *N Engl J Med* 1987;316:780–789, 844–852
29. Spirito P, Maron BJ: Significance of left ventricular outflow tract cross-sectional area in hypertrophic cardiomyopathy: A two-dimensional echocardiographic assessment. *Circulation* 1983;67:1100–1108
30. Fighali S, Krajcer Z, Edelman S, Leachman RD: Progression of hypertrophic cardiomyopathy into a hypokinetic left ventricle: Higher incidence in patients with midventricular obstruction. *J Am Coll Cardiol* 1987;9:288–294
31. Falicov RE, Resnekov L: Midventricular obstruction in hypertrophic obstructive cardiomyopathy: New diagnostic and therapeutic challenge. *Br Heart J* 1977;39:701–705
32. Kuhn H, Mercier J, Köhler E, Frenzel H, Hort W, Loogen F: Differential diagnosis of hypertrophic cardiomyopathies: Typical (subaortic) hypertrophic obstructive cardiomyopathy, atypical (midventricular) hypertrophic obstructive cardiomyopathy and hypertrophic non-obstructive cardiomyopathy. *Eur Heart J* 1983;4(suppl F):93–102
33. McIntosh CL, Greenberg GJ, Maron BJ, Leon ML, Cannon RO III, Clark RE: Clinical and hemodynamic results after mitral valve replacement in patients with obstructive hypertrophic cardiomyopathy. *Ann Thorac Surg* 1989;47:236–244
34. Krajcer Z, Leachman RD, Cooley DA, Ostajic M, Coronado R: Mitral valve replacement and septal myectomy in hypertrophic cardiomyopathy: Ten-year follow-up in 80 patients. *Circulation* 1989;80(suppl I):I-57–I-64
35. McIntosh CL, Maron BJ: Current operative treatment of obstructive hypertrophic cardiomyopathy. *Circulation* 1988; 78:1–9
36. Cooley DA, Leachman RD, Hallman GL, Gerami S, Hall RJ: Idiopathic hypertrophic subaortic stenosis: Surgical treatment including mitral valve replacement. *Arch Surg* 1971;103: 606–609

KEY WORDS • hypertrophic cardiomyopathy • echocardiography • mitral valve • papillary muscle • obstruction

Appearance of or Persistence of Severe Mitral Regurgitation Without Left Ventricular Outflow Obstruction After Partial Ventricular Septal Myotomy-Myectomy in Hypertrophic Cardiomyopathy

Charles Stewart Roberts, MD, S. David Gertz, MD, Heinrich G. Klues, MD, Richard O. Cannon III, MD, Barry J. Maron, MD, Charles L. McIntosh, MD, and William Clifford Roberts, MD

At the National Heart, Lung, and Blood Institute from 1959 through October 1989, 626 patients underwent operative treatment of obstructive hypertrophic cardiomyopathy: ventricular septal myotomy-partial myectomy alone in 539 patients; mitral valve replacement alone in 68 patients; and both procedures, not necessarily simultaneously, in 27 patients. The septal myotomy-myectomy procedure in most patients provided clinical improvement, but in some patients the results of this procedure have been unsatisfactory and reoperation has been performed.[1] In the 27 patients who underwent reoperation after septal myotomy-myectomy, the indication was persistent left ventricular outflow obstruction in 24 patients[2] and pure mitral regurgitation, without outflow obstruction, in 3 patients. This report describes certain clinical and morphologic features in the latter 3 patients.

Certain clinical and operative findings in the 3 patients are summarized in Table I. All 3 patients had peak systolic pressure gradients at rest or with provocation between left ventricle and systemic artery >50 mm Hg before the myotomy-myectomy operation, and 1 patient (no. 2) had a large (61 mm Hg) gradient across the right ventricular outflow tract. All 3 patients also had mitral regurgitation before the myotomy-myectomy operation performed through an aortotomy. Mitral regurgitation in patient 1 was only mild before the myotomy-myectomy operation but severe afterwards; in patient 2, mitral regurgitation was severe both before and after the initial operation (Figure 1), and in patient 3 it was of moderate degree before myotomy-myectomy and severe afterwards. All 3 patients had complete relief of left ventricular outflow obstruction by the myotomy-myectomy operation; nevertheless, severe symptoms of cardiac dysfunction persisted. At reoperation, ruptured mitral chordae tendineae were found in patients 1 and 2 and severe posterior mitral leaflet systolic anterior motion in patient 3. In none of the 3 patients was the mitral anulus dilated. The operatively excised mitral valves are shown in Figure 2. After mitral replacement, symptoms of cardiac dysfunction less-

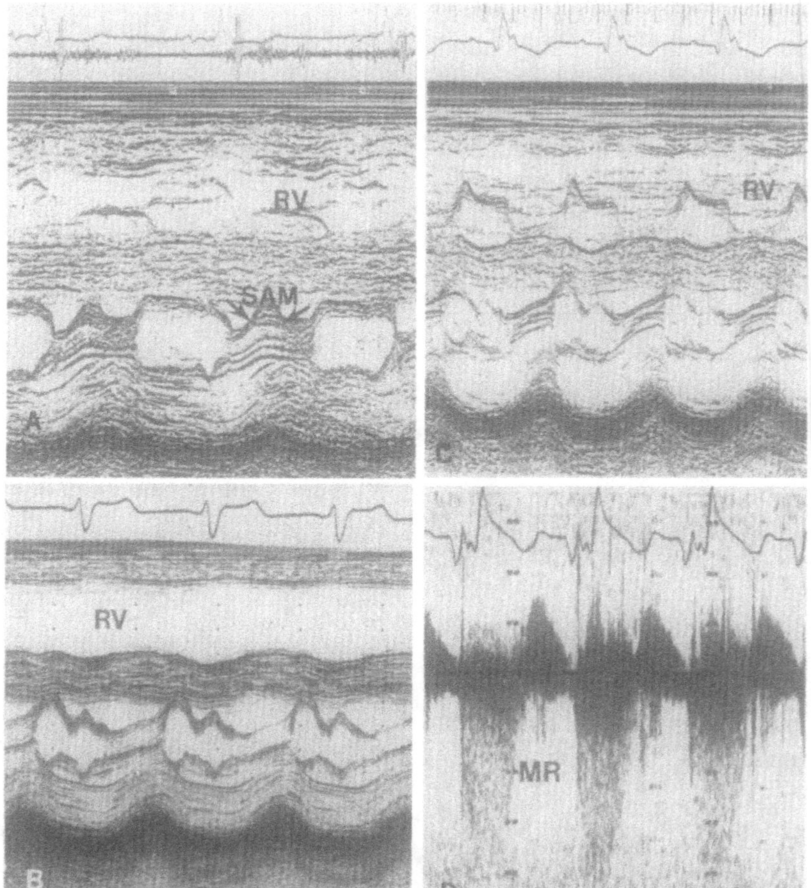

FIGURE 1. M-mode echocardiograms from patient 2 (CW). *A*, preoperative. Systolic anterior motion (SAM) of the mitral valve with mitral valve–septal contact. *B and C*, 6 and 25 months after septal myotomy-myectomy operation. SAM is now absent and the ventricular septum is thinner. *D*, postoperative. Continuous-wave Doppler tracing obtained from left ventricular apex showing mitral regurgitation (MR). RV = right ventricle.

From the Surgery, Pathology, and Cardiology Branches, National Heart, Lung, and Blood Institute, National Institutes of Health, Bethesda, Maryland. Manuscript received July 9, 1991; revised manuscript received and accepted August 14, 1991.

TABLE I Observations in Three Patients with Hypertrophic Cardiomyopathy Who Had Ventricular Myotomy–Myectomy for Left and/or Right Ventricular Outflow Obstruction Followed Later by Mitral Valve Replacement for Pure Mitral Regurgitation

	Patient 1 (MS)				Patient 2 (CW)				Patient 3 (AM)			
	Before M&M	Six Months After M&M	Shortly Before MVR	Six Months After MVR	Before M&M	Six Months After M&M	Shortly Before MVR	Six Months After MVR	Before M&M	Six Months After M&M	Shortly Before MVR	Six Months After MVR
Age (years)	23	23	34	34	22	22	24	25	55	55	60	60
Functional class (I–IV) (NYHA)	3	1	3	2	3	2	3	2	4	2	4	2
Atrial fibrillation	0	0	0	0	0	0	0	0	+	+	+	+
Echocardiographic findings												
Systolic anterior motion	+	–	0	–	+	0	0	–	+	0	0	–
Right ventricular cavity (mm)	28	–	35	34	30	36	42	40	22	30	29	28
Left atrial cavity (mm)	56	–	66	64	46	55	55	60	45	50	62	57
Left ventricular cavity (mm) (s/d)	38/–	–	50/38	50/40	31/21	41/24	46/34	45/	38/24	42/32	42/30	44/32
Ascending aorta (mm)	33	–	32	32	26	28	29	–	25	25	28	29
Ventricular septum (mm)	21	–	10	10	34	19	14	–	21	11	12	12
Left ventricular free wall (mm)	14	–	14	14	18	18	18	–	10	10	10	10
Intravascular pressures (mm Hg)												
Pulmonary artery wedge, V (m)	12 (9)	14 (11)	26 (18)	10 (7)	20 (15)	36 (29)	–	–	25 (18)	–	30 (24)	32 (21)
Right ventricle (s/d)	28/6	26/6	33/7	26/9	95/18	56/24	–	–	48/4	–	65/12	67/18
Pulmonary artery (s/d)	26/18	26/10	33/12	26/4	34/24	57/29	–	–	48/20	–	65/30	67/25
Left ventricle (s/d)	90/13	110/28	93/22	95/6	125/20	102/37	–	–	150/6	–	122/17	115/16
Aorta (s/d)	90/55	120/60	93/57	100/58	125/78	115/75	–	–	96/60	–	122/60	120/60
LV–aorta peak systolic gradient												
Rest	0	0	0	0	0*	0	–	–	54	–	0	0
Provocation	91	0	0	0	70	0	–	–	96	–	–	0
Cardiac index (liters/min/m^2)	2.9	2.9	1.7	2.6	2.9	1.8	–	–	1.9	–	2.7	1.7
Mitral regurgitation (0.4+), LV cine	1+	–	4+	1+	3+	3+	3+	–	2+	–	3+	0
Interval (mo) M&M to MVR		128					25			73		
Interval (mo) MVR to March 1990				44				21 →				97‡ →
Date of M&M (month–year)	11–1975	–	–	–	6–1986	–	–	–	2–1976	–	–	–
Date of MVR (month–year)	–	–	7–1986	–	–	–	6–1988	–	–	–	2–1982	–
Type (size [mm]) substitute valve	–	–	B-S (27)	–	–	–	SJM (31)	–	–	–	Hancock (27)	–
Operative findings												
Weight VS excised (g)	9.6	–	–	–	10.2†	–	–	–	0.6	–	–	–
Ruptured mitral CT	–	–	+	–	–	–	0	–	–	–	0	–
Prolapsed PML	–	–	0	–	–	–	0	–	–	–	+	–
Thickened AML + CT	–	–	+	–	–	–	+	–	–	–	+	–

*Immediately before provocation, peak systolic gradient at rest was 50 mm Hg. Note that this patient had a 61 mm Hg systolic pressure gradient at rest between right ventricle and a major pulmonary artery.
†Includes myocardium from both right and left ventricular outflow tracts.
‡This patient died suddenly 97 months after mitral valve replacement. A necropsy was not performed.
AML = anterior mitral leaflet; B-S = Bjork-Shiley prosthesis; cine = cineangiography; CT = chordae tendineae; LV = left ventricular; M&M = myotomy and myectomy (partial); MVR = mitral valve replacement; NYHA = New York Heart Association classification; PML = posterior mitral leaflet; s/d = peak systolic/end diastolic; SJM = St. Jude Medical prosthesis; V = peak V wave; VS = ventricular septum; – = no information available or not done.

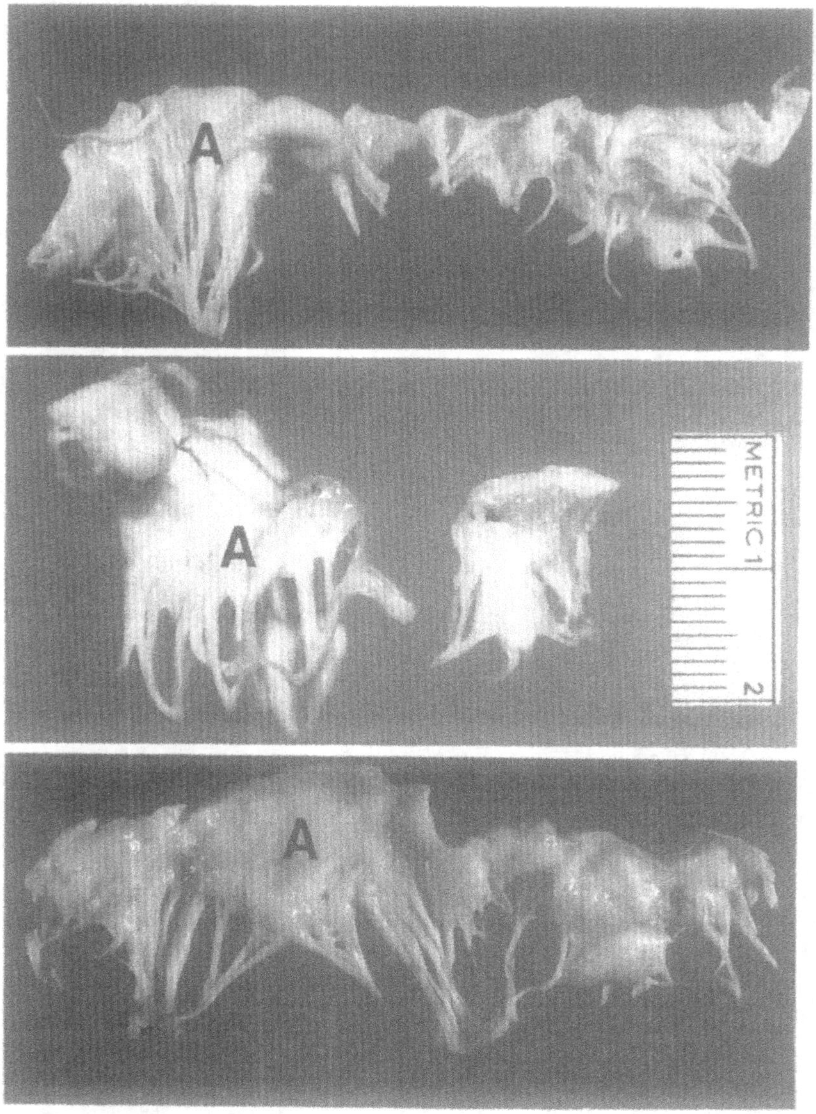

FIGURE 2. Operatively excised mitral valves from each of the 3 patients. *Upper,* patient 1 (MS) showing ruptured chordae tendineae from the anterior half of the anterior (A) mitral leaflet. A portion of the posterior leaflet is elongated. *Middle,* patient 2 (CW). Chordae from the anterior (A) half of the anterior leaflet also are absent (ruptured). *Bottom,* patient 3 (AM). No chordae are ruptured or missing but a portion of posterior leaflet is elongated. The *bottom* photograph is reproduced with permission from the American Heart Association, from Maron BJ, Harding AM, Spirito P, Roberts WC, and Waller BF. Systolic anterior motion of the posterior mitral leaflets: a previously unrecognized cause of dynamic subaortic obstruction in patients with hypertrophic cardiomyopathy. *Circulation* 1983;68:282–293.

ened by 1 New York Heart Association functional class in patients 1 and 2 and by 2 functional classes in patient 3 late postoperatively.

Almost every patient who undergoes ventricular septal myotomy-myectomy for left ventricular outflow obstruction has some degree of mitral regurgitation preoperatively. This operative procedure usually reduces the degree of mitral regurgitation, and it also usually relieves left ventricular outflow obstruction.[3] Reoperation is seldom necessary in obstructive hypertrophic cardiomyopathy and when it is performed, the indication is usually persistent left ventricular outflow obstruction. Rare is the postoperative patient who has pure mitral regurgitation producing significant symptoms without any associated left ventricular outflow obstruction. Such was the case, however, in our 3 patients.

The causes of the worsening or persistence of pure mitral regurgitation in patients 1 and 2 appear to have been inadvertent severance of several mitral chordae tendineae at the time of the myotomy-myectomy operation. This technical complication was unrecognized at operation. Retrospective review of the intraoperative echocardiogram before and after the septal myectomy, however, clearly indicates that several chordae tendineae were severed. Patient 3 was known to have systolic anterior motion of a portion of posterior mitral leaflet before myotomy-myectomy and this systolic anterior motion persisted after the initial operation. Why the mitral regurgitation worsened, however, after relief of left ventricular outflow obstruction was not discernible from study of the operatively excised mitral valve.

This study indicates that damage may occur to the mitral valve at the time of ventricular septectomy-septotomy in obstructive hypertrophic cardiomyopathy, and that this damage may cause worsening of or persistence of mitral regurgitation postoperatively.

1. McIntosh CL, Maron BJ. Current operative treatment of obstructive hypertrophic cardiomyopathy. *Circulation* 1988;78:487–495.

2. Roberts CS, McIntosh CL, Brown PS Jr, Cannon RO III, Gertz SD, Clark RE. Reoperation for persistent outflow obstruction in hypertrophic cardiomyopathy. *Ann Thorac Surg* 1991;51:455–460.

3. Cooper MM, Tucker E, McIntosh CL, Cannon RO III, Clark RE. Effect of left ventricular septal myectomy on concurrent mitral regurgitation. *Ann Thorac Surg* 1989;48:251–256.

Severe Mitral or Aortic Valve Regurgitation, or Both, Requiring Valve Replacement for Infective Endocarditis Complicating Hypertrophic Cardiomyopathy

WILLIAM C. ROBERTS, MD, FACC, JOAN C. KISHEL, MD, CHARLES L. McINTOSH, MD, FACC, RICHARD O. CANNON III, MD, FACC, BARRY J. MARON, MD

Bethesda, Maryland

Certain clinical and morphologic findings are described in 11 patients with hypertrophic cardiomyopathy complicated by infective endocarditis that produced severe mitral or aortic valve regurgitation, or both, necessitating valve replacement. All 11 patients had changes in the operatively excised valve or valves characteristic of healed infective endocarditis. The infection involved only the mitral valve in seven patients, only the aortic valve in three patients and both valves in one patient.

Study of the operatively excised mitral valves indicated that the healed vegetations were located most commonly on the left ventricular aspects of the anterior mitral leaflet, indicating that vegetation had formed at contact points of this leaflet with mural endocardium of the left ventricular outflow tract. In all 11 patients, the infective endocarditis either worsened preexisting valve regurgitation or initiated valve regurgitation and led to worsened signs and symptoms of cardiac dysfunction, necessitating valve replacement. Functional class improved in the nine patients who survived 7 to 101 months after valve replacement.

Hypertrophic cardiomyopathy appears to be a factor predisposing to infective endocarditis. Patients with hypertrophic cardiomyopathy should receive prophylactic antibiotic therapy during procedures that predispose to infective endocarditis.

(J Am Coll Cardiol 1992;19:365–71)

From 1961 through October 1989, 626 patients with hypertrophic cardiomyopathy underwent a cardiac operation at the Surgery Branch of the National Heart, Lung, and Blood Institute: partial septotomy/septectomy alone in 539 patients (86%); septotomy/septectomy followed later by mitral valve replacement in 19 patients (3%) and mitral valve replacement alone in 68 patients (11%). Of the 87 patients undergoing mitral valve replacement with or without septotomy/septectomy, mitral valve replacement was performed because of severe left ventricular outflow obstruction unassociated with severe thickening of the ventricular septum in 65 patients; damage to either the mitral or aortic valve at the time of earlier septotomy/septectomy in 5 patients; inability to wean the patient from cardiopulmonary bypass after septotomy/septectomy in 3 patients; severe regurgitation of uncertain etiology in 3 patients; and valvular regurgitation caused by or worsened by infective endocarditis in 11 patients. This report describes certain clinical and morphologic cardiac findings in the 11 patients with hypertrophic cardiomyopathy with severe mitral or aortic valvular regurgitation, or both, from infective endocarditis.

From the Pathology, Cardiology and Surgery Branches, National Heart, Lung, and Blood Institute, National Institutes of Health, Bethesda, Maryland.

Manuscript received May 8, 1991; revised manuscript received July 15, 1991, accepted July 29, 1991.

Address for reprints: William C. Roberts, MD, Building 10, Room 2N258, NHLBI-NIH, Bethesda, Maryland 20892.

Methods

Clinical characteristics (Tables 1 to 3). All 11 patients had clear clinical evidence of hypertrophic cardiomyopathy: 1) each had evidence of left ventricular hypertrophy on both the electrocardiogram (ECG) and the M-mode echocardiogram; 2) immediately before cardiac valve replacement, only 1 patient had a dilated left ventricular cavity as determined by left ventricular angiography and the dilation was of mild degree; 3) none had a history of systemic hypertension and, with one exception, all had systemic arterial indirect pressure recordings ≤140 mm Hg systolic and ≤90 mm Hg diastolic (Patient 3 had a systemic arterial direct pressure of 160/90 mm Hg recorded immediately before valve replacement, but other pressures recorded were normal); 4) although cardiac index was normal in only four of nine patients in whom it was recorded, the other five had evidence of severe valvular regurgitation (worsened by infective endocarditis) at the time of the recording; 5) the maximal thickness of the ventricular septum was greater than that of the left ventricular free wall in all patients before either valve replacement or partial ventricular septotomy/septectomy; and 6) all patients had hemodynamic documentation of subaortic obstruction at some time.

Characteristics of infective endocarditis. All 11 patients had evidence of active infective endocarditis at some time (Fig. 1 to 7). Ten patients had a typical clinical illness of active infective endocarditis. Of the nine patients with one

Table 1. Clinical and Morphologic Features in 11 Patients Having Valve Replacement for Valvular Regurgitation Due to or Worsened by Infective Endocarditis Complicating Hypertrophic Cardiomyopathy

Pt No.	Age (yr) at VR/ Gender	Diagnosis of HCM		NYHA Functional Class (I-IV)			Septotomy/Septectomy (7 patients)				Follow-Up After Valve Replacement (mo)	NYHA Class at Latest Follow-Up	Interval IE to VR (mo)	Type Valve Prosthesis		Morphology of Operatively Excised Valve				
																MV			AV	
		Before IE	After IE	Just Before IE	After IE	Just Before VR	Before IE	After IE	Before VR	With VR				MV (size)	AV (size)	Calcium	P	RCT	Calcium	P
1	12/M	+	0	II	IV	IV	0	0	0	0	7	I	17	SE	–	+	+	+	–	–
2	25/M	+	0	II	III	III	+	+	0	+	21	I	10	H (27 mm)	–	+	+	+	–	–
3	43/M	+	0	II	III	III	0	0	0	0	10	II	19	H (25 mm)	–	+	+	+	–	–
4	46/M	–	–	–	–	III	0	+	0	+	101	III	–	H (25 mm)	–	0	+	+	–	–
5	63/M	+	0	III	IV	IV	0	0	0	0	90	II	8	H (31 mm)	–	+	+	+	–	–
6	64/M	0	+	II	II	III	0	0	0	0	18	I	156	H (31 mm)	–	+	+	+	–	–
7	71/M	+	0	II	III	IV	0	–	+	0	30 days	Dead	204	H (31 mm)	–	+	+	+	–	–
8	51/M	0	+	I	IV	IV	0	–	0	+	72	I	3	–	SE (9A)	–	–	–	+	+
9	52/F	+	0	II	III	III	0	–	0	+	33	II	7	–	SE (9A)	–	–	–	+	+
10	54/F	0	+	I	III	IV	0	+	0	+	12	I	60	–	H (21 mm)	–	–	–	0	+
11	58/M	+	0	III	IV	IV	0	+	+	0	3 days	Dead	168	H (2[illegible] mm)	H (23 mm)	+	+	+	0	+

AV = aortic valve; F = female; H = Hancock; HCM = hypertrophic cardiomyopathy; IE = infective endocarditis; M = male; MV = mitral valve; NYHA = New York Heart Association; P = perforation or indentation (deficiency of leaflet tissue); Pt = patient; RCT = ruptured chordae tendineae; SE = Starr-Edwards; VR = valve replacement; 0 = absent or negative; + = present or positive; – = no information available or not applicable.

clinical episode of active infective endocarditis, the interval between active infective endocarditis and valve replacement ranged from 3 to 204 months (mean 54, median 17). This interval was <1 year in four patients. Patient 11 (Table 1) had two episodes of active infective endocarditis that occurred 168 and 27 months, respectively, before valve replacement (Fig. 7). Only the second episode caused clinical worsening of this patient's cardiac status. Patient 4 apparently never had a clinical illness diagnosed as active infective endocarditis, but examination of the operatively excised mitral valve disclosed a large deficit in the anterior mitral leaflet adjacent to several ruptured chordae tendineae, anatomic findings diagnostic of healed infective endocarditis (1). Of the 11 patients, 9 had active infective endocarditis before they were admitted to the National Institutes of Health; 1 had active infective endocarditis treated at another hospital, but hypertrophic cardiomyopathy had previously been diagnosed at the National Institutes of Health; and 1 patient had active infective endocarditis while hospitalized at the National Institutes of Health. Diagnosis of hypertrophic cardiomyopathy had been established previously in 7 of the 10 patients with a clinical illness diagnosed as active infective endocarditis; it was made in the other 3 patients after active infective endocarditis had healed. In five patients, a factor other than hypertrophic cardiomyopathy predisposing to infective endocarditis was apparent: dental procedures in Patients 4 and 5, cardiac catheterization in Patients 6 and 10 and opiate addiction in Patient 11.

During active infective endocarditis, information regarding the results of blood cultures were known in eight patients: in two, the blood cultures were negative and in six a bacterium was identified (alpha streptococcus in Patients 7, 10 and 11; group D streptococcus in two patients [nonenterococcal in Patient 2 and enterococcus in Patient 6]; and *Cardiobacterium hominis* in Patient 4). All 11 patients, however, had anatomic deficiencies of mitral or aortic valve cusps, and in those with infective endocarditis involving the mitral valve, there were associated ruptured chordae tendineae. The 10 patients with clear clinical evidence of active infective endocarditis received appropriate antibiotic treatment, and by the time of valve replacement, the infection had healed in all 10 patients. The M-mode echocardiogram immediately before valve replacement showed "echo densities" compatible with healed vegetations in four of seven patients in whom healed infective endocarditis involved the mitral valve and two of four in whom it involved the aortic valve.

Valvular regurgitation caused by infective endocarditis. Active infective endocarditis worsened the symptomatic status in nine patients by at least one New York Heart Association functional class. It also increased the intensity of the precordial systolic murmur (mitral regurgitation) in three of three patients in whom this information was known and caused the appearance of a basal diastolic murmur in all four patients with aortic regurgitation. Despite the appearance or worsening of valvular regurgitation, the left ventric-

Table 2. M-Mode Echocardiographic Data Before and After Operation in the 11 Patients With Infective Endocarditis Complicating Hypertrophic Cardiomyopathy and Requiring Valve Replacement

Pt No.	Interval Echo to VR (days)	Wall Thickness (mm)		Cavity (mm)			FS (%)	Echo Density		Flail		SAM
		VSd	LVd	LVd	LVs	LA		MV	AV	MV	AV	
1	9 (MVR)	20	13	41	18	45	56	+	0	+	0	+
	PO	16	10	37	18	35	51	–	0	–	0	–
2												
3	78 (MVR)	17	14	36	16	56	55	0	0	+	0	+
	PO	—	—	—	—	—	—	–	–	–	–	–
4	12 (MVR)	19	15	40	18	40	55	0	0	0	0	–
	PO	15	—*	—*	—*	57	—	–	0	–	0	–
5	65 (MVR)	32	14	46	28	55	19	±	0	0	0	+
	PO	14	—	—	—	57	—	–	0	–	0	–
6	16 (MVR)	26	13	56	38	68	32	+	0	0	0	+
	PO	—	—	—	—	—	—	–	–	–	–	–
7	33 (MVR)	—	—	—	—	72	—	0	0	±	0	–
	PO	—	—	—	—	63	—	–	0	–	0	–
8	8 (AVR)	20	13	40	22	43	45	0	+	0	–	0
	PO	10	10	—*	—*	40	—	0	–	0	–	0
9	37 (AVR)	26	14	44	22	49	50	0	+	0	+	0
	PO†		11	51	29	45	43	0	–	0	–	0
10	41 (AVR)	24	13	53	41	60	23	0	0	0	0	–
	PO	11	11	—*	—*	52	—	0	–	0	–	0
11	16 (MVR, AVR)	—	—	—	—	54	—	0	0	0	0	0
	PO	—	—	—	—	—	—	–	–	–	–	–

*Paradoxical movement; †ventricular septal defect created at operation. AV = aortic valve; AVR = aortic valve replacement; d = end-diastole; Echo = echocardiography; FS = fractional shortening; LA = left atrium; LV = left ventricle; MV = mitral valve; MVR = mitral valve replacement; PO = after operation; s = peak systole; SAM = systolic anterior motion of the anterior mitral leaflet; VS = ventricular septum – = not applicable; other abbreviations as in Table 1.

Table 3. Hemodynamic and Angiographic Data Immediately Before and ≥6 Months After Valve Replacement in 11 Patients With Infective Endocarditis Complicating Hypertrophic Cardiomyopathy

Pt No.	Time of Cath (mo PO)	PA* (s/d)	RV* (s/d)	RA* (m)	Mean PAW*	LA*		LV* (s/d)	SA* (s/d)	LV-SA psg*	MR by LV Cine (0–4+)	AR by AA Cine (0–4+)	CAD by Cine	CI
						a	v							
1	Pre-VR	66/40	65/16	7	25	36	38	180/25	118/60	62	4+	—	—	3.8
	PO (6)	32/14	32/4	4	9	16	0	130/12	125/65	5	—	—	—	2.2
2	Pre-VR	80/40	80/18	18	45	AF	50	138/24	138/60	0	4+	1+	—	2.1
3	Pre-VR	88/40	88/14	11	32	32	44	140/30	114/65	26	4+	0	0	1.8
	PO (6)	44/20	44/6	4	14	16	12	150/14	158/88	0	0	0	—	3.3
4	Pre-VR	90/40	90/10	8	30	27	40	165/32	120/70	45	3+	—	0	2.0
5	Pre-VR†	50/25	50/10	5	15	—	—	245/40	160/90	85	3+	—	—	3.7
	PO (10)‡	—	120/30	19	35	23	55	130/24	130/65	0	2+	0	—	2.0
	PO (21)	60/25	60/9	17	24	—	32	—	—	—	—	—	—	2.5
6	Pre-VR	45/23	45/8	4	20	28	36	110/10	105/70	5	3+	—	—	2.5
	PO (6)	—	24/5	3	—	—	—	105/6	105/60	0	0	—	—	2.3
7	Pre-VR	50/25	50/5	6	31	AF	50	120/20	130/75	0	4+	—	§	1.5
8	Pre-VR	85/35	85/12	—	38	AF	55	120/14	120/60	0	4+	—	—	—
9	Pre-VR	50/25	50/15	6	27	40	45	164/34	86/40	78	1+	3+	0	—
	PO (12)	24/11	24/7	4	6	13	8	115/16	110/65	5	—	—	—	2.0
10	Pre-VR	60/30	65/15	9	20	10	22	200/28	130/68	70	1+	2+	0	3.1
	PO (8)	—	—	—	16	20	28	165/20	105/55	0	—	—	—	4.4
	PO (58)	30/12	30/5	6	12	—	—	—	120/70	—	—	—	—	—
11	Pre-VR	55/30	55/6	5	17	25	20	240/30	100/30	140	3+	3+	0	1.7
	PO (76)	75/35	75/36	15	31	28	44	150/24	145/85	5	3+	1+	0	2.1

*Pressures in mm Hg. †Cardiac catheterization (Cath) 36 months before valve replacement. ‡peribasilar bioprosthetic communication found by left ventricular cineangiography (Cine) and it was operatively closed after this cardiac catheterization procedure. §This patient was the only one with significant coronary narrowing and he had aortocoronary bypass grafting in addition to valve replacement (VR). a = a wave; AA = ascending aorta; AF = atrial fibrillation; AR = aortic regurgitation; CAD = coronary artery narrowing >50% in diameter of >1 major artery; CI = cardiac index in liters/min per m^2; LA = left atrium; LV = left ventricle: MR = mitral regurgitation; PA = pulmonary artery; PAW = pulmonary artery wedge; PO = after operation (months); Pre = before; psg = peak systolic gradient; Pt = patient; RA = right atrium; RV = right ventricle; SA = systemic artery; s/d = peak systole/end-diastole; v = v wave.

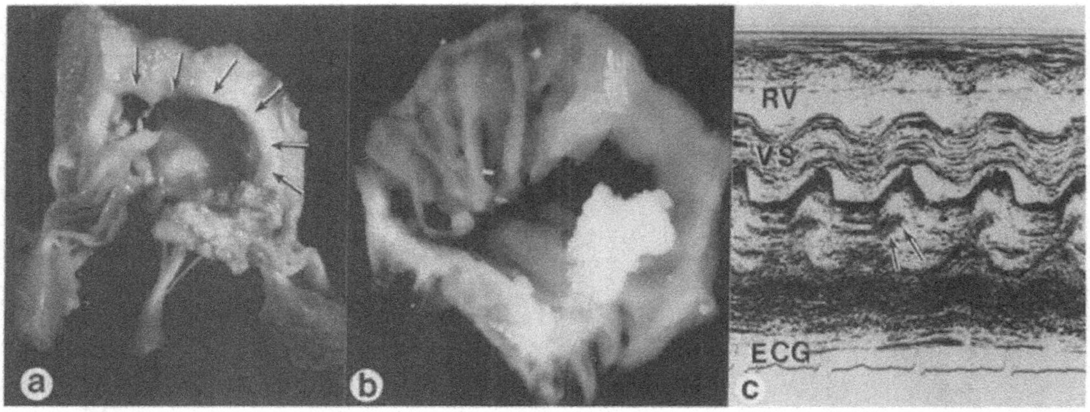

Figure 1 (above). Patient 1. Operatively excised mitral valve. **a,** Leaflets, chordae tendineae and attached papillary muscles showing loss of tissue in the posterior leaflet and absence of chordae tendineae (**arrows**). A large deposit of calcium is present and is better seen in **b,** a radiograph of the excised valve. **c,** M-mode echocardiogram taken shortly before mitral valve replacement, showing thickening and impaired mobility of the anterior mitral leaflet and fluttering (**arrows**) of the posterior leaflet. ECG = electrocardiogram; RV = right ventricular cavity; VS = ventricular septum.

Figure 2 (below). Patient 2. Operatively excised mitral valve (**a, b,** and **c**) and M-mode echocardiogram (**d**). **a,** Radiograph of the opened valve. The **arrows** point to a calcific deposit. **b** and **c,** Close-up views of the atrial aspect of a portion of both leaflets. The anterior leaflet contains two perforations (**solid arrows**) and the posterior leaflet one perforation (**dashed arrow**). **d,** Typical echocardiogram in hypertrophic cardiomyopathy with asymmetric thickening of the anterior ventricular septum (VS). The **arrows** point to dense echoes of the thickened anterior mitral leaflet, which contacts the ventricular septum in diastole. Mild mitral systolic anterior motion is present (*). PW = posterior wall; RV = right ventricular cavity.

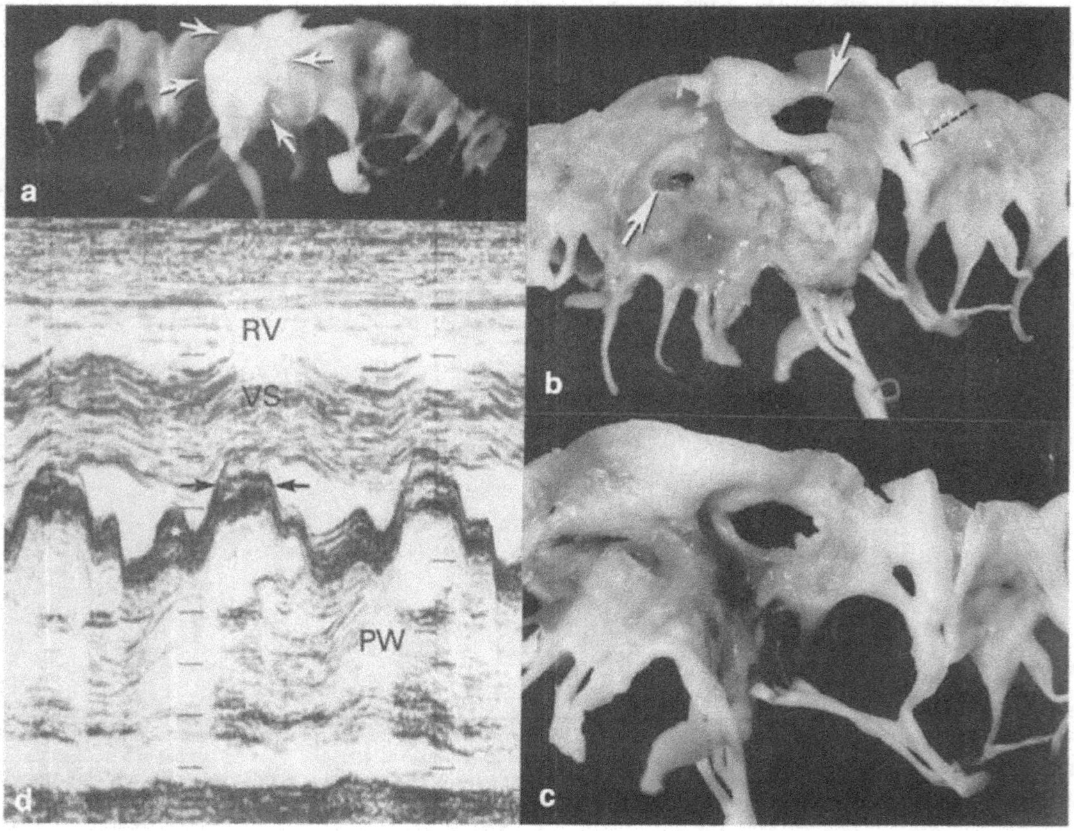

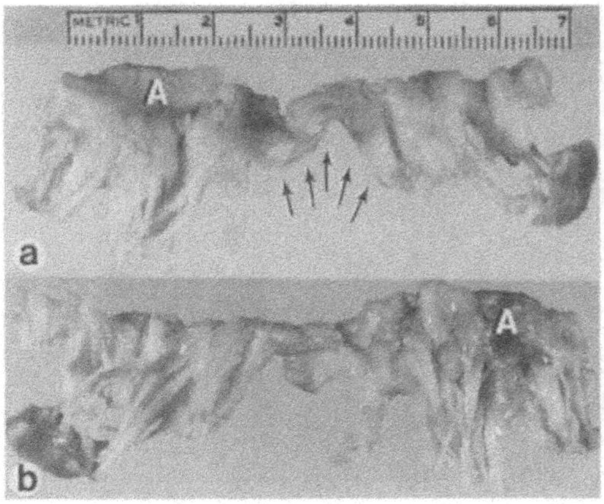

Figure 3. Patient 3. Opened mitral valve. **a,** Atrial surface. **b,** Ventricular surface. The arrows designate the area where chordae tendineae are missing (ruptured) and a site where a portion of the leaflet is absent (destroyed by the previous infection). A = anterior mitral leaflet.

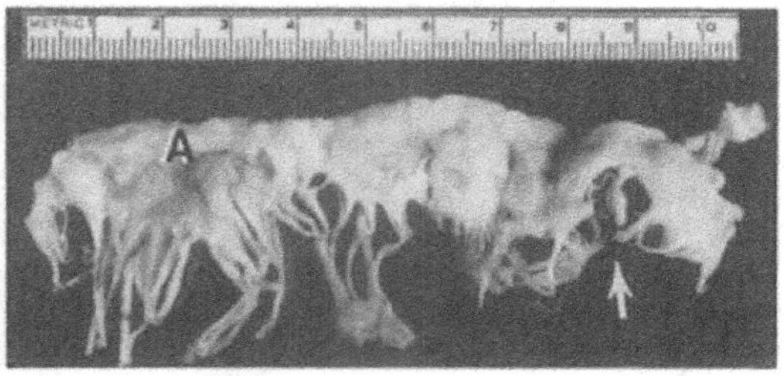

Figure 5. Patient 6. Opened mitral valve from its atrial aspect, showing a large indentation (arrow) in the posterior leaflet. Both anterior (A) and posterior leaflets are thickened by fibrous tissue. The indentation represents a site of previous vegetation.

Figure 4. Patient 5. Opened mitral valve from its atrial aspect, showing a large perforation (arrow) in the anterior leaflet (A) with adjacent focal calcific deposits. The perforation represents a site where vegetation had been present.

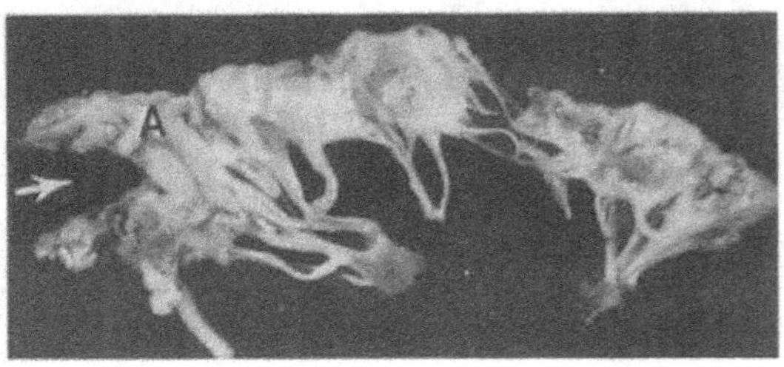

ular cavity was of normal size on the echocardiogram immediately before valve replacement in nine of nine patients; left ventricular angiograms in the other two patients disclosed mild left ventricular cavity dilation in one of them. The degree of valvular regurgitation immediately before valve replacement in each of the 11 patients was severe: in the 7 patients with isolated mitral valve replacement, the degree of mitral regurgitation by left ventricular angiography was either 3+/4+ or 4+/4+, in the 3 patients with isolated aortic valve replacement, the degree of aortic regurgitation by aortic root angiography was 3+/4+ in 2 and 2+/4+ in 1; in the single patient with replacement of both left-sided cardiac valves, the degree of mitral regurgitation was 4+/4+ and aortic regurgitation, 1+/4+.

Effect of infective endocarditis on the left ventricular outflow pressure gradient. Active infective endocarditis involving the mitral valve was associated with a decrease in the peak systolic pressure gradient between the left ventricle and a systemic artery. In the three patients who had cardiac catheterization before and after active infective endocarditis, the peak systolic pressure gradient decreased from 90 to 62 mm Hg in Patient 1, from 100 to 5 mm Hg in Patient 4 and from 76 to 55 mm Hg in Patient 6.

Results of cardiac valve replacements. Valve replacement was successful in nine patients. The other two patients (Patients 7 and 11), each of whom died within 30 days of valve replacement, were the only patients who had had partial septectomy and septotomy before cardiac valve replacement. Of the nine hospital survivors after valve replacement (combined with partial septotomy and septectomy in four), eight were in functional class I or II and one was in class III when seen 6 to 21 months after valve replacement, whereas preoperatively three had been in functional class III and five in functional class IV. Cardiac catheterization was performed 6 to 21 months (mean 14) after valve replacement in seven of the nine long-term survivors (Table 3). In three of the seven patients, no left ventricular outflow tract obstruction was present preoperatively and the postoperative study disclosed no pressure gradient between the left ventricle and a systemic artery during peak systole. In the other four patients, the peak systolic pressure gradient before valve replacement (combined with partial septotomy and septectomy in three patients) decreased from an average of 74 mm Hg (range 62 to 85) preoperatively to ≤5 mm Hg postoperatively.

Discussion

Major findings of present study. Although 30 reports describing one or more patients (19 were single case studies) with hypertrophic cardiomyopathy and infective endocarditis have appeared (cases tabulated by Alessandri et al. [2]), the presence of infective endocarditis was confirmed anatomically (2–11) only in 15 of the reported 56 cases and in none was the type of valvular damage illustrated. The present study analyzed 11 patients from the same center with

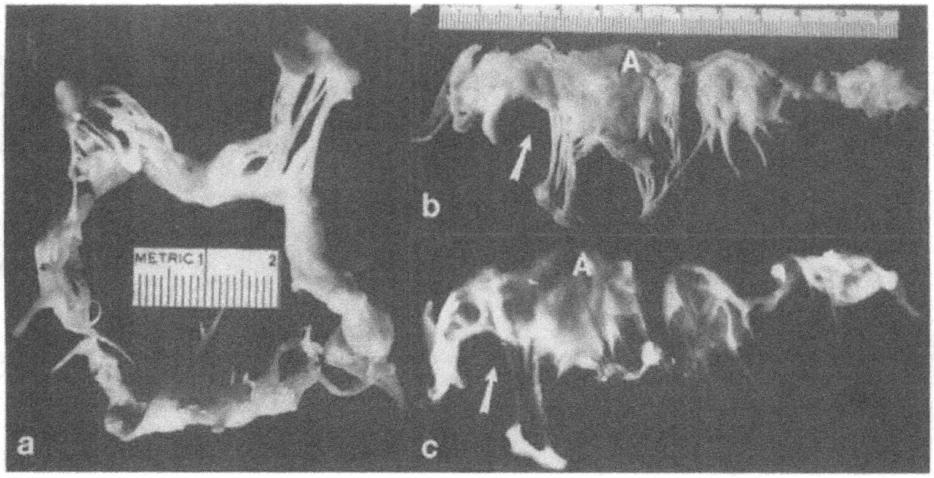

Figure 6. Patient 7. **a,** Unopened mitral valve. **b,** Opened mitral valve showing its atrial aspect. The arrow points to an indentation at the junction of the anterior (A) and posterior leaflets. Several chordae tendineae are missing (ruptured) at this site. **c,** Radiograph of the opened mitral valve. Several calcific deposits are present in the annular region of the posterior leaflet.

hypertrophic cardiomyopathy complicated by infective endocarditis necessitating replacement of one or more cardiac valves in each, and in each the operatively excised valve was studied. It is apparent that infective endocarditis should be recognized as a complication of hypertrophic cardiomyopathy and that the latter predisposes to infective endocarditis. The frequency with which the complication occurs is unclear. The present study suggests that among patients with hypertrophic cardiomyopathy with mitral or aortic valve regurgitation, or both, severe enough to warrant valve replacement, infective endocarditis often is responsible for the severe regurgitation. Of the 87 patients with hypertrophic cardiomyopathy who underwent valve replacement at our institution, 11 underwent this procedure because of damage by infective endocarditis. None of the other operatively excised valves had cusp perforations or tears or ruptured chordae tendineae and therefore it is unlikely that any of these other patients had had infective endocarditis at any time.

Location of the vegetations in infective endocarditis complicating hypertrophic cardiomyopathy. The most frequent site of vegetations in patients with hypertrophic cardiomyopathy is the mitral valve and specifically its anterior leaflet. It is this leaflet, of course, which tends to contact the mural endocardium of the ventricular septum during one or both phases of the cardiac cycle and it is likely that vegetations form at these contact sites. Of our 11 patients, 8 had vegetations that left telltale residua of infective endocarditis on the mitral valve (1 also had damage to the aortic valve, but the damage was not diagnostic of healed infective endocarditis [1]) and 3 had both clinical and anatomic evidence of damage to one or more aortic valve cusps by infective endocarditis. The vegetations on the anterior mitral leaflet appear to have been on their ventricular aspects, unlike those in most patients with active infective endocarditis involving the mitral valve. The mechanism of formation of aortic valve vegetations in patients with hypertrophic cardiomyopathy is unclear. In three of our four patients having aortic valve replacement, the left ventricular aortic

Figure 7. Patient 8. Three-cusped aortic valve with severe destruction of one of the three cusps by the infective process.

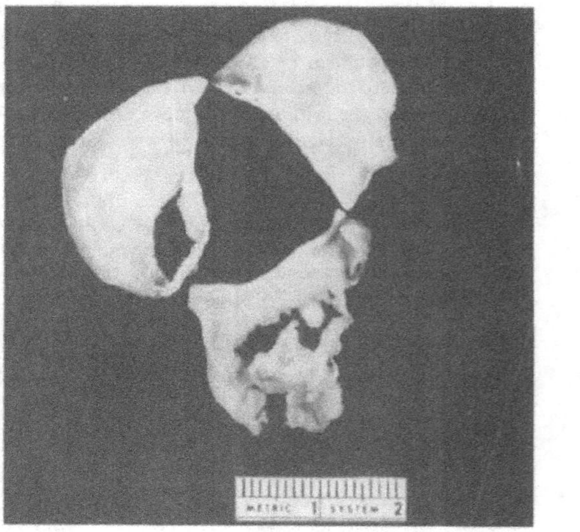

peak systolic pressure gradient was high (70, 78 and 140 mm Hg, respectively), whereas only one of the seven patients with isolated mitral valve replacement had a left ventricular outflow pressure gradient of this magnitude. The vegetations on the aortic valve appear to have been located on the ventricular aspects of these cusps, the usual location of vegetations on this valve.

Valvular regurgitation after infective endocarditis in hypertrophic cardiomyopathy. The present study shows that infective endocarditis complicating hypertrophic cardiomyopathy can result in serious consequences. In all 11 patients, the symptomatic status was unequivocally worsened by active infective endocarditis that healed. Additionally, the intensity of the precordial systolic murmur increased in the patients with infective endocarditis involving the mitral valve, and infective endocarditis involving the aortic valve caused the appearance of a murmur of aortic regurgitation, which was confirmed in each by angiography. The degree of valvular regurgitation was severe in all 11 patients; however, despite the severe degree of regurgitation, the left ventricular cavity immediately before valve replacement was not dilated in any patient on M-mode echocardiography and was only mildly dilated in one of two patients studied by angiography.

Benefit of valve replacement. Despite recognized potential complications of mitral valve replacement in patients with hypertrophic cardiomyopathy (12), the present study indicates that valve replacement for infective endocarditis complicating hypertrophic cardiomyopathy may result in a striking diminution or disappearance of previous symptoms of cardiac dysfunction.

References

1. Roberts WC, Buchbinder NA. Healed left-sided infective endocarditis: a clinicopathologic study of 59 patients. Am J Cardiol 1977;40:876–88.
2. Alessandri N, Pannarale G, del Monte F, Moretti F, Marino B, Reale A. Hypertrophic obstructive cardiomyopathy and infective endocarditis: a report of seven cases and a review of the literature. Eur Heart J 1990;11:1041–8.
3. Nagle JP. Idiopathic hypertrophic subaortic stenosis and bacterial endocarditis. JAMA 1967;200:643–5.
4. Vecht RJ, Oakley CM. Infective endocarditis in three patients with hypertrophic obstructive cardiomyopathy. Br Med J 1968;2:455–9.
5. Caramanian M, Joly F, Fouchard J, Guerinon J. Endocardite infectieuse sur stenose musculaire hypertrophique du ventricule gauche. Arch Mal Coeur 1971;64:1117–31.
6. Chretien EH, Limas C, Garagusi VF. Association of bacterial endocarditis in idiopathic hypertrophic subaortic stenosis. South Med J 1973;66:269–72.
7. Wang K, Gobel FL, Gleason DF. Bacterial endocarditis in idiopathic hypertrophic subaortic stenosis. Am Heart J 1975;89:359–65.
8. Heret JF, Jandin M, Rigaud M, et al. Endocardite a staphyloccque dore au cours d'une cardiomyopathie obstructive. Arch Mal Coeur 1977;70:1227–32.
9. Greenland P, Murphy GW. Acute valvular insufficiency complicating hypertrophic obstructive cardiomyopathy. Chest 1979;75:182–3.
10. LeJemtel TH, Factor SM, Koenigsberg M, O'Reilly M, Frater R, Sonnenblick EH. Mural vegetations at the site of endocardial trauma in infective endocarditis complicating idiopathic hypertrophic subaortic stenosis. Am J Cardiol 1979;44:569–74.
11. Pueyo JM, Shahin A, Benazet JM, Camaeno AM, San Miguel JG. Endocarditis infecciosa en estenosis subaortica hipertrofica idiopatica: a proposito de una observacion. Med Clin Barcelona 1981;76:129–31.
12. Roberts WC. Operative treatment of hypertrophic obstructive cardiomyopathy: the case against mitral valve replacement. Am J Cardiol 1973;32:377–81.

Diversity of Structural Mitral Valve Alterations in Hypertrophic Cardiomyopathy

Heinrich G. Klues, MD; Barry J. Maron, MD;
Allen L. Dollar, MD; and William C. Roberts, MD

Background. **Hypertrophic cardiomyopathy (HCM) is characterized by an asymmetrically hypertrophied left ventricle and is regarded as a disease of cardiac muscle.**

Methods and Results. **To assess the possibility that the mitral valve itself may be involved in the disease process, we studied mitral valves from 94 patients with HCM and 45 normal control subjects. The area of the mitral leaflets was increased in patients with HCM compared with control subjects (12.9±3.7 versus 8.7±2.0 cm²; $p<0.001$). For the overall group of patients, this increase was largely caused by an increase in anterior leaflet length (2.2±0.5 cm for HCM versus 1.8±0.3 cm for control subjects; $p<0.001$), because circumference did not differ between the two groups. Mitral leaflet area was increased (≥12.0 cm²) in 55 (58%) of the 94 valves. In 12 of these 55 valves, both the anterior and posterior leaflets were enlarged; the other 43 valves had asymmetrical or segmental enlargement of either the anterior leaflet (36 patients) or a portion of posterior leaflet (seven patients). In addition, nine patients had a congenital malformation of the mitral apparatus in which one or both papillary muscles inserted directly into anterior mitral leaflet (mitral valve area was normal in seven of the nine).**

Conclusions. **Sixty-two (66%) of 94 mitral valves had a constellation of structural malformations, including increased leaflet area and elongation of the leaflets or anomalous papillary muscle insertion directly into anterior mitral leaflet. These findings expand the morphological definition of HCM by demonstrating that the disease process is not confined to cardiac muscle but rather many patients also have structural abnormalities of the mitral valve that are unlikely to be acquired or secondary to mechanical factors. (*Circulation* 1992;85:1651–1660)**

KEY WORDS • hypertrophy • cardiomyopathies • valves • genetics • left ventricle

Hypertrophic cardiomyopathy (HCM) is considered to be a primary disease of cardiac muscle characterized by a diverse morphological and clinical spectrum.[1–7] It is generally accepted as a basic tenet of HCM that left ventricular hypertrophy represents both the gross anatomic marker and is probably the principal determinant of the clinical and pathophysiological features of the disease.[2–8] Most morphological reports of HCM have described the mitral valve as being intrinsically normal, with only focal secondary thickening of the leaflets and chordae tendineae.[1,2,6,9,10] Anecdotal descriptions, however, have suggested that the mitral valve may be congenitally abnormal in some patients with HCM.[11–16] To resolve this issue, we systematically examined mitral valves in a large number of patients with HCM.

Methods

Selection of Case Material

Patients with HCM. The files of the Pathology Branch from 1982 to 1989 were reviewed. Eighty-two mitral valves previously excised surgically from patients with HCM had been accessioned; 66 had been removed intact and were in suitable condition for study. Of the 66 valves, one had morphological features of mitral prolapse[17–21] and was excluded, reducing the number of operative specimens to 65. These valves had been surgically excised from severely symptomatic patients with HCM undergoing mitral valve replacement to relieve obstruction to left ventricular outflow[15,22–24]; each operation had been performed by the same surgeon (Dr. Charles L. McIntosh). Each mitral valve specimen consisted of both leaflets, the attached chordae tendineae, and in some instances portions of the papillary muscles. To include mitral valves from patients with nonobstructive HCM, as well as patients with obstruction who had not undergone mitral valve replacement, 29 heart specimens with HCM also were selected from the files of the Pathology Branch by virtue of suitable condition for study and a recent complete hemodynamic or echocardiographic evaluation. Of these 29 patients, seven died after ventricular septal myotomy/myectomy (four within 30 days of operation and three later). None of the other 22 had a cardiac operation; 11 died suddenly, seven of progressive congestive heart failure and four of noncardiac causes. Mitral valves were excised from these 29 hearts (as well as 45 controls), with care taken to remove the leaflets from their circumferential attachments along the annular margin, leaving a 2–3-mm border as done by the

From the Pathology and Cardiology Branches, National Heart, Lung, and Blood Institute, National Institutes of Health, Bethesda, Md.

Address for correspondence: Barry J. Maron, MD, Cardiology Branch, National Institutes of Health, Building 10, Room 7B-15, Bethesda, MD 20892.

Received May 13, 1991; revision accepted January 7, 1992.

surgeon in excising the valves at operation. Thus, the 65 mitral valves removed at surgery and the 29 removed after death constitute the overall study group of 94 valves.

In each study patient, diagnosis of HCM was based on the presence of a hypertrophied nondilated left ventricle in the absence of another cardiac or systemic disease capable of producing the magnitude of hypertrophy present in that patient[8]; in addition, each patient had typical necropsy and/or clinical features of HCM.[2–8] The magnitude of the left ventricular outflow gradient was assessed at cardiac catheterization in 89 of 94 patients, including all 65 with mitral valve replacement. In the other five patients, basal left ventricular outflow gradients were estimated by Doppler echocardiography.[25,26] Of these five patients, four had no evidence of basal outflow obstruction; each was also judged to be free of significant provocable obstruction on the basis of the absence of ventricular septal endocardial plaque and the presence of nonthickened mitral leaflets at necropsy.[2,4,6]

Patients were classified as obstructive if the subaortic peak systolic pressure gradient was >30 mm Hg under basal conditions and/or with provocative maneuvers or as nonobstructive if the subaortic gradient was absent under basal conditions and <30 mm Hg with provocation (Table 1).

Control patients. Mitral valves from 45 consecutively studied patients with entirely normal hearts, both functionally and anatomically, were chosen as control subjects (Table 1). All 45 patients died from noncardiac conditions. In each control patient, heart weight was ≤350 g in men and ≤300 g in women. The 45 patients ranged in age from 15 to 74 years (mean, 45); 24 were men, and 21 were women.

Morphometry

Mitral valves were fixed in 10% buffered formalin after their removal at operation. Valves were introduced to the fixative freely without stretching or manipulation. Tissue specimens were placed in an opened position on a cutting board and extended to full length (i.e., circumference) with the atrial aspect exposed. Usually it was necessary to affix the opened valve directly to the board with pins to flatten the specimen.

The following morphological measurements (Figure 1)[27] were made directly from the mitral valve specimen: 1) circumference of the valve annulus measured along its margin of attachment; 2) and 3) maximum lengths of anterior and posterior leaflets (from attachment margin to free edge); 4) thickness of the anterior leaflet; 5) weight of the excised valve; and 6) areas of the leaflets, both together and separately. To assess mitral leaflet area (in square centimeters), borders of the opened valves were traced with a fine-tipped pen on an acetate overlay. The areas of the leaflets were then planimeterized. Maximal thickness of anterior leaflet was measured with an adjustable caliper. Mitral valves were weighed on a scale accurate to 0.1 g.

Reproducibility

Interobserver and intraobserver variability for measurement of mitral leaflet area was tested in a subset of 20 valves (14 with HCM and six normal control subjects). To determine interobserver variability, two observers (H.G.K. and A.L.D.) independently measured the mitral valves. To determine intraobserver variability, one observer (H.G.K.) measured mitral leaflet area on two occasions 4 months apart.

Histology

Twenty-two mitral valves from patients with HCM (10 obstructive and 12 nonobstructive) and 12 from normal control subjects were studied by light microscopy. Longitudinal sections were taken in the midportion of the anterior leaflet as well as in the most elongated portion of the posterior leaflet in 22 valves. Tissue was embedded in paraffin and sectioned at 6 μm. Two histology sections were prepared: one was stained by the Movat method and one with hematoxylin and eosin. The extent of mucopolysaccharide deposition was assessed in qualitative terms from the histological sections.

Statistical Analyses

Data were expressed as mean±SD. Differences in morphological measurements between groups of patients were assessed by unpaired Student's t test. Proportions were compared by the χ^2 test, and other selected comparisons were assessed with one-way ANOVA. Relations between selected parameters or variables were assessed by linear regression analysis. A stepwise regression analysis[28] was used to determine the association between mitral leaflet area and several clinical and morphological variables in patients with HCM and in normal controls (i.e., age, sex, body height and weight, heart weight, previous ventricular septal myotomy/myectomy, left ventricular wall thickness and end-diastolic cavity dimension, magnitude of mitral regurgitation, left ventricular systolic pressure, and outflow gradient).

Results

Group Analysis of Mitral Valve Morphology

Mitral leaflet area. In the 94 patients with HCM, the mitral leaflet area ranged from 6.3 to 23.0 cm^2 (mean, 12.9±3.7 cm^2) and significantly exceeded that of normal control subjects (4.7–13.0 cm^2; mean, 8.7±2.0 cm^2; $p<0.001$) (Figures 2 and 3; Table 1). In 44 (47%) of the 94 valves, total leaflet area exceeded that of the largest control valve. Mitral leaflet area was significantly smaller in valves removed from patients at surgery (12.0±3.5 cm^2) than in those obtained at necropsy (14.6±3.3 cm^2; $p<0.001$) (Tables 2 and 3).

Valve length. In patients with HCM, the lengths of the anterior and posterior leaflets were 1.0–3.4 cm (mean, 2.2±0.5 cm) and 0.7–2.4 cm (mean, 1.4±0.4 cm), respectively, and both significantly exceeded values for normal controls (Figure 4; Table 1).

Valve circumference. Mitral valve circumference was similar in the overall group of 94 patients with HCM (5.5–12.8 cm; mean, 8.5±1.7 cm) and in normal controls (6.4–9.5 cm; mean, 8.2±2.8 cm; $p>0.05$) (Figure 5; Table 1).

Mitral valve weight and thickness. Mitral valves from patients with HCM were thicker and heavier than those from controls (by about 2:1) (Table 1).

Table 1. Clinical, Hemodynamic, and Morphometric Data in Patients With HCM and in Normal Controls

	All HCM patients	Control subjects	*p*	Obstructive group	Nonobstructive group	*p*
Patients (*n*)	94	45	. . .	77 (82%)	17 (18%)	. . .
Surgically excised valves	65	0	. . .	65	0	. . .
Age (mean±SD years) (range)	43±15 (15–77)	45±17 (15–74)	NS	45±15 (15–77)	34±12 (18–54)	NS
Male:female, *n* (%)	48 (51%): 46 (49%)	24 (53%): 21 (47%)	NS	41 (53%): 36 (47%)	7 (41%): 10 (59%)	NS
Systemic hypertension	6 (6%)	0	NS	5 (6%)	1 (6%)	NS
One or more major coronary arteries narrowed >50% (angiography), *n* (%)	13 (14%)	0	<0.01	12 (16%)	1 (6%)	<0.01
LV-SA gradient (mm Hg)*						
Basal	52±47	. . .	. . .	69±43	0	<0.001
Provoked	85±55	. . .	. . .	110±36	5±8	<0.001
Operation						
MVR	52 (55%)	0	. . .	52 (68%)	0	. . .
M&M	7 (7%)†	0	. . .	7 (9%)†	0	. . .
M&M plus MVR	13 (10%)†	0	. . .	13 (17%)†	0	. . .
New York Heart Association functional class:						
I	7 (7%)	45	<0.001	1 (1%)	6 (35%)	<0.001
II	8 (9%)	0		6 (8%)	2 (12%)	
III	70 (74%)	0		61 (79%)	9 (53%)	
IV	9 (10%)	0		9 (12%)	0	
Echo measurements (mm)						
Septal thickness	21±6	. . .	. . .	20±5	24±8	<0.05
Free wall thickness	14±4	. . .	. . .	13±4	16±5	<0.05
Mitral valve measurements						
Areas (cm^2)						
Anterior leaflet	5.9±1.7	4.3±1.0	<0.001	5.7±1.7	6.7±1.4	<0.05
Posterior leaflet	2.6±1.1	1.7±0.5	<0.001	2.5±1.1	2.9±1.0	NS
Total leaflet	12.9±3.7	8.7±2.0	<0.001	12.4±3.7	14.4±3.2	<0.05
Circumference (cm)	8.5±1.7	8.2±2.8	NS	8.2±1.6	9.8±1.5	<0.001
Lengths (cm)						
Anterior leaflet	2.2±0.5	1.8±0.3	<0.001	2.1±0.5	2.4±0.3	<0.01
Posterior leaflet	1.4±0.4	1.1±0.2	<0.001	1.4±0.4	1.6±0.4	<0.05
Weight (g)	2.0±0.7	1.0±0.3	<0.001	2.1±0.7	1.3±0.6	<0.001
Thickness, anterior leaflet (mm)	2.1±0.9	1.1±0.4	<0.001	2.4±0.8	1.0±0.4	<0.001
Valves with increased area (>12.0 cm^2), *n* (%)	55 (59%)	1 (2%)	<0.001	40 (52%)	15 (88%)	<0.01
Valves with papillary muscle insertion, *n* (%)	9 (10%)	1 (2%)	<0.01	9 (12%)	0	NS
Heart weight (g)‡	597±164	271±45	<0.001	673±127	543±167	<0.05

HCM, hypertrophic cardiomyopathy; LV-SA, left ventricle to systemic artery; MVR, mitral valve replacement; M&M, ventricular septal myotomy/myectomy.

*Determined by cardiac catheterization in 89 patients (95%) and by Doppler echocardiography in five patients (5%).

†Twenty patients with a previous ventricular septal myotomy/myectomy showed no difference in anterior, posterior, and total mitral leaflet area, circumference, lengths of anterior and posterior leaflets, valve weight, and thickness of anterior leaflet compared with the remaining 57 obstructed patients without myotomy/myectomy.

‡Heart weight available only in the 29 necropsy patients.

. . . , Not applicable or complete data not available.

Individual Patient Analysis of Mitral Valve Morphology

Mitral valve size. Mitral leaflet area exceeded the 95th percentile of the normal control valves (≥12.0 cm^2) in 55 (59%) of 94 patients and was <12.0 cm^2 in the other 39 (41%). Consequently, the 55 mitral valves ≥12.0 cm^2 were considered to be increased in size, while the other valves were judged to be of normal size. Also, mitral leaflet area exceeded the greatest value in the control group (i.e., 13.0 cm^2) in 44 (47%) of 94 patients (Figure 3). In 36 of the 55 enlarged valves, only the anterior leaflet was increased in size (area>5.0 cm^2; normal <4.6

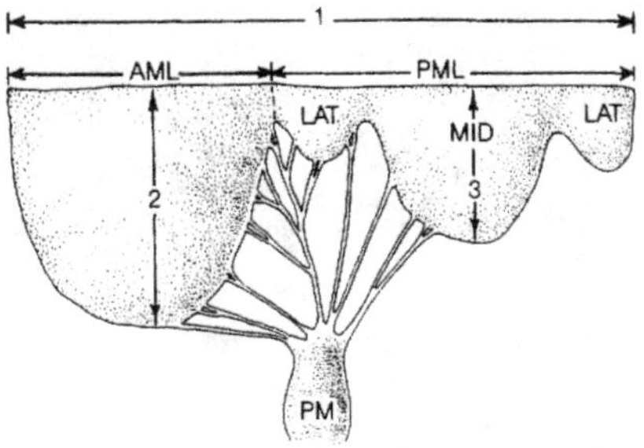

FIGURE 1. *Schematic of an opened normal mitral valve showing anterior (AML) and posterior (PML) mitral valve leaflets. Posterior leaflet is composed of two lateral (LAT) scallops and a middle (MID) scallop. 1, Total circumference of valve along annular margin; 2 and 3, lengths of anterior and posterior leaflets. Anatomic demarcation of anterior mitral leaflet from posterior leaflet was made visually, usually by identification of insertion of a fanlike arrangement of commissural chordae between the two.*[27] *PM, papillary muscle.*

cm^2); in seven other valves, only the posterior leaflet was increased in size (area >2.5 cm^2; normal <1.9 cm^2), often caused by segmental elongation of one scallop of the leaflet (length 85–113% of anterior leaflet length); in the remaining 12 valves both mitral leaflets were enlarged.

Mitral valves were without the morphological features of mitral valve prolapse,[17–21] such as ballooning and redundancy of the leaflets, increased annular circumference, and apparent elongation of the chordae tendineae. Analysis of Movat-stained histological sections showed that none of the patients with HCM studied had increased amounts of mucopolysaccharide compared with normal control subjects.

Anomalous papillary muscle insertion. In nine of the 94 patients with HCM (each with basal outflow obstruction), the head of one or both papillary muscles inserted directly into the ventricular aspect of anterior mitral leaflet, involving the anterolateral or posteromedial commissural region but also extending to adjacent portions of the leaflets (Figure 6).[29] Chordae tendineae were absent in the region of anomalous papillary muscle insertion but appeared normal in other areas. Mitral leaflet size was normal (<12.0 cm^2) in seven and mildly increased in two (12.2 and 13.0 cm^2).

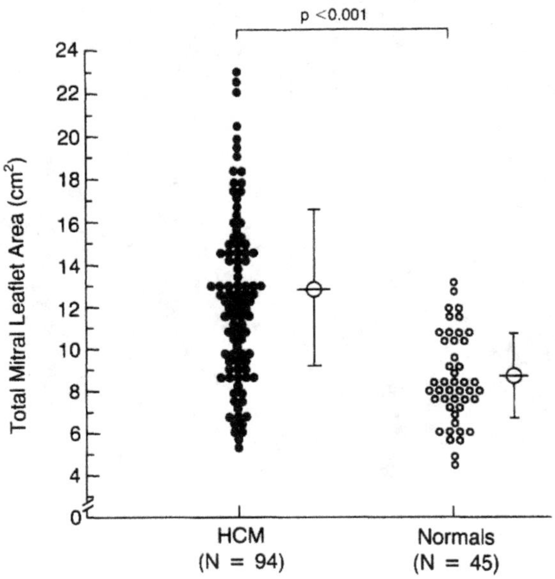

FIGURE 2. *Scatterplot of total area of mitral valve leaflets in patients with hypertrophic cardiomyopathy (HCM) and normal controls.*

Reproducibility

Analysis of interobserver variability showed small differences in mitral leaflet area between the two observers (0.56±1.4 cm^2). Linear regression analysis relating the two measurements showed a correlation coefficient of 0.91. Analysis of intraobserver variability also showed small differences in mitral leaflet area between the two observations (0.25±0.9 cm^2); linear regression analysis showed a correlation coefficient of 0.97.

Other Valvular Abnormalities

Scallops. Of the 94 mitral valves, 34 (36%) had an increased number of posterior leaflet scallops (either four or five) that were of similar size; the circumference and mitral valve area of these 34 valves (8.9±1.6 cm and 12.9±3.4 cm^2, respectively) did not differ significantly from those of the other 60 valves (8.4±1.6 cm and 12.3±3.2 cm^2, respectively). In contrast, only two of the 45 control valves (4%) had more than three posterior leaflet scallops ($p<0.001$).

Fibrous thickening. Of the 94 patients, 38 had no or only focal thickening of the anterior mitral leaflet (usually at the free leaflet edge) that occupied <50% of total leaflet area. In the other 56 valves, the fibrous thickening was more diffuse, often involved most of the leaflet, and was judged to be of secondary origin.[2,6,9]

Markedly different patterns of fibrous thickening were observed in obstructive and nonobstructive patients. The 17 nonobstructive patients had either no or only mild focal thickening; each of the 77 patients with obstruction had mild or diffuse thickening ($p<0.001$). In the subgroup of 38 study patients with no or mild focal anterior leaflet thickening, mitral leaflet area (13.9±3.7 cm^2) exceeded that of normal control subjects (8.7±2.0 cm^2; $p<0.001$) (Table 4).

Comparison of Obstructive and Nonobstructive Patients

When the 17 patients without outflow obstruction were compared with the combined obstructive group of 77 patients (12 necropsy and 65 surgical), nonobstructive patients proved to have larger leaflet area, circumference, and length (Table 1).

Relation of Mitral Valve Size to Clinical and Morphological Features

The relation of mitral valve area to clinical and pathological variables was analyzed by stepwise regression analysis separately for patients with mitral valve replacement and those studied at necropsy. In patients with mitral valve replacement, leaflet area was inversely related to female sex and directly related to body height ($p=0.041$ and $p=0.014$, respectively; multiple $r^2=0.24$); in necropsy patients, leaflet area was inversely related only to female sex ($p<0.001$). In both analyses, the body

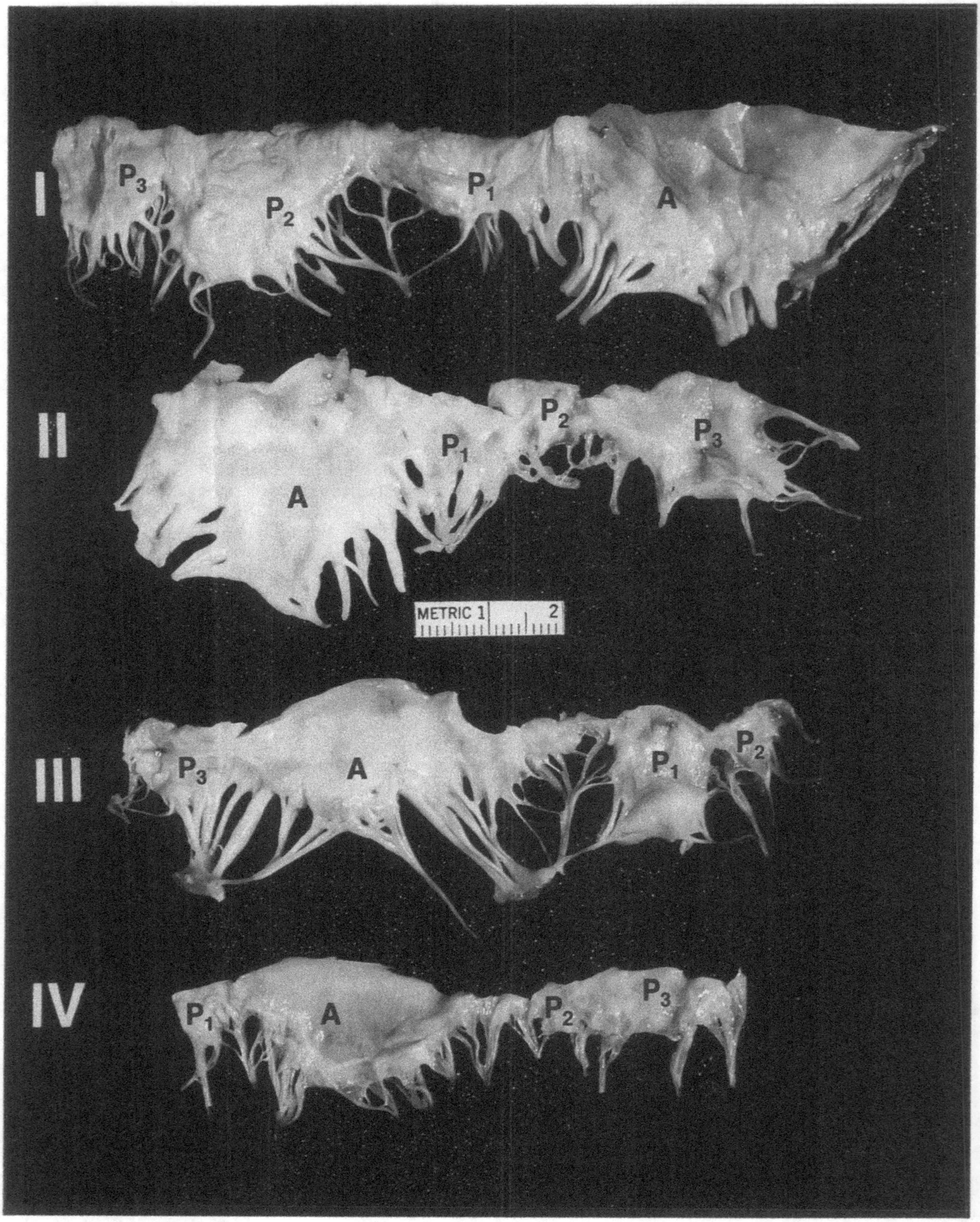

FIGURE 3. *Photographs of mitral valves from three patients with obstructive hypertrophic cardiomyopathy aged 31, 29, and 60 years (I, II, and III) and from a normal control patient without cardiovascular disease (IV) showing variation in valvular size and structure. Valves have been opened with the circumference displayed in a horizontal orientation, exposing the atrial surface. I, Large valve (area, 22 cm^2) in which both the anterior (A) and posterior (P) leaflets are greatly elongated and increased in area. II, Large valve in which increased valve size (area, 18 cm^2) is caused primarily by elongation and enlargement of the anterior leaflet. III, Segmental elongation and increased area confined to a lateral scallop of posterior mitral leaflet, which has virtually the same length as the normal-size anterior leaflet. IV, Valve is normal in area (i.e., 11 cm^2), length, and thickness.*

Table 2. Comparison of Patients With HCM Who Had Mitral Valves Removed Surgically With Those With Mitral Valves Removed at Necropsy

	Mitral valves removed surgically	Mitral valves removed at necropsy	p
Patients (n)	65 (69%)	29 (31%)	...
Age (mean±SD years)	47±14	36±14	<0.001
Male:female, n (%)	32 (49%):33 (51%)	17 (59%):12 (41%)	NS
LV-SA peak systolic gradient (mm Hg)			
Basal	71±45	24±34	<0.001
Provoked	111±37	33±48	<0.001
New York Heart Association functional class			
I	0	7	<0.001
II	3	5	
III/IV	62	17	
Echo measurements			
Septal thickness (mm)	19±4	25±7	<0.001
Free wall thickness (mm)	13±3	16±5	<0.001
Mitral valve measurements			
Areas (cm^2)			
Anterior mitral leaflet	5.4±1.5	7.0±1.6	<0.001
Posterior mitral leaflet	2.4±1.1	3.0±1.0	<0.02
Total leaflets	12.0±3.5	14.6±3.3	<0.001
Circumference (cm)	8.0±1.5	9.7±1.6	<0.001
Lengths (cm)			
Anterior mitral leaflet	2.0±0.5	2.5±0.3	<0.001
Posterior mitral leaflet	1.3±0.4	1.6±0.4	<0.001
Weight (g)	2.2±0.7	1.6±0.7	<0.001
Thickness (mm) (anterior leaflet)	2.4±0.8	1.4±0.9	<0.001

HCM, hypertrophic cardiomyopathy; LV-SA, left ventricle to systemic artery.
. . . , Not applicable.

height and/or gender accounted for only 24% of the observed variability in mitral valve area.

The relation between mitral leaflet area and heart weight in patients with HCM was not significant; correlation coefficients were 0.36 (p=0.054), although there was a significant correlation between these two parameters in normal controls (correlation coefficient, 0.40; p=0.01). For the overall group, there was no linear relation between mitral leaflet area and either age, magnitude of mitral regurgitation or outflow tract gradient, left ventricular cavity size, or wall thickness. Sixteen female patients >50 years old had the smallest mitral valves, with leaflet areas significantly less than those for the other 78 patients (11.0±2.5 versus 13.2±3.8 cm^2; p<0.05).

Histological Findings

Valves from patients with obstructive HCM had histological changes judged to be secondary in origin. Normal leaflet architecture remained largely intact, although the thickness of the fibrosa was markedly increased because of increased amounts of fibrous tissue that appeared in a pattern of parallel layers with varying density. In contrast, the spongiosa layer was decreased in thickness, with reduced amounts of elastic fibers. Patients with nonobstructive HCM had a histological mitral valve structure similar to that of the control subjects.

Discussion

Hypertrophic cardiomyopathy is generally regarded as an inheritable disease of cardiac muscle.[3-5,30] Most pathophysiological consequences of HCM have been ascribed largely to the asymmetrically thickened left ventricular muscle, which is the most characteristic morphological marker of this disease.[1,2,4-6,31-33] For many years, the mitral valve has been known to play an important role in hemodynamic alterations by producing systolic anterior motion, midsystolic contact with the ventricular septum, and consequently dynamic obstruction to left ventricular outflow.[11,16,34-40] The question of whether or not the mitral valve is altered as part of the basic disease process in HCM has never been studied systematically or resolved. Indeed, most previously reported observations made either at necropsy or surgery have described the mitral valve as virtually free of intrinsic disease (although often secondarily thickened).[1,2,6,9,10] Isolated observations in selected patients with HCM, however, have described structural abnormalities of the mitral valve that appear to be congenital and are associated with systolic anterior motion and outflow obstruction.[11-16]

The findings of the present study of almost 100 mitral valves removed at necropsy or at surgery provide substantial evidence for important structural abnormalities of the mitral valve in HCM that do not appear to be of

TABLE 3. Patients With HCM and Obstruction to Left Ventricular Outflow: Comparison of Mitral Valves Removed Surgically With Those Removed at Necropsy

	Mitral valves removed surgically	Mitral valves removed at necropsy	*p*
Patients (*n*)	65	12	. . .
Age (mean±SD years)	47±14	38±16	NS
Male:female, *n* (%)	32 (49%):33 (51%)	9 (75%):3 (25%)	NS
LV-SA peak systolic gradient (mm Hg)			
Basal	71±45	60±26	NS
Provoked	111±37	102±26	NS
New York Heart Association functional class			
I	0	1	<0.01
II	3	3	
III/IV	62	8	
Echo measurements			
Septal thickness (mm)	19±4	27±5	<0.001
Free wall thickness (mm)	13±3	17±5	<0.05
Mitral valve measurements			
Areas (cm^2)			
Anterior mitral leaflet	5.4±1.5	7.4±1.7	<0.001
Posterior mitral leaflet	2.4±1.1	3.1±1.1	NS
Total leaflets	12.0±3.5	14.8±3.7	<0.05
Circumference (cm)	8.0±1.5	9.6±1.8	<0.01
Lengths (cm)			
Anterior mitral leaflet	2.0±0.5	2.6±0.3	<0.001
Posterior mitral leaflet	1.3±0.4	1.6±0.4	<0.05
Weight (g)	2.2±0.7	2.1±0.5	NS
Thickness (mm) (anterior leaflet)	2.4±0.8	2.0±1.0	NS

HCM, hypertrophic cardiomyopathy; LV-SA, left ventricle to systemic artery.
. . . , Not applicable.

acquired origin. Indeed, these observations would appear to expand the basic morphological definition of HCM, and representing an evolution of the precept that this disease is structurally confined to cardiac muscle. Mitral leaflet area was significantly greater in our patients with HCM than in control patients without car-

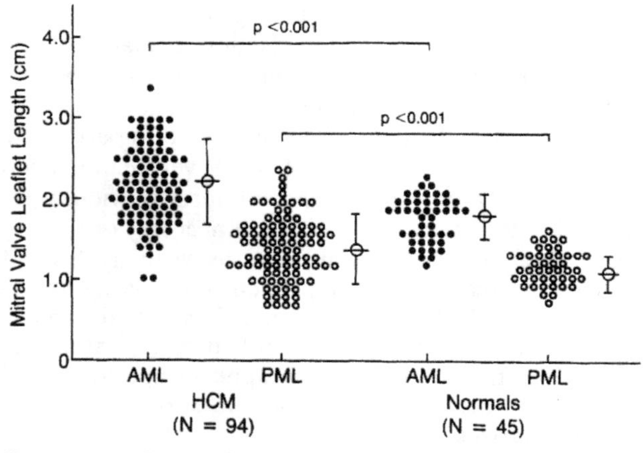

FIGURE 4. *Scatterplot of mitral valve leaflet lengths shown separately for both anterior (AML) and posterior mitral leaflets (PML) in patients with hypertrophic cardiomyopathy (HCM) and normal controls.*

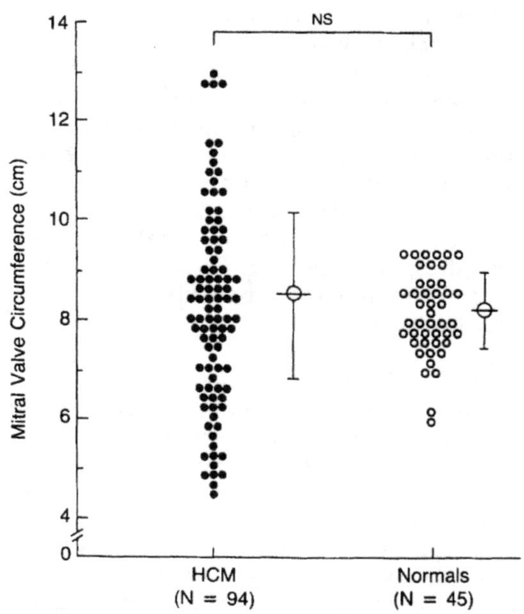

FIGURE 5. *Scatterplot of mitral valve circumference in patients with hypertrophic cardiomyopathy (HCM) and normal controls.*

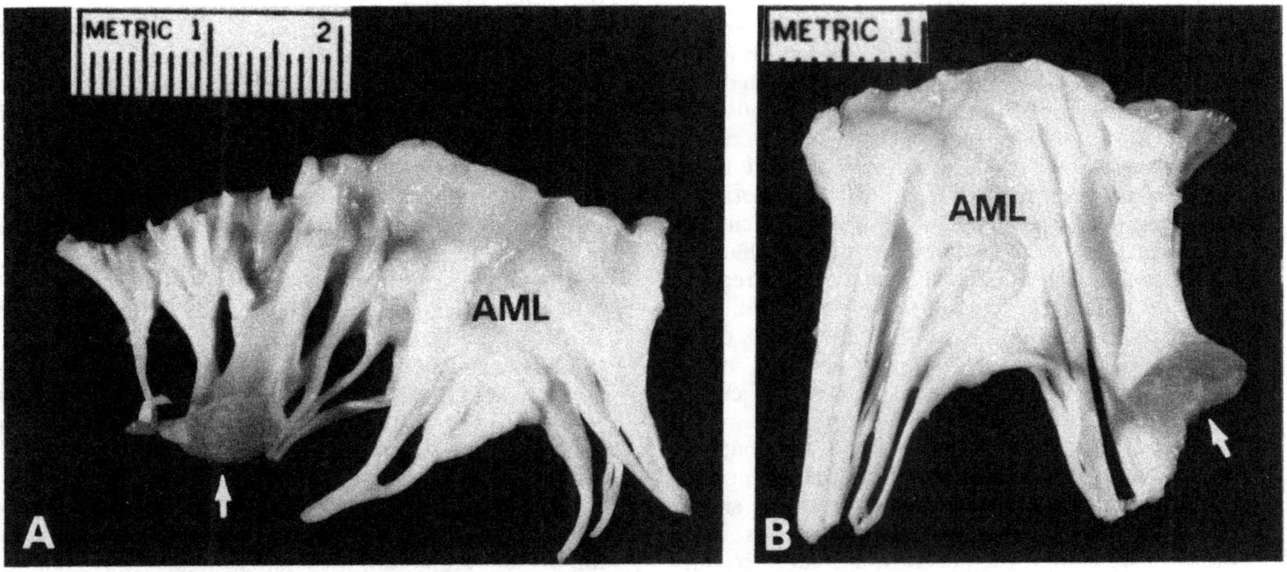

FIGURE 6. *Photographs of mitral valve specimens (with ventricular aspect exposed) excised at operation from a 31-year-old man* (panel A) *and a 62-year-old woman* (panel B), *both with obstructive HCM, showing anomalous papillary muscle insertion directly into anterior mitral leaflet. Panel A: Papillary muscle (arrow) insertion is largely confined to the area of the posteromedial commissure but spares the distal margin of anterior leaflet. Panel B: Papillary muscle (arrow) inserts into the anterolateral commissural region and also occupies substantial portions of the anterior mitral leaflet (AML).*

diovascular disease. The patients with HCM also showed considerable variability with respect to mitral valve structure and size. About 60% of all mitral valves were enlarged (some up to twice the normal leaflet area), and only about 40% were within the 95% confidence limits of the normal control valves (<12.0 cm^2). For the overall group of patients with HCM, the increased mitral leaflet size was largely a result of an increase in leaflet length (from margin of attachment to free margin).

In addition to increased overall mitral valve size, leaflet elongation, and asymmetrical (segmental) enlargement of either the anterior or a portion of the posterior leaflet, other structural malformations of the

TABLE 4. Comparison of Control Subjects and Patients With HCM Having No or Mild Focal Fibrous Mitral Valve Thickening

	Control subjects	HCM with no or mild focal fibrous thickening	p
Patients (n)	45	38	...
Age (mean±SD years)	45±17	38±14	<0.05
Male:female, n (%)	24 (53%):21 (47%)	24 (53%):21 (47%)	NS
New York Heart Association functional class			
I	45	6	<0.001
II	0	4	
III/IV	0	28	
Heart weight (g)	271±45	561±161	<0.001
Mitral valve measurements			
Areas (cm^2)			
Anterior mitral leaflet	4.3±1.0	6.5±1.7	<0.001
Posterior mitral leaflet	1.7±0.5	2.8±1.1	<0.001
Total leaflets	8.7±2.0	13.9±3.7	<0.001
Circumference (cm)	8.2±2.8	9.3±1.7	<0.001
Lengths (cm)			
Anterior mitral leaflet	1.8±0.3	2.4±0.5	<0.001
Posterior mitral leaflet	1.1±0.2	1.5±0.4	<0.001
Weight (g)	1.0±0.3	1.6±0.7	<0.001
Thickness (mm) (anterior leaflet)	1.1±0.4	1.3±0.5	NS

HCM, hypertrophic cardiomyopathy; LV-SA, left ventricle to systemic artery.
. . . , Not applicable.

mitral valve were found that are not readily explained as secondary or acquired abnormalities. About 10% of the patients studied had a congenital malformation of the mitral apparatus characterized by direct insertion of one or both papillary muscles into anterior mitral leaflet.[29,41] Thus, two thirds of our study patients had increased mitral leaflet size or a structural valve malformation that is likely to have been present from birth. Furthermore, multiple regression analysis of a variety of clinical, morphological, and hemodynamic parameters that theoretically could have influenced mitral leaflet area and shape showed that the combined impact of all such variables accounted for no more than about 25% of the observed variability in valve size. In addition, mitral leaflet enlargement could not be explained on the basis of fibrous thickening alone (secondary to traumatic septal contact), because our subset of 38 study patients with either no or minimal mitral valve thickening nevertheless had mitral valve areas that were also significantly greater than those of the normal controls.

Although we cannot exclude with absolute certainty the hypothesis that other undefined mechanical factors related to the complex left ventricular geometry in HCM influenced mitral valve structure, it is difficult to conceive of secondary mechanisms by which malformations such as direct anomalous papillary muscle insertion into anterior mitral leaflet or particularly enlarged and elongated mitral leaflets (>13 cm^2 in area) could have been acquired. Even if some of the mitral valve abnormalities described in the present report are not primary, our findings would nevertheless represent a major conceptual departure by expanding the basic morphological definition of HCM beyond the ventricular myocardium to the mitral valve.

The size of the mitral leaflets does not, however, appear to be the sole determinant of outflow obstruction in patients with HCM. Indeed, in those patients without outflow obstruction, mean mitral leaflet area was actually slightly greater than in patients with obstruction; also, more than 70% of the nonobstructive patients had enlarged valves, and there was no identifiable relation between the magnitude of outflow gradient and mitral leaflet area. The explanation for the absence of outflow obstruction in some patients with enlarged valves probably lies with the observation that variables other than mitral leaflet area and length may also be important determinants of obstruction – e.g., increased ejection velocity,[25,26,35] reduced outflow tract area,[39] anterior displacement of mitral valve and papillary muscles within the left ventricular cavity,[40,42–44] and probably also basal ventricular septal thickness.[43] Undoubtedly, mitral valve systolic anterior motion (and outflow obstruction) results from a complex interplay between a number of these variables, in addition to mitral valve size.

In the present study, we have demonstrated considerable variability in mitral valve structure among patients with HCM. However, the mitral valve alterations identified are not unique to this disease. Patients with mitral valve prolapse, for example, also have increased mitral leaflet size.[17–21] Increased leaflet area in "floppy" mitral prolapse valves, however, is associated with distinctive morphological features not present in our HCM valves, such as leaflet ballooning, elongated chordae, and excessive mucopolysaccharide deposition.[17–20] Furthermore, valves producing mitral prolapse also show a marked increase in circumference[21] not characteristic of most mitral valves in HCM. Finally, preoperative echocardiograms recorded in each of our 65 patients with mitral valve replacement did not show evidence of mitral valve prolapse motion pattern. Therefore, there is no convincing evidence that the structurally abnormal mitral valves present in our patients represent examples of the primary floppy mitral valve, itself an uncommon occurrence in patients with HCM.[45]

The findings of the present study also have potentially relevant implications with regard to the pathogenesis of HCM. Recently, mutations in the gene that encodes for the heavy chains of cardiac myosin (localized to chromosome 14) have been identified in members of families with HCM.[46–48] However, to date, not all families with HCM studied appear to show this abnormality,[49] and therefore the broad morphological spectrum and clinical heterogeneity of HCM ultimately may not be explained solely by a myosin defect. Indeed, the findings of the present study that focus on structural valve abnormalities represent an evolution in our understanding of the complex nature of HCM and raise the possibility that the disease process is not limited to myocardium (and a defect in myosin) in all patients.

Acknowledgment

We wish to recognize the expert photographic assistance of Mr. Michael Spencer.

References

1. Teare D: Asymmetrical hypertrophy of the heart in young adults. *Br Heart J* 1958;20:1–8
2. Roberts CS, Roberts WC: Morphologic features, in Zipes DP, Rowlands DJ (eds): *Progress in Cardiology* 2/2. Philadelphia, Pa, Lea & Febiger, 1989, pp 3–32
3. Braunwald E, Lambrew CT, Rockoff SD, Ross J Jr, Morrow AG: Idiopathic hypertrophic subaortic stenosis: I. A description of the disease based upon an analysis of 64 patients. *Circulation* 1964; 30(suppl IV):IV-3–IV-119
4. Wigle ED, Sasson Z, Henderson MA, Rudd TD, Fulop J, Rakowski H, Williams WG: Hypertrophic cardiomyopathy: The importance of the site and the extent of hypertrophy: A review. *Prog Cardiovasc Dis* 1985;28:1–83
5. Maron BJ, Bonow RO, Cannon RO, Leon MB, Epstein SE: Hypertrophic cardiomyopathy: Interrelation of clinical manifestations, pathophysiology, and therapy. *N Engl J Med* 1987;316: 780–789, 844–852
6. Olsen EG: Anatomic and light microscopic characterization of hypertrophic obstructive and nonobstructive cardiomyopathy. *Eur Heart J* 1983;4(suppl F):1–6
7. Maron BJ, Roberts WC: Quantitative analysis of cardiac muscle cell disorganization in the ventricular septum of patients with hypertrophic cardiomyopathy. *Circulation* 1979;59:689–706
8. Maron BJ, Epstein SE: Hypertrophic cardiomyopathy: A discussion of nomenclature. *Am J Cardiol* 1979;43:1242–1244
9. Morrow AG, Roberts WC, Ross J Jr, Fisher RD, Behrendt DM, Mason DT, Braunwald E: Obstruction to left ventricular outflow: Current concepts of management and operative treatment. *Ann Intern Med* 1968;69:1255–1286
10. Roberts WC: Operative treatment of hypertrophic obstructive cardiomyopathy: The case against mitral valve replacement. *Am J Cardiol* 1973;32:377–381
11. Maron BJ, Harding AM, Spirito P, Roberts WC, Waller BF: Systolic anterior motion of the posterior mitral leaflet: A previously unrecognized cause of dynamic subaortic obstruction in patients with hypertrophic cardiomyopathy. *Circulation* 1983;68:282–293
12. Bjork VO, Hutquist G, Lodin H: Subaortic stenosis produced by an abnormally placed anterior mitral leaflet. *J Thorac Cardiovasc Surg* 1969;41:659–669
13. Moro E, ten Cate FJ, Hugenholtz PG, Roelandt J: Genesis of systolic anterior motion of the mitral valve in hypertrophic cardio-

myopathy: An anatomical or dynamic event? *Eur Heart J* 1987;8: 1312–1321
14. Mikami T, Hashimoto M, Kudo T, Sugawara T, Sakamoto S, Yasuda H: Mitral valve and its ring in hypertrophic cardiomyopathy: A mechanism creating surplus mitral leaflet involved in systolic anterior motion. *Jpn Circ J* 1988;52:597–603
15. Ellis JG, Terneny OJ, Winters WL, Leachman RD: The critical role of the mitral valve leaflet in hypertrophic subaortic stenosis and amelioration of the disease by mitral valve replacement. *Chest* 1971;9:378–382
16. Fix P, Moberg A, Soderberg H, Karnell J: Muscular subvalvular aortic stenosis: An abnormal anterior mitral leaflet possibly the primary factor. *Acta Radiol* 1964;2:177–193
17. Angelini A, Becker AE, Anderson RH, Davies MJ: Mitral valve morphology: Normal and mitral valve prolapse, in Boudoulas H, Wooley CF (eds): *Mitral Valve Prolapse and the Mitral Valve Prolapse Syndrome.* New York, Futura Publishing Co, Inc, 1988, pp 13–53
18. Pomerance A: Ballooning deformity (mucoid degenerations) of atrioventricular valves. *Br Heart J* 1969;31:343–351
19. Popp RL, Winkle RA: Mitral valve prolapse syndrome. *JAMA* 1976;236:867–870
20. Davies MJ, Moore BP, Braimbridge MV: The floppy mitral valve: Study of incidence, pathology, and complications in surgical, necropsy, and forensic material. *Br Heart J* 1978;40:468–481
21. Waller BF, Morrow AG, Maron BJ, Del Negro AA, Kent KM, McGrath FJ, Wallace RB, McIntosh CL, Roberts WC: Etiology of clinically isolated, severe, chronic, pure mitral regurgitation: Analysis of 97 patients over 30 years of age having mitral valve replacement. *Am Heart J* 1982;104:276–288
22. McIntosh CL, Greenberg GJ, Maron BJ, Leon MB, Cannon RO III, Clark RE: Clinical and hemodynamic results after mitral valve replacement in patients with obstructive hypertrophic cardiomyopathy. *Ann Thorac Surg* 1989;47:236–244
23. Krajcer Z, Leachman RD, Cooley DA, Ostajic M, Coronado R: Mitral valve replacement and septal myectomy in hypertrophic cardiomyopathy: Ten-year follow-up in 80 patients. *Circulation* 1989;80(suppl I):I-57–I-64
24. Cooley DA, Leachman RD, Wukasch DC: Diffuse muscular subaortic stenosis: Surgical treatment. *Am J Cardiol* 1973;31:1–6
25. Yock PG, Hatle L, Popp RL: Patterns and timing of Doppler-detected intracavitary and aortic flow in hypertrophic cardiomyopathy. *J Am Coll Cardiol* 1986;8:1047–1058
26. Sasson Z, Yock PG, Hatle LK, Aldermann EL, Popp RL: Doppler echocardiographic determination of the pressure gradient in hypertrophic cardiomyopathy. *J Am Coll Cardiol* 1988;11:752–756
27. Ranganathan N, Lam JHC, Wigle ED, Silver MD: Morphology of the human mitral valve: II. The valve leaflets. *Circulation* 1970;41: 459–467
28. Draper N, Smith H: The stepwise regression procedure, in Draper N, Smith H (eds): *Applied Regression Analysis,* ed 3. New York, John Wiley & Sons, Inc, 1981, pp 307–311
29. Klues HG, Roberts WC, Maron BJ: Anomalous insertion of papillary muscle directly into anterior mitral leaflet in hypertrophic cardiomyopathy. *Circulation* 1991;84:1188–1197
30. Maron BJ, Nichols PF III, Pickle LW, Wesley YE, Mulvihill JJ: Patterns of inheritance in hypertrophic cardiomyopathy: Assessment by M-mode and two-dimensional echocardiography. *Am J Cardiol* 1984;53:1087–1094
31. Martin RP, Rakowski H, French J, Popp RL: Idiopathic hypertrophic subaortic stenosis viewed by wide-angle, phased-array echocardiography. *Circulation* 1979;59:1206–1217
32. Shapiro LM, McKenna WJ: Distribution of left ventricular hypertrophy in hypertrophic cardiomyopathy: A two-dimensional echocardiographic study. *J Am Coll Cardiol* 1983;2:437–444
33. Maron BJ, Gottdiener JS, Epstein SE: Patterns and significance of distribution of left ventricular hypertrophy in hypertrophic cardiomyopathy: A wide-angle, two-dimensional echocardiographic study of 125 patients. *Am J Cardiol* 1981;48:418–428
34. Shah PM, Taylor RD, Wong M: Abnormal mitral valve coaptation in hypertrophic obstructive cardiomyopathy: Proposed role in systolic anterior motion of mitral valve. *Am J Cardiol* 1981;48: 258–262
35. Shah PM, Gramiak R, Kramer DH: Ultrasound location of left ventricular outflow obstruction in hypertrophic obstructive cardiomyopathy. *Circulation* 1969;40:3–11
36. Maron BJ, Epstein SE: Clinical significance and therapeutic implications of the left ventricular outflow tract pressure gradient in hypertrophic cardiomyopathy. *Am J Cardiol* 1986;58:1093–1096
37. Spirito P, Maron BJ: Pattern of systolic anterior motion of the mitral valve in hypertrophic cardiomyopathy: Assessment by two-dimensional echocardiography. *Am J Cardiol* 1984;54:1039–1046
38. Rodger JC: Motion of mitral apparatus in hypertrophic cardiomyopathy with obstruction. *Br Heart J* 1976;38:732–737
39. Simon AL, Ross J, Gault JH: Angiographic anatomy of the left ventricle and mitral valve in idiopathic hypertrophic subaortic stenosis. *Circulation* 1967;36:852–867
40. Henry WL, Clark CE, Griffith JM, Epstein SE: Mechanism of left ventricular outflow obstruction in patients with obstructive asymmetric septal hypertrophy (idiopathic hypertrophic subaortic stenosis). *Am J Cardiol* 1975;35:337–345
41. Roberts WC, Cohen LS: Left ventricular papillary muscles: Description of the normal and a survey of conditions causing them to function abnormally. *Circulation* 1972;46:138–154
42. Wigle ED, Adelman AG, Auger P, Marquis Y: Mitral regurgitation in muscular subaortic stenosis. *Am J Cardiol* 1969;24:698–706
43. Spirito P, Maron BJ: Significance of left ventricular outflow tract cross-sectional area in hypertrophic cardiomyopathy: A two-dimensional echocardiographic assessment. *Circulation* 1983;67: 1100–1108
44. Jiang L, Levine RA, King ME, Weyman AE: An integrated mechanism for systolic anterior motion of the mitral valve in hypertrophic cardiomyopathy based on echocardiographic observations. *Am Heart J* 1987;113:633–644
45. Petrone RK, Klues HG, Panza JA, Peterson E, Maron BJ: Coexistence of mitral valve prolapse in a consecutive group of 528 patients with hypertrophic cardiomyopathy assessed by echocardiography. *J Am Coll Cardiol* (in press)
46. Jarcho JA, McKenna WJ, Pare PJA, Solomon SD, Holcombe RF, Dickie S, Levi T, Donis-Keller H, Seidman JG, Seidman CE: Mapping a gene for familial hypertrophic cardiomyopathy to chromosome 14q1. *N Engl J Med* 1989;321:1372–1378
47. Tanigawa G, Jarcho JA, Kass S, Solomon SD, Vosberg HP, Seidman JG, Seidman CE: A molecular basis for familial hypertrophic cardiomyopathy: An α/β cardiac myosin heavy chain hybrid gene. *Cell* 1990;62:991–998
48. Geisterfer-Lowrance AA, Kass S, Tanigawa G, Vosberg HP, McKenna WJ, Seidman CE, Seidman JG: A molecular basis for familial hypertrophic cardiomyopathy: A β cardiac myosin heavy chain gene missense mutation. *Cell* 1990;62:999–1006
49. Solomon SD, Jarcho JA, McKenna WJ, Geisterfer-Lowrance A, Germain R, Salerni R, Seidman JG, Seidman CE: Familial hypertrophic cardiomyopathy is a genetically heterogenous disease. *J Clin Invest* 1990;86:993–999

Relation Between Extent of Cardiac Muscle Cell Disorganization and Left Ventricular Wall Thickness in Hypertrophic Cardiomyopathy

Barry J. Maron, MD, James K. Wolfson, MD, and William C. Roberts, MD

The presence of numerous, abnormally arranged, cardiac muscle cells distributed widely throughout the hypertrophied left ventricular (LV) wall has been considered a characteristic, morphologic feature of patients dying of hypertrophic cardiomyopathy (HC) and also probably a determinant of impaired LV compliance. However, the relation between such regions of myocardial cell disarray and the magnitude of wall thickness in the same areas of the left ventricle has not been defined. Therefore, the present study was undertaken in which LV wall thickness and the percent area of myocardium disorganized were systematically compared in the same tissue section. No correlation was identified between wall thickness and the amount of myocardium disorganized in the same tissue sections, either when calculated separately for the ventricular septum, and anterolateral and posterior free walls, or when expressed for all 3 regions combined.

Therefore, in patients with HC: (1) disorganized myocardial architecture is not confined to greatly thickened portions of the LV wall, but regions of the left ventricle with normal or only mildly increased thickness may also be disordered; and (2) whereas both LV wall thickening and cellular disorganization are manifestations of the primary cardiomyopathic process, these 2 morphologic features do not appear to be directly related with regard to their extent and distribution within the LV wall. These observations will potentially enhance understanding of the relation between LV structure and compliance in HC.

(Am J Cardiol 1992;70:785–790)

From the Pathology and Cardiology Branches, National Heart, Lung, and Blood Institute, National Institutes of Health, Bethesda, Maryland. Manuscript received December 27, 1991; revised manuscript received and accepted June 1, 1992.

Address for reprints: Barry J. Maron, MD, National Heart, Lung, and Blood Institute, National Institutes of Health, Building 10, Room 7B-15, Bethesda, Maryland 20892.

Hypertrophic cardiomyopathy (HC) is a primary cardiac disease characterized by an asymmetrically hypertrophied but nondilated left ventricle.[1] Disorganized arrangement of cardiac muscle cells has been recognized to be an important morphologic feature of the ventricular architecture in this disease.[2–13] It has also been generally accepted that in HC the thickest portions of the left ventricular (LV) wall are most likely to contain disordered myocardial cells. However, this relation between the magnitude of LV wall thickness and the degree of cardiac muscle cell disorganization has not been systematically investigated in HC. Therefore, the present investigation was performed using histologic sections obtained at necropsy from 31 patients with HC.

METHODS

Selection of patients: The cardiovascular registry of the National Heart, Lung, and Blood Institute was reviewed, and 31 hearts were included in the present study group. Each patient fulfilled our basic anatomic definition of HC with an asymmetrically hypertrophied nondilated left ventricle in the absence of another cardiac or systemic disease capable of producing the magnitude of LV hypertrophy present in that patient.[1] In 25 of 31 patients, typical clinical, hemodynamic, angiocardiographic and operative findings of HC[14,15] were also present; the other 6 had no cardiovascular evaluation during life, and sudden death was the first definitive manifestation of cardiac disease.[14–16]

The 31 study patients ranged in age from 11 to 61 years (mean 34); 16 (51%) were male. Before death, 9 patients were asymptomatic, 9 mildly symptomatic, and 13 severely symptomatic. Nineteen patients had the obstructive form of HC (outflow gradient ≥30 mm Hg during basal conditions or with provocative maneuvers), 6 were nonobstructive (gradient <30 mm Hg during basal conditions or with provocation), and the remaining 6 did not have cardiac catheterization. In the 25 patients with hemodynamic studies, maximal basal or provocable gradients ranged from 0 to 175 mm Hg (average 81).

Eighteen patients died suddenly (3 from progressive congestive heart failure, 8 at operation or cardiac catheterization, 1 of stroke, and 1 by suicide). Heart weights were 270 to 1,020 g (mean 592 ± 171) for the 24 adult patients (488 ± 111 g in 12 women, and 695 ± 160 g in 12 men). In the 7 children (aged 11 to 17 years), heart weights were 270 to 530 g.

Preparation of specimens: In each, full thickness tissue blocks were obtained from the LV wall in the transverse plane perpendicular to the long axis of the ventricle (approximately half the distance between the apex and the base of the aortic valve) in the following 3 sites: (1) ventricular septum, (2) anterolateral free wall approximately 2 cm lateral to the left anterior descending coronary artery, and (3) posterior free wall between the papillary muscles. The tissue was imbedded in paraffin, sectioned at 6 μ thickness and stained with hematoxylin and eosin.

Maximal wall thickness was measured in each LV section from the fixed and stained tissue specimen with the use of calipers. Measurements were obtained perpendicular to the endocardial surfaces of the wall; care was taken to exclude trabeculae, papillary muscles, crista supraventricularis muscle and the endocardial contact plaque[17] from these measurements. Furthermore, tissue sections with transmural or extensive replacement fibrosis were excluded from this study.[18]

Definition and classification of abnormal cardiac muscle cell arrangement: Cardiac muscle cell disorganization was classified into 2 major types (Figure 1). Type I disorganization was the most frequent and usually consisted of areas of myocardium in which adjacent cells were aligned perpendicularly or obliquely to each other, forming tangled masses or "pinwheel" configurations. Although most of these lesions were small, the size of individual foci of disorganization varied greatly. Alternatively, type I disorganization comprised relatively broad bundles of muscle cells that were oriented at oblique or perpendicular angles to each other; cells within these bundles were, however, normally arranged.

Type II disorganization consisted of relatively narrow (usually 1 or 2 cells wide) longitudinally cut bundles of cells that were interlaced in various directions among larger groups of transversely cut cells (that appeared circular). This type of disorganization gave the myocardium a distinctive, "swirled" appearance.

Abnormally arranged cardiac muscle cells were not considered representative of true disorganization if present in the following areas where cells normally converge at acute angles: (1) at or near the junction of the ventricular septum with the left and right ventricular free walls; (2) in trabeculations; (3) in or at the edges of

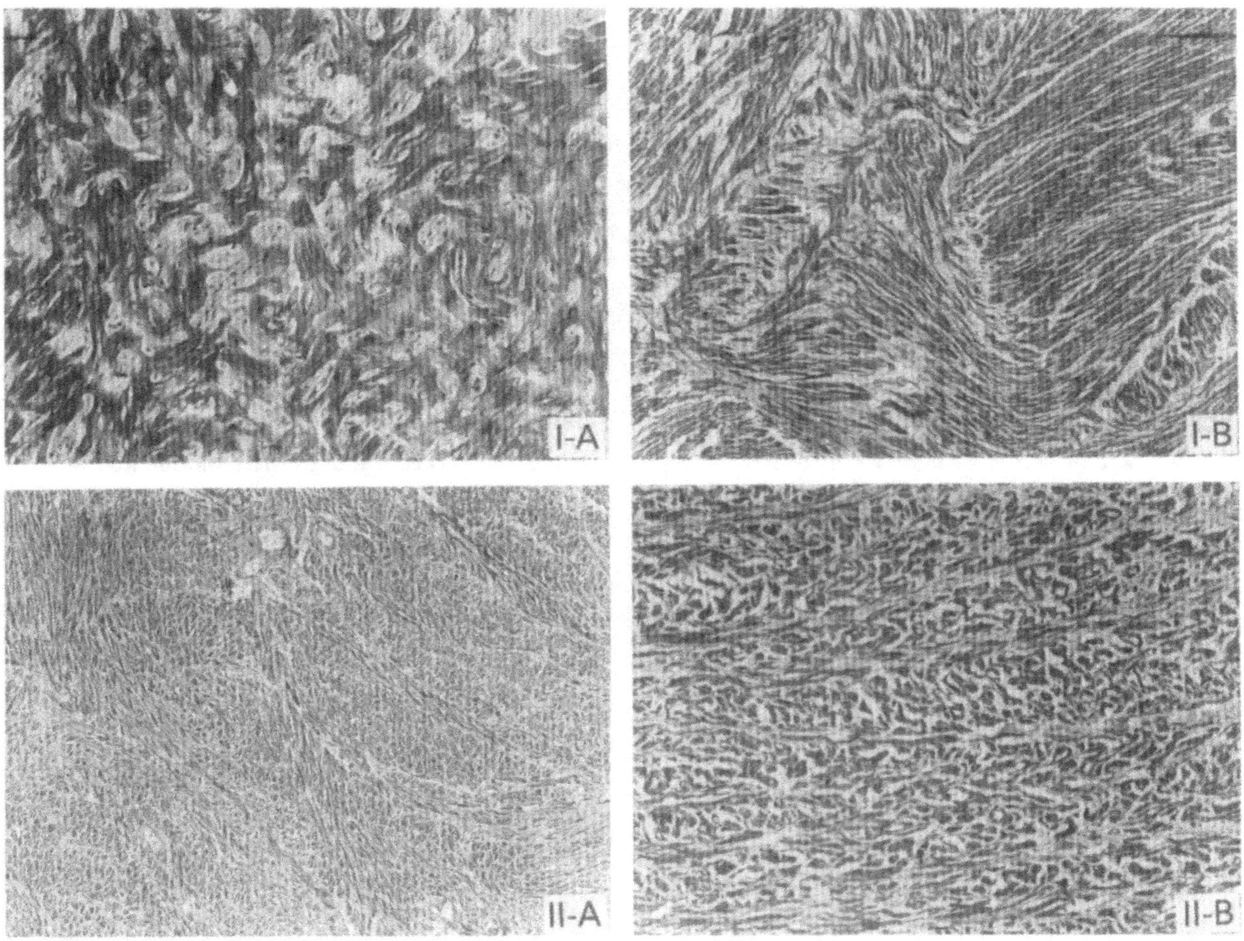

FIGURE 1. Patterns of cardiac muscle cell disorganization present in left ventricular myocardium from patients with hypertrophic cardiomyopathy. Type I exclusively involves cardiac muscle cells cut longitudinally. The most frequent pattern, designated here as type I-A, consisted of areas of myocardium in which adjacent cardiac muscle cells were aligned perpendicularly or oblique to each other. In type I-B, relatively broad bundles of muscle cells were oriented at oblique or perpendicular angles to each other. Type II involves cells cut either longitudinally or transversely. Type II-A consisted of relatively narrow bundles of cardiac muscle cells interlaced in various directions among other, larger groups of cells. Type II-B was similar except that disorganized bundles of cells were more linear in orientation. (Hematoxylin-eosin stain: I-A $\times$ 130, I-B and II-A $\times$ 40, II-B $\times$ 80; reduced by 26%.)

areas of fibrosis; (4) at points of convergence of major muscle bundles; or (5) adjacent to interstitial spaces containing blood vessels.

We did not attempt to assess the degree to which cells were malaligned in a given area of tissue. Disorganization was judged only to be present or absent and its severity was expressed in terms of extent.

Quantitation of cardiac muscle cell arrangement: A previously described technique[9] was used to quantitatively assess the extent to which cardiac muscle cell disorganization was present in each tissue section. Histologic sections were photographed and the images were enlarged to occupy 30 × 40 inch positive prints. A transparent cellulose overlay was then placed on the print. Areas of myocardium occupied by disorganized cardiac muscle cells were outlined on the overlay with a marking pen. We often could not obtain this assessment exclusively and directly from the print, and frequently had to reexamine the original tissue section with a light microscope to reliably identify the disorganized area. Furthermore, areas in which cardiac muscle cells were cut either longitudinally or transversely were demarcated; regions of fibrosis (replacement, interstitial and the endocardial contact plaque), artifacts of tissue preparation or large interstitial spaces with blood vessels were also outlined and ultimately excluded from the analysis. The transparent overlay was then removed from the print and photographed, and the image was reproduced (with substantial reduction) as a 5 × 7 inch positive print. Each area into which the tissue section had been divided was outlined separately with a fine-point marking pen on ordinary tablet paper. The area of each outlined silhouette was then quantitated using a video planimetry system.

Areas of tissue sections studied were 5.9 ± 2.7 cm^2 for the ventricular septum, 3.8 ± 1.8 cm^2 for the anterolateral free wall, and 2.8 ± 1.3 cm^2 for the posterior free wall.

Formulas used in quantitative calculations of cardiac muscle cell arrangement: The formulas used to calculate the percent area of tissue section occupied by disorganized cardiac muscle cells were as follows (the area of myocardium "at risk" for disorganization is in the denominator of both equations):

$$\% \text{ area of type I disorganization} = \frac{D_I}{L + D_I} \times 100$$

$$\% \text{ area of type II disorganization} = \frac{D_{II}}{L + T + D_{II}} \times 100$$

where L = area occupied by longitudinally cut but normally arranged cells, T = area occupied by transversely cut cells, D_I = area occupied by type I disorganization, and D_{II} = area occupied by type II disorganization. Percent disorganization plotted for each tissue section was the value for type I or II disorganization, whichever was greater. Values for types I and II disorganization could not be combined in patients with both types, because this calculation often resulted in a marked underestimation of the overall extent of disorganization present in a given tissue section.

Statistical analyses: Data were expressed as mean ± SD. Morphologic measurements between groups of patients were assessed by unpaired Student's *t* test. The relation between percent area of tissue section disorganized and LV wall thickness was assessed by linear regression analysis.

RESULTS

Left ventricular wall thickness: Measurement of LV wall thickness was greatest for the ventricular septum, ranging from 14 to 40 mm (mean 22). Anterolateral and posterior wall thicknesses were similar; anterolateral was 10 to 30 mm (mean 18), and posterior was 11 to 27 mm (mean 17). Wall thicknesses <15 mm were considered normal or virtually normal; such measurements were present in 1 ventricular septal tissue section, and 8 anterolateral and 10 posterior free wall sections.

Cardiac muscle cell disorganization: VENTRICULAR SEPTUM: The extent of cellular disorganization was greatest in the ventricular septum. The percent area of septum disorganized ranged from 0 to 95% (mean 40). Some disorganization was present in 30 patients (97%); disorganization constituted 5 to 24% of the relevant part of the tissue section in 8 patients (26%) and 25 to 49% in 6 patients (19%), and was particularly extensive involving ≥50% of the section in 13 patients (42%).

ANTEROLATERAL FREE WALL: Substantial cardiac muscle cell disorganization was also identified in the anterolateral free wall, with the percent area of tissue section disorganized ranging from 0 to 94% (mean 33). Some disorganization was present in 25 patients (81%); disorganization constituted 5 to 24% of the relevant part of the tissue section in 9 patients (29%) and 25 to 49% in 2 patients (6%), and was particularly extensive involving ≥50% of the section in 11 patients (36%).

POSTERIOR FREE WALL: In the posterior free wall, the percent area of tissue section disorganized ranged from 0 to 95% (mean 31). Some disorganization was present in 23 patients (74%); disorganization constituted 5 to 24% of the relevant part of the tissue section in 5 patients (19%) and 25 to 49% in 6 patients (19%), and was particularly extensive involving ≥50% of the section in 5 patients (16%).

In the 19 tissue sections studied (septum, and anterolateral and posterior free walls) with wall thickness <15 mm, the extent of cardiac muscle cell disorganization was 0 to 94% (mean 40 ± 32). In the 6 sections >30 mm in thickness, the extent of cellular disorganization was similar (range 9 to 59%, mean 36 ± 18; p >0.05). In 28 tissue sections with <5% disorganization, wall thicknesses were 12 to 19 mm (mean 18 ± 4); in 28 sections with ≥50% disorganization, wall thicknesses were similar (range 11 to 40 mm, mean 19 ± 7; p >0.05).

Relation between left ventricular wall thickness and extent of cardiac muscle cell disorganization: Comparison of LV wall thicknesses and percent area disorganized in the same tissue sections showed no correlation, either when calculated separately for the ventricular

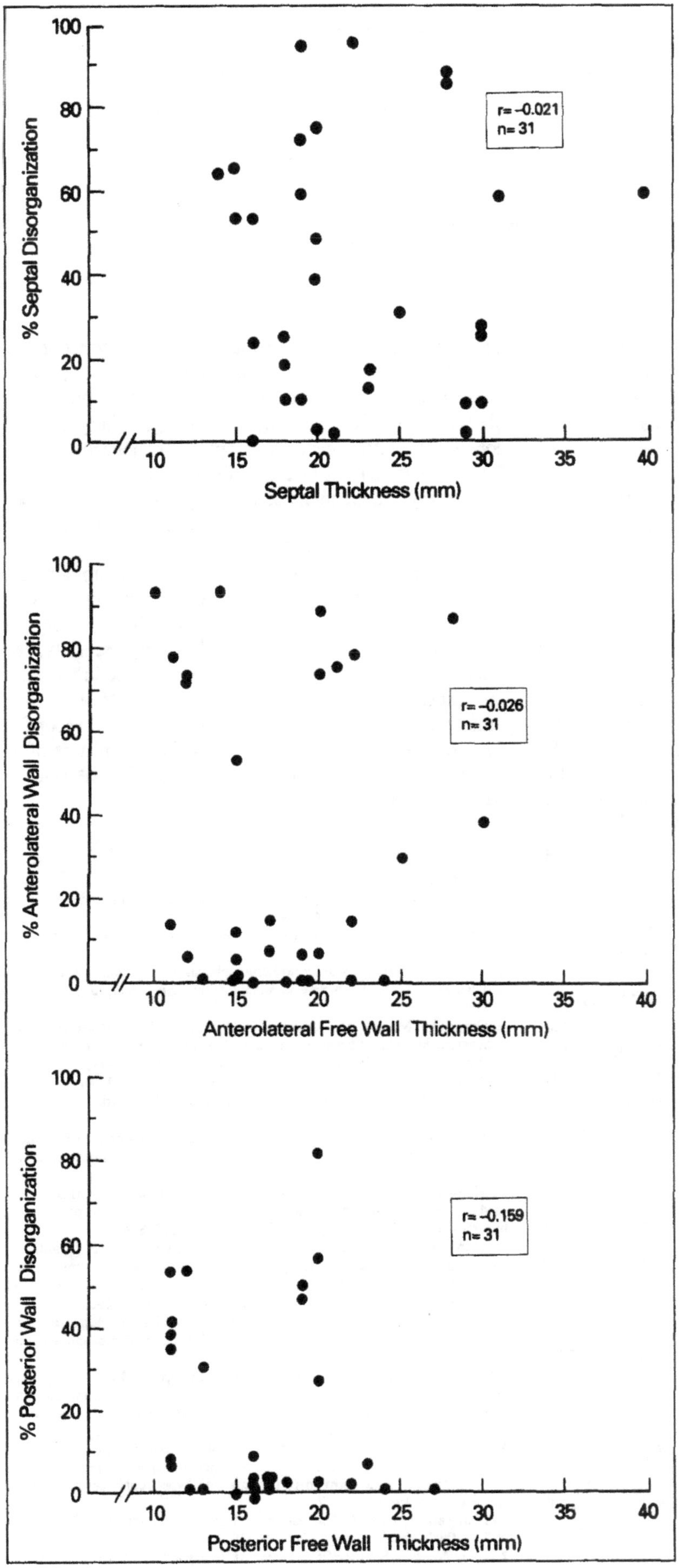

FIGURE 2. Relation between left ventricular wall thickness (in 3 sites) and extent of cardiac muscle cell disorganization in same tissue section from 31 patients with hypertrophic cardiomyopathy.

TABLE I Relation Between Cardiac Muscle Cell Disorganization and Left Ventricular Wall Thickness in 31 Patients with Hypertrophic Cardiomyopathy

LV Site	No. of Pts.	% Area Disorganized	Wall Thickness (mm)	r Value	Slope
Ventricular septum	31	40 ± 30 (0–95)	22 ± 6 (14–40)	−0.021	−0.101
Anterolateral free wall	31	33 ± 36 (0–94)	18 ± 5 (10–30)	−0.026	−0.188
Posterior free wall	31	19 ± 23 (0–81)	17 ± 4 (11–27)	−0.159	−0.863
All combined	93	31 ± 31 (0–95)	19 ± 5 (10–40)	−0.063	−0.342

LV = left ventricular.

septum, and anterolateral and posterior free walls (Figure 2), or when expressed for all 3 regions combined (Table I); correlation coefficients ranged from −0.021 to −0.159. Furthermore, no correlation was evident between LV wall thickness and either type I or II disorganization when assessed separately. No correlation was evident between total percent cellular disorganization and basal LV outflow gradient in the 25 patients with hemodynamic studies (r = −0.08).

DISCUSSION

We previously demonstrated that in patients dying of HC, disorganization of cardiac muscle cells is usually widely distributed throughout the LV wall.[6–10] The findings of the present study extend those observations and show that disordered myocardial architecture is not confined to greatly thickened portions of the ventricular myocardium, and that conversely, regions of normal or only mildly increased wall thickness also may be disorganized. For the overall group of patients studied, there was absolutely no statistical relation between the magnitude of LV wall thickness and the extent to which cardiac muscle cells within the same tissue section were disorganized, regardless of the particular region of the LV wall assessed (i.e., ventricular septum, or anterolateral or posterior free wall).

The clear inference of the data is that whereas both LV wall thickening and cellular disorganization appear to be manifestations of the primary cardiomyopathic process in HC,[15] these 2 morphologic features are not linked with respect to their extent and distribution. Our observation that LV segments of normal or only mildly increased thickness may have substantial regions of disorganization demonstrates that even the least hypertrophied portions of the LV wall may also be considered part of the primary myopathic process. This finding deviates from the previous morphologic perception that it is primarily the greatly hypertrophied portions of hearts with HC that show abnormal myocardial architecture.[19,20]

The significance of the disordered myocardial architecture characteristic of HC is uncertain, although it has been suggested that it may have an important role in producing increased ventricular chamber stiffness and impaired relaxation.[14,15,21] If myocardial disorganization has such pathophysiologic significance, then the present data would suggest that abnormalities in compliance may involve normal or relatively thin segments of the wall (as well as those with greater wall thickness), in sharp contrast to the widely held concept that impaired compliance in HC is closely related to particularly substantial LV wall thickening.[14,21] However, the observations in the percent morphologic study are also consistent with previous Doppler echocardiographic findings[22] that LV diastolic filling abnormalities in HC are largely independent of the magnitude of LV hypertrophy, and are also frequent in patients with only mild and localized hypertrophy.

We could not assess with precision the impact that connective tissue formation had on the relation between LV wall thickness and the extent of cellular disorganization in the same tissue section. First, by necessity, sections with substantial scarring[23–25] were excluded from the present analysis (because assessment of cardiac muscle cell arrangement was precluded), and second, a detailed quantitative assessment of the magnitude of interstitial, perivascular and replacement fibrosis was not part of the study design.

REFERENCES

1. Maron BJ, Epstein SE. Hypertrophic cardiomyopathy: a discussion of nomenclature. *Am J Cardiol* 1979;43:1242–1244.

2. Teare D. Asymmetrical hypertrophy of the heart in young adults. *Br Heart J* 1958;20:1–8.

3. Olsen EG. Anatomic and light microscopic characterization of hypertrophic obstructive and non-obstructive cardiomyopathy. *Eur Heart J* 1983;4(suppl F):1–8.

4. Ferrans VJ, Morrow AG, Roberts WC. Myocardial ultrastructure in idiopathic hypertrophic subaortic stenosis: a study of operatively excised left ventricular outflow tract muscle in 14 patients. *Circulation* 1972;45:769–792.

5. Sutton MSJ, Lie JT, Anderson KR, O'Brien PC, Frye RL. Histopathological specificity of hypertrophic obstructive cardiomyopathy. Myocardial fibre disarray and myocardial fibrosis. *Br Heart J* 1980;44:433–443.

6. Maron BJ, Roberts WC. Hypertrophic cardiomyopathy and cardiac muscle cell disorganization revisited: relation between the two and significance. *Am Heart J* 1981;102:95–110.

7. Maron BJ, Anan TJ, Roberts WC. Quantitative analysis of the distribution of cardiac muscle cell disorganization in the left ventricular wall of patients with hypertrophic cardiomyopathy. *Circulation* 1981;63:882–894.

8. Maron BJ, Sato N, Roberts WC, Edwards JE, Chandra RS. Quantitative analysis of cardiac muscle cell disorganization in the ventricular septum: comparison of fetuses and infants with and without congenital heart disease and patients with hypertrophic cardiomyopathy. *Circulation* 1979;60:685–696.

9. Maron BJ, Roberts WC. Quantitative analysis of cardiac muscle cell disorganization in the ventricular septum of patients with hypertrophic cardiomyopathy. *Circulation* 1979;59:689–706.

10. Maron BJ, Epstein SE. Hypertrophic cardiomyopathy. Recent observations regarding the specificity of three hallmarks of the disease: asymmetric septal hypertrophy, septal disorganization, and systolic anterior motion of the anterior mitral leaflet. *Am J Cardiol* 1980;45:141–154.

11. Isner JM, Maron BJ, Roberts WC. Comparison of amount of cardiac-muscle-cell disorganization in operatively-excised septectomy specimens to amount observed at necropsy in 18 patients with hypertrophic cardiomyopathy. *Am J Cardiol* 1980;46:42–47.

12. Fujiwara H, Kawai C, Hamashima Y. Myocardial fascicle and fiber disarray in 25 μ-thick sections. *Circulation* 1979;59:1293–1298.

13. Van Noorden S, Olsen EGJ, Pearse AGE. Hypertrophic obstructive cardiomyopathy, a histological, histochemical, and ultrastructural study of biopsy material. *Cardiovasc Res* 1971;5:118–131.

14. Wigle ED, Sasson Z, Henderson MA, Ruddy TD, Fulop J, Rakowski H, Williams WG. Hypertrophic cardiomyopathy. The importance of the site and the extent of hypertrophy. A review. *Prog Cardiovasc Dis* 1985;28:1–83.

15. Maron BJ, Bonow RO, Cannon RO, Leon MB, Epstein SE. Hypertrophic cardiomyopathy: Interrelation of clinical manifestations, pathophysiology and therapy. *N Engl J Med* 1987;780–789 and 844–852.

16. McKenna WJ, Camm AJ. Sudden death in hypertrophic cardiomyopathy: assessment of patients at high risk. *Circulation* 1989;80:1489–1492.

17. Roberts CS, Roberts WC. Morphologic features. In: Zipes DP, Rowlands DJ, eds. Progress in Cardiology 2/2. Philadelphia: Lea & Febiger, 1989:3–22.

18. Maron BJ, Epstein SE, Roberts WC. Hypertrophic cardiomyopathy and transmural myocardial infarction without significant atherosclerosis of the extramural coronary arteries. *Am J Cardiol* 1979;43:1086–1102.

19. Henry WL, Clark CE, Epstein SE. Asymmetric septal hypertrophy (ASH): echocardiographic identification of the pathognomonic anatomic abnormality of IHSS. *Circulation* 1973;47:225–233.

20. Epstein SE, Henry WL, Clark CE, Roberts WC, Maron BJ, Ferrans VJ, Redwood DR, Morrow AG. Asymmetric septal hypertrophy. *Ann Intern Med* 1974;81:650–680.

21. Goodwin JF. Congestive and hypertrophic cardiomyopathies: a decade of study. *Lancet* 1970;1:731–739.

22. Spirito P, Maron BJ. Relation between extent of left ventricular hypertrophy and diastolic filling abnormalities in hypertrophic cardiomyopathy. *J Am Coll Cardiol* 1990;15:808–813.

23. Factor SM, Butany J, Sole MJ, Wigle ED, Williams WC, Rojkind M. Pathologic fibrosis and matrix connective tissue in the subaortic myocardium of patients with hypertrophic cardiomyopathy. *J Am Coll Cardiol* 1991;17:1343–1351.

24. Tanaka M, Fujiwara H, Onodera T, Wu D-J, Hamashima Y, Kawai C. Quantitative analysis of myocardial fibrosis in normals, hypertensive hearts, and hypertrophic cardiomyopathy. *Br Heart J* 1986;55:575–581.

25. Maron BJ, Wolfson JK, Epstein SE, Roberts WC. Intramural ("small vessel") coronary artery disease in hypertrophic cardiomyopathy. *J Am Coll Cardiol* 1986;8:545–557.

Myocardial Disarray at Junction of Ventricular Septum and Left and Right Ventricular Free Walls in Hypertrophic Cardiomyopathy

Toshiro Kuribayashi, MD, and William C. Roberts, MD

The abnormality of the myocardium in hearts with hypertrophic cardiomyopathy (HC) was assessed regarding whether the muscle bundle in the midwall layer maintains its normal circular and continuous orientation surrounding the left ventricular (LV) cavity. Forty-seven autopsied hearts with HC were examined. The LV wall midway between the base and apex was divided into 6 segments in the transverse plane. Histologically, the circular orientation was destroyed largely or completely due to marked fascicle disarray in 77% of the anterior and posterior junctional segments. In 33% of the middle portion of the ventricular septum and in 34% of the anterior and posterior portions of the LV free wall, the midwall layer showed disarray of muscle fibers or small fascicles. In contrast, the lateral LV free wall was devoid of disarranged fibers in its midwall layer. Myocardial fibrosis usually was predominant in the portion where disarray was marked. There were deep tissue clefts often in the area of junction. In 11 hearts (7 from patients aged >65 years), the circular unit was intact in almost every segment, as it was in 9 of 10 control hearts. The destruction of the circular unit in the area of septal-free wall junctions in most patients with HC is a previously undescribed morphologic feature of HC. This discontinuity may result from retention of an abnormal fetal myocardial architecture in which the septal latitudinal muscle was continuous with the right ventricular free wall.

(Am J Cardiol 1992;70:1333–1340)

From the Pathology Branch, National Heart, Lung, and Blood Institute, National Institutes of Health, Bethesda, Maryland. Dr. Kuribayashi was supported in part by Meiji Institute of Health Science, Odawara, Japan. Manuscript received March 11, 1992; revised manuscript received July 8, 1992, and accepted July 9.

Address for reprints: Toshiro Kuribayashi, MD, Department of Anatomy, Kyoto Prefectural University of Medicine, Kawaramachi-Hirokoji, Kamigyo-Ku Kyoto, 602, Japan.

Since the report by Teare[1] on hypertrophic cardiomyopathy (HC), myocardial disarray has generally been considered a characteristic morphologic feature of this condition.[2–6] Various kinds of myocardial disarray have been demonstrated in hearts with HC, including disarray of myofilaments, myofibrils, fibers and fascicles.[1–6] The disarray, however, has lost its specificity for HC owing to its presence in some normal hearts and in hearts with various other diseases, particularly congenital heart disease.[7–17] In the present study, myocardial architecture was examined from a new point of view. In normal hearts, the muscle fiber orientation across the left ventricular (LV) wall approximately midway between the base and apex changes gradually from the endocardium to the epicardium, or to the right-sided endocardium, with latitudinal fibers predominating in the midwall layer, and longitudinal or oblique fibers on its inner and outer sides. The midwall latitudinal fiber bundle is smoothly continuous between the LV free wall and ventricular septum, constituting a circular unit surrounding the LV cavity.[18–20] Thus, the LV midwall muscle bundle of hearts with HC was assessed to determine if it deviated from the normal circular orientation, and if so, to what degree.

METHODS

Subjects: We examined 47 necropsy hearts of patients with HC and without severe LV fibrosis (Table I). Certain clinical and morphologic findings have been described elsewhere.[21] Patients included 25 males aged 11 to 71 years (mean 30 ± 16), and 22 females aged 16 to 83 years (mean 42 ± 34); 8 patients were aged >65 years. Nine of 13 patients with cardiac catheterization had LV outflow tract obstruction at rest or with provocation. Ten normal hearts also were examined.

Tissue preparation: The LV wall was cut transversely midway between the base and apex, and divided into 6 segments (Figure 1): anterior and posterior areas of junction, middle portion of the ventricular septum between the 2 junctions, and anterior, posterior and lateral segments of the LV free wall (the latter including the area immediately posterior to the anterior papillary muscle and most distant from both junctions). All 47 hearts contained the anterior or posterior junctional segment, or both, but did not always contain all 6 segments. The lateral segment of all hearts available appeared obviously intact on macroscopic observation. Hence, the segment was sampled for tissue sections from 19 hearts with HC, the junctional segments of which macroscopically displayed severe derangement. Tissue sections (5 to 7 microns in thickness) were made

TABLE I Clinical and Gross Morphologic Data in 47 Patients with Hypertrophic Cardiomyopathy	
Age (year)	11–83 (40 ± 21)
Male/female	25/22
Family history	
Positive	6
Unclear	43
Mode of death	
Sudden	29 (62%)
Cardiac	6 (13%)
Noncardiac	9 (19%)
Unknown	3 (6%)
History of systemic hypertension*	5 (11%)
Heart weight (g)	250–1,250 (524 ± 206)
Ventricular septum thicker than free wall	34 (72%)
Left ventricular outflow	
Obstruction	9 (19%)
No obstruction	4 (9%)
Unknown	34 (72%)
Left ventricular cavity dilatation	11 (23%)
Epicardial coronary artery disease	3 (6%)

*Systolic pressure >140 mm Hg or diastolic pressure >90 mm Hg, or both; pressure gradient >30 mm Hg at rest or with provocation.

parallel to the transverse plane and stained with Masson's trichrome.

Assessment of myocardial abnormality: In each of the 6 wall segments, the assessment was performed by microscopic observation under a magnification of ×8 to 20. The extent to which the midwall fiber bundle deviated from the circular orientation was graded as follows: 0, individual muscle fibers in the midwall layer were normally arranged (Figures 2A, 3D, 4D and 5B); 1+, muscle fibers in the midwall layer were slightly deviated from parallel alignment mainly due to the development of side branches, but the fiber bundle as a whole had clear circular orientation (Figures 3B and 4C); 2+, muscle fibers and small fascicles in the midwall layer were considerably disarranged, but the latitudinal muscle bundle as a whole maintained a circular orientation (Figures 2D, 3C and 4B); 3+, muscle fibers or fascicles, or both, in the midwall layer were highly disarranged, and there was no circular unit of muscle bundle (Figures 2B, 2C, 3A and 4A).

Fibrosis in the midwall layer was graded as follows: 0, no fibrosis; 1+, increased interstitial fibrosis; and 2+,

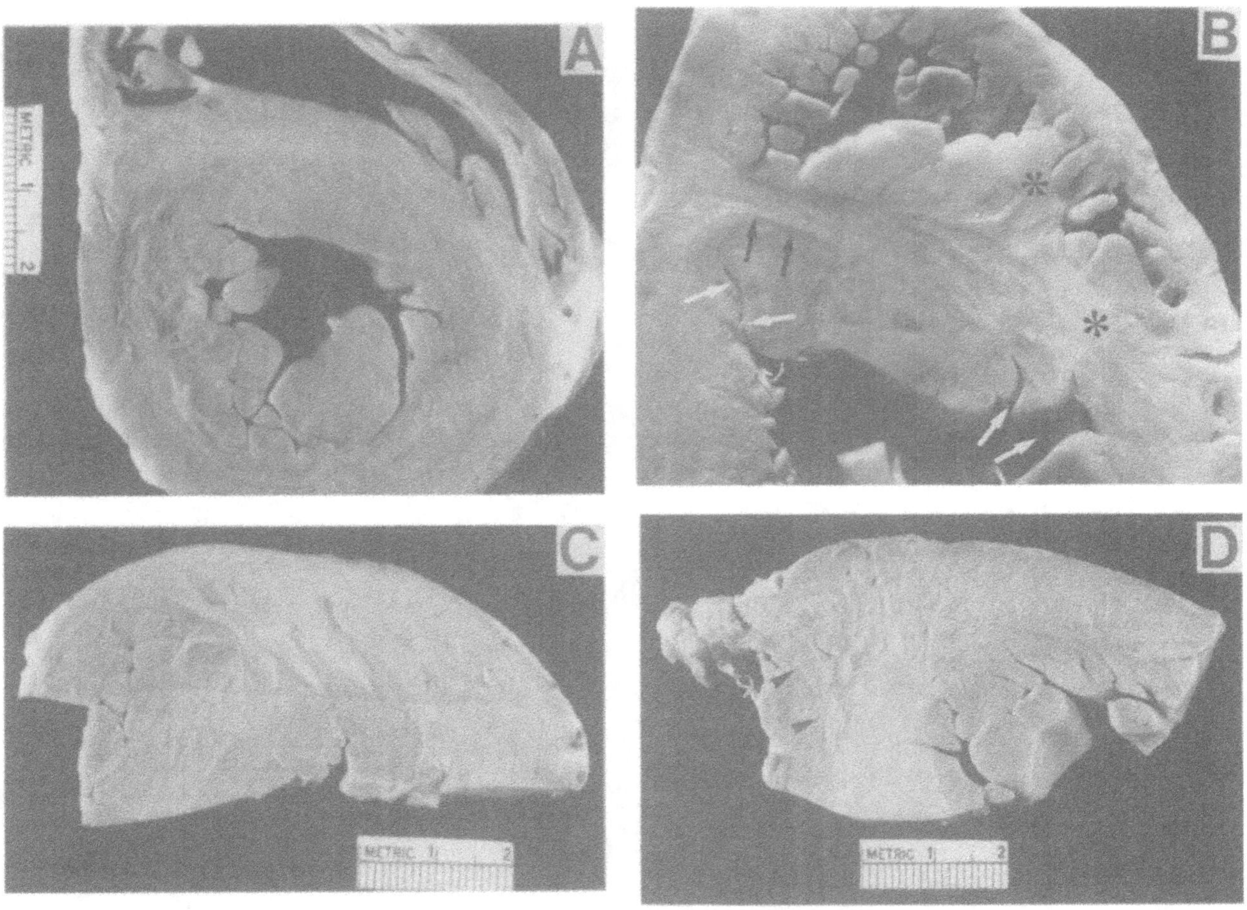

FIGURE 1. Transversely cut surface of ventricular wall approximately midway between base and apex. *A,* normal heart. *B to D,* hearts with hypertrophic cardiomyopathy. A, circular muscle layer through midwall, which is smoothly continuous between ventricular septum and left ventricular free wall. *B,* in area of anterior junction on right side, ventricular septum comprises 2 components *(asterisks)*: 1 continuous with right ventricular free wall and the other with left ventricular free wall, the 2 being separated by a large tissue cleft. In area of posterior junction, there is fiber bundle oriented from septal midwall toward right ventricle *(black arrows)*. There are deep endocardial notches in junctional areas *(white arrows)*. *C,* posterior half of heart. In area of junction between septum and left ventricle, there are fiber fascicles oriented perpendicularly to circular direction surrounding left ventricle. *D,* posterior junction. There is fiber bundle that is continuous between ventricular septum and right ventricular free wall *(arrowheads)*.

focal replacement scars of various sizes (Figure 2C). In addition, tissue clefts of unknown nature lined with endothelium often were present in the area of junction and were graded as follows: 0, no cleft; 1+, <3 clefts; and 2+, clefts present in mesh-like fashion (Figure 5A). Endocardial notches partly due to large trabeculae carneae (Figure 1B), which also were not rare in the junctional areas of hearts with HC, were not considered to be the tissue cleft.

Furthermore, histologic features were assessed separately in the small area of junction between the ventricular septum and right ventricular free wall, because this area appeared somewhat different from other areas in that pathologic changes were not rare in normal control hearts (Figure 5B). The deviation of individual muscle fibers from parallel alignment and the presence of interstitial fibrosis or scars each were given scores of 0 to 2+ according to severity.

Statistical analysis: The grade of abnormalities between hearts with HC and normal hearts were compared by the Mann-Whitney test. The grade of abnormalities between the 6 portions of the hearts with HC was compared by either chi-square or Fisher's exact test, as appropriate.

RESULTS

Normal hearts: The midwall muscle layer almost always formed a smooth circular unit surrounding the LV cavity macroscopically and microscopically (Figures 1A, 2A and 6A, and Table II). In the small area of junctions between the ventricular septum and right ventricular free wall, myocyte disarray and fibrosis were not rare in control hearts, although the severity was significantly lower than in the hearts with HC (Table III). Furthermore, the disarray and fibrosis in this portion of the normal heart did not extend to the middle circular muscle bundle (Figures 5B and 6A).

Hearts with hypertrophic cardiomyopathy: The cut surface of hearts with HC usually did not have the smooth continuity between the ventricular septum and LV free wall; there often was a fiber bundle directed from the ventricular septum toward the right ventricular free wall (Figure 1, B to D). The histology of the junctional area revealed fascicle disarray, with individu-

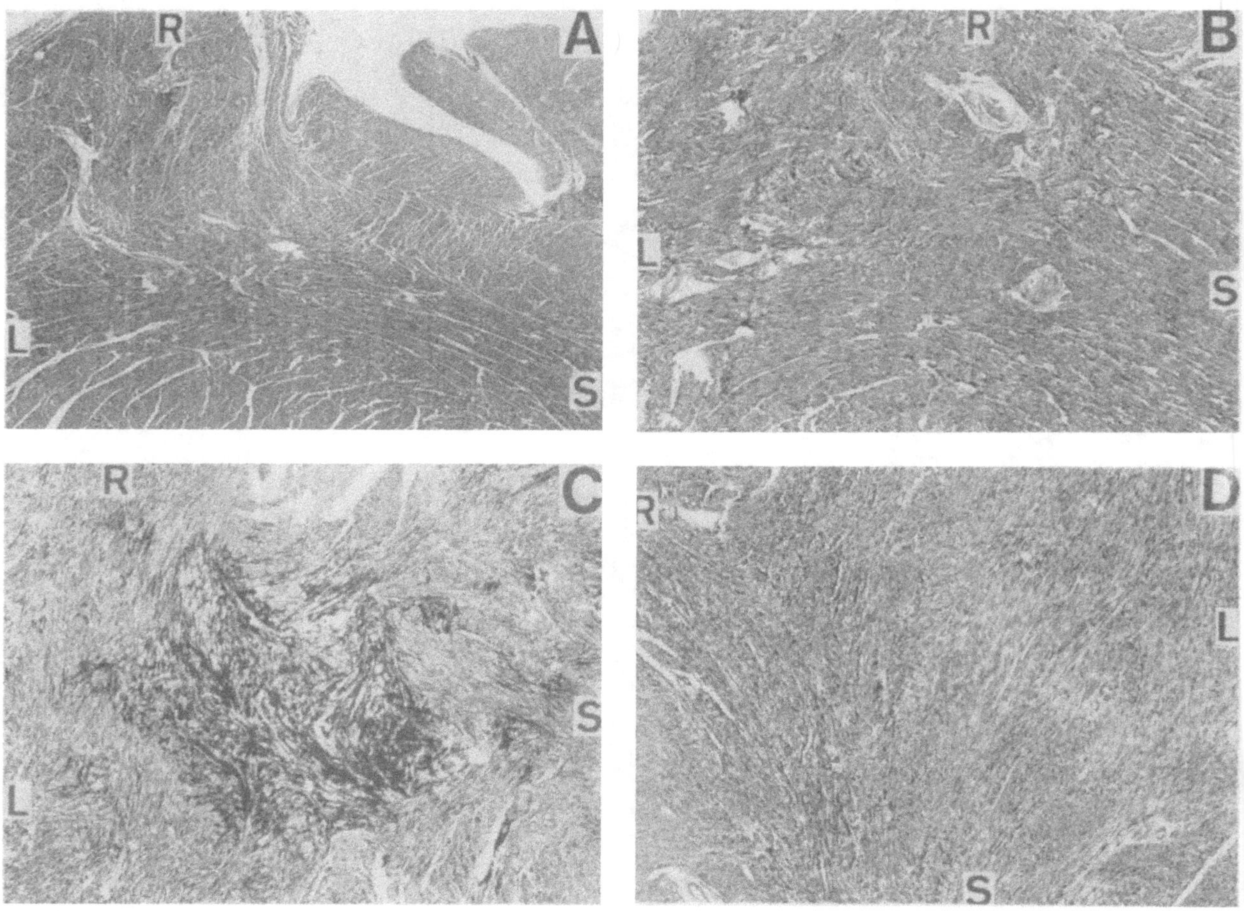

FIGURE 2. Left (L) and right (R) ventricular free walls, and ventricular septum (S). ***A*, posterior area of junction from same heart as in Figure 1A. Muscle fibers in midwall layer are aligned parallel to each other and oriented along circular direction surrounding left ventricle. *B to D*, hearts with hypertrophic cardiomyopathy. *B*, posterior area of junction. Normally oriented latitudinal muscle fiber bundles in left ventricular free wall and S are involved in fascicle disarray and lose their continuity at junction. *C*, posterior junctional area. There is large focal or replacement fibrosis at junction, with marked fascicle disarray of middle latitudinal muscle layer on both septal and left ventricular sides. *D*, from same specimen as in Figure 1D. *Left*, there is fiber fascicle oriented from S to right ventricular free wall. *Right*, myocardial disarray and replacement fibrosis disturbing circular orientation of muscle bundle. Original magnification: A, C and D ×8, and B ×14; reduced by 30%.**

al fibers in each fascicle usually having an almost parallel alignment (Figures 2, B to D, 3A, 4A and 6B), a type previously described in the study by Maron and Roberts.[3] There was a grade 2+ or 3+ abnormality in 66 of 86 junctional segments (77%) (Table II).

The ventricular septal segment had a grade 2+ abnormality in 31% of cases, but grade 3+ in only 2% (Table II). Disarray in the midwall layer of the ventricular septal segment usually was of muscle fibers or small fascicles (Figures 3B, 4B and 6B), with development of side or oblique branching from individual myocytes. In approximately half of hearts with HC, the location of the septal latitudinal muscle bundle deviated rightward due to preponderance of the left-sided longitudinal fiber layer; sometimes it was divided into several fascicles parallel to each other, with longitudinal fibers intervening between them.

In the anterior and posterior LV segments also, myocardial diarray of the midwall layer was mostly of muscle fibers or small fascicles, or both (Figures 3C, 4C and 6B). The grade of abnormality did not significantly differ from that in the middle ventricular septum (Table II).

The lateral LV walls were devoid of disarray in the midwall layer, even when a grade 3+ abnormality was present in the junctional areas (Figures 3D, 4D and 6B; Table II). Thus, there usually was a gradient of abnormality of the bundle from the junctional area toward the middle ventricular septum and LV lateral wall (Figure 6B).

Myocardial disarray was not rare in the layers on both sides of the midwall layer in which muscle fibers were oriented longitudinally. Disarray in these layers occurred in combination with a significant abnormality of the midwall layer (Figures 3C, 4, A to C, and 6B). Mild disarray of longitudinal muscle fibers was also seen in the portion where the papillary muscles or large trabeculae carneae were attached (Figure 6).

Interstitial and focal fibrosis also was most marked in the junctional segments (Table II). In 39 segments (45%), relatively large foci of fibrosis covered the entire width of the midwall layer at the junction between the ventricular septum and LV free wall; in 12 (14%), it was present as an isolated lesion in contact with or surrounded by severe fascicle disarray (Figure 2C). This type of fibrosis could easily be identified as a whitish

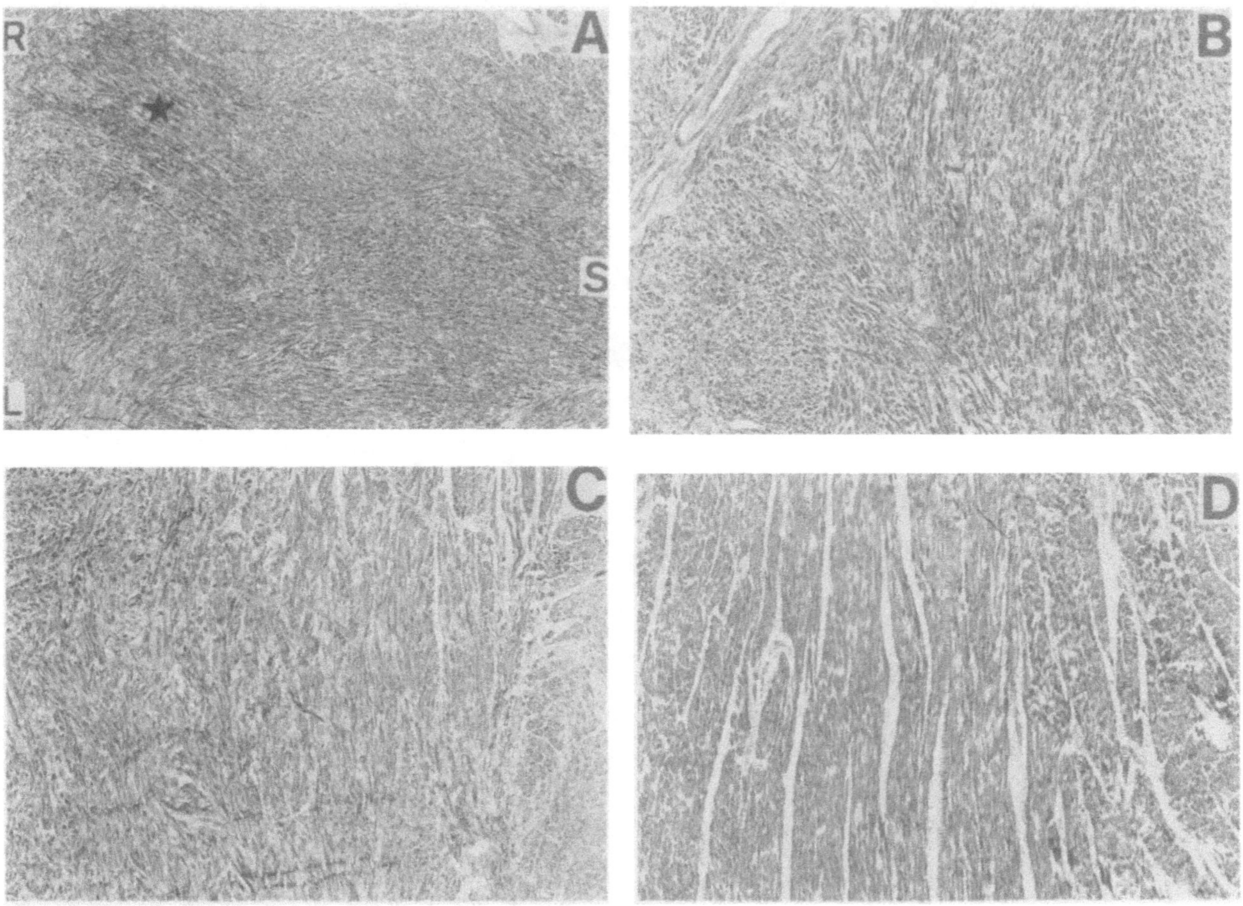

FIGURE 3. All panels are from same heart as in Figure 1B. *A,* posterior junction. Relatively large fascicles are oriented perpendicularly or obliquely to each other, and circular component surrounding left ventricle is lacking at all. There is a fascicle oriented from septal midwall toward right ventricle *(asterisk),* which corresponds to that identified by *black arrows* in Figure 1B. *B,* middle ventricular septum (S). *C,* posterior left ventricular free wall (L). *B and C,* alignment of individual muscle fibers or small fascicles in midwall layer is considerably deviated from parallelism to each other, but muscle bundle of layer as a whole maintains clear circular orientation. *C,* there is disarray in longitudinal muscle layer on *left* (epicardial side). *D,* lateral left ventricular free wall, with midwall layer showing neither muscle fiber disarray nor deviation from circular orientation. R = right ventricular free wall. Original magnification: A ×10, B and D ×20, and C ×14; reduced by 30%.

spot on the cut surface of the formalin-fixed hearts. Interstitial fibrosis also was frequent in the midwall layer of the junctional area, ventricular septum, and anterior and posterior LV free wall. The lateral LV free wall segments contained little fibrous tissue (Figures 3D and 4D).

Deep tissue clefts were restricted in the junctional segments, with a predominance in the anterior one (Table II). They were mainly located in the subepicardial layer (Figure 5A), occasionally involving the midwall layer. The walls of the clefts were lined with a simple-layered endothelium. The adjacent myocardium usually had marked fascicle disarray.

Histology of the right ventricular transverse sections revealed that fiber disarray was present in the latitudinal layer and that its hypertrophy was mainly due to thickening of the inner layer in which muscle fibers were oriented longitudinally (Figure 5, C to D).

In 11 of 47 hearts with HC (23%), the abnormality of myocardial architecture was graded 0 or 1+ in all 6 LV wall segments, although their mean heart weight (506 g) was similar to other groups with a grade 2+ or 3+ abnormality (Table I). The 11 patients comprised 7 females (aged 47 to 83 years) and 4 males (aged 14 to 71 years, mean 60); 7 patients were aged >65 years. The mean age of the 26 patients with a grade 3+ abnormality was 25 years. Of the aforementioned 11 patients, none had family history of HC, 4 died suddenly (1 had coronary artery disease), 5 died from noncardiac causes, 2 died of congestive heart failure, 3 had history of systemic hypertension, and 5 had ventricular septa thicker than the LV free wall. Only 2 of the 11 patients had a grade 2+ fibrosis in the junctional segments associated with that in other segments. The grade of abnormal continuity did not differ between patients with and without LV outflow obstruction.

DISCUSSION

The findings in this study were obtained by macroscopic inspection of the transversely cut surfaces of the heart and by low-magnification microscopic observation of the tissue sections. In 36 of 47 hearts with HC (77%), the circular muscular layer surrounding the LV cavity was destroyed by fiber and fascicle disarray (Figure 6). Whittaker et al[22] found a similar result. Considering the functional importance of the circular unit for the generation of LV pressure,[19,20] this abnormality of myocardial architecture should add another significant pathologic aspect to HC.

It is widely accepted that myocardial disarray usually is present in normal hearts also, particularly in the area of junction.[3,6,7,10,15–18,21,22] This led to the exclusion

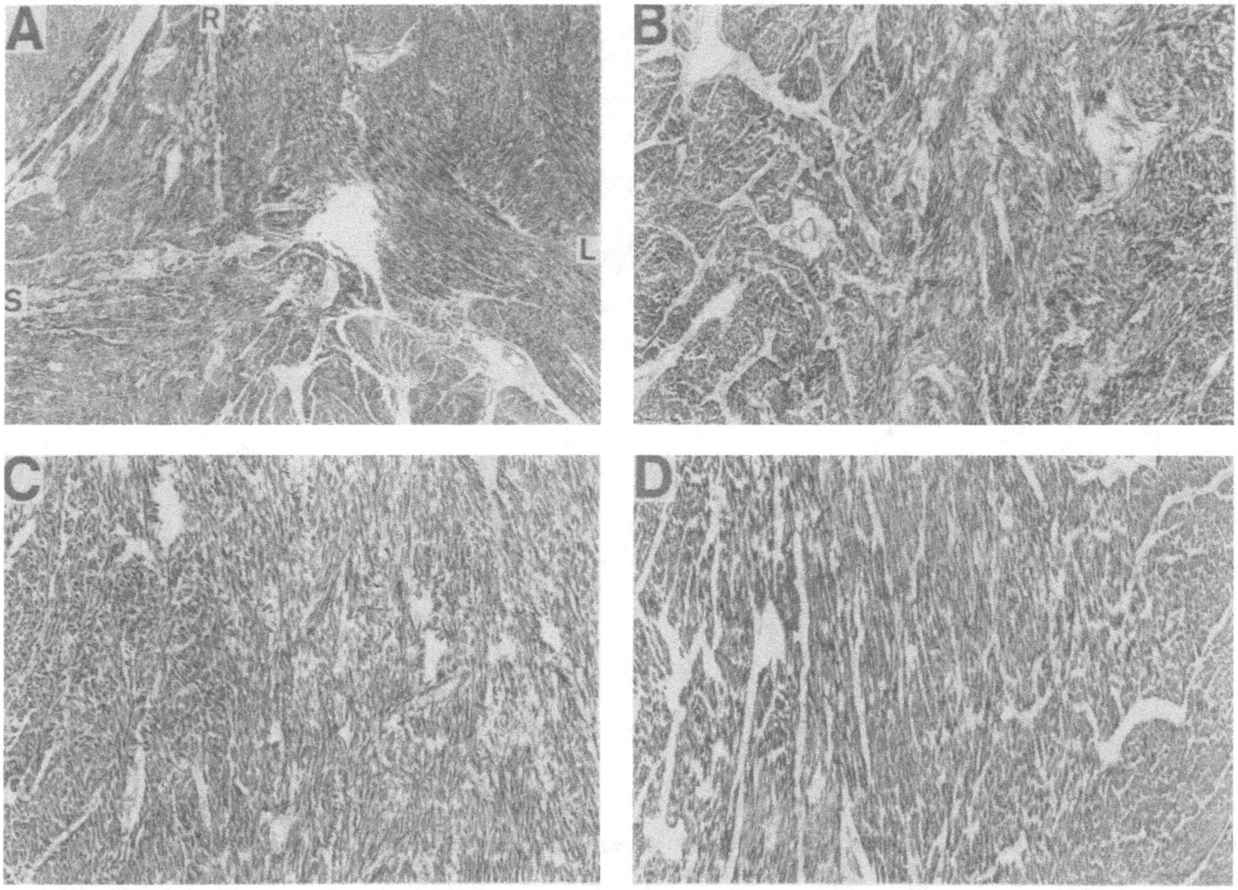

FIGURE 4. All panels are from same heart as in Figure 1C. *A,* posterior area of junction. There is no circular unit of muscle bundle between ventricular septum (S) and left ventricular free wall (L) due to severe fascicle disarray. *B,* middle portion of ventricular septum. *C,* posterior portion of L. *B and C,* circular orientation is maintained despite presence of considerable fiber disarray. Disarray is present in longitudinal muscle layers on both sides of the midwall layer. *D,* lateral L showing normal myocardial architecture. R = right ventricular free wall. Original magnification: A ×10, and B to D ×20; reduced by 30%.

of this area from quantitative estimation of myocardial disarray in previous studies.[3,22] The present study demonstrated that disarray in normal hearts was almost always restricted in the small area of junction between the ventricular septum and right ventricular free wall, with rare involvement of the LV midwall muscle layer. However, the area of junction in many hearts with HC showed disarray of relatively large fascicles in the midwall layer. It was previously described that fascicle disarray in hearts with HC is usually present in the midwall layer[3,22] and in or near the area of junction.[6]

Myocardial fibrosis also was most marked in and near the area of junction. Fibrosis is often associated with disarray in hearts with ischemia or HC.[3,17,23] The present study showed that severe disarray was often present predominantly in these areas of junction even in the absence of fibrosis, and hence disarray in hearts with HC may not necessarily be secondary to fibrosis.

Teare,[1] and James and Marshall[24] reported that deep tissue clefts were present in 2 of 8 and 7 of 22 hearts with HC, respectively. They also found that the clefts were always lined with endothelium similar to normal endocardium and occasionally continuous with the right or LV cavity, or both, but not with vessels.

It is unlikely that a synchronous muscle contraction would occur in the area of junction in the presence of these abnormalities; they may disturb the transmission of electrical activation and have a mechanical influence on the sequence and efficacy of muscle contraction, leading to the derangement of both the contraction phase and the tension direction.[24,25] The absence of synchronism here should affect the orientation of muscle fibers contiguous with this area, with the effect decreasing as the muscle fibers become distant. The normal orientation of muscle fibers is believed to need the presence of a properly fixed polarity; when the chordae are disconnected from the mitral valve, the papillary muscle develops muscle fiber disarray.[8] Furthermore, it has been suggested that myocytes and myofibrils are aligned in accordance with direction of a linear force induced by contraction of a group of muscle cells.[17,26]

The situation in which the continuity of midwall muscle bundle between the LV free wall and ventricular septum is disturbed by fascicle disarray, fibrosis and tissue clefts is similar to that in WKY/NCrj (Wistar Kyoto) normotensive rats.[27] The study of rats suggested that the discontinuity may result from an abnormal myocardial architecture in the fetus in which the septal

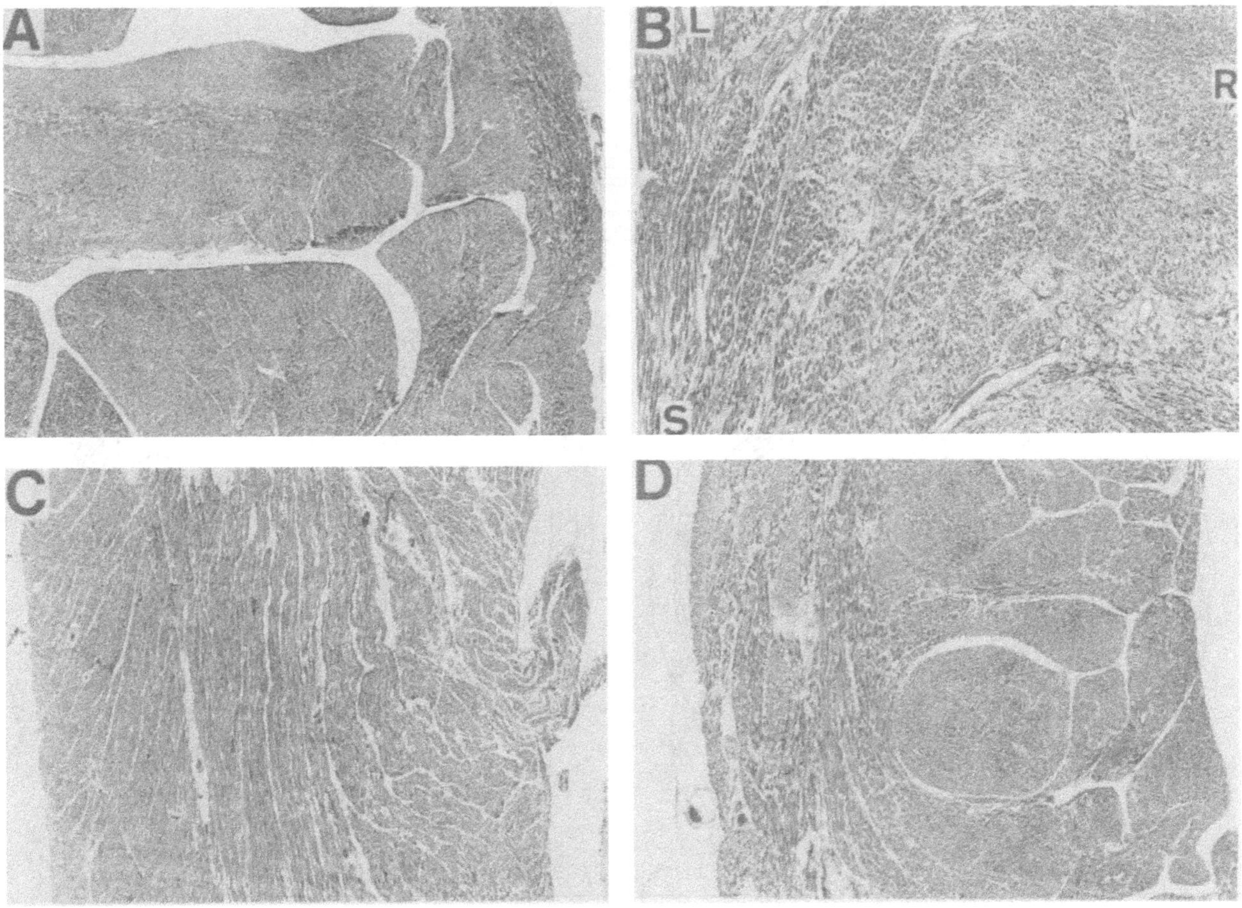

FIGURE 5. ***A,*** **anterior area of junction from heart with hypertrophic cardiomyopathy. Mesh-like tissue clefts with marked fascicle disarray in adjacent myocardium.** ***B,*** **normal heart. In area of junction between ventricular septum (S) and right ventricular free wall (R), there are muscle fiber disarray and interstitial fibrosis.** ***Left,*** **smoothly oriented middle latitudinal muscle fibers.** ***C,*** **right ventricle from normal heart. Muscle fiber orientation is similar to that in left ventricle, with latitudinal fibers in midwall layer and longitudinal fibers on both sides.** ***D,*** **right ventricle from same heart as in Figure 1C. Latitudinal fibers show disarray. Wall thickening is mainly due to thickening of inner layer that consists of longitudinal fibers. L = left ventricular free wall. Original magnification: A ×7, B ×16, C ×27, and D ×12; reduced by 30%.**

latitudinal muscle bundle was continuous with the right ventricular free wall.[28] The abnormal rightward continuity, once establishd before birth, may be difficult to remedy because myocytes lose their proliferating capacity soon after birth; the discontinuity may develop as an expression of the failure of postnatal conversion of the continuity from the rightward to the leftward. This speculation may be valid in the present human hearts

TABLE II Semiquantification of Abnormal Myocardial Architecture, Fibrosis and Tissue Clefts in Various Ventricular Wall Segments

	Anterior Area of Junction (%)		Posterior Area of Junction (%)		Middle Ventricular Septum (%)		Left Ventricular Free Wall (%)					
							Anterior		Posterior		Lateral	
	HC (n = 41)	N (n = 10)	HC (n = 45)	N (n = 10)	HC (n = 45)	N (n = 10)	HC (n = 39)	N (n = 10)	HC (n = 43)	N (n = 10)	HC (n = 19)	N (n = 10)
Myocardial architecture grade												
0	7	5	16	6	38	9	36	7	44	10	89	10
1+	15	4	9	3	29	1	28	3	23	0	11	0
2+	20	1	25	1	31	0	33	0	30	0	0	0
3+	58	0	51	0	2	0	2	0	2	0	0	0
Versus N	$p < 0.01$		$p < 0.01$		$p < 0.01$		$p < 0.05$		$p < 0.01$		NS	
Versus VS	$p < 0.001$		$p < 0.001$				NS		NS		$p < 0.001$	
Fibrosis grade												
0	12	7	18	6	56	9	36	9	53	9	84	10
1+	41	3	38	4	29	1	26	1	33	1	16	0
2+	47	0	44	0	16	0	38	0	14	0	0	0
Versus N	$p < 0.01$		$p < 0.01$		$p < 0.05$		$p < 0.01$		$p < 0.05$		NS	
Versus VS	$p < 0.001$		$p < 0.001$				$p < 0.05$		NS		$p < 0.05$	
Tissue cleft grade												
0	44	9	80	10								
1+	22	1	11	0								
2+	34	0	9	0								
Versus N	$p < 0.01$		NS									
Versus PJ	$p < 0.01$											

Number of sampled specimens in HC group is smaller than number of patients (47), because all 6 segments could not be sampled from all hearts. Incidence of each grade was expressed as percentage in HC groups, but as number in normal groups.
HC = hearts with hypertrophic cardiomyopathy; N = normal control hearts; NS = not significant; PJ = posterior area of junction; VS = middle ventricular septum.

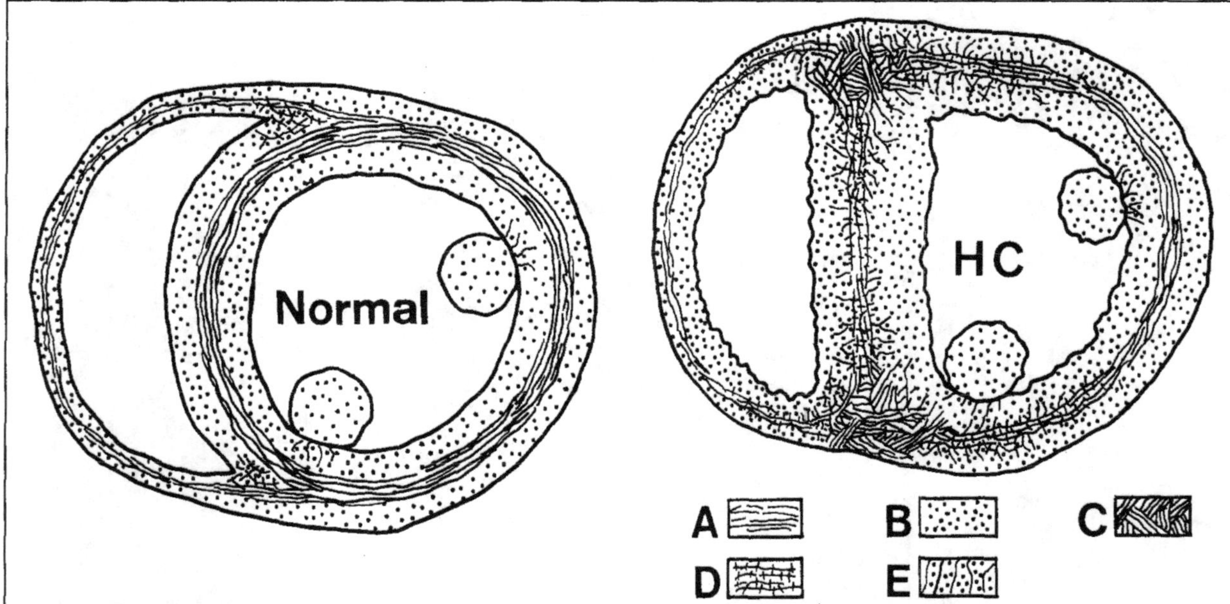

FIGURE 6. *Diagrams* showing myocardial architecture of ventricular walls in midventricular transverse plane of normal heart and one with hypertrophic cardiomyopathy (HC). Anterior surface of heart is on *top*. *A*, latitudinal fiber layer that is smoothly continuous surrounding left ventricular cavity in normal heart. *B*, longitudinal fiber layer that is well developed on left side of ventricular septum and in inner layer of right ventricular free wall in heart with HC. *C*, fascicle disarray that is marked in area of junction of 3 ventricular walls in heart with HC. *D*, fiber disarray that is marked in portion adjacent to fascicle disarray, but relieved as it becomes distant from junctional areas. *E*, disarray in longitudinal fiber layer, which is present in continuity with fascicle or fiber disarray in midwall latitudinal layer. Disarray in normal heart is restricted in small area of junction between ventricular septum and right ventricular free wall and area adjacent to papillary muscles.

TABLE III Myocyte Disarray and Fibrosis in the Small Area of Junction Between the Ventricular Septum and Right Ventricular Free Wall

	Anterior Junction (%)		Posterior Junction (%)	
	HC (n = 36)	N (n = 10)	HC (n = 42)	N (n = 10)
Myocyte disarray grade				
0	6	2	7	3
1+	33	6	45	6
2+	61	2	48	1
Versus N	$p < 0.05$		$p < 0.05$	
Fibrosis grade				
0	11	6	14	7
1+	47	3	55	2
2+	42	1	31	1
Versus N	$p < 0.01$		$p < 0.01$	

Abbreviations as in Table II.

with HC, many of which had fiber fascicles obviously directed from the ventricular septum toward the right (Figures 1, B to D, 2D, 3A and 4A).

Recently, a subset of HC with relatively good prognosis was reported to occur predominantly in elderly patients.[29-31] The apical 4-chamber view of 2-dimensional echocardiograms revealed that the elderly patients had an ovoid contour of the LV cavity, whereas a younger group had a crescent-shaped LV cavity and an ovoid-shaped right ventricle due to a reversed septal curvature.[30] Unlike the young patients, the elderly ones had good systolic leftward excursion of the ventricular septum.[31] A reversed septal curvature and crescent-shaped LV cavity are also found in many autopsied hearts with HC when they are cut longitudinally.[14,21] This may in part correspond to the present findings expressed in the transverse plane, in which the septal latitudinal muscle bundle was not continuous with the left, but was directed toward the right. Therefore, the 11 HC hearts with an intact circular unit (also obtained mainly from elderly patients) may correspond to the subset of HC with an ovoid LV cavity.

Acknowledgment: We are grateful to Michael Spencer for expert photographic assistance.

REFERENCES

1. Teare D. Asymmetrical hypertrophy of the heart in young adults. *Br Heart J* 1958;20:1–8.

2. Roberts WC, Ferrans VJ. Pathologic aspects of certain cardiomyopathies. *Circ Res* 1974;34 and 35 (suppl II):128–144.

3. Maron BJ, Roberts WC. Quantitative analysis of cardiac muscle cell disorganization in the ventricular septum in patients with hypertrophic cardiomyopathy. *Circulation* 1979;59:689–706.

4. McKenna WJ, Stewart JT, Nihoyannopoulos P, McGinty F, Davies MJ. Hypertrophic cardiomyopathy without hypertrophy: two families with myocardial disarray in the absence of increased myocardial mass. *Br Heart J* 1990:63: 287–290.

5. Ferrans VJ, Morrow AG, Roberts WC. Myocardial ultrastructure in idiopathic hypertrophic subaortic stenosis. A study of operatively excised left ventricular outflow tract muscle in 14 patients. *Circulation* 1972;45:769–792.

6. Fujiwara H, Kawai C, Hamashima T. Myocardial fascicle and fiber disarray in 25 μ-thick sections. *Circulation* 1979;59:1293–1298.

7. van der Bel-Kahn J. Muscle fiber disarray in common heart diseases. *Am J Cardiol* 1977;40:355–364.

8. Pirolo JS, Hutchins GM, Moore GW, Weisfeldt ML. Myocyte disarray develops in papillary muscles released from normal tension after mitral valve replacement. *Circulation* 1982;66:841–846.

9. Bulkley BH, Weisfeldt ML, Hutchins GM. Asymmetric septal hypertrophy and myocardial fiber disarray. Features of normal, Developing, and malformed hearts. *Circulation* 1977;56:292–298.

10. Kawai S, Okada R, Kitamura K, Suzuki A, Saito H. A morphometrical study of myocardial disarray associated with right ventricular outflow tract obstruction. *Jpn Circ J* 1984;48:445–456.

11. Maron BJ, Clark CE, Henry WL, Fukuda T, Edwards JE, Mathews EC, Redwood DR, Epstein SE. Prevalence and characteristics of disproportionate ventricular septal thickening in patients with acquired or congenital heart disease. Echocardiographic and morphologic findings. *Circulation* 1977;55:489–496.

12. Becu L, Sommerville J, Gallo A. 'Isolated' pulmonary valve stenosis as part of more wide spread cardiovascular disease. *Br Heart J* 1976;38:472–482.

13. Somerville J, Becu L. Congenital heart disease associated with hypertrophic cardiomyopathy. *Br Heart J* 1978;40:1034–1039.

14. Hutchins GM, Bulkley GH. Catenoid shape of the interventricular septum: possible cause of idiopathic hypertrophic subaortic stenosis. *Circulation* 1978; 58:392–297.

15. Becker AE, Caruso G. Myocardial disarray. A critical review. *Br Heart J* 1982;47:527–538.

16. Wigle ED, Silver MD. Myocardial fiber disarray and ventricular septal hypertrophy in asymmetrical hypertrophy of the heart. *Circulation* 1978;58: 398–402.

17. Ferrans VJ, Rodriguez ER. Specificity of light and electron microscopic features of hypertrophic obstructive and nonobstructive cardiomyopathy. Qualitative, quantitative and etiologic aspects. *Eur Heart J* 1983;4(suppl I):9–22.

18. Greenbaum RA, Ho SY, Gibson DG, Becker AE, Anderson RH. Left ventricular fibre architecture in man. *Br Heart J* 1981;45:248–263.

19. Kuribayashi T, Furukawa K, Katsume H, Ijichi H, Ibata Y. Regional differences of myocyte hypertrophy and three-dimensional deformation of the heart. *Am J Physiol* 1986;250:H378–H388.

20. Phillips CA. Left ventricular work and power: circumferential, radial and longitudinal components. Mathematical derivation with left ventricular dysfunction. *J Biomech* 1982;15:427–440.

21. Roberts CS, Roberts WC. Morphologic features. In: Zipes DP, Rowlands DJ, eds. Progress in Cardiology 2/2 (Hypertrophic cardiomyopathy). Philadelphia, London: Lea & Febiger, 1989:3–32.

22. Whittaker P, Romano T, Silver MD, Boughner DR. An improved method for detecting and quantifying cardiac muscle disarray in hypertrophic cardiomyopathy. *Am Heart J* 1989;118:341–346.

23. Anderson KR, St J Sutton MG, Lie JT. Histopathological types of cardiac fibrosis in myocardial disease. *J Pathol* 1979;128:79–85.

24. James TN, Marshall TK. De Subitaneis Morbitus. XII. Asymmetrical hypertrophy of the heart. *Circulation* 1975;51:1149–1166.

25. Brutsaert DL. Nonuniformity: a physiologic modulator of contraction and relaxation of the normal heart. *J Am Coll Cardiol* 1987;9:341–348.

26. Manasek FJ. Histogenesis of the embryonic myocardium. *Am J Cardiol* 1970;25:149–168.

27. Kuribayashi T, Mizuta T, Shimoo K, Kubota Y, Katsume H, Nakagawa M, Ibata Y. Spontaneously occurring hypertrophic cardiomyopathy in the rat. II. Distribution of, and correlations between, various cardiac abnormalities in the WKY/NCrj and its related strains. *Jpn Circ J* 1988;52:1156–1170.

28. Kuribayashi T, Shimoo K, Nakamura T, Hamaoka K, Nakagawa M, Ibata Y, Mizuta T, Komeda T, Nagaoka A. Tetralogy of Fallot, cardiac hypertrophy, pulmonary hypertension, and anomalies of great vessels in fetuses and neonates of WKY/NCrj rats. *Pediatr Res* 1990;28:429–436.

29. Fay WP, Taliercio CP, Ilstrup DM, Tajik AJ, Gersh BJ. Natural history of hypertrophic cardiomyopathy in the elderly. *J Am Coll Cardiol* 1990;16:821–826.

30. Lever HM, Karam RF, Currie PJ, Healy BP. Hypertrophic cardiomyopathy in the elderly: distinctions from the young based on cardiac shape. *Circulation* 1989;79:580–589.

31. Lewis JF, Maron BJ. Elderly patients with hypertrophic cardiomyopathy: a subset with distinctive left ventricular morphology and progressive clinical course late in life. *J Am Coll Cardiol* 1989;13:36–45.

Morphologic Basis for Obstruction to Right Ventricular Outflow in Hypertrophic Cardiomyopathy

Barry J. Maron, MD,* Charles L. McIntosh, MD, PhD, Heinrich G. Klues, MD, Richard O. Cannon III, MD, and William C. Roberts, MD†

The mechanism by which obstruction to right ventricular (RV) outflow occurs in patients with hypertrophic cardiomyopathy (HC) is not well understood. To clarify this issue, 5 severely symptomatic patients (aged 18 to 55 years, mean 30) with HC and marked subpulmonic obstruction (basal peak systolic pressure gradients 60 to 118 mm Hg) were studied. Four patients also had obstruction to left ventricular outflow (maximal basal or provocable pressure gradient 12 to 110 mm Hg). The RV outflow obstruction in each patient resulted from greatly hypertrophied musculature comprised of crista supraventricularis, moderator band or trabeculae. Operative resection of portions of this muscle resulted in abolition or substantial reduction of the RV outflow gradient (to 0 to 11 mm Hg) in the 3 patients with both pre- and postoperative hemodynamic studies. The left ventricular wall and ventricular septum also were massively thickened (32 to 40 mm) in each patient. These findings support the view that marked RV outflow tract obstruction in patients with HC is due to greatly hypertrophied RV muscle, and that operative resection will relieve the outflow gradients and normalize RV systolic pressure. The muscular RV hypertrophy causing obstruction appeared to constitute a primary and excessive hypertrophic process involving both ventricles.

(Am J Cardiol 1993;71:1089–1094)

Many patients with hypertrophic cardiomyopathy (HC) have dynamic obstruction to left ventricular outflow due to systolic anterior motion of the mitral valve, and midsystolic contact between the mitral leaflets and ventricular septum.[1–5] Substantial right ventricular (RV) outflow tract pressure gradients also may occur (although infrequently) in HC[6–19] and are usually associated with subaortic gradients.[8–10,12–15,17,19] To determine the mechanism of RV outflow obstruction, we studied at operation or necropsy, or both, 5 patients with HC who had marked obstruction to RV outflow.

METHODS

Selection of patients: The case records of the Cardiology and Pathology Branches were reviewed. Five adults with HC were identified who fulfilled the following inclusion criteria: (1) RV outflow tract peak systolic pressure gradient >50 mm Hg at catheterization; and (2) RV anatomy assessed directly at operation (n = 4) and by gross visual inspection at necropsy (n = 3). Each patient had a hypertrophied, nondilated left ventricle in the absence of another cardiac or systemic disease.[20]

Echocardiography: Echocardiographic studies were performed in 3 patients, using commercially available instruments with 2.25 or 2.50 MHz transducers. Two-dimensional images were obtained in standard cross-sectional planes[21]; M-mode echocardiograms were derived from 2-dimensional images under direct anatomic visualization.

RESULTS

Demographics: The 5 study patients (all men) ranged in age from 18 to 55 years (mean 30) at operation or death. All 5 patients had had substantial symptoms of cardiac dysfunction (Table I). Four patients had evidence of genetic transmission of HC to first-degree relatives,[22] including 3 with family history of sudden cardiac death; 1 of the latter patients had a brother with HC who had left ventricular outflow tract obstruction.[16]

Preoperative hemodynamics (Table I): In each patient, peak systolic pressure gradients between the RV body and outflow tract under basal conditions ranged from 60 to 118 mm Hg (average 76) (Figure 1). Each gradient was recorded by pullback withdrawal of the catheter from the pulmonary trunk to right ventricle. RV systolic pressures ranged from 82 to 135 mm Hg.

Four patients also had obstruction to left ventricular outflow; subaortic gradients were recorded under basal conditions in 3 patients (50, 82 and 110 mm Hg) and

From the Cardiology, Surgery and Pathology Branches, National Heart, Lung, and Blood Institute, National Institutes of Health, Bethesda, Maryland. Manuscript received July 24, 1992; revised manuscript received November 20, 1992, and accepted November 23.

*Present address: Minneapolis Heart Institute Foundation, Division of Cardiovascular Research, 920 East 28th Street, Minneapolis, Minnesota 55407.

†Present address: Baylor Cardiovascular Institute, Baylor University Medical Center, 3701 Junius Street, P.O. Box E010, Dallas, Texas 75246.

Address for reprints: Barry J. Maron, MD, Cardiology Branch, National Institutes of Health, Building 10, Room 7B-15, Bethesda, Maryland 20892.

only after provocation with isoproterenol infusion in 1 (40 mm Hg). The remaining patient had no pressure gradient under basal conditions, but provocative maneuvers were not performed.

Right ventricular anatomy: Morphology of the RV outflow tract was assessed at operation in the 4 patients at the time of right ventriculotomy and muscular resection (and also at necropsy in 2 of them), and only at necropsy in the 1 who had myotomy-myectomy without right ventriculotomy. Based on direct visual inspection of outflow tract anatomy, greatly hypertrophied myocardium was observed, which decreased RV cavity size (Figure 2). In 4 patients, the crista supraventricularis muscle (both the septal and parietal limbs) was enor-

TABLE I Clinical and Morphologic Findings in Five Patients with Hypertrophic Cardiomyopathy and Marked Obstruction to Right Ventricular Outflow

	1 (CW)	2 (FR)	3 (CZ)	4 (DP)	5 (GK)
Age (year)*	28	28	21	18	55
NYHA functional class (preop/postop)	3/2	3/2	4/—	3/1	3/—
Syncope	+	0	+	0	+
Exertional dyspnea	0	+	+	+	+
Chest pain	0	+	+	+	+
LV-SA peak systolic gradient (mm Hg) (preop/postop)					
Basal	50/0	82/40	12/—	0/—	110/0
Provocation	70/10	104/104	40/—	—/—	150/—
Systolic anterior motion, mitral valve (preop/postop)†	3+/0	4+/1+	0/—	—/—	—/—
RV-PA peak systolic gradient (mm Hg) (preop/postop)					
Basal	60/0	60/11	77/—	118/0	65/—
Provocation	—	—	–	–	80/—
Right ventricle (s/d) (mm Hg)	95/18	82/1	115/15	135/7	86/6
Left ventricle (s/d) (mm Hg)	148/20	180/10	140/24	108/4	230/10
LV contractility (angiogram)	↑	Normal	↑	—	—
Cardiac index (L/min/m^2) (preop/postop)	2.8/1.7	2.6/3.1	2.8/—	4.1/4.1	2.5/—
Family history of HC	+	+	0	+	+
Echocardiographic dimensions (mm)					
LV thickness					
Anterior septum	35	37	35	40‖	32‖
Posterior septum	30	29	35	—	—
Lateral free wall	25	19	22	—	—
Posterior free wall	12	14	15	19	18
Cavity					
LV (end-diastole)	42	34	40	—	—
Left atrium	52	40	42	—	—
Electrocardiogram					
RV hypertrophy	0	0	0	+	0
T-wave inversion	0	+ (I, AVL, V_6)	+ (I, AVL, V_5, V_6)	+	0
LV hypertrophy	0	0	0	0	0
Q waves	+ (I, AVL)	+ (V_1–V_3)	0	+ (II, III, AVF)	+ (I, AVL)
↓ right precordial lead voltage	0	0	0	+	+
LA/RA enlargement	+/+	+/0	0/0	0/0	+/+
Right BBB/left AFB	+/+	+/+	+/+	0/0	0/+
Operation					
Myotomy-myectomy (or myotomy)	+‡	+	+	0	+
RV resection	+	+	+	+	0
Age (year)	23	22	21	13	55
RV muscle resected					
Moderator band	+	+	+	0	0
Crista supraventricularis	+	0	+	+	+
Trabeculations	0	0	0	+	0
Weight of resected myocardium (g)					
Ventricular septum	3.5	3.5	1.2	0	0
Right ventricle	10.2	2.2	20.0	—	0
RV wall thickness (mm)	16	7	18	—	10
Outcome	Alive	Alive	Dead (1 day postop)	Died suddenly (5 years postop)	Dead (7 days postop)
Ventricular septal histology					
Cellular disorganization	+§	0§	+	+	+
Abnormal intramural arteries	+§	0§	+	0	+

*Current or at death.

†Classification of mitral valve systolic anterior motion as assessed from M-mode echocardiogram[2]: 0 = absent; 1+ = present with the minimum distance between mitral valve and ventricular septum during systole > 10 mm; 2+ = without mitral-septal contact, but with a distance < 10 mm between mitral valve and septum during systole; 3+ = brief mitral-septal contact (< 30% of echocardiographic systole); and 4+ = prolonged apposition of mitral valve with septum (> 30% of echocardiographic systole).

‡Underwent mitral valve replacement for moderately severe mitral regurgitation 2 years after myotomy-myectomy.

§Only surgical specimens available; all others based on necropsy observations.

‖Died before era of echocardiography; wall thickness measurements were obtained at necropsy.

AFB = anterior fascicular block; BBB = bundle branch block; LV = left ventricular; NYHA = New York Heart Association; PA = pulmonary artery; postop = postoperative; preop = preoperative; RA = right atrial; RV = right ventricular; SA = systemic artery; s/d = peak systole/end-diastole; — = data not available or not applicable; + = present; 0 = absent; ↑ = increased; ↓ = decreased.

mously thickened, as was the moderator band and other RV trabeculae; the RV free wall[23] was thickened in all 5 patients (Figure 2). In 1 patient, RV hypertrophy appeared to preferentially involve the moderator band.

Two-dimensional echocardiogram (Figure 3) and RV angiogram showed a small or normal-sized RV cavity. In addition, echo-dense structures (or filling defects) were identified in the mid-cavity or outflow tract regions that were consistent with severely hypertrophied intraventricular trabeculae, muscle bands or crista supraventricularis (Figure 4).

Operative procedures: In 3 of 4 patients with evidence of obstruction to left ventricular outflow, a standard septal myotomy-myectomy operation (Morrow procedure)[24,25] was performed through an aortotomy; 1.2 to 3.5 g of muscle was resected from the ventricular septum (Figures 3 and 4). One other patient had septal myotomy alone. In 3 of 4 patients with myotomy-myectomy (or myotomy alone), a right ventriculotomy also was performed at the same operation (Figures 3 and 5). In the remaining patient, only a right ventriculotomy was performed (without prior myotomy-myectomy). Thus, in all 4 study patients with right ventriculotomy, substantial portions of greatly hypertrophied RV muscle (believed by the surgeon to be obstructive to outflow) were resected (2.2 to 20.0 g), including crista and moderator band in 2 patients, crista and greatly hypertrophied trabeculae in 1, and moderator band alone in 1; the removal of muscle substantially enlarged RV outflow tract size (Figures 2 to 5). In patient 1, after surgery, the RV cavity was dilated and showed impaired contractility and decreased cardiac output (Table I).

Postoperative hemodynamics: In 3 patients, a postoperative cardiac catheterization was performed; the basal RV outflow tract gradient was eliminated in 2 patients and was 11 mm Hg in the third (Figure 1). Similarly, in the same 3 patients, the basal left ventricular outflow gradient was abolished in 2 and reduced to 40 mm Hg in 1 patient.

Left ventricular hypertrophy: Assessment by echocardiography and at necropsy showed that all 5 patients had a particularly marked and diffuse pattern of left ventricular hypertrophy (Figures 3 and 5). The thickness of the anterior portion of the ventricular septum ranged from 32 to 40 mm; substantial portions of the posterior ventricular septum and anterolateral free wall also were also greatly thickened. Heart weights (3 specimens) ranged from 660 to 1,070 g (normal ≤400).

Electrocardiograms (Table I): Electrocardiograms showed several abnormalities, and no single pattern was characteristic. Three patients had combined right bundle branch and left anterior fascicular block, and 1 other had left anterior fascicular block alone; 4 had prominent Q waves.

DISCUSSION

This study focuses on the mechanism by which marked obstruction to RV outflow occurs in patients with HC. Subpulmonic gradients in HC usually occur in association with left ventricular outflow tract obstruction[8–10,12–15,17,19,26,27]; 4 of 5 patients had biventricular obstruction. All 5 severely symptomatic patients with HC were selected for study solely because they had marked RV outflow tract gradients. Based on hemodynamic, angiographic, operative and necropsy observations, the RV outflow gradients in these patients appeared to result from the excessive hypertrophy and increased mass of RV muscular components (most frequently and prominently the crista supraventricularis). Therefore, in contrast to left ventricular outflow obstruction in HC (which is characteristically dynamic and due to mitral valve systolic anterior motion),[1–5] RV outflow gradients in HC are the result of a static and fixed muscular impediment to outflow. These observations differ from previous speculations that RV outflow obstruction in patients with HC is produced by the projection of the hypertrophied ventricular septum into the RV cavity[7,17,19] or by systolic anterior motion of a tricuspid valve leaflet.[28]

Postoperative hemodynamic studies showed that the subpulmonic gradients were abolished or greatly reduced after portions of the hypertrophied RV muscular structures were resected at operation. This finding substantiates that these muscular components were responsible for the RV outflow gradients measured before op-

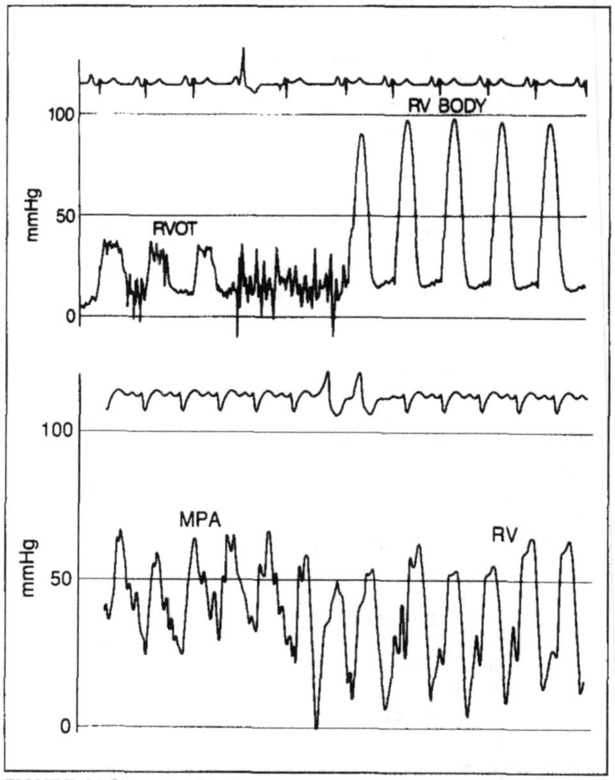

FIGURE 1. Changes in right heart pressure recordings associated with operative resection of hypertrophied right ventricular (RV) muscles in a 28-year-old man with hypertrophic cardiomyopathy and biventricular obstruction (patient 1; Table I). *Top,* preoperative pullback of catheter from RV body to RV outflow tract (RVOT) shows intraventricular peak systolic pressure gradient of 60 mm Hg. *Bottom,* postoperative pullback of catheter from the main pulmonary artery (MPA) to RV body shows that the RV outflow tract pressure gradient has been abolished. Pulmonary hypertension is present postoperatively due to elevation in left ventricular filling pressures.

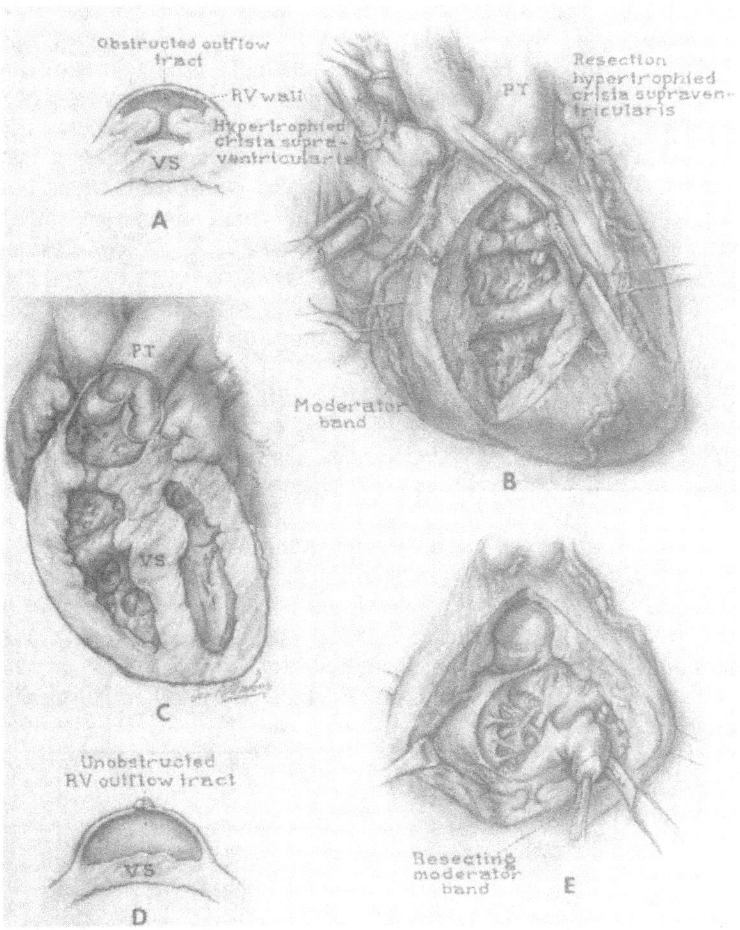

FIGURE 2. Right ventricular (RV) anatomy in 21-year-old man (patient 3; Table I) with hypertrophic cardiomyopathy who had marked obstruction to RV outflow (outflow gradient 77 mm Hg). *A, B, D, and E,* as viewed by the surgeon through right ventriculotomy at the time of muscular resection (i.e., of hypertrophied crista supraventricularis and moderator band). *C,* diagrammatic portrayal of preoperative cardiac anatomy showing asymmetric ventricular septal (VS) thickening and hypertrophy of RV structures (including crista supraventricularis, moderator band and RV free wall) compromising the effective size of the cavity. PT = pulmonary trunk.

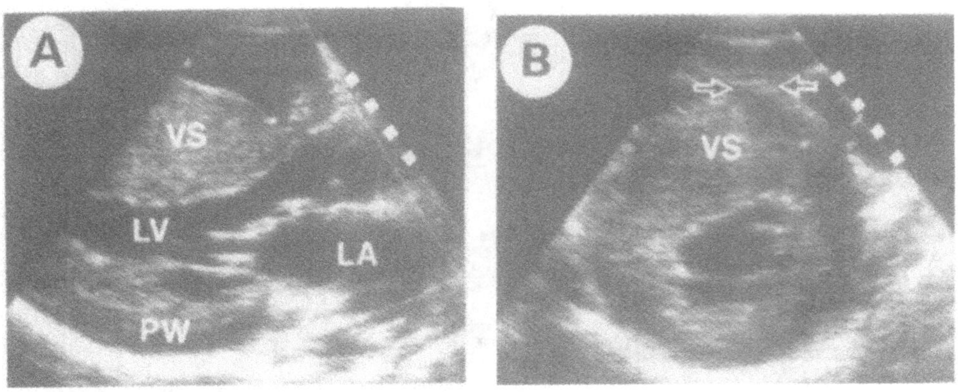

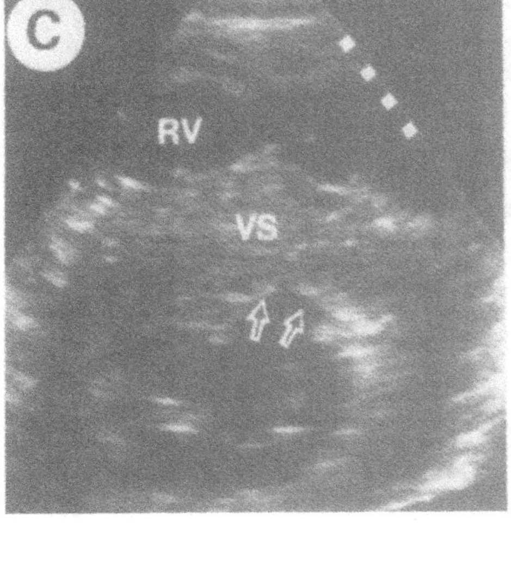

FIGURE 3. Preoperative *(A and B)* and postoperative *(C),* stop-frame, 2-dimensional echocardiograms obtained in a 21-year-old man with hypertrophic cardiomyopathy and biventricular outflow obstruction (patient 3; Table I). *A,* parasternal long-axis view showing asymmetric thickening of ventricular septum (VS) that appears to bulge into both the left (LV) and right (RV) ventricular outflow tracts, and reduces the effective size of each cavity. *B,* short-axis view at chordal level showing hypertrophy of anterior and posterior portions of septum that bulge into RV outflow tract and appear to obliterate the RV cavity at this level *(arrows).* *C,* short-axis view obtained intraoperatively at same level as in *B* after the resection of portions of moderator band and crista supraventricularis muscle. The RV cavity at this level appears dilated compared with that in *B.* There is also evidence of the ventricular septal myotomy-myectomy *(arrows).* Calibration marks are 1 cm apart. LA = left atrium; PW = posterior left ventricular free wall.

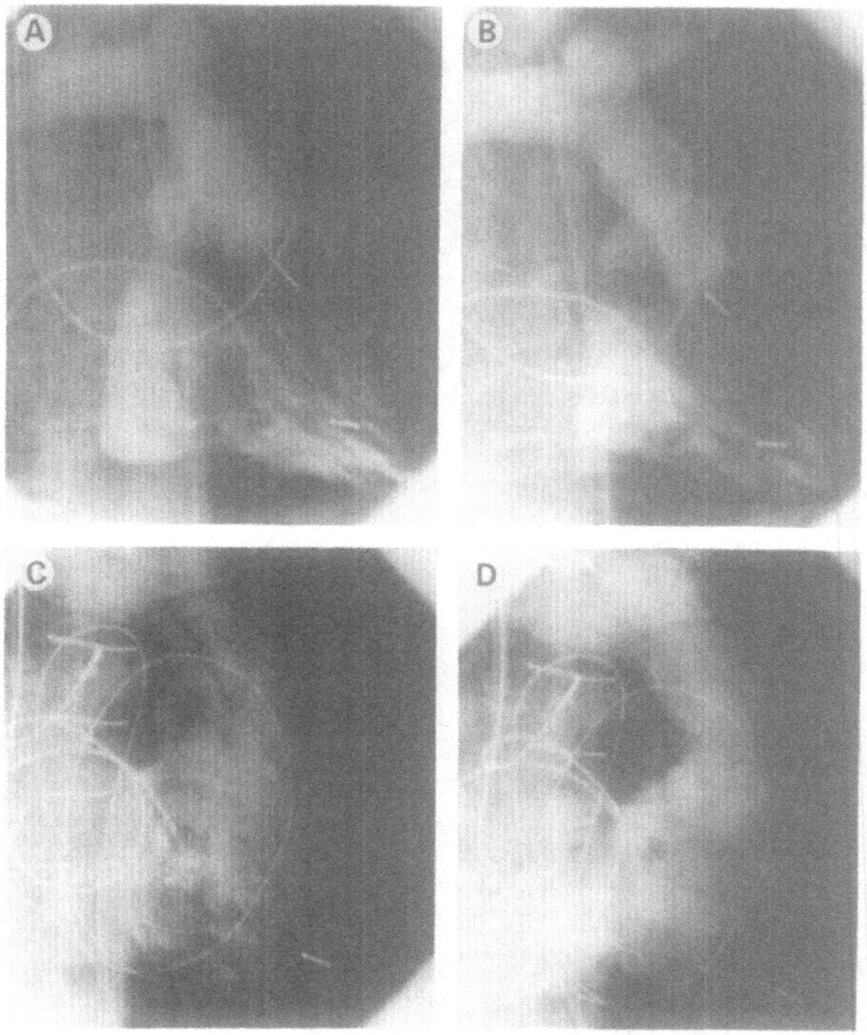

FIGURE 4. Right ventricular angiocardiograms obtained in the anteroposterior projection preoperatively *(A and B)* and postoperatively *(C and D)* in a 28-year-old man with hypertrophic cardiomyopathy and marked obstruction to right ventricular outflow. *(A and C* are diastolic, and *B and D* are systolic*)*. *A and B*, large radiolucent filling defects are evident in the mid-cavity. *C and D*, after resection of portions of crista supraventricularis and moderator band musculature, the filling defects are no longer evident.

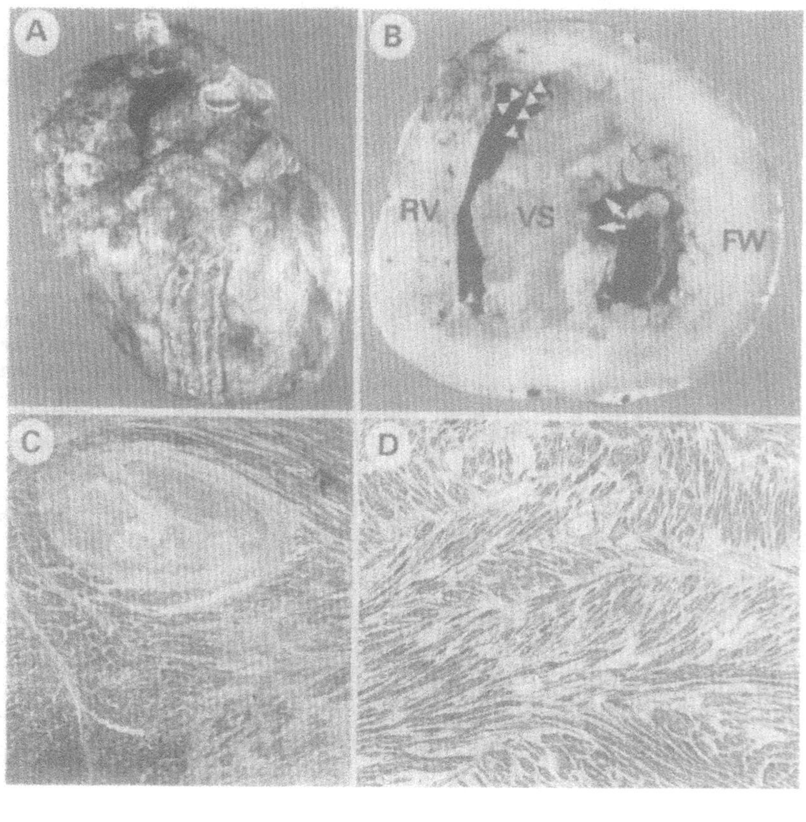

FIGURE 5. Necropsy findings in 21-year-old man with hypertrophic cardiomyopathy and biventricular outflow tract obstruction who died 1 day postoperatively (patient 3; Table I). *A*, external view of the heart that was greatly increased in mass (weight 1,070 g). *B*, transverse section showing marked asymmetric hypertrophy of ventricular septum (VS) with respect to the left ventricular free wall (FW), markedly increased right ventricular (RV) wall thickness, and reduced size of both RV and left ventricular cavities. The sites of the operative resection of muscle from RV *(arrowheads)* and left ventricular *(arrows)* outflow tracts are evident. Discoloration of ventricular septum is probably the result of an intraoperative myocardial infarction. *C*, abnormal intramural coronary artery with thickened wall and apparently narrowed lumen (hematoxylin–eosin stain ×40; reduced by 37%). *D*, chaotic arrangement of cardiac muscle cells in which adjacent cells are arranged at oblique and perpendicular angles to each other (hematoxylin–eosin stain ×60; reduced by 37%).

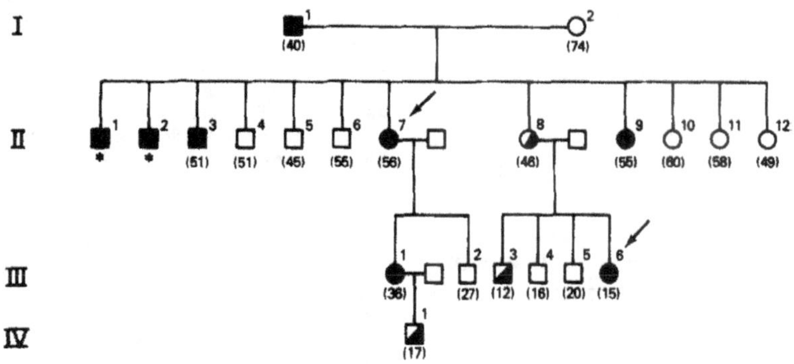

Fig. 1. Pedigree of the family. *Solid symbols* = sudden death probably or definitely due to hypertrophic cardiomyopathy; *half-filled symbols* = alive with hypertrophic cardiomyopathy that was identified by echocardiography or cardiac catheterization or both; *clear symbols* = evaluated with M-mode echocardiographic studies and considered free of hypertrophic cardiomyopathy. However, two-dimensional echocardiography was not performed and therefore it was not possible to exclude the possibility that hypertrophy was present in areas of the left ventricle inaccessible to M-mode echocardiography. *Circles* = female subjects; *squares* = male subjects. Patient's ages (years) are shown in *parentheses* below the symbols; patient's identification numbers are to the *upper right* of the symbols. Arrows indicate the index patient (No. II.7) and her niece (No. III.6); the hearts of these two patients are shown in Fig. 2. ★ = died in infancy due to unknown causes.

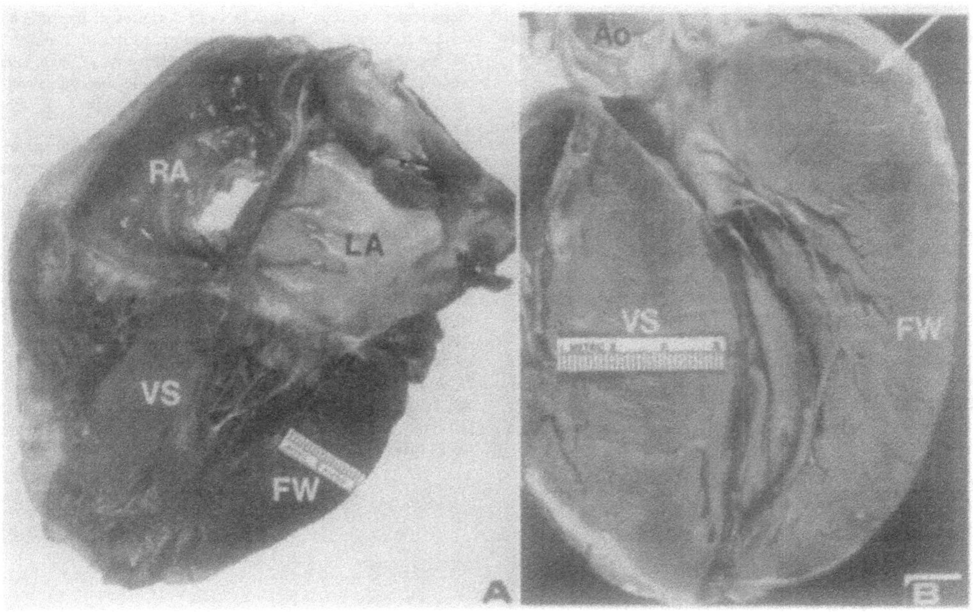

Fig. 2. Hearts of two family members showing contrasting distribution and magnitude of left ventricular hypertrophy. *A*, Index patient with symmetric but relatively mild left ventricular wall thickening and a small left ventricular cavity. *Ao* = aorta; *LA* = left atrium, *RA* = right atrium. *B*, Patient No. III.6, the 15-year-old niece of the index case. The ventricular septum *(VS)* is markedly hypertrophied (35 mm) and is disproportionately thickened with respect to the left ventricular free wall *(FW)*. Note that the distribution of hypertrophy in that portion of the free wall shown is not uniform. The posterobasal left ventricular free wall behind the posterior mitral leaflet *(arrow)* is much thicker (33 mm) than the portions of free wall located more caudad.

Six family members closely related to the index case also were identified as having HC by echocardiography or at necropsy. Patient No. III.6, a niece of the index case, died suddenly at 15 years of age without having previously experienced cardiac symptoms; no cardiac evaluation had been performed during life. In contrast to the index case, patient III.6 showed at necropsy an asymmetric pattern of LV hypertrophy and more marked ventricular wall thickening (Fig. 2, *B*). Maximal septal thickness was 36 mm; substantial portions of the LV free wall were only 12 mm in thickness (septal–free wall thickness ratio = 3.0) (Fig. 2, *B*). The heart weighed 550 gm, almost twice that of the eration and also demonstrates a suitable surgical approach to this abnormality. However, 1 patient had a dilated RV cavity with impaired contractility after operative resection of substantial amounts (10 g) of RV muscle, suggesting that excessive removal of muscle may have deleterious effects on RV function.

In all 5 patients, RV hypertrophy was associated with massive left ventricular hypertrophy. Left ventricular wall thickening was marked and diffuse, involving most of the ventricular septum and free wall; septal thickness was >30 mm in each patient and ranged up to 40 mm.[29] Consequently, the muscular RV hypertrophy causing the outflow tract obstruction appeared to constitute part of a primary and excessive hypertrophic process involving both ventricles.

We made no effort to estimate the prevalence of subpulmonic gradients in the overall population of patients with HC. Relatively small (5 to 25 mm Hg) RV outflow tract gradients occur frequently in patients with HC.[5,26,27] Although this study does not examine the etiology of such small gradients, we presume that the underlying mechanisms responsible are likely to be similar to those for the larger RV outflow tract gradients described in the present report.

1. Shah PM, Gramiak R, Kramer DH. Ultrasound location of left ventricular outflow obstruction in hypertrophic obstructive cardiomyopathy. *Circulation* 1969;40:3–11.
2. Pollick C, Rakowski H, Wigle DE. Muscular subaortic stenosis: the quantitative relationship between systolic anterior motion and pressure gradient. *Circulation* 1984;69:43–49.
3. Spirito P, Maron BJ. Patterns of systolic anterior motion of the mitral valve in hypertrophic cardiomyopathy: assessment by two dimensional echocardiography. *Am J Cardiol* 1984;54:1039–1046.
4. Maron BJ, Bonow RO, Cannon RO, Leon MB, Epstein SE. Hypertrophic cardiomyopathy: interrelation of clinical manifestations, pathophysiology, and therapy. *N Engl J Med* 1987;316:780–789 and 844–852.
5. Wigle DE, Sasson Z, Henderson MA, Ruddy TD, Fulop J, Rakowski H, Williams WG. Hypertrophic cardiomyopathy. The importance of the site and extent of hypertrophy. A review. *Prog Cardiovasc Dis* 1985;28:1–83.
6. Asin Cardiel E, Alonso M, Delcan JL, Menarguez L. Echocardiographic sign of right sided hypertrophic obstructive cardiomyopathy. *Br Heart J* 1978;40:1321–1324.
7. Barr PA, Celermajer JM, Bowdler JD, Cartmill TB. Idiopathic hypertrophic obstructive cardiomyopathy causing severe right ventricular outflow tract obstruction in infancy. *Br Heart J* 1973;35:1109–1115.
8. Bevegard S, Jonsson B, Karlof I. Low subvalvular aortic and pulmonic stenosis caused by asymmetrical hypertrophy and derangement of muscle bundles of the ventricular wall. *Acta Medica Scand* 1973;172:269–283.
9. Botti G, Tagliavini S, Bonatti V, Aurier E. Isolated hypertrophic obstructive cardiomyopathy of the right ventricle. *G Ital Cardiol* 1979;9:170–181.
10. Cohen J, Effat H, Goodwin JF, Oakley CM, Steiner RE. Hypertrophic obstructive cardiomyopathy. *Br Heart J* 1964;26:16–32.
11. Goodwin JF, Hollman A, Cleland WP, Teare D. Obstructive cardiomyopathy simulating aortic stenosis. *Br Heart J* 1960;22:403–414.
12. Grosse-Brockhoff F, Loogen F. Infundibular pulmonary stenosis in chronic left ventricular cardiopathy. *Dtsch Med Wochenschr* 1962;87:525–530.
13. Lockhart A, Charpentier A, Bourdarias JP, Ben Ismail M, Ourback P, Scebat L. Right ventricular involvement in obstructive cardiomyopathies. Hemodynamic studies in 13 cases. *Br Heart J* 1966;28:122–133.
14. Maron BJ, Edwards JE, Henry WL, Clark CE, Bingle GJ, Epstein SE. Asymmetric septal hypertrophy (ASH) in infancy. *Circulation* 1974;50:809–820.
15. Maron BJ, Tajik AJ, Ruttenberg HD, Graham TP, Atwood GF, Victorica BE, Lie JT, Roberts WC. Hypertrophic cardiomyopathy in infants: clinical features and natural history. *Circulation* 1982;65:7–17.
16. Morrow AG, Fisher RD, Fogarty TJ. Isolated hypertrophic obstruction to right ventricular outflow. *Am Heart J* 1969;77:814–817.
17. Taylor RR, Bernstein L, Jose AD. Obstructive phenomena in ventricular hypertrophy. *Br Heart J* 1964;26:193–198.
18. Von Doenhoff LJ, Nanda NC. Obstruction within the right ventricular body: two-dimensional echocardiographic features. *Am J Cardiol* 1983;51:1498–1501.
19. Wigle ED, Heimbecker RO, Gunton RW. Idiopathic ventricular septal hypertrophy causing muscular subaortic stenosis. *Circulation* 1962;26:325–340.
20. Maron BJ, Epstein SE. Hypertrophic cardiomyopathy: a discussion of nomenclature. *Am J Cardiol* 1979;43:1242–1244.
21. Tajik AJ, Seward JB, Hagler DJ, Mair DD, Lie JT. Two-dimensional real-time ultrasonic imaging of the heart and great vessels. *Mayo Clin Proc* 1978;53:271–303.
22. Maron BJ, Nichols PF, Pickle LW, Wesley YE, Mulvihill JJ. Patterns of inheritance in hypertrophic cardiomyopathy: assessment by M-mode and two-dimensional echocardiography. *Am J Cardiol* 1984;53:1087–1094.
23. McKenna WJ, Kleinebenne A, Nihoyannopoulos P, Foale R. Echocardiographic measurement of right ventricular wall thickness in hypertrophic cardiomyopathy: relation to clinical and prognostic features. *J Am Coll Cardiol* 1988;11:351–358.
24. Morrow AG, Reitz BA, Epstein SE, Henry WL, Conkle DM, Itscoitz SB, Redwood DR. Operative treatment in hypertrophic subaortic stenosis: techniques and the results of pre and postoperative assessments in 83 patients. *Circulation* 1975;52:88–102.
25. Maron BJ, Epstein SE, Morrow AG. Symptomatic status and prognosis of patients after operation for hypertrophic obstructive cardiomyopathy: efficacy of ventricular septal myotomy and myectomy. *Eur Heart J* 1983;4(suppl F):175–185.
26. Frank S, Braunwald E. Idiopathic hypertrophic subaortic stenosis. Clinical analysis of 126 patients with emphasis on the natural history. *Circulation* 1968;37:759–788.
27. Braunwald E, Lambrew CT, Morrow AG, Pierce GE, Rockoff SD, Ross J. Idiopathic hypertrophic subaortic stenosis: I. A description of the disease based upon an analysis of 64 patients. *Circulation* 1964;29 and 30(suppl IV):IV-3–119.
28. Brik H, Meller J, Bahler AS, Herman MV, Teichholz LE. Systolic anterior motion of the tricuspid valve in idiopathic hypertrophic subaortic stenosis. *J Clin Ultra* 1978;6:121–124.
29. Louie EK, Maron BJ. Hypertrophic cardiomyopathy with extreme increase in left ventricular wall thickness: Clinical significance, functional and morphologic features. *J Am Coll Cardiol* 1986;8:57–65.

Coexistence of Sudden Cardiac Death and End-Stage Heart Failure in Familial Hypertrophic Cardiomyopathy

GABRIELA M. HECHT, MD, HEINRICH G. KLUES, MD, WILLIAM C. ROBERTS, MD, FACC, BARRY J. MARON, MD, FACC

Bethesda, Maryland

Objectives. **The purpose of this study was to determine the occurrence of sudden cardiac death or end-stage heart failure, two phases of the natural history of hypertrophic cardiomyopathy, in closely related relatives.**

Background. **Hypertrophic cardiomyopathy is a genetically transmitted cardiac disease with a particularly diverse clinical and morphologic spectrum. Premature death usually occurs either suddenly or as a result of progressive congestive heart failure.**

Methods. **We describe seven families with genetically transmitted hypertrophic cardiomyopathy that were studied with echocardiography or necropsy, or both, and were selected because they were known to include relatives who had incurred either premature sudden cardiac death or the end-stage phase of the disease.**

Results. **The seven families comprised 128 relatives; 26 died suddenly, and 9 developed end-stage heart failure (including 2 with heart transplantation) associated with left ventricular cavity enlargement, wall thinning or decreased contractility, alone or in combination, as well as loss of outflow obstruction. Patients who died suddenly did so at younger ages (23 ± 10 years) than did patients who died or required heart transplantation in the end-stage phase of hypertrophic cardiomyopathy (42 ± 8 years, p < 0.001).**

Conclusions. **This study demonstrates that family members with hypertrophic cardiomyopathy, despite a common genetic substrate, may exhibit markedly diverse and distinct expressions of the natural history of their disease, which occur at widely separated periods of life.**

(J Am Coll Cardiol 1993;22:489–97)

Hypertrophic cardiomyopathy is a primary cardiac disease that is usually genetically transmitted as an autosomal dominant trait (1–4). Recently, mutations in the beta-cardiac myosin heavy chain gene have been identified in members of families with hypertrophic cardiomyopathy (5–7), as responsible for the disease.

The natural history of hypertrophic cardiomyopathy is characteristically variable and includes patients who remain clinically stable and relatively symptom free for long periods of time (8–13), as well as those who experience premature death that is sudden (1,2,14–20) or due to progressive end-stage heart failure characterized by left ventricular cavity enlargement, wall thinning or decreased ejection fraction, or any combination of these abnormalities (21–28). However, the occurrence of such strikingly diverse clinical profiles in closely related patients with hypertrophic cardiomyopathy has not been fully appreciated. This study examines such distinctive clinical variability in several selected families known to have genetically transmitted hypertrophic cardiomyopathy.

From the Cardiology and Pathology Branches, National Heart, Lung, and Blood Institute, National Institutes of Health, Bethesda, Maryland.

Manuscript received September 17, 1992; revised manuscript received January 19, 1993, accepted January 27, 1993.

Address for correspondence: Barry J. Maron, MD, Cardiovascular Research Division, Minneapolis Heart Institute, 920 East 28th Street, Minneapolis, Minnesota 55407.

Methods

Selection of pedigrees. The pedigrees of seven index cases with hypertrophic cardiomyopathy, evaluated at the National Heart, Lung, and Blood Institute, were selected for the present study on the basis of the following criteria: 1) hypertrophic cardiomyopathy was documented in relatives in two or more generations; 2) at least one relative had died suddenly and prematurely (i.e., before age 40 years) of hypertrophic cardiomyopathy; and 3) at least one relative was documented to have had the end-stage phase of the disease (21–28).

Definitions. *Hypertrophic cardiomyopathy* was defined as the demonstration by echocardiography or angiography or at necropsy of an asymmetrically hypertrophied, nondilated left ventricle in the absence of another cardiovascular or systemic disease that could itself produce left ventricular hypertrophy (29). Family members who died suddenly and unexpectedly before age 40 years (but in whom these morphologic features could not be documented definitively because of incomplete echocardiographic, angiographic or necropsy data) were also judged to have died of hypertrophic cardiomyopathy.

End-stage hypertrophic cardiomyopathy was defined as that phase representing an evolution from the typical asymmetrically hypertrophied and nondilated left ventricle (with normal or increased systolic function) (29) to a disease state characterized by left ventricular wall thinning, cavity en-

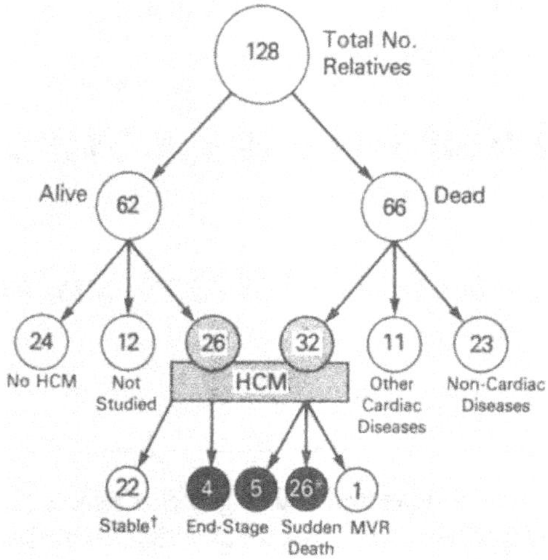

Figure 1. Flow diagram showing clinical outcome in the 128 relatives studied in the seven families with hypertrophic cardiomyopathy (HCM). *Includes 16 patients in whom the diagnosis of hypertrophic cardiomyopathy was documented by echocardiography, angiography or necropsy and also 10 other relatives without definitive anatomic documentation who died suddenly and unexpectedly before age 40 years and were assumed to have had hypertrophic cardiomyopathy for the purpose of this study. †Includes asymptomatic as well as symptomatic patients with hypertrophic cardiomyopathy but without evidence of the end-stage phase. MVR = mitral valve replacement.

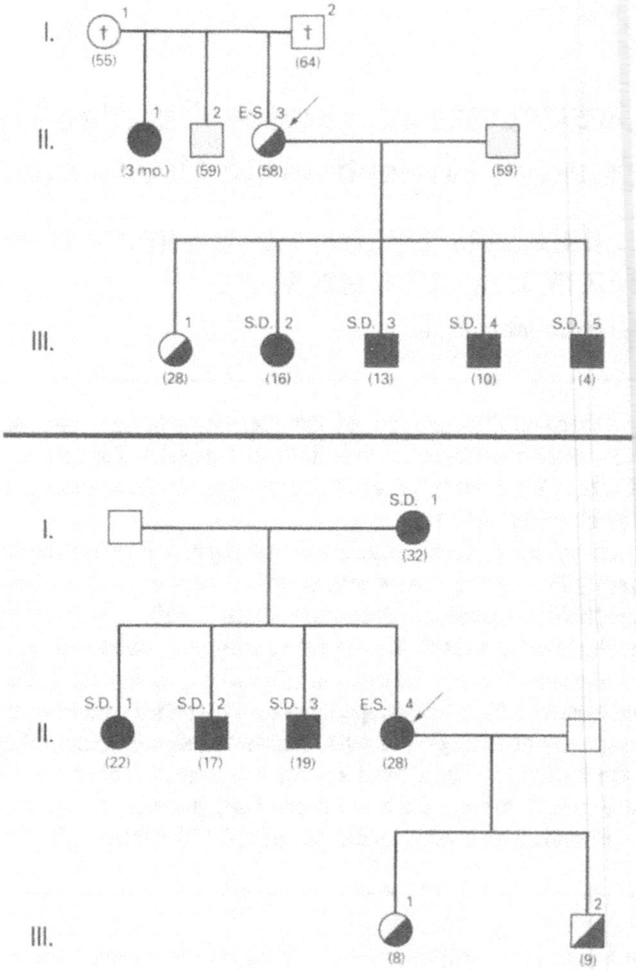

Figure 2. Pedigrees C. (top panel) and St. (bottom panel), in which family members experienced sudden cardiac death and the end-stage phase of hypertrophic cardiomyopathy. **Black symbols** = death due to hypertrophic cardiomyopathy; **black-and-white symbols** = alive but affected with hypertrophic cardiomyopathy; **gray symbols** = no evidence of hypertrophic cardiomyopathy by echocardiography; **white symbols** = subject not evaluated by echocardiography; **circles** = female relatives; **squares** = male relatives; **arrow** = propositus; † = death due to noncardiac causes or apparently cardiac in origin, but insufficient data available to judge whether hypertrophic cardiomyopathy was present. Patient ages in years are shown in **parentheses**. Roman numerals indicate generations; arabic numerals indicate relatives within a generation. E-S = end-stage hypertrophic cardiomyopathy; S.D. = sudden death due to hypertrophic cardiomyopathy.

largement or impaired systolic function (i.e., ejection fraction ≤45%) (30), or any combination of these abnormalities, and associated with clinical evidence of progressive congestive heart failure in the absence of hemodynamically significant coronary artery disease. In each study patient with the end-stage phase, these morphologic and functional abnormalities were documented by serial observations with echocardiography or contrast or radionuclide angiography or at necropsy. Specifically, of the nine relatives identified as having the end-stage phase, four patients fulfilled all three diagnostic criteria (left ventricular wall thinning, cavity enlargement and decreased ejection fraction); three of these four patients also showed a decrease in the basal outflow gradient. Two other patients in the end-stage phase had cavity enlargement and impaired systolic function without wall thinning, and the remaining three patients had impaired systolic function.

Echocardiography. Echocardiograms were obtained with commercially available instruments using 2.25- or 3.0-MHz transducers. Two-dimensional echocardiographic images were obtained in several cross-sectional planes by using standard transducer positions (31). M-mode echocardiograms were derived from two-dimensional images under direct anatomic visualization. The magnitude and distribution of left ventricular hypertrophy were assessed as previously described (32). Other cardiac dimensions were measured according to the recommendations of the American Society of Echocardiography (33).

Assessment of hemodynamic state. The magnitude of left ventricular outflow obstruction under basal conditions was assessed at cardiac catheterization (17 patients) or was estimated from the M-mode echocardiogram on the basis of the magnitude and duration of systolic anterior motion of the mitral valve (3 patients) (34). In those patients without cardiac catheterization or echocardiography, the absence of a left ventricular outflow tract plaque at necropsy was considered to be evidence that basal outflow tract obstruction was not present (35). Outflow obstruction was considered to be present if the measured or estimated subaortic gradient was >30 mm Hg.

Statistical methods. Data are expressed as mean value ± SD. Differences between group means were assessed using

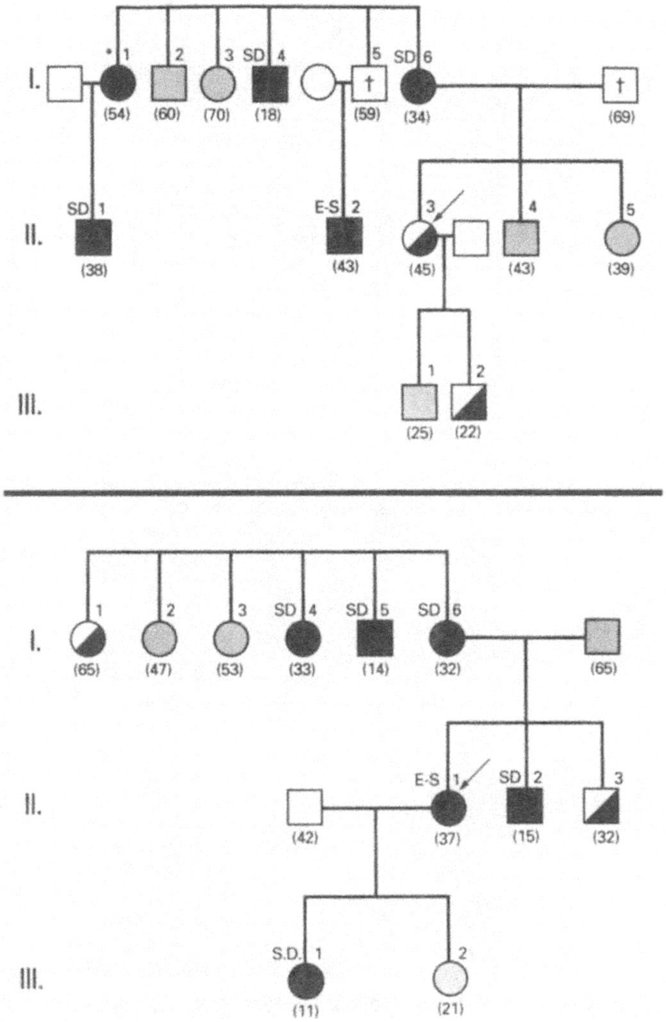

Figure 3. Pedigrees K. (top panel) and S. (bottom panel). Because of practical considerations with regard to the substantial size of this family, the entire pedigree K. is not depicted here; the excluded portion includes four relatives who died suddenly. *In pedigree K., this patient died 1 day after mitral valve replacement. Abbreviations and symbols as in Figure 2.

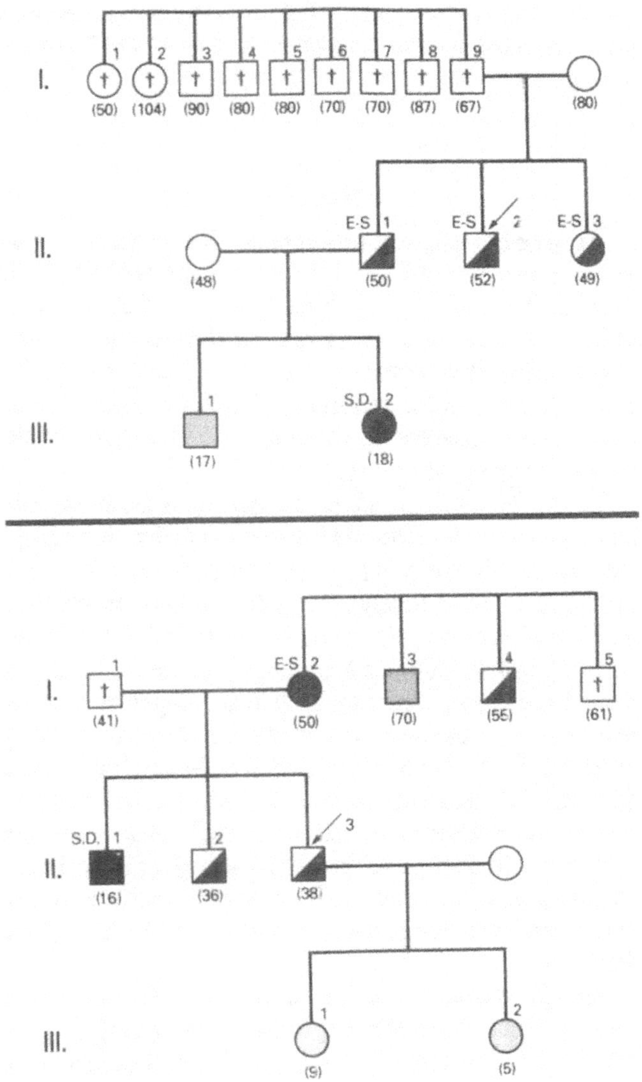

Figure 4. Pedigrees B. (top panel) and R. (bottom panel). In pedigree B., patients II.1. and II.2. underwent heart transplantation because of severe heart failure due to end-stage hypertrophic cardiomyopathy. Abbreviations and symbols as in Figure 2.

Figure 5. Pedigree E. Patients II.1. and II.2. with hypertrophic cardiomyopathy underwent ventricular septal myotomy–myectomy, 9 and 2 years, respectively, before death. Abbreviations and symbols as in Figure 2.

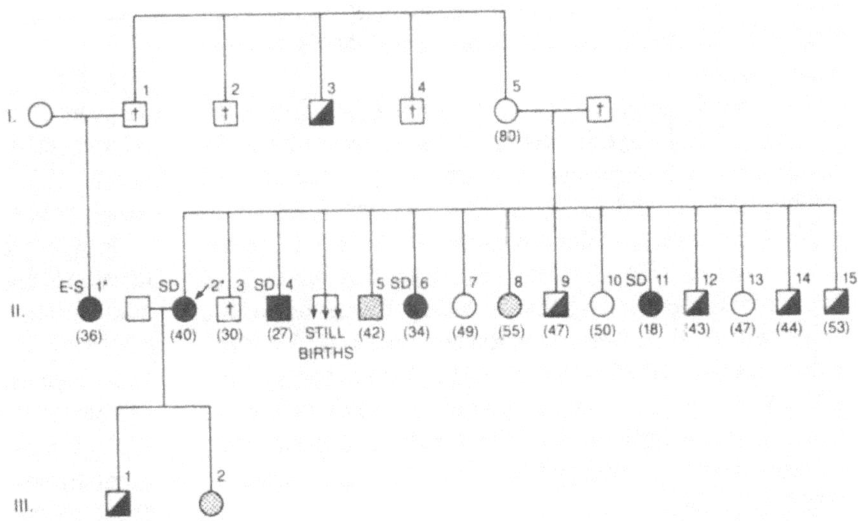

the unpaired Student t test; differences between proportions were analyzed by the chi-square or Fisher exact test, as appropriate.

Results

Analysis of pedigrees: pooled data. The seven study pedigrees comprise a total of 128 family members (Fig. 1). Of these 128 relatives, 62 are currently alive, and 66 have died. Of the 62 survivors, 26 have been documented to have hypertrophic cardiomyopathy, and 24 are known to be free of the disease; in the remaining 12 relatives, the available data were insufficient to determine whether hypertrophic cardiomyopathy was present.

Of the 26 surviving affected relatives, 4 are in the end-stage phase of hypertrophic cardiomyopathy, including 2 who ultimately underwent heart transplantation (at age 46 and 52 years, respectively). Of the 66 nonsurviving relatives, 32 died of hypertrophic cardiomyopathy. Of these 32 persons, 26 had sudden death (including 16 whose death was documented by echocardiography, angiography or necropsy and 10 without anatomic documentation who died before age 40 years). Five other relatives died of end-stage heart failure, whereas the remaining patient died after mitral valve replacement performed to relieve outflow obstruction and symptoms. In summary, among the seven study pedigrees, 26 relatives with hypertrophic cardiomyopathy died suddenly, and 9 evolved to the end-stage phase (5 are dead, and 4 are alive).

Individual pedigree analyses of (Fig. 2 to 5). *Pedigree C. (Fig. 2).* Four of five offspring of the index case (III.2., 3., 4. and 5.) died suddenly of hypertrophic cardiomyopathy at ages 4 to 16 years; none had experienced cardiac symptoms before death. Only one of the offspring (III.1.) has survived, a 28-year old affected woman, who remains virtually asymptomatic. The mother (II.3.) is also known to have hypertrophic cardiomyopathy. She first experienced mild exertional symptoms of angina and dyspnea at age 35 years; however, at age 55 years (10 years after her fourth child had died suddenly), she developed symptomatic deterioration associated with left ventricular wall thinning and cavity enlargement (Fig. 6).

Pedigree St. (Fig. 2). The index patient (II.4.) died at age 28 years of end-stage hypertrophic cardiomyopathy while awaiting heart transplantation. Each of her three affected siblings (II.1., 2. and 3.) died suddenly at age 17, 19 and 22 years, respectively, as did her mother (I.1) at age 32 years.

Pedigree K. (Fig. 3). Seven relatives died suddenly of hypertrophic cardiomyopathy, including the mother of the index patient. A severely symptomatic cousin (II.2.) of the propositus (II.3.) died in the end-stage phase at age 43 years while awaiting heart transplantation; 25 years before his death from heart failure, this patient had also experienced a cardiac arrest after running from which he was successfully resuscitated (36).

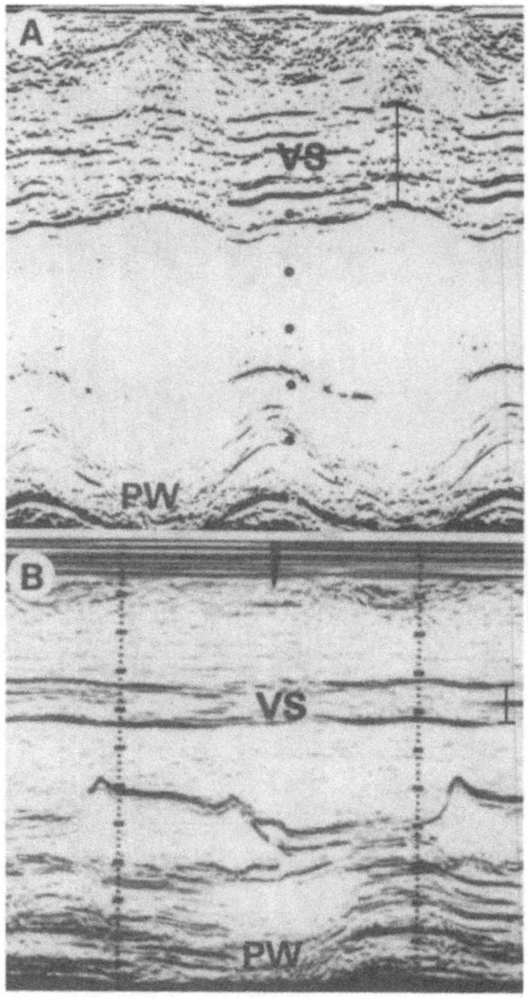

Figure 6. Two M-mode echocardiograms from the propositus of pedigree C. in Figure 2 (II.3. and also Patient 9 in Table 2), who showed clinical and morphologic evidence of end-stage hypertrophic cardiomyopathy. **A,** Tracing obtained at age 50 years, when the patient had only mild symptoms. The ventricular septum (VS) is asymmetrically thickened (17 mm) with respect to the posterior free wall (PW); the left ventricle is nondilated (48 mm in end-diastole) and percent fractional shortening is normal (33%). **B,** Tracing obtained at age 58 years when the patient had moderately severe symptoms. The ventricular septum has thinned considerably (to 10 mm); the left ventricle is now dilated (59 mm in end-diastole) and percent fractional shortening is markedly decreased (19%).

Pedigree S. (Fig. 3). The index patient (II.1.) died at age 37 years in the end-stage phase of the disease; five other relatives died suddenly between ages 11 and 32 years (I.4., 5. and 6.; II.2. and III.1.), including the mother, brother and daughter of the index patient.

Pedigree B. (Fig. 4). Three siblings (II.1., 2. and 3.) developed end-stage heart failure; two of these (II.1. and 2.) had marked replacement scarring and ventricular enlargement (Fig. 7) and underwent heart transplantation at age 46 and 52 years, respectively, because of severe congestive symptoms unresponsive to medical treatment; the third (II.3.) is now 49 years of age and severely symptomatic. An asymptomatic affected daughter of one of the siblings with end-stage heart failure (III.2.) died suddenly at age 18 years

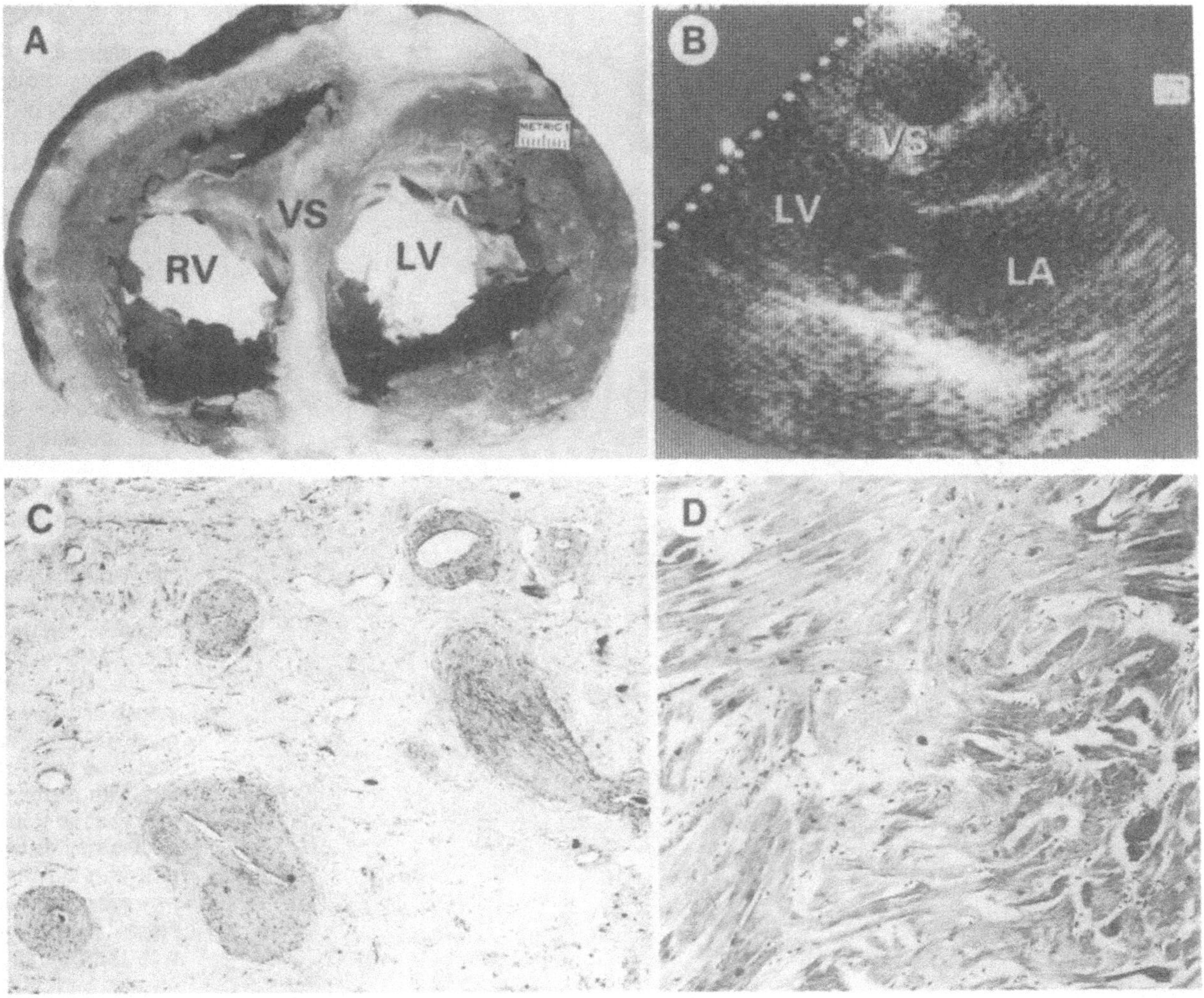

with a markedly hypertrophied, nondilated left ventricle (Fig. 8).

Pedigree R. (Fig. 4). The mother of the index patient (I.2.) died at age 50 years of heart failure after developing evidence of the end-stage phase. Of her three sons, one (II.1.) died suddenly at age 16 years, whereas the other two (II.2. and II.3.) are alive with only mild symptoms.

Pedigree E. (Fig. 5). The index patient (II.2.) and three siblings (II.4., 6. and 11.) died suddenly of hypertrophic cardiomyopathy at ages 18 to 40 years. The index patient underwent ventricular septal myotomy–myectomy 2 years before death for alleviation of outflow obstruction and symptoms. A cousin of this patient (II.1.) also underwent myotomy-myectomy but later developed the end-stage phase and died at age 36 years.

Clinical and morphologic comparisons. *Age and gender.* The 26 patients who died suddenly ranged in age from 4 to 40 years (mean 23 ± 10) (Table 1). Nine other patients who developed the end-stage phase of hypertrophic cardiomyopathy ranged in age (at time of death, most recent evaluation or heart transplantation) from 28 to 58 years (Table 2). Data were then analyzed, excluding the two study patients with end-stage phase who have survived to date without transplantation. The remaining seven patients who either died or underwent heart transplantation were significantly older than those relatives who died suddenly (42 ± 8 vs. 23 ± 10 years, $p < 0.001$). There was no significant difference with respect to gender between these two subgroups (i.e., 14 [54%] of 26 patients with sudden cardiac death were female, as were 6 [67%] of 9 patients with end-stage disease).

Figure 7. End-stage hypertrophic cardiomyopathy in a 46-year old man (II.1. from pedigree B in Fig. 4 and Patient 7 in Table 2). **A,** Transverse section of the heart obtained after heart transplantation, showing extensive scarring and thinning of the ventricular septum (VS), which extends into the anterior and posterior free wall. The left ventricular (LV) cavity appears enlarged. RV = right ventricle. **B,** Stop-frame echocardiogram in parasternal long-axis view (obtained 2 weeks before heart transplantation), showing relatively mild (18 mm) wall thickening confined to the basal anterior ventricular septum. The left atrium (LA) is enlarged (65 mm). **C** and **D,** Photomicrographs of left ventricular myocardium. **C,** Showing several abnormal coronary arteries with markedly thickened walls and a narrowed lumen, dispersed in an area of replacement fibrosis. Hematoxylin-eosin ×45, reduced by 20%. **D,** Showing bundles of hypertrophied cardiac muscle cells arranged in a chaotic pattern, with adjacent cells oriented in oblique and perpendicular angles to each other. Hematoxylin-eosin ×30, reduced by 20%.

Ventricular septal thickness (Tables 1 and 2). Among the 26 family members who died suddenly, ventricular septal

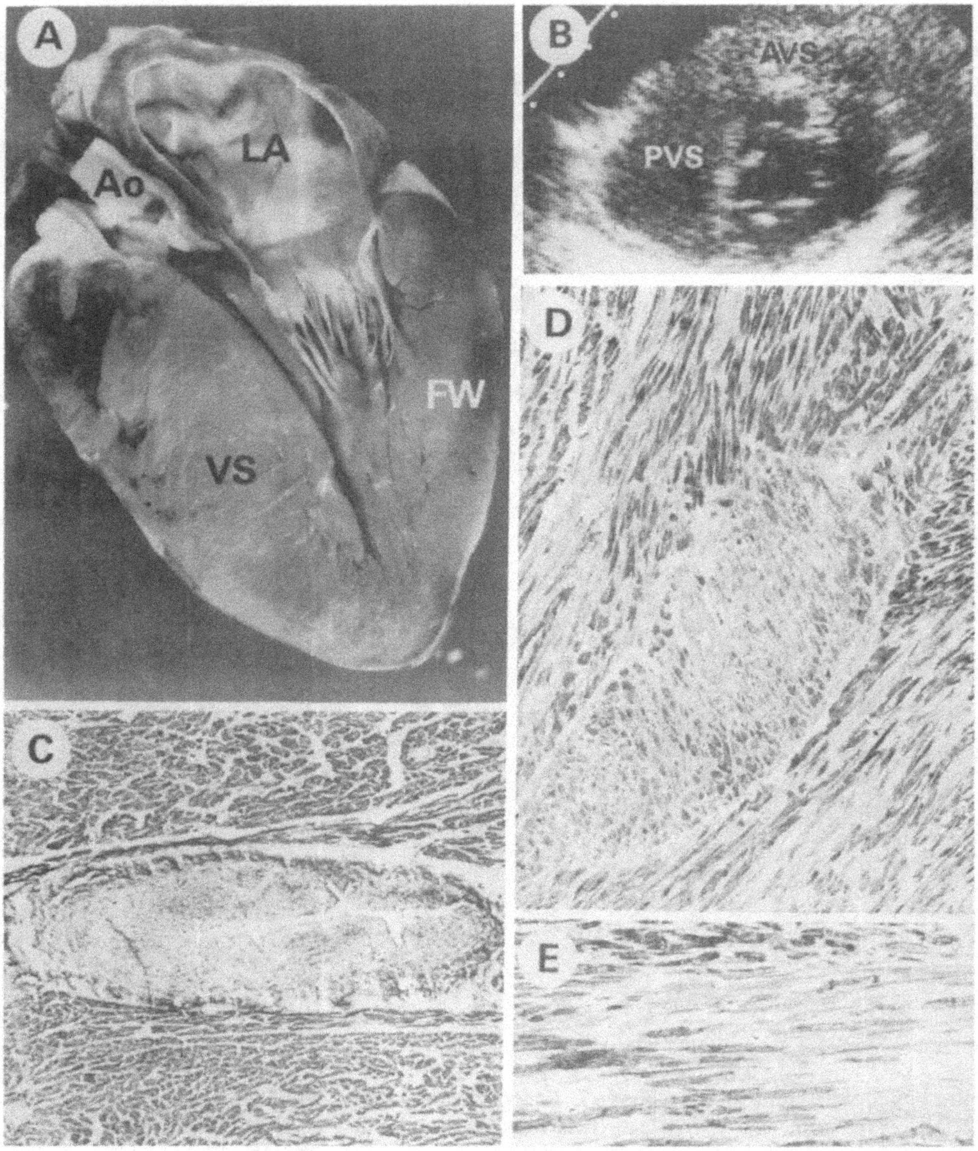

Figure 8. Necropsy and echocardiographic findings in a previously asymptomatic 18-year old woman (III.2. from pedigree B. in Fig. 4 and Patient 9 in Table 1) who died suddenly at home after running up a flight of stairs. **A,** Gross heart specimen shows the ventricular septum (VS) to be markedly increased in thickness, bulging into the left ventricular outflow tract and left ventricular cavity, which is reduced in size. Ao = aorta; FW = left ventricular free wall; LA = left atrium. **B,** Parasternal short-axis echocardiographic view from the same patient, obtained 8 months before death. Left ventricular wall thickening is substantial, with the predominant region of hypertrophy identified in the posterior portion of the ventricular septum (PVS), which measures up to 40 mm in thickness; calibration dots are 1 cm apart. AVS = anterior ventricular septum. **C, D,** and **E,** Photomicrographs of left ventricular myocardium. **C,** Showing an abnormally thickened intramural coronary artery with narrowed lumen. Hematoxylin-eosin ×50, reduced by 20%. **D,** Showing disorganized architecture with adjacent bundles of hypertrophied cardiac muscle cells arranged in a disorganized fashion with the centrally located bundle oriented perpendicularly to the adjacent groups of cells. Hematoxylin-eosin ×100, reduced by 20%. **E,** Showing an area of replacement fibrosis. Hematoxylin-eosin ×50, reduced by 20%.

thickness judged suitable for quantitative analysis was available in 10; these values ranged from 16 to 40 mm (mean 27 ± 7). Of the nine relatives who progressed to the end-stage phase of the disease, septal thickness data from the initial echocardiographic study (before the development of marked congestive symptoms) were judged suitable for such an analysis in six patients and the values were significantly lower than values in the patients who died suddenly (range 16 to 25 mm, mean 19 ± 4, p = 0.04).

Obstruction to left ventricular outflow. In nine of the patients who died suddenly, basal outflow gradient was measured at cardiac catheterization or estimated from the M-mode echocardiogram; gradients ranged from 0 to 63 mm Hg (average 25) (Table 1). In the nine relatives who evolved to the end-stage phase of the disease, basal outflow gradient at initial evaluation ranged from 0 to 80 mm Hg (average 30); in each of the four patients with an initial outflow gradient ≥40 mm Hg, the gradient decreased to zero during the end-stage phase (Table 2).

Histologic findings. Left ventricular myocardium sufficient for histologic analysis was available in 10 of the study patients who died of hypertrophic cardiomyopathy (7 with sudden cardiac death and 3 with death in the end-stage phase of the disease). In each of these 10 patients, one or two characteristic abnormal features of hypertrophic cardiomyopathy were identified (37,38), including disorganization of hypertrophied cardiac muscle cells (Fig. 7D and 8D), areas of replacement fibrosis (Fig. 7C and 8E) and intramural coronary arteries with thickened walls and apparently narrowed lumen, situated near or within areas of fibrosis (Fig. 7C and 8C). In the one family (pedigree B.) in which histologic observations were available in three relatives, findings characteristic of hypertrophic cardiomyopathy were documented in two brothers (both of whom underwent heart

Table 1. Clinical and Morphologic Data in Family Members With Hypertrophic Cardiomyopathy Who Died Suddenly*

Pt No./ Initials	Pedigree	Age at Death (yr)/Gender	FC	Circumstances of Death		Maximal LV Thickness (mm)		Heart Wt. (g)	LV Histology†			Basal LVOT Gradient (mm Hg)‡
				Sedentary	Active	Echo	Necropsy		CMC Disorg	Fibrosis	IMCA	
1/D.C.	C. III.5	4/M	I	+			§	75	–	–	–	–
2/S.C.	C. III.4	10/M	I		+		§	–	–	–	–	–
3/R.S.	S. III.1	11/F	II		+	30		–	–	–	–	15
4/D.C.	C. III.3	13/M	I		+		23	375	–	–	–	–
5/R.P.	S. II.2	15/M	II		+	§		–	–	–	–	30
6/K.C.	C. III.2	16/F	I		+		21	310	+	0	0	0
7/G.R.	R. II.1	16/M	II		+	§		–	–	–	–	–
8/R.W.	St. II.2	17/M	I	+			25	800	–	+	–	–
9/C.B.	B. III.2	18/F	I		+	40		540	+	+	+	0
10/K.W.	St. II.3	19/M	II	+			§	960	–	–	–	–
11/S.S.	K.‖	26/F	II		+		23	500	+	0	+	63¶
12/H.P.	S. I.6	32/F	III	+			§	420	–	–	–	50
13/V.B.	S. I.4	33/F	III	+**			30	470	+	+	+	0
14/E.W.	St. I.1	32/F	I	+**			16	580	–	+	–	–
15/J.S.	K. II.1	38/M	I		+		25	560	+	+	+	0
16/C.E.	E. II.2	40/F	III	+		33		–	–	–	–	64

*Includes 16 of the 26 study patients with sudden cardiac death in whom documentation of hypertrophic cardiomyopathy was available, but excludes the 10 patients with sudden death before age 40 years in whom definitive documentation of hypertrophic cardiomyopathy was not available. †Histologic features of left ventricle consistent with hypertrophic cardiomyopathy (i.e., cardiac muscle cell disorganization estimated >5% of tissue section [37], areas of substantial matrix connective tissue or replacement fibrosis [38] or >1 intramural coronary artery with thickened walls and narrowed lumen [38]). ‡Measured at cardiac catheterization or estimated from M-mode echocardiogram (34); §Hypertrophied nondilated left ventricle at necropsy, cardiac catheterization or echocardiography, consistent with hypertrophic cardiomyopathy (29), but quantitative expression of wall thickness not available. ‖Not depicted in Figure 3. ¶Midventricular muscular gradient. **Died during sleep. CMC Disorg = cardiac muscle cell disorganization; Echo = echocardiography; F = female; FC = functional class (New York Heart Association); IMCA = abnormal intramural coronary arteries; LV = left ventricular; LVOT = left ventricular outflow tract; M = male; Pt. = patient; Wt. = weight; + = present; 0 = absent; – = data not available.

transplantation because of end-stage hypertrophic cardiomyopathy), as well as the offspring of one of these brothers who died suddenly at age 18 years.

In the three patients with end-stage hypertrophic cardiomyopathy in whom an intact gross heart specimen was available for detailed analysis, marked transmural replacement fibrosis was present in the ventricular septum and in portions of the free wall (Fig. 7, A and C, and Patients 6 to 8 in Table 2).

Discussion

Natural history of hypertrophic cardiomyopathy. Hypertrophic cardiomyopathy is a primary cardiac disease for which a broad morphologic and clinical spectrum has been documented in numerous reports (1,2,32). Sudden and unexpected cardiac death may occur at a wide range of ages but occurs most commonly early in life, between age 12 and 35 years (15–20). Alternatively, other patients with hypertrophic cardiomyopathy (usually about 25 to 50 years old) may become severely symptomatic or die by virtue of developing an altogether dissimilar clinical course characterized by progressive heart failure and left ventricular wall thinning, cavity enlargement or decreased systolic function, or a combination of these abnormalities (21–24), as well as the loss of outflow obstruction unassociated with coronary artery disease (39). Such patients in this end-stage phase represent a distinctive part of the natural history of hypertrophic cardiomyopathy that is distinguished from the more typical circumstance in this disease in which congestive heart failure is associated with a small left ventricular cavity and intact systolic function (1,2).

Relation of clinical outcome to genetic substrate. The present study was designed to document the principle (utilizing several retrospectively selected pedigrees) that in hypertrophic cardiomyopathy, diverse profiles of the natural history, such as sudden cardiac death and end-stage progression of the disease, may occur even among closely related patients who share an identical genetic substrate. These two divergent expressions of hypertrophic cardiomyopathy largely occurred at different periods of life. In one study pedigree, the mother (and index patient) was virtually asymptomatic until age 50 years, at which time she developed progressive congestive symptoms associated with left ventricular wall thinning and cavity enlargement; in contrast, four of her five offspring had previously died suddenly before age 17 years without experiencing previous cardiac symptoms. In a related circumstance, two patients who ultimately developed end-stage hypertrophic cardiomyopathy during midlife had each survived an unexpected cardiac arrest years earlier (at a time when the left ventricle was nondilated); hence, occasional patients with hypertrophic

Table 2. Clinical and Morphologic Data in Family Members With End-Stage Hypertrophic Cardiomyopathy

			Initial Evaluation						Most Recent Evaluation						Outcome	
Pt. No./ Initials	Pedigree	Gender	Age (yr)	FC	Maximal LV Thickness (mm)	LVED (mm)	LVSF* (%)	Basal LVOT Gradient (mm Hg)	Age (yr)	FC	Maximal LV Thickness (mm)	LVED (mm)	LVSF* (%)	Basal LVOT Gradient (mm Hg)	Alive	Dead
1/M.S.	St. II.4	F	23	II	16	48	28[e]	0	28	III	15	48	44[r]	0		+
2/A.B.†	E. II.1	F	27	II	24	38	47[e]	80	35	III–IV	20	45	24[r]	0		+
3/L.S.	S. II.1	F	16	II	18	42	74[r]	17	37	III	13	52	35[r]	0		+
4/K.J.‡	K. II.2	M	18	I	25	49	36[e]	10	43	III–IV	14	60	26[r]	0		+
5/S.B.	B. II.3	F	18	I	§	NL§	NL§	70	49	III	16	38	40[r]	0	+	
6/M.P.‖	R. I.2	F	40	II	17	NL§	NL§	0	50	III	15	58	19[e]	0		+
7/G.B.‖	B. II.1	M	15	I	§	NL§	NL§	57	50	III–IV‖	18	55	25[r]	0	+**	
8/C.B.‖	B. III.2	M	21	I–II	§	NL§	NL§	40	52	III–IV¶	21	48	26[r]	0	+††	
9/V.C.	C. II.3	F	37	II	17	48	33[e]	0	58	III	10	59	40[r]	0	+	

*Normal left ventricular systolic function was defined as ≥45% ejection fraction with radionuclide angiography (30) and ≥25% fractional shortening with echocardiography. †Hypertrophic cardiomyopathy initially diagnosed at age 27 years after cardiac arrest from which patient was successfully resuscitated; underwent ventricular septal myotomy-myectomy 1 month after arrest. ‡First evidence of disease was cardiac arrest (at age 18 years), from which patient was successfully resuscitated. §Hypertrophied nondilated left ventricle consistent with hypertrophic cardiomyopathy (29), but quantitative expression of wall thickness, chamber size and/or systolic function not available. ‖Histologic features of left ventricle consistent with hypertrophic cardiomyopathy (i.e., cardiac muscle cell disorganization estimated >5% of tissue section [37], areas of substantial matrix connective tissue or replacement fibrosis [38] or >1 intramural coronary artery with thickened walls and narrowed lumen [38]. ¶Functional class before cardiac transplantation. **Cardiac transplantation at age 46 years. ††Cardiac transplantation at age 52 years. [e]Assessed with echocardiography. [r]Assessed with radionuclide angiography. F = female; FC = functional class (New York Heart Association); LV = left ventricular; LVED = left ventricular end-diastolic dimension; LVOT = left ventricular outflow tract; LVSF = left ventricular systolic function; M = male; Pt = patient; + = present; 0 = absent.

cardiomyopathy may have both aborted sudden cardiac death and end-stage progression within their lifetime.

The profiles of the pedigrees reported here raise certain considerations with regard to the genetic nature of hypertrophic cardiomyopathy. At present, it is uncertain whether the diverse clinical presentations of hypertrophic cardiomyopathy occurring in those relatives identified in the present study have implications with respect to the primary genetic defect and mutations in the beta-cardiac myosin heavy chain gene (5–7); this is a retrospective clinical investigation, and characterization of the underlying genetic abnormality in the families studied was beyond our initial intent and study design.

We should also emphasize that our criteria for identification of the end-stage phase of hypertrophic cardiomyopathy were relatively strict and confined to those patients with available serial documentation of left ventricular wall thinning, cavity enlargement or decrease in ejection fraction. Consequently, it is possible that other members of the families in this study who manifested congestive heart failure could have also had the end-stage phase, although validation of the precise changes in left ventricular function and dimensions was lacking. Therefore, it is possible that the coexistence of the end-stage phase and sudden cardiac death in pedigrees with hypertrophic cardiomyopathy may be more common than is currently perceived.

References

1. Wigle ED, Sasson Z, Henderson MA, et al. Hypertrophic cardiomyopathy. The importance of the site and the extent of hypertrophy. A review. Prog Cardiovasc Dis 1985;28:1–83.
2. Maron BJ, Bonow RO III, Cannon RO, Leon MB, Epstein SE. Hypertrophic cardiomyopathy: interrelations of clinical manifestations, pathophysiology, and therapy. N. Engl J Med 1987;316:780–9, 844–52.
3. Maron BJ, Nichols PF III, Pickle LW, Wesley YE, Mulvihill JJ. Patterns of inheritance in hypertrophic cardiomyopathy: assessment by M-mode and two-dimensional echocardiography. Am J Cardiol 1984;53:1087–94.
4. Ciró E, Nichols PF III, Maron BJ. Heterogeneous morphologic expression of genetically transmitted hypertrophic cardiomyopathy. Two-dimensional echocardiographic analysis. Circulation 1983;67:1227–33.
5. Jarcho JA, McKenna W, Pare JAP, et al. Mapping a gene for familial hypertrophic cardiomyopathy to chromosome 14 q1. N Engl J Med 1989;321:1372–8.
6. Hejtmancik JF, Brink PA, Towbin J, et al. Localization of the gene for familial hypertrophic cardiomyopathy to chromosome 14 q1 in a diverse US population. Circulation 1991;83:1592–7.
7. Watkins H, Rosenzweig A, Hwang D-S, et al. Characteristics and prognostic implications of myosin missense mutations in familial hypertrophic cardiomyopathy. N Engl J Med 1992;326:1108–14.
8. Frank S, Braunwald E. Idiopathic hypertrophic subaortic stenosis. Clinical analysis of 126 patients with emphasis on the natural history. Circulation 1968;37:759–88.
9. Shah PM, Adelman AG, Wigle ED, et al. The natural (and unnatural) history of hypertrophic cardiomyopathy. Circ Res 1974;35(suppl II):II-179–95.
10. McKenna W, Deanfield J, Faruqui A, England D, Oakley C, Goodwin J. Prognosis in hypertrophic cardiomyopathy: role of age and clinical, electrocardiographic and hemodynamic features. Am J Cardiol 1981;47:532–8.
11. Koga Y, Itaya K, Toshima H. Prognosis in hypertrophic cardiomyopathy. Am Heart J 1984;108:351–9.
12. Spirito P, Chiarella F, Carratino L, Berisso MZ, Bellotti P, Vecchio C. Clinical course and prognosis of hypertrophic cardiomyopathy in an outpatient population. N Engl J Med 1989;320:749–55.
13. Hecht GM, Panza JA, Maron BJ. Clinical course of middle-aged asymptomatic patients with hypertrophic cardiomyopathy. Am J Cardiol 1992;69:935–40.
14. McKenna WJ, England D, Doi YL, Deanfield JE, Oakley C, Goodwin JF. Arrhythmia in hypertrophic cardiomyopathy. I: influence on prognosis. Br Heart J 1981;46:168–72.
15. Maron BJ, Lipson LC, Roberts WC, Savage DD, Epstein SE. "Malignant" hypertrophic cardiomyopathy: identification of a subgroup of

families with unusually frequent premature death. Am J Cardiol 1978;41:1133–40.

16. Maron BJ, Roberts WC, Epstein SE. Sudden death in hypertrophic cardiomyopathy: a profile of 78 patients. Circulation 1982;65:1388–94.
17. McKenna WJ, Camm AJ. Sudden death in hypertrophic cardiomyopathy. Assessment of patients at high risk. Circulation 1989;80:1489–92.
18. Maron BJ, Roberts WC, McAllister HA, Rosing DR, Epstein SE. Sudden death in young athletes. Circulation 1980;62:218–29.
19. Spirito P, Maron BJ. Relation between extent of left ventricular hypertrophy and occurrence of sudden cardiac death in hypertrophic cardiomyopathy. J Am Coll Cardiol 1990;15:1521–6.
20. Maron BJ, Fananapazir L. Sudden cardiac death in hypertrophic cardiomyopathy. Circulation 1992;85(suppl I):I-57–63.
21. Fujiwara H, Onodera T, Tanaka M, et al. Progression from hypertrophic obstructive cardiomyopathy to typical dilated cardiomyopathy-like features in the end-stage. Jpn Circ J 1984;48:1210–4.
22. ten Cate FG, Roelandt J. Progression to left ventricular dilatation in patients with hypertrophic obstructive cardiomyopathy. Am Heart J 1979;97:762–5.
23. Fighali S, Krajcer Z, Edelman S, Leachman RD. Progression of hypertrophic cardiomyopathy into a hypokinetic left ventricle: higher incidence in patients with mid-ventricular obstruction. J Am Coll Cardiol 1987;9:288–94.
24. Spirito P, Maron BJ, Bonow RO, Epstein SE. Occurrence and significance of progressive left ventricular wall thinning and relative cavity dilatation in hypertrophic cardiomyopathy. Am J Cardiol 1987;60:123–9.
25. Spirito P, Maron BJ, Bonow RO, Epstein SE. Severe functional limitation in patients with hypertrophic cardiomyopathy and only mild localized left ventricular hypertrophy. J Am Coll Cardiol 1986;8:537–44.
26. Spirito P, Maron BJ. Absence of progression of left ventricular hypertrophy in adult patients with hypertrophic cardiomyopathy. J Am Coll Cardiol 1987;9:1013–7.
27. Spirito P, Lakatos E, Maron BJ. Degree of left ventricular hypertrophy in patients with hypertrophic cardiomyopathy and chronic atrial fibrillation. Am J Cardiol 1992;69:1217–22.
28. Maron BJ, Epstein SE, Roberts WC. Hypertrophic cardiomyopathy and transmural myocardial infarction without significant atherosclerosis of the extramural coronary arteries. Am J Cardiol 1979;43:1086–102.
29. Maron BJ, Epstein SE. Hypertrophic cardiomyopathy: a discussion of nomenclature. Am J Cardiol 1979;43:1242–4.
30. Bonow RO, Bacharach SL, Green MV, et al. Impaired left ventricular diastolic filling in patients with coronary artery disease: assessment with radionuclide angiography. Circulation 1981;64:315–23.
31. Tajik AJ, Seward JB, Hagler DJ, Mair DD, Lie JT. Two-dimensional real-time ultrasonic imaging of the heart and great vessels. Mayo Clin Proc 1978;53:271–303.
32. Maron BJ, Gottdiener JS, Epstein SE. Patterns and significance of distribution of left ventricular hypertrophy in hypertrophic cardiomyopathy: a wide-angle, two-dimensional echocardiographic study of 125 patients. Am J Cardiol 1981;48:418–28.
33. Sahn DJ, DeMaria A, Kisslo J, Weyman A. The committee on M-mode standardization of the American Society of Echocardiography: recommendations regarding quantitation in M-mode echocardiography: results of a survey of echocardiographic methods. Circulation 1978;58:1072–83.
34. Pollick C, Rakowski H, Wigle ED. Muscular subaortic stenosis: the quantitative relationship between systolic anterior motion and the pressure gradient. Circulation 1984;69:43–9.
35. Roberts CS, Roberts WC. Morphologic features. In: Zipes DP, Rollins DJ, eds. Progress in Cardiology. Philadelphia: Lea & Febiger, 1989:3–32.
36. Ciró E, Maron BJ. Unusual long-term survival following cardiac arrest in hypertrophic cardiomyopathy. Am Heart J 1983;105:145–7.
37. Maron BJ, Anan TJ, Roberts WC. Quantitative analysis of the distribution of cardiac muscle cell disorganization in the left ventricular wall of patients with hypertrophic cardiomyopathy. Circulation 1981;63:882–94.
38. Maron BJ, Wolfson JK, Epstein SE, Roberts WC. Intramural ("small vessel") coronary artery disease in hypertrophic cardiomyopathy. J Am Coll Cardiol 1986;8:545–57.
39. Ciró E, Maron BJ, Bonow RO, Cannon RO III, Epstein SE. Relation between marked changes in outflow tract gradient and disease progression in hypertrophic cardiomyopathy. Am J Cardiol 1984;53:1103–9.

Echocardiographic Assessment of Mitral Valve Size in Obstructive Hypertrophic Cardiomyopathy

Anatomic Validation From Mitral Valve Specimen

Heinrich G. Klues, MD; Michael A. Proschan, PhD; Allan L. Dollar, MD; Paolo Spirito, MD; William C. Roberts, MD; and Barry J. Maron, MD

Background. **In patients with hypertrophic cardiomyopathy, obstruction to left ventricular outflow is produced by systolic anterior motion of the mitral valve. In many of these patients, the mitral leaflets are elongated and increased in overall size. Mitral valve size may be responsible, in part, for the presence and magnitude of the outflow gradient and the pattern of systolic anterior motion of the leaflets. It may also influence the effectiveness of ventricular septal myotomy-myectomy in relieving subaortic obstruction. Therefore, the present study was undertaken to determine whether mitral valve dimensions could be assessed in quantitative terms from the echocardiogram in patients with hypertrophic cardiomyopathy.**

Methods and Results. **A group of 37 patients with hypertrophic cardiomyopathy was selected for this study by virtue of having a high-quality transthoracic or intraoperative echocardiogram suitable for certain quantitative measurements from stop-frame images as well as a morphologically intact mitral valve specimen (removed during surgery). Seven measurements of mitral valve dimensions were obtained from the two-dimensional and M-mode echocardiograms. A univariate regression analysis identified the mitral valve opening area as the best single predictor of actual mitral leaflet area measured from the specimen (r^2=.75; r=.87). The linear relation between mitral valve opening area as assessed by two-dimensional echocardiography and actual mitral leaflet area measured from the mitral valve specimen accounted for approximately 75% of the variability in mitral leaflet area. With such statistical models, it was possible to reliably identify from the echocardiogram enlarged mitral valves (≥12.0 cm^2) in 16 of 19 patients (84%) and normal-sized valves in 15 of 18 patients (83%).**

Conclusions. **In a selected group of patients with obstructive hypertrophic cardiomyopathy, a model derived from a regression analysis of quantitative echocardiographic measurements permitted (with good precision) estimation of actual mitral leaflet area and consequently overall mitral valve size and the discrimination of enlarged from normal-sized mitral valves. (*Circulation* 1993;88:548-555)**

Key Words • mitral valve • cardiomyopathies • echocardiography

In patients with hypertrophic cardiomyopathy, the systolic anterior motion of the mitral valve and its contact with the ventricular septum are the principal determinants of obstruction to left ventricular outflow.[1-14] Recent morphological studies of mitral valves removed at surgery or autopsy from patients with hypertrophic cardiomyopathy have shown that the majority of these valves have a variety of structural alterations, including increased leaflet area and segmental enlargement of the valve.[14] Mitral valve size and leaflet length also appear, in selected patients, to be a determinant of the presence and magnitude of the subaortic gradient,[13-16] the pattern of systolic anterior motion responsible for that gradient,[11-13] and whether outflow obstruction is effectively relieved by ventricular septal myotomy-myectomy.[17]

Because of the clinical implications of mitral valve size in hypertrophic cardiomyopathy and the fact that there have been few systematic attempts at assessing mitral leaflet dimensions in patients with cardiac disease using echocardiography,[15,18-21] we considered it desirable to develop a quantitative method for estimating mitral valve size from the echocardiogram prospectively during life. In the present study, the availability of both echocardiograms and mitral valve specimens from the same patients with obstructive hypertrophic cardiomyopathy afforded us the unique opportunity to validate quantitative echocardiographic measurements of mitral valve size in this disease.

Methods

Selection of Study Patients

The cardiovascular registry of the Pathology Branch from 1982 through 1989 was reviewed, and 77 mitral valve specimens that had been removed intact at surgery or autopsy from patients with obstructive hyper-

Received June 25, 1992; revision accepted March 24, 1993.

From the Pathology (H.G.K., A.L.D., W.C.R.), Cardiology (B.J.M., P.S.), and Biostatistics Research Branches (M.A.P.), National Heart, Lung, and Blood Institute, National Institutes of Health, Bethesda, Md.

Correspondence to Minneapolis Heart Institute Foundation, 920 E 28th St, Ste 40, Minneapolis, MN 55407 (Dr Maron).

trophic cardiomyopathy[14] were judged to be in suitable condition for morphometric study. Nine of these 77 valves were excluded because they had direct papillary muscle insertion into the anterior mitral leaflet.[22] The remaining 68 mitral valves were free of any other intrinsic valve abnormalities, such as floppy mitral valve.[23-27] Of these 68 patients, 12 were excluded because they did not have preoperative echocardiographic studies. Of the remaining 56 patients, 37 were selected for the final study group by virtue of having a preoperative transthoracic or intraoperative echocardiogram judged (by the consensus of two independent observers, H.G.K. and A.L.D.) to be of satisfactory technical quality for the present investigation (ie, they permitted selected quantitative measurements of the mitral valve to be made from stop-frame echocardiographic images with reasonable precision). In 25 of the 37 study patients, the transthoracic echocardiograms were of high technical quality and were used preferentially for analysis. In the other 12 patients, the intraoperative echocardiogram was used because the transthoracic echocardiogram was judged to be inadequate to make the measurements necessary for the present study. In the 25 patients with transthoracic echocardiographic studies, the time interval between echocardiogram and mitral valve replacement was 1 to 86 days (mean, 34 days).

Control Patients

Mitral valves from 45 consecutively studied patients with entirely normal hearts, both functionally and anatomically, were chosen as controls, solely for the purpose of determining the normal limits for mitral leaflet area measured from the surgical specimen. In each control patient, heart weight was 350 g or less in men and 300 g or less in women. The 45 controls ranged in age from 15 to 74 years (mean, 45 years); 24 were men, and 21 were women. The age and sex distributions in the controls did not significantly differ from those in the study group.

Characterization of Study Patients

The 37 study patients ranged in age from 15 to 69 years (mean, 45±14); 19 were men, and 18 were women. In each patient, the diagnosis of hypertrophic cardiomyopathy was based on the presence of a hypertrophied, nondilated left ventricle in the absence of another cardiac or systemic disease capable of producing the magnitude of hypertrophy present in that patient.[28] In addition, each patient had typical clinical features of hypertrophic cardiomyopathy[1,2,29] and severe symptoms of cardiac dysfunction (New York Heart Association functional class III or IV). Maximal ventricular septal thickness assessed by echocardiography ranged from 17 to 30 mm (mean, 24±3 mm), and left ventricular end-diastolic dimension ranged from 30 to 55 mm (mean, 41±6 mm).

Each patient had undergone left-heart catheterization within 3 months of the operation. Basal left ventricular outflow gradients ranged from 0 to 165 mm Hg (average, 79±42 mm Hg), including 26 with subaortic gradients of more than 50 mm Hg. Each of the 11 patients with gradients of less than 50 mm Hg under basal conditions had gradients of more than 50 mm Hg (range, 90 to 160 mm Hg; average, 110±19 mm Hg) with provocative maneuvers (ie, isoproterenol infusion, Valsalva maneuver, and amyl nitrite inhalation).

Mitral Valve Morphometry

Mitral valves were fixed in 10% buffered formalin after their removal at surgery. Valves were introduced to the fixative freely, without stretching or manipulation. Tissue specimens were placed in an opened position on a cutting board and extended to their full length with the atrial aspect exposed. Quantitative morphological measurements were made directly from the mitral valve specimen of the circumference of the valve, measured along its margin of attachment; maximum length of the anterior leaflet, from annular margin to free edge; and the area of the combined anterior and posterior mitral leaflets.

To assess overall mitral leaflet area, borders of the opened valves were traced onto an acetate overlay and then planimeterized using a digital tape (Micro DigiPad 1212).

Echocardiographic Techniques

Transthoracic two-dimensional echocardiograms were performed with an Advanced Technology Laboratory Mark 500 or a Hewlett-Packard Sonos 500 Instrument, using 2.25-, 2.5-, or 3.5-MHz transducers. Two-dimensional echocardiographic images were obtained in a number of cross-sectional planes by using standard transducer positions, as previously described.[30]

Intraoperative echocardiograms were obtained just before cardiopulmonary bypass, using a commercially available Hewlett Packard ultrasound unit with a 3.5- to 5.0-MHz transducer enclosed in a sterile sleeve.[31] A small amount of ultrasound transmission gel was placed between the transducer head and sleeve, and the transducer was positioned directly on the surface of the right ventricle of the beating heart. Standard long-axis and short-axis planes were achieved and recorded on ½-in. videotape. M-mode echocardiograms were derived from two-dimensional images under direct anatomic visualization.

Echocardiographic Measurements

Mitral valve opening area. A continuous scan from aorta to left ventricle in the parasternal short-axis view was used to identify a representative stop-frame image at the cross-sectional level where both the anterior and the posterior mitral leaflets could be visualized and where the mitral valve opening area was greatest during diastole (usually near the tips of the leaflets).[6] With this image, the circumferential innermost margins of the mitral valve were traced onto a plastic transparency, and the outlined area (mitral valve opening area) was then planimeterized using an Apple McIntosh SE computer. The diastolic mitral valve circumference was derived from the calculation of the opening area (Fig 1).

In addition, the maximal internal transverse and horizontal diameters of the mitral valve opening area were measured from the innermost margins of the circumference of the mitral opening area. To enhance the accuracy of these measurements, the outline of mitral valve opening area was routinely verified by reviewing the videotape in slow motion and single-frame modes against the background of the traced stop-frame.

Anterior mitral leaflet length. Length of the anterior mitral leaflet was measured from the standard paraster-

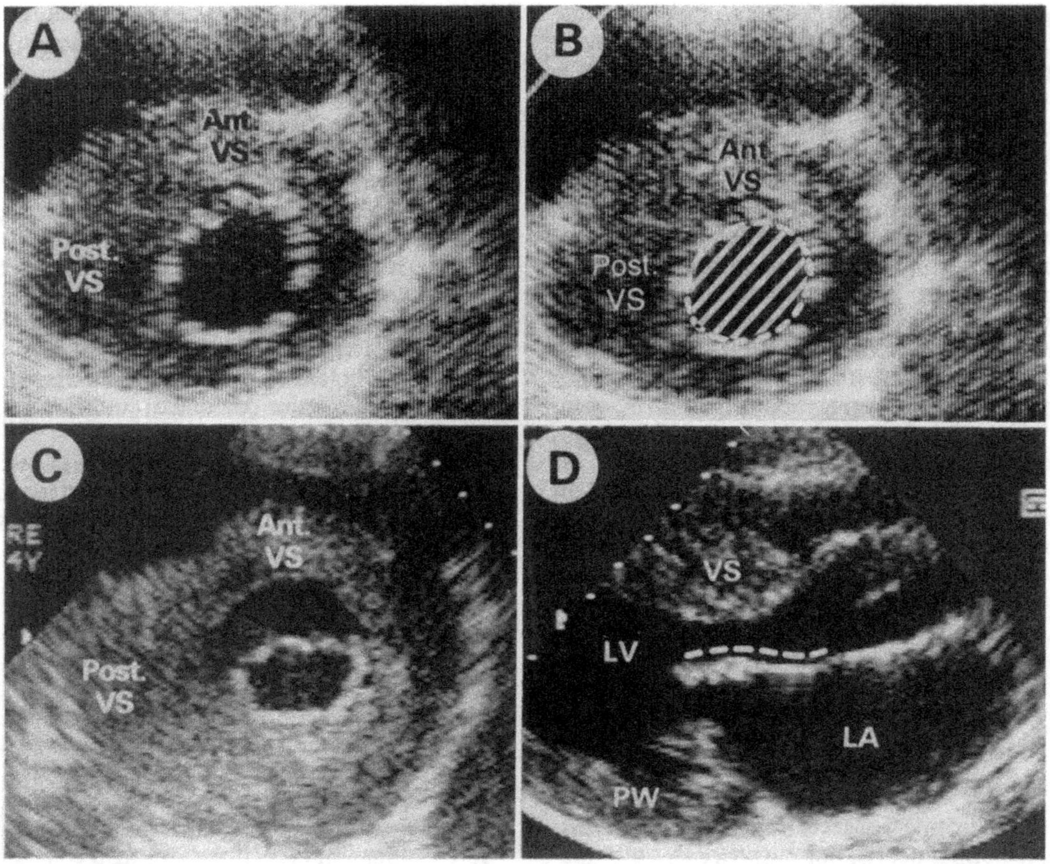

FIG 1. *Representative diastolic stop-frame two-dimensional echocardiographic images illustrating the mitral valve measurements made in the study patients with hypertrophic cardiomyopathy: mitral valve opening area and circumference in the short-axis view (A, B, and C) and anterior leaflet length (broken line) in the parasternal long-axis view (D). A and B, Same stop-frame; the area and circumference of the mitral valve are demarcated only in B. C, From another patient in whom mitral valve opening is considerably less than that evident in A and B. Ant. VS indicates anterior ventricular septum; LA, left atrium; LV, left ventricle; post. VS, posterior ventricular septum; PW, posterior wall; and VS, ventricular septum.*

nal long-axis image (with the ultrasound beam transsecting the center of the left ventricular cavity) during mid diastole and with the leaflet maximally extended, as the distance from the junction between the anterior leaflet and the posterior aortic wall ("hinge-point") to the tip of the leaflet (Fig 1). To aid in verifying the site of these landmarks and particularly in distinguishing mitral leaflet from chordae tendineae, the videotape was reviewed several times in slow motion and single-frame modes against the background of the measured stop-frame. Anterior mitral leaflet length was measured from the parasternal long-axis view (rather than the apical four-chamber) because our judgment and experience indicated that the anatomic limits of the leaflet were best perceived in that cross-sectional plane.

Left ventricular outflow tract cross-sectional area. Left ventricular outflow tract area was measured using a previously described method.[6] In brief, a continuous scan from aorta to left ventricle in the parasternal short-axis identified a representative stop-frame image at the level where both mitral leaflets could be visualized; outflow tract area was measured at this level at the onset of systole (ie, on the first frame showing the mitral valve closed). From this image, the innermost margins of the outflow tract were traced onto a plastic transparency, and the outlined area was then planimeterized (in a fashion similar to that described above for mitral valve opening area).

Other cardiac dimensions. Left ventricular end-diastolic and end-systolic dimensions and left atrial size were obtained from the M-mode echocardiogram according to the criteria of the American Society of Echocardiography.[32] Measurement of transverse mitral valve diameter, defined as the maximal diastolic separation of the anterior and posterior mitral leaflets (at the level of the leaflet tips), was also obtained from standard M-mode echocardiographic tracings.

Reproducibility

Interobserver and intraobserver variability for the measurement of mitral valve opening area was assessed in all 37 patients, using the method of Bland and Altman.[33] To determine interobserver variability, two observers (H.G.K. and A.L.D.) independently measured the mitral valve opening area from the two-dimensional videotape without prior knowledge of the morphological data obtained from the surgical specimens and without preselection of particular portions of the videotape. To determine intraobserver variability, one observer (H.G.K.) measured mitral valve opening area in the same fashion on two occasions (2 months apart, without preselection of portions of the videotape).

Statistical Analysis

Data are expressed as mean±SD. Initially, a linear regression analysis was used to define the single echocardiographic predictor that best estimated mitral leaflet area, using actual mitral leaflet area (measured from the surgical specimen) as the dependent variable, and each of seven echocardiographic measurements as independent variables (see "Statistical Appendix"). Subsequently, a regression analysis[34] was performed with echocardiographic measurements added singly in a stepwise fashion to determine whether the percentage of explained variability in mitral leaflet area could be increased. As a result of that analysis, the measurement of mitral valve opening area was then incorporated into regression equations that expressed the best possible echocardiographic estimation of actual mitral leaflet area. Because of the technical differences between transthoracic and intraoperative echocardiography, we independently analyzed the data in the two subgroups of patients studied by these respective techniques, thereby generating a separate regression equation for each.

Cross-validation method[35] was used to assess the degree of error likely to occur when the regression equation for predicting mitral leaflet area from the echocardiographic measures was applied to future and similar patients with hypertrophic cardiomyopathy. Specifically, cross-validation assesses how well a calculated regression line predicts a data point that has been removed from the analysis (and therefore has not been used to fit that line). Therefore, in cross-validation (as it applies to the present analysis), a single data point consisting of mitral valve opening area and actual mitral leaflet area was deleted from the analysis. The best regression line was then fit to the remaining data to determine how reliable that equation was in predicting the omitted data point. This procedure was repeated (in turn) after reintroducing the omitted data point and eliminating another, until all 37 data points had been assessed by regression analysis.

Results

Mitral Valve Morphometry

In the 37 study patients, total mitral leaflet area ranged from 7.3 to 22.4 cm^2 (mean, 12.4±3.5 cm^2). Of the 37 patients, 19 (51%) had increased leaflet area exceeding the 95% confidence limits for normal leaflet area (≥12.0 cm^2)[14]; the remaining 18 patients had normal leaflet size (area of less than 12.0 cm^2). Increased mitral leaflet area in the 19 patients was due to both increased leaflet length (2.2±0.5 versus 1.9±0.4 cm for normal-sized valves; P<.05) and increased circumference (8.9±1.4 versus 7.2±1.0 cm for normal-sized valves; P<.001).

Echocardiographic Findings

Mitral valve opening area measured from the echocardiogram in the overall group of 37 patients ranged from 1.6 to 6.9 cm^2 (mean, 3.4±1.2 cm^2) and was significantly larger in the 19 patients with increased mitral leaflet area (as measured from surgical specimens) than in the 18 patients with normal-sized mitral leaflets (4.2±1.0 versus 2.6±0.8 cm^2; P<.001). Also, anterior mitral leaflet length as assessed by echocardiography was longer in patients with enlarged valves (2.5±0.4 cm) than in patients with normal-sized valves (2.2±0.2 cm; P<.001).

Left ventricular outflow tract area measured from the echocardiogram in the 37 patients ranged from 0.6 to 5.0 cm^2 and was larger in the 19 patients with increased leaflet area (3.3±1.0 cm^2) than in those 18 patients with normal leaflet area (2.0±0.6 cm^2; P<.001).

Other echocardiographic dimensions were also significantly greater in patients with enlarged valves compared with those with normal-sized valves. These included circumference of the mitral valve opening area (9.7±1.4 cm in enlarged versus 8.1±1.3 cm in normal-sized valves; P<.01), horizontal diameter of the mitral valve opening area (2.7±0.5 versus 2.3±0.6 cm; P<.05), and mitral valve transverse diameter obtained from the M-mode echocardiogram (3.0±0.4 versus 2.2±0.4 cm; P<.001) and from the two-dimensional echocardiogram (2.4±0.4 versus 2.1±0.4 cm).

Comparison of Data Obtained With Transthoracic and Intraoperative Echocardiography

The 25 patients with transthoracic and the 12 patients with intraoperative echocardiograms were analyzed separately for the correlation between mitral valve opening area (assessed by echocardiography) and actual mitral leaflet area (measured from the surgical specimen); squared correlations were .67 (r=.82) and .86 (r=.93), respectively. Comparing the slopes of the regression lines relating mitral valve opening area with mitral leaflet area in these two subgroups showed a difference that was not statistically significant (P=.08).

Relation Between Actual Mitral Leaflet Area and Echocardiographic Variables

Univariate regression analysis, using actual mitral leaflet area as the dependent variable, showed mitral valve opening area to be the best single echocardiographic predictor of actual mitral leaflet area for the 37 study patients; the squared correlation (r^2) for this variable was .75 (r=.87) (Table 1). Thus, approximately 75% of the variability in actual mitral leaflet area could be explained by this single variable.

Treating mitral leaflet area as the dependent variable (see "Statistical Appendix"), the other seven echocardiographic variables were added into the stepwise regression model to determine whether a further increase in the percentage of explained variability for actual leaflet area could be achieved. Variability in mitral leaflet area was increased only marginally by adding these independent variables; therefore, mitral valve opening area was chosen to be the only variable to remain in the model (Fig 2).

This analysis resulted in the following final equations. For patients with transthoracic echocardiograms,

$$\text{MLA}=4.64+2.17\times\text{MVOA}$$

For patients with intraoperative echocardiograms,

$$\text{MLA}=2.19+3.06\times\text{MVOA}$$

where MLA is mitral leaflet area, MVOA is mitral valve opening area, 4.64 and 2.19 reflect the intercept, and 2.17 and 3.06 are the slopes.

TABLE 1. Relation Between Actual Mitral Leaflet Area and Echocardiographic Variables in a Univariate Regression Model

Echocardiographic variables	r^2	r	P
MVOA (cm^2)	.75	.87	<.0001
Circumference of MVOA (cm)	.58	.76	<.0001
Transverse diameter of MVOA (cm)*	.52	.72	<.0001
Anterior mitral leaflet length (cm)	.49	.70	<.001
Left ventricular outflow tract area (cm^2)	.48	.69	<.001
Transverse diameter of MVOA (cm)	.31	.56	<.001
Horizontal diameter of MVOA (cm)	.27	.52	<.001

MVOA indicates mitral valve opening area.
*Obtained from the M-mode echocardiogram; all other variables were measured from the two-dimensional echocardiogram.

Identification of Normal or Increased Mitral Leaflet Area by Echocardiography

Using the mitral leaflet area estimated from the regression equations, echocardiography correctly predicted mitral leaflet area to be normal (<12.0 cm^2) in 15 of 18 patients (83%) but incorrectly overestimated leaflet area in the other three patients with normal valve size (Fig 3). Similarly, echocardiography correctly predicted mitral leaflet area to be enlarged (≥12.0 cm^2) in 16 of 19 patients (84%) but incorrectly underestimated leaflet area in the other three patients.

Reproducibility

Interobserver variability. The difference between the two observers for measurement of mitral valve opening area was compared with the average of the two measurements for each of the 37 patients. The mean difference between the measurements of the two observers was 0.20±0.38 cm^2; these differences appeared to be relatively constant across the range of values calculated for mitral valve opening area.

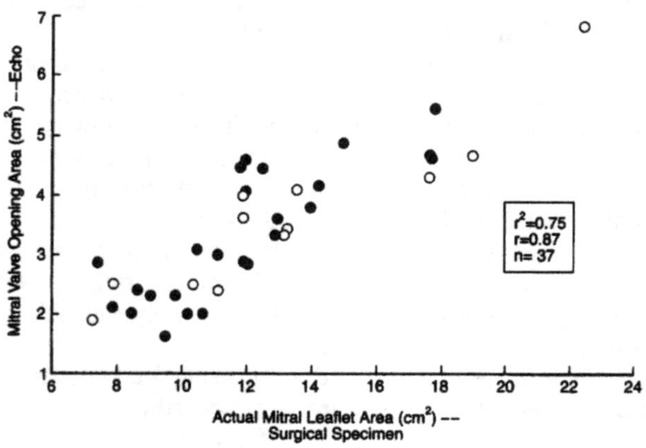

FIG 2. *Scatterplot of relation between mitral valve opening area measured from the two-dimensional echocardiogram and actual mitral leaflet area measured from the surgical specimen in 37 patients with hypertrophic cardiomyopathy. Data are from 25 patients studied with transthoracic echocardiography (●) and 12 patients with intraoperative echocardiography (○).*

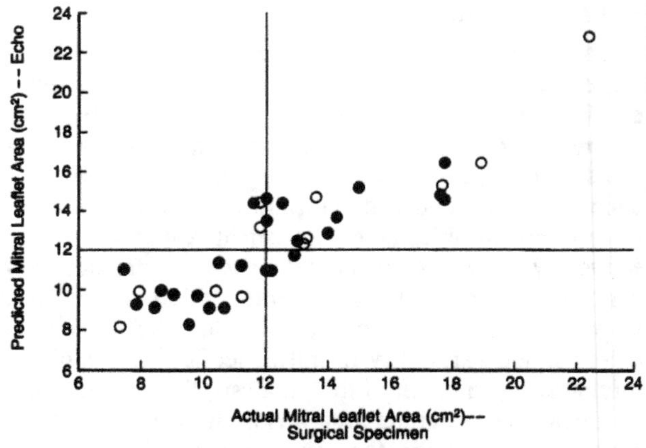

FIG 3. *Scatterplot of relation between actual mitral leaflet area measured from the surgical specimen and leaflet area predicted from two-dimensional echocardiography (using regression analysis) in 37 patients with hypertrophic cardiomyopathy. Data are from 25 patients studied with transthoracic echocardiography (●) and 12 patients with intraoperative echocardiography (○). Mitral leaflet area was estimated using separate regression equations for the transthoracic and intraoperative echocardiograms (see text for details).*

Intraobserver variability. The difference between the two measurements of mitral valve opening area made by the same observer was compared with the average of the two measurements for each of the 37 patients. The mean difference between the two measurements was 0.05±0.17 cm^2; these differences appeared to be relatively constant across the range of values calculated for mitral valve opening area.

Cross-Validation Analysis

In each of the 37 study patients, differences between the actual mitral leaflet area measured from the surgical specimen and that predicted from two-dimensional echocardiography were compared with the actual mitral leaflet area using the cross-validation method.[34] Differences between actual and predicted mitral leaflet area were 2.0 cm^2 or less in 27 of the 37 patients (73%) and 2.5 cm^2 or less in 30 patients (81%). Also, the error in prediction proved to be relatively constant across the wide range of actual mitral leaflet areas.

Discussion

The impetus for designing the present study was our relatively recent appreciation that mitral valve structure is abnormal in many patients with hypertrophic cardiomyopathy and that such alterations may have important clinical implications. For example, in a recent morphometric study of mitral valves removed at surgery or autopsy from almost 100 patients with hypertrophic cardiomyopathy, about 60% showed an increase in leaflet area as well as a variety of patterns of valve enlargement and elongation.[14] Indeed, increased mitral leaflet size, in association with reduced left ventricular outflow tract size and increased ventricular septal thickness, appears to be an important morphological determinant of the presence and magnitude of the subaortic gradient,[13-15] the pattern of mitral valve systolic anterior

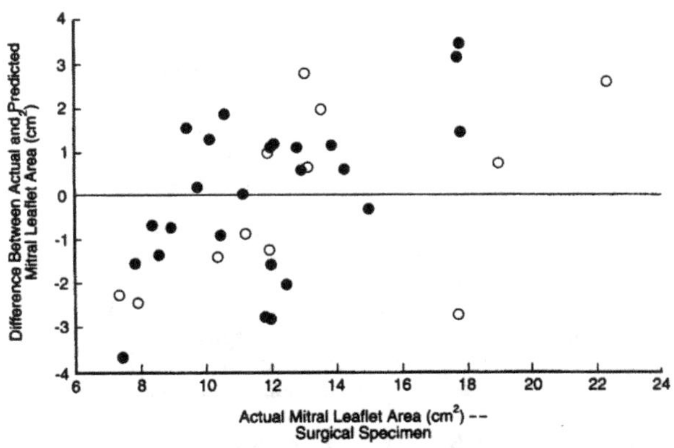

FIG 4. *Scatterplot of difference between the actual mitral leaflet area measured from the surgical specimen and that predicted from two-dimensional echocardiography (using regression analysis) plotted against actual mitral leaflet area, using the cross-validation method[34] in the 37 study patients with hypertrophic cardiomyopathy. This analysis estimates the application of the present data to a theoretical future and similar population of patients with hypertrophic cardiomyopathy. Data are from 25 patients studied with transthoracic echocardiography* (●) *and 12 patients with intraoperative echocardiography* (○).

motion,[11-13,16] and the likelihood that the systolic anterior motion and outflow obstruction will be relieved by myotomy-myectomy.[17] Recognition that the mitral valve is greatly increased in size may alter surgical strategy in selected patients with hypertrophic cardiomyopathy. For example, such an enlarged mitral valve may predispose to residual systolic anterior motion of the valve leaflets into an apparently adequate myotomy-myectomy trough, resulting in persistent postoperative systolic septal contact and outflow obstruction. Therefore, in such patients, more extensive muscular resection,[17,31] suture plication of the mitral valve in addition to myotomy-myectomy,[17] or even mitral valve replacement alone[31,36] may be necessary to achieve the desired hemodynamic result. For these reasons, it was important to determine the reliability of echocardiography in the quantitative assessment of mitral valve size in patients with hypertrophic cardiomyopathy.

To date, few attempts have been made to use quantitative echocardiographic measurements in assessing mitral valve structure and motion in patients with hypertrophic cardiomyopathy[15] or other cardiac diseases.[18-21] One of the reasons for the lack of investigative activity in this area has been the unavailability of a gold standard (ie, mitral valve specimens) to validate the echocardiographic measurements of mitral valve dimensions. Indeed, the unique facet of the present study is the availability of suitable mitral valve specimens and echocardiographic recordings in the same patients, which permitted direct comparisons.

We incorporated morphometric and quantitative echocardiographic data from these patients into a regression analysis and formulated an equation that estimated mitral leaflet area from the echocardiographic measures with good precision. This statistical model identified mitral valve opening area as the strongest single predictor of actual mitral leaflet area. About 75% of the variability in actual mitral leaflet area was explained by this single echocardiographic measurement alone. Also, using the estimation of mitral leaflet area from our statistical model, we were able to discriminate normal-sized from enlarged mitral valves in individual patients with reasonable reliability (ie, in more than 80% of patients). It should be pointed out that the regression equations derived in this study may not apply in precise terms to all other clinical settings, due to expected variability in patient selection, instrumentation, and measurement technique. However, the results of our cross-validation statistical analysis suggests that it would not be unreasonable to apply, with acceptable error, the data from the present study patients to other

TABLE 2. Morphological and Echocardiographic Dimensions in 37 Patients With Obstructive Hypertrophic Cardiomyopathy and Normal-Sized or Enlarged Mitral Valve Leaflets

		Actual mitral leaflet area (cm^2)		
	Complete study group	Normal-sized (<12.0)	Enlarged (≥12.0)	*P*
No. of patients (%)	37	18 (49)	19 (51)	–
Actual mitral leaflet dimensions				
Total leaflet area (cm^2)	12.4±3.5	9.8±1.6	14.9±3.0	–
Leaflet circumference (cm)	8.1±1.5	7.2±1.0	8.9±1.4	<.001
Anterior leaflet length (cm)	2.0±0.5	1.9±0.4	2.2±0.5	<.05
Echocardiographic mitral valve dimensions				
MVOA (cm^2)	3.4±1.2	2.6±0.8	4.2±1.0	<.001
Anterior leaflet length (cm)	2.4±0.4	2.2±0.2	2.5±0.4	<.001
Circumference of MVOA (cm)	8.9±1.6	8.1±1.3	9.7±1.4	<.01
Transverse diameter (cm)	2.3±0.5	2.1±0.4	2.4±0.4	<.05
Transverse diameter (cm)*	2.6±0.6	2.2±0.4	3.0±0.4	<.001
Horizontal diameter (cm)	2.5±0.6	2.3±0.6	2.7±0.5	<.05
Left ventricular outflow tract area (cm^2)	2.7±1.1	2.0±0.6	3.3±1.0	<.001

MVOA indicates mitral valve opening area.
*Obtained from the M-mode echocardiogram; all other variables were measured from the two-dimensional echocardiogram.

theoretical future and similar patients with hypertrophic cardiomyopathy.

Our data were obtained in a highly selected study population that, for the purposes of this investigation, (1) included only those patients in whom the mitral valve specimen was in suitable condition for morphometry and (2) either a transthoracic or intraoperative echocardiogram was available that permitted quantitative assessment of a variety of dimensions from stop-frame, two-dimensional images and the M-mode echocardiogram. Therefore, although virtually all of the transthoracic echocardiographic studies considered for (or included in) our study group were clinically satisfactory and of sufficient diagnostic quality, some were less than optimal for the unique design of the present study, which required quantitative measurements of several ventricular and valvular dimensions. It was for these reasons that the intraoperative echocardiogram was used in about one third of the final study group. Mitral leaflet area estimated from the intraoperative echocardiograms did not, however, differ significantly from that derived from the standard transthoracic echocardiograms in the same patients.

The results of the present investigation establish for the first time an important principle, namely, that it is possible to assess mitral valve size and dimensions from the echocardiogram with reasonable precision and also discriminate large from normal-sized valves in individual patients with hypertrophic cardiomyopathy. Such measurements may have important clinical implications by improving our understanding of the pathophysiology of outflow obstruction as well as in designing the most effective surgical strategy to relieve outflow obstruction.

References

1. Maron BJ, Bonow RW, Cannon RO, Leon MB, Epstein SE. Hypertrophic cardiomyopathy: interrelation of clinical manifestations, pathophysiology, and therapy. *N Engl J Med.* 1987;316: 780-789, 844-852.
2. Wigle ED, Sasson Z, Henderson MA, Ruddy TD, Fulop J, Rakowski H, Williams WG. Hypertrophic cardiomyopathy: the importance of the site and the extent of hypertrophy: a review. *Prog Cardiovasc Dis.* 1985;28:1-83.
3. Shah PM, Gramiak R, Kramer DH. Ultrasound location of left ventricular outflow obstruction in hypertrophic obstructive cardiomyopathy. *Circulation.* 1969;40:3-11.
4. Shah PM, Taylor RD, Wong M. Abnormal mitral valve coaptation in hypertrophic obstructive cardiomyopathy: proposed role in systolic anterior motion of mitral valve. *Am J Cardiol.* 1981; 48:258-262.
5. Spirito P, Maron BJ. Patterns of systolic anterior motion of the mitral valve in hypertrophic cardiomyopathy: assessment by two-dimensional echocardiography. *Am J Cardiol.* 1984;54:1039-1046.
6. Spirito P, Maron BJ. Significance of left ventricular outflow tract cross-sectional area in hypertrophic cardiomyopathy: a two dimensional echocardiographic assessment. *Circulation.* 1983;67:1100-1108.
7. Popp RL, Harrison DC. Ultrasound in the diagnosis and evaluation of therapy of idiopathic hypertrophic subaortic stenosis. *Circulation.* 1969;40:905-914.
8. Yock PG, Hatle L, Popp RL. Patterns and timing of Doppler-detected intracavitary and aortic flow in hypertrophic cardiomyopathy. *J Am Coll Cardiol.* 1986;8:1047-1058.
9. Pollick C, Rakowski H, Wigle ED. Muscular subaortic stenosis: the quantitative relationship between systolic anterior motion and the pressure gradient. *Circulation.* 1984;69:43-49.
10. Maron BJ, Epstein SE. Clinical significance and therapeutic implications of the left ventricular outflow tract pressure gradient in hypertrophic cardiomyopathy. *Am J Cardiol.* 1986;58:1093-1096.
11. Maron BJ, Harding AM, Spirito P, Roberts WC, Waller BF. Systolic anterior motion of the posterior mitral leaflet: a previously unrecognized cause of dynamic subaortic obstruction in patients with hypertrophic cardiomyopathy. *Circulation.* 1983;68:282-293.
12. Jiang L, Levine RA, King ME, Weyman AE. An integrated mechanism for systolic anterior motion of the mitral valve in hypertrophic cardiomyopathy based on echocardiographic observations. *Am Heart J.* 1987;113:633-644.
13. Klues HG, Roberts WC, Maron BJ. Morphologic determinants of echocardiographic patterns of mitral valve systolic anterior motion in obstructive hypertrophic cardiomyopathy. *Circulation* 1993;87: 1570–1579.
14. Klues HG, Maron BJ, Dollar AL, Roberts WC. Diversity of structural mitral valve alterations in hypertrophic cardiomyopathy. *Circulation.* 1992;85:1651-1660.
15. Grigg LE, Wigle ED, Williams WG, Daniel LB, Rakowski H. Transesophageal Doppler echocardiography in obstructive hypertrophic cardiomyopathy: Clarification of pathophysiology and importance in intraoperative decision-making. *J Am Coll Cardiol.* 1992;20:42-52.
16. Lewis JF, Maron BJ. Elderly patients with hypertrophic cardiomyopathy: a subset with distinctive left ventricular morphology and progressive clinical course late in life. *J Am Coll Cardiol.* 1989;13: 36-45.
17. McIntosh CL, Maron BJ, Cannon RO, Klues HG. Initial results of combined anterior mitral leaflet plication and ventricular septal myotomy-myectomy for relief of left ventricular outflow tract obstruction in patients with hypertrophic cardiomyopathy. *Circulation.* 1992;86(suppl II):II-60-II-67.
18. Pini R, Devereux RB, Greppi B, Roman MJ, Hochreiter C, Kramer-Fox R, Niles NW, Kligfield P, Erlebacher JA, Borer JS. Comparison of mitral valve dimensions and motion in mitral valve prolapse with severe mitral regurgitation to uncomplicated mitral valve prolapse and to mitral regurgitation without mitral valve prolapse. *Am J Cardiol.* 1988;62:257-263.
19. Pini R, Greppi B, Roman MJ, Kramer-Fox R, Devereux RB. Time-motion reconstruction of mitral leaflet motion from two-dimensional echocardiography in mitral valve prolapse. *Am J Cardiol.* 1991;68:215-220.
20. Pini R, Greppi B, Kramer-Fox R, Roman MJ, Devereux RB. Mitral valve dimensions and motion and familial transmission of mitral valve prolapse with and without mitral leaflet billowing. *J Am Coll Cardiol.* 1988;12:1423-1431.
21. Weissman NJ, Pini R, Roman MJ, Kramer-Fox R, Anderson HS, Devereux RB. In vivo mitral valve morphology and motion in mitral valve prolapse. *Clin Res.* 1992;40:364A. Abstract.
22. Klues HG, Roberts WC, Maron BJ. Anomalous insertion of papillary muscle directly into the anterior mitral leaflet in hypertrophic cardiomyopathy: significance in producing left ventricular outflow obstruction. *Circulation.* 1991;84:1188-1197.
23. Dollar AL, Roberts WC. Morphologic comparison of patients with mitral valve prolapse who died suddenly with patients who died from severe valvular dysfunction or other conditions. *J Am Coll Cardiol.* 1991;17:921-931.
24. Davies MJ, Moore BP, Braimbridge MV. The floppy mitral valve. Study of incidence, pathology, and complications in surgical, necropsy, and forensic material. *Br Heart J.* 1978;40:468-481.
25. Chester E, King RA, Edwards JE. The myxomatous mitral valve and sudden death. *Circulation.* 1983;67:632-639.
26. Waller BF, Morrow AG, Maron BJ, McIntosh CL, Del Negro AA, Kent KM, Wallace RB, Roberts WC. Etiology of clinically isolated, severe, chronic, pure mitral regurgitation: analysis of 97 patients over 30 years of age having mitral valve replacement. *Am Heart J.* 1982;104:276-288.
27. Marks AR, Choong CY, Sanfilippo AJ, Ferre M, Weyman AE. Identification of high-risk and low-risk subgroups of patients with mitral valve prolapse. *N Engl J Med.* 1989;320:1031-1036.
28. Maron BJ, Epstein SE: Hypertrophic cardiomyopathy: a discussion of nomenclature. *Am J Cardiol.* 1979;43:1242-1244.
29. Maron BJ, Gottdiener JS, Epstein SE. Patterns and significance of distribution of left ventricular hypertrophy in hypertrophic cardiomyopathy: a wide angle, two-dimensional echocardiographic study of 125 patients. *Am J Cardiol.* 1981;48:418-428.
30. Tajik AJ, Seward JB, Hagler DJ, Mair DD, Lie JT. Two-dimensional real-time ultrasonic imaging of the heart and great vessels. *Mayo Clin Proc.* 1978;53:271-303.
31. McIntosh CL, Maron BJ. Current operative treatment of obstructive hypertrophic cardiomyopathy. *Circulation.* 1988;78:487-495.
32. Sahn D, DeMaria A, Kisslo J, Weyman A. Recommendations regarding quantitation in M-mode echocardiography: results of a survey of echocardiographic measurements. *Circulation.* 1978;58: 1072-1083.

33. Bland JM, Altman DG. Statistical methods for assessing agreement between two methods of clinical measurement. *Lancet.* 1986; 1:307-310.
34. Draper N, Smith H, eds. *Applied Regression Analysis,* ed 2. New York: John Wiley & Sons, 1981:307-311.
35. Efron B, Gong G. A leisure look at the bootstrap, the jackknife, and cross-validation. *Am Stat.* 1983;37:36-48.
36. McIntosh CL, Greenberg G, Maron BJ, Leon MB, Cannon RO, Clark RE: Clinical and hemodynamic results after mitral valve replacement in patients with obstructive hypertrophic cardiomyopathy. *Ann Thorac Surg.* 1989;47:236-244.
37. Draper NR, Smith H, eds. *Applied Regression Analysis,* ed 2. New York: John Wiley & Sons, 1981:47-51.

Statistical Appendix

Mitral leaflet area (MLA) is measured from the anatomic specimen with very little error, whereas mitral valve opening area (MVOA) could not be measured from the two-dimensional echocardiogram with nearly the same precision. Therefore, the most relevant regression equation would relate MVOA to MLA rather than vice versa. That is, if x=MLA and y=MVOA, the most natural regression equation is:

$$(1) \qquad y=\alpha_0+\alpha_1 x+\delta$$

where α_0 and α_1 are the intercept and slope, respectively, and δ is a random error. However, we wish to predict x=MLA from a given value of y=MVOA, which is opposite to the way in which the Equation 1 is usually used. One way to accomplish this is to apply inverse regression.[37p47] However, this method entails the concept of fiducial limits, which is not universally accepted. Nevertheless, in some instances, this technique is the only alternative. An example would be in the calibration of a measuring instrument using standard objects of known dimensions that are chosen in some systematic way and therefore cannot be regarded as a random sample. However, we believe that it is reasonable to regard the present data as a random sample of actual MLAs. Under this assumption, we are justified in inverting the regression equation so that the actual MLA is conditioned on the measured MVOA:

$$(2) \qquad \text{MLA}=\beta_0+\beta_1\,\text{MVOA}+\text{e}$$

where β_0 and β_1 are the intercept and slope, respectively, and e is a random error. We can therefore regard MLA as the dependent variable in the regression analysis and use standard regression methodology.

Clinicopathologic Features of Hypertrophic Cardiomyopathy Managed by Cardiac Transplantation

Jamshid Shirani, MD,* Barry J. Maron, MD,† Richard O. Cannon III, MD, Sheyda Shahin, and William C. Roberts, MD‡

Clinical records, electrocardiographic, echocardiographic, hemodynamic and radionuclide data, and the operatively excised hearts were reviewed in 10 patients (aged 19 to 46 years, mean 35) who had cardiac transplantation for hypertrophic cardiomyopathy. Severe congestive heart failure unassociated with outflow obstruction was the indication for transplantation in 9 patients. During a pretransplantation period ranging from 45 to 312 months (mean 137) in these 9 patients, pulmonary artery wedge pressure increased from 19 ± 9 to 27 ± 7 mm Hg, left ventricular ejection fraction decreased from 51 ± 11% to 41 ± 1%, left ventricular end-diastolic dimension increased from 42 ± 6 to 48 ± 4 mm, and total 12-lead QRS voltage decreased from 209 ± 50 to 156 ± 41 mm. In these 9 patients, the explanted hearts had dilated left ventricular cavities, and 8 had left ventricular scars without significant narrowing of the epicardial coronary arteries. The tenth patient had a nondilated left ventricular cavity and had transplantation because of recurrent, refractory syncope. Of the 10 patients, 3 died within the first month, and another died 8 months after transplantation. The remaining 6 patients have survived 20 to 54 months (mean 39) after transplantation and are in functional class I or II.

(Am J Cardiol 1993;72:434–440)

Approximately 3,000 cardiac-transplantations were performed worldwide in 1990.[1] In adults, idiopathic dilated cardiomyopathy is the most common indication for cardiac transplantation, closely followed by atherosclerotic coronary artery disease. Only 1 report describing clinicopathologic features in 2 patients having cardiac transplantation for hypertrophic cardiomyopathy (HC) has appeared.[2] During the last 15 years, 12 patients with HC studied at the National Heart, Lung, and Blood Institute have had cardiac transplantation, and in 10 of them, the explanted hearts have been examined by us. This report describes clinicopathologic findings in the latter 10 patients.

METHODS

Study patients: The files of the Pathology Branch of the National Heart, Lung, and Blood Institute were searched for cases coded as having "idiopathic hypertrophic subarotic stenosis" or "hypertrophic cardiomyopathy." Of the 229 cases so coded between the years 1975 and 1992, 10 had heart transplantation and are the subjects of this report.

Sources of the data: Although patients were studied clinically in the Cardiology Branch of the National Heart, Lung, and Blood Institute, the transplantation procedures were performed at medical centers other than the National Institutes of Health. The hearts in the 10 patients, however, were submitted to the Pathology Branch of the National Heart, Lung, and Blood Institute for study. The hearts, which came from 10 different medical centers, were initially examined by WCR and subsequently by JS. The clinical records, electrocardiograms, echocardiograms, hemodynamic data, photographs of the explanted hearts, and microscopic slides of the hearts were reviewed in all 10 patients. Follow up data were obtained by contacting the centers where the cardiac transplantation operations were performed.

Statistical analysis: Data are expressed as mean ± SD. Differences between means were determined using the unpaired or paired Student *t* test where appropriate.

RESULTS

Clinical observations: AGE, SYMPTOMS AND TREATMENT: Pertinent clinical findings in the 10 patients are summarized in Table I. The age at onset of symptoms of cardiac dysfunction ranged from 12 to 32 years (mean 22); the estimated age at the onset of left ventricular dilatation, which occurred in 9 patients, ranged from 18 to 45 years (mean 29), and cardiac transplantation was performed at ages 19 to 46 years (mean 35), a mean of 15 years from the onset of symptoms of cardiac dysfunction

From the Pathology and Cardiology Branches, National Heart, Lung, and Blood Institute, National Institutes of Health, Bethesda, Maryland.
Manuscript received and accepted March 9, 1993.

*Division of Cardiology, Department of Medicine, Medical College of Virginia, Richmond, Virginia 23298.

†Cardiovascular Research Division, Minneapolis Heart Institute Foundation, Minneapolis, Minnesota 55407.

‡Baylor Cardiovascular Institute, Baylor University Medical Center, Dallas, Texas 75246.

TABLE I Clinical, Hemodynamic and Ventriculographic Findings in 10 Patients with Cardiac Transplantation for Hypertrophic Cardiomyopathy

Pt.	Age at: Onset of Symptoms	Age at: Diagnosis	Age at: Estimated Onset of Left Ventricular Enlargement	Age at: Cardiac Transplant	Sex	FH of HC	AP	CHF	Sy	Interval Study to Transplant (mos)	RA (mean)	RV (s/d)	PA (s/d)	PAW (mean)	LV (s/d)	SA (s/d)	LV-SA Psg: At Rest	LV-SA Psg: With Provocation	CI (L/min/m²)	MR (1–3+)	Dilated LV	Radionuclide Ventriculography: Interval to Transplant (mos)	Radionuclide Ventriculography: LVEF (%)
1	12	12	18	19	M	+	+	+	0	24	18	51/—	60/30	32	117/15	116/85	0	—	2.0	+	0	9	48
										9	22	50/20	50/30	28	108/24	120/76	0	—	1.8	++	+	—	—
2	18	21	—	24	F	0	0	+	+	34	5	22/2	13/5	5	100/10	120/65	0	14	3.3	0	0	33	72
										8	3	22/6	22/8	9	110/12	105/59	20	64	3.4	+	0	30	65
3	16	16	22	27	M	0	0	+	0	89	—	—	—	—	108/20	108/65	0	0	—	0	0	68	66
										3	22	45/20	45/35	29	—	110/70	—	—	2.6	—	—	63	64
4	17	17	31	33	F	0	0	+	0	156	3	36/4	27/12	13	84/12	96/54	0	—	3.4	0	0	—	—
										27	7	50/9	50/19	28	95/23	95/68	0	—	2.0	—	+	—	—
5	23	23	33	36	M	+	+	+	+	120	3	32/5	34/14	15	105/18	100/60	0	60	1.9	0	0	37	67
										34	—	45/23	55/26	30	—	—	—	—	—	—	—	—	—
6	19	22	36	37	F	0	0	+	+	175	6	50/15	50/21	24	105/17	105/70	0	0	2.8	+	0	4	40
										4	6	47/8	44/20	32	110/17	120/60	0	10	2.9	++	+	2	41
7	32	36	36	40	M	+	0	+	0	48	12	60/16	65/30	20	110/28	110/80	0	—	1.3	0	+	35	38
										—	—	—	—	—	—	—	—	—	—	—	—	7	30
8	29	17	39	42	M	+	+	+	0	312	3	20/3	20/9	8	145/15	95/55	50	110	2.5	0	0	66	53
										151	4	36/12	28/10	12	160/27	110/60	50	85	3.3	0	0	11	39
9	20	36	41	45	F	+	+	+	0	—	—	—	—	—	—	—	—	—	—	—	—	67	53
										25	16	70/21	70/35	36	140/21	155/88	0	—	1.8	—	—	4	44
10	16	19	45	46	M	+	+	+	0	276	—	—	—	—	—	—	60	—	—	0	0	38	43
										2	4	48/4	44/22	23	96/24	110/60	0	0	2.8	+	+	3	29
Totals	12–32 (20 ± 6)	12–36 (22 ± 8)	18–45 (28 ± 8)	19–46 (35 ± 9)	Men = 6/10	6/10	5/10	10/10	3/10 *	I = 137 vs II = 29	7 ± 6 vs 11 ± 8	39/8† vs 45/14	38/17 vs 45/22	17 ± 9† vs 25 ± 9	109/17 vs 117/21	106/67 vs 115/67	—	—	2.5 ± 0.8 vs 2.6 ± 0.6	2/9 vs 4/5	1/9 vs 4/6	40 vs 17	53 ± 12† vs 45 ± 15

*I (upper row) and II (lower row) represent the mean values for the first and second studies, respectively.
†p<0.05.
AP = angina pectoris; CHF = congestive heart failure; CI = cardiac index; F = female; FH = family history; HC = hypertrophic cardiomyopathy; LV = left ventricle; LVEF = left ventricular ejection fraction; M = male; MR = mitral regurgitation; PA = pulmonary artery; PAW = pulmonary artery wedge; Psg = peak systolic gradient; RA = right atrium; RV = right ventricle; SA = systemic artery; s/d = systolic/diastolic; Sy = syncope.

TABLE II Electrocardiographic Findings in 10 Patients with Cardiac Transplantation for Hypertrophic Cardiomyopathy

Pt.	Interval Study to Transplant (months)	Rhythm	Rate (beats/min)	Intervals (ms) PR	QRS	QTc	QRS Voltage (mm) I	II	III	aVR	aVL	aVF	V_1	V_2	V_3	V_4	V_5	V_6	Total 12-lead	Conduction Abnormality
1	45	S	60	16	8	42	8	24	21	16	12	21	17	22	35	44	44	27	291	0
	10	AF	63	—	12	—	12	12	17	18	12	14	13	8	9	14	15	12	146	RBBB, LPFB
2	57	S	88	18	8	44	18	21	12	23	10	18	22	33	45	51	34	26	313	0
	39	S	72	19	8	40	23	34	15	27	11	23	29	44	46	44	41	41	378	0
3	68	AF	100	—	8	—	12	14	7	12	8	8	5	14	16	23	20	10	149	0
	4	AF	70	—	16	—	10	11	15	4	10	13	3	8	13	13	14	7	121	Pacemaker
4	23	S	54	24	16	34	20	33	7	21	33	16	7	8	5	10	14	12	186	IVCD
	—	AF	—	—	—	—	—	—	—	—	—	—	—	—	—	—	—	—	—	—
5	33	S	50	26	16	39	5	13	18	7	11	14	9	17	23	42	24	34	219	LBBB
	15	AF	80	—	9	—	6	5	11	2	8	8	7	5	12	12	21	12	109	0
6	89	AF	70	—	14	—	19	21	7	19	9	12	8	23	22	15	7	6	168	Pacemaker
	24	AF	70	—	15	—	12	14	14	12	12	12	10	19	26	24	9	8	172	Pacemaker
7	48	S	65	26	12	44	5	12	11	6	7	11	12	21	26	18	27	21	177	IVCD
	23	S	61	29	15	50	3	10	9	5	5	8	10	22	21	13	21	18	145	IVCD
8	169	S	80	14	12	51	11	22	28	7	20	24	14	31	27	9	11	10	214	IVCD
	125	AF	70	—	14	—	6	18	20	5	13	16	13	29	28	24	17	12	201	IVCD
9	78	S	60	20	8	39	12	19	24	10	17	19	23	41	33	32	23	18	271	0
	40	S	64	22	9	36	7	17	19	9	12	16	24	46	27	23	15	12	227	0
10	—	S	—	—	—	—	—	—	—	—	—	—	—	—	—	—	—	—	—	—
	2	S	60	30	22	54	5	7	8	5	6	7	13	25	19	12	11	12	130	IVCD
Totals	I = 66	S = 8/10	70 ± 16	21	11	42	13	20	15	13	14	16	13	25	26	27	23	18	221 ± 58†	
*	vs	vs	vs	vs	vs	vs	vs	vs	vs	vs	vs	vs	vs	vs	vs	vs	vs	vs	vs	
	II = 31	4/10	68 ± 6	25	14	45	9	14	14	10	10	13	14	23	22	20	18	15	181 ± 83	

*I (upper row) and II (lower row) represent the mean values for the first and second 12-lead electrocardiograms, respectively.
†$p < 0.05$.
AF = atrial fibrillation; IVCD = interventricular conduction delay; LBBB = left bundle branch block; LPFB = left posterior fascicular block; RBBB = right bundle branch block; S = sinus.

TABLE III Echocardiographic and Cardiac Morphologic Findings in 10 Patients with Cardiac Transplantation for Hypertrophic Cardiomyopathy

Pt.	Interval Study to Transplant (months)	Dimensions (mm)				Thickness (mm)			Heart Weight (g)	Thickness (mm)		Dilatation (1–3+)		LVOT Plaque	Thickened AML	Epi-cardial CAD	Gross Fibrosis (1–3+)		Myofiber Disarray in VS	Thickened IMCA	Follow-Up		
		LA	LVDd	LVDs	FS (%)	VS	LVFW	SAM		VS	LVFW	LV	RV				VS	LVFW			Year Transplant Performed	Months After Trans-plant	Outcome
1	41	39	36	27	25	15	15	0	385	20	15	+	+	0	0	0	0	0	+	+	1988	43	FC I
	21	55	45	33	27	13	13	0															
2	34	37	30	15	50	29	30	0	650	34	32	0	0	0	0	0	0	0	+	+	1988	52	FC I–II
	8	44	31	16	48	31	35	+															
3	57	50	32	22	31	22	13	0	340	20	20	+	+	0	0	0	+	+	+	+	1985	<1	Died (rejection)
	14	54	42	29	31	20	10	0															
4	—	—	—	—	—	—	—	—	340	15	14	+	+	0	0	0	+++	+++	+	+	1977	1	Died (toxo-plasmosis)
	27	—	—	—	—	15	11	0															
5	37	38	44	24	45	19	13	+	390	17	11	+	+	0	0	0	+++	+++	+	+	1979	<1	Died (rejection)
	11	50	48	27	44	16	10	+															
6	95	54	40	26	35	14	11	0	290	17	13	+	+	0	0	0	+	+	+	+	1988	54	FC II
	4	54	45	34	24	14	10	0															
7	48	52	52	43	17	17	9	0	310	19	11	+	+	0	0	0	+++	+++	+	+	1987	8	Died (rejection)
	4	56	53	45	15	14	8	0															
8	143	43	42	28	33	22	12	+	455	18	13	+++	+++	+	+	0	+++	++	+	+	1990	20	FC I
	126	44	45	30	33	17	11	+															
9	89	30	48	38	21	15	11	—	350	15	11	+	+	0	0	0	+	+	+	+	1989	39	FC I–II
	40	56	48	40	17	12	10	0															
10	58	52	43	34	21	23	15	0	480	18	18	+++	+++	+	+	0	+++	++	+	+	1985	27	FC I
	2	58	55	38	31	17	10	0															
Totals *	I = 67 vs II = 28	44 ± 8† vs 52 ± 5	41 ± 7 vs 46 ± 7	29 ± 9 vs 32 ± 8	31 ± 11 vs 30 ± 11	20 ± 5 vs 17 ± 5	14 ± 6 vs 12 ± 8	2/10 vs 3/10	290–650 (400 ± 110)	19 ± 5 (19 ± 7)	16 ± 6 (16 ± 9)	9/10	9/10	2/10	2/10	0/10	8/10	8/10	10/10	10/10			

*I (upper row) and II (lower row) represent mean values for the first and second echocardiograms, respectively.
AML = anterior mitral leaflet; CAD = atherosclerotic coronary artery disease; FC = New York Heart Association functional class; FS = fractional shortening; IMCA = intramural coronary arteries; LA = left atrial; LV = left ventricular; LVD (d and s) = left ventricular dimension (in diastole and systole); LVFW = left ventricular free wall; LVOT = left ventricular outflow tract; RV = right ventricular; SAM = systolic anterior motion of the anterior mitral leaflet; VS = ventricular septal.

and 13 years from the diagnosis of HC. All patients had signs and symptoms of left ventricular failure, and 9 had cardiac failure refractory to medical therapy. Patient 2 (Table I) had cardiac transplantation for recurrent syncope. In 4 patients (nos. 2, 3, 6 and 10), a permanent pacemaker had been placed, and 2 (nos. 5 and 8) had undergone ventricular septal myotomy and myectomy.

CARDIAC CATHETERIZATION (TABLE I): Only 1 patient (no. 2) had normal right-sided pressures. In 3 patients (nos. 2, 8 and 10), a pressure gradient was present be-

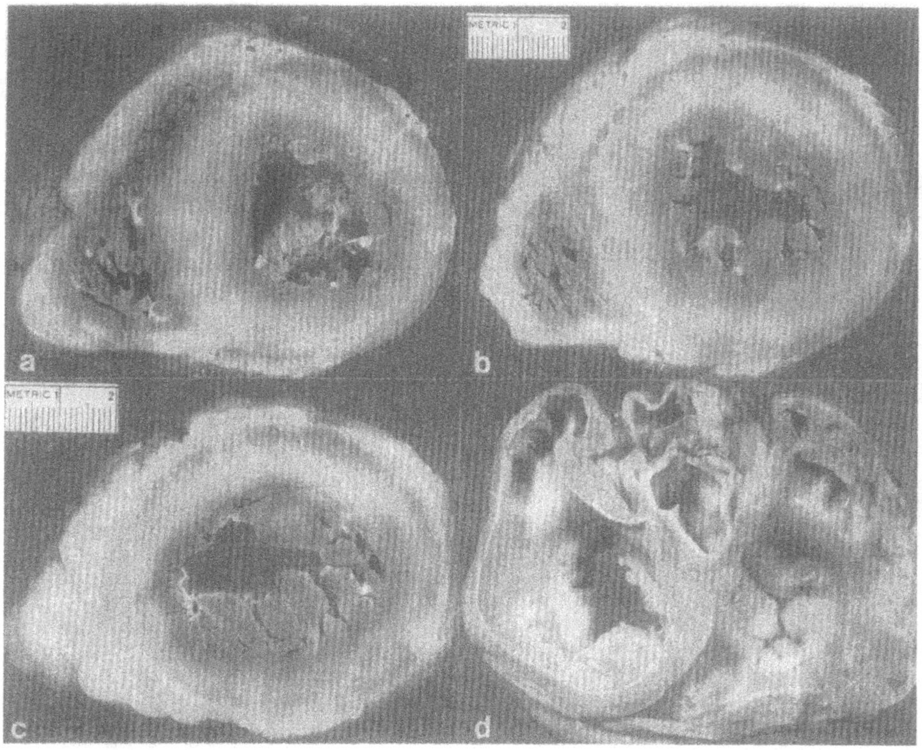

FIGURE 1. Heart of a 40-year-old man (pt. 7) with hypertrophic cardiomyopathy who had cardiac transplantation for refractory congestive heart failure. *a*, *b*, and *c*, views of the cardiac ventricles at different levels, showing a dilated left ventricle and grossly visible scars in the ventricular septum and the left ventricular free wall. *d*, view of the cardiac atria from above, showing dilated cavities and thickened walls.

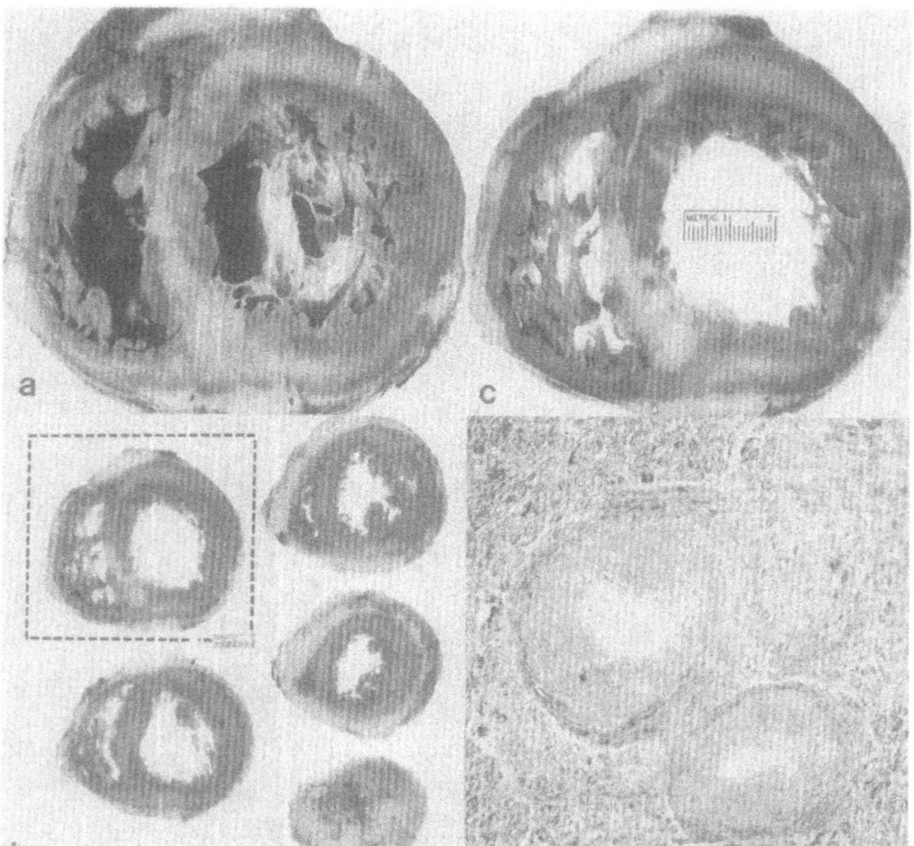

FIGURE 2. Heart of a 42-year-old man (pt. 8) with hypertrophic cardiomyopathy and progressive systolic dysfunction. *a*, view of the basal portion of the cardiac ventricles. *b*, transverse section of the cardiac ventricles. A close-up of the section *in brackets* is shown in *c*. The ventricular cavities are dilated, and the septum and portions of the left and right ventricular walls are scarred. *d*, photomicrograph of intramural coronary arteries in the ventricular septum showing thickened walls and narrowed lumens. Movat stain × 100; reduced by 24%.

tween the left ventricle and ascending aorta during peak systole; this gradient was 50 and 60 mm Hg in patients 8 and 10, respectively. In patient 10, myotomy and myectomy were performed, and in patient 8, the peak systolic gradient was absent at the second cardiac catheterization when the left ventricle was markedly dilated, and the left ventricular ejection fraction was 29%. In 8 patients in whom the results of a second cardiac catheterization were available, the right atrial, right ventricular, pulmonary arterial and pulmonary artery wedge pressures had increased compared with the results at the first study over a mean time span of 108 months. The cardiac index did not change significantly between the 2 studies. More patients had mitral regurgitation at the second left ventricular cineangiogram than at the first (2 of 9 vs 4 of 5). The left ventricular cavity was dilated in 1 of 9 patients at the first study and in 4 of 6 at the second.

RADIONUCLIDE VENTRICULOGRAPHY (TABLE I): The left ventricular ejection fraction, assessed by radionuclide ventriculography, decreased from a mean of 53 to 45% ($p \leq 0.05$) in 2 studies performed a mean of 40 and 17 months, respectively, before transplantation in 7 patients.

ELECTROCARDIOGRAPHIC FINDINGS (TABLE II): Comparison of the 12-lead electrocardiographic recordings obtained at a mean of 66 and 31 months before transplantation showed an increase in the prevalence of atrial fibrillation (from 2 of 10 to 6 of 10 patients, respectively), and a significant decrease in the total 12-lead QRS voltage (from a mean of 221 to 181 mm, respectively; $p < 0.05$).

FIGURE 3. Heart of a 46-year-old man (pt. 10) with hypertrophic cardiomyopathy, progressive congestive heart failure, systolic dysfunction (left ventricular ejection fraction 29%) and total 12-lead QRS voltage of 130 mm. Views of the cardiac ventricles *(a, b, and c)* showing markedly dilated cavities and extensive scars, which involve the ventricular septum more than the left and right ventricular free walls.

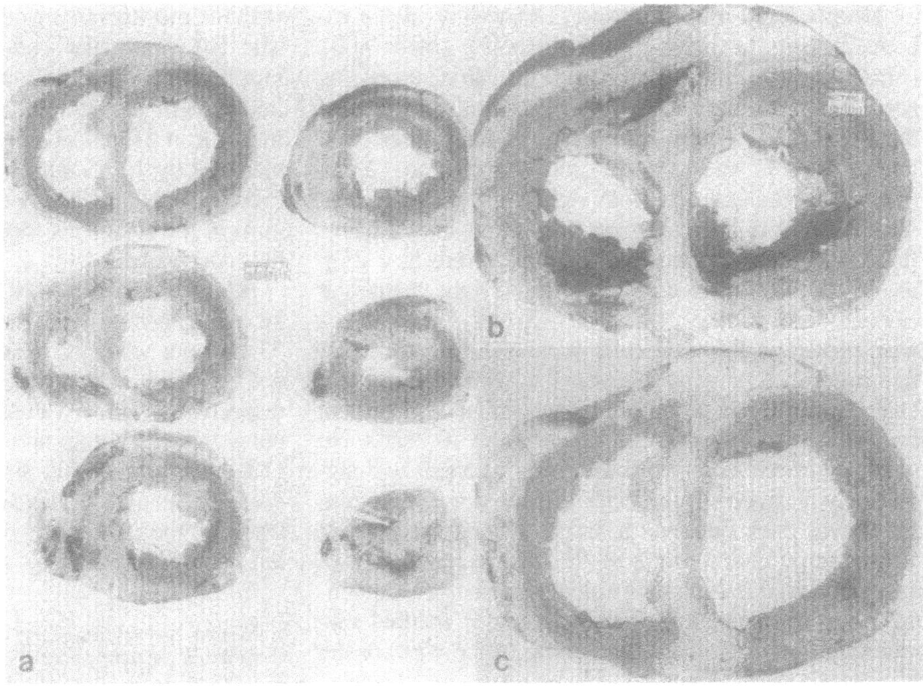

FIGURE 4. Heart of a 24-year-old woman (pt. 2) with hypertrophic cardiomyopathy and recurrent, refractory syncope. Transverse sections of cardiac ventricles show no cavity dilatation, and greatly thickened walls. The myocardium is free of grossly visible lesions.

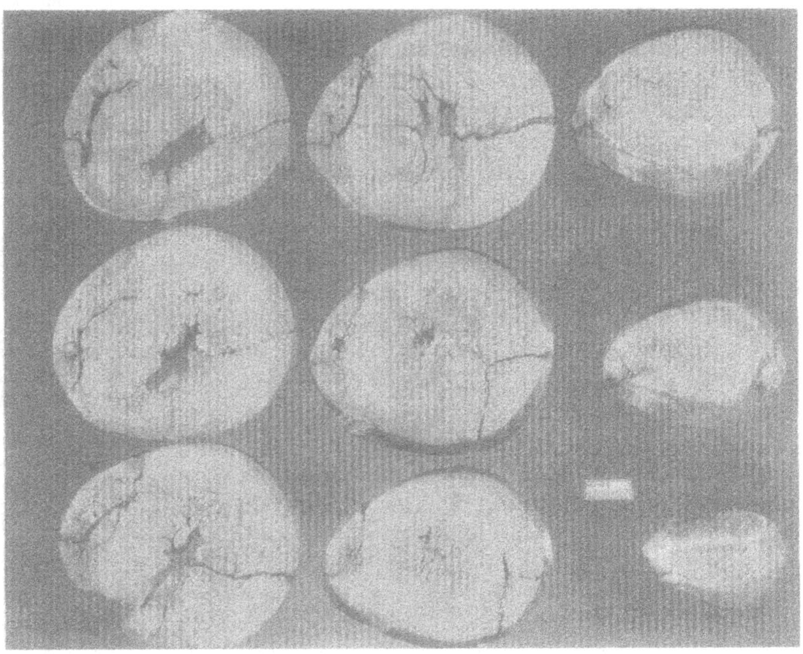

ECHOCARDIOGRAPHIC FINDINGS (TABLE III): The left atrial, and left ventricular systolic and diastolic dimensions increased from a mean of 44, 29 and 41 mm to 52, 32 and 46 mm, respectively, in a mean interval of 39 months before transplantation. In the same period, the thickness of the ventricular septum decreased from a mean of 20 to 17 mm, and that of the left ventricular free wall from 14 to 12 mm.

OUTCOME OF TRANSPLANTATION (TABLE III): Three of 10 patients died within the first month after transplantation: 2 because of rejection of the implanted homograft, and 1 of infection due to *Toxoplasma gondii*. Another patient died 8 months after transplantation, because of rejection. The remaining 6 patients have survived 20 to 54 months (mean 39) after transplantation and are in New York Heart Association functional class I or II.

Morphologic observations: The weight of the explanted hearts ranged from 290 to 650 g (mean 400). (This weight excludes portions of the atria, ascending aorta and pulmonary trunk.) The maximal thickness of the ventricular septum and left ventricular free wall ranged from 15 to 34 mm (mean 19) and 11 to 32 mm (mean 16), respectively. Both right and left ventricular cavities were dilated by gross inspection in 9 patients (Figure 1): mild to moderate in 7 and severe in 2 (Figures 2 and 3). In 1 heart, both left and right ventricular cavities were small (Figure 4). Grossly visible scars were present in the ventricular septa and left ventricular free walls in 8 patients (Figures 1 to 3), and they were extensive in 5. Histologically, myocardial replacement and interstitial fibrosis were present in all 10 hearts. No major epicardial coronary artery in any patient was significantly narrowed. In 2 hearts, the anterior mitral valve leaflet was thickened, and a fibrous plaque was present on the mural endocardium of the ventricular septum in apposition to this leaflet. Histologic sections of the ventricular septum in all 10 patients showed marked myofiber disorganization and thickening of the walls of the intramural coronary arteries (Figure 2).

DISCUSSION

Indications for transplantation: Of the 10 patients, 9 had transplantation because of refractory congestive heart failure. In each of these patients, the left ventricular cavities dilated during the pretransplantation period (left ventricular end-diastolic dimension from 42 ± 6 to 48 ± 4 mm; $p < 0.05$), left ventricular ejection fraction decreased (from $51 \pm 11\%$ to $41 \pm 13\%$; $p < 0.05$), total 12-lead QRS voltage decreased (from 209 ± 50 to 156 ± 40 mm; $p < 0.05$), the ventricular septa thinned (from 18 ± 4 to 15 ± 2 mm; $p < 0.01$), and the left ventricular free wall thinned (from 12 ± 2 to 10 ± 1 mm; $p < 0.05$). The remaining patient (no. 2), a 24-year-old woman, had transplantation for recurring syncope that began at age 19. The syncope was refractory to antiarrhythmic medications and placement of a cardiac pacemaker, but was eliminated by transplantation. In the last 8 months before transplantation, she had daily syncope. She was the only patient among the 10 with a nondilated ventricular cavity, without progressive ventricular wall thinning, without progressive decrease in total 12-lead QRS voltage and, with one other exception (no. 1), without ventricular wall scarring.

Left ventricular dilatation and wall thinning: In adults with HC, the occurrence of severe heart failure in the absence of outflow obstruction is often marked by an increase in the left ventricular end-diastolic dimension, and thinning of the ventricular septum and left ventricular free wall.[3–7] The prognosis for such patients is poor.[8] In 7 of our patients, the left ventricular diastolic dimension, as measured by M-mode echocardiography, increased by 1 to 12 mm (mean 6). The largest increase in left ventricular cavity size occurred in the 2 patients with the most severe myocardial scarring (nos. 8 and 10). The left ventricular end-diastolic dimension was >52 mm (upper limit of normal for adults) in 2 patients. The thickness of the ventricular septum decreased by 2 to 6 mm (mean 3) in 7 patients, and that of the left ventricular wall by 1 to 5 mm (mean 2) in 8 patients. The ventricular septal thickness decreased the most (5 and 6 mm) in the 2 patients (nos. 8 and 10, respectively) with the most scarring.

Electrocardiographic findings: In a study by Dollar and Roberts,[9] the mean total 12-lead QRS voltage in 57 patients with HC was 205 and 155 mm for those without and with transmural left ventricular scars, respectively. Those values are comparable to those of our 9 patients before and after the onset of left ventricular enlargement (209 and 156 mm, respectively). The decrease in total 12-lead QRS voltage in our patients was, for the most part, proportional to the severity of left ventricular scarring.

1. Kriett JM, Kaye MP. The registry of the international society of heart and lung transplantation: eight official report-1991. *J Heart Lung Transplant* 1991;10:491–498.
2. Warren SE, Cohen LH, Schoen FJ, Mudge GH, Lorell BH. Advanced diastolic heart failure in familial hypertrophic cardiomyopathy managed with cardiac transplantation. *J Applied Cardiol* 1988;3:415–422.
3. ten Cate FJ, Roelandt J. Progression of the left ventricular dilatation in patients with obstructive hypertrophic cardiomyopathy. *Am Heart J* 1979;97:762–765.
4. Fujiwara H, Onodera T, Tanaka M, Shirane H, Kato H, Yoshikawa J, Osakada S, Sasayama S, Kawai C. Progression from hypertrophic obstructive cardiomyopathy to typical dilated cardiomyopathy-like features in the end stage. *Jpn Circ J* 1984;48:1210–1214.
5. Funakoshi M, Imamura M, Sasaki J, Fujimo M, Kawano T, Sasaki Y, Nakashima Y, Motooka T, Fukuda F, Imagawa M, Hiroki T, Arakawa K. Seventeen year follow-up of a patient with hypertrophic cardiomyopathy which progressed to dilated cardiomyopathy. *Jpn Heart J* 1984;25:805–809.
6. Spirito P, Maron BJ. Absence of progression of left ventricular hypertrophy in adult patients with hypertrophic cardiomyopathy. *J Am Coll Cardiol* 1987;9:1013–1017.
7. Spirito P, Maron BJ, Bonow RO, Epstein SE. Severe functional limitation in patients with hypertrophic cardiomyopathy and only mild localized left ventricular hypertrophy. *J Am Coll Cardiol* 1986;8:537–544.
8. Spirito P, Maron BJ, Bonow RO, Epstein SE. Occurrence and significance of progressive left ventricular wall thinning and relative cavity dilatation in hypertrophic cardiomyopathy. *Am J Cardiol* 1987;60:123–129.
9. Dollar AL, Roberts WC. Usefulness of total 12-lead QRS voltage compared with other criteria for determining left ventricular hypertrophy in hypertrophic cardiomyopathy: analysis of 57 patients studied at necropsy. *Am J Med* 1989;87:377–381.

Comparison of Morphologic Findings in Spontaneously Occurring Hypertrophic Cardiomyopathy in Humans, Cats and Dogs

Si-Kwang Liu, DVM, PhD, William C. Roberts, MD, and Barry J. Maron, MD

Morphologic features of spontaneously occurring hypertrophic cardiomyopathy (HC) were compared in 38 humans, 51 cats and 10 dogs. Asymmetric hypertrophy of the ventricular septum, marked disorganization of cardiac muscle cells, abnormal intramural coronary arteries and myocardial fibrosis were each present in the ventricular septum of human, feline, and canine forms of HC; these abnormalities were generally more severe and most frequently identified in humans. Asymmetric left ventricular hypertrophy (based on the calculated septal-to-free wall thickness ratio) was most common in humans (31 of 38 [81%]) and dogs (8 of 10 [80%]), as compared with cats (16 of 51 [31%]; p <0.001) with HC; in all 3 species, hypertrophy was often diffuse, involving substantial portions of the anterolateral and posterior free walls, and the ventricular septum. Marked septal disorganization (≥5% of the tissue section) was present in 35 patients (92%), but in only 14 cats (27%) and 2 dogs (20%) (p <0.001). Abnormal intramural coronary arteries occurred with similar frequency in the ventricular septum of patients (n = 25; 66%), cats (n = 38; 74%) and dogs (n = 6; 60%) (p <NS). Moderate-to-severe septal fibrosis was identified more commonly in humans (15 of 38 [39%]) than in animals (13 of 61 [21%]; p <0.001). In all 3 species, abnormal intramural coronary arteries were most commonly observed within or at the margins of areas of fibrous tissue. These morphologic findings describe spontaneously occurring models of HC in cats and dogs with substantial structural similarities to the well-recognized disease entity in humans.

(Am J Cardiol 1993;72:944–951)

From the Department of Pathology, The Animal Medical Center, New York, New York, and the Pathology Branch, National Heart, Lung, and Blood Institute, National Institutes of Health, Bethesda, Maryland. Manuscript received February 22, 1993; revised manuscript received and accepted June 7, 1993.

Address for reprints: Si-Kwang Liu, DVM, PhD, Department of Pathology, The Animal Medical Center, 510 East 62nd Street, New York, New York 10021.

Hypertrophic cardiomyopathy (HC) is a primary (and often familial) cardiac disease in which the most characteristic morphologic feature is a hypertrophied, nondilated left ventricle,[1] and the myocardium typically shows bizarre and disorganized cellular architecture, abnormal small intramural coronary arteries and increased amounts of matrix or replacement fibrosis.[2–23] Although HC has been a well-recognized and extensively studied clinical and pathologic entity in patients since 1958,[2,14,15] a morphologically similar condition occurring spontaneously in cats[24,25] and dogs[26,27] has only more recently been identified. The present study extends our morphologic observations to the canine and feline forms of HC, and compares certain structural hallmarks of this disease observed at necropsy.

METHODS

Selection of case material: The cardiovascular registry of the Pathology Department of The Animal Medical Center was reviewed for a 2-year period. During that time, 189 cats and 177 dogs with cardiac disease were examined at necropsy; the hearts of 51 cats and 10 dogs were identified as having HC. Of 61 animals, 50 (82%) were male. Cats with HC were most commonly of the domestic shorthair breed (n = 39 [77%]); in addition, 7 (14%) were Persian, 4 (8%) were Siamese, and 1 (1%) was Maine Coon. Four dogs were German shepherds, and 1 each was a Doberman pinscher, Airedale, French poodle, Great Dane, bulldog and Boston terrier. In the 61 animals, death was sudden in 23 (38%), due to heart failure with or without thromboembolism in 33 (54%), and due to noncardiac causes in 5 (8%).

Case records of the Pathology Branch of the National Heart, Lung, and Blood Institute were reviewed also, and 38 hearts with HC that previously underwent detailed histologic characterization were selected for comparative study.[5–11,15,23,28] Patients were aged 11 to 53 years (mean 26); 17 (45%) were male. Five patients had symptoms of cardiac dysfunction; 15 had been asymptomatic, and sudden death was the first definitive manifestation of their cardiac disease. Death was sudden in 22 patients, due to congestive heart failure in 5, during or shortly after operation in 8, and a result of cerebrovascular accident, suicide or cardiac catheterization in 1 each. Of 25 patients with cardiac catheterization, 16 had obstruction to left ventricular outflow (gradient ≥30 mm Hg under basal or provocable conditions), and the other 9 were nonobstructive.

The diagnosis of HC in all 99 hearts studied was based on the presence of a hypertrophied nondilated left ventricle in the absence of another cardiac or systemic disease (such as systemic hypertension, aortic valvular stenosis or coronary artery disease) capable of producing the magnitude of hypertrophy present in that patient.[1] The hearts of 60 cats, 25 dogs and 83 human patients that died of cardiac diseases other than HC, or of noncardiac causes and had normal hearts, both structurally and functionally, were studied for the purposes of selected morphologic comparisons (Table I).

Preparation of tissue: In each of the 273 humans, cats and dogs studied (99 with HC, and 174 controls), full-thickness tissue blocks were obtained from the left ventricular wall in the transverse plane perpendicular to the long axis of the left ventricle, approximately one half the distance between the apex and base of the aortic valve, in the: (1) ventricular septum, (2) anterolateral free wall approximately 2 cm lateral to the left anterior descending coronary artery, and (3) posterior free wall between the papillary muscles. Tissue was imbedded in paraffin, sectioned at 6 μ thickness, and stained with hematoxylin and eosin or Movat's pentachrome.

Left ventricular wall thicknesses were measured in formalin-fixed gross specimens perpendicular to the endocardial surfaces. Trabeculae, papillary muscles, crista supraventricular muscle and the endocardial contact plaques were excluded from these measurements.

Definition and classification of abnormal cardiac muscle cell arrangement: Cardiac muscle cell disorganization was classified into 2 major types. Type I disorganization, the most common, consisted of areas of myocardium in which adjacent cells were aligned perpendicularly or obliquely to each other, forming tangled masses or "pinwheel" configurations. Alternatively, type I disorganization appeared as relatively broad bundles of muscle cells oriented at oblique or perpendicular angles to each other; cells within these bundles were normally arranged.

Type II disorganization consisted of relatively narrow, longitudinally cut bundles of cells that were interlaced in various directions among larger groups of transversely cut cells (which appeared circular). This type of disorganization gave the myocardium a distinctive "swirled" appearance.

Abnormally arranged cardiac muscle cells were not considered representative of true disorganization if present in areas where cells normally converge at acute angles: (1) junction of ventricular septum with ventricular free walls; (2) trabeculations; (3) edges of areas of fibrosis; (4) points of convergence of major muscle bundles; or (5) adjacent to interstitial spaces.

Quantitation of cardiac muscle cell arrangement: A previously described technique was used to quantitatively assess the extent to which cardiac muscle cell disorganization was present in each tissue section.[7–9] Histologic sections were photographed, and the images were enlarged to occupy 30 × 40 inch positive prints. A transparent cellulose overlay was placed over the print. Areas of myocardium occupied by disorganized cardiac muscle cells were outlined. The transparent overlay was then reproduced as a 5 × 7 inch photograph. Areas into which the tissue section had been divided were outlined separately with a fine-point marking pen on tablet paper and quantitated using a video planimetry system; the percent area of tissue section occupied by disorganized cardiac muscle cells calculated with respect to the area of myocardium "at risk" for disorganization.

TABLE I Cardiac Diseases in 168 Control Patients or Animals

Disease	Cats	Dogs	Humans
Aortic valve disease	0	0	17
Coronary heart disease	0	0	15
Mitral valve disease	0	0	10
Systemic hypertension	0	0	8
Dilated (congestive) cardiomyopathy	16	3	6
Primary pulmonary hypertension	0	0	6
Pulmonary valve stenosis	0	0	3
Aortic & mitral valve disease	0	0	2
Supravalvular aortic stenosis	2	0	2
Ventricular septal defect	0	1	2
Discrete subaortic stenosis	0	2	1
Malformation mitral valve complex	3	2	0
Dysplasia of tricuspid valve	3	2	0
Normal heart	36	15	11
Total	60	25	83

Analysis of intramural coronary arteries: Assessment of intramural coronary artery anatomy was confined to those small vessels (<1,500 μ diameter in humans, and <1,200 μ in animals) that were viewed in cross section (transverse cut) without obvious obliquity and did not appear to be branches of intramural vessels, or portions of a "tunneled" epicardial vessel. Small coronary arteries present in trabeculae or papillary muscles were excluded from this analysis. Sections were considered abnormal with >1 abnormal intramural coronary artery in humans and 1 or more arteries in animals.

Analysis of myocardial fibrosis: The extent of fibrous tissue formation was assessed qualitatively in each tissue section. Mild fibrosis was judged to be present when an isolated small scar or prominent interstitial fibrous tissue, or both, was identified; severe fibrosis consisted of replacement scarring occupying substantial portions of the tissue section. Moderate fibrosis was intermediate in extent between the mild and severe grades.

Statistical methods: Data were expressed as mean ± SEM. Differences between means were assessed by Student's unpaired *t* test and 1-way analysis of variance.

RESULTS

Heart weights: Heart weights were 19 to 33 g (28.0 ± 0.5 SEM) in the 51 cats, and 98 to 385 g (231 ± 23) in the 10 dogs. Heart weight in relation to body weight was significantly greater in cats (6.4 ± 0.1 g/kg) and dogs (9.6 ± 0.3 g/kg) with HC than in normal control cats (4.8 ± 0.1 g/kg; p <0.001) and dogs (6.6 ± 0.3 g/kg; p <0.001). Heart weights were 300 to 1,002 g (548 ± 35) in the 28 adult patients with HC, and 270 to 650 g (457 ± 36) in the 10 children aged <18 years.

Ventricular septal thickness (Figure 1 and Table II): Maximal ventricular septal thickness was 9.0 ± 0.2 mm in the 51 cats, and 19 ± 2 in the 10 dogs with HC, and was significantly greater in these cats and dogs than in their respective controls with normal hearts (5.0 ± 0.2 and 12.0 ± 0.5 mm; p <0.001). Ventricular septal thickness in each patient with HC exceeded the generally accepted upper limits for necropsy measurements (i.e., 15 mm). In the 10 children (age <18 years), septal thickness was 17 to 38 mm (mean 24).

Left ventricular free wall thickness (Table II): ANTEROLATERAL WALL: Wall thicknesses in cats (9.0 ± 0.1 mm) and dogs (18 ± 1.5 mm) with HC were significantly greater than in their respective controls (6.0 ± 0.3 and 15 ± 0.7 mm; $p < 0.01$). Anterolateral wall thickness was >15 mm in 23 patients with HC.

POSTERIOR WALL: Wall thicknesses in cats (8.0 ± 0.1 mm) and dogs (15 ± 0.7 mm) with HC were significantly greater than in their respective controls (6.0 ± 0.2 and 13 ± 0.6 mm; $p < 0.001$ and < 0.05). Posterior wall thickness was ≥15 mm in 24 patients with HC.

Asymmetric hypertrophy of the ventricular septum (defined as ventricular septal–to–posterior free wall thickness ratio ≥1.3 in patients,[10] and ≥1.1 in cats and dogs[24,26,27]) was present in 31 of 38 patients with HC (81%) and in 8 of 10 dogs (80%), but only 16 of 51 cats (31%) ($p < 0.001$) (Figures 1 and 2).

Cardiac muscle cell disorganization (Figure 3 and Table III): VENTRICULAR SEPTUM: Percent area of cellular disorganization in the ventricular septum was signifi-

TABLE II Left Ventricular Wall Thickness in Cats, Dogs and Humans with Hypertrophic Cardiomyopathy

	Ventricular Septum (mm)	LV Free Wall (mm) Anterolateral	LV Free Wall (mm) Posterior	VS/PW
Cats (n = 51)	9.0 ± 0.2	9.0 ± 0.1	8.0 ± 0.1	1.10 ± 0.03
	(6–12)	(7–11)	(6–11)	(0.8–1.6)
Dogs (n = 10)	19.0 ± 2.3	18.0 ± 1.5	15.0 ± 0.7	1.30 ± 0.04
	(13–22)	(11–23)	(10–19)	(1.0–1.5)†
Humans (n = 38)	25 ± 1	18.0 ± 0.9	16.0 ± 0.7	1.8 ± 0.2
	(17–44)	(10–30)	(9–27)	(0.8–2.6)*

*Significantly greater than in cats and dogs ($p < 0.005$).
†Significantly greater than in cats ($p < 0.01$).
LV = left ventricular; VS/PW = ventricular septal–to–posterior free wall thickness ratio.

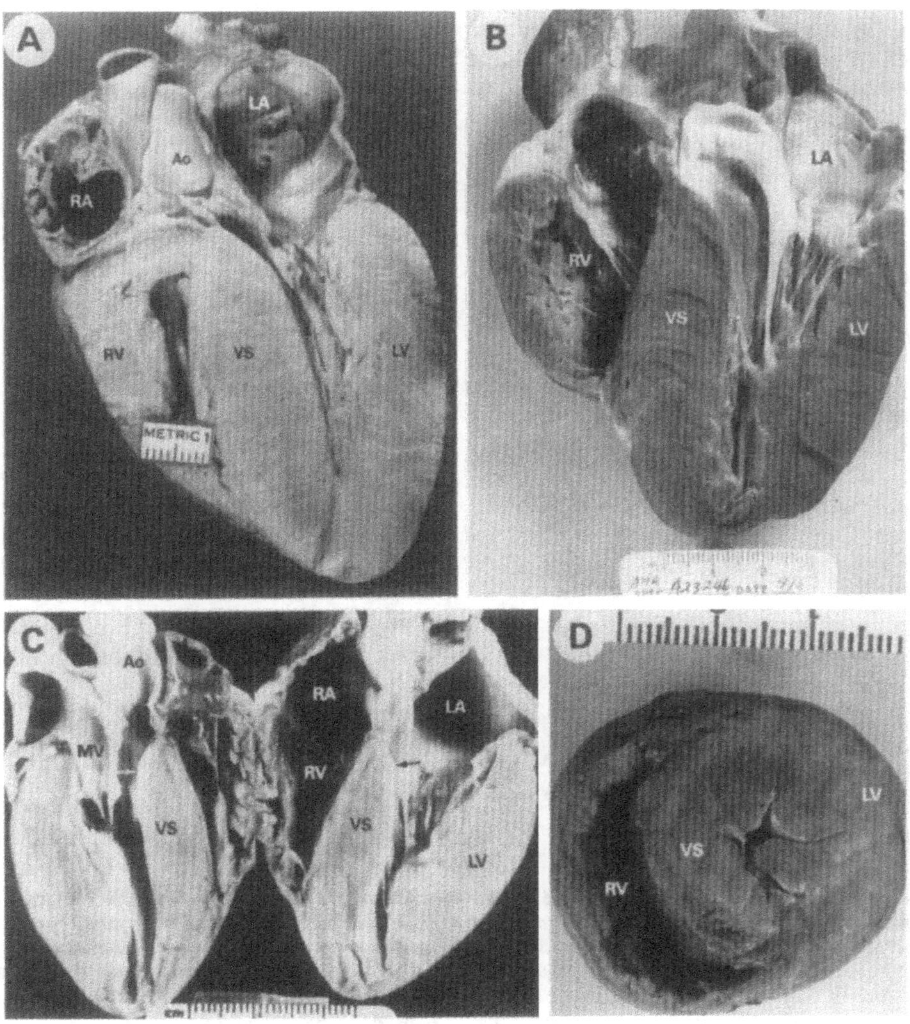

FIGURE 1. Gross morphologic features of hearts from a human and animals with hypertrophic cardiomyopathy. Displayed in longitudinal *(A, B and C)* and transverse *(D)* sections. *A,* 7-year-old child showing marked asymmetric hypertrophy of ventricular septum (VS) in relation to left ventricular (LV) free wall, very small LV cavity and dilated left (LA) and right (RA) atria. *B,* 7-year-old German shepherd dog. Heart is similar in appearance to the human in *panel A* with asymmetric VS hypertrophy. *C,* 3-year-old domestic shorthair cat. Bisected heart shows relatively mild pattern of asymmetric septal hypertrophy. Small LV cavity, and enlarged left and right atria. An endocardial contact plaque on VS in the LV outflow tract is present *(arrows)*. *D,* 13-year-old domestic shorthair cat; asymmetric hypertrophy of VS in relation to LV free wall is shown in distal portion of left ventricle. The cavity appears particularly small, and papillary muscles are also greatly hypertrophied. Ao = aorta; MV = mitral valve; RV = right ventricle.

cantly greater in patients with HC than in cats and dogs ($p < 0.001$). Disorganization was identified in 37 of 38 patients (97%), but less commonly in 15 of 51 cats (30%) and in 2 of 10 dogs (20%) ($p < 0.001$) (Figure 2). Similarly, septal disorganization comprising ≥5% of the relevant portions of tissue section was present in 35 of 38 patients with HC (92%), in 14 of 51 cats (27%) and in 2 of 10 dogs (20%) ($p < 0.001$). Particularly extensive cellular disorganization (≥25%) was evident in 25 humans (66%), but in only 7 cats (14%) and no dogs ($p < 0.001$) (Figure 3).

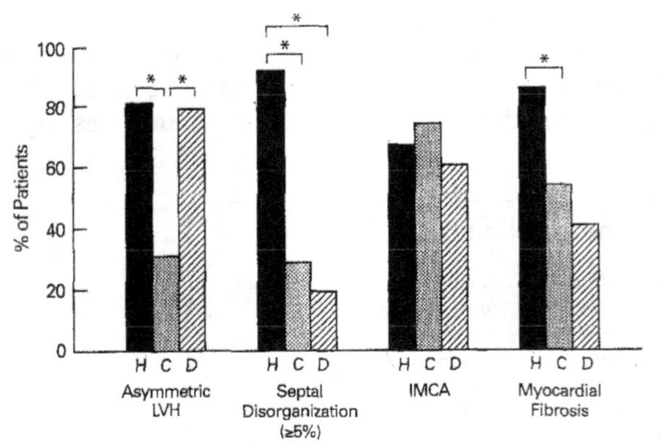

FIGURE 2. Frequency of occurrence of 4 morphologic hallmarks of hypertrophic cardiomyopathy in humans (H), cats (C) and dogs (D). *Asterisks,* comparison achieved statistical significance ($p < 0.001$). Histologic data for cellular disorganization, abnormal intramural coronary arteries (IMCA) and myocardial fibrosis are presented for ventricular septum only. LVH = left ventricular hypertrophy.

In each patient with HC, septal disorganization was predominantly of the type I pattern; in 22 of 37, foci were present in which adjacent cardiac muscle cells were aligned perpendicularly and obliquely to each other (Figure 3A). The size of these individual foci of dis-

TABLE III Left Ventricular Cellular Disorganization* in Cats, Dogs and Humans with Hypertrophic Cardiomyopathy

	Ventricular Septum (%)	LV Free Wall (%) Anterolateral	Posterior
Cats (n = 51)	7.0 ± 1.9 (0–47)†	1.5 ± 0.6 (0–29)†	1.0 ± 0.4 (0–22)†
Dogs (n = 10)	3.0 ± 1.7 (0–14)	1.0 ± 0.7 (0–8)	0
Humans (n = 38)	38.0 ± 3.4 (0–95)‡	37.0 ± 5.3 (0–94)‡	19.0 ± 4.1 (0–93)‡

*Expressed as that percentage of the relevant portions of the tissue section comprised of disorganized cardiac muscle cells.[9]
†Significantly greater than in dogs ($p < 0.01$).
‡Significantly greater than in cats and dogs ($p < 0.001$).
LV = *left ventricular.*

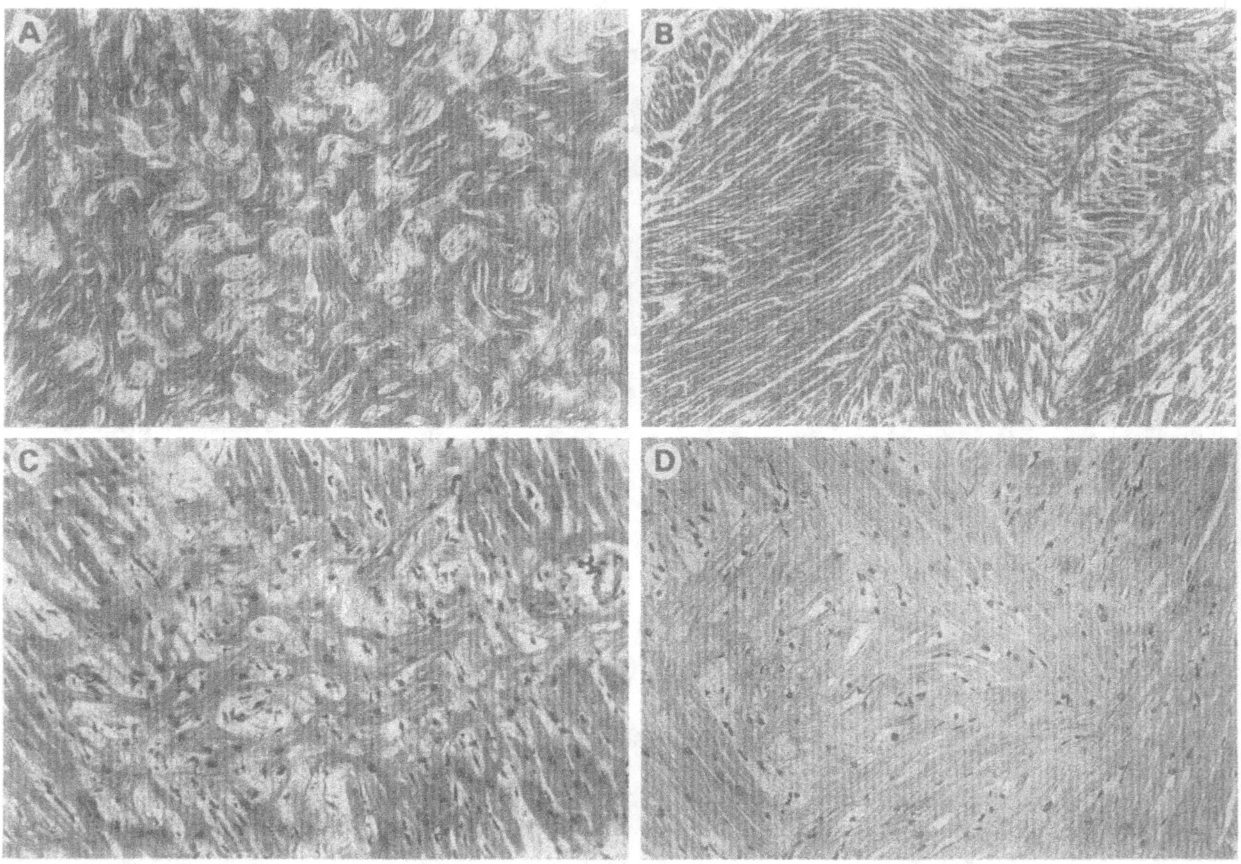

FIGURE 3. Distorted ventricular septal architecture in humans *(A and B)* and cats *(C and D)* with hypertrophic cardiomyopathy. *A,* markedly disordered arrangement of cardiac muscle cells with adjacent cells arranged at perpendicular and oblique angles to each other. *B,* cellular disorganization in which broad bundles of cardiac muscle cells are arranged at oblique or perpendicular angles; cells within these bundles are normally arranged. *C,* tangled arrangement of cardiac muscle cells in a cat; pattern is similar to that characteristic of humans *(A). D,* disordered arrangements of bundles of myocardial cells in a cat, similar to that in the human *(B).* (Hematoxylin-eosin stains, original magnification ×100, reduced by 25%.)

organization showed great variability, but most were relatively small. The other 15 patients had type I disorganization in which broad bundles of cells were oriented at oblique and perpendicular angles (Figure 3B). Type II disorganization also was present in 5 patients.

In animals with HC, type I disorganization involving foci of adjacent cardiac muscle cells also predominated (Figure 3C). These areas of disorganization varied considerably in size, but were usually smaller than in patients with HC. Cats often showed a distinctive "swiss

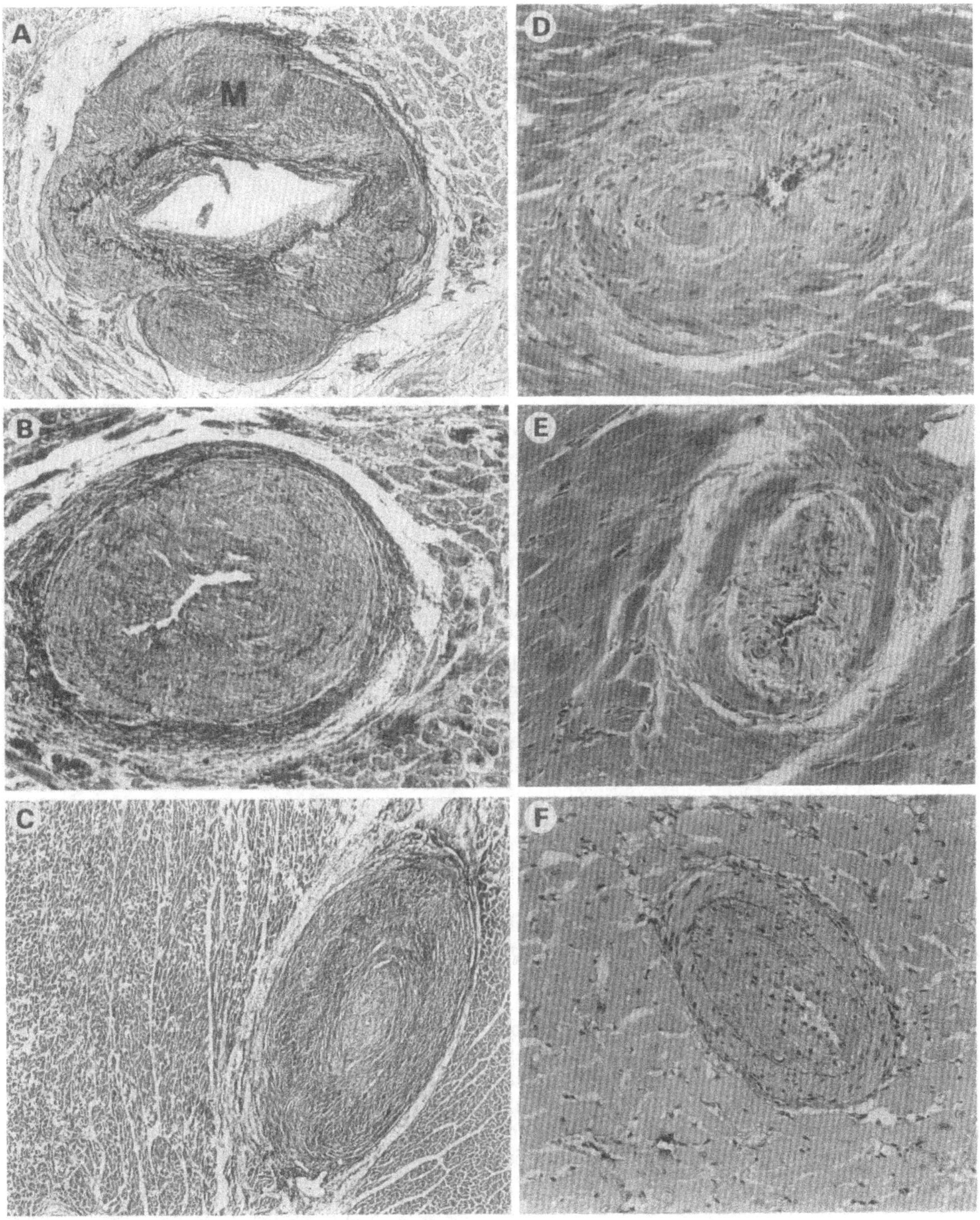

FIGURE 4. Histologic abnormalities of intramural coronary arteries in humans and animals with hypertrophic cardiomyopathy. *A*, human artery with an apparently narrowed lumen and thickened wall due primarily to medial (M) hypertrophy. (Hematoxylin-eosin stain, original magnification ×50, reduced by 23%.) *B and D to F*, feline arteries with very narrowed (or virtually obliterated) lumen and thickened wall, which appeared to be due primarily to proliferation of smooth muscle cells and connective tissue elements in both the media and intima. (Hematoxylin-eosin, Tyson's elastic or Masson's trichrome stain, original magnification ×100, ×150, ×200 and ×200, respectively; reduced by 23%.) *C*, canine artery with an obliterated lumen and markedly thickened wall, which appeared to include intimal and medial proliferation of smooth muscle cells, elastic fibers and fibrous connective tissue. (Tyson's elastic stain, original magnification ×50, reduced by 23%.)

TABLE IV Left Ventricular Cellular Disorganization* in Cats, Dogs and Humans with Hypertrophic Cardiomyopathy as Compared with Controls

	Ventricular Septum (%)	LV Free Wall (%) Anterolateral	Posterior
Cats			
HC (n = 51)	7.0 ± 1.9†	1.5 ± 0.6†	1.0 ± 0.4
Controls (n = 60)	0.3 ± 0.2	0	0
Dogs			
HC (n = 10)	3.0 ± 1.7†	0.8 ± 0.2	0
Controls (n = 25)	0	0	0
Humans			
HC (n = 38)	38.0 ± 3.4†	37.0 ± 5.3†	19.0 ± 4.1†
Controls (n = 83)	2.0 ± 0.9	9.4 ± 1.5	1.5 ± 0.5

*Expressed as that percentage of the relevant portions of the tissue section comprised of disorganized cardiac muscle cells.[9]
†Significantly greater than controls (p <0.001).
HC = hypertrophic cardiomyopathy; LV = left ventricular.

cheese'' myocardial architecture, characterized by multiple small foci of cell-to-cell disarray (Figure 3C). Extent of septal, anterolateral and posterior wall disorganization was significantly greater in patients, dogs and cats than in their respective controls (Table IV).

LEFT VENTRICULAR FREE WALL: Mean area of cellular disorganization in both the anterolateral and posterior wall was significantly greater in patients than in cats or dogs (p <0.001) (Table III). When analyzed with regard to individual subjects, extent of disorganization was greater in humans than in cats and dogs for both free wall sections (p <0.001) (Figure 2).

Intramural coronary arteries (Figure 4 and Table V): In humans (Figure 4A), abnormal arteries were characterized by increased size and thickened walls. Usually, the lumen appeared narrowed. Thickening of the arterial wall was due to thickening of both media and intima, and the thickening resulted particularly from increases in smooth muscle cells, fibrous tissue, elastic fibers and mucoid deposits (acid mucopolysaccharide). In animals (Figure 4, B to F), the thickening of the arterial wall resulted primarily from increased connective tissue elements (and to a much lesser extent smooth muscle cells) in the intima and media.

Abnormal intramural coronary arteries (ranging in number from 2 to 6) were identified in ventricular septal tissue sections with similar frequency in all 3 species (i.e., in 25 of 38 patients with HC [66%], in 38 of 51 cats [74%] and in 6 of 10 dogs [60%]) (Figure 2). Abnormal intramural coronary arteries were most common in the ventricular septum in all 3 species, but were also identified in each of the 3 tissue sites in 4 patients, 18 cats and 2 dogs. In each of the species with HC, abnormal arteries were significantly more common than in their respective controls (i.e., 3 of 60 cats [5%], 1 of 25 dogs [4%], and 5 of 68 previously reported human controls [7%][23]; all p <0.001).

Myocardial fibrosis (Figure 5): Areas of substantial interstitial fibrous tissue or replacement fibrosis of varying sizes were much more common in patients with HC (33 of 38 [86%]) than in either cats (27 of 51 [53%]) or dogs (4 of 10 [40%]; p <0.001) (Figure 2). In addi-

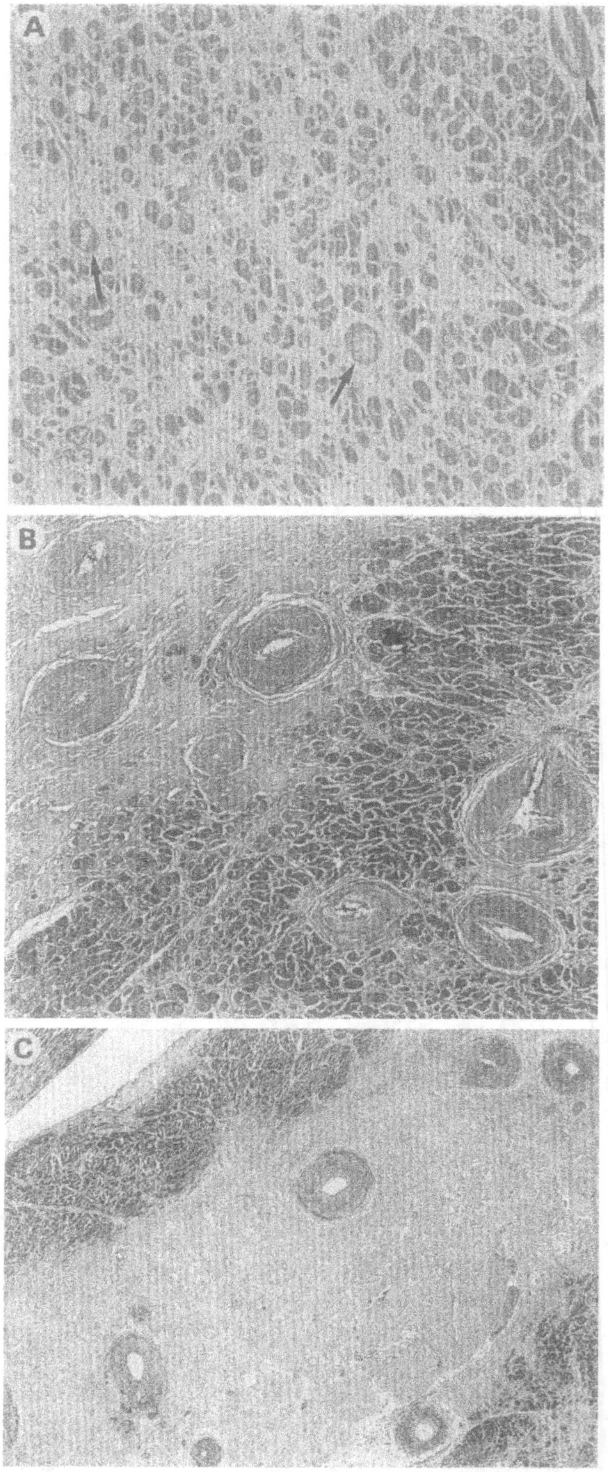

FIGURE 5. Myocardial fibrosis and relation to abnormal intramural coronary arteries in a bulldog *(A)* and humans *(B and C)* with hypertrophic cardiomyopathy. *A,* cardiac muscle cells embedded in framework of fibrous connective tissue; a few intramural coronary arteries are evident *(arrows).* (Masson's trichrome stain, original magnification ×50, reduced by 30%.) *B,* numerous abnormal intramural coronary arteries are present in a region of fibrosis *(top left),* as well as in an adjacent area of myocardium that is not scarred *(bottom right).* (Hematoxylin-eosin, original magnification ×100, reduced by 30%.) *C,* an area of substantial scarring in which several abnormal intramural coronary arteries are present. (Hematoxylin-eosin, original magnification ×55, reduced by 30%.)

TABLE V Abnormal Intramural Coronary Arteries in Left Ventricular Wall of Cats, Dogs and Humans with Hypertrophic Cardiomyopathy

	IMCAs in Patients	IMCAs in Tissue Sections	Ventricular Septum*	LV Free Wall (%)*	
				Anterolateral	Posterior
Cats	38/51 (74%)	82/153 (53%)	3.0 ± 0.4 (2–6)	1.0 ± 0.2 (0–3)	1.0 ± 0.3 (0–4)
Dogs	7/10 (70%)	14/30 (46%)	2.3 ± 0.4 (1–3)	1.0 ± 0.3 (0–2)	0.5 ± 0.2 (0–1)
Humans	28/38 (74%)	50/114 (44%)	5.0 ± 1.3 (0–50)†	1.4 ± 0.3 (0–8)†	0.5 ± 0.2 (0–4)

*Expressed as an absolute number of abnormal IMCAs/tissue section.
†Significantly greater than in cats and dogs ($p < 0.05$).
IMCAs = intramural coronary arteries; LV = left ventricular.

tion, fibrosis believed to be moderate to severe was evident in 15 patients (39%), but in only 13 of 61 animals (21%) ($p = 0.05$).

Relation between abnormal coronary arteries and myocardial fibrosis (Figure 5): In patients with HC, myocardial fibrosis was absent or mild in 85 of the 114 total left ventricular tissue sections, and moderate to severe in the other 29. Abnormal intramural coronary arteries (usually within or at the margins of areas of fibrosis) were significantly more common in tissue sections with moderate-to-severe fibrosis (12 of 29 [41%]) than in those with no or mild fibrosis (5 of 85 [6%]; $p < 0.001$). In animals with HC, fibrosis was absent or mild in 157 of the 183 tissue sections, and moderate to severe in 26; abnormal intramural coronary arteries were significantly more common in sections with moderate or severe fibrosis (15 of 26 [57%]) than in those with no or mild fibrosis (27 of 157 [17%]; $p < 0.001$).

DISCUSSION

This report compares particular morphologic features of HC in patients[2–10] with those in various breeds of cats and dogs[24–27] with spontaneously occurring cardiac disease that appears similar to the human disease entity. Both cats and dogs had each of the 4 morphologic hallmarks of left ventricular muscle described in patients with this disease (i.e., asymmetric patterns of wall thickening,[1–3,10,14,15,28–30] disorganization of cardiac muscle cells,[4–13] abnormal intramural coronary arteries[18,22,23] and myocardial fibrosis[17,18,21–23]). When analyzed separately, however, the frequency with which each abnormality occurred differed substantially among the 3 species.

Asymmetric patterns of left ventricular hypertrophy (based on the calculated septal–to–free wall thickness ratio) were much more common in patients and dogs than in cats; in all 3 species, hypertrophy was often diffuse, involving substantial portions of the anterolateral and posterior free walls, as well as the ventricular septum. Cardiac muscle cell disorganization was observed to be much more frequent and extensive in patients than in either cats or dogs, but was much more likely to be limited to the septum in animals. Abnormal intramural coronary arteries, with thickened walls and narrowed lumens, occurred with relatively equal frequency in both humans and animals, although fibrous tissue formation was more common in humans. In both humans and animals, abnormal intramural coronary arteries were present more commonly in tissue sections with moderate-to-severe fibrosis, and these arteries were usually evident within or at the margins of areas of fibrosis.[18,23] This association between myocardial fibrosis and abnormal intramural coronary arteries implies a causal relation, and suggests that small vessel abnormalities in both animals and humans with HC are of pathophysiologic significance, and constitute a form of "small vessel disease" that may produce or contribute to myocardial ischemia and necrosis.[23]

The findings of this study show that primary cardiac diseases that are phenotypically similar in many respects to HC in humans, also occur in cats and dogs. However, there is substantial morphologic variability among the species; consequently, spontaneously occurring feline and canine HC cannot be viewed as morphologically identical to the human disease entity.

1. Maron BJ, Epstein SE. Hypertrophic cardiomyopathy: a discussion of nomenclature. *Am J Cardiol* 1979;43:1242–1244.

2. Teare D. Asymmetrical hypertrophy of the heart in young adults. *Br Heart J* 1958;20:1–8.

3. Olsen EG. Anatomic and light microscopic characterization of hypertrophic obstructive and nonobstructive cardiomyopathy. *Eur Heart J* 1983;4(suppl F):1–8.

4. Ferrans VJ, Morrow AG, Roberts WC. Myocardial ultrastructure in idiopathic hypertrophic subaortic stenosis: a study of operatively excised left ventricular outflow tract muscle in 14 patients. *Circulation* 1972;45:769–792.

5. Sutton MSJ, Lie JT, Anderson KR, O'Brien PC, Frye RL. Histopathological specificity of hypertrophic obstructive cardiomyopathy. Myocardial fibre disarray and myocardial fibrosis. *Br Heart J* 1980;44:433–443.

6. Maron BJ, Roberts WC. Hypertrophic cardiomyopathy and cardiac muscle cell disorganization revisited: relation between the two and significance. *Am Heart J* 1981;102:95–110.

7. Maron BJ, Anan TJ, Roberts WC. Quantitative analysis of the distribution of cardiac muscle cell disorganization in the left ventricular wall of patients with hypertrophic cardiomyopathy. *Circulation* 1981;63:882–894.

8. Maron BJ, Sato N, Roberts WC, Edwards JE, Chandra RS. Quantitative analysis of cardiac muscle cell disorganization in the ventricular septum: Comparison of fetuses and infants with and without congenital heart disease and patients with hypertrophic cardiomyopathy. *Circulation* 1979;60:685–696.

9. Maron BJ, Roberts WC. Quantitative analysis of cardiac muscle cell disorganization in the ventricular septum of patients with hypertrophic cardiomyopathy. *Circulation* 1979;59:689–706.

10. Maron BJ, Epstein SE. Hypertrophic cardiomyopathy. Recent observations regarding the specificity of three hallmarks of the disease: asymmetric septal hypertrophy, septal disorganization, and systolic anterior motion of the anterior mitral leaflet. *Am J Cardiol* 1980;45:141–154.

11. Isner JM, Maron BJ, Roberts WC. Comparison of amount of cardiac-muscle-cell disorganization in operatively-excised septectomy specimens to amount observed at necropsy in 18 patients with hypertrophic cardiomyopathy. *Am J Cardiol* 1980;46:42–47.

12. Fujiwara H, Kawai C, Hamashima Y. Myocardial fascicle and fiber disarray in 25 μ-thick sections. *Circulation* 1979;59:1293–1298.

13. Van Noorden S, Olsen EGJ, Pearse AGE. Hypertrophic obstructive cardiomyopathy, a histological histochemical, and ultrastructural study of biopsy material.

Cardiovasc Res 1971;5:118–131.
14. Wigle ED, Sasson Z, Henderson MA, Ruddy TD, Fulop J, Rakowski H, Williams WG. Hypertrophic cardiomyopathy. The importance of the site and the extent of hypertrophy. A review. *Prog Cardiovasc Dis* 1985;28:1–83.
15. Maron BJ, Bonow RO, Cannon RO, Leon MB, Epstein SE. Hypertrophic cardiomyopathy: interrelation of clinical manifestations, pathophysiology and therapy. *N Engl J Med* 1987;316:780–789, 844–852.
16. McKenna WJ, Camm AJ. Sudden death in hypertrophic cardiomyopathy: assessment of patients at high risk. *Circulation* 1989;80:1489–1492.
17. Roberts CS, Roberts WC. Morphologic features. In: Zipes DP, Rowlands DJ, eds. *Progress in Cardiology* 2/2. Philadelphia: Lea & Febiger, 1989:3–22.
18. Maron BJ, Epstein SE, Roberts WC. Hypertrophic cardiomyopathy and transmural myocardial infarction without significant atherosclerosis of the extramural coronary arteries. *Am J Cardiol* 1979;43:1086–1102.
19. Goodwin JF. Congestive and hypertrophic cardiomyopathies: a decade of study. *Lancet* 1970;1:731–739.
20. Spirito P, Maron BJ. Relation between extent of left ventricular hypertrophy and diastolic filling abnormalities in hypertrophic cardiomyopathy. *J Am Coll Cardiol* 1990;15:808–813.
21. Factor SM, Butany J, Sole MJ, Wigle ED, Williams WC, Rojkind M. Pathologic fibrosis and matrix connective tissue in the subaortic myocardium of patients with hypertrophic cardiomyopathy. *J Am Coll Cardiol* 1991;17:1343–1351.
22. Tanaka M, Fujiwara H, Onodera T, Wu D-J, Hamashima Y, Kawai C. Quantitative analysis of myocardial fibrosis in normals, hypertensive hearts, and hypertrophic cardiomyopathy. *Br Heart J* 1986;55:575–581.
23. Maron BJ, Wolfson JK, Epstein SE, Roberts WC. Intramural ("small vessel") coronary artery disease in hypertrophic cardiomyopathy. *J Am Coll Cardiol* 1986;8: 545–557.
24. Liu SK, Maron BJ, Tilley LP. Feline hypertrophic cardiomyopathy: gross anatomic and quantitative histologic features. *Am J Pathol* 1981;102:388–395.
25. Tilley LP, Liu S K, Gilbertson SR, Wagner BM, Lord PF. Primary myocardial disease in the cat. *Am J Pathol* 1977;87:493–522.
26. Liu S K, Maron BJ, Tilley LP. Hypertrophic cardiomyopathy in the dog. *Am J Pathol* 1979;94:497–508.
27. Liu S K, Hsu FS, Lee RCT. An Atlas of Cardiovascular Pathology. Taiwan: Pig Research Institute 1989:198–227.
28. Roberts WC, Ferrans VJ. Pathologic anatomy of the cardiomyopathies. *Hum Pathol* 1975;6:287–342.
29. Maron BJ, Gottdiener JS, Epstein SE. Patterns and significance of the distribution of left ventricular hypertrophy in hypertrophic cardiomyopathy: a wide-angle, two-dimensional echocardiographic study of 125 patients. *Am J Cardiol* 1981;48: 418–428.
30. Maron BJ. Asymmetry in hypertrophic cardiomyopathy: the septal to free wall thickness ratio revisited. *Am J Cardiol* 1985;55:835–838.

Circadian Variability in the Occurrence of Sudden Cardiac Death in Patients With Hypertrophic Cardiomyopathy

BARRY J. MARON, MD, FACC, JULIE KOGAN, MD, MICHAEL A. PROSCHAN, PHD, GABRIELA M. HECHT, MD, WILLIAM C. ROBERTS, MD, FACC

Minneapolis, Minnesota and Bethesda, Maryland

Objectives. **The present study examined whether sudden death in patients with hypertrophic cardiomyopathy occurred with a particular pattern of frequency throughout the day.**

Background. **Previous investigators have shown a circadian distribution in the occurrence of sudden death and other cardiovascular events in patients with atherosclerotic coronary artery disease. Sudden death is also an important feature of the natural history of patients with hypertrophic cardiomyopathy.**

Methods. **The study group comprised 94 patients with a time of death (or cardiac arrest) that could be ascertained accurately to the nearest hour. This hourly distribution was analyzed by harmonic regression.**

Results. **Sudden death did not occur uniformly or randomly throughout the day. Rather, it was distributed in a bimodal pattern that conformed to a two-harmonic regression model. A disproportionate number of sudden deaths (43 [46%] of 94) occurred in the first peak in midmorning between 7 AM and 1 PM. The second peak of sudden death was less distinct but was in the early evening, between 8 PM and 10 PM. This periodicity in occurrence of sudden cardiac death was not evident for the days of the week or months of the year and, furthermore, did not appear to be influenced by other clinical variables, such as age, gender, severity of symptoms, subaortic gradient or left ventricular wall thickness. Sudden death occurred most commonly during periods of severe exertion (37 [39%] of 94).**

Conclusions. **Sudden death in hypertrophic cardiomyopathy demonstrates a bimodal pattern of circadian variability over the 24-h day, with a prominent midmorning peak similar to that described in patients with coronary artery disease, and a less striking early-evening peak of occurrence. These findings suggest that temporally related physiologic changes, possibly in the electrical vulnerability of the myocardial substrate, may play a role in the sudden death of patients with hypertrophic cardiomyopathy.**

(J Am Coll Cardiol 1994;23:1405–9)

Several previous investigations in patients with coronary artery disease have demonstrated a circadian periodic rhythm with respect to the distribution and occurrence of acute cardiovascular events, such as sudden cardiac death and nonfatal acute myocardial infarction (1–11). These studies have identified peak frequencies of occurrence after awakening in the morning (1–5,8–10) and occasionally in the early evening as well (6,7,11), providing potential clinical clues with regard to mechanisms underlying sudden cardiac death in patients with ischemic heart disease.

Sudden death is also an important feature of the natural history of patients with hypertrophic cardiomyopathy (12–18), a genetically transmitted primary cardiac disease in which a number of pathophysiologic mechanisms have been proposed as causes of cardiac arrest (13,14,17–23). The present study examined whether the occurrence of sudden death in hypertrophic cardiomyopathy was randomly distributed throughout the day or, alternatively, was clustered in a periodic pattern.

From the Cardiovascular Research Division, Minneapolis Heart Institute Foundation, Minneapolis, Minnesota and Cardiology and Pathology Branches, National Heart, Lung, and Blood Institute and Biostatistics Research Branch, National Institutes of Health, Bethesda, Maryland.

Manuscript received August 30, 1993; revised manuscript received December 9, 1993, accepted December 17, 1993.

Address for correspondence: Dr. Barry J. Maron, Cardiovascular Research Division, Minneapolis Heart Institute Foundation, 920 E. 28th Street, Suite 40, Minneapolis, Minnesota 55407.

Methods

Selection of patients. The registry of the Pathology Branch and the case records of the Cardiology Branch, National Heart, Lung, and Blood Institute, were reviewed, and 135 patients with hypertrophic cardiomyopathy were identified who had either died suddenly and unexpectedly or had experienced cardiac arrest from which they were successfully resuscitated under fortuitous circumstances (for simplicity we will refer to both as sudden death). Of the 135 patients, 41 were excluded by virtue of the following: 1) presence of severe and progressive congestive symptoms associated with evidence of the "end-stage" phase (24); 2) previous cardiac operation; 3) noncardiovascular death or circumstances that were sufficiently unclear to raise substantial doubt as to whether the patient's death was cardiac in origin; 4) in-hospital death; 5) presence of associated "floppy" mitral valve; and 6) time of sudden death or cardiac arrest that could not be ascertained to the nearest hour by retrospective telephone contact with witnesses, persons in close contact with the deceased, surviving relatives or attending physician or, alternatively, by analysis of the death certificate or autopsy report. The latter exclusion criteria included six patients who had been found dead in the early morning hours but for whom it was not possible to determine retrospectively with reasonable precision the actual time of death.

The remaining 94 patients constitute the final study group. On the basis of echocardiographic and necropsy findings, each of these patients met our diagnostic criteria for hypertrophic cardiomyopathy (i.e., hypertrophied, nondilated left ventricle in the absence of another cardiac or systemic disease capable of producing the magnitude of hypertrophy present in that patient) (25). Study patients ranged in age from 8 to 62 years (mean age 28 years); 67 were <25 years old (71%); 57 were men (61%) and 37 were women (39%).

Statistical analyses. Harmonic regression (Fourier) analysis was utilized to assess the hourly distribution of sudden deaths and to ascertain whether these events occurred uniformly (i.e., randomly) throughout the 24-h day or were more frequent at certain times than at others. First, the data were tested for uniformity against a single harmonic regression model for one peak of occurrence of sudden death. Subsequently, the distribution of sudden death events was analyzed with a double-harmonic model for two peaks of occurrence (24). The model was

$$\sqrt{N} = \beta_0 + \beta_1 \cos(2\pi t/24) + \beta_2 \sin(2\pi t/24) + \beta_3 \cos(4\pi t/24) + \beta_4 \sin(4\pi t/24) + e,$$

where, N = the number of events in each hourly interval; t = the midpoint of the hourly interval; and e = a random error. Each cosine and sine pair represents one harmonic and, therefore this model incorporates two harmonics. By convention, deaths at or after midnight and before 1:00 AM (i.e., midnight to 12:59 AM) were considered to have occurred during the first hour of the day; deaths at or after 1:00 AM and before 2:00 AM were judged to be in the second hour, and so on.

Occurrence of sudden death also was tested by harmonic regression against other measures of periodicity, such as the days of the week and the months (and seasons) of the year. To ascertain whether the circadian pattern was related to administration of cardioactive medications or occurrence of cardiac arrest, data were analyzed by dividing the 24-h day into four quadrants suggested by the overall data (i.e., 1 AM to 6:59 AM, 7 AM to 12:59 PM, 1 PM to 6:59 PM and 7 PM to 12:59 AM) and then applying a standard chi-square test comparing the frequency of each event within these quadrants.

Results

Hourly distribution of sudden death. The hourly distribution of events is presented in Figure 1. Sudden death occurred at least once in 21 of the 24 h with no deaths occurring between 1 AM and 2 AM, 4 AM and 5 AM and 6 AM and 7 AM; sudden death occurred most commonly between 9 AM and 10 AM, noon and 1 PM and 8 PM and 9 PM. Visual inspection of the hourly distribution of events suggested a prominent midmorning peak comprising the 6 h between 7 AM and 1 PM (43 [46%] of 94 patients) and also a less distinct early evening peak between 8 PM and 10 PM. Therefore, these two peaks of sudden death were ~12 h apart, with troughs in event activity during the early morning and afternoon hours. Deaths in the morning peak were more frequent in number by a factor of 1.8 than during the next-frequent 6-h period of the day.

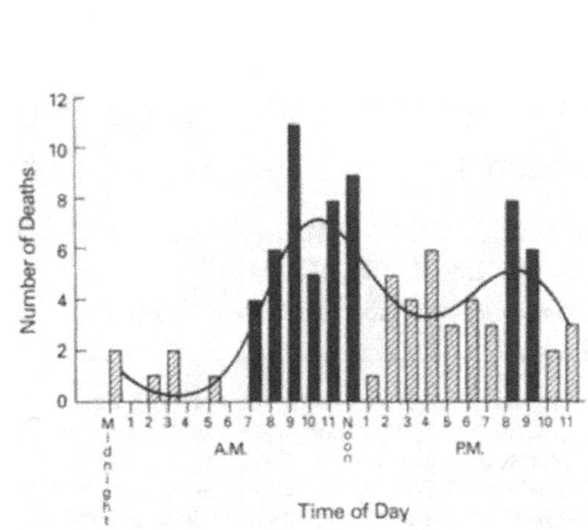

Figure 1. Histogram showing hourly distribution of sudden cardiac death events throughout the day in 94 patients with hypertrophic cardiomyopathy. Superimposed line denotes the bimodal pattern (double-harmonic model) with a prominent early peak between 7 AM and 1 PM and a secondary peak in the early evening, most evident between 8 PM and 10 PM.

Harmonic regression analysis substantiated that the occurrence of sudden cardiac death was not uniformly or randomly distributed throughout the day. These data showed that a single peak constituted a statistically significant improvement over a uniform distribution of events ($p = 0.01$). Adding a second harmonic for another peak yielded a statistically significant ($p = 0.012$) improvement in the fit of the data. Therefore, the best fitting model for the distribution of sudden cardiac death throughout the day contained two peaks (Fig. 1), as expressed by the equation

$$\sqrt{N} = 1.760 - 0.584 \cos(2\pi t/24) - 0.487 \sin(2\pi t/24) + 0.258 \cos(4\pi t/24) - 0.573 \sin(4\pi t/24).$$

A number of other clinical and morphologic features identified in the study patients (i.e., age, presence or magnitude of symptoms, administration of beta-adrenergic receptor blocking agents, maximal left ventricular wall thickness and heart weight) had no impact on the hourly circadian pattern. Patients with nonobstructive hypertrophic cardiomyopathy died more frequently in the morning (7 AM to

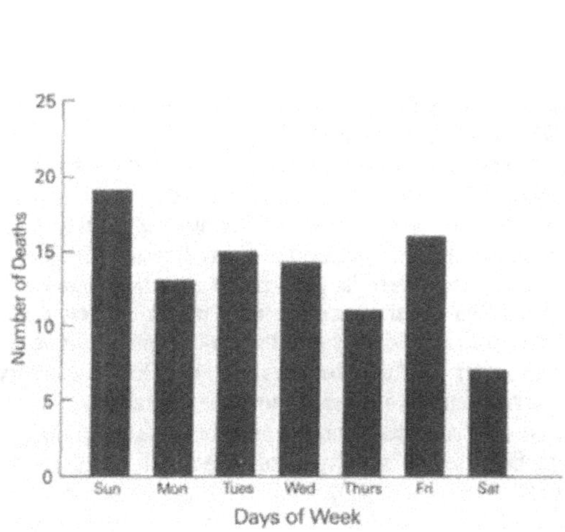

Figure 2. Daily distribution of sudden cardiac death events throughout the week showing a uniform pattern of occurrence in 94 patients with hypertrophic cardiomyopathy.

1 PM) although the level of statistical significance was borderline ($p = 0.048$).

Harmonic regression analysis showed the occurrence of sudden death to be consistent with a uniform distribution throughout the days of the week. Sudden death events were also uniformly distributed throughout the 12 months and four seasons of the year (Fig. 2 and 3).

In addition, we specifically analyzed the particular impact on the hourly circadian distribution of sudden cardiac death potentially created by the exclusion of six patients from the analysis because they had been found dead in bed in the early morning hours and in whom it was not possible to determine retrospectively with reasonable precision the actual time of death. We addressed this issue in two ways. First, we considered all possibilities for distributing the six deaths across the six hourly intervals between midnight and 6 AM. For each, we tested for a two-harmonic circadian pattern versus uniformity using all the actual and hypothetically generated data. When the hypothetic hour of death for each of the six patients is calculated, there are $6^6 = 46,656$ possibilities (many of which generate the same hourly totals). For example, if Patients 1 to 5 died between midnight and 1:00 AM, and Patient 6 died between 3 AM and 4 AM, the six hourly totals would be 5, 0, 0, 1, 0 and 0; the same hourly totals would result if Patient 1 had died between 3 AM and 4 AM and Patients 2 to 6 had died between midnight and 1 AM. Of the total 46,656 generated data sets, in 98.6% the p value for testing the two-harmonic model against uniformity was < 0.05. Furthermore, the largest p value was only 0.058, occurring when the hypothetically generated data assigned two deaths to each of the intervals 2 AM to 3 AM, 3 AM to 4 AM and 4 AM to 5 AM. Therefore, even if the precise times of death had been known for the six patients in question, these data would not have changed measurably the present findings or conclusions.

Second, we also addressed this issue by restricting analysis to those deaths occurring in the hours between 6 AM and 11:59 PM, and performed the harmonic regression only on those data. The two-harmonic model (with two peaks) remained a significant improvement over both uniformity ($p = 0.044$) and a single-harmonic model ($p = 0.019$).

Clinical profile. Of the 94 study patients, 59 were asymptomatic, 26 had mild symptoms (New York Heart Association functional class II), and 7 had marked symptoms (class III). In two patients the symptomatic state just before death could not be established with certainty. A substantial proportion of patients (38 [40%] of 94) were taking cardioactive medications (i.e., beta-adrenergic blocking agents, verapamil or a variety of antiarrhythmic agents) before death; specifically 26 of these 38 patients were taking standard doses of one of a variety of beta-blockers alone or in combination with other drugs.

Sudden death occurred during sedentary or mild activities in 27 patients (including 2 during sleep), moderate physical activity in 30 and severe exertion in 37 (including 10 competitive athletes, of whom 5 died during sport activity). Hemodynamic state had been assessed at cardiac catheterization in 60 of the 94 patients: 25 had left ventricular outflow tract obstruction under basal conditions (gradient >30 mm Hg, range 35 to 160), whereas the remaining 35 patients were nonobstructive (basal gradient <30 mm Hg).

Maximal left ventricular wall thicknesses ranged from 13 to 55 mm (mean thickness 26 mm), and heart weights ranged from 270 to 970 g (mean weight 512 g). Four patients had associated atherosclerotic coronary artery disease, and two had a history of relatively mild systemic hypertension.

Figure 3. Monthly distribution of sudden cardiac death events throughout the year showing a uniform pattern of occurrence in 94 patients with hypertrophic cardiomyopathy.

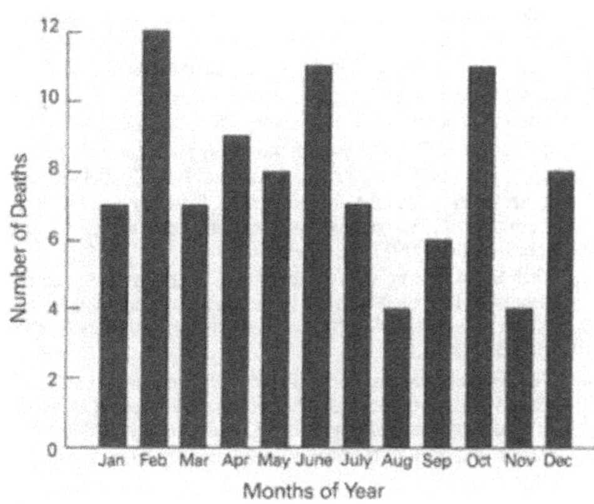

Discussion

Circadian variability. Epidemiologic studies have demonstrated that several unfavorable and usually unpredictable cardiovascular events, such as sudden cardiac death, nonfatal acute myocardial infarction due to coronary thrombosis

(1–11), transient, silent episodes of myocardial ischemia (2,27) and stroke (28), do not occur randomly throughout the day; rather, they occur with increased frequency after awakening during the morning hours (usually 6:00 AM to noon). Indeed, circadian rhythms have also been documented for a number of physiologic variables, such as heart rate, blood pressure, platelet aggregability, blood fibrinolytic activity and plasma catecholamines, suggesting that such variables may trigger cardiovascular events (1,2,29).

In this study of patients with hypertrophic cardiomyopathy, the findings also show a circadian pattern in the occurrence of sudden cardiac death (and cardiac arrest). Hypertrophic cardiomyopathy is a primary cardiac disease in which sudden death appears to be largely related to primary arrhythmias or several other mechanisms (13–19,22,23). Specifically, our harmonic regression analysis of 94 patients with hypertrophic cardiomyopathy showed a midmorning peak of occurrence of sudden death between 7 AM and 1 PM, comprising almost one-half of all patients studied, similar to that reported in patients with coronary artery disease (1–9) or stroke (28). We also identified a secondary, less distinct peak of sudden death in the early evening, principally between 8:00 PM and 10:00 PM, similar to that reported previously in some patient groups with acute myocardial infarction (6,7).

Mechanisms of sudden death. This study does not address directly the underlying mechanisms responsible for the circadian periodicity of sudden cardiac death that we observed in patients with hypertrophic cardiomyopathy. Hypertrophic cardiomyopathy is a disease with a diverse morphologic and clinical expression (15,16), in which a number of pathophysiologic mechanisms for sudden death have been proposed (13,14,17–23). Consequently, our study group undoubtedly includes patients exhibiting a variety of such underlying mechanisms and predisposing variables, including primary ventricular and supraventricular arrhythmias, conduction abnormalities, dynamic subaortic obstruction and small-vessel vasoconstriction with myocardial ischemia (13,14,17–23). The circadian pattern of sudden death in hypertrophic cardiomyopathy described here may well offer clues to the causative processes responsible for these events. For example, arrhythmias have been incriminated as important pathways by which sudden death may be mediated in patients with hypertrophic cardiomyopathy (13–19,22,23,30). Also, studies of patients with or without cardiac disease (and unassociated with acute myocardial infarction) have reported diurinal variation in the occurrence of ventricular or supraventricular ectopic activity, with peak occurrence in the morning (31–34). Consequently, it is reasonable to speculate that sudden cardiac death in hypertrophic cardiomyopathy may be related to a circadian variability in the occurrence of arrhythmias. The vulnerability of the arrhythmogenic myocardial substrate in hypertrophic cardiomyopathy (14) may predispose certain patients with this disease to electrical instability and potentially lethal arrhythmias in the morning hours, possibly related to surges in catecholamines and sympathetic nervous system activity associated with waking and rising (1,2,27,35).

Approximately 40% of the patients in this analysis died suddenly during active periods of the day while engaged in moderate to severe exertion. This finding raises the possibility that a causal association exists between activity levels and cardiac arrest in hypertrophic cardiomyopathy, that substantial physical activity may trigger sudden death in these patients (36) and that the lack of uniformity in death times over 24 h may be a result of a lack of uniformity of activity times. However, it should be pointed out that we can only offer speculation on this point because our knowledge is confined to the activity status specifically at the time of death; we cannot judge either the proportion of the day during which marked exertion took place or the activity patterns at other times of the day or on previous days.

Limitations of study design. The relatively small size of our study group was unavoidable because hypertrophic cardiomyopathy and the occurrence of sudden death in such patients are uncommon. This factor limited the power of the subgroup analysis, in which the potential impact of a number of clinical and morphologic variables on the hourly circadian pattern was assessed. However, there are advantages implicit in an investigation of this scope in that it permitted us to validate the cardiac diagnosis with a high degree of specificity and limit the study group to witnessed cardiac arrests in which the time of death could be assessed with considerable precision (often aided by direct interviews with witnesses or surviving family members). This is in contrast to other retrospective studies in which circadian variability was identified in larger patient populations that necessarily utilized less precise methods of data acquisition to estimate time of death and onset of myocardial infarction or to establish the cardiac diagnosis (3,4,9,28).

References

1. Muller JE, Tofler GH, Stone PH. Circadian variation and triggers of onset of acute cardiovascular disease. Circulation 1989;79:733–43.
2. Quyyumi AA. Circadian rhythms in cardiovascular disease. Am Heart J 1990;120:726–33.
3. Willich SN, Levy D, Rocco MB, Tofler GH, Stone PH, Muller JE. Circadian variation in the incidence of sudden cardiac death in the Framingham Heart Study population. Am J Cardiol 1987;60:801–6.
4. Muller JE, Ludmer PL, Willich SN, et al. Circadian variation in the frequency of sudden cardiac death. Circulation 1987;75:131–8.
5. Muller JE, Stone PH, Turi ZG, et al. Circadian variation in the frequency of onset of acute myocardial infarction. N Engl J Med 1985;313:1315–22.
6. Thompson DR, Blandford RL, Sutton TW, Marchant PR. Time of onset of chest pain in acute myocardial infarction. Int J Cardiol 1985;7:139–46.
7. Hjalmarson A, Gilpin EA, Nicod P, et al. Differing circadian patterns of symptom onset in subgroups of patients with acute myocardial infarction. Circulation 1989;80:267–75.
8. Willich SN, Linderer T, Wegscheider K, Leizorovicz A, Alamercery I, Schroder R. Increased morning incidence of myocardial infarction in the ISAM study: Absence with prior beta-adrenergic blockade. Circulation 1989;80:853–8.
9. Ridker PM, Manson JE, Buring JE, Muller JE, Hennekens CH. Circadian variation of acute myocardial infarction and the effect of low-dose aspirin in a randomized trial of physicians. Circulation 1990;82:897–902.
10. Aronow WS, Ahn C. Circadian variation of primary cardiac arrest or

sudden cardiac death in patients aged 62 to 100 years (mean 82). Am J Cardiol 1993;71:1455–6.

11. Peters RW, Zoble RG, Liebson PR, Pawitan Y, Brooks MM, Proschan M. Identification of a secondary peak in myocardial infarction onset 11 to 12 hours after awakening: the Cardiac Arrhythmia Suppression Trial (CAST) Experience. J Am Coll Cardiol 1993;22:998–1003.
12. Maron BJ, Roberts WC, Epstein SE. Sudden death in hypertrophic cardiomyopathy: profile of 78 patients. Circulation 1982;65:1388–94.
13. McKenna WJ, Camm AJ. Sudden death in hypertrophic cardiomyopathy: Assessment of patients at high risk. Circulation 1989;80:1489–92.
14. Maron BJ, Fananapazir L. Sudden cardiac death in hypertrophic cardiomyopathy. Circulation 1992;85 suppl 1:I-57–63.
15. Wigle ED, Sasson Z, Henderson MA, et al. Hypertrophic cardiomyopathy: The importance of the site and the extent of hypertrophy: a review. Prog Cardiovasc Dis 1985;28:1–83.
16. Maron BJ, Bonow RO, Cannon RO, Leon MB, Epstein SE. Hypertrophic cardiomyopathy: interrelation of clinical manifestations, pathophysiology, and therapy. N Eng J Med 1987;316:780–9, 844–52.
17. McKenna WJ, England D, Doi JL, Deanfield JE, Oakley CM, Goodwin JF. Arrhythmia in hypertrophic cardiomyopathy: I. influence of prognosis. Br Heart J 1981;46:168–72.
18. Maron BJ, Savage DD, Wolfson JK, Epstein SE. Prognostic significance of 24-hour ambulatory electrocardiographic monitoring in patients with hypertrophic cardiomyopathy: a prospective study. Am J Cardiol 1981; 48:252–7.
19. Nicod P, Polikar R, Peterson KL. Hypertrophic cardiomyopathy and sudden death. N Engl J Med 1988;318:1255–7.
20. Spirito P, Maron BJ. Relation between extent of left ventricular hypertrophy and occurrence of sudden cardiac death in hypertrophic cardiomyopathy. J Am Coll Cardiol 1990;15:1521–6.
21. Saumarez RC, Camm AJ, Panagos A, et al. Ventricular fibrillation in hypertrophic cardiomyopathy is associated with increased fractionation of paced right ventricular electrograms. Circulation 1992;86:467–74.
22. Stafford WJ, Trohman RG, Bilsker M, Zaman L, Castellanos A, Myerberg RJ. Cardiac arrest in an adolescent with atrial fibrillation and hypertrophic cardiomyopathy. J Am Coll Cardiol 1986;7:701–4.
23. Fananapazir L, Tracy CM, Leon MB, et al. Electrophysiologic abnormalities in patients with hypertrophic cardiomyopathy: a consecutive analysis in 155 patients. Circulation 1989;80:1259–68.
24. Spirito P, Maron BJ, Bonow RO, Epstein SE. Occurrence and significance of progressive left ventricular wall thinning and relative cavity dilatation in patients with hypertrophic cardiomyopathy. Am J Cardiol 1987;60:123–9.
25. Maron BJ, Epstein SE. Hypertrophic cardiomyopathy: a discussion of nomenclature. Am J Cardiol 1979;43:1242–4.
26. Bliss CI: Statistics in Biology. vol 2. New York: McGraw-Hill, 1979.
27. Rocco MB, Barry J, Campbell S, et al. Circadian variation of transient myocardial ischemia in patients with coronary artery disease. Circulation 1987;75:395–400.
28. Marler JR, Price TR, Clark GL, et al. Morning increase in onset of ischemic stroke. Stroke 1989;20:473–6.
29. Tofler GH, Stone PH, MacLure M, et al. and the MILIS study group. Analysis of possible triggers of acute myocardial infarction (the MILIS study). Am J Cardiol 1990;66:22–7.
30. Spirito P, Watson RM, Maron BJ. Relation between extent of left ventricular hypertrophy and occurrence of ventricular tachycardia in hypertrophic cardiomyopathy. Am J Cardiol 1987;60:1137–42.
31. Raeder EA, Hohnloser SH, Graboys TB, Podrid PJ, Lampert S, Lown B. Spontaneous variability and circadian distribution of ectopic activity in patients with malignant ventricular arrhythmia. J Am Coll Cardiol 1988; 12:656–61.
32. Siegel D, Black DM, Seeley DG, Hulley SB. Circadian variation in ventricular arrhythmias in hypertensive men. Am J Cardiol 1992;69: 344–7.
33. Kupari M, Koskinen P, Leinonen H. Double-peaking circadian variation in the occurrence of sustained supraventricular tachyarrhythmias. Am Heart J 1990;120:1364–9.
34. Rostagno C, Taddei T, Paladini B, Modesti PA, Utari P, Bertini G. The onset of symptomatic atrial fibrillation and paroxysmal supraventricular tachycardia is characterized by different circadian rhythms. Am J Cardiol 1993;71:453–5.
35. Linsell CR, Lightman SL, Mullen PE, Brown MJ, Causon RC. Circadian rhythms of epinephrine and norepinephrine in man. J Clin Endocrinol Metab 1985;60:1210–5.
36. Mittleman MA, Maclure M, Tofler GH, Sherwood JB, Goldberg RJ, Muller JE. Triggering of acute myocardial infarction by heavy physical exertion. N Engl J Med 1993;329:1677–83.

Hypertrophic Cardiomyopathy With Left Ventricular Apical Diverticulum

Barry J. Maron, MD, Robert G. Hauser, MD, and William C. Roberts, MD

Hypertrophic cardiomyopathy (HC) is a diverse disease with many morphologic manifestations.[1] One of the least common of these features is an aneurysm or diverticulum that develops in the apical portion of the left ventricle and is often associated with midcavity muscular narrowing and outflow obstruction.[2–6] We have encountered 3 such patients with apical left ventricular (LV) protrusions. A description of the clinical and structural features in this subgroup of patients with HC is the purpose of this communication.

• • •

Case 1. L.N., a 2-month-old boy, developed severe respiratory difficulties at home and was rushed to the hospital. An echocardiogram disclosed asymmetric thickening of the ventricular septum; the ventricles contracted vigorously, the left atrium was dilated, and systolic anterior motion of the mitral valve was absent. He died shortly after the echocardiogram was recorded. Autopsy revealed asymmetric LV hypertrophy, typical of HC, as well as evidence of midcavity muscular narrowing (Figure 1).

Case 2. B.J., a 19-year-old woman, was found to have a precordial murmur at age 6. She was asymptomatic until age 17 (22 months before death), when she developed fever, supraventricular arrhythmias, and α streptococcal septicemia 2 months after a dental procedure. Because of marked deterioration in effort tolerance, cardiac catheterization was performed (16 months before death). A peak systolic pressure gradient of 162 mm Hg was recorded between the left ventricle (260/20) and the ascending aorta (98/75), and a 34 mm Hg gradient between the right ventricle (62/12) and the pulmonary trunk (28/20). A left ventricular cineangiocardiogram was typical of HC, although the LV apex was not visualized. Mitral regurgitation was mild. The coronary arteries appeared normal with aortic root injection. Electro-

From the Minneapolis Heart Institute Foundation, Minneapolis, Minnesota, and the Baylor Cardiovascular Institute, Baylor University Medical Center, Dallas, Texas. Manuscript received June 12, 1995; revised manuscript received and accepted January 10, 1996.

Address for reprints: Barry J. Maron, MD, Minneapolis Heart Institute Foundation, 920 E. 28th Street, Suite 40, Minneapolis, Minnesota 55407.

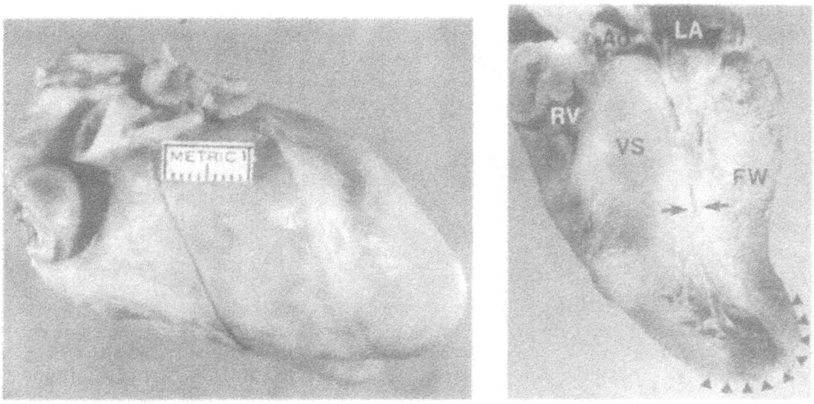

FIGURE 1. Case 1. *Left,* exterior of the heart showing an apical left ventricular bulge. *Right,* longitudinal view showing the ventricular septum (VS) to be much thicker than the left ventricular free wall (FW), with maximal thickening and greatest narrowing of the cavity (*arrows*) located about midway between the aortic valve and the apex. The wall of the apical bulge is shown as consisting of myocardium (*arrowheads*). The mitral leaflets are mildly thickened, but there is no mural endocardial thickening in the left ventricular outflow tract in apposition to anterior mitral leaflet. Ao = aorta; LA = left atrium; RV = right ventricle. (Reproduced with permission from Roberts CS and Roberts WC. Morphologic features [of hypertrophic cardiomyopathy]. *Progr Cardiol* 1989;2:3–32).

cardiography showed biventricular hypertrophy. At surgery (septal myotomy and myectomy), performed 9 days before death, an LV apical aneurysm was observed. Autopsy (NIH A70-278) showed the apical diverticulum, midcavity muscular narrowing, as well as the myotomy-myectomy site (Figure 2). The heart weighed 730 g, and the ventricular septum was asymmetrically thickened with respect to the LV free wall.

Case 3. T.C., a 43-year-old man, developed progressive exertional dyspnea 9 months before death. Echocardiography disclosed severe thickening largely confined to the midportion of the ventricular septum (wall thickness 25 mm) and LV free wall, and LV papillary muscles. Systolic anterior motion of the anterior mitral valve was absent. Angiography (Figure 3) showed striking "dumbbell" deformation of the LV cavity with marked muscular midcavity systolic constriction. Cephalad to the muscular constriction was a normally contracting chamber with end-diastolic dimension of 53 mm and caudally, a greatly enlarged, akinetic and dyskinetic chamber. Moderate mitral regurgitation was present. LV pressure in the apical region was 225/20 mm Hg, just

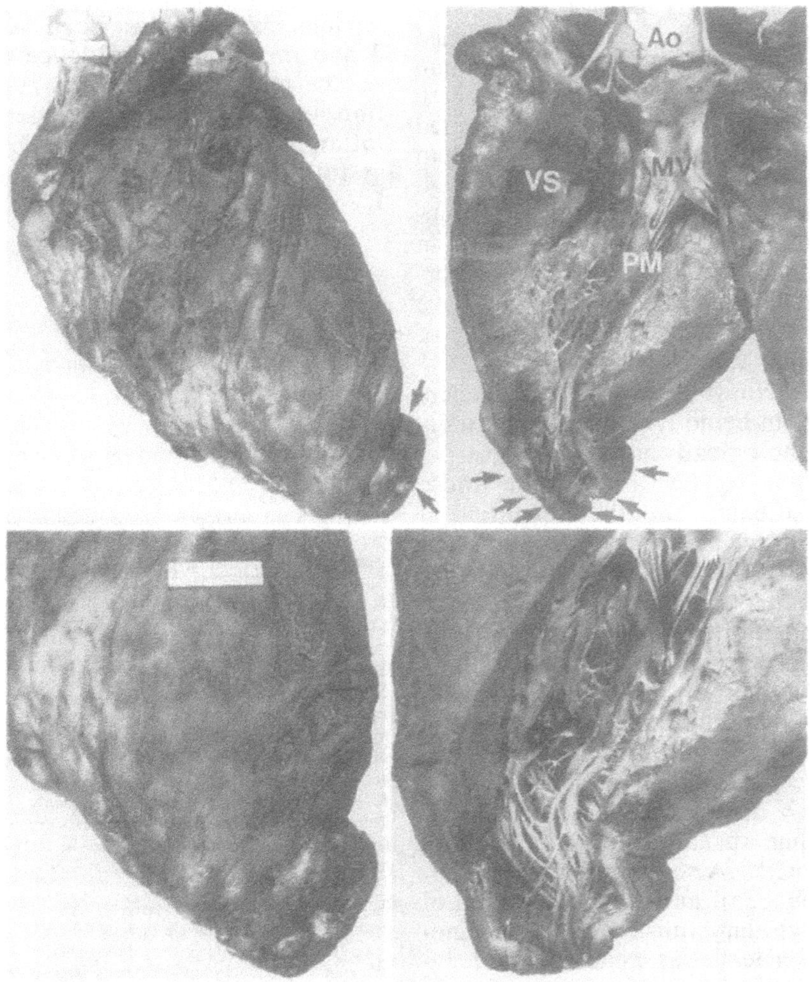

FIGURE 2. Case 2. *Upper left,* exterior of the heart showing a large apical left ventricular bulge (*arrows*). *Upper right,* opened left ventricle, showing the apical bulge (*arrows*) as well as the serrated myotomy-myectomy site in ventricular septum (VS) just caudal to the aortic valve. *Lower left,* close-up external view of the apical bulge. *Lower right,* opened apical diverticulum, showing that its wall consists of myocardium. Ao = aorta; MV = mitral valve; PM = papillary muscle; VS = ventricular septum. (Reproduced with permission from Roberts WC and Ferrans VJ. Pathologic anatomy of the cardiomyopathies: idiopathic dilated and hypertrophic types, infiltrative types, and endomyocardial disease with and without eosinophilia. *Human Pathol* 1975;6:287–342.)

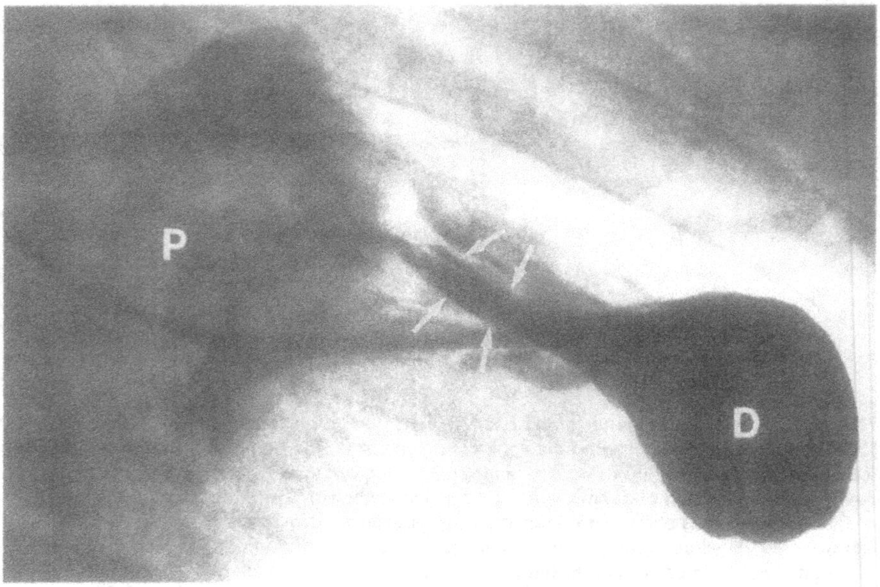

FIGURE 3. Case 3. Left ventricular angiogram showing severe midcavity constriction (*arrows*) due to substantial muscular hypertrophy producing marked outflow obstruction (in the absence of mitral valve systolic anterior motion). Distal (D) and proximal (P) left ventricular cavities are evident adjacent to the midventricular narrowing; the distal cavity is aneurysmal and akinetic/dyskinetic but without evidence of mural thrombus.

caudal to the aortic valve was 125/10, and in the aorta, 108/59 mm Hg. Peak systolic outflow gradient across the midcavity was 100 mm Hg. Pulmonary arterial pressure was 57/28 mm Hg (mean 40). Electrocardiography showed anterolateral and inferior T-wave inversion and intraventricular conduction delay. The patient developed angina pectoris, dyspnea even at rest, orthopnea, nocturnal dyspnea, peripheral edema, and syncope. He was treated with an angiotensin-converting enzyme inhibitor, digoxin, diltiazem, nifedipine, propranolol, disopyramide, hydro-chlorothiazide, warfarin, and amiodarone (for atrial fibrillation and nonsustained ventricular tachycardia). He underwent bypass grafting of the right coronary artery and also septal muscular resection. On the fourth postoperative day, cardiac arrest occurred, followed by anoxic encephalopathy. He died 2 weeks later.

• • •

Each of the 3 patients described here had HC and apical LV bulges that could be regarded as either aneurysms or diverticula. We prefer the term diverticula because the walls enclosing the apical protrusions (at least in the 2 study patients who had autopsies) consisted entirely of myocardium, and not fibrotic tissue as is the case with LV aneurysm occurring as a consequence of acute myocardial infarction.

The mechanism of formation of the apical diverticula is uncertain. It is possible that the extremely high pressure in the apical portions of the left ventricle (260 and 225 mm Hg in the 2 study patients who had cardiac catheterization) simply caused bulging of the thinnest and most vulnerable portion of the LV wall, i.e., the apex. Because the LV outflow was severely obstructed (peak pressure gradients 162 mm Hg [case 2] and 100 mm Hg [case 3]), this high pressure was exerted toward the apex, and a diverticulum was the result. Particularly high systolic LV pressure in HC is unusual at any age but particularly in childhood, and therefore its occurrence at a youthful age may have been a factor in the remodeling of the LV wall.

Not only was there evidence, both hemodynamically and morphologically, of severe obstruction to LV outflow in these patients, but the location of intraventricular obstruction appeared to be in the midcavity rather than at a more cephalad position corresponding to the margins of the mitral leaflets.[1,6] Neither of the 2 patients with echocardiograms had systolic anterior motion of the mitral leaflets, additional evidence that the LV obstruction was more caudal than usual for patients with HC.[1,6] Also, there was no evidence of anomalous insertion of papillary muscle onto the anterior leaflet as a cause of midcavity obstruction in these patients.[7] It is possible that formation of diverticula in our patients was related in some way to the caudal site of muscular subaortic obstruction in the midcavity area.

In summary, 3 patients with HC and LV apical diverticula of various sizes are described. All 3 had morphologic evidence of severe midventricular obstruction, including 2 with documentation of greatly elevated LV systolic pressure and marked LV outflow pressure gradients.

1. Maron BJ, Bonow RO, Cannon RO, Leon MB, Epstein SE. Hypertrophic cardiomyopathy: interrelation of clinical manifestations, pathophysiology, and therapy. *N Engl J Med* 1987;316:780–789 and 844–852.

2. Ando H, Imaizumi T, Urabe Y, Takeshita A, Nakamura M. Apical segmental dysfunction in hypertrophic cardiomyopathy: subgroup with unique clinical features. *J Am Coll Cardiol* 1990;16:1579–1588.

3. Fighali S, Krajcer Z, Edelman S, Leachman RD. Progression of hypertrophic cardiomyopathy into a hypokinetic left ventricle: higher incidence of patients with midventricular obstruction. *J Am Coll Cardiol* 1987;9:288–294.

4. Falicov RE, Resnekov L, Bharati S, Lev M. Mid-ventricular obstruction: a variant of obstructive cardiomyopathy. *Am J Cardiol* 1976; 37:432–437.

5. Maron BJ, Bonow RO, Seshagiri TN, Roberts WC, Epstein SE. Hypertrophic cardiomyopathy with ventricular septal hypertrophy localized to the apical region of the left ventricle (apical hypertrophic cardiomyopathy). *Am J Cardiol* 1982;49:1838–1848.

6. Wigle ED, Sasson Z, Henderson MA, Ruddy TD, Fulop J, Rakowski H, Williams WG. Hypertrophic cardiomyopathy: the importance of the site and extent of hypertrophy—a review. *Prog Cardiovasc Dis* 1985;28:1–83.

7. Klues HG, Roberts WC, Maron BJ. Anomalous insertion of papillary muscle directly into anterior mitral leaflet in hypertrophic cardiomyopathy: significance in producing left ventricular outflow obstruction. *Circulation* 1991;84:1188–1197.

Comparison of Clinical and Morphologic Cardiac Findings in Patients Having Cardiac Transplantation for Ischemic Cardiomyopathy, Idiopathic Dilated Cardiomyopathy, and Dilated Hypertrophic Cardiomyopathy

Thomas A. Waller, MD,* William L. Hiser, MD,† John E. Capehart, MD, and William C. Roberts, MD

This article compares intergroup and intragroup clinical and morphologic findings in patients with ischemic cardiomyopathy (IC), idiopathic dilated cardiomyopathy (IDC), and dilated hypertrophic cardiomyopathy (HC) undergoing cardiac transplantation (CT). Few previous publications have described findings in native hearts explanted at the time of CT. The explanted heart in 92 patients having CT was examined in uniform manner with particular attention to the sizes of the ventricular cavities and the presence of and extent of ventricular scarring. Of the 92 hearts examined, 47 had IC, 35 had IDC, and 10 had dilated HC. Although considerable degrees of intragroup variation occurred, the mean degree of left ventricular dilatation was similar among the patients with IC, IDC, and dilated HC. All patients with IC had left ventricular free wall scarring more extensive than that involving the ventricular septum, but the intragroup variation in the amounts of scarring was considerable. Nine of the 10 patients with dilated HC also had ventricular wall scarring, but it was more extensive in the ventricular septum than in the left ventricular free wall and involvement of the right ventricular wall also was present. Eight (23%) of the 35 IDC patients also had grossly visible ventricular scars but they were small and only 1 of the 8 had coronary narrowing and that was not in the distribution of the scarring. Narrowing of 1 or more epicardial coronary arteries >75% in cross-sectional area by plaque was present in all 47 IC patients, in 8 of the 35 IDC patients (7 had no ventricular scars), and in none of the 10 dilated HC patients. Coronary angiography was the major clinical tool allowing separation of the IC, IDC, and HC patients. Coronary angiography did not detect narrowing in any of the 8 patients with IDC who were found to have coronary narrowing on anatomic study. Thus, among patients with IC, IDC, and dilated HC having CT, distinctive anatomic features allow separation of patients with IC, IDC, and dilated HC, but within each group considerable variation in left ventricular cavity size and extent of ventricular scarring occurs.

(Am J Cardiol 1998;81:884–894)

Cardiac transplantation (CT) has become a recognized therapy for the treatment of patients with irreversible and intractable heart failure. Each year approximately 3,000 patients have CT worldwide.[1] We have studied in uniform fashion the recipient's native explanted heart in 92 patients having CT for 1 of 3 different conditions: ischemic cardiomyopathy (IC), idiopathic dilated cardiomyopathy (IDC), and dilated hypertrophic cardiomyopathy (HC). Review of previously published articles on CT surprisingly have provided few details of native hearts excised at the time of CT. This report describes various morphologic features in these hearts explanted for these 3 conditions and correlates electrocardiographic, echocardiographic, and hemodynamic findings with the morphologic changes.

From the Departments of Medicine, Cardiothoracic Surgery, and Pathology, and the Baylor Cardiovascular Institute, Baylor University Medical Center, Dallas, Texas. Manuscript received November 18, 1997; revised manuscript received and accepted January 6, 1998.

Address for reprints: William C. Roberts, MD, Baylor Cardiovascular Institute, Baylor University Medical Center, 3500 Gaston Avenue, Dallas, Texas 75246.

*Present address: 1600 Coit Road, Suite 301, Plano, Texas 75075.

†Present address: Section of Cardiology, Department of Medicine, University of Nebraska Medical Center, Omaha, Nebraska 68198.

PATIENTS STUDIED AND METHODS

Sources of cases: Of the 92 patients, the cardiac transplant operation was performed at Baylor University Medical Center in 58 (63%) from March 1, 1993, until June 2, 1997. Each heart was examined, weighed (each on the same accurate scales), and described initially by WCR. Most were reexamined by TAW and WLH. The remaining 34 recipient hearts (37%) were submitted to the Pathology Branch of the National Heart, Lung, and Blood Institute in Bethesda, Maryland, from 1977 until 1993. The submitting institutions were Fairfax Hos-

TABLE I Clinical and Morphologic Findings in the 47 Patients With Ischemic Cardiomyopathy

Patient Demographics				Morphology						Laboratory			Echocardiogram	
Pt. No.	Age (yr)	Sex	Interval (mo) S→CT	HW (g)	BW (kg)	T	CABG (grafts)	CA >75%↓	LVMD (cm)	H (%)	TC (mg/dl)	TG (mg/dl)	LVEDD (cm)	LVESD (cm)
1	42	M	12	325	70	0	0	4	5.5	44	308	138	—	—
2	43	M	5	380	64	0	0	3	7.0	23	241	286	—	—
3	43	M	60	450	—	+(LV)	0	1	5.5	—	308	—	—	—
4	43	M	6	—	—	0	0	2	—	—	—	—	—	—
5	45	M	8	475	76	0	0	1	6.5	30	135	50	7.4	6.4
6	45	M	—	305	—	0	+(4)	4	4.0	—	—	—	—	—
7	46	F	4	365	73	0	+(4)	3	—	41	126	243	5.0	4.0
8	46	M	14	—	74	0	+(1)	3	—	50	168	—	—	—
9	49	M	8	351	58	0	+(3)	4	5.0	38	252	74	6.2	5.5
10	49	M	24	490	72	0	0	3	6.5	39	167	188	8.0	—
11	50	M	15	345	91	0	0	1	5.0	43	162	316	6.2	4.8
12	50	M	84	570	89	0	+(1)	3	6.0	42	125	115	6.5	5.8
13	50	M	30	395	78	0	0	3	6.5	30	180	97	5.5	4.8
14	51	M	11	440	73	0	+(2)	4	—	34	247	278	6.9	6.3
15	51	M	30	565	71	+(LV)	0	3	5.0	40	242	115	—	—
16	51	M	36	503	72	0	+(3)	3	5.0	46	155	54	7.0	6.0
17	51	M	7	450	70	0	0	2	5.5	32	194	90	—	—
18	52	M	41	510	75	0	+(2)	3	4.0	32	334	296	8.0	7.0
19	52	M	24	565	—	0	+(3)	3	5.0	—	240	—	—	—
20	53	M	6	260	—	0	0	3	—	33	260	658	4.3	2.9
21	53	M	11	535	96	0	+(4)	3	6.3	42	264	—	—	—
22	54	M	1	500	—	0	0	3	—	—	226	—	—	—
23	55	M	108	490	74	0	+(3)	4	5.5	37	158	156	6.0	5.5
24	55	M	—	430	—	0	+(3)	3	—	—	—	—	—	—
25	56	M	240	520	85	0	+(3)	2	6.0	43	204	180	6.5	—
26	56	M	15	430	82	0	0	4	6.0	39	280	501	—	—
27	56	F	60	385	50	0	0	3	6.0	30	219	168	6.2	5.7
28	56	M	33	720	103	0	0	2	7.9	31	240	123	7.4	6.2
29	56	M	36	—	—	0	+(4)	4	—	—	—	—	—	—
30	57	M	24	415	77	0	0	3	5.5	37	183	96	6.5	5.0
31	57	M	144	535	90	0	+(2)	3	6.5	34	227	147	8.0	—
32	57	M	4	—	—	0	+(4)	3	—	31	174	—	—	—
33	57	M	1	—	—	0	0	1	—	—	—	—	—	—
34	58	M	11	352	75	0	+(4)	4	—	35	281	147	4.3	3.8
35	58	M	56	580	99	0	+(4)	1	3.5	38	267	170	—	—
36	58	M	12	590	70	0	+(4)	4	6.6	37	132	—	—	—
37	59	M	8	390	—	0	0	1	5.5	—	—	—	7.0	6.5
38	59	M	13	490	88	0	+(3)	3	5.3	35	105	65	6.5	5.1
39	60	M	21	365	72	+(LV)	0	2	6.0	42	146	69	7.5	6.0
40	60	M	31	610	74	0	0	2	6.0	30	131	106	6.0	—
41	61	M	12	690	94	0	+(4)	3	6.5	39	198	147	5.7	4.2
42	61	M	47	385	77	0	+(4)	3	6.7	36	202	73	6.4	6.1
43	62	F	120	480	66	0	0	3	6.5	35	161	232	7.8	7.1
44	62	M	24	503	68	0	0	2	6.5	40	217	—	8.8	7.2
45	63	M	13	450	84	0	+(3)	3	4.5	33	209	83	6.0	4.8
46	63	M	36	750	80	0	0	3	6.3	42	—	—	—	—
47	65	M	1	280	—	0	0	3	5.0	—	—	—	—	—

*When not in atrial fibrillation.

AF = atrial fibrillation; BBB = bundle branch block; BW = body weight; CABG = coronary artery bypass graft; CHB = complete heart block; CI = cardiac index; CT = cardiac transplantation; H = hematocrit; HW = heart weight; L = left; LAD = left atrial diameter; LV = left ventricle; LVEDD = left ventricular end-diastolic diameter; LVEF = left ventricular ejection fraction; LVESD = left ventricular end systolic diameter; LVFW = left ventricular free wall; LVMD = left ventricular maximum diameter; MR = mitral regurgitation; PAW = pulmonary artery wedge; R = right; RA = right atrium; RV = right ventricle; S = symptoms; SA = systemic arterial; s/d = peak systole/end diastole; T = thrombus; TC = total cholesterol; TG = triglyceride; TR = tricuspid regurgitation; VSW = ventricular septal width; VT = ventricular tachycardia; + = positive or present; 0 = negative or absent; — = no information available.

pital, Fairfax, Virginia; Medical College of Virginia, Richmond, Virginia; Georgetown University Medical Center, George Washington University Medical Center, and Washington Hospital Center, all in Washington, DC. During this time WCR was Chief of the Pathology Branch and he examined each heart and also histologic sections of the heart prepared in the same manner as the cases studied at Baylor University Medical Center. Nine of the 10 cases having dilated HC have been reported previously elsewhere.[2]

Methods of examining the recipient hearts: The hearts in each of the 92 patients were examined and described initially by WCR. The cardiac ven-

TABLE I (Continued)

Echocardiogram							Electrocardiogram				Pressures (mm Hg)						
LAD (cm)	VSW (cm)	LVFW (cm)	MR (0–4)	TR (0–4)	LVEF (%)	BBB	Total QRS Voltage (mm)	AF	VT	PR (>200 ms)	SA (s/d)	LV (s/d)	RV (s/d)	PA (s/d)	RA (mean)	PAW (mean)	CI (L/min/m^2)
—	—	—	2	2	15	0	120	0	0	0	106/70	—	36/3	36/14	0	19	2.7
—	—	—	—	—	28	+(L)	129	0	0	0	121/60	—	29/2	25/14	1	10	—
—	—	—	—	—	8	—	—	—	—	—	—	—	—	—	—	—	—
—	—	—	—	—	10	0	—	0	0	0	—	—	—	—	—	—	—
5.0	1.2	1.3	2	2	20	0	101	+	+	AF	100/60	—	47/15	46/23	5	27	2.4
—	—	—	—	—	—	—	—	—	—	—	—	—	—	—	—	—	—
4.0	1.2	1.1	—	—	23	0	131	0	+	0	146/79	115/24	31/3	35/10	3	7	3.1
—	—	—	—	—	30	+(L)	83	0	+	0	120/80	130/28	—	—	—	—	—
4.6	0.5	1.0	4	4	15	0	188	0	0	0	100/78	92/3	30/10	33/13	3	10	2.1
4.5	—	—	3	2	20	0	220	0	0	0	142/80	—	58/9	48/21	4	27	1.8
5.2	0.7	0.7	4	1	37	0	97	+	+	+*	118/94	—	39/9	39/17	4	19	2.2
3.0	1.0	1.0	1	1	25	+(L)	120	0	0	+	100/60	—	34/1	34/19	8	14	1.5
4.0	—	—	—	0	20	0	87	0	+	0	118/76	—	21/7	25/8	2	7	1.9
4.2	0.8	0.9	0	0	22	+(L)	201	0	+	0	114/76	117/25	52/6	42/23	3	26	—
—	—	—	—	—	15	0	180	0	0	0	100/70	93/13	31/6	26/	3	5	3.3
4.5	0.8	1.0	2	0	25	0	74	+	0	AF	92/60	—	46/11	39/24	8	22	2.9
—	—	—	3	—	—	0	86	0	0	0	84/66	77/23	65/14	67/32	13	24	1.2
4.5	0.9	0.9	3	0	15	0	138	+	0	0*	121/52	—	25/1	23/8	3	8	—
—	—	—	—	—	15	+(R)	—	0	—	—	—	—	—	55/30	—	27	—
3.3	—	1.0	0	0	—	0	91	0	+	0	125/60	125/40	—	64/22	12	24	2.4
—	—	—	—	—	11	—	—	—	—	—	140/90	—	—	—	—	—	—
—	—	—	—	—	15	—	—	—	—	—	—	—	—	—	12	12	—
4.0	1.0	1.0	2	0	20	+(R)	152	0	0	0	116/74	112/39	—	34/15	—	12	2.0
—	—	—	—	—	—	—	—	—	—	—	—	—	—	—	—	—	—
5.0	—	—	3	3	25	0	133	0	0	+	100/60	—	58/15	55/26	15	30	2.0
—	—	—	—	—	20	0	184	0	0	0	116/57	—	32/11	28/13	5	9	2.5
—	—	—	4	2	13	0	159	0	0	+	100/56	—	—	35/20	—	14	2.7
5.3	1.3	1.3	3	3	20	0	97	+	+	+*	97/56	—	59/4	61/25	3	19	2.6
—	—	—	—	—	—	—	—	—	—	—	—	—	—	—	—	—	—
4.5	1.0	1.0	1	0	28	0	86	0	0	0	110/60	98/7	41/6	30/2	0	5	2.5
5.0	0.8	0.8	3	2	25	0	234	0	+	+	95/60	—	34/7	33/10	5	7	2.2
—	—	—	—	—	—	0	108	0	0	0	120/60	120/25	37/8	38/20	—	7	—
—	—	—	—	—	—	—	—	—	+	—	—	—	—	—	—	—	—
4.1	1.4	1.6	—	—	40	0	115	0	0	0	—	—	21/8	19/7	6	7	2.2
5.0	—	—	2	2	30	0	154	0	0	0	120/80	—	22/7	47/7	1	9	2.4
—	—	—	—	—	10	—	—	—	—	—	100/60	—	47/14	47/28	15	27	2.0
—	—	—	2	—	15	—	—	0	+	—	98/70	—	—	25/12	3	8	—
5.1	1.2	1.1	3	1	19	—	—	—	—	—	103/70	—	60/14	56/33	12	26	1.9
4.5	1.0	1.0	2	0	20	+(R)	70	0	0	+	112/82	—	50/11	46/24	13	28	1.8
5.0	1.1	1.1	4	3	15	0	128	+	+	AF	105/62	—	—	50/29	9	30	2.5
4.1	1.0	1.0	—	—	25	+(L)	132	0	+	+	138/55	—	28/5	20/6	2	4	—
4.4	0.8	0.7	3	3	15	0	98	+	+	+*	94/62	95/14	32/9	32/13	5	12	1.7
4.8	0.7	0.9	1	0	15	+(L)	172	0	0	0	110/59	106/10	30/5	23/11	2	10	2.7
4.1	1	1.1	4	2	8	+(L)	—	0	—	—	90/60	90/26	—	40/16	—	18	2.5
4.6	1.2	1.2	0	0	20	+(CHB)	94	+	0	CHB	100/60	—	43/12	44/19	13	22	2.8
—	—	—	—	3	—	—	—	—	—	—	160/90	160/44	50/10	50/30	7	24	2.4
—	—	—	—	—	30	0	97	0	0	+	140/80	140/40	45/14	45/28	10	30	—

*When not in atrial fibrillation.

AF = atrial fibrillation; BBB = bundle branch block; BW = body weight; CABG = coronary artery bypass graft; CHB = complete heart block; CI = cardiac index; CT = cardiac transplantation; H = hematocrit; HW = heart weight; L = left; LAD = left atrial diameter; LV = left ventricle; LVEDD = left ventricular end-diastolic diameter; LVEF = left ventricular ejection fraction; LVESD = left ventricular end systolic diameter; LVFW = left ventricular free wall; LVMD = left ventricular maximum diameter; MR = mitral regurgitation; PAW = pulmonary artery wedge; R = right; RA = right atrium; RV = right ventricle; S = symptoms; SA = systemic arterial; s/d = peak systole/end diastole; T = thrombus; TC = total cholesterol; TG = triglyceride; TR = tricuspid regurgitation; VSW = ventricular septal width; VT = ventricular tachycardia; + = positive or present; 0 = negative or absent; — = no information available.

tricles were cut into transverse slices about 1 cm in width beginning at the cardiac apex and extending to about 2 cm caudal to the posterior atrioventricular sulcus. The cuts were made parallel to the posterior atrioventricular sulcus. The maximum internal diameter of the left ventricular cavity, either left to right or anterior to posterior, was determined and recorded. The specimen was weighed after removing any intracavity blood or thrombus and any noncardiac epicardial attachments. The heart weight included only portions of the atrial walls and atrial septum. The major epicardial coronary arteries were incised transversely at varying intervals, usually 5-mm ones, throughout their courses. At least 4

TABLE II Clinical and Morphologic Findings in the 35 Patients With Idiopathic Dilated Cardiomyopathy

Patient Demographics				Morphology						Laboratory			Echocardiogram	
Pt. No.	Age (yr)	Sex	Interval (mo) S→CT	HW (g)	BW (kg)	F	T	CA >75%↓	LVMD (cm)	H (%)	TC (mg/dl)	TG (mg/dl)	LVEDD (cm)	LVESD (cm)
1	14	M	5	355	66	0	0	0	—	33	111	85	8.5	7.5
2*	25	M	4	480	—	0	0	0	—	31	116	70	7.7	7.4
3†	25	F	1	—	81	0	0	0	6.5	—	—	—	—	—
4	26	M	2	401	68	0	+(LV)	0	5.0	33	157	107	6.9	6.7
5	26	M	—	890	—	+	0	0	—	—	—	—	—	—
6	28	F	23	371	84	0	0	0	5.5	40	203	170	7.5	6.0
7	28	F	3	280	62	0	0	0	5.0	39	180	200	6.0	—
8	28	F	7	385	56	0	0	0	7.0	33	151	62	6.8	6.4
9	32	M	—	501	75	0	0	0	—	—	—	—	—	—
10	36	F	42	290	57	0	0	0	6.3	31	138	57	5.7	4.8
11	45	F	132	380	77	0	0	0	5.0	40	140	105	7.0	6.5
12	46	M	—	525	—	0	0	1	—	—	—	—	—	—
13	47	M	21	605	78	+	0	0	7.0	33	143	95	8.1	7.4
14	48	F	168	320	64	0	0	0	3.5	34	154	177	—	—
15	48	M	12	450	82	0	0	1	4.5	42	252	183	6.0	—
16	50	F	48	450	79	0	0	0	4.5	41	146	306	—	—
17	51	M	25	285	92	+	0	0	4.0	27	121	70	6.2	5.0
18	53	F	11	425	64	0	0	1	—	42	125	110	—	—
19	53	F	276	505	67	+	0	0	6.0	35	158	223	7.2	6.2
20	53	M	47	630	78	0	0	0	6.8	31	135	121	6.1	—
21	54	F	37	625	56	+	0	0	7.6	37	179	104	9.7	8.3
22	55	F	22	325	67	0	0	0	6.0	41	213	172	6.0	4.9
23	55	M	11	455	—	0	0	2	—	—	200	—	7.3	—
24	57	F	28	580	68	+	0	0	6.0	38	213	108	7.1	6.7
25	57	F	92	485	53	0	0	0	6.0	36	245	198	7.0	6.0
26	58	F	10	330	59	0	0	0	—	40	—	—	—	—
27	59	F	59	550	66	0	0	0	5.5	40	207	156	6.5	—
28	61	M	24	545	94	0	0	0	6.5	39	192	187	6.0	—
29	61	M	9	435	73	0	0	2	5.5	48	165	236	6.9	6.0
30§	62	M	20	450	74	0	0	0	6.0	40	181	109	—	—
31	62	F	24	425	—	0	0	0	5.9	39	155	100	—	—
32	63	F	86	475	45	+	0	0	6.0	36	137	67	7.0	6.0
33	64	F	55	325	51	+	0	2	5.5	33	192	397	6.1	5.7
34	64	F	22	310	78	0	0	0	3.5	39	179	183	7.0	6.0
35	66	F	300	515	51	0	0	3	5.0	35	207	61	7.0	—

*This patient had a history of androgen use and was a weightlifter.
†This patient developed symptoms of IDC during her third trimester of pregnancy.
‡When not in atrial fibrillation.
§This patient had hyperthyroidism.
CA = coronary arteries; F = fibrosis; G = gender; other abbreviations as in Table I.

hematoxylin-eosin stained sections of left ventricular myocardium (including ventricular septum) were prepared from the heart of each patient and examined with a microscope.

Other cases studied during the same time period: In the time period during which the heretofore mentioned 92 recipient hearts were studied, an additional 8 others also were examined and studied morphologically in similar fashion. Of these 8 other patients, 4 had valvular heart disease necessitating valve replacement, including 1 with associated atherosclerotic coronary artery disease and previous myocardial infarction. All 4 had dilated ventricles. One patient had combined heart/lung transplant because of severe pulmonary hypertension from sarcoidosis and she also had dilated ventricular cavities. One patient had significant narrowing of 3 major coronary arteries but no grossly visible myocardial scars and normal-sized ventricular cavities despite poor left ventricular function clinically. This patient also had recurring ventricular arrhythmias. One patient was treated with adriamycin for sarcoma and subsequently developed a dilated cardiomyopathy. The final patient had HC but nondilated ventricular cavities and nonscarred ventricular walls; she had CT because of severe recurring ventricular arrhythmias despite the presence of an implantable cardiac defibrillator. Of these 8 cases, 5 were studied in the Pathology Branch of the National Heart, Lung, and Blood Institute, and the other 3 at Baylor University Medical Center. These 8 patients with "other cardiac conditions" will not be further discussed in this article.

Methods of collecting clinical data: The hospital records were reviewed in each of the 92 patients. Most of the echocardiographic data were taken from the echocardiographic reports in the hospital charts.

TABLE II (Continued)

Echocardiogram						Electrocardiogram					Pressures (mm Hg)						
LAD (cm)	VS (cm)	LVFW (cm)	MR (0–4)	TR (0–4)	LVEF (%)	BBB	Total QRS Voltage (mm)	AF	VT	PR (>200 ms)	SA (s/d)	LV (s/d)	RV (s/d)	PA (s/d)	RA (mean)	PAW (mean)	CI (L/min/m²)
—	—	—	—	—	10	0	207	0	0	0	78/57	87/29	30/10	34/22	8	23	1.4
5.8	0.8	0.8	—	—	10	0	130	0	0	0	100/80	112/11	46/2	42/23	—	17	—
—	—	—	—	—	—	+(R)	—	0	—	0	—	—	—	—	—	—	—
5.0	0.9	1.0	4	4	25	0	130	+	+	0†	88/57	87/20	41/7	41/20	3	17	2.9
—	—	—	—	—	—	—	—	—	—	—	—	—	—	—	—	—	—
5.0	0.8	0.8	2	0	25	+(L)	173	0	+	0	130/80	—	38/3	37/6	2	16	—
3.0	—	—	0	2	15	+(L)	121	0	0	0	128/60	—	16/6	13/	0	3	2.5
4.2	0.8	1.0	3	3	26	+(L)	146	0	0	0	102/66	—	—	38/24	9	20	2.0
—	—	—	2	—	—	—	—	—	—	—	—	—	—	—	—	—	—
—	—	—	3	3	37	0	217	0	0	0	100/86	98/11	34/5	34/14	4	14	3.4
5.2	0.8	0.9	1	2	20	0	64	0	0	0	90/60	—	28/0	28/10	3	6	2.7
—	—	—	—	—	9	—	—	—	+	—	—	—	—	69/34	32	46	—
5.8	0.7	1.0	3	3	15	0	307	+	0	AF	111/70	—	78/20	76/26	11	38	3.0
—	—	—	2	0	28	0	142	0	0	0	106/58	101/2	32/5	22/13	5	8	2.8
4.7	1.0	1.0	—	—	40	0	81	+	0	AF	96/78	93/16	51/17	53/34	16	31	2.5
—	—	—	3	2	16	0	—	0	0	0	90/65	—	55/10	45/22	10	22	2.4
4.7	0.7	0.8	2	4	25	0	60	+	0	AF	100/65	—	27/16	34/22	23	24	2.0
—	—	—	3	—	20	+(L)	164	0	0	0	114/75	110/25	43/13	39/21	9	30	1.6
5.3	1.2	1.2	2	1	13	+(L)	203	0	0	0	112/80	103/24	24/7	39/13	3	18	2.3
4.5	1.0	1.0	4	3	15	+(R)	53	0	+	0	92/55	104/43	42/6	51/29	15	31	1.3
5.3	0.8	1.0	4	3	20	+(L)	160	+	+	0‡	85/60	—	43/15	45/31	9	28	1.6
4.1	0.8	0.9	2	0	20	0	153	0	0	0	90/70	88/21	33/7	23/18	1	11	2.5
—	—	—	3	—	14	+(L)	149	0	0	0	80/56	80/25	45/15	40/22	10	25	1.5
4.3	1.0	1.0	2	0	14	+(L)	166	0	0	0	112/82	—	47/7	47/17	13	17	1.7
4.5	1.0	1.0	2	1	20	+(L)	236	0	0	+	118/80	—	49/7	50/28	5	32	2.0
—	—	—	4	—	25	0	—	0	+	+	128/50	128/12	55/4	55/23	4	27	3.7
4.8	—	—	0	0	23	+(R)	121	0	0	0	104/56	103/15	42/5	42/12	4	19	3.0
5.0	—	—	2	2	30	0	86	+	+	AF	92/60	90/19	52/5	54/25	11	30	1.8
6.2	0.8	0.8	2	3	15	0	201	0	0	0	150/80	126/29	30/5	28/12	3	15	3.2
—	—	2	3	20	0	0	86	0	0	0	114/64	108/24	37/3	37/11	4	18	3.3
—	—	—	3	3	19	+(L)	—	0	0	0	—	—	11/6	—	2	4	1.8
4.5	1.0	1.0	1	0	10	+(CHB)	168	0	0	CHB	120/62	—	30/9	36/15	2	11	2.8
4.1	1.1	1.2	2	0	10	+(L)	223	+	+	0‡	95/58	—	39/3	39/9	0	11	2.9
4.0	1.1	1.0	1	1	25	0	109	0	0	0	110/74	132/16	23/5	21/9	3	5	3.1
6.0	—	—	4	3	15	0	120	+	0	AF	96/60	—	35/15	42/25	—	22	—

*This patient had a history of androgen use and was a weightlifter.

†This patient developed symptoms of IDC during her third trimester of pregnancy.

‡When not in atrial fibrillation.

§This patient had hyperthyroidism.

CA = coronary arteries; F = fibrosis; G = gender; other abbreviations as in Table I.

When certain items were missing or unclear, the last echocardiogram before CT was reviewed by TAW. Each of the electrocardiograms were reviewed by TAW and the total 12-lead QRS voltage was measured by a method described elsewhere,[3] and other electrocardiographic findings also were recorded. Most data derived at cardiac catheterization were those present in the final cardiac catheterization record in the hospital chart. Where data were missing the original pressure tracings were reviewed. The interval from initial onset of symptoms of cardiac dysfunction or myocardial ischemia to CT was determined from first onset of angina or acute myocardial infarction in the case of IC, and from onset usually of evidence of heart failure or a ventricular arrhythmia in the case of IDC or dilated HC.

Statistical analysis: Differences between groups were determined by 2-tailed Student's *t* test or chi-square analysis (SPSS for MS Windows, version 6.1). Because the 3 groups differed in size, the Levine technique was used to test for nonhomogeneity of variances. When the degree of heterogeneity was not significant ($p > 0.05$), 1-way analysis of variance was performed to determine the differences in groups. When the Levine test was significant, Kruskal Wallis 1-way analysis of variance was used. Significance was defined as $p < 0.05$. When the results were significant, Fisher's LSD post hoc analysis was employed to determine which of the differences in group means accounted for the significance. The Tamhane's T2 post hoc analysis was used after finding a significance with Kruskal Wallis. Chi square was used to determine differences in groups when the dependent variable was measured at the nominal level (e.g., gender).

TABLE III Clinical and Morphologic Data in the 10 Patients With Dilated Hypertrophic Cardiomyopathy

Demographics				Morphology			Echocardiogram								Electrocardiogram				Pressures (mm Hg)					
Pt No.	Age (yr)	Sex	Interval (mo) S→CT	HW (g)	F	LVMD (cm)	LVEDD (cm)	LVESD (cm)	LAD (cm)	VSW (cm)	LVFW (cm)	MR (0–4)	TR (0–4)	LVEF (%)	BBB	Total QRS Voltage (mm)	AF	PR >200 ms	SA (s/d)	LV (s/d)	RV (s/d)	RA (mean)	PAW (mean)	CI (L/min/m²)
1	19	M	84	385	0	—	4.5	3.3	5.5	1.3	1.3	3	0	48	+(R)	146	+	AF	120/76	108/24	50/20	22	28	1.8
2	27	M	132	340	+	—	4.2	2.9	5.4	2.0	1.0	0	0	64	0	121	+	AF	110/70	108/20	45/20	22	29	2.6
3	33	F	192	340	+	—	—	—	—	1.5	1.1	0	0	—	—	—	0	—	95/68	95/23	50/9	7	28	2.0
4	36	M	156	390	+	—	4.8	2.7	5.0	1.6	1.0	0	0	67	0	109	+	AF	—	105/18	45/23	—	30	—
5	37	F	216	290	+	—	4.5	3.4	5.4	1.4	1.0	3	0	41	0	172	+	AF	120/60	110/17	47/8	6	32	2.9
6	40	M	96	310	+	3.8	5.3	4.5	5.6	1.4	0.8	0	0	30	0	145	+	+*	110/80	110/28	60/16	12	20	1.3
7	42	M	156	455	+	4.5	4.5	3.0	4.4	1.7	1.1	0	0	39	0	201	+	AF	110/60	160/27	36/12	4	12	3.3
8	43	F	36	220	+	5.0	3.7	2.5	5.0	1.8	1.3	3	2	60	0	287	0	0	100/60	—	41/17	15	27	1.3
9	45	F	300	350	+	—	4.8	4.0	5.6	1.2	1.0	—	0	44	0	227	0	+	155/88	140/21	70/21	16	36	1.8
10	46	M	360	480	+	5.1	5.5	3.8	5.8	1.7	1.0	2	0	29	0	130	0	+	110/60	96/24	48/4	4	23	2.8

* When not in atrial fibrillation.
Abbreviations as in Tables I and II.

DEFINITIONS

Ischemic cardiomyopathy[4]: These patients had hearts with dilated ventricular cavities, 1 or more grossly visible transmural scars in the left ventricular free wall with or without similar scars in the ventricular septum and right ventricular free wall, narrowing >75% in cross-sectional area by atherosclerotic plaque of 1 major (right, left anterior descending and left circumflex) epicardial coronary artery, normal or nearly normal cardiac valves, and absent inflammatory, giant, neoplastic cells or nonfibrous myocardial infiltrates (such as amyloid). The intramural coronary arteries were normal.

Idiopathic dilated cardiomyopathy[5]: These patients had dilated ventricular cavities, normal or nearly normal cardiac valves, normal epicardium, and no inflammatory, giant, or neoplastic cells or infiltrates (such as amyloid) in the cardiac walls. The epicardial coronary arteries were usually normal; a few patients had atherosclerotic plaques including some in whom the plaques narrowed the lumen >75% in cross-sectional areas in 1 or more major epicardial coronary arteries. The patients with associated coronary narrowing, however, either had no myocardial scars or (1 patient) a very small scar. The intramural coronary arteries were normal.

Dilated hypertrophic cardiomyopathy[2]: These patients had dilated ventricular cavities but past clinical evidence of nondilated cavities. Transmural scarring of the ventricular septum with or without scarring of the left and right ventricular free walls was present in all but 1 patient. The ventricular septum at sometime in the past or presently was thicker than the left ventricular free wall; typical myofiber disorganization was present in the ventricular septum, and the intramural coronary arteries were abnormal (on histologic study).[6]

RESULTS

Of the 92 cases, 47 had IC (Table I), 35 had IDC (Table II), and 10 had dilated HC (Table III) (Figures 1 to 12). Various comparative findings in each of these 3 groups are summarized in Table IV. The mean ages of the 3 groups were different (IC = 54; IDC = 47, and HC = 37 years) ($p < 0.001$). The percentage of men in each of the 3 groups was different: IC 94% (44 of 47); IDC 40% (14 of 35); and dilated HC 60% (6 of 10) ($p < 0.001$). The mean intervals from onset of symptoms of cardiac dysfunction and/or myocardial ischemia to CT were significantly longer in the dilated HC group (173 months) than in the IC (24 months) and IDC (51 months) groups ($p < 0.001$). The mean heart weights of the IC and IDC groups were similar (467 and 455 g) and heavier than those in the HC group (351 g) ($p < 0.02$). The mean body weights of each of the 3 groups were different (77.2 vs 69.0 vs 59.5 kg) ($p < 0.03$). By definition, 100% of the 47 patients with IC had relatively large transmural left ventricular scars with or without ventricular septal scars, and 9 (90%) of the 10 HC patients had transmural ventricular septal scars with or without

TABLE IV Comparison of Findings in Patients With Ischemic Cardiomyopathy (IC), Idiopathic Dilated Cardiomyopathy (IDC), and Dilated Hypertrophic Cardiomyopathy (HC) Having Cardiac Transplantation (CT)

	Etiology		
	IC (n = 47)	IDC (n = 35)	HC (n = 10)
Morphology			
Age (yr)	54 ± 6*	47 ± 15**	37 ± 9**
Men	44 (94%)*	14 (40%)*	6 (60%)*
Women	3 (6%)*	21 (60%)*	4 (40%)*
Duration of symptoms to CT (mos)	34 ± 45**	51 ± 73**	173 ± 99*
Heart weight (g) (mean): men/women	471/410**	501/418**	393/300*
Body weight (kg) (mean): men/women	79/63	78/61	53/60
LV or ventricular septal necrosis	4 (9%)	0	0
LV or ventricular septal fibrosis	47 (100%)*	8 (23%)*	9 (90%)*
LV or right ventricular thrombus	3 (6%)	1 (3%)	0
LV mural plaque	31 (66%)*	25 (74%)*	2 (20%)*
Epicardial CAs narrowed >75% in CSA	47 (100%)*	7 (20%)*	0*
LV diameter (cm)	5.8 ± 0.9	5.6 ± 1.0	4.6 ± 0.6
Laboratory			
Hematocrit	37% ± 6%	37% ± 4%	41% ± 4%
Total cholesterol (mg/dl)	207 ± 57*	170 ± 37*	141 ± 36*
Triglycerides (mg/dl)	176 ± 132	146 ± 79	60 ± 34
Electrocardiogram			
Interval study to CT (mo)	3 ± 4**	4 ± 4**	28 ± 39*
Heart rate (beats/min)	83 ± 17	96 ± 23***	68 ± 6***
Bundle branch block	11/36 (31%)*	15/31 (48%)*	1 (10%)*
Total 12-lead QRS voltage (mm)	129 ± 43	149 ± 59	171 ± 58
Atrial fibrillation	8/37 (22%)	8/32 (25%)	6 (60%)
PR Interval >0.20 sec.	10/30 (33%)*	2/26 (8%)*	3/4 (75%)*
Ventricular tachycardia	14/36 (39%)	7/31 (23%)	3 (30%)
Echocardiogram			
Interval study to CT (mo)	7.7 ± 6.3**	9.1 ± 12.2**	26.6 ± 37.3*
LV end-diastole (cm)	6.6 ± 1.1**	6.9 ± 0.9**	4.6 ± 0.5*
LV end-systole (cm)	5.5 ± 1.1*	6.3 ± 0.9*	3.3 ± 0.7*
LA cavity (cm)	4.5 ± 0.6***	4.8 ± 0.8	5.3 ± 0.4***
Ventricular septum (cm)	1.0 ± 0.2**	0.9 ± 0.3**	1.6 ± 0.3*
LV free wall (cm)	1.0 ± 0.2	0.9 ± 0.3	1.1 ± 0.2
Mitral regurgitation 3+ or 4+/4+	13/26 (50%)	12/29 (41%)	3/9 (33%)
Tricuspid regurgitation 3+ or 4+/4+	6/26 (23%)	11/25 (44%)	0
LV ejection fraction	20% ± 7%**	19% ± 8%**	45% ± 14%*
Hemodynamics			
Interval study to CT (mo)	3 ± 5	3 ± 3	31 ± 45
Systemic artery (mm Hg) (s/d)	113/68	104/67	114/69
Left ventricle (mm Hg) (s/d)	111/24	99/18	117/23
Right ventricle (mm Hg) (s/d)	40/8	38/8	49/14
Pulmonary artery (mm Hg) (s/d)	39/18	40/20	49/24
Right Atrial mean (mm Hg)	6 ± 5***	8 ± 7	12 ± 7***
Pulmonary artery wedge (mm Hg)	17 ± 9***	20 ± 10	26 ± 6***
Cardiac index (L/min/m^2) (mean)	2.3 ± 0.5	2.4 ± 0.7	2.2 ± 0.7
Right ventricular end-diastole >6 mm Hg	20/31 (65%)	15/30 (50%)	9 (90%)
Pulmonary artery peak systole >40 mm Hg	15/38 (39%)*	14/31 (45%)*	9 (90%)*
Pulmonary artery wedge mean >12 mm Hg	21/39 (54%)*	26/32 (81%)*	9 (90%)*
Cardiac index >2.5 L/min/m^2	8/30 (27%)	13/28 (46%)	4/9 (44%)

— = all 3 numbers are significantly different (p < 0.05).
*—** = one (*) of the 3 numbers is significant different.
— = 2 of the 3 numbers are significantly different.
CAs = coronary arteries; CSA = cross-sectional area; other abbreviations as in Table I.

left ventricular free wall scars; in contrast, 8 (23%) of the 35 IDC patients had left ventricular scars and in each they were small. Only 4 patients had left ventricular thrombi: 3 with IC and 1 with IDC. By definition, 1 or more major epicardial coronary arteries were narrowed >75% in cross-sectional area at some point by atherosclerotic plaque in 100% of the IC patients, but similar, much less extensive narrowing by plaque was present in 1 or more epicardial coronary arteries in 20% (7 of 35) of the IDC group; none of the dilated HC patients had significant narrowing of any of the epicardial coronary arteries. The mean maximal internal diameters of the left ventricular cavities in each of the 3 groups was similar (5.8 vs 5.6 vs 5.0 cm).

The IC group had higher average serum total cholesterol levels (207 mg/dl) than either the IDC (170 mg/dl) or the HC (183 mg/dl) group (p <0.02). The average serum triglyceride levels were insignificantly different among the 3 groups.

On their last electrocardiogram or Holter monitoring before CT, the frequency of atrial fibrillation and runs of ventricular tachycardia were similar in the 3 groups. The frequency of prolonged (>0.20 second) PR intervals was higher in the HC group (75%) than in either the IDC (8%) or IC (33%) group (p = 0.03).

By echocardiogram, the left ventricular end-diastolic and peak systolic cavity sizes were similar in the IC and IDC groups (6.6 and 5.5 cm; 6.9 and 6.3 cm, respectively) and smaller in the HC group (4.6 and 3.3 cm) (p <0.001). The mean left atrial cavity size was significantly smaller in the IC group (4.5 cm), and larger in the HC group (5.3 cm) (p <0.001). The mean thickness of the ventricular septum was similar to that of the left ventricular free wall in both the IC and IDC groups (1.0 and 0.9 cm), but the septum was thicker than the free wall (1.6 vs 1.1 cm) in the HC group and significantly thicker than the ventricular septum of the IC and IDC groups (p <0.001). The mean ejection fraction was similar in the IC and IDC groups (20% and 19%) but significantly higher in the HC group (45%) (p <0.001).

By cardiac catheterization, the right atrial mean pressure was significantly less in the IC group (6

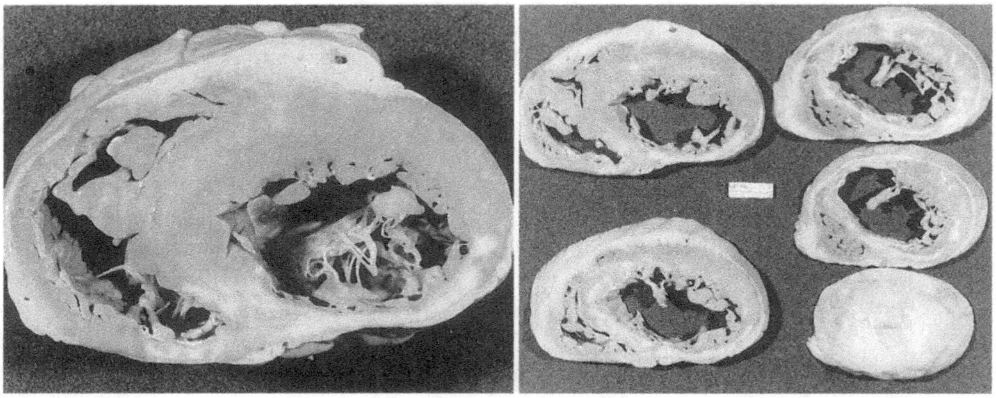

FIGURE 1. Patient #13, Table I. Transverse section exposing the cephalad portion of the heart (*left*) and 1-cm-thick slices of the caudal portion of the heart (*right*) in a 50-year-old man (BUMC #S96-674) with IC. The posterior portion of the left ventricle, ventricular septum, and right ventricle are scarred and thinned basally and apically and also apically the anterior, lateral, and septal walls are scarred.

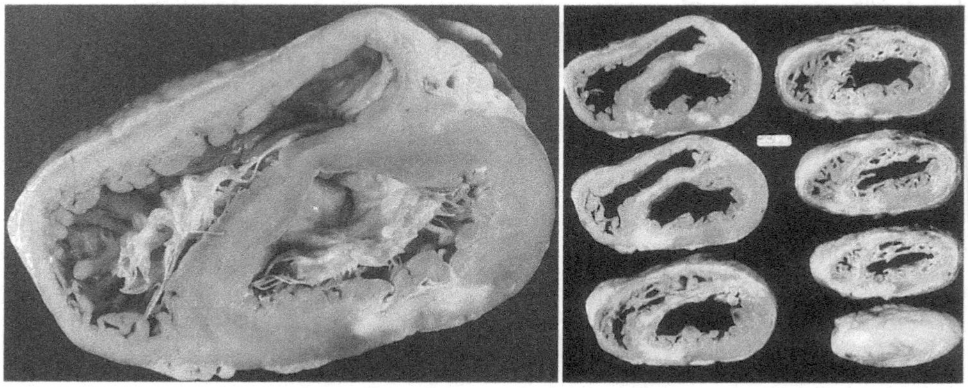

FIGURE 2. Patient #17, Table I. Transverse section exposing the cephalad portion (*left*) and caudal slices (*right*) of the heart in a 51-year-old man (BUMC #S96-10318) with IC. A distant posterior scar is present basally and the scarring apically is circumferential and associated with extensive wall thinning.

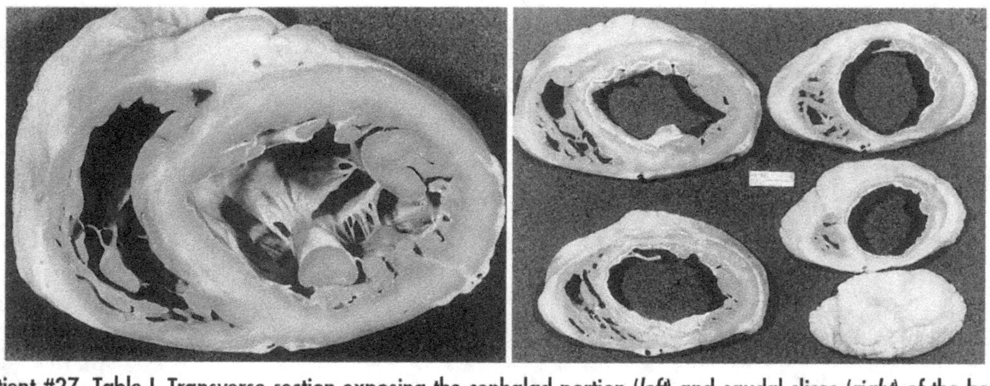

FIGURE 3. Patient #27, Table I. Transverse section exposing the cephalad portion (*left*) and caudal slices (*right*) of the heart in a 56-year-old woman (BUMC #S 95-9546) with IC. Some scarring is present in the central portion of the ventricular septum (left) and circumferentially in the more apical portions (right), which are also severely thinned.

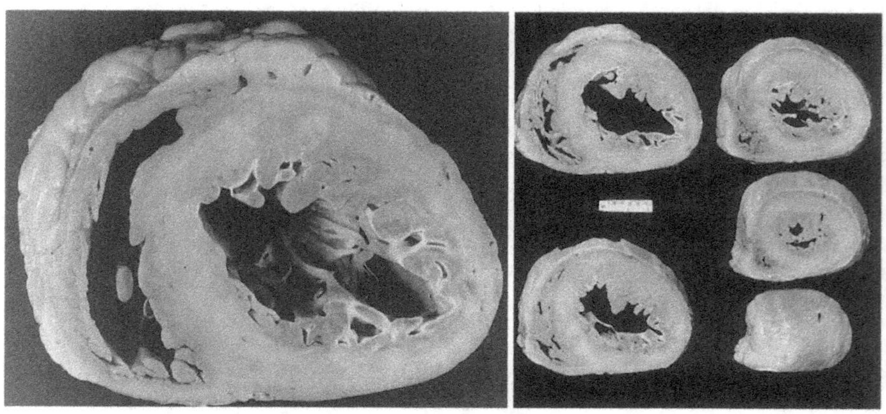

FIGURE 4. Patient #26, Table I. Transverse section exposing the basal portion (*left*) and caudal slices (*right*) of the heart in a 56-year-old man (BUMC #S95-274) with IC. Scarring and thinning is mainly localized to the lateral wall.

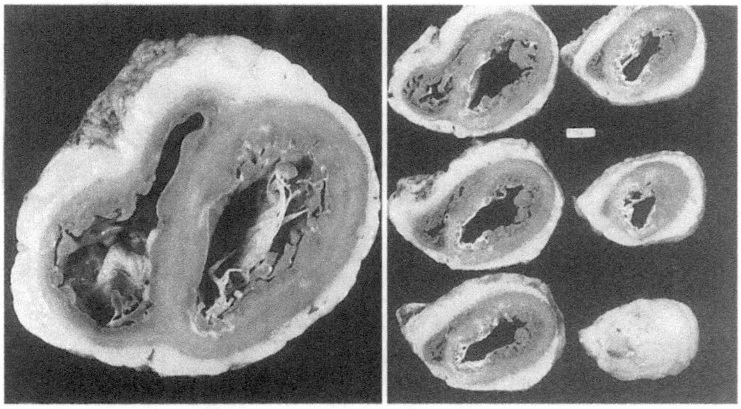

FIGURE 5. Patient #41, Table I. Transverse section exposing the cephalad portion (*left*) and transverse slices of caudal portion (*right*) in a 61-year-old man (BUMC #S96-12855) with IC. A small posterior wall scar is seen basally and more apically the scar extends into the ventricular septum and anterior free wall.

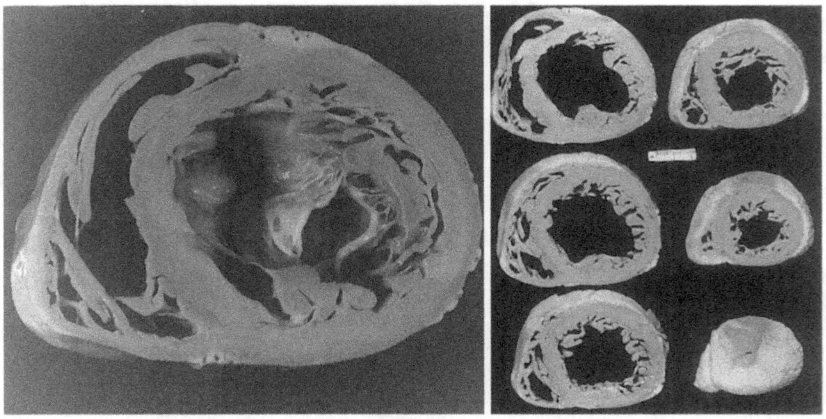

FIGURE 6. Patient #10, Table II. Transverse section exposing the cephalad portion (*left*) and transverse slices of the caudal portion (*right*) of the heart in a 36-year-old woman (BUMC #S95-15071) with IDC. Both ventricular cavities are enormously dilated and the walls are free of scars.

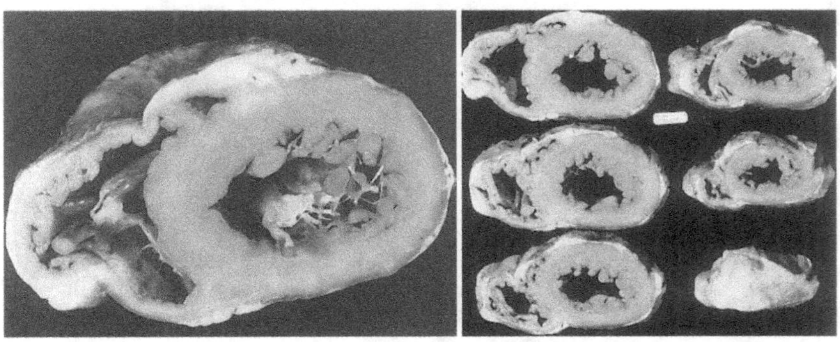

FIGURE 7. Patient #15, Table II. Transverse section exposing the cephalad portion (*left*) and transverse slices of the caudal portion (*right*) of the heart in a 48-year-old man (BUMC #S96-12962) with IDC. The ventricular cavities are moderately dilated and the walls are devoid of scars.

mm Hg) than in the dilated HC group (12 mm Hg) ($p = 0.04$). Similarly, the pulmonary artery wedge pressure was significantly less in the IC group (17 mm Hg) than in the dilated HC group (26 mm Hg) ($p = 0.01$). The percentage of patients with pulmonary artery peak systolic pressures >40 mm Hg and pulmonary artery wedge pressures >12 mm Hg was smallest in the IC group (39% and 54%), intermediate in the IDC group (45% and 81%), and highest in the dilated HC group (90%) ($p < 0.05$).

DISCUSSION

Although numerous reports have appeared describing cardiac morphologic findings *after* CT (i.e., those in the donor heart),[7,8] few reports have appeared describing morphologic findings in the native heart (i.e., the one excised at the time of CT). Indeed, we found only 7 publications[2,9–14] that described in any detail features of the operatively excised native heart, and in only 2 of these publications[2,9] was 1 or more gross photographs of a native heart presented. In 4 reports,[9,10,12–14] photomicrographs of certain features in the native hearts were presented.

The present study compares cardiac morphologic and clinical findings in operatively excised native hearts in 3 different conditions. Although the hearts in each of the 3 conditions were distinctly different morphologically and these differences were readily discernible from examination of the operatively excised heart, considerable intragroup morphologic variation occurred. The intragroup amounts of scarring in the left ventricular free wall and ventricular septum, for example, varied considerably among patients in the IC group and also within the dilated HC group. Furthermore, the amounts of intragroup ventricular cavity dilatation varied considerably.

Despite the clear intergroup anatomic differences among the 3 groups of patients, clinically there were considerably fewer differences in clinical characteristics. The clinical presentation, electrocardiographic, echocardiographic, and hemodynamic features usually were not specific in separating patients in one group from another group. Coronary angiography was the key clinical tool separating patients in one group from another. Although 7 patients in the IDC group had narrowing of 1 or more major epicardial coronary

FIGURE 8. Patient #16, Table II. Transverse section exposing the cephalad portion (*left*) and transverse slices of the caudal portion (*right*) of heart in a 50-year-old woman (87S-8929) with IDC. Both ventricular cavities are severely dilated and the walls are devoid of scars.

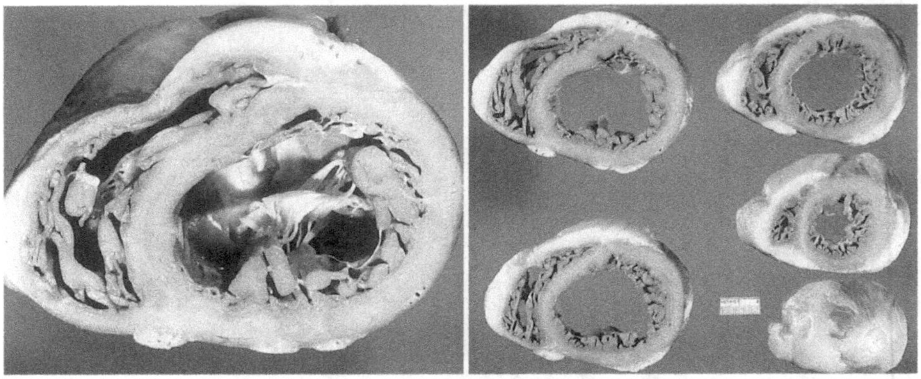

FIGURE 9. Patient #17, Table II. Transverse section exposing the cephalad portion (*left*) and slices of the caudal portion (*right*) in a 51-year-old man (BUMC #S96-05417) with IDC. A small scar is present in the anterior wall (*left*). The ventricles are moderately dilated.

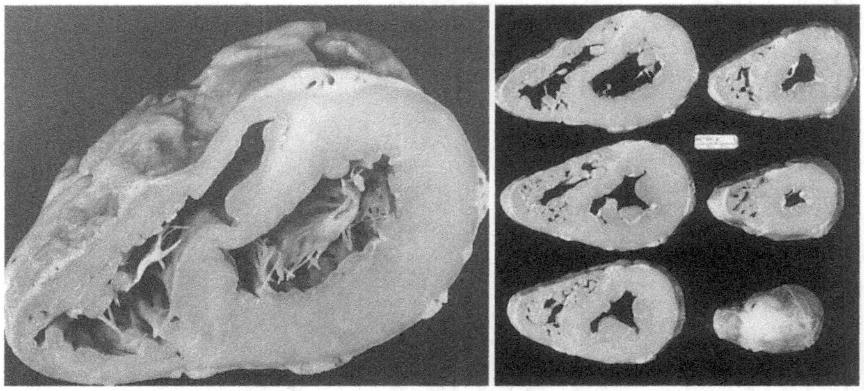

FIGURE 10. Patient #29, Table II. Transverse cut exposing the cephalad portion (*left*) and slices of the caudal portion (*right*) of the heart in a 61-year-old man (BUMC #S95-07656) with IDC. This patient also had narrowing >75% in cross-sectional area of 2 of the 3 major epicardial coronary arteries. Angiographically, however, before CT, no coronary narrowing of significance was noted. No ventricular scars are present.

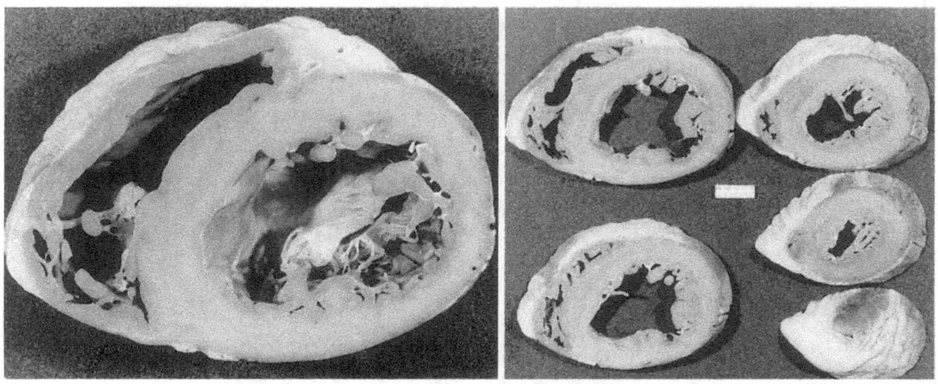

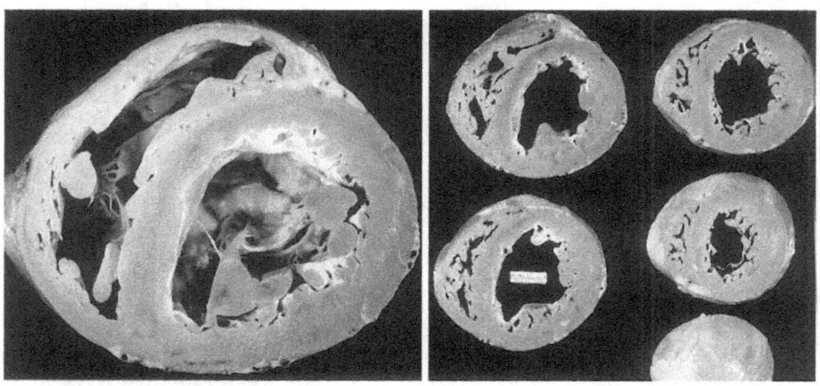

FIGURE 11. Patient #31, Table II. Transverse section exposing the cephalad portion (*left*) and transverse slices of the caudal portion (*right*) of heart in a 62-year-old woman (#91S-11353) with IDC. The ventricles are severely dilated and the walls are free of scars. The left ventricular endocardium is focally thickened by fibrous tissue, probably the result of organization of intracardiac thrombi.

arteries on anatomic examination, coronary angiography before CT had not detected such narrowings. In contrast, all 47 patients with IC had angiographic documentation of severe narrowings in 1 or more major epicardial coronary arteries before CT.

Acknowledgment: We are indebted to J. Carolyn Bank, PhD, for providing statistical support, John F. Dixon, MSN, RN, for creating a patient database program for analyzing data, Bonnie Martinez for photographic support, and Linda B. Maddox for secretarial support.

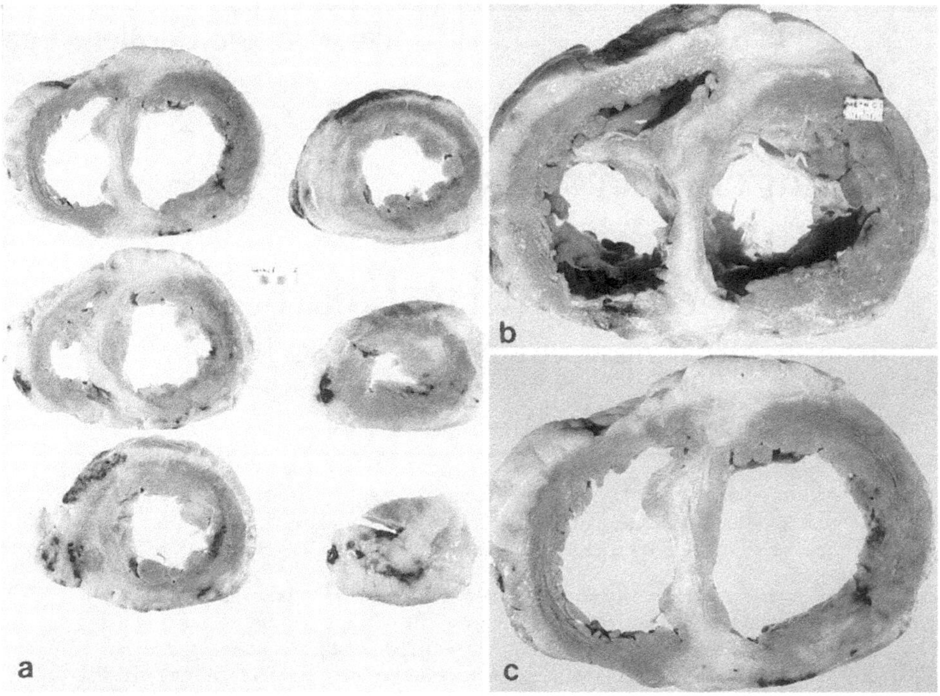

FIGURE 12. Patient #10, Table III. Transverse cuts exposing the caudal portions (*a*) and cephalad portions (*b,c*) of the heart in a 46-year-old man with dilated HC. The ventricular cavities are severely dilated, the ventricular septum is severely scarred and thinned. Small scars are present in the posterior walls of both right and left ventricles. The major epicardial coronary arteries were not significantly narrowed. (Reproduced with permission from reference 4).

1. Hosenpud JD, Novick RJ, Bennett LE, Keck BM, Fiol B, Daily OP. The registry of the International Society for Heart and Lung Transplantation: Thirteenth Official report-1996. *J Heart Lung Transplant* 1996;15:661–674.

2. Shirani J, Maron BJ, Cannon RO III, Shahin S, Roberts WC. Clinicopathologic features of hypertrophic cardiomyopathy managed by cardiac transplantation. *Am J Cardiol* 1993;72:434– 440.

3. Siegel RJ, Roberts WC. Electrocardiographic observations in severe aortic valve stenosis: correlative necropsy study to clinical, hemodynamic, and ECG variables demonstrating relation of 12– lead QRS amplitude to peak systolic transaortic pressure gradient. *Am Heart J* 1982;103:210–221.

4. Ross MR, Roberts WC. Severe atherosclerotic coronary artery disease, healed myocardial infarction and chronic congestive heart failure: analysis of 81 patients studied at necropsy. *Am J Cardiol* 1986;57:44– 50.

5. Roberts WC, Siegel RJ, McManus BM. Idiopathic dilated cardiomyopathy: analysis of 152 necropsy patients. *Am J Cardiol* 1987;60:1340–1355.

6. Roberts CS, Roberts WC. Morphologic features (of hypertrophic cardiomyopathy). Progress in Cardiology 2/2; Zipes DP, Rowlands DJ, eds. Philadelphia: Lea & Febiger, 1989:3–32.

7. Arbustini E, Dal Bello B, Morbini P, Grasso M, Diegoli M, Fasani R, Pilotto A, Bellini O, Pellegrini C, Martinelli L, Campana C, Gavazzi A, Specchia G, Vigano M, Roberts WC. Frequency and characteristics of coronary thrombosis in the epicardial coronary arteries after cardiac transplantation. *Am J Cardiol* 1996; 78:795–800.

8. Arbustini E, Roberts WC. Morphologic observation in the epicardial coronary arteries and their surroundings late after cardiac transplantation (Allograft vascular disease). *Am J Cardiol* 1996;78:814–820.

9. Keren A, Billingham ME, Weintraub D, Stinson EB, Popp RL. Mildly dilated congestive cardiomyopathy. *Circulation* 1985;72:302– 309.

10. Schaper J, Froede R, Hein S, Buck A, Hashizume H, Speiser B, Friedl A, Bleese N. Impairment of the myocardial ultrastructure changes of the cytoskeleton in dilated cardiomyopathy. *Circulaion* 1991;83:504–514.

11. Becker AE, Heijams CD, Essed CE. Chronic non-ischemic congestive heart disease and endomyocardial biopsies. Worth the extra? *Eur Heart J* 1991;12: 218–223.

12. Ardehali A, Laks H, Drinkwater DC, Ziv ET, Sorensen TJ, Hamilton MA, Warner-Stevenson L, Moriguchi JB, Kobashigawa JA, edited by Terasaki and Cecka. Cardiac transplantation at UCLA. *Clinical Transpl* 1993:119–127.

13. Beltrami CA, Finato N, Rocco M, Feruglio GA, Puricelli C, Cigola E, Sonnenblick EH, Olivetti G, Anversa P. The cellular basis of dilated cardiomyopathy in humans. *J Mol Cell Cardiol* 1995;27:291–305.

14. Narula J, Haider N, Virmani R, DiSalvo TG, Kolodgie FD, Hajjar RJ, Schmidt U, Semigran MJ, Dec GW, Khaw B-A. Apoptosis in myocytes in end-stage heart failure. *N Engl J Med* 1996;335:1182–1189.

Morphology and Significance of the Left Ventricular Collagen Network in Young Patients With Hypertrophic Cardiomyopathy and Sudden Cardiac Death

Jamshid Shirani, MD, FACC,* Ruth Pick, MD,† William C. Roberts, MD, FACC,‡ Barry J. Maron, MD, FACC§

Bronx, New York; Chicago, Illinois; Dallas, Texas; Minneapolis, Minnesota

BACKGROUND Hypertrophic cardiomyopathy (HCM) is a primary cardiac disease with a diverse clinical spectrum, in which many of the abnormal structural and pathophysiologic features are consequences of inappropriate left ventricular hypertrophy.

METHODS We analyzed the amount, distribution and structure of the cardiac collagen network in transmural sections of the ventricular septum (thickness 17 to 40 mm, mean 25 mm) in 16 previously asymptomatic children and young adults with HCM (11 to 31 years of age, mean 20 years) who died suddenly. The morphologic appearance and volume fractions of interstitial (matrix) and perivascular (adventitial) collagen were analyzed with polarization microscopy and computerized videodensitometry in picrosirius red-stained sections. Findings were compared with 16 structurally normal hearts, 5 with systemic hypertension and 6 infants who died of HCM.

RESULTS Adults and young children with HCM had an eightfold greater amount of matrix collagen compared with normal controls (14.1 ± 8.8% vs. 1.8 ± 1% of the tissue section; $p < 0.0001$), and a threefold increase compared with patients with systemic hypertension (4.5 ± 1.3%; $p < 0.001$) and infants with HCM (4.0 ± 2.4%; $p < 0.001$). Compared with normal controls and hypertensives, adults and young children (and infants) with HCM showed increased numbers and thickness of each collagen fiber component of the matrix (perimysial coils, pericellular weaves and struts), which were often arranged in disorganized patterns. In HCM patients, the amount of collagen was not a consequence of other clinical, demographic and morphologic disease variables.

CONCLUSIONS Left ventricular collagen matrix in young, previously asymptomatic patients with HCM who died suddenly is morphologically abnormal and substantially increased in size. The enlarged matrix collagen compartment is present in HCM at an early age, further expands during growth, is partially responsible for increased ventricular septal thickness and likely represents a primary morphologic abnormality in this disease. These findings support the view that the complex HCM disease process is not confined to sarcomere protein abnormalities, but also involves connective tissue elements. (J Am Coll Cardiol 2000;35:36–44) © 1999 by the American College of Cardiology

Hypertrophic cardiomyopathy (HCM) is a primary and genetically transmitted cardiac disease with a heterogeneous clinical and morphologic profile (1–3). Recently, considerable attention has focused on several mutations in genes encoding proteins of the cardiac sarcomere, including β-myosin heavy chain, cardiac troponin-T, troponin-I, α-tropomyosin and myosin-binding protein-C (3–6). Indeed, in HCM, many prominent and characteristic structural alterations, such as left ventricular (LV) wall thickening (7) and disorganization of cardiac muscle cells (8,9), directly involve proteins of the sarcomere.

However, other common pathologic features of HCM, such as the thickened and narrowed intramural coronary arteries (1,10), elongated mitral valve leaflets (11–13), congenital malformations of the mitral apparatus (14) and myocardial fibrosis (15–20), largely involve connective tissue elements. Thus, we have examined the possibility that in HCM an expanded LV collagen matrix is involved in this process (19) and may contribute to the abnormally increased

From the *Departments of Medicine (Division of Cardiology) and Pathology, Albert Einstein College of Medicine, Bronx, New York; †Cardiac Morphology Laboratory, Michael Reese Hospital and Medical Center, Chicago, Illinois; ‡Baylor Cardiovascular Institute, Baylor University Medical Center, Dallas, Texas; and §Minneapolis Heart Institute Foundation, Minneapolis, Minnesota.

Manuscript received December 18, 1997; revised manuscript received July 8, 1999; accepted September 10, 1999.

Abbreviations and Acronyms

HCM = hypertrophic cardiomyopathy
LV = left ventricle (ventricular)

LV wall thickness, the sine qua non of this disease (7). Consequently, the present study analyzes the morphologic appearance and extent of the collagen matrix in patients with HCM who had died suddenly in comparison with several control groups.

METHODS

Patient population. The 16 study patients were selected from the HCM registry of the Pathology Branch of the National Heart, Lung, and Blood Institute. Each heart met the morphologic definition of HCM, that is, a hypertrophied, nondilated LV in the absence of another cardiac or systemic disease capable of producing the magnitude of hypertrophy present (7). Patients were selected by virtue of the following inclusion criteria: 1) age <35 years at the time of death; 2) absence of symptoms or evidence of cardiac dysfunction during life; 3) sudden and unexpected, out-of-hospital death as the only clinical manifestation of HCM; 4) absence of myocardial scarring on gross visual inspection; and 5) absence of cross-sectional luminal narrowing ≥75% by atherosclerosis of a major epicardial coronary artery.

The control groups consisted of: 1) 16 adults (20 to 78 years; mean 43 ± 18 years) with structurally normal hearts who died of noncardiovascular causes (all related to trauma); 2) five nondiabetic adults (39 to 55 years, mean 46 ± 7 years) with LV hypertrophy as a consequence of long-standing and severe systemic hypertension in the absence of significant atherosclerotic coronary artery narrowing, who died of noncardiovascular causes (trauma in four and cerebral hemorrhage in one); and 3) six infants with HCM who were stillborn or died of congestive heart failure (1 to 146 days of age; mean 71 ± 63 days).

Gross examination. After fixation in 10% phosphate-buffered formaldehyde, each heart was sectioned transversely (i.e., perpendicular to the long axis of the LV), from apex to base, at approximately 1 cm intervals. Maximal ventricular septal and LV free wall thicknesses were measured perpendicular to the endocardial surfaces of the wall (excluding papillary muscles and trabeculae).

Preparation of specimens for histologic studies. A transmural section of ventricular septum, taken at the mid-LV cavity level in the area of maximal wall thickness, was removed for histomorphologic examination, taking care to exclude the LV outflow tract fibrous plaque (Fig. 1). Each specimen was embedded in paraffin, sectioned at 5-μm thickness and stained with hematoxylin and eosin and picrosirius red (Pfaltz and Bauer; Stamford, Connecticut). Stained sections were utilized for quantitative analysis of collagen content and the extent of cardiac muscle cell disorganization.

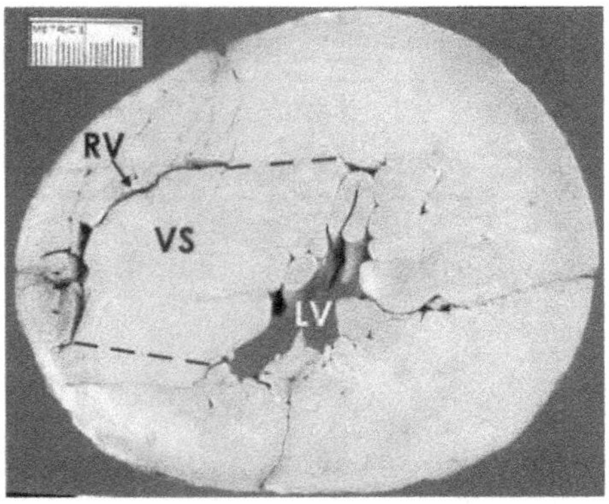

Figure 1. Cross section of the heart at mid-left ventricular **(LV)** cavity level from a 21-year-old patient with HCM showing the site from which tissue blocks were taken from ventricular septum **(VS)** for histologic examination (inside broken line). RV = right ventricle.

Qualitative and quantitative assessment of collagen. Morphology of interstitial (matrix) and perivascular (adventitial) collagen was assessed from the picrosirius red-stained sections with polarization microscopy. Picrosirius red is a collagen-specific stain that also enhances the natural birefringence of the collagen fibrils under polarized light and permits identification of various components of the matrix collagen (perimysial coils, pericellular weaves and struts) (21,22).

Collagen volume fractions were quantified in tissue sections using a semi-automated computerized image analysis system (Quantimet 520; Cambridge Laboratories, Inc., Cambridge, Massachusetts), similar to the technique described by Hoyt et al. (23). Analysis was performed with a standard light microscope and a mounted video camera system connected to a host computer and a digitizer. First, by systematically scanning each microscopic slide (at a magnification of 7.8×), a composite digitized image was obtained. The volume fraction of interstitial collagen was then calculated as the area occupied by connective tissue divided by the sum of the areas occupied by connective tissue and cardiac muscle cells. Intramural vessels, perivascular collagen, endocardium and trabeculae were excluded from this particular analysis.

Perivascular collagen was defined as that collagen in the adventitia of those intramural coronary arteries identified by picrosirius red staining. This volume fraction was calculated by dividing the sum of all perivascular collagen by the total area of the tissue section.

Quantitation of cardiac muscle cell disorganization. The area of ventricular septum occupied by disorganized cardiac muscle cells was measured using the method described by Maron and Roberts (9). Briefly, hematoxylin and eosin-stained sections were magnified to occupy a 30 × 40 in. positive print, over which a transparent cellulose overlay was

Table 1. Demographic and Morphologic Findings in Infants, Children and Young Adults With Hypertrophic Cardiomyopathy: Patients With Systemic Hypertension and Normal Controls

Parameters	HCM Children/Young Adults	HCM Infants	Hypertension	Normal Controls
No. patients	16	6	5	16
Age, years (mean, range)	20 ± 7 (11–31)	0.2 ± 0.2	46 ± 7 (39–55)	43 ± 18 (20–78)
Male, no. (%)	10 (62%)	4 (67%)	3 (60%)	8 (50%)
Heart weight, g	518 ± 156 (320–970)	—*	438 ± 38 (387–489)	305 ± 56 (195–390)#
Ventricular septal thickness, mm	27 ± 7 (17–40)	17 ± 7 (8–30)	16 ± 1 (15–17)	12 ± 2 (10–15)
LV free wall thickness, mm	15 ± 3 (9–20)	8 ± 3 (3–13)	16 ± 1 (14–17)	12 ± 1 (10–15)
Septum/free wall ratio	1.9 ± 0.5 (0.9–2.7)	2.1 ± 0.5 (1.4–2.7)	1.0 ± 0.1 (0.9–1.1)	1.0 ± 0.1 (0.8–1.2)
Area of septum examined, cm^2	5.2 ± 2.0 (2.1–9.1)	2.3 ± 0.5 (1.4–3.0)	4.4 ± 0.4 (3.9–4.9)	3.5 ± 0.8 (2.7–5.0)
Percent area of disorganized cells	53 ± 20 (12–88)	25 ± 8 (17–34)	2 ± 1 (0–3.9)	2 ± 1 (0.1–4.2)
Collagen volume fraction:				
Total	16.7 ± 9.1 (5.8–30.6)†	7.0 ± 3.0 (3.7–12.5)‡	8.2 ± 1.8 (6.1–9.9)§	4.0 ± 1.6 (1.7–7.6)
Interstitial	14.1 ± 8.8 (4.5–27.7)‖	4.0 ± 2.4 (1.3–7.8)	4.5 ± 1.3 (2.7–6.2)¶	1.8 ± 1.0 (0.6–3.6)
Perivascular	2.6 ± 1.0 (1.0–4.6)	3.0 ± 1.0 (2.2–4.7)	3.7 ± 1.4 (2.0–5.8)	2.2 ± 1.0 (1.1–4.3)
Percent of total collagen:				
In interstitial space	81 ± 11 (56–95)	53 ± 15 (35–71)	55 ± 12 (42–68)	44 ± 13 (19–64)
In perivascular space	19 ± 11 (5–44)	47 ± 15 (29–65)	45 ± 12 (32–58)	56 ± 13 (36–81)

*Data not available; †<0.0001 and <0.005 vs. normals and hypertensives, respectively; ‡<0.01 vs. normals; §0.006 vs. normals; ‖<0.001 to <0.0001 vs. HCM infants, hypertensives and normals; ¶<0.01 vs. normals; #<0.005 vs. normals.

HCM = hypertrophic cardiomyopathy; LV = left ventricular.

placed. Each area of myocardium occupied by disorganized cardiac muscle cells was outlined separately on the overlay with a marking pen, and the silhouettes were then quantified using a video-planimetry system. Percent area of disorganized cardiac muscle cells was calculated as the ratio of the area occupied by disorganized cells to the area occupied by disorganized cells and longitudinally cut but normally arranged cells (9).

Statistical analyses. Data are expressed as mean ± standard deviation. Differences between continuous variables were assessed with the unpaired Student *t* test. Chi-square or Fisher exact tests compared proportions. Selected variables were compared using linear regression analysis. Univariate regression analysis assessed the degree to which collagen amount was associated with particular clinical, demographic and morphologic disease parameters.

RESULTS

Normal control subjects. GROSS AND HISTOLOGIC FINDINGS (TABLE 1). Heart weights were 195 to 390 g (mean 305 ± 56 g) and within normal limits in each subject (<350 g in women; <400 g in men). Ventricular septal and LV free wall thicknesses were 10 to 15 mm (mean 12 ± 2 mm). Scattered small foci of disorganized cardiac muscle cells, present in each subject, occupied 2 ± 1% of septal tissue sections.

ASSESSMENT OF COLLAGEN FIBER MORPHOLOGY. The collagen matrix in normal controls consisted of an orderly arrangement of thin "spring-like" perimysial coils (Fig. 2A and B) that coursed parallel to the long axis of the cardiac muscle cells and were connected through transversely oriented struts to a fine network of pericellular weaves (Fig. 2A and B) encircling the sarcolemma of individual muscle cells. In addition, lateral surfaces of adjacent muscle cells were also interconnected by thin, transversely oriented struts (Fig. 2A and B).

COLLAGEN VOLUME FRACTION (TABLE 1; FIG. 3). Total collagen volume in septal tissue sections was 4.0 ± 1.6%. Volume fractions of interstitial (matrix) and perivascular collagen were 1.8 ± 1.0% and 2.2 ± 1.0%, respectively, and interstitial/perivascular collagen ratio was 0.81. Interstitial collagen was evenly distributed throughout the middle, inner (adjacent to LV) and outer (adjacent to right ventricle) one-thirds of the septal tissue sections (35 ± 3%, 35 ± 3% and 31 ± 4%, respectively).

Children and young adults with HCM. GROSS AND HISTOLOGIC FINDINGS (TABLE 1). Heart weights were 320 to 970 g (mean 518 ± 156 g), and increased relative to age and gender in each patient. Ventricular septal and free wall thicknesses were 17 to 40 mm (mean 27 ± 7 mm) and 9 to 20 mm (mean 15 ± 3 mm), respectively. Extensive cardiac muscle cell disorganization was present in each patient, occupying 53 ± 20% of the septal tissue section. Cellular disorganization involved areas of myocardium of varying size in which adjacent longitudinally sectioned cells (or bundles of cells) were aligned perpendicularly and obliquely, or in which longitudinally sectioned cells were interlaced among transversely oriented cells. Microscopic areas of replacement fibrosis were not observed.

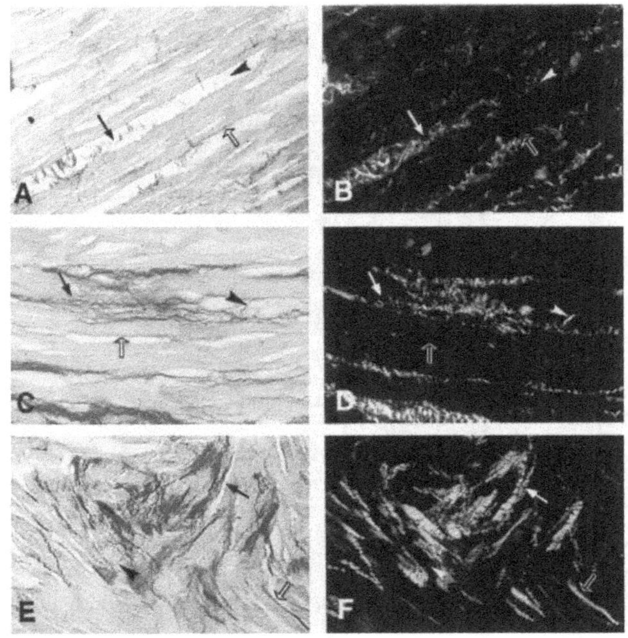

Figure 2. Ventricular septal tissue sections from a normal control, age 36 years **(A and B)** and a 31-year-old patient with HCM who died suddenly **(C–F)**. All sections are stained with picrosirius red and viewed at the same magnification (×400) using standard light **(left panels)** or polarization **(right panels)** microscopy. **A and B:** Structurally normal heart. Thin collagen fibers are stained red **(A)** and appear green-to-yellow under polarized light **(B)**. Various components of the normal collagen matrix are visualized consisting of the perimysial coils **(solid arrows)**, pericellular weaves **(open arrows)** and intercellular struts **(triangles)**. **C and D:** HCM in an area of normally arranged and longitudinally sectioned cardiac muscle cells. All components of the collagen matrix are increased in amount and differ morphologically from controls. The perimysial coils **(solid arrows)** are thickened and appear to be stretched (reduced degree of coiling). Pericellular weaves **(open arrows)** and struts **(triangles)** are abundant and thickened. **E and F:** HCM in an area of disorganized cardiac muscle cells. Perimysial coils **(solid arrows)**, pericellular weaves **(open arrows)** and struts **(triangles)** are significantly increased in amount and are also arranged in a markedly disorganized pattern.

ASSESSMENT OF COLLAGEN MORPHOLOGY (TABLE 2). Although variation was evident among patients, in sharp contrast to normal controls, HCM hearts showed a marked increase in the number and thickness of all fiber components of the collagen matrix (Figs. 2C–F and 4). The perimysial fibers appeared particularly thickened and straighter than normal with a loss of their normal "spring-like" coiled configuration (Fig. 2C and D). Pericellular weaves formed dense networks of thickened fibers encasing cardiac muscle cells in substantial portions of ventricular septum and were particularly evident in association with cardiac muscle cells sectioned transversely (Fig. 4). Fiber components of the matrix showed a disorganized arrangement compared with normals, particularly in areas of cardiac muscle cell disarray. Therefore, when compared with normal controls as well as to hypertensives, the appearance of these collagen fiber types was markedly abnormal, both in areas of disorganized myocytes (Fig. 2E and F) and normal myocardial architecture (Fig. 2C and D).

In addition, dense perivascular collagen encased numerous abnormal intramural coronary arteries with apparently narrowed lumen and thickened walls (with media containing abundant collagen) (Figs. 5 and 6).

COLLAGEN VOLUME FRACTION (TABLE 1; FIG. 3). Total collagen volume in the ventricular septal tissue sections was 16.7 ± 9.1%, significantly exceeding that in the normal controls (4.0 ± 1.6%), hypertensives (8.2 ± 1.8%) and HCM infants (7.0 ± 3.0%) ($p < 0.0001$). Volume fraction of the matrix collagen was 14.1 ± 8.8%, also significantly exceeding normal controls (1.8 ± 1.0%), hypertensives (4.5 ± 1.3%) and HCM infants (4.0 ± 2.4%). This represented an eightfold increase in matrix collagen compared with normal controls, and a threefold increase with respect to hypertensives. Interstitial collagen was distributed disproportionately in the middle one-third of the transmural tissue sections (49 ± 9%), compared with either the inner (34 ± 13%) or outer (17 ± 12%) one-thirds ($p < 0.001$).

Volume fraction of perivascular collagen was 2.6 ± 1.0% in children and young adults with HCM, and did not differ significantly from that in any control group. Therefore, the highest proportion of collagen identified was in the interstitial compartment, with an interstitial/perivascular collagen ratio of 5.4.

Patients with systemic hypertension. GROSS AND HISTOLOGIC FINDINGS. Heart weights were 387 to 489 g (mean 438 ± 38 g) and were increased in each (>350 g in women and >400 g in men). Septal and free wall thicknesses were 15 to 17 mm (mean 16 ± 1 mm) and 14 to 17 mm (mean 16 ± 1 mm), respectively. Scattered small foci of disorganized cardiac muscle cells, present in four patients, occupied 2 ± 1% of the tissue sections. Microscopic areas of replacement fibrosis were not observed.

QUALITATIVE ASSESSMENT OF COLLAGEN. Within the interstitial space, intercellular struts, pericellular weaves and perimysial coils appeared more abundant and thicker than normal, but with ordered arrangement. Abundant perivascular collagen surrounded intramural coronary arteries, a few of which showed thickened walls with increased medial collagen.

COLLAGEN VOLUME FRACTION (TABLE 1; FIG. 3). Total and interstitial collagen volume in patients with hypertension were significantly greater than normal but less than in children and adults with HCM. Interstitial collagen appeared evenly distributed throughout the middle, inner and outer one-thirds of tissue sections. Interstitial/perivascular collagen ratio was only 1.2, and the perivascular collagen volume fraction did not differ from normals.

Infants with HCM. GROSS AND HISTOLOGIC FINDINGS. Ventricular septal and LV free wall thicknesses ranged 8 to 30 mm (mean 17 ± 7 mm) and 3 to 13 mm (mean 8 ±

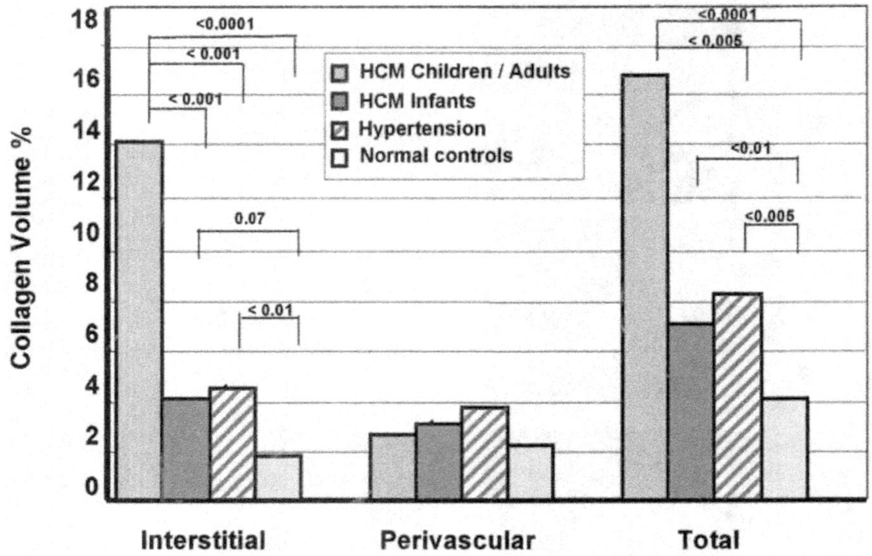

Figure 3. Volume fractions of interstitial, perivascular and total collagen compartments in ventricular septal tissue sections from children and young adults with HCM, compared with controls with structurally normal hearts, patients with systemic hypertension and secondary left ventricular hypertrophy and infants with HCM. Significant differences are present between the groups in total and interstitial, but not perivascular, collagen volume fraction.

3 mm), respectively. Extensive disorganization of myocytes was present in each infant, occupying 25 ± 8% of the tissue section. Small microscopic foci of replacement fibrosis were evident in each heart.

QUALITATIVE ASSESSMENT OF COLLAGEN. Alterations in collagen fiber morphology, consisting of thickening and increased numbers of struts, weaves and perimysial coils (also with stretching of the coils), were similar to that of children and adults with HCM. Collagen fibers also appeared disorganized in their arrangement, particularly in areas of abnormal myocyte arrangement. Similar to the older patients with HCM, areas of dense perivascular collagen encased numerous abnormal intramural coronary arteries with apparently narrowed lumen, thickened walls and increased medial collagen.

Table 2. Correlation Coefficients Relating Demographic and Clinical Parameters to Amount of Collagen in Tissue Sections From 16 Children and Young Adults with Hypertrophic Cardiomyopathy

	Collagen Volume Fractions (%)		
Parameters	Total	Interstitial	Pervivascular
Age (yrs)	0.21 (0.56)	0.22 (0.57)	0.009 (0.97)
Heart weight (g)	0.33 (0.22)	0.33 (0.21)	0.07 (0.80)
Septal thickness (mm)	0.44 (0.09)	0.42 (0.10)	0.34 (0.20)
Percent cellular disorganization	0.15 (0.58)	0.17 (0.54)	−0.12 (0.67)
Media area/total area of intramural coronary arteries	0.32 (0.23)	0.30 (0.25)	0.24 (0.62)

Numbers shown in table are r values from univariate analyses; appropriate p values appear in parentheses.

COLLAGEN VOLUME FRACTION (TABLE 1; FIG. 3). Total and interstitial collagen volume in HCM infants was significantly less than in children and adults with HCM but

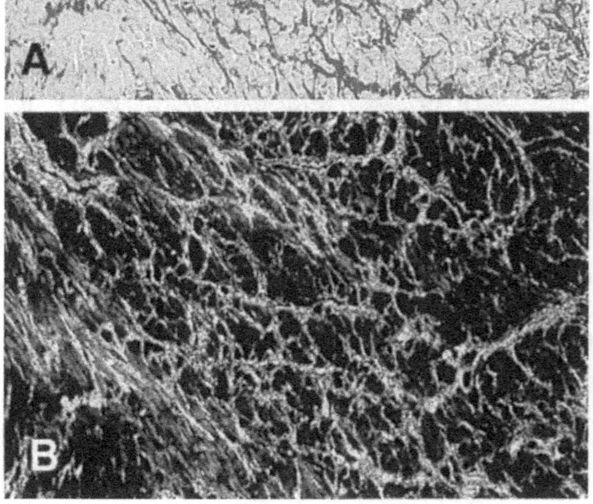

Figure 4. Transversely cut cardiac muscle cells in ventricular septum from a 17-year-old patient with HCM, stained with picrosirius red and viewed by light **(A)** and polarization **(B)** microscopy. The myoctes show characteristic encasement within a dense network of matrix collagen. (Magnification ×100.)

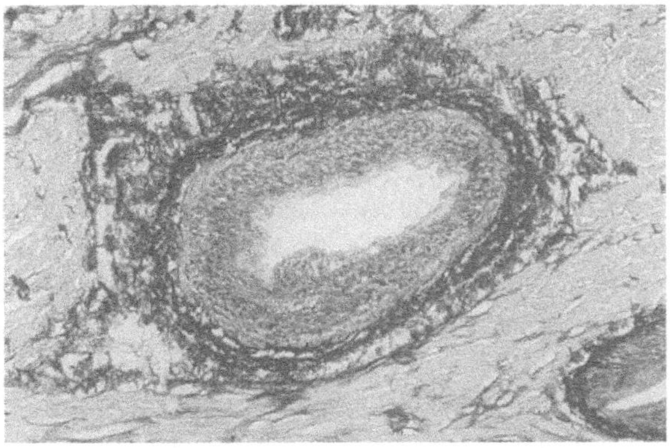

Figure 5. High-power view of a transversely cut abnormal intramural coronary artery in a ventricular septal tissue section from a 28-year-old patient with HCM. Picrosirius red stain shows dense perivascular (adventitial) collagen, as well as increased amounts of collagen in the thickened media. (Magnification ×100.)

greater than in normal (adult) controls (although for interstitial volume, p was only 0.07). The interstitial/perivascular collagen ratio was 1.3, and the perivascular collagen volume fraction in HCM infants did not differ from the other groups.

Relation of amount of collagen to clinical and morphologic features (Table 2). By univariate analysis, for hearts of the children and young adults with HCM, no statistically significant relation was identified between the total or interstitial collagen volume fractions and several clinical and morphologic parameters: age, gender, heart weight, percent of section occupied by disorganized cells and wall thickness of intramural arteries. Only the relation between total collagen and septal thickness approached statistical significance ($r = 0.44$; $p = 0.09$; Table 2).

DISCUSSION

Collagen matrix in HCM. The cardiac collagen matrix, the fibrillar collagen network comprising the interstitium of the heart, represents the structural skeletal framework of the myocardium composed of pericellular, intercellular and fascicular connective tissue (22). In the present study, we demonstrated that this collagen network in the ventricular septum of children and adults with HCM (who died suddenly as the first clinical manifestation of their disease) was substantially greater in size and differed considerably in morphologic appearance when compared with controls without evidence of cardiovascular disease as well as patients with systemic hypertension and secondary LV hypertrophy (24–27). For example, the calculated volume fraction of interstitial collagen was about eight times greater than that of normal controls (and three times greater than that of hypertensives), and comprised about 15% (up to 27%) of the transmural septal tissue sections. Consequently, thickening of the ventricular septum in HCM (7) is not solely due to increased size or number of myocytes, but is also in part a consequence of the substantial expansion of the collagen matrix.

Furthermore, in contrast to the more orderly arrangement of fine collagen fibrils in normal hearts, or in the hypertrophied hearts of patients with hypertension, the fibrillar collagen in our patients with HCM was characteristically more numerous and thickened and was frequently arranged in disorganized patterns.

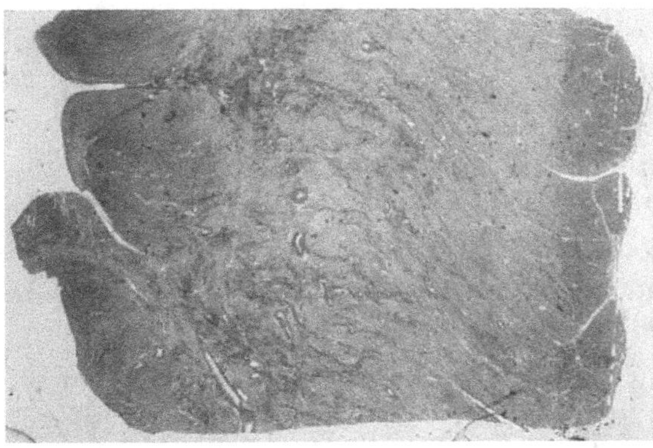

Figure 6. Low-power view of ventricular septal tissue section from a 20-year-old patient with HCM stained with picrosirius red showing widely distributed interstitial collagen. Volume fraction of interstitial collagen in this patient was 18%. Abnormal intramural coronary arteries with thickened walls are also visible. (Magnification ×6.)

Matrix collagen expansion as a primary abnormality. Several of our observations suggest that the excess amount and disorganized architecture of matrix collagen in HCM may represent a primary abnormality of ventricular structure, rather than a secondary consequence of cardiac muscle cell hypertrophy or other factors. First, the expanded size of the collagen matrix in HCM as compared with secondary LV hypertrophy (i.e., systemic hypertension) and normals proved to be largely independent of all potentially relevant morphologic or clinical disease variables (such as heart weight, septal thickness, age and gender). In addition, we found no consistent relationship among our patients between the amount of interstitial collagen and disorganization of myocardial architecture, suggesting that the size of the interstitium is independent of (and not determined by) disordered myocyte architecture (26). Second, infants with HCM who died <5 months of age had already showed greater than normal amounts of total and interstitial collagen. The additional finding that these infants had 3.5 times less collagen than older children and adults with HCM also suggests a remodeling process in which LV interstitial collagen compartment expands as the ventricular wall thickens during childhood with accelerated growth and development (28). Third, the morphologic appearance and architectural organization of individual collagen fibrils in HCM that constitute the complex connective tissue framework of the matrix differed distinctly from that in normal hearts and those from patients with severe hypertension and LV hypertrophy. Finally, the distribution of interstitial collagen across the transmural tissue sections in adults and young children with HCM was atypical by virtue of its concentration in the central portion of the wall rather than in those areas adjacent to the left and right ventricular cavities.

Clinical significance of collagen matrix. The expanded collagen matrix compartment in the ventricular septum can potentially explain certain clinical and functional features of HCM. While HCM is frequently associated with impaired LV relaxation and filling (1–3,29–31), there is some evidence that diastolic dysfunction is largely unrelated to the magnitude or distribution of LV hypertrophy (30), suggesting a contributory role for factors other than myocyte hypertrophy. Indeed, it is possible that the expanded and morphologically abnormal collagen matrix in HCM may affect the rate and extent of myocyte relaxation and filling of the LV chamber. Also, the increased amounts of collagen present in the perivascular compartment of these patients provide a possible structural explanation for the impaired coronary vasodilator reserve and myocardial ischemia described in HCM (in the absence of epicardial coronary artery disease) (32,33).

Prior studies of collagen. Previous studies have addressed the general issue of fibrosis in HCM (15–20,24). The vast majority of these were, however, largely concerned with pathologic scars (replacement fibrosis) (20), and assessed fibrosis by semiquantitative grading methods (15–18,24), utilized small tissue samples from the LV obtained by biopsy or at operation (19,24) or did not focus on the interstitial (matrix) collagen compartment with collagen-specific staining techniques (15–18,24). In contrast, in the present study, we specifically analyzed interstitial and perivascular collagen in a quantitative fashion using picrosirius staining, and in large transmural tissue sections representative of the LV (exclusive of pathologic scarring). We minimized the chances of encountering replacement fibrosis, however, by limiting our study to a relatively homogeneous group of young patients who died suddenly as the first manifestation of HCM in whom congestive symptoms and cardiac dysfunction were absent.

Of note, Factor et al. (19) described the matrix connective tissue morphology in surgically resected specimens of myocardium from patients with HCM using collagen-specific staining (silver impregnation method). However, the small tissue specimens removed at myotomy-myectomy were not of sufficient size to permit quantitation of the volume fraction of the interstitial compartment as described here, nor to be certain whether the observed collagen abnormalities were truly representative of the LV. Also, because these observations were confined to severely symptomatic patients (who had undergone operation), tissue samples included pathologic scarring as well as interstitial fibrosis.

Our observation that interstitial collagen in HCM was more extensive than in normal hearts or in patients with systemic hypertension and secondary LV hypertrophy differs from that of some other reports in which the size of the interstitial compartment in HCM was described as similar to normals (15) or hypertensives (16,24), probably due to the use of less precise methods of collagen quantitation utilizing other than collagen-specific stains. Most of these studies (15–18,20,24,34) employed staining techniques (such as Masson's trichrome) that permit examination of pathologic fibrosis rather than the thin collagen fibers of the matrix (35). On the other hand, other authors have reported that the quantities of fibrous tissue in HCM significantly exceed that in the hearts of hypertensive patients (17,19). Also, some prior studies have shown greater than normal amounts of fibrous tissue in hearts with aortic stenosis (36).

Methodology utilized. Picrosirius red staining used in the present study has proved to be a reliable method for quantifying the amount of collagen in myocardial tissue. Indeed, assessment of the volume fraction of myocardial collagen by this technique has been shown to correlate with the hydroxyproline content of tissue (27). Sirius red F_3BA is a strong anionic dye with an elongated molecule and six sulphonic acid groups, which at low pH binds to lysine and hydroxyproline (21), the major components of the collagen molecule. Picric acid prevents staining of noncollagenous elements, and therefore, picrosirius red selectively stains collagen. Other histologic stains (such as hematoxylin and eosin or Masson's trichrome) do not stain matrix components selectively, and consequently may underestimate the amount of collagen in tissue sections (35). The computerized videodensitometry method we used to quantitate collagen content in tissue sections has been shown to be more accurate than other techniques, such as visual grading or point counting-grid methods (23,35).

Polarization microscopy in combination with picrosirius red staining is a powerful method for the morphologic assessment of the collagen matrix. Consequently, even very thin collagen fibers can be identified in tissue sections stained with picrosirius red and viewed by polarization microscopy. Although collagen fiber structure has also been studied by the silver impregnation technique (37) and electron microscopy (38), these techniques do not permit the quantification of myocardial collagen within tissue sections.

Significance of findings to basic molecular defects in HCM. HCM is a primary cardiac disease with a heterogeneous clinical and morphologic expression for which disease-causing mutations in five major genes, each encoding proteins of the cardiac sarcomere, have been identified (1,3–6). These laboratory observations have suggested a unifying principal by which HCM can be regarded as a single etiological entity and a disease of the sarcomere (3–5). However, the present findings describing an expanded and morphologically abnormal collagen matrix compartment in HCM are consistent with the view that the phenotypic expression of HCM is not limited to the abnormal structure and arrangement of cardiac muscle cells (1,9). Indeed, several other prominent morphologic features of HCM also importantly involve connective tissue elements. For example, enlargement and elongation of the mitral valve leaflets (11–13) may be particularly marked in many patients, independent of the magnitude of LV hypertrophy. In addition, the "small vessel disease" in patients with HCM, characterized by numerous intramural coronary arteries with apparently narrowed lumen and thickened walls due to medial hypertrophy (10,29), is probably responsible, in part, for impaired coronary reserve and myocardial ischemia (30,31).

These morphologic abnormalities prominently involving connective tissue elements, which are common in HCM, suggest that the phenotypic expression of this disease may be importantly influenced by factors other than the many reported disease-causing mutations in genes encoding sarcomeric proteins (1,3–6), such as modifier genes (possibly angiotensin-I converting enzyme genotypes) (4–6), or presently undefined environmental variables.

Reprint requests and correspondence: Dr. Jamshid Shirani, The Jack D. Weiler Hospital of the Albert Einstein College of Medicine, 1825 Eastchester Road, Room W1-70K, Bronx, New York 10461. E-mail: jshirani@montefiore.org.

REFERENCES

1. Maron BJ. Hypertrophic cardiomyopathy. Lancet 1997;350:127–33.
2. Wigle ED, Sasson Z, Henderson MA, et al. Hypertrophic cardiomyopathy: the importance of the site and extent of hypertrophy—a review. Progr Cardiovasc Dis 1985;28:1–83.
3. Spirito P, Seidman CE, McKenna WJ, Maron BJ. The management of hypertrophic cardiomyopathy. N Engl J Med 1997;336:775–85.
4. Maron BJ, Moller JH, Seidman CE, et al. Impact of laboratory molecular diagnosis on contemporary diagnostic criteria for genetically transmitted cardiovascular diseases: hypertrophic cardiomyopathy, long-QT syndrome, and Marfan syndrome. Circulation 1998;98: 1460–71.
5. Schwartz K, Carrier L, Guicheney P, Komajda M. Molecular basis of familial cardiomyopathies. Circulation 1995;91:532–40.
6. Marian AJ, Roberts R. Recent advances in the molecular genetics of hypertrophic cardiomyopathy. Circulation 1995;92:1336–47.
7. Klues HG, Schiffers A, Maron BJ. Phenotypic spectrum and patterns of left ventricular hypertrophy in hypertrophic cardiomyopathy: morphologic observations and significance as assessed by two-dimensional echocardiography in 600 patients. J Am Coll Cardiol 1995;26:1699–708.
8. Teare D. Asymmetrical hypertrophy of the heart in young adults. Br Heart J 1958;20:1–18.
9. Maron BJ, Roberts WC. Quantitative analysis of cardiac muscle cell disorganization in the ventricular septum of patients with hypertrophic cardiomyopathy. Circulation 1979;59:689–706.
10. Maron BJ, Wolfson JK, Epstein SE, Roberts WC. Intramural ("small vessel") coronary artery disease in hypertrophic cardiomyopathy. J Am Coll Cardiol 1986;8:545–57.
11. Klues HG, Maron BJ, Dollar AL, Roberts WC. Diversity of structural mitral valve alterations in hypertrophic cardiomyopathy. Circulation 1992;85:1651–60.
12. Grigg LE, Wigle ED, Williams WG, Daniel LB, Rakowski H. Transesophageal Doppler echocardiography in obstructive hypertrophic cardiomyopathy: clarification of pathophysiology and importance in intraoperative decision-making. J Am Coll Cardiol 1992;20:42–52.
13. Jiang L, Levine RA, King ME, Weyman AE. An integrated mechanism for systolic anterior motion of the mitral valve in hypertrophic cardiomyopathy based on echocardiographic observations. Am Heart J 1987;113:633–44.
14. Klues HG, Roberts WC, Maron BJ. Anomalous insertion of papillary muscle directly into anterior mitral leaflet in hypertrophic cardiomyopthy: significance in producing left ventricular outflow obstruction. Circulation 1991;84:1188–97.
15. Sutton MGStJ, Lie JT, Anderson KR, O'Brien PC, Frye RL. Histo-pathological specificity of hypertrophic obstructive cardiomyopathy. Br Heart J 1980;44:433–43.
16. Fujiwara H, Hoshino T, Yamana K, Fujiwara M, Hamashima Y, Kawai C. Number and size of myocytes and amount of interstitial space in the ventricular free wall in hypertrophic cardiomyopathy. Am J Cardiol 1983;52:818–23.
17. Tanaka M, Fujiwara H, Onodera T, Wu DJ, Hamashima Y, Kawai C. Quantitative analysis of myocardial fibrosis in normals, hypertensive hearts, and hypertrophic cardiomyopathy. Br Heart J 1986;55:575–81.
18. Unverferth DV, Baker PB, Pearce LI, Lautman J, Roberts WC. Regional myocyte hypertrophy and increased interstitial myocardial fibrosis in hypertrophic cardiomyopathy. Am J Cardiol 1987;59: 932–6.
19. Factor SM, Butany J, Sole MJ, Wigle ED, Williams WC, Rojkind M. Pathologic fibrosis and matrix connective tissue in subaortic myocardium of patients with hypertrophic cardiomyopathy. J Am Coll Cardiol 1991;17:1343–51.
20. Maron BJ, Epstein SE, Roberts WC. Hypertrophic cardiomyopathy and transmural myocardial infarction without significant atherosclerosis of the extramural coronary arteries. Am J Cardiol 1979;43:1086–102.
21. Janqueira LCU, Bignolas G, Brentani RR. Picrosirius red staining plus pola rization microscopy, a specific method for collagen detection in tisssue sections. Histochemical J 1979;11:447–55.
22. Weber KT. Cardiac interstitium in health and disease: the fibrillar collagen network. J Am Coll Cardiol 1989;13:1637–52.
23. Hoyt RH, Erickson E, Collins SM, Skorton DJ. Computer-assisted quantitation of myocardial fibrosis in histologic section. Arch Pathol Lab Med 1984;108:280–3.
24. Sugihara N, Genda A, Shimizu M, et al. Quantitation of myocardial fibrosis and its relation to function in essential hypertension and hypertrophic cardiomyopathy. Clin Cardiol 1988;11:771–8.
25. Pearlman ES, Weber KT, Janicki JS, et al. Muscle fiber orientation and connective tissue content in the hypertrophied human heart. Lab Invest 1982;46:158–64.
26. Tanaka M, Fujiwara H, Onodera T, et al. Pathogenetic role of myocardial fiber disarray in the progression of cardiac fibrosis in normal hearts, hypertensive hearts and hearts with hypertrophic cardiomyopathy. Jp Circ J 1987;51:624–30.
27. Weber KT, Brilla CG. Pathological hypertrophy and cardiac interstitium. Fibrosis and renin-angiotensin-aldosterone system. Circulation 1991;83:1849–65.
28. Maron BJ, Spirito P, Wesley YE, Arce J. Development and progression of left ventricular hypertrophy in children with hypertrophic cardiomyopathy. N Engl J Med 1986;315:610–4.
29. Maron BJ, Spirito P, Green KJ, Wesley YE, Bonow RO, Arce J. Noninvasive assessment of left ventricular diastolic function by pulsed Doppler echocardiography in patients with hypertrophic cardiomyopathy. J Am Coll Cardiol 1987;10:733–42.
30. Spirito P, Maron BJ. Relation between extent of left ventricular hypertrophy and diastolic filling abnormalities in hypertrophic cardiomyopathy. J Am Coll Cardiol 1990;15:808–13.
31. Pak PH, Maughan WL, Baughman KL, Kass DA. Marked discordance between dynamic and passive diastolic pressure-volume relations in idiopathic hypertrophic cardiomyopathy. Circulation 1996;94:52–60.
32. Cannon RO III, Rosing DR, Maron BJ, et al. Myocardial ischemia in patients with hypertrophic cardiomyopathy: contribution of inadequate vasodilator reserve and elevated left ventricular filling pressures. Circulation 1985;71:234–43.
33. Koga Y, Yamaguchi R, Ogata M, Kihara K. Toshima H. Decreased coronary vasodilatory capacity in hypertrophic cardiomyopathy determined by split-dose thallium-dipyridamole myocardial scintigraphy. Am J Cardiol 1990;65:1134–9.
34. Maron BJ, Spirito P. Implications of left ventricular remodeling in hypertrophic cardiomyopathy. Am J Cardiol 1998;81:1339–44.

35. Whittaker P, Kloner RA, Boughner DR, Pickering JG. Quantitative assessment of myocardial collagen with picrosirius red staining and circularly polarized light. Bas Res Cardiol 1994;89:397–410.
36. Cheitlin MD, Robinowitz M, McAllister H, Hoffman JIE, Bharati S, Lev M. The distribution of fibrosis in the left ventricle in congenital aortic tenosis and coarctation of the aorta. Circulation 1980;62:823–30.
37. Robinson TF, Cohen-Gould L, Factor SM. Skeletal framework of mammalian heart muscle. Arrangement of inter- and pericellular connective tissue structures. Lab Invest 1983;49:482–98.
38. Robinson TF, Factor SM, Capasso JM, Wittenberg BA, Blumenfeld OO, Seifter S. Morphology, composition and function of struts between cardiac myocytes of rat and hamster. Cell Tissue Res 1987;249:247–55.

Sudden Cardiac Arrest in Hypertrophic Cardiomyopathy in the Absence of Conventional Criteria for High Risk Status

Barry J. Maron, MD[a,*], Martin S. Maron, MD[b], John R. Lesser, MD[a], Robert G. Hauser, MD[a], Tammy S. Haas, RN[a], Caitlin J. Harrigan, BA[c,d], Evan Appelbaum, MD[c,d], Michael L. Main, MD[e], and William C. Roberts, MD[f]

Two patients with hypertrophic cardiomyopathy are reported from the recent experience of the Hypertrophic Cardiomyopathy Center of the Minneapolis Heart Institute Foundation, demonstrating limitations in the risk stratification algorithm currently used for this disease. One patient, an asymptomatic 21-year-old male college student, was prophylactically implanted with a cardioverter-defibrillator. This decision was based largely on the presence of apparent extensive myocardial fibrosis identified by contrast-enhanced cardiovascular magnetic resonance imaging, currently not considered a risk factor in this disease. Fifteen months later, ventricular fibrillation was interrupted by an appropriate defibrillator shock. The other patient, an asymptomatic 15-year-old male subject without any apparent high-risk markers, died suddenly at home. Necropsy examination of the heart identified scarring confined to portions of both left ventricular papillary muscles, possibly representing a substrate for ventricular tachyarrhythmias. In conclusion, these 2 cases demonstrate that present strategies for assessing high-risk status in hypertrophic cardiomyopathy are inadequate to identify all such patients. However, while the anecdotal nature of these observations cannot yet justify altering the general guidelines for implantation of defibrillators for the primary prevention of sudden death related to hypertrophic cardiomyopathy, 1 of our 2 cases suggests a future role for contrast-enhanced cardiovascular magnetic resonance in the risk stratification of this complex disease.
(Am J Cardiol 2008;101:544–547)

The current risk stratification algorithm used in hypertrophic cardiomyopathy (HC) has proved to be an effective guide for the identification of high-risk patients eligible for the prophylactic use of implantable cardioverter-defibrillators (ICDs) and the primary prevention of sudden death.[1,2] Although the true frequency of sudden death in young patients with HC without acknowledged risk factors is unknown, it is believed to be a rare occurrence.[3,4] We present 2 patients, unique in the experience of the 15-year-old Hypertrophic Cardiomyopathy Center at the Minneapolis Heart Institute Foundation, who within the previous 12 months had unexpected cardiac arrest in the *absence* of risk markers sufficient to definitively document high-risk status.

Case Descriptions

Patient 1, a 21-year-old asymptomatic college student, had been followed for 10 years after the fortuitous identification of HC at 11 years of age (Table 1). At 21 years of age, cardiovascular magnetic resonance (CMR) was performed as part of a routine annual evaluation. Left ventricular (LV) hypertrophy was

Table 1
Clinical comparison of 2 patients with hypertrophic cardiomyopathy and sudden cardiac arrest

Variable	Patient 1	Patient 2
Age (yrs)	21	16
Gender	Male	Male
Drugs	Atenolol (25 mg)	0
Electrocardiographic abnormalities	0	+
Maximum LV thickness (mm)	21	18
Location of maximum thickness	Ventricular septum (anterior)	LV free wall (anterior)
LV delayed enhancement by CMR	+	0
LV outflow gradient at rest	0	0
Systolic anterior motion (at rest)	0	0
Exercise LV outflow gradient (mm Hg)	105	0
Ejection fraction (%)	80	77
Left atrial dimension (mm)	44	41
LV cavity at end-diastole (mm)	50	40
Mitral regurgitation	+ (mild)	0
Ventricular ectopy on Holter recording	+	0

[a]Hypertrophic Cardiomyopathy Center, Minneapolis Heart Institute Foundation, Minneapolis, Minnesota; [b]Hypertrophic Cardiomyopathy Center, Division of Cardiology, Tufts-New England Medical Center; [c]Perfuse Core Laboratory and Data Coordinating Center and [d]Department of Medicine (Cardiovascular Division), Beth Israel Deaconess Medical Center, Harvard Medical School, Boston, Massachusetts; [e]Mid-America Heart Institute, St. Luke's Hospital, Kansas City, Missouri; [f]Baylor Heart and Vascular Institute, Baylor University Medical Center, Dallas, Texas.
Manuscript received August 17, 2007; revised manuscript received and accepted September 21, 2007.

*Corresponding author: Tel: 612-863-3996; fax: 612-863-3875.

E-mail address: hcm.maron@mhif.org (B.J. Maron).

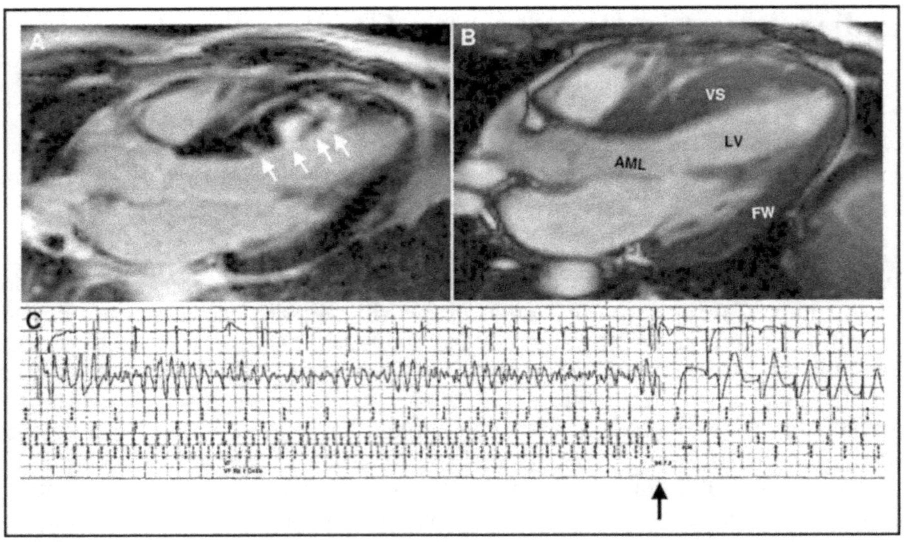

Figure 1. Patient 1: a 21-year-old man with HC and ventricular septal scarring who survived an episode of cardiac arrest. *(A)* CMR long-axis contrast-enhanced image showing a bright area of transmural delayed enhancement occupying a substantial proportion of septum *(arrows)*. *(B)* Same CMR cross-sectional image without contrast showing relatively mild thickening of ventricular septum (VS; 21 mm). *(C)* Intracardiac electrocardiogram from the patient recorded during the event. Ventricular fibrillation was interrupted by defibrillation shock *(arrow)*, thereby restoring sinus rhythm. AML = anterior mitral leaflet; FW = free wall of left ventricle; LV = left ventricular cavity.

confined to the anterior portion of ventricular septum (thickness 21 mm). Mitral valve systolic anterior motion and LV outflow obstruction were absent at rest (Figure 1). Of particular note, after the infusion of gadolinium, an extensive area of transmural delayed enhancement was demonstrated, occupying 27% of the ventricular septum and 11% of overall LV wall myocardium (Figure 1).

This patient showed no evidence of high-risk status on the basis of conventional risk factor analysis. Although his father is known to have HC, there is no family history of premature HC-related sudden death. Blood pressure response to exercise was appropriate. Drug treatment was atenolol 25 mg/day. A 24-hour ambulatory (Holter) electrocardiogram showed 94 premature ventricular complexes and an isolated, brief 3-beat burst of nonsustained ventricular tachycardia (170 beats/min), itself judged insufficient evidence to establish high-risk status in this patient.

After discussion with the patient and family about the concern for potential malignant arrhythmias posed by the transmural septal scar, the mutual decision was reached to implant an ICD prophylactically. Fifteen months later, the patient was awakened from sleep by an appropriate defibrillator shock that terminated ventricular fibrillation and immediately restored sinus rhythm (Figure 1).

Patient 2, an asymptomatic male subject, was initially evaluated at 15 years of age (Table 1). Two-dimensional echocardiography showed borderline LV wall thickness of 13 mm in the anterior portion of ventricular septum and 14 mm in the contiguous portion of anterior LV free wall; mitral valve systolic anterior motion and obstruction to LV outflow were absent at rest, associated with distal LV cavity obliteration in systole. CMR established the diagnosis of HC by demonstrating more prominent segmental hypertrophy of the basal anterior portion of the LV free wall (18 mm)[5] (Figure 2). After the infusion of gadolinium, there was no evidence of delayed enhancement in the LV wall (Figure 2).

Patient 2 also did not have demonstrable evidence of high-risk status. There was no history of syncope or family history of HC-related premature sudden death. Blood pressure response to exercise was normal, and 24-hour ambulatory (Holter) electrocardiography showed no ventricular or supraventricular ectopy. He did not take cardioactive drugs. Nine months later, he collapsed at home suddenly and subsequently was found to be in ventricular fibrillation in the emergency department. Organized heart rhythm was restored briefly, but he became asystolic, was never responsive, and died 1 hour later.

Examination of the heart showed (Figure 2) a weight of 428 g (upper 95th percentile 380 g); maximal ventricular septal and LV free wall thicknesses were 18 mm. Small focal mural endocardial plaques were present on the LV aspect of the ventricular septum caudal to and in apposition to the anterior mitral leaflet. By visual inspection, the atrial cavities were considered to be of normal size, and the LV chamber was small. None of the major epicardial coronary arteries tunneled within the ventricular septum or LV free wall myocardium. On the basis of histopathologic examination of 10 transverse sections of the left ventricle (5 each from the septum and the free wall), neither replacement fibrosis or myocyte disarray was identified (Figure 2).

Grossly visible replacement scarring was present in the apical portions of the anterolateral and posteromedial papillary muscles, as also shown in histopathologic sections (Figure 2). A few intramural coronary arteries had thickened walls, and interstitial fibrosis appeared in appropriate amounts. Contraction band necrosis was marked in several sections (this finding was attributed to the lack of myocardial oxygenation from the time of the cardiac arrest to discontinuation of resuscitative efforts [1 hour]).

Comments

The 2 patients with HC reported here demonstrate that the current strategy for assessing high-risk status in HC, al-

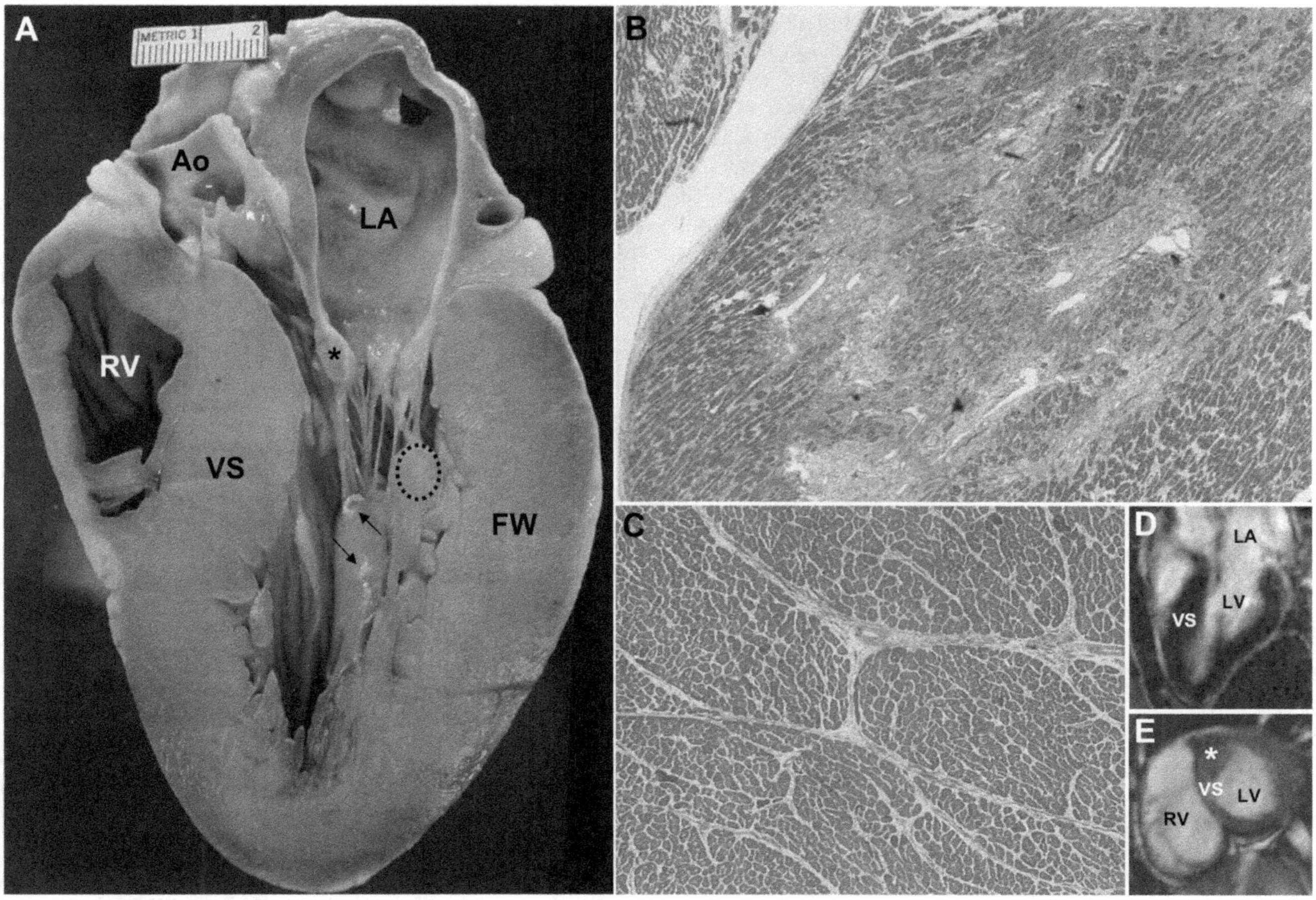

Figure 2. Morphologic findings in a 15-year-old male patient with HC and sudden unexpected death. *(A)* Gross specimen cut longitudinally showing thickened ventricular septum (VS) and left ventricular free wall (FW), small LV cavity, and absence of grossly visible myocardial scarring of the LV wall. A scar is evident in the apex of the head of the posteromedial papillary muscle *(dotted circle)*. Two areas of mural endocardial fibrosis are present on the other head of the posteromedial papillary muscle *(arrows)*, presumably due to distal cavity obliteration in ventricular systole. The distal portion of the anterior mitral leaflet is thickened *(asterisk)* in apposition to a mural endocardial plaque on VS. *(B)* Low-power photomicrograph of anterolateral papillary muscle in the apical portion showing extensive replacement scarring *(areas stained in blue*; Masson's trichrome stain × 40). *(C)* Photomicrograph of histologic section of VS showing absence of disarray and replacement fibrosis (Masson's trichrome stain × 40). *(D)* CMR 10-mm contiguous slice after gadolinium contrast in long axis (similar to the cross section of gross heart specimen in *A*), showing absence of delayed enhancement. *(E)* CMR basal 10-mm short-axis slice showing LV wall thickening confined to anterior FW segment *(asterisk)*. CMR was obtained 9 months before sudden death. Ao = aorta; LA = left atrium; RV = right ventricle.

though useful as a guide to selecting patients for prophylactic ICD therapy,[1–4] nevertheless is not precise and harbors certain limitations.[1,4] Such experiences underscore the importance of defining additional criteria for the selection of young high-risk patients who would benefit from ICD implantation. This is a crucial consideration, given that ICDs have proved effective and reliable in terminating potentially lethal ventricular tachyarrhythmias in HC.[1–3,6]

Patient 1 was the initial patient in our experience in whom the CMR finding of delayed enhancement, presumed to represent widespread myocardial fibrosis,[7,8] itself led to the implantation of a defibrillator and ultimately to a lifesaving device intervention. By exercising the judgment in this particular patient that extensive delayed enhancement represented a likely substrate for ventricular tachyarrhythmias, the clinical course was altered and sudden death prevented. Although definitive data are presently lacking in HC, contrast-enhanced CMR, with its capability for the in vivo detection of potentially arrhythmogenic myocardial scarring, could offer additional important information leading to the identification of increased risk status in select patients with HC.[9] Nevertheless, the recognition of delayed enhancement as an acknowledged independent risk factor for sudden death in HC must await long-term, CMR-based studies in large patient populations. The decision to implant an ICD in patient 1 for primary prevention was based on the available clinical information, particularly the concern that extensive delayed enhancement could represent the substrate for ventricular tachyarrhythmias.

Case 2 is notable for the sudden death of a young patient in the absence of any clinical or necropsy markers of increased risk for such an event. This patient did not demonstrate any of the 5 acknowledged primary prevention risk factors in HC[1,3,4,10] and was the first such young patient to die under these circumstances in the 15-year experience of the Hypertrophic Cardiomyopathy Center at the Minneapolis Heart Institute Foundation, which now includes the evaluation of almost 1,000 patients. Furthermore, at autopsy, there was no evidence of either previous myocardial ischemia with replacement scarring[11,12] or myocyte disarray,[13] nor coronary artery bridging,[14] all potential markers for an unstable electrical substrate and potentially lethal ventricular tachyarrhythmias in HC.

The sole finding of potential clinical relevance to this patient's sudden death was extensive fibrosis of both papillary muscles. Recently, similar papillary muscle scars (unassociated with evidence of fibrosis in the LV wall) have been identified by contrast-enhanced CMR in some patients with HC.[15] Such pathology has also been observed not uncommonly at autopsy in patients dying of other cardiac diseases or anemia (e.g., sickle-cell disease, leukemia).[16–18] However, it is unresolved as to whether isolated papillary muscle scars (presumably due to focal myocardial ischemia) can in fact represent an arrhythmogenic focus. Nevertheless, the identification of papillary muscle fibrosis in our patient dying suddenly of HC (without any of the conventional risk factors) raises an unavoidable speculation of whether such areas of myocardial scarring could have triggered lethal arrhythmias.

To date, there has been no histopathologic correlation with contrast-enhanced CMR findings in patients with HC who have died suddenly or were not in the end-stage phase of the disease.[8,19] Therefore, the present CMR and histologic observations in patient 2 offer an important validation for delayed enhancement, by documenting that contrast-enhanced CMR accurately described the absence of myocardial fibrosis throughout the LV wall proper in this patient (i.e., by the lack of delayed enhancement).

In contrast, the CMR findings in patient 2 were inconclusive with regard to scar formation in the papillary muscles (despite gross and histopathologic evidence of fibrosis in the apical portion of both muscles). Therefore, the observations in this patient underscore that the delayed enhancement imaging strategy used here was not sufficient to reliably detect myocardial scars in the papillary muscles, raising the future consideration of acquiring thinner contiguous slices (5 to 7 mm) or using higher resolution imaging for this purpose.

1. Maron BJ, Spirito P, Shen W-K, Haas TS, Formisano F, Link MS, Epstein AE, Almquist AK, Daubert JP, Lawrenz T, et al. Outcomes of patients with implantable cardioverter-defibrillators for prevention of sudden cardiac death in hypertrophic cardiomyopathy. *JAMA* 2007;298:405–412.
2. Maron BJ, Shen W-K, Link MS, Epstein AE, Almquist AK, Daubert JP, Bardy GH, Favale S, Rea RF, Boriani G, et al. Efficacy of implantable cardioverter-defibrillators for the prevention of sudden death in patients with hypertrophic cardiomyopathy. *N Engl J Med* 2000;342:365–373.
3. Maron BJ, McKenna WJ, Danielson GK, Kappenberger LJ, Kuhn HJ, Seidman CE, Shah PM, Spencer WH, Spirito P, ten Cate FJ, Wigle ED. American College of Cardiology/European Society of Cardiology clinical expert consensus document on hypertrophic cardiomyopathy. A report of the American College of Cardiology Task Force on Clinical Expert Consensus Documents and the European Society of Cardiology Committee for Practice Guidelines Committee to Develop an Expert Consensus Document on Hypertrophic Cardiomyopathy. *J Am Coll Cardiol* 2003;42:1687–1713.
4. Elliott PM, Poloniecki J, Dickie S, Sharma S, Monserrat L, Varnava A, Mahon NG, McKenna WJ. Sudden death in hypertrophic cardiomyopathy: identification of high risk patients. *J Am Coll Cardiol* 2000;36:2212–2218.
5. Rickers C, Wilke NM, Jerosch-Herold M, Casey SA, Panse P, Panse N, Weil J, Zenovich AG, Maron BJ. Utility of cardiac magnetic resonance imaging in the diagnosis of hypertrophic cardiomyopathy. *Circulation* 2005;112:855–861.
6. Jayatilleke I, Doolan A, Ingles J, McGuire M, Booth V, Richmond DR, Semsarian C. Long-term follow-up of implantable cardioverter-defibrillator therapy for hypertrophic cardiomyopathy. *Am J Cardiol* 2004;93:1192–1194.
7. Kim RJ, Judd RM. Gadolinium-enhanced magnetic resonance imaging in hypertrophic cardiomyopathy: in vivo imaging of the pathologic substrate for premature cardiac death? *J Am Coll Cardiol* 2003;41:1568–1572.
8. Moon JC, Reed E, Sheppard MN, Elkington AG, Ho SY, Burke M, Petrou M, Pennell DJ. The histologic basis of late gadolinium enhancement cardiovascular magnetic resonance in hypertrophic cardiomyopathy. *J Am Coll Cardiol* 2004;43:2260–2264.
9. Moon JC, McKenna WJ, McCrohon JA, Elliott PM, Smith GC, Pennell DJ. Toward clinical risk assessment in hypertrophic cardiomyopathy with gadolinium cardiovascular magnetic resonance. *J Am Coll Cardiol* 2003; 41:1561–1567.
10. Maron BJ. Hypertrophic cardiomyopathy: a systematic review. *JAMA* 2002;287: 1308–1320.
11. Maron BJ, Wolfson JK, Epstein SE, Roberts WC. Intramural ("small vessel") coronary artery disease in hypertrophic cardiomyopathy. *J Am Coll Cardiol* 1986;8:545–557.
12. Basso C, Thiene G, Corrado D, Buja G, Melacini P, Nava A. Hypertrophic cardiomyopathy and sudden death in the young: pathologic evidence of myocardial ischemia. *Hum Pathol* 2000;31:988–998.
13. Maron BJ, Roberts WC. Quantitative analysis of cardiac muscle cell disorganization in the ventricular septum of patients with hypertrophic cardiomyopathy. *Circulation* 1979;59: 689–706.
14. Yetman AT, McCrindle BW, MacDonald C, Freedom RM, Gow R. Myocardial bridging in children with hypertrophic cardiomyopathy—a risk factor for sudden death. *N Engl J Med* 1998;339:1201–1209.
15. Harrigan CJ, Appelbaum E, Gibson CM, Udelson JE, Manning WJ, Maron BJ, Maron MS. Evidence for papillary muscle involvement in hypertrophic cardiomyopathy by cardiac magnetic resonance (abstr). *J Cardiovasc Magn Reson* 2007;9:428.
16. Roberts WC, Cohen LS. Left ventricular papillary muscles. Description of the normal and a survey of conditions causing them to be abnormal. *Circulation* 1972;46:138–154.
17. Marcus FI, Gomez L, Glancy DL, Ewy GA, Roberts WC. Papillary muscle fibrosis in primary myocardial disease. *Am Heart J* 1969; 77:681–685.
18. Berezowski K, Mautner GC, Roberts WC. Scarring of the left ventricular papillary muscles in sickle-cell disease. *Am Heart J* 1992; 70:1368–1370.
19. Papavassiliu T, Schnabel P, Schröder M, Borggrefe M. CMR scarring in a patient with hypertrophic cardiomyopathy correlates well with histological findings of fibrosis. *Eur Heart J* 2005;26:2395.

The First Patient Clinically Diagnosed With Hypertrophic Cardiomyopathy

Barry J. Maron, MD[a,*], Robert O. Bonow, MD[b], Lisa Salberg[c], William C. Roberts, MD[d], and Eugene Braunwald, MD[e]

It has now been 50 years since the initial clinical description of hypertrophic cardiomyopathy. In this regard, it is noteworthy that the first patient diagnosed with this disease has survived to date in good health with an active and productive lifestyle—albeit with heart transplantation necessitated by an aggressive disease course with progression to the end-stage phase. **(Am J Cardiol 2008;102:1418–1420)**

It has been emphasized that hypertrophic cardiomyopathy (HC) is a complex cardiac disease consistent with extended (and often normal) longevity.[1–4] This outcome may evolve either because the disease itself does not produce major complications (i.e., sudden arrhythmic death, intractable heart failure, or embolic stroke)[1,5,6] or because disease consequences occur, but are controlled, reversed, or prevented by major treatment interventions such as implantable cardioverter-defibrillators, surgical septal myectomy, or heart transplantation.[7–9] Recently, we were reminded of this paradigm in HC by an unexpected event. Mr. Claude Brady (of Arlington, Virginia), the first patient clinically identified with HC, emerged on the 50th anniversary of his diagnosis at the recent 11th annual patients' meeting of the Hypertrophic Cardiomyopathy Association in Morristown, New Jersey (Figure 1).

Case Description

The initial suspicion that Mr. Brady had cardiac disease was at 11 years of age, when a local physician heard a precordial murmur, which was attributed at that time to a "family trait" (i.e., the "Brady heart"). Several aunts and uncles had died of heart failure, believed to be due to rheumatic fever. In 1959, at 22 years of age, Mr. Brady presented to the Clinical Center of the National Institutes of Health (Bethesda, Maryland) with exertional dyspnea and fatigue.

His 2 siblings had heart murmurs, and many members of his father's family were said to have heart murmurs. Several of these had died suddenly in childhood or during early adult life. Notably, a grade IV/VI midsystolic murmur was heard at the fourth left intercostal space and apex associated with a prominent left ventricular (LV) lift. Electrocardiography showed right-axis deviation and incomplete right bundle branch block.

One of the investigators (E.B.) made the clinical diagnosis of idiopathic hypertrophic subaortic stenosis (IHSS), now called HCM. Right and retrograde left-sided cardiac catheterization was performed, and a peak systolic outflow gradient of 40 mm Hg was recorded between the LV cavity and the subaortic area, confirming the precatheterization diagnosis (Figure 2). During a subsequent attempted passage of the catheter into the left ventricle for angiography, ventricular fibrillation occurred. Immediate thoracotomy, cardiac massage, and defibrillation were required to restore sinus rhythm, and the postoperative course was unremarkable.

Comments

Thus, Mr. Brady became the index patient for a new disease, which insofar as we know had not previously been diagnosed clinically[10–12] and has captured our attention and intense interest over the subsequent 5 decades.[1] In addition, Mr. Brady's brother and sister were also identified with IHSS, underscoring from the onset the familial nature of this disease.[1,10,12]

Over the next several years, Mr. Brady experienced gradual clinical deterioration, with progressive, unrelenting heart failure and eventually LV systolic dysfunction, recognized as the "burned-out" or "end stage" of HC.[5] In June 1989, at 52 years of age, he underwent successful heart transplantation at The Johns Hopkins Hospital. He is now 71 years old, with his donor heart of 19 years. Mr. Brady's brother (George) underwent heart transplantation for the same reason 4 years earlier at 45 years of age, making the Bradys, insofar as we know, the only siblings who have received donor hearts in the United States for any condition. It is perhaps odd that the first 2 patients identified clinically with IHSS (Claude and George Brady) ultimately developed a very uncommon clinical profile and course of the disease (i.e., the end-stage phase, which has a prevalence of only 2%), characterized morphologically by widespread myocardial scarring[5,13] (Figure 3).

Mr. Brady is now healthy and vigorous, and has been particularly active in promoting heart transplantation as the founder of 2 organizations: Transplant Recipients

[a]Hypertrophic Cardiomyopathy Center, Minneapolis Heart Institute Foundation, Minneapolis, Minnesota; [b]Northwestern University Feinberg School of Medicine, Chicago, Illinois; [c]Hypertrophic Cardiomyopathy Association, Hibernia, New Jersey; [d]Baylor Heart and Vascular Institute, Dallas, Texas; and [e]TIMI Study Group, Brigham and Women's Hospital, Boston, Massachusetts. Manuscript received July 18, 2008; revised manuscript received and accepted August 4, 2008.

*Corresponding author: Tel: 612-863-3996; fax: 612-863-3875.

E-mail address: hcm.maron@mhif.org (B.J. Maron).

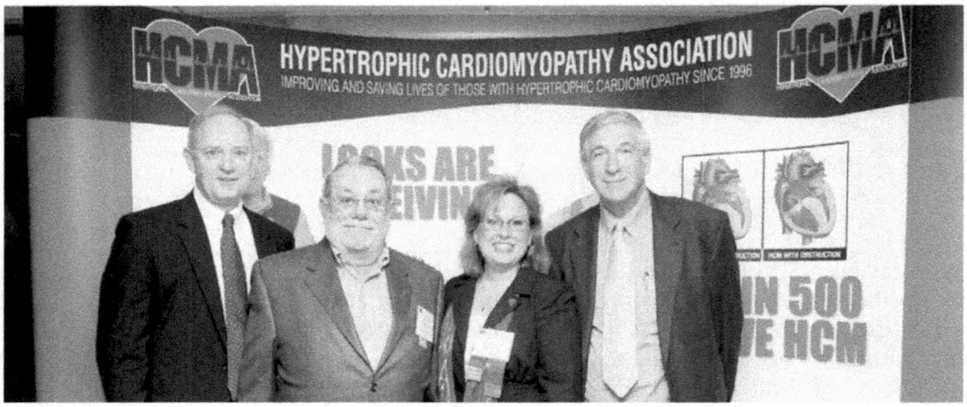

Figure 1. Photograph taken at the 11th annual patients' meeting of the Hypertrophic Cardiomyopathy Association (HCMA) on May 31, 2008. *Left to right* Dr. Robert O. Bonow (past president, American Heart Association), Claude Brady, Lisa Salberg (president, HCMA), and Dr. Barry Maron.

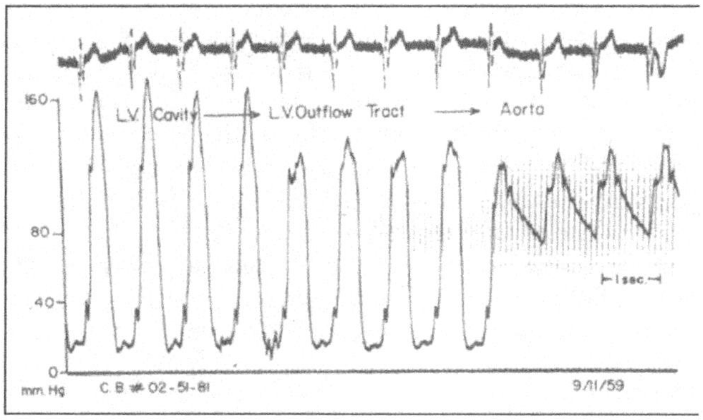

Figure 2. Mr. Brady's continuous pullback pressure tracing, recorded as the catheter was withdrawn from the LV cavity through the outflow tract across the aortic valve and into the aorta. Reproduced with permission from *Am J Med.*[12]

International Organization, Inc. (National Capital Chapter), as well as Transplant Awareness, Inc. As the "IHSS" index case, Claude Brady has taught us a great deal, not only about HC but also the important principle that patients with this sometimes profound hereditary condition can by virtue of their attitudes, perceptions, and fortitude (in conjunction with contemporary management strategies) ultimately prevail against substantial odds.

1. Maron BJ, McKenna WJ, Danielson GK, Kappenberger LJ, Kuhn HJ, Seidman CE, Shah PM, Spencer WH, Spirito P, ten Cate FJ, Wigle ED. American College of Cardiology/European Society of Cardiology clinical expert consensus document on hypertrophic cardiomyopathy. A report of the American College of Cardiology Task Force on Clinical Expert Consensus Documents and the European Society of Cardiology Committee for Practice Guidelines Committee to Develop an Expert Consensus Document on Hypertrophic Cardiomyopathy. *J Am Coll Cardiol* 2003;42:1687–1713.
2. Maron BJ, Casey SA, Poliac LC, Gohman TE, Almquist AK, Aeppli DM. Clinical course of hypertrophic cardiomyopathy in a regional United States cohort. *JAMA* 1999;281:650–655.

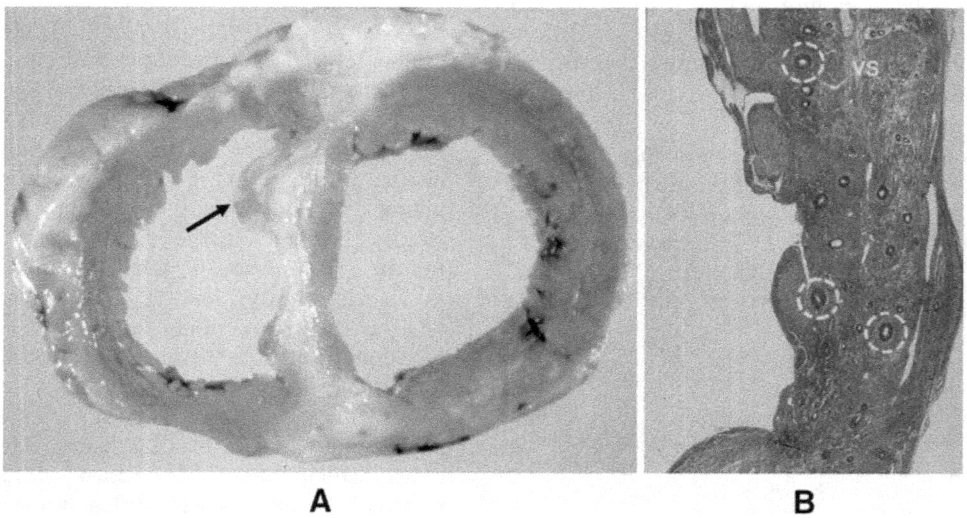

Figure 3. The "Brady heart." *(A)* Gross and extensive transmural myocardial scarring and thinning of the ventricular septum *(yellow areas)*. A localized area of hypertrophy in the anterior septum persists *(arrow)*. *(B)* Photomicrograph (elastic van Gieson stain, 3×) of septal histopathology showing transmural fibrosis *(stained blue)* with small areas of viable myocardium along the endocardial borders *(stained red)*. Abnormal intramural coronary arteries with thickened walls and narrowed lumen ("small-vessel disease"), responsible for bursts of "silent" myocardial ischemia, are present within the area of scarring *(broken circles)*. Reproduced with permission from *Am J Cardiol.*[13]

3. Maron BJ. Hypertrophic cardiomyopathy: a systematic review. *JAMA* 2002;287:1308–1320.
4. Maron BJ, Casey SA, Hauser RG, Aeppli DM. Clinical course of hypertrophic cardiomyopathy with survival to advanced ages. *J Am Coll Cardiol* 2003;42:882–888.
5. Harris KM, Spirito P, Maron MS, Zenovich AG, Formisano F, Lesser JR, Mackey-Bojack S, Manning WJ, Udelson JE, Maron BJ. Prevalence, clinical profile and significance of left ventricular remodeling in the end-stage phase of hypertrophic cardiomyopathy. *Circulation* 2006;114:216–225.
6. Maron BJ, Olivotto I, Bellone P, Conte MR, Cecchi F, Flygenring BP, Casey SA, Gohman TE, Bongioanni S, Spirito P. Clinical profile of stroke in 900 patients with hypertrophic cardiomyopathy. *J Am Coll Cardiol* 2002;39:301–307.
7. Maron BJ, Spirito P, Shen W-K, Haas TS, Formisano F, Link MS, Epstein AE, Almquist AK, Daubert JP, Lawrenz T, et al. Implantable cardioverter-defibrillators and prevention of sudden cardiac death in hypertrophic cardiomyopathy. *JAMA* 2007;298:405–412.
8. Ommen SR, Maron BJ, Olivotto I, Maron MS, Cecchi F, Betocchi S, Gersh BJ, Ackerman MJ, McCully RB, Dearani JA, et al. Long-term effects of surgical septal myectomy on survival in patients with obstructive hypertrophic cardiomyopathy. *J Am Coll Cardiol* 2005;46:470–476.
9. Shirani J, Maron BJ, Cannon RO, Shahin S, Roberts WC. Clinicopathologic features of hypertrophic cardiomyopathy managed by cardiac transplantation. *Am J Cardiol* 1993;72:434–440.
10. Morrow AG, Braunwald E. Functional aortic stenosis: a malformation characterized by resistance to left ventricular outflow without anatomic obstruction. *Circulation* 1959;20:181–189.
11. Braunwald E, Lambrew GT, Morrow AG, Pierce GE, Rockoff SD, Ross J. Idiopathic hypertrophic subaortic stenosis. American Heart Association Monograph #10. *Circulation* 1964;29&30(suppl):4–212.
12. Braunwald E, Morrow AG, Cornell WP, Aygen MM, Hilbish TF. Idiopathic hypertrophic subaortic stenosis: clinical, hemodynamic and angiographic manifestations. *Am J Med* 1960;29:924–945.
13. Maron BJ, Epstein SE, Roberts WC. Hypertrophic cardiomyopathy and transmural myocardial infarction without significant atherosclerosis of the extramural coronary arteries. *Am J Cardiol* 1979;43:1086–1102.

From the Editor

Fifty Years of Hypertrophic Cardiomyopathy†

In 1869, Liouville[1] and Hallopeau[2] each reported a patient who probably had hypertrophic cardiomyopathy (HC). The 2 investigators noted striking hypertrophy of the ventricular septum, and each considered the left ventricular outflow tract to be obstructed by the hypertrophied septal muscle; Hallopeau noted thickening of the anterior mitral leaflet in his 69-year-old patient.

In 1907, Schmincke[3] described severe hypertrophy of the ventricular septum in the hearts of 2 women aged 50 and 56 years. In addition to the septal thickening, the left ventricular free wall in each patient was severely hypertrophied. Schmincke considered the ventricular septal hypertrophy to be primary and of congenital origin, leading to obstruction to left ventricular ejection and to secondary hypertrophy of the left ventricular free wall.

After Schmincke's[3] report in 1907, a period of nearly 50 years elapsed before another probable report of this disease appeared. In 1952, Davies[4] described a family in which many members had heart disease and histories of sudden death and systolic precordial murmurs. At necropsy, the heart of 1 patient showed "diffuse sub-aortic stenosis" associated with left ventricular hypertrophy. Davies described an area of fibrosis of 4 cm^2 in the left ventricular outflow tract opposite the anterior mitral leaflet, a lesion highly suggestive of HC.

In 1957, Brock[5] operated on a 63-year-old woman thought to have a valvular aortic stenosis and systematic hypertension. At operation, however, the aortic valve was normal, and no obstruction to left ventricular outflow was encountered by dilating instruments, despite direct pressure tracings showing subvalvular obstruction. The patient died shortly after the operation, and necropsy showed a hypertrophied, nondilated left ventricular cavity and no subaortic fibrous stricture.

Although the cases reported by Liouville,[1] Hallopeau,[2] Schmincke,[3] Davies,[4] and Brock[5] were probable examples of HC, the comparative thicknesses of the ventricular septum and left ventricular free wall were not described by any of them. The first unequivocal description of HC was by Teare[6] in London, reported in the *British Heart Journal* in January 1958. Although Brock's clinical report was published in *Guy's Hospital Reports* in the final quarterly issue of 1957, Teare's report had been received by the journal in January 1957, before Brock operated on his patient, and Brock's publication did not appear, until 1958 although the date on the issue was 1957. Thus, it is fair to credit Teare with the first detailed anatomic description and to credit Brock with the first description of the functional nature of this entity. Teare described gross and histologic cardiac findings in 9 patients aged 14 to 45 years (average 26; 2 female, 7 male), 8 of whom died suddenly. Although he did not give measurements of the thicknesses of the ventricular septum and left ventricular free wall, Teare clearly indicated and illustrated that the septum was thicker than the left ventricular free wall and, indeed, called the condition asymmetrical hypertrophy of the heart. He considered the localized septal hypertrophy to be a "benign tumor" or "hamartoma." Teare observed on histologic examination "bizarre arrangements of muscle bundles" and "considerable variation in size" of the myocardial fibers in the ventricular septum. He also noted a similar disordered arrangement of muscle bundles in the adjacent anterior free wall of the left ventricle. In 1 patient, the posterior left ventricular free wall "appeared thinner than normal," and histologic examination of it showed normal arrangement and uniform size of the myocardial fibers. Although 1 of his 9 patients underwent valvulotomy for suspected mitral stenosis (this was the only patient in his study who had not died suddenly), there were no descriptions of the mitral valve, no mention of mural endocardial thickening in the left ventricular outflow tract, and no comments regarding the sizes of the various cardiac

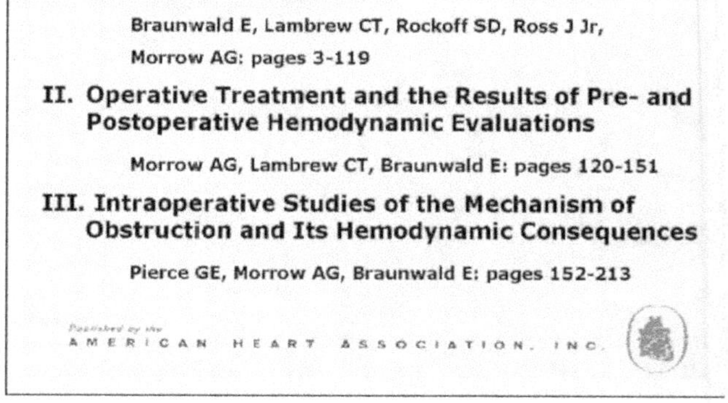
American Heart Association Monograph Number Ten

Idiopathic Hypertrophic Subaortic Stenosis

I. A Description of the Disease Based Upon an Analysis of 64 patients

Braunwald E, Lambrew CT, Rockoff SD, Ross J Jr, Morrow AG: pages 3-119

II. Operative Treatment and the Results of Pre- and Postoperative Hemodynamic Evaluations

Morrow AG, Lambrew CT, Braunwald E: pages 120-151

III. Intraoperative Studies of the Mechanism of Obstruction and Its Hemodynamic Consequences

Pierce GE, Morrow AG, Braunwald E: pages 152-213

Published by the AMERICAN HEART ASSOCIATION, INC.

Figure 1. The 1964 monograph of 213 pages by Braunwald et al.[8–10]

Manuscript received November 6, 2008; revised manuscript received and accepted November 7, 2008.

†A modified version of this piece was presented on October 4, 2008, at a scientific symposium sponsored by the Eugene Braunwald Endowment for the Advancement of Cardiovascular Discovery and Care at the Brigham and Women's Hospital, Boston, Massachusetts.

Table 1
Cardiac findings in hypertrophic cardiomyopathy divided by presence or absence of cardiac operation

Characteristic	Cardiac Operation		
	0 (n = 153)	+ (n = 77)	Total (n = 230)
Dilated atria	98%	100%	99%
Increased heart weight	95%	96%	96%
Nondilated left ventricle	82%	75%	80%
Thickened anterior mitral leaflet	66%	94%	75%
Mural plaque, LV outflow tract	60%	93%	71%
VS larger than left ventricle	71%	63%	68%
Transmural scarring, VS and/or LV wall	42%	43%	42%
Disorganization, cardiac myocytes	95%	95%	95%
Intramural coronary disease	83%	83%	83%
Interstitial fibrosis, VS and LV wall	90%	90%	90%

LV = left ventricular; VS = ventricular septum.

Table 2
Gross cardiac findings by 3 age groups in 153 patients with hypertrophic cardiomyopathy without cardiac operations

Characteristic	Age Group (yrs)		
	≤10 (n = 15)	11–70 (n = 124)	>70 (n = 14)
Dilated atria	95%	100%	100%
Increased heart weight	80%	98%	86%
Nondilated left ventricle	73%	81%	93%
Thickened anterior mitral leaflet	27%	66%	100%
Mural plaque, LV outflow tract	27%	78%	100%
VS larger than left ventricle	73%	71%	79%
Transmural scarring, VS and/or LV wall	0%	45%	50%

LV = left ventricular; VS = ventricular septum.

Table 3
Complications of hypertrophic cardiomyopathy

- Death: sudden and nonsudden
- Atrial dilatation: atrial fibrillation
- Mitral valve disease: mitral regurgitation
  - Fibrous thickening (anatomic systolic anterior motion)
  - Insertion, papillary muscle, into leaflet
  - Rupture of chordae tendineae
  - Prolapse
  - Annular calcification
  - Infective endocarditis
  - Papillary muscle calcification
- Myocardial infarction: left ventricular dilation
- Left ventricular apical diverticulum
- Pulmonary hypertension
  - Aneurysm pulmonary arteries
  - Ossific nodules, lungs
- Heart block and bundle branch block

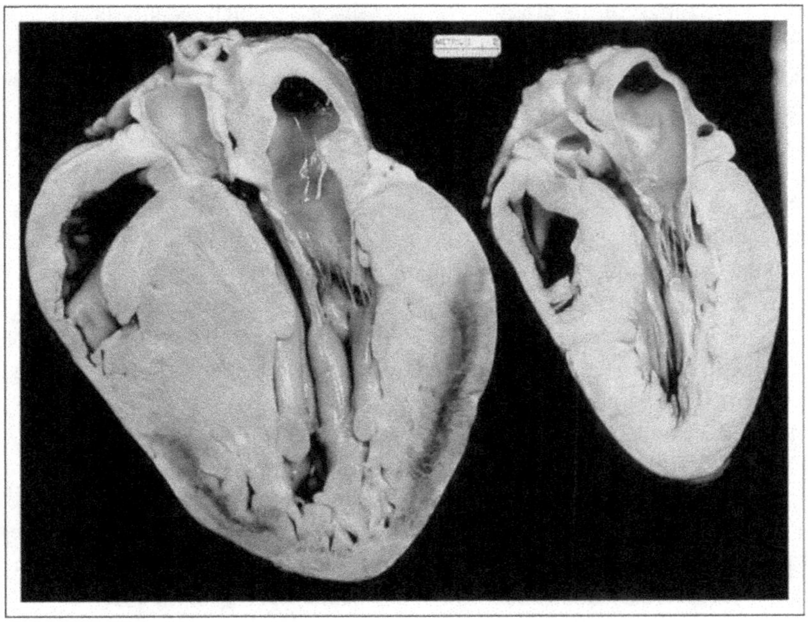

Figure 2. The hearts of 2 15-year-old male patients with HC, each of whom died suddenly. The heart on the *left* weighed 1,415 g, and the ventricular septum was much thicker than the left ventricular free wall. The heart on the right weighed 425 g, and the thicknesses of the ventricular septum and left ventricular free wall were similar.

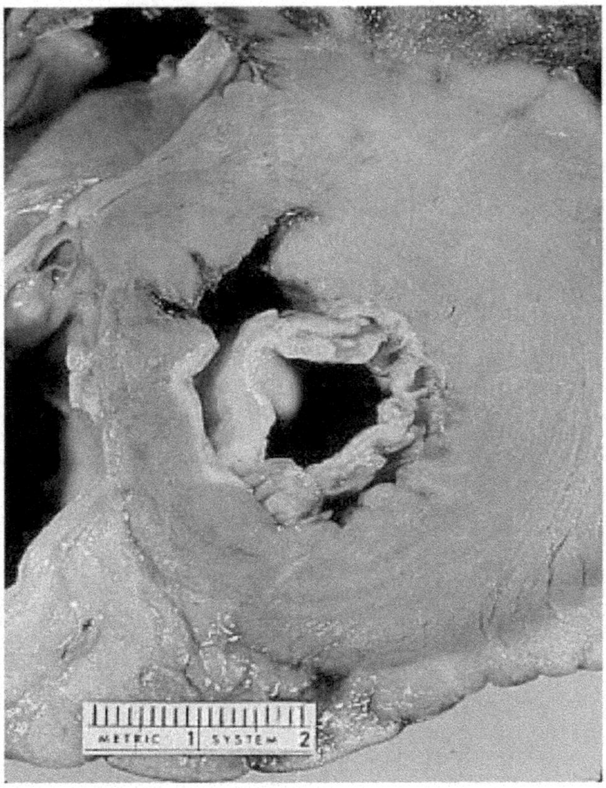

Figure 3. Heart of a patient who underwent partial ventricular septectomy and septotomy for HC. The septal mural endocardium and anterior mitral leaflet were thickened by fibrous tissue. The thickening represents the anatomic equivalent of systolic anterior motion of the anterior mitral leaflet.

chambers. Teare's report, however, established HC as a distinct entity.

Although these heretofore-mentioned reports, mainly necropsy ones, likely represent examples of the disease, HC was put on the clinical screen by Braunwald et al[7] in 1960, and by 1964, Braunwald et al[8–10] had reported extensive clinical and operative studies on 64 of these patients (Figure 1). This American Heart Association monograph included 213 pages of original work! No condition in the annals of medicine had been described so extensively in such a short period of time, and Dr. Braunwald deserves the credit. Indeed, as Dr. William Osler emphasized, "In science the credit goes to the man who convinces the world, not to the man to whom the idea first occurred."

Dr. Albert Schweitzer opined that "as we acquire more knowledge, things do not become more comprehensive, but more mysterious." Certainly this statement is applicable to HC as it has unfolded in the past 50 years.

Listed in Table 1 are morphologic features of 230 patients with HC studied at autopsy by the same investigator from 1959 to the present time.[11] The diversity of anatomic findings has altered the definition of this condition on several occasions. Essentially, none of the 10 morphologic features occurs in all patients. The ventricular septum is thicker than the left ventricular free wall in about two-thirds

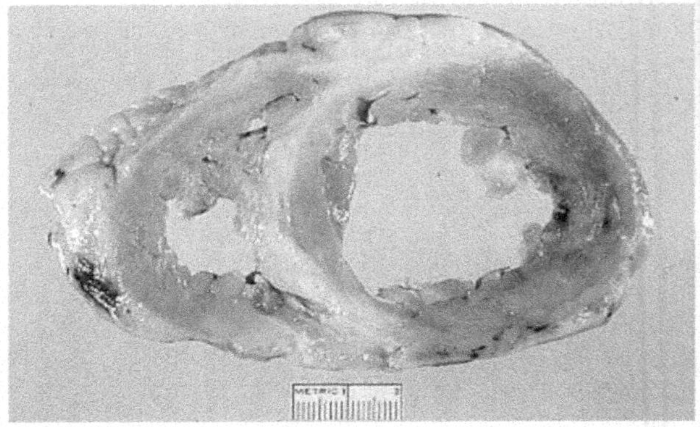

Figure 4. Transverse slice of the cardiac ventricles in a 46-year-old man with HC who developed extensive ventricular septal scarring and dilatation of both ventricular cavities. The resulting severe heart failure prompted cardiac transplantation. Reproduced with permission from *Am J Cardiol*.[22]

of patients, not 100%, as some originally thought. Cardiac mass is usually, but not always, increased.[12] This condition has produced the largest hearts known to humankind.[13]

Figure 2 shows the hearts of 2 15-year-old male patients with HC.[13,14] Both patients died suddenly. The heart on the left weighed 1,415 g, the heaviest I have ever seen. The ventricular septum was much thicker than the left ventricular free wall. The heart on the right weighed 425 g, or 30% of the heart on the left. The ventricular septum and left ventricular free wall were of similar thickness. Yet the 2 patients had the same condition, namely, HC.

The congenital condition, according to Dr. Barry Maron,[15] is present in 1 of 500 humans (the same prevalence, incidentally, as familial hyperlipidemia[16]). It can be manifested in newborns or not until the nonagenarian age group (Table 2).[15,17] It is of course a congenital heart disease, which usually is not manifested until adulthood.[18]

HC has many complications, and some are listed in Table 3. Sometimes a complication is the first clinical manifestation of the condition.

Figure 3 shows a heart in which the myectomy-myotomy procedure was performed. The operation was devised by Dr. Andrew G. Morrow,[9] who performed 299 of these operations and who himself had the disease. This operation is not for the occasional heart surgeon, which is 1 reason I predict that it will eventually vanish. Mitral valve replacement is not the proper operation, except in patients with very damaged mitral valves from infective endocarditis.[19,20]

Figure 4 shows the heart of a patient with HC who developed extensive ventricular septal scarring with ventricular cavity dilation, an occurrence, according to Dr. Maron, in 2% of these patients.[21] These patients are candidates for cardiac transplantation.[22]

In summary, HC was put on the diagnostic and therapeutic map by Dr. Braunwald and his colleagues[7–10] in the early 1960s. Much additional information, of course, has been learned subsequently. This condition produces the largest myofibers of any condition with or without the stimulus of ventricular outflow obstruction or elevation of ventricular peak systolic pressures. The ultimate therapy, in my view, will involve an agent that reduces myofiber size. Whether myofiber number is increased in HC remains unclear.

William Clifford Roberts, MD
Baylor Heart and Vascular Institute
Baylor University Medical Center
Dallas, Texas

1. Liouville H. Rétrécissement cardiaque sous aortique. *Gazette Med Paris* 1869;24:161–163.
2. Hallopeau M. Rétrécissement ventriculo-aortique. *Gazette Med Paris* 1869;24:683–684.
3. Schmincke A. Ueber linkseitigue muckulöse conusstenosen. *Dtsch Med Wochenschr* 1907;33:2082.
4. Davies LG. Familial heart disease. *Br Heart J* 1952;14:206–212.
5. Brock R. Functional obstruction of the left ventricle (acquired aortic subvalvular stenosis). *Guys Hosp Rep* 1957;106:221–238.
6. Teare D. Asymmetrical hypertrophy of the heart in young adults. *Br Heart J* 1958;20:1–18.
7. Braunwald E, Morrow AG, Cornell WP, Aygen MM, Hilbish TF. Idiopathic hypertrophic subaortic stenosis. Clinical, hemodynamic and angiographic manifestations. *Am J Med* 1960;29:924–925.
8. Braunwald E, Lambrew CT, Rockoff SD, Ross J Jr, Morrow AG. I. A description of the disease based upon an analysis of 64 patients. *Am Heart Assoc Monogr* 1964;10:IV3–IV119.
9. Morrow AG, Lambrew CT, Braunwald E. Operative treatment and the results of pre- and postoperative hemodynamic evaluations. *Am Heart Assoc Monogr* 1964;10:IV120–IV151.
10. Pierce GE, Morrow AG, Braunwald E. Intraoperative studies of the mechanism of obstruction and its hemodynamic consequences. *Am Heart Assoc Monogr* 1964;10:IV152–IV213.
11. Roberts CS, Roberts WC. Morphologic features (of hypertrophic cardiomyopathy). In: Zipes DP, Rowlands DJ, eds. Progress in Cardiology. Philadelphia, Pennsylvania: Lea & Febiger, 1989:3–32.
12. Olivotto I, Maron MS, Autore C, Lesser JR, Rega L, Casolo G, DeSantis M, Quarta G, Nistri S, Cecchi F, Salton CJ, Udelson JE, Manning WJ, Maron BJ. Assessment and significance of left ventricular mass by cardiovascular magnetic resonance in hypertrophic cardiomyopathy. *J Am Coll Cardiol* 2008; 52:559–566.
13. Roberts CS, Roberts WC. Hypertrophic cardiomyopathy as a cause of massive cardiomyopathy (>1000 g). *Am J Cardiol* 1989;64:1209–1210.
14. Maron BJ, Maron MS, Lesser JR, Hauser RG, Haas TS, Harrigan CJ, Appelbaum E, Main ML, Roberts WC. Sudden cardiac arrest in hypertrophic cardiomyopathy in the absence of conventional criteria for high risk status. *Am J Cardiol* 2008;101:544–547.
15. Maron BJ. Hypertrophic cardiomyopathy. A systemic review. *JAMA* 2002;287:1308–1320.
16. Brown MS, Goldstein JL. How LDL receptors influence cholesterol and atherosclerosis. *Sci Am* 1984;251:58–66.
17. Maron BJ, Tajik AJ, Ruttenberg HD, Graham TP, Atwood GF, Vitorica BE, Lie JT, Roberts WC. Hypertrophic cardiomyopathy in infants. Clinical features and natural history. *Circulation* 1982;65: 7–17.
18. Roberts WC. Congenital cardiovascular abnormalities usually silent until adulthood. In: Roberts WC, ed. Adult Congenital Heart Disease. Philadelphia, Pennsylvania: F.A. Davis, 1987:717–727.
19. Roberts WC. Operative treatment of hypertrophic obstructive cardiomyopathy. The case against mitral valve replacement. *Am J Cardiol* 1973;32:377–381.
20. Roberts WC, Kishel JC, McIntosh CL, Cannon RO III, Maron BJ. Severe mitral or aortic valve regurgitation, or both, requiring valve replacement for infective endocarditis complicating hypertrophic cardiomyopathy. *J Am Coll Cardiol* 1992;19:365–371.
21. Hecht GM, Klues HG, Roberts WC, Maron BJ. Coexistence of sudden cardiac death and end-stage heart failure in familial hypertrophic cardiomyopathy. *J Am Coll Cardiol* 1993;22:489–497.
22. Shirani J, Maron BJ, Canon RO III, Sheyda S, Roberts WC. Clinicopathologic features of hypertrophic cardiomyopathy managed by cardiac transplantation. *Am J Cardiol* 1993;72:434–440.

expert roundtable »

Alcohol Ablation or Ventricular Septal Myotomy/Myectomy for Severe Obstructive Hypertrophic Cardiomyopathy?

Moderated by **William Roberts, MD**[1]
Discussants: **Joseph Dearani, MD**[2] and **Barry Maron, MD**[3]

The following Expert Roundtable Discussion was held on March 12, 2010. Dr. William Roberts from the Baylor Heart and Vaslar Institute moderated the topic "Alcohol Ablation or Ventricular Septal Myotomy/Myectomy for Severe Obstructive Hypertrophic Cardiomyopathy?" with Drs. Joseph Dearani from the Mayo Clinic and Barry Maron from the Hypertrophic Cardiomyopathy Center at the Minneapolis Heart Institute participating.

The discussion focused primarily on: (1) hypertrophic cardiomyopathy (HC) and prevalence of left ventricular outflow obstruction, (2) therapeutic plan for patients with HC, including beta blocker therapy, alcohol ablation and surgical myectomy, (3) gradients for determining suitability for surgery, (4) technique of performing surgical myectomy, (5) post-surgical follow-up patient care, (5) effectiveness of myectomy surgery on patient quality of life, (6) considerations for using alcohol septal ablation, and (7) probability of installing an ICD post surgery. (*Med Roundtable Cardiovasc Ed.* 2010;1(2):128–133) ©2010 FoxP2 Media, LLC

From the Baylor Heart and Vascular Institute, Dallas, TX[1]*; the Hypertrophic Cardiomyopathy Center, Minneapolis Heart Institute Foundation, Minneapolis, MN*[2]*; and the Mayo Clinic, Rochester, MN*[3]
Address for correspondence: William Roberts, MD, Baylor Heart and Vascular Institute, 600 Gaston Avenue, Dallas, Texas 75246
E-mail: wc.roberts@baylorhealth.edu
Published online: www.themedicalroundtable.com • Search for ID: CV0032

DR. ROBERTS: Although several case reports and very small series of cases had been reported earlier, hypertrophic cardiomyopathy (HC) was really put on the screen 50 years ago when Braunwald and Morrow reported their first experiences. At the time obstruction to left ventricular outflow was believed to be universal in the condition, and they called it IHSS, or idiopathic hypertrophic subaortic stenosis. Morrow in 1960 devised the ventricular septal myotomy-myectomy procedure, and it proved quite successful in most patients. In 1995, another procedure to reduce or eliminate the outflow gradient was introduced, namely alcohol septal ablation, and it has been employed in hundreds of patients in the last 15 years.

Today we will discuss both of these gradient-reducing procedures, the advantages and disadvantages of each. I'm William C. Roberts, and I'm the Executive Director of the Baylor Heart and Vascular Institute at Baylor University Medical Center in Dallas, Texas. With me are Dr. Barry Maron, who is Director of the Hypertrophic Cardiomyopathy Center in Minneapolis at the Minneapolis Heart Institute Foundation, and Dr. Joseph A. Dearani, who is a cardiovascular surgeon at the Mayo Clinic in Rochester, Minnesota, and the person there who does most of the HC myectomy operations. May we start with you, Dr. Maron? How often do patients with HC have left ventricular outflow obstruction either at rest or with exercise?

DR. MARON: Left ventricular outflow tract obstruction is very common in the overall disease. If you combine those patients with obstruction at rest with those who have obstruction only with physiologic provocation such as exercise, then the percentage could be as high as 75%. Therefore, hypertrophic cardiomyopathy can be regarded as a predominantly obstructive disease which comes full circle, of course, back to the original descriptions of IHSS by Dr. Braunwald that you mentioned.

DR. ROBERTS: You follow a large number of patients with HC. What is your general plan? What percent of these individuals do you send to surgery to do a ventricular septal myotomy-myectomy? Do you send any patients to have alcohol septal ablation? What is the effect of medical therapy alone on the outflow gradient?

DR. MARON: Medical therapy is not usually effective in reducing the outflow gradient. Neither beta blockers nor verapamil have proven to be of value in reducing resting obstruction. The only exception to that would be the possibility that beta blocker therapy can minimize or reduce physiologically provocable outflow tract obstruction with exercise. The concept of reducing the gradient to reduce symptoms continues to require invasive intervention. We call this *septal reduction* to encompass both surgical myectomy, which is a gold standard, and the alternative in very select patients, which is alcohol septal ablation.

The overall percentage of patients who are referred to surgery, of course, depends some on the referral patterns that are operative, but it is a very small percentage of the overall HC patient population who become eligible. These would be those patients who progress in terms of heart failure, usually to New York Heart Association functional class 3 or 4. We are talking about a patient subset here, which is characterized by severe exertional dyspnea. Putting this into real-life terms, it is a patient who cannot walk comfortably for one block on level ground or one flight of stairs.

If patients meet that symptomatic threshold—that is, no longer benefit from and are refractory to drug therapy (which can include beta blockers, verapamil, possibly disopyramide or diuretics), then they become candidates to have the mechanical obstruction or impedance to left ventricular outflow reversed. Obstructive HC is a reversible form of heart failure because it is due to mechanical obstruction, i.e., systolic anterior motion of the mitral valve, and mitral septal contact. So the concept of surgical myectomy—which goes back, as you alluded, to 1960 and Andrew G. Morrow at the National Institutes of Health—is a procedure which removes obstruction and normalizes left ventricular pressures. That dramatically reduces the level of symptoms which patients incur, and it very often returns them to normal activity.

DR. ROBERTS: You do not refer a patient for the operative procedure unless they are quite symptomatic, New York Heart Association 3 or 4?

DR. MARON: Right, the only exception to this would be in children. The principle of the New York Heart Association functional class III doesn't hold as well for them because young children are rarely allowed to progress to that level of limitation. In that age group, surgery is often performed much earlier. Whether it should be performed in asymptomatic children or not is controversial, but it is a question that arises in some young patients because most cardiac surgery for congenital heart disease is, of course, in asymptomatic patients.

DR. ROBERTS: What if the patient has a very high gradient on provocation only, and no gradient at rest, but is quite symptomatic?

DR. MARON: That patient is an operative candidate as well, because the symptoms of heart failure that patients experience occur during exertion. Placing that patient on the treadmill (the Bruce protocol) and eliciting a gradient as well as symptoms during exercise, makes a reasonable connection between the gradient with exercise and external symptoms. Traditionally, those patients have benefitted in a similar fashion as the larger group of patients with rest obstruction.

DR. ROBERTS: What if the patient has a 90 mm peak systolic pressure gradient between the left ventricle and aorta and is asymptomatic?

DR. MARON: It is a subgroup that has always been difficult to manage or make decisions for. I'll put it in a historical context. When myectomy surgery was associated with a higher operative mortality, (5%-8%), which takes us back maybe 25 years, then there was a bias, of course, against operating on asymptomatic or mildly symptomatic patients. Operative mortality today is quite different than 5 decades ago. At centers experienced with the myectomy operation, as Dr. Dearani will be able to tell us, 30-day mortality following surgery is now <1%. It has been more than a decade, for example, at the Mayo Clinic since a patient undergoing a surgical septal myectomy has died as a result of the surgery.

Myectomy has become one of the safest open-heart operations. The question that is sometimes debated now is whether that fact should alter the level of symptoms that would justify surgical myectomy. However, clinical practice at this time is still to reserve surgery for severely symptomatic obstructive patients, because cardiac surgery is always associated with an unpredictable small risk.

DR. ROBERTS: When I was at NIH with you, Barry, Glen Morrow told me he did 299 myotomy-myectomy procedures for patients with HC. As you indicated, the operative mortality at that time over 25 years ago was about 8%, and a few of those patients developed ventricular septal defects. When you say the operative mortality for this procedure now is <1%, you're talking about the operative mortality by a surgeon like Dr. Dearani, who does this procedure many times a year, not once a year as happens it seems to me in many parts of the country. Dr. Dearani, how do you do this procedure, and how do you get such a low mortality and presumably morbidity from the procedure?

DR. DEARANI: Before I answer that I'd like to make a brief comment about the two issues that you just described that are important to me as a surgeon when I'm seeing a patient and discussing the risks and benefits of myectomy. You made a comment about rest gradient versus provocable gradient. For me as a surgeon, there are many patients whom I operate on that have minimal or no pressure gradient between the LV and the aorta at rest, but a substantial gradient with provocation. A thorough echocardiogram should include a rest gradient and some provocative maneuver (amylnitrate or Valsalva) to see what the gradient is with the provocation since this is such a dynamic problem that is dependent on their hydration status, their medical program, etc. At any point in time you can change the echo findings depending upon these variables. It is important to me to know what the provocative gradient is since this usually correlates with exertion. There are many patients who have surgery who have a minimal gradient at rest, but have a considerable gradient with provocation.

The second issue that you commented on was the asymptomatic patient. It should be pointed out that asymptomatic may not mean asymptomatic if they have an abnormal exercise test. Many patients will tell you that they do not have any symptoms, but on exercise, they often have markedly reduced exercise capacity. To me that's not an asymptomatic patient. If they have normal exercise tolerance and report no symptoms, then this is a truly asymptomatic patient. Since many of these patients live a very limited lifestyle, they may appear to be asymptomatic, but with exercise examination they perform poorly indicating that they are not really asymptomatic.

With regard to the operation, the cardiac surgical community has the impression that septal myectomy is not a terribly difficult operation and that many cardiac surgeons can do it. I would say is that it's a hard operation to do well. There is an increasing number of patients being considered for repeat myectomy, and it's usually because the first myectomy was an inadequate myectomy. Looking down the aortic root and carving out the inside of the left ventricle can be quite an intimidating endeavor for a surgeon who's not used to doing it. The risk of aortic valve injury, the risk of mitral valve injury, the risk of ventricular septal defect or heart block is a very real problem for somebody who is not used to doing it.

In addition, the myectomy that we do now is different than the myectomy that Dr. Morrow described some 50 years ago where the myectomy was more limited. We've learned over the last 20 years that the myectomy needs to be much broader, particularly as you get further into the ventricle. This issue of ventricular septal defect that you touched on in the early days resulted from this notion that it was important to focus the myectomy and thinning of the septum right at the base of the heart. This would increase your risk of ventricular septal defect (VSD), and you would just move the point of obstruction a little further into the ventricle. The focus in the current era of myectomy surgery is to make the myectomy wider as you go further in the ventricle.

It is important for the myectomy to be comprehensive opposite the mitral valve and the subvalvular apparatus, including resection of muscle opposite the papillary muscles, opposite the chordae, and opposite the anterior leaflet of the mitral valve. In addition, the extended version of the myectomy also involves limited resection of muscle along the left ventricular free wall extending around toward the anterior mitral valve leaflet. This is very different than what Dr. Morrow discussed many years ago where the myectomy was confined to the basal septum. Now, the extended myectomy includes removing muscle along the left ventricular free wall and a broader resection at the midventricular level.

> ***"It is very common for these patients to report New York Heart Association functional class 1 after myectomy—that is, they can do virtually anything..."***
>
> *– Barry Maron, MD*

Thus, in the current era, the myectomy is a much more comprehensive myectomy than was done in the early years, and the mortality is reportedly low in the hands of surgeons and experienced centers that take care of many patients with hypertrophic cardiomyopathy. It's not an everyday operation for the vast majority of busy cardiac surgeons. The learning curve is steep. And to put it in perspective, it is very difficult for me to teach a resident how to do this operation. In fact, I find it to be one of the hardest operations to teach a resident because you can't see what's being done by the person you are helping. The only person who can see is the person who's holding the knife and performing the myectomy. It's very difficult to coach somebody through it because you can't see at the same time they're doing it to help him/her them navigate where the knife should be going. For all of these reasons, it's an operation that I think is vulnerable to problems when it gets in inexperienced hands. In experienced hands, like everything else, you get good at it, and the mortality and morbidity gets to be quite low.

DR. ROBERTS: How many of these operations do you do a year?

DR. DEARANI: There are two of us at the Mayo Clinic (Dr. Hartzell Schaff and me) who routinely perform the myectomies, and we do between 150 and 200 a year. We each do approximately 75 to 100 cases annually. Our total experience now approaches 2000 cases. Of course, my mentor and predecessor, Dr. Gordon Danielson, was also largely involved with this operation. He helped introduce some of the extended resection maneuvers.

DR. ROBERTS: When I was at the NIH, I saw the portions of ventricular septum that Dr. Morrow would excise in patients with HC. Early on (in the 1960s and 1970s) he excised as much as 15 grams or so, but toward the end of his career, he would take out only about 2 grams. Also, I think toward the end of his career he did more myotomy than myectomy. I would agree that the thickest portion of the ventricular septum is not just below the aortic valve, but is indeed about halfway between the aortic valve and the apex of the left ventricle. How much myocardium do you excise, Dr. Dearani, in your HC patients?

DR. DEARANI: That question is asked by both physicians and patients. It depends on the thickness of the ventricular septum. When the septum is 3–5 cm thick, the amount of muscular resection is substantial. Many grams can come out. In contrast, those with a septum 1.5 cm thick have small amounts of septum excised. In fact, our approach here has been that if they have dynamic left ventricular outflow tract obstruction, which is sort of one of the principle findings with this diagnosis, we always do a myectomy. The magnitude of the myectomy is lessened if the septum is thin. Somebody with a 1.5 cm septum may not have even a gram of muscle excised, whereas somebody who has a septum that's up to 5 cm or more will have multiple grams of muscle excised.

In general, I like to have the remaining septum, particularly at the base of the heart, to be anywhere from 0.5 to 1 cm in thickness.

DR. ROBERTS: Dr. Dearani, when you say you take out some of the muscle of the left ventricular free wall, what do you mean?

DR. DEARANI: It's the posterolateral wall. It's the segment of lateral free wall that is between the anterior leaflet of the mitral valve and the commissure between the left and the right coronary cusps. I begin the myectomy in the middle of the noncoronary cusp, maybe just slightly to the right, being careful of the conduction tissue. Once moving beyond the commissure between the left and the right cusps, this becomes the lateral free wall of the left ventricle and it is not ventricular septum anymore. In many of these patients, as you know, the hypertrophy involves more than just the ventricular septum. If the free wall is also quite hypertrophied, there is an opportunity to enlarge the outflow tract by resecting muscle in this area as well.

DR. ROBERTS: You see these patients after operation for about 30 days and then send them back to their cardiologist.

DR. DEARANI: In our practice at the Mayo Clinic, we have many out of town patients. In general, they're in the hospital about five days, and when they get discharged, many of them will stay in town for a few days and we will see them prior to their departure from Rochester. When they get home they usually follow up with their home medical physician within a week or two. If somebody lives within driving distance of the Mayo Clinic, they usually come back for a followup visit within that first 4-6 weeks.

> ***"...myotomy-myectomy is the gold standard, but there are a lot of cardiologists around the world now who love injecting alcohol into those septal arteries."***
>
> *– William Roberts, MD*

We keep track of them in our database, and all patients who have had cardiac surgery here, not just the myectomy patients. It's the exception rather than the rule that I would see most of the patients 30-days postoperatively. Many of them are back home by then, and if it's far away they don't make a trip back here for a follow-up visit unless there's a concern that needs to be addressed.

DR. ROBERTS: Dr. Maron, what happens to these patients after ventricular myotomy-myectomy? How many lose their symptoms? How many have the outflow gradient completely obliterated? I remember at NIH virtually all of the patients had left bundle branch block immediately after the procedure. What happens to these patients? You follow them all.

DR. MARON: Surgical myectomy is the gold standard based on the consensus in the cardiovascular community. In other words, it is the primary treatment option. The reason that consensus has been reached is surgical myectomy has proven over this considerable period of time to be highly beneficial in improving the quality of life of patients. Relief of the mechanical impedance to left ventricular outflow normalizes left ventricular systolic pressures and returns these patients to normal or near-normal functional capacity. Very often, as Dr. Dearani will tell you, it is very common for these patients to report New York Heart Association functional class 1 after myectomy—that is, they can do virtually anything, and it makes sense if one understands the basic effect of surgical myectomy.

The second benefit in addition to improvement in quality of life has to do with survival. We published a paper based on the Mayo Clinic operative experience with Dr. Dearani in which Steve Ommen is the first author, showing that many years after surgical myectomy patients had a survival that was equivalent to and did not differ significantly from the general US population. A control group—and I should indicate this was not a randomized study—of patients who had obstruction to left ventricular outflow and were not operated on had a total mortality that was very different. The percentages for total mortality were 83% for the operated patients and 61% for the nonoperated patients. For cardiovascular mortality only, the operated patients (after more than a decade on the average post-myectomy) had a cardiovascular survival rate of 93%. We've learned a lot about long-term effects of surgery that we didn't know before, and the myectomy operation improves quality of life as well as survival, and may allow patients with obstructive HCM who have had surgical myectomy to achieve normal or near-normal longevity.

DR. ROBERTS: Dr. Maron, patients go on the Internet a lot now, and I'm sure some of your patients read about alcohol septal ablation. You talk to them about that alternative procedure. What is your view on alcohol septal ablation? You have stressed that myotomy-myectomy is the gold standard, but there are a lot of cardiologists around the world now who love injecting that alcohol into septal arteries.

DR. MARON: The interventional community has aggressively promoted alcohol septal ablation as a treatment option over the last 15 years. I think Dr. Dearani and I have similar views, and that is that we're we are pleased that there is an alternative to surgical myectomy for those very few patients who require it. The alcohol ablation has been shown to reduce the outflow gradient, and any technique that reduces gradient will probably reduce heart failure symptoms in obstructive HC.

However, the key issue is, are these equivalent procedures? I believe the evidence is that they are not. That argument begins with the principle that alcohol ablation produces a transmural myocardial infarct (intentionally) which occupies 10% on average of the left ventricular wall and as much as 30% of ventricular septum. This is not a small matter. Alcohol ablation is an unusual technique, which has to be considered as such because it is highly destructive to myocardial tissue.

The controversy, which at this time is not completely resolved, has to do with the potential for lethal ventricular tachyarrhythmia that would emanate from that alcohol induced transmural scar. About 10% of patients after alcohol ablation have life-threatening ventricular tachyarrhythmias, which may trigger sudden death. The scar can be arrhythmogenic, at least in some patients. This is one of the reasons that surgical myectomy is regarded as the primary treatment option for most severely symptomatic patients with obstruction.

Now, the exceptions to that could be, for example, patients of advanced age, who, for one reason or another, would not be good operative candidates. For example, any patient who has a morbid fear of open-heart surgery could benefit from the alternative alcohol ablation because no surgeon or cardiologist would want to refer a patient to myectomy who looked upon the operation in that way. Patients with associated diseases, particularly those that elevate the potential risk to surgery could be candidates for alcohol ablation.

"The strategy of, we can use surgery as plan B if plan A, septal alcohol ablation, doesn't work out is really not a good one"
- Joseph Dearani, MD

But the primary issue is age, because if the infarct potentially promotes risk for sudden death and arrhythmia, then patients who are older would be preferred, since they have shorter risk periods. The idea of alcohol ablation in young patients, and this procedure has been performed in patients as young as age 4, doesn't make a lot of sense to many of us who take care of patients with hypertrophic cardiomyopathy.

DR. DEARANI: Another point should be made about the issue of septal alcohol ablation, which I think the patient community and the medical community oftentimes don't realize. There are many patients sent for ventricular septal myotomy/myectomy who have already had a septal alcohol ablation. The rationale is, let's begin with this less invasive technique, and if it doesn't work out, we can then consider surgery. There are a couple of major problems with that strategy. The first is that the risk of myectomy after septal alcohol ablation is not less than 1%. It is definitely higher.

The second issue relates to the comment made earlier about a left bundle branch block with septal myectomy. We haven't mentioned this except in passing, but if the septal myectomy is extended as we do it in the current era, most patients will end up with a left bundle branch block. Importantly, with septal alcohol ablation, many patients will get a right bundle branch block, or they will get complete heart block right after that procedure. Consequently, if myectomy is performed after septal alcohol ablation, many of those patients will require a pacemaker after surgery (if they do not already have one). Also, many of those patients will end up needing a defibrillator because of the preexisting presence of an infarct.

The strategy of, we can use surgery as plan B if plan A, septal alcohol ablation, doesn't work out is really not a good one, since the operative risk is increased and the need for an ICD after surgery increases substantially. In our experience more than 50% will require a device, but in many cases it can approach 90% or more depending upon the nature of the preoperative rhythm.

DR. ROBERTS: Good point. Barry. What about dual chamber pacing? Does anybody do that anymore to lessen the gradient?

DR. MARON: Virtually no one, although I must say it's still popular in Japan, so there are pockets of interest in dual chamber pacing because perhaps other treatments such as surgery or alcohol ablation are not popular in a culture.

I wanted to make one other point; Joe would agree with this. Another limitation of alcohol ablation in addition to the consequence of the scar has to do with ablation and myectomy not providing the same exposure to left ventricular outflow tract anatomy. Alcohol ablation is limited, of course, to the course of the septal perforator that is chosen by the operator for injection.

As we all agree, and Dr. Dearani has described this in some detail, the anatomy of the left ventricular outflow tract is complex in hypertrophic cardiomyopathy, particularly in certain patients, and the extended myectomy that he described has the obvious advantage of direct operative visualization to take into account that structural diversity. The alcohol ablation doesn't have that capability or advantage because, as I have mentioned, it is performed based on the course and distribution of the artery chosen to inject the alcohol. I guess the bottom line to all of this is that these are not at all equal or equivalent procedures.

DR. DEARANI: Another comment worth making about septal alcohol ablation has to do with the anatomy of the outflow tract. There are two anatomic issues that are extremely important and can help guide management. Approximately 5% and at times up to 8% of patients who are referred to the HC clinic at the Mayo Clinic do not have HC, but fixed subaortic stenosis which can only be treated with surgery. Septal alcohol ablation will not treat subaortic stenosis because of the fibrous membrane in the outflow tract.

The second issue regarding anatomy is that there are frequently concomitant abnormalities with the mitral valve, myxomatous abnormalities that would require mitral valve repair, and, other anatomical abnormalities such as, direct insertions of papillary muscles into the anterior leaflet of the mitral valve, accessory papillary muscles, and abnormal chordal attachments into the left ventricular outflow tract. A cardiologist that is thinking about these anatomical issues when an echocardiogram is being performed on a patient with a presumed diagnosis of HC has a responsibility to identify these findings. Importantly, if they are found to be present, then people are not candidates for septal alcohol ablation. They can only be properly treated with surgery so that these other anatomic abnormalities can be addressed at the same time. Of course, if there is myxomatous or ruptured chordae of the mitral valve, then it would need to be addressed at the time of surgery in addition to the myectomy.

DR. ROBERTS: You mean replacing the mitral valve?

DR. DEARANI: No, repairing the mitral valve. The role of mitral valve replacement in the current era is limited to complex mitral valve disease which would include rheumatic mitral valve stenosis and/or stenosis regurgitation where successful mitral valve repair would be unlikely. In this situation, it would be preferable to replace the valve, treating both the problem of outflow tract obstruction and mitral pathology. In this country rheumatic valvular heart disease is not common. Consequently, in an experienced center, the need to resort to mitral valve replacement is going to be less than 2% of the time to treat obstructive hypertrophic cardiomyopathy.

DR. ROBERTS: Dr. Maron has described insertion of one papillary muscle directly into the anterior mitral leaflet, and that does occur in an occasional HC patient. Also, these patients have an increased frequency of infective endocarditis that can tear up the mitral valve. It seems to me that possibly those patients might be candidates for mitral replacement.

DR. DEARANI: Yes.

DR. ROBERTS: Gentlemen, I think we've done it. The conclusion is that the ventricular myotomy-myectomy operation remains the gold standard assuming that the surgery is done by someone who is a student of HC and does a lot of these procedures, not the occasional cardiac surgeon. You would both agree with that, I presume?

DR. MARON AND DR. DEARANI: Yes.

Continue the Discussion:
www.TheMedicalRoundtable.com/Discuss

Dramatically Different Phenotypic Expressions of Hypertrophic Cardiomyopathy in Male Cousins Undergoing Cardiac Transplantation With Identical Disease-Causing Gene Mutation

William C. Roberts, MD[a,b,d,*], Carey Camille Roberts[d], Jong Mi Ko, BA[d], Paul A. Grayburn, MD[b,d], Anumeha Tandon, MD[b], Johannes J. Kuiper, MD[b], John E. Capehart, MD[c], and Shelley A. Hall, MD[b]

Described herein are certain findings in 2 male cousins who underwent cardiac transplantation for severe heart failure (HF), one of the diastolic type (ejection fraction ≈65%), and one of the systolic type (ejection fraction ≈20%), both the consequence of hypertrophic cardiomyopathy (HC), and each had identical disease-causing gene mutations. The implanted heart in one had normal-sized ventricular cavities and no grossly visible ventricular wall lesions (except in one papillary muscle) and the other patient had severely dilated ventricular cavities and multiple extensive ventricular wall scars. The heart mass and the age of onset of symptoms was similar in each patient. A number of other family members had evidence of HC. **(Am J Cardiol 2013;111:1818–1822)**

Hypertrophic cardiomyopathy (HC) is a genetically transmitted cardiac disease with a diverse variety of clinical and morphologic manifestations. Its frequency of 1 in 500 persons is similar to that of familial hypercholesterolemia.[1] Some patients with HC remain asymptomatic or nearly so throughout a long life; others die suddenly, usually prematurely; many have symptoms related to left ventricular outflow obstruction and once the obstruction is relieved the symptoms vanish or at least decrease in frequency, and some patients develop end-stage HF that can be relieved only by cardiac transplantation (CT).[2–4] Recently, we encountered 2 male cousins with HC, both of whom underwent CT, and examination of the recipient heart disclosed nearly opposite morphologic features of the disease although both had identical disease-causing gene mutations. A description of certain findings in them is the purpose of this report.

Patient Descriptions

Pertinent clinical and morphologic findings in the 2 patients are tabulated in Table 1. The pedigrees of the family are illustrated in Figure 1. Both were African American men, one had CT at age 45 and the other, at age 48 years. One became symptomatic from HF about 6 years before CT, the other 7 years, before CT. Both had class IV HF. Each also had one or more episodes of syncope, atrial fibrillation, and runs of ventricular tachycardia. Neither had a precordial murmur. Neither had obstruction to outflow from either the right or left ventricle. Both had normal epicardial coronary arteries. The left ventricular ejection fractions were strikingly different. In case #1 it was ≈65%, and in case #2, ≈20%. Both patients had elevated pulmonary arterial pressures. Both had cardiac defibrillators implanted several years before CT. Patient #2 had a left ventricular assist device. Echocardiograms before CT are shown in Figures 2–4.

[a]Department of Pathology, [b]Department of Internal Medicine, Division of Cardiology, [c]Department of Cardiothoracic Surgery, and [d]Baylor Heart and Vascular Institute, Baylor University Medical Center, Dallas, Texas. Manuscript received September 19, 2012; revised manuscript received and accepted February 6, 2013.

See page 1822 for disclosure information.

*Corresponding author: Tel: 214-820-7911; fax: 214-820-7533.

E-mail address: wc.roberts@baylorhealth.edu (W.C. Roberts).

Table 1
Certain clinical and morphologic findings in the 2 African American male cousins who underwent cardiac transplantation for end-stage heart failure secondary to hypertrophic cardiomyopathy

Variable	Case #1	Case #2
Age (yrs) at cardiac transplantation	45	48
Age (yrs) onset symptoms	39	41
Heart failure class IV	+	+
Chest pain	0	+
Syncope	+	+
Precordial murmur	0	0
Atrial fibrillation	+	+
Ventricular tachycardia	+	+
Body mass index (Kg/m^2)	26.5	30.6
Left ventricular ejection fraction	65%	20%
Cardiac index (l/min/m^2)	1.3	1.8
Pulmonary artery peak systolic pressure (mm Hg)	82	56
Coronary narrowing by angiogram	0	0
Left ventricular assist device inserted	0	+
Heart weight (g)	410	410
Scars (0-4+), left ventricular wall and ventricular septum	0*	+(4+)
Dilated right ventricle	0	+
Dilated left ventricle	0	+
Mitral valve	normal	normal
Mural endocardial thickening in the left ventricular outflow tract in apposition to anterior mitral leaflet	0	0
Mitral annular calcium	3+/4+	0
Abnormal intramural coronary arteries	0	+

* Scarring in one left ventricular papillary muscles.

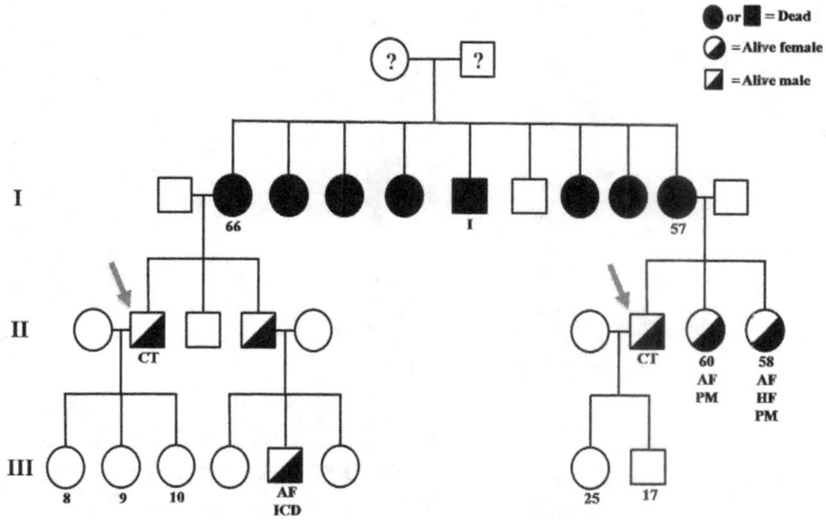

Figure 1. Pedigree of the family of case #1 *(left)* and case #2 *(right)*. Whether or not the grand parents had heart disease is unclear but 8 of their 9 children died of heart disease, several of them suddenly and prematurely, and others from heart failure of varying durations. The *arrows* designate the 2 patients described herein. The numbers represent the ages at death or presently (2012). AF = atrial fibrillation; CT = cardiac transplantation; HF = heart failure; I = stillbirth; ICD = intracardiac defibrillator; PM = pacemaker.

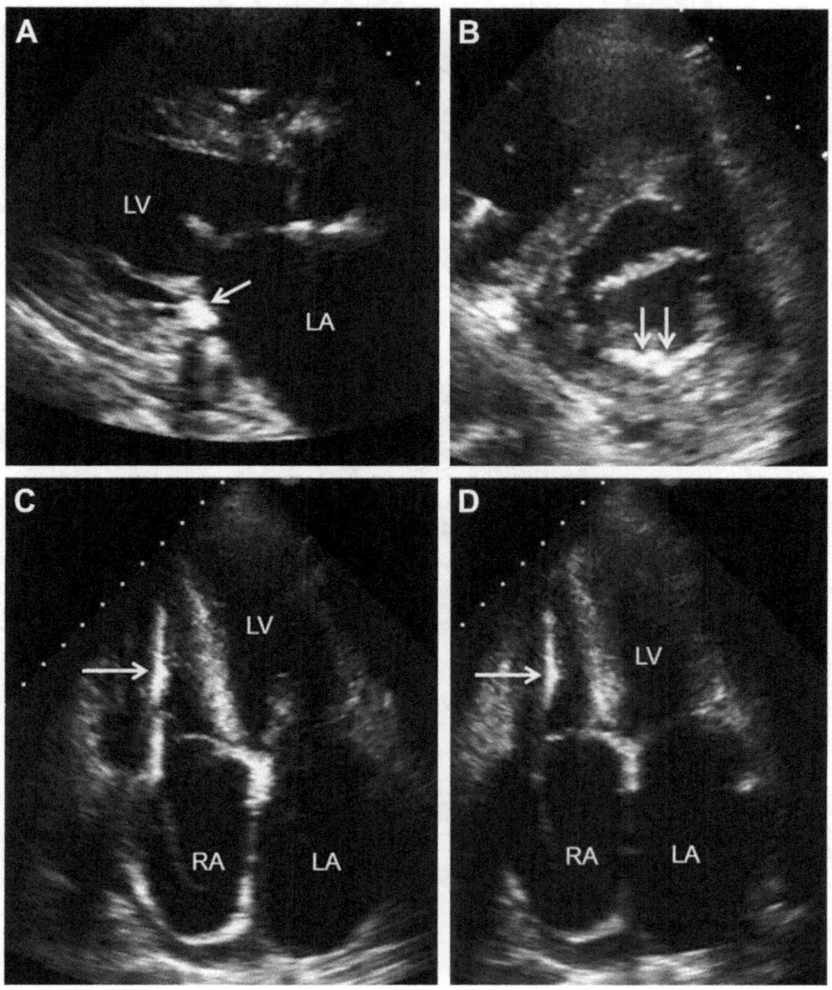

Figure 2. Echocardiogram in patient #1. *(A)* Parasternal long-axis view showing a very dilated left atrium (LA) and a non-dilated left ventricle (LV). The *arrow* points to calcium in the mitral annular area. *(B)* Parasternal short-axis view of the ventricles. The *arrows* again point to calcium deposits in the mitral valve area. *(C)* Four-chamber view during ventricular diastole. The *arrow* points to the intracardiac defibrillator catheter. *(D)* Four-chamber view in ventricular systole. Cavity size is much smaller than in diastole, consistent with a left ventricular ejection fraction of ≈65%.

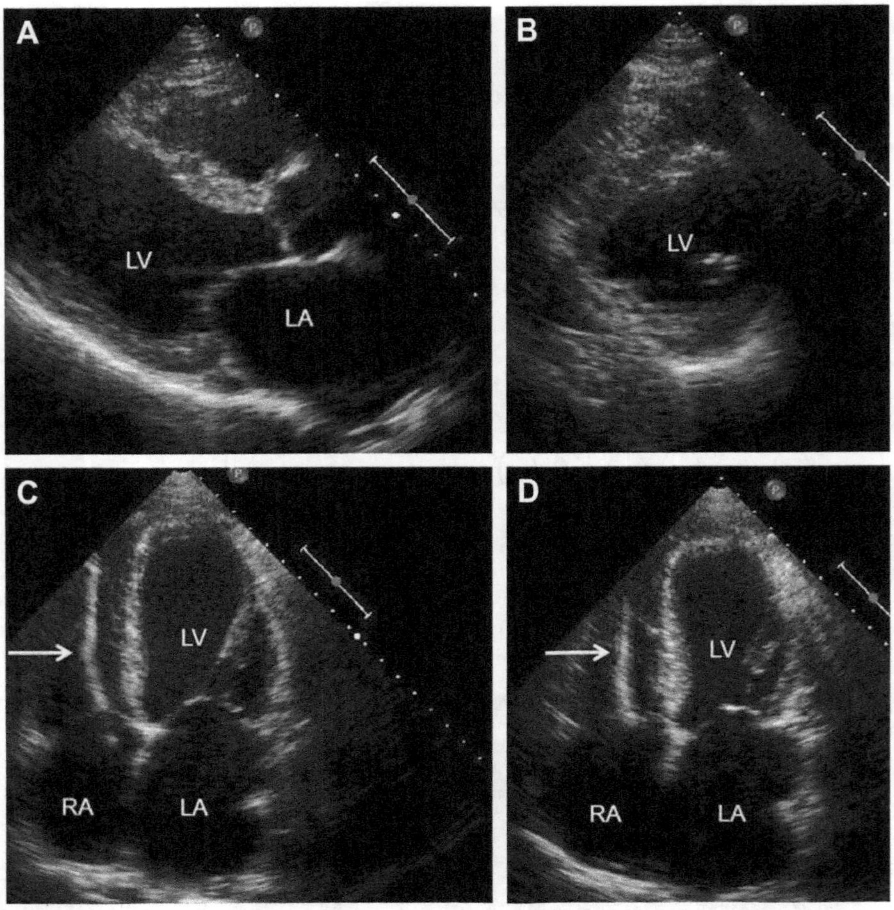

Figure 3. Echocardiogram is patient #2. *(A)* Parasternal long-axis view showing very dilated left ventricle (LV) and left atrium (LA). *(B)* Parasternal short-axis view of the left ventricle. *(C)* Four-chamber view showing the very dilated left ventricles in ventricular diastole with its thin walls. The *arrow* points to the implanted intracardiac defibrillator catheter. RA = right atrium. *(D)* Same view in ventricular systole, with minimal change in ventricular size and wall thickness indicative of markedly depressed systolic function.

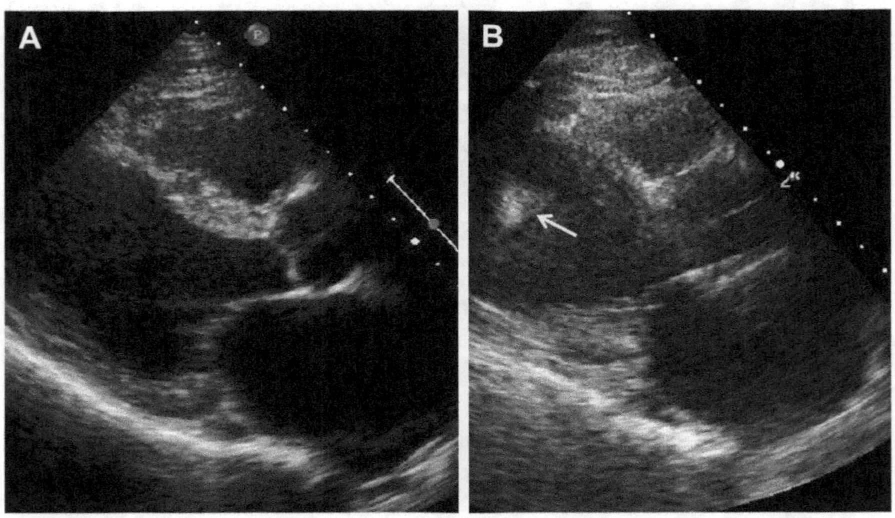

Figure 4. Echocardiogram in patient #2 before *(A)* and after *(B)* insertion of a left ventricular assist device *(arrow)*. The size of the left ventricular cavity is larger before than after insertion of the device.

The explanted heart in each patient weighed 410 g (portions of the atrial walls are not included in the weight) (Figures 5 and 6). Both hearts contained excessive subepicardial adipose tissue. In case #1, neither cardiac ventricles was dilated. Except for one left ventricular papillary muscle, no grossly visible myocardial scars were

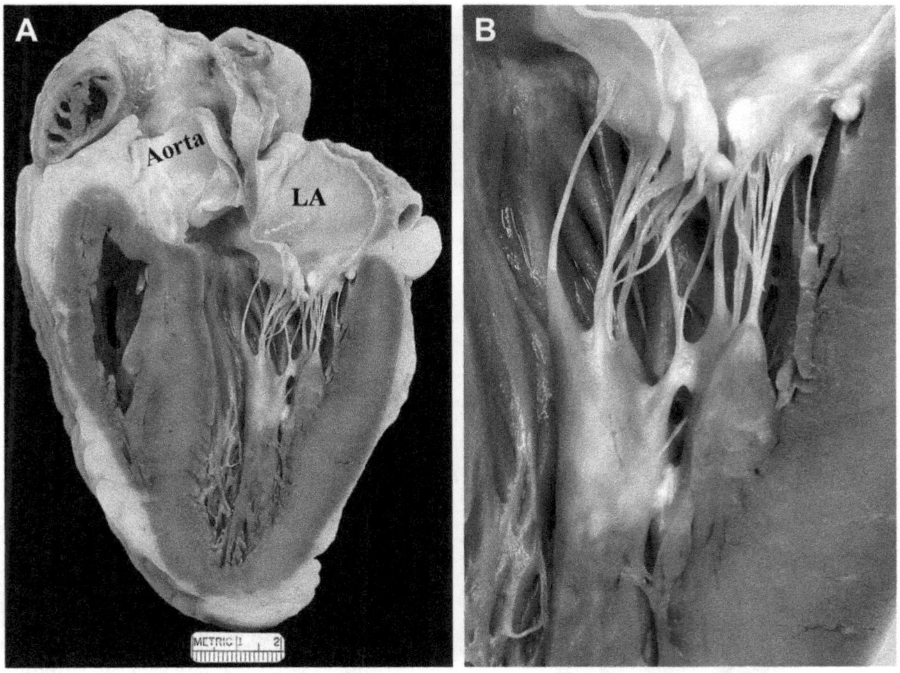

Figure 5. Case #1. *(A)* Longitudinal view of the left ventricle, right ventricular outflow tract, aortic valve, mitral valve, and left atrium. The thickness of the ventricular septum is a bit greater than that of the left ventricular free wall. The apical portion of the posteromedial papillary muscle is scarred. Calcium is present in the mitral annular region. *(B)* Close-up of the scarred papillary muscle.

present. In case #2, in contrast, there was extensive, usually transmural, scarring of the left ventricular free wall and ventricular septum with some scarring also in the right ventricular free wall. The ventricular cavities were dilated in case #2 but not as dilated as would have occurred had not a left ventricular assist device been inserted 29 months earlier. Neither patient had mural endocardial thickening in the ventricular septum in apposition to the anterior mitral leaflet, the anatomic feature of systolic anterior motion of the anterior mitral leaflet with septal contact. Patient #1, but not patient #2, had calcium in the mitral annular region.[5] Histologic study demonstrated considerable enlargement of the myocardial fibers in both patients. The intramural coronary arteries in patient #2 were increased in number and size and the lumens in many were narrowed. The quantity of interstitial fibrous tissue between myofibers was increased in both patients.

Several months after CT, both patients had blood samples (in EDTA) sent to Gene Dx (207 Perry Parkway, Gaithersburg, Maryland 20877) for "hypertrophic cardiomyopathy panel" analysis. Both patients had the p.Arg 186Gln (CGG>GAG)(R186Q) mutation in exon 8 of the troponin I (TNN13) gene (NM_000363.4), confirming that both patients had the identical disease-causing gene mutation despite strikingly different phenotypic expressions.

Discussion

Although HC is a genetically transmitted disease with an autosomal dominant trait, the penetrance into the family of the 2 cousins described herein is particularly striking. Some family members died suddenly, usually prematurely, others developed severe heart failure, and others developed various arrhythmias and conduction disturbances with intracardiac pacemakers and implantable intracardiac defibrillators implanted.

Cardiac transplantation for patients with HC is relatively infrequent, and most patients with HC having CT have severe systolic heart failure and no obstruction to either left or right ventricular outflow. Warren and colleagues[6] in 1988 appear to have been the first to describe CT for HC. Both of their patients had severe diastolic heart failure with normal sized ventricular cavities, apparently similar to our patient #1. Shirani and colleagues[7] in 1993 described 10 patients with HC who had CT and all of them had severe systolic heart failure with severe left ventricular and ventricular septal scarring, similar to that in our patient #2. Hecht and associates[8] in the same year described 2 patients with end-stage systolic heart failure who underwent CT. Contu and colleagues[9] in 2004 described 14 patients with HC who underwent CT, 13 of whom underwent CT for severe heart failure, presumably systolic in type, and 1 for malignant ventricular arrhythmias. Biagini and associates[10] in 2008 described 18 patients with HC who underwent CT, 17 of whom had severe systolic heart failure and severely dilated ventricular cavities and 1 of whom had severe diastolic heart failure with normal sized ventricular cavities. Maron and colleagues[11] in 2010 acquired data from the United Network of Organ-Sharing Registry and found among 26, 706 patients $\geq$18 years of age having CT that 303 (1%) had CT for HC. Among those 303 patients it is unclear how many had systolic or diastolic HF. They found that survival after CT was at least similar to that in non-HC patients having CT and maybe better. And finally, Kato and colleagues[12] in 2012 described 41 patients with HC who underwent CT, 39 (95%) for "refractory heart failure" and 2

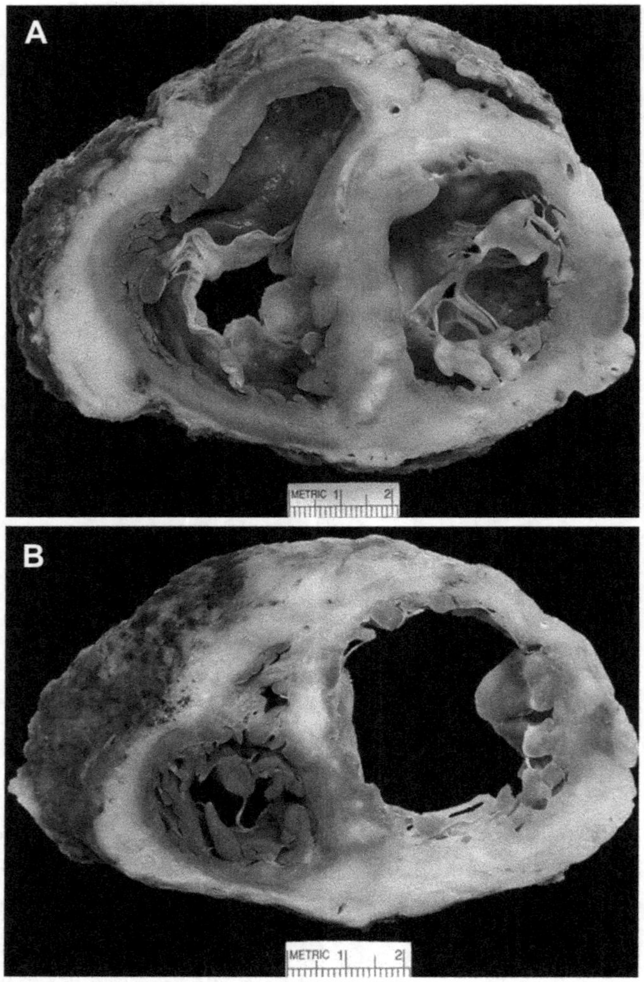

Figure 6. Case #2. Basal portion of the heart *(A)* and more caudal portion *(B)* showing extensive scarring in the left ventricular free wall and ventricular septum and scarring in the moderator band of the right ventricle. Both ventricular cavities dilated.

from "recurrent ventricular arrhythmias." Prior to CT only 14 (34%) of the 41 patients had a dilated left ventricular cavity (left ventricular end-diastolic dimension >55 mm) and 27 patients (66%) had smaller left ventricular cavities. Survival of their 41 HC patients after CT was better than that for their 771 non-HC patients. Thus, CT is a useful procedure for the relatively small percentage of patients with HC who develop end-stage HF or refractory ventricular arrhythmias unassociated with left or right ventricular outflow obstruction.

Acknowledgment: We thank Ms. Carolyn Q. Alexander RN, BSN, for arranging the acquisition of the genetic tests in each of the 2 patients.

Disclosures

The authors have no conflicts of interest to disclose.

1. Maron BJ, Gardin JM, Flack JM, Gidding SS, Kurosaki TT, Bild DE. Prevalence of hypertrophic cardiomyopathy in a general population of young adults: echocardiographic analysis of 4111 subjects in the CARDIA study. *Circulation* 1995;92:785–789.
2. Maron BJ. Hypertrophic cardiomyopathy. *Lancet* 1997;350:127–133.
3. Spirito P, Seidman CE, McKenna WJ, Maron BJ. The management of hypertrophic cardiomyopathy. *New Eng J Med* 1997;366:775–785.
4. Maron BJ, Maron MS, Wigle ED, Bruanwald E. The 50-year history, controversy, and clinical implication of left ventricular outflow tract obstruction in hypertrophic cardiomyopathy. From idiopathic cardiomyopathy subaortic stenosis to hypertrophic cardiomyopathy. *J Am Coll Cardiol* 2009;54:191–200.
5. Motamed HE, Roberts WC. Frequency and significance of mitral anular calcium in hypertrophic cardiomyopathy: analysis of 200 necropsy patients. *Am J Cardiol* 1987;60:877–884.
6. Warren SE, Cohn LH, Schoen FJ, Mudge GH Jr, Lorell BH. Advanced diastolic heart failure in familial hypertrophic cardiomyopathy managed with cardiac transplantation. *J Appl Cardiol* 1988;3:415–422.
7. Shirani J, Maron BJ, Cannon RO III, Shahin S, Roberts WC. Clinicopathologic features of hypertrophic cardiomyopathy managed by cardiac transplantation. *Am J Cardiol* 1993;72:434–440.
8. Hecht GM, Heinrich GK, Roberts WC, Maron BJ. Coexistence of sudden cardiac death and end-stage heart failure in familial hypertrophic cardiomyopathy. *J Am Coll Cardiol* 1993;22:489–497.
9. Coutu M, Parrault LP, White M, Pelletier GB, Racine N, Poirier NC, Carrier M. Cardiac transplantation for hypertrophic cardiomyopathy: a valid therapeutic option. *J Heart Lung Transplant* 2004;43:413–417.
10. Biagini E, Spirito P, Leone O, Piccio FM, Coccolo F, Ragni L, Lofiego C, Grigioni F, Potena L, Rocchi G, Bacchi-Reggiani L, Boriani G, Prandstraller D, Arbustini E, Branzi A, Rapezzi C. Heart transplantation in hypertrophic cardiomyopathy. *Am J Cardiol* 2008;101:387–392.
11. Maron MS, Kalsmith BM, Udelson JE, Li W, DeNofrio D. Survival after cardiac transplantation in patients with hypertrophic cardiomyopathy. *Circ Heart Fail* 2010;3:574–579.
12. Kato TS, Takayama H, Yoshizawa S, Morboe C, Schulze PS, Farr M, Naka Y, Mancini D, Maurer MS. Cardiac transplantation in patients with hypertrophic cardiomyopathy. *Am J Cardiol* 2012;110:568–574.

Advanced Heart Failure With Preserved Systolic Function in Nonobstructive Hypertrophic Cardiomyopathy

Under-Recognized Subset of Candidates for Heart Transplant

Ethan J. Rowin, MD; Barry J. Maron, MD; Michael S. Kiernan, MD; Susan A. Casey, RN; David S. Feldman, MD; Katarzyna M. Hryniewicz, MD; Raymond H. Chan, MD; Kevin M. Harris, MD; James E. Udelson, MD; David DeNofrio, MD; William C. Roberts, MD; Martin S. Maron, MD

Background—In hypertrophic cardiomyopathy (HCM), heart transplant has been predominantly confined to patients with systolic dysfunction. An underappreciated HCM subset comprises patients with preserved left ventricular (LV) systolic function who may also require consideration for transplantation. Therefore, we sought to define the clinical profile and occurrence of advanced heart failure among patients with nonobstructive HCM and preserved systolic function.

Methods and Results—Databases from 2 referral centers comprising 2100 HCM patients were interrogated. Forty-six nonobstructive HCM patients (2.2%) either received or were listed for heart transplant, including 20 with normal systolic function (ejection fraction ≥50%). At transplant listing, these 20 patients were 42±13 years old, each in New York Heart Association functional class III/IV with ejection fraction of 62±7%. LV was hypertrophied with maximum wall thickness of 22±4 mm and nondilated (end-diastolic dimension, 39±7 mm). Cardiovascular magnetic resonance in 10 (of 15) patients showed no or minimal fibrosis (≤5% LV mass). Elevated LV end-diastolic or pulmonary capillary wedge pressure, consistent with diastolic dysfunction, was present in 15 patients (75%). LV filling was impaired by echocardiographic measures in all patients, including a restrictive inflow pattern in 8 (40%). In 2 patients, traditional criteria for transplant were absent, including peak V_{O_2} >14 mL/kg/min. Heart transplantation was performed in 12 patients with each alive and without cardiovascular symptoms, 2.3±1.7 years later.

Conclusions—A previously under-recognized segment of the broad HCM clinical spectrum consists of nonobstructive patients with advanced heart failure, in the presence of preserved systolic function, for whom heart transplant is the sole definitive therapeutic option. **(*Circ Heart Fail*. 2014;7:967-975.)**

Key Words: diastolic dysfunction ■ heart transplantation ■ hypertrophic cardiomyopathy

Sudden death has perhaps been the most visible adverse consequence of hypertrophic cardiomyopathy (HCM).[1–4] However, with the increased use of the implantable cardioverter defibrillator for primary prevention,[5–8] heart failure progression and death are emerging prominently within the natural history of HCM and with regard to strategies for disease management.[9–12] In this regard, heart transplantation has, by convention, been confined predominantly to those HCM patients evolving into the end-stage phase, characterized by left ventricular (LV) systolic dysfunction (ejection fraction [EF] <50%).[13–17] However, within the diverse HCM phenotypic spectrum, we have recently recognized a subgroup of nonobstructive patients with severe drug-refractory heart failure symptoms, but nevertheless have preserved LV systolic function; without other therapeutic options, these patients become candidates for heart transplant. Therefore, we take this opportunity to characterize the presentation, clinical profile, and outcome of this largely under-recognized subset within the HCM patient population.

Clinical Perspective on p 975

Methods

Patient Selection

HCM patient databases of 2 referral centers, Minneapolis Heart Institute Foundation (Minneapolis, MN) and Tufts Medical Center (Boston, MA), were accessed. Patients with HCM who had undergone heart transplant or were listed for transplant (2004–2013) were included. Patients who met the following criteria constitute the preserved LV systolic function study population: (1) EF ≥50%; (2) New York Heart Association (NYHA) functional class III/IV, refractory to maximum medical management; (3) LV outflow gradient <30 mm Hg

Received April 7, 2014; accepted September 15, 2014.

From the Department of Medicine, Hypertrophic Cardiomyopathy Center, Division of Cardiology, Tufts Medical Center, Boston, MA (E.J.R., M.S.K., J.E.U., D.D., M.S.M.); Department of Medicine, the Hypertrophic Cardiomyopathy Center, Minneapolis Heart Institute Foundation, Minneapolis, MN (B.J.M., S.A.C., D.S.F., K.M.H., K.M.H.); Departments of Medicine (Cardiovascular Division) and Radiology, Beth Israel Deaconess Medical Center, Boston, MA (R.H.C.); and Department of Pathology and Medicine, Baylor University Medical Center, Dallas, TX (W.C.R.).

Guest Editor for this article was Douglas L. Mann, MD.

The Data Supplement is available at http://circheartfailure.ahajournals.org/lookup/suppl/doi:10.1161/CIRCHEARTFAILURE.114.001435/-/DC1.

Correspondence to Martin S. Maron, MD, Tufts Medical Center, No. 70, 800 Washington St, Boston, MA 02111. E-mail mmaron@tuftsmedicalcenter.org at rest and with physiological (exercise) provocation. Patients with LV outflow obstruction who underwent septal reduction therapy and subsequently developed advanced heart failure were excluded (n=7).

Initial clinical evaluation was the first clinical assessment obtained at either participating institution. Transplant listing was defined as date of acceptance on the UNOS (united network for organ sharing) heart transplant list.[18] Most recent evaluation was obtained during clinic visit or by telephone interview. This study has been reviewed and approved by Institutional Review Boards of the participating institutions, Allina Health Systems and Tufts Medical Center, permitting use of patient medical information for research. All authors had full access and took responsibility for integrity of the data and agreed to the article as written.

Definitions

HCM Diagnosis

HCM diagnosis was made by echocardiographic and cardiovascular magnetic resonance (CMR) documentation of a hypertrophied and nondilated left ventricle (wall thickness ≥15 mm in adults), at some time during their clinical course, in the absence of another cardiac or systemic disease capable of producing a similar magnitude of hypertrophy.[1]

Heart Failure

Advanced heart failure was defined as symptom limitation to New York Heart Association (NYHA) functional class III or IV, characterized predominately by exertional dyspnea (with or without chest pain). Global LV systolic dysfunction (by convention, end-stage HCM) was arbitrarily defined by EF <50% at rest.[2,15] Patients with EF ≥50% were designated as preserved LV systolic function.[2]

Echocardiography

Transthoracic echocardiographic studies were performed with commercially available instruments 2.3±6.1 months before transplant listing. Magnitude of LV hypertrophy, left-atrial, and LV end-diastolic dimensions were obtained as previously described.[19] Mitral regurgitation was graded as mild, moderate, or severe by combined analysis of jet area, width, and spectral Doppler intensity. EF was calculated from 2-dimensional echocardiographic images with the modified Simpson rule formula or area-length method.

LV outflow tract obstruction because of systolic anterior motion of the mitral valve with septal contact was imaged in the apical views with continuous wave Doppler. Patients without an LV outflow gradient under basal conditions underwent exercise echocardiography performed with symptom-limited Bruce protocol. LV outflow tract gradient was reassessed immediately after exercise.[19]

Mitral inflow velocity and annular tissue Doppler indices signals were obtained, as previously described.[20] Peak pulsed Doppler velocities were assessed to determine early (E) and late (A) diastolic flow across the mitral valve. Tissue Doppler index of the mitral annulus was obtained from the apical 4-chamber view, and peak early tissue Doppler velocities of the septal mitral annulus (e′) were analyzed. Diastolic dysfunction was classified according to previous consensus recommendations.[20] Echocardiographic measures of diastolic function were not assessed in 2 patients because of presence of atrial fibrillation at the time of study.

Cardiovascular Magnetic Resonance

CMR studies were performed with a 1.5 Tesla clinical CMR scanner in 15 patients, while 5 patients did not undergo CMR examination because of a previously implanted implantable cardioverter defibrillator. Breath-hold cine steady state free precession sequences were performed in horizontal long axis, vertical long axis, and contiguous short axis slices with full coverage of LV and slice thickness of 10 mm with no gap. Short-axis cine stack was obtained parallel to atrioventricular groove, covering the entire LV chamber.

Late gadolinium enhancement (LGE) images were acquired 10 to 15 minutes after intravenous administration of 0.2 mmol/kg gadolinium-DTPA (Magnevist, Schering;Berlin Germany) using breath-held segmented inversion recovery sequence acquired in same orientations as the cine images. The LV short-axis stack of LGE images was first assessed visually for presence of LGE. Quantification of LGE was then performed on all LGE-positive studies by manually adjusting a grayscale threshold to define areas of visually identified LGE. These areas were then summed to generate a total volume of LGE and expressed as a proportion of total LV myocardium (%LGE).

Cardiopulmonary Stress Test

Cardiopulmonary stress testing was performed in 17 patients with symptom-limited erect treadmill exercise testing using a standard ramp protocol with simultaneous respiratory gas analysis. Peak oxygen consumption (Vo_2) was defined as the maximum Vo_2 achieved during exercise, expressed in ml/min/kg. Predicted % Vo_2 relative to patient age and sex was calculated according to established guidelines.[18]

Invasive Hemodynamics

Hemodynamic studies were performed on cardioactive medications, 1.9±3.1 months before transplant listing. Right atrial, pulmonary artery, pulmonary capillary pressures, and LV end-diastolic pressures were measured at end expiration and taken as the average of ≥3 beats. Cardiac output was determined by the Fick method using directly measured saturations and oxygen consumption and indexed to body surface area (cardiac index). Hemodynamic measurements were obtained with exercise in 3 patients in whom LV filling pressures were normal under resting conditions (mean PA pressure ≤25 mmHg and PCWP≤15 mmHg), and peak Vo_2 was >14 mL/min/kg. An exercise protocol was performed by outstretched arm adduction lifting of 4 pound weights until fatigue, with hemodynamic parameters measured after peak exercise and at 1 minute recovery.

Statistical Analysis

Data are displayed as mean± SD for continuous variables and as proportions for categorical variables. Student's *t* test or Wilcoxon rank-sum test assessed statistical significance for continuous variables and χ^2 or Fisher's exact tests for categorical variables. *P* values <0.05 were considered significant and 2-sided where appropriate. Statistical analyses were performed with SAS for Windows version 9.3 (SAS Institute Inc, Cary, NC).

Results

Prevalence, Demographics, and Clinical Profile

Of the 2100 HCM patients in the cohort, 46 (2.2%) had been transplanted, listed for transplant, or died while awaiting transplantation. Of these 46 patients, 26 (1.2%) had systolic dysfunction (EF <50%) and were considered to be in the end-stage phase of HCM, while the other 20 patients (1.0%) had preserved EF ≥50% and constitute the study group (prevalence, 9.5 per 1000 HCM patients; Figure 1 and Table 1).

Among the 20 study patients (11 men), initial HCM diagnosis was at 32±15 years of age (range 12–61) and onset of heart failure symptoms at 35±16 years (Figure 2). Patients were listed for transplant at 42±13 years (range 16–66; Tables 2 and 3). Duration between symptom onset and listing was 8.0±8.9 years, including 6 patients listed <2 years after symptom onset and 9 patients ≥5 years after symptoms developed.

Among the 20 nonobstructive HCM patients with preserved LV systolic function, 12 underwent transplant at a mean age of 42±16 years (220±181 days after listing), including 4 patients <30 years of age, 5 patients between 40 and 49 years, and 3 patients >50 years. Time on the waiting list before transplantation ranged from 21 to 615 days (mean, 0.6±0.5 years).

In 14 of the 20 patients, ≥1 family member was known to have HCM, including 5 (25%) with a first-degree relative who developed end-stage HCM (EF=34±2%). Two of the family

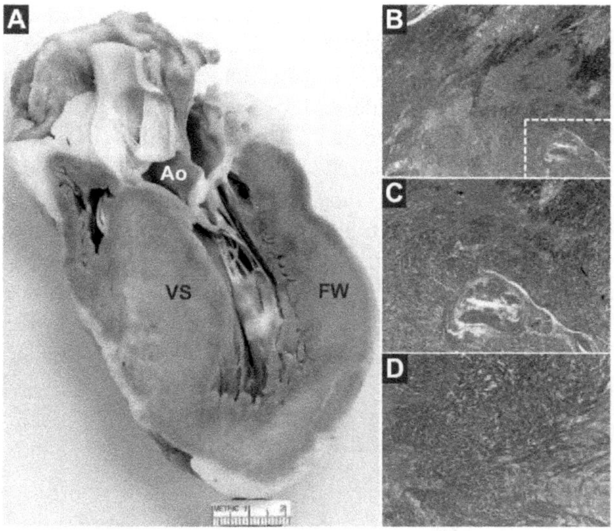

Figure 1. Explanted gross heart sectioned longitudinally (**A**) and histopathology (**B–D**) from a 50-year-old woman who underwent transplant for progressive severe heart failure refractory to pharmacological therapy in the presence of preserved left ventricular systolic function (EF=65%; No. 15 in Table 2). **A**, Ventricular septal thickness is marked (30 mm), left ventricular cavity is small, and distribution of hypertrophy is asymmetrical. Heart weight is 450 g. Patchy scarring (white areas) is visible in the septum, left ventricular free wall near the apex and in both papillary muscles. **B**, Area of myocardial scar (stained blue) in ventricular septum adjacent to an abnormal intramural coronary artery evident in the box at lower right. Original magnification 20×. **C**, A higher power micrograph of intramural coronary artery with thickened wall (media) and narrowed lumen, shown in panel B. Original magnification 40×. **D**, Area of viable myocardium (stained red) with cardiac muscle cells arranged in disorganized patterns. Original magnification 40×. Ao indicates aorta; FW, free wall; and VS, ventricular septum. Masson trichome stain for **B–D**.

members in the end-stage (mothers of patients Nos. 6 and 8) required heart transplant at 51 and 58 years of age, respectively, whereas the remaining 3 relatives in end-stage are alive, symptomatic, but without transplant.

A variety of pathogenic sarcomeric protein mutations were identified in 6 of 9 patients who underwent genetic testing: MYH7 (n=3), ACTC1 (n=1), TNNI (n=1), and TPM1 (n=1; Tables 2 and 3), including 1 patient with a family member in the end stage with the identical mutation (MYH7 Arg723Cys; patient No. 1).

Phenotypic Expression

Based on echocardiography, CMR, and pathological examination of explanted hearts (n=8), each patient had a hypertrophied, thick-walled LV in the presence of a nondilated ventricular cavity. Maximum LV wall thickness (usually in ventricular septum) was 22±4 mm (range, 15–34 mm) by echocardiography, including 4 patients with 25 to 29 mm and 2 patients with massive hypertrophy, that is, ≥30 mm (Figures 1 and 3). LV cavity size was small, 39±7-mm end-diastolic dimension (range, 29–52 mm, and ≤40 mm in 10 patients). Left atrial diameter was 46±8 (range, 31–57 mm). EF was 62±7% (range, 55–70%), including 6 patients with an EF of 70% and 5 with EF of 55%.

Coronary artery patency was examined by arteriogram or CT angiography in 18 of 20 patients and by examination of the explanted heart in the other 2. Atherosclerotic coronary artery disease (ie., ≥50% luminal narrowing in ≥1 epicardial vessels) was absent in each patient. Three patients had a history of angina responsible for functional limitation, considered to be HCM-related.

Table 1. Demographic and Clinical Variables of 20 HCM Patients with Preserved Systolic Function and 26 End-Stage HCM Patients With or Considered for Heart Transplantation

Variable	Preserved LV Systolic Function, EF ≥50% (n=20)	End-stage HCM EF <50% (n=26)	*P* Value
Male, n (%)	11 (55%)	15 (58%)	0.86
Age at HCM diagnosis, y	32±15	28±15	0.44
Age at development of NYHA III/IV symptoms, y	35±16	33±16	0.78
Age at transplant listing, y	42±13	42±13	0.98
Family history of HCM, n (%)	14 (70%)	16 (62%)	0.56
Family history of end-stage HCM, n (%)	5 (25%)	5 (19%)	0.88
EF, %	62±7	39±12	0.0001‡
LVED, mm	39±7	50±9	0.0001‡
LA dimension, mm	46±8	49±11	0.30
Maximal LV wall thickness, mm	22±4	18±4	0.003‡
Diastolic dysfunction*			
Grade I (impaired relaxation)	4 (22%)	3 (19%)	0.81
Grade II (pseudonormal)	6 (33%)	8 (50%)	0.32
Grade III (restrictive)	8 (45%)	5 (31%)	0.43
E/e′	12±4	13±5	0.64
Peak Vo_2, ml/kg/min	14.6±5.6	12.2±3.3	0.12
Presence of LGE on CMR, n (%)	10/15 (66%)†	5/6 (83%)†	0.47
Extent of LGE on CMR, %	9±8	13±10	0.07
Invasive hemodynamics			
RA pressure, mm Hg	12±9	12±7	0.95
Mean PA pressure, mm Hg	31±11	28±9	0.27
PCWP, mm Hg	22±7	19±9	0.33
Cardiac index, L/min/m² (Fick Method)	2.2±0.7	2.1±0.5	0.71
Outcome			
Heart transplant	12 (60%)	15 (58%)	0.88
Death awaiting transplant	2 (10%)	6 (23%)	0.26
Active on transplant list	6 (30%)	5 (19%)	0.41

Values as mean±standard deviation, or number (% of subjects), when applicable.

CMR indicates cardiac MRI; EF, ejection fraction; HCM, hypertrophic cardiomyopathy; LA, left atrium; LGE, late gadolinium enhancement; LV, left ventricular; LVED, left ventricular end-diastolic dimension; NYHA, New York Heart Association; PA, pulmonary artery; PCWP, pulmonary capillary wedge pressure; RA, right atrium; and VO_2, peak oxygen consumption.

*Diastolic function available in 18 patients with preserved systolic function and 16 patients in the end stage.

†Out of 15 patients with preserved LV systolic function and 6 patients in the end-stage phase who underwent cardiovascular magnetic resonance.

‡indicates $P<0.01$.

Hemodynamics

Evidence of increased LV filling pressure, consistent with diastolic dysfunction, was present at cardiac catheterization

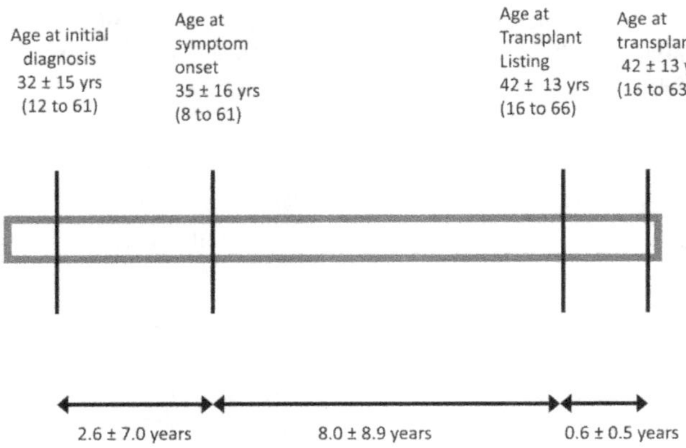

Figure 2. Timeline representing the clinical course of patients with nonobstructive hypertrophic cardiomyopathy, preserved left ventricular systolic function, and progression to advanced heart failure symptoms.

under basal conditions in 15 patients (75%), including LV end-diastolic pressure >15 mmHg in 5 patients (range, 20–30) and pulmonary capillary wedge pressure >15 mmHg in 8 patients without left heart catheterization (>25 mmHg in 6; Tables 2 and 3). In 2 patients, pressures were normal at rest, but increased substantially at peak exertion (wedge pressure, 26 and 28 mmHg). With echocardiography, diastolic dysfunction was assessed in 13 patients in sinus rhythm, each with impaired LV filling patterns: restrictive (Grade III) in 8, pseudonormal (Grade II) in 3, and impaired relaxation (Grade I) in 2.

Of the 5 remaining study patients, each had normal LV filling pressures at rest. Invasive hemodynamic assessment with exercise was not performed in 4 (because of particularly severe functional limitation), and in 1 patient, LV filling pressures were normal at rest and with exercise. However, in each of these 5 patients, there was evidence of diastolic dysfunction by echocardiography (Grade I in 2 and Grade II in 3).

Pathology/Myocardial Fibrosis

Explanted Hearts

Native explanted hearts were available for gross and histological examination in 8 patients (Figure 1). Heart weight was increased in each (508±94 g in males and 418±61 g in females), including two >500 g. In each, histopathology showed cardiac muscle cell disorganization and abnormal

Table 2. Clinical and Demographic Data From 20 Patients With HCM and Preserved Systolic Function Listed for Heart Transplant

Patient	Gender	Age at TP Listing, y	Age at Dx, y	Age at 1st HF Symptoms, y	Time From Listing to TP, y	History of Atrial Fibrillation	Family Hx HCM	NSVT	Genetic Testing	LVED, mm	LA Dimension, mm	Max LV Thickness, mm	EF, %	Mitral Regurgitation (0–4+)
1	F	16	12	12	0.64	N	Y; ES	N	MYH7* Arg723Cys	30	36	20	60	1+
2	M	20	20	19	1.13	Ch-AF	N	N	…	47	55	18	55	1+
3	M	22	12	22	1.68	N	N	Y	MYH7 Arg719Trp	49	49	21	55	1+
4	F	28	12	12	0.44	P-AF	Y	N	MYH7†	29	42	23	60	0
5	F	33	25	32	…	N	N	N	TNNI3 Ala157Val	39	34	18	60	1+
6	F	40	24	8	0.29	Ch-AF	Y: ES, TP	N	…	35	54	25	70	1+
7	M	41	27	29	…	P-AF	N	N	TPM1 Glu96Asp	29	42	24	70	1+
8	M	41	25	37	…	N	Y: ES, TP	N	…	41	47	34	60	1+
9	F	41	23	22	0.44	P-AF	N	N	…	38	53	27	70	1+
10	F	43	41	42	…	N	Y: SD	N	…	33	39	26	70	1+
11	M	44	39	38	…	N	Y	Y	…	45	44	23	70	0
12	M	45	37	42	0.21	Ch-AF	Y	N	…	31	49	21	55	1+
13	M	46	43	44	1.21	P-AF	Y	Y	…	44	52	21	65	1+
14	M	48	47	48	0.69	P-AF	Y: ES	N	…	52	48	17	60	0
15	F	50	39	49	0.17	N	Y: SD	N	ACTC Ala323Val	47	36	30	65	0
16	F	51	20	28	…	P-AF	Y	N	…	42	57	21	65	2+
17	M	54	44	46	…	P-AF	Y	N	…	41	46	15	55	1+
18	F	57	29	48	0.28	P-AF	Y	N	…	29	53	16	65	1+
19	M	63	58	58	0.06	N	Y: ES, SD	Y	…	35	31	21	70	1+
20	M	66	61	61	…	Ch-AF	N	Y	…	46	56	26	55	2+

ACTC indicates α cardiac actin 1; Ch-AF, chronic atrial fibrillation; Dx, diagnosis; EF, ejection fraction; ES, end stage HCM; HCM, hypertrophic cardiomyopathy; HF, heart failure; LA, left atrium; LV, left ventricular; LVED, left ventricular end-diastolic dimension; MYH7, β myosin heavy chain; NSVT, nonsustained ventricular tachycardia; SD, sudden cardiac death; TNNI3, cardiac troponin I; TPM1, tropomyosin 1 α; and TP, transplant.

*Identical disease causing mutation identified in the patient's father with end-stage HCM.

†Double mutation in MYH7:Arg719Trp, His581Arg (1 inherited from father, 1 from mother).

Table 3. Clinical and Outcome Data for 20 Patients With HCM and Preserved Systolic Function Listed for Heart Transplant

Patient	E/A	E/E′	Deceleration Time, ms	Diastolic Filling Pattern, Grade	Peak Vo_2, ml/min/kg	LGE on CMR, %	RA Pressure, mm Hg	PA Pressure S/D (mean), mm Hg	PCWP Pressure, mm Hg	LV end Diastolic Pressure, mm Hg	Fick CO; CI, L/min; L/min/m²	Inotrope as Bridge to Transplant	Outcome
1	1.3	9.8	170	II	20.1*	0	4	29/13 (20)	14‖	...	3.1;2.4	Mil	TP;Alive
2	2.8	10.7	140	III	22.8*	0	34	60/40 (47)	30	...	2.4;1.3	Mil	TP; Alive
3	2.0	7.8	160	II	12.5	...	4	46/21 (31)	23	...	8.0;4.0	Mil	TP; Alive
4	2.7	6.1	166	III	9.6	0	11	43/23 (30)	21	30	1.4;0.9	...	TP; Alive†
5	0.8	8.6	180	I	24.6	0	7	26/13 (18)	15‡	...	4.0;2.3	...	TL: Status 2
6	1.7	8.6	200	II	...	4.4	8	50/21 (32)	20	...	3.6;1.9	...	TP; Alive§
7	1.8	13.5	140	III	18.6*	1.1	11	38/23 (30)	20	...	4.0;1.8	...	TL: Status 2
8	1.8	13.7	160	II	14.0	...	7	34/3 (25)	15‖	10	3.4;1.9	...	Died on TL
9	...	24	167	...	16.1	2.0	7	54/22 (36)	26	...	4.2;2.7	Mil	TP; alive
10	0.8	12.6	240	I	16.2	4.7	12	32/18 (22)	14¶	...	5.4;2.8	...	TL: Status 2
11	3.1	10.6	94	III	...	2.5	31	69/36 (50)	31	26	7.0;2.9	...	Died on TL#
12	3.1	17.4	100	III	10.1	21.0	11	51/27 (35)	23	...	4.4;2.1	Mil	TP; Alive
13	0.7	9.0	210	I	10.0	1.8	5	29/13 (20)	11‖	9	5.9;2.7	...	TP: Alive†
14	1.4	14.0	271	II	9.5	7.9	7	50/24 (41)	26	30	2.9;1.4	...	TP; Alive†
15	1.5	9.2	184	II	...	...	5	23/12 (16)	11‖	15	4.5;2.7	Mil+Dob	TP; Alive
16	3.5	16.7	132	III	9.3	...	10	40/20 (27)	25	20	3.2;1.6	...	TL: Status 2
17	2.0	16.8	120	III	8.6	...	15	71/39 (50)	35	...	2.6;1.6	Mil	TL: Status 1b
18	2.7	13.0	140	III	6.7	0	22	47/30 (35)	30	...	3.1;1.4	Mil	TP; Alive**
19	1.0	11.4	221	I	19.3	7.2	5	26/12 (16)	15‡	...	5.7;2.7	Mil+Dob	TP; Alive
20	...	14.2	120	...	20.4	18	17	52/26 (35)	26	20	4.0/2.0	...	TL: Status 2

CI indicates cardiac Index; CMR, cardiac MRI; CO, cardiac output; Dob, dobutamine; HCM, hypertrophic cardiomyopathy; LGE, late gadolinium enhancement; LV, left ventricular; LVED, left ventricular end-diastolic dimension; Mil, milrinone; PA, pulmonary artery; PCWP, pulmonary capillary wedge pressure; RA, right atrium; S/D, peak systolic/end diastolic; TL, transplant list; TP, transplant; and VO_2, peak oxygen consumption.

*<50% predicted for age.

†Received transplant as exception status.

‡Normal resting LV filling pressures but abnormal exercise hemodynamic (mean PA pressure >30, WP >25).

§Nipride used to optimize hemodynamics as bridge to transplant.

‖Normal resting LV filling pressures, invasive exercise hemodynamic not obtained.

¶Normal resting and exercise LV filling pressures (mean PA ≤30, WP ≤25).

#VAD placed as bridge to transplant.

**Intra-aortic balloon pump placed as bridge to transplant.

intramural coronary arteries typical of HCM.[1] With gross and histopathologic examination, fibrosis was absent or minimal in 5 hearts (Figure 1), whereas moderate-to-extensive diffuse amounts of patchy nontransmural myocardial fibrosis was evident in ventricular septum and lateral wall of 3 hearts.

Percent LGE

Myocardial fibrosis was assessed by contrast-enhanced CMR in 15 patients (Figure 3). LGE was absent in 5 and present in 10 occupying 9±8% of LV mass (range 1.8%–21%), with 5 minimal and focal (<5% of LV mass) and 3 extensive/diffuse (≥15% of LV mass).

Atrial Fibrillation

Atrial fibrillation was present in 12 patients, paroxysmal in 8 and persistent in 4. Attempts to restore and maintain sinus rhythm were unsuccessful with both electric cardioversion and antiarrhythmic drugs (ie, amiodarone [n=8], dofetilide [n=3], disopyramide [n=3], dronedarone [n=1], and sotalol [n=1]). In 7 patients, isolated pulmonary vein radiofrequency ablation was unsuccessful in restoring and maintaining sinus rhythm. Although heart failure symptoms were exacerbated in atrial fibrillation, all patients were in NYHA functional class III heart failure even when in sinus rhythm.

Pharmacological and Mechanical Support

Efforts to control heart failure symptoms and chest pain with drug treatment were unsuccessful in all patients, including administration of β-blockers and calcium channel blockers (n=20), diuretics (n=14), angiotensin-converting enzyme inhibitor or angiotension receptor blocker (n=7), aldosterone inhibitor (n=2), or ranolazine/nitrates (n=2). In addition, inotropic therapy (milrinone, n=7; combination milirinone and dobutamine, n=2) was administered to 9 patients. In-hospital support was necessary in 2 patients because of particularly unstable hemodynamic profiles using an LV-assist device in 1 (Thoratec Percutaneous Ventricular Assist Device, Pleasanton, CA) for management of refractory cardiogenic shock with end-organ dysfunction[21] and an intra-aortic balloon pump for persistently low cardiac index (despite inotropic therapy) in 1.

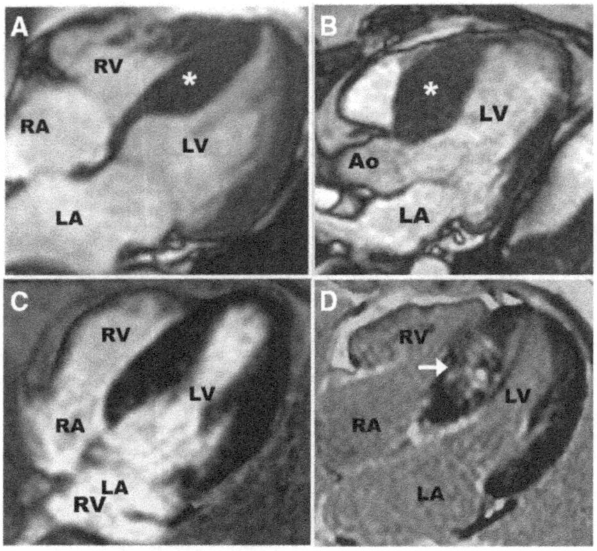

Figure 3. Cardiac MRI images of 3 nonobstructive hypertrophic cardiomyopathy patients with preserved systolic function and 1 patient in the end-stage phase with systolic dysfunction (EF<50%), each of whom either received heart transplant or are currently listed for transplant. **A**, Four-chamber long-axis image from a 41-year-old man genotyped to a pathogenic sarcomere mutation (TPM1 Glu 96 Asp) with normal systolic function (EF=70%), small LV cavity (end-diastolic diameter=29 mm), and septal thickness of 24 mm (asterisk; patient No. 7, Tables 2 and 3). **B**, Three-chamber long-axis image in a 63-year-old man with EF of 60% and ventricular septal hypertrophy (21 mm; asterisk) who required inotropic support with intravenous milrinone and dobutamine before heart transplant (patient No. 19). **C**, Four-chamber long-axis contrast-enhanced image demonstrating absence of late gadolinium enhancement (LGE; ie.,fibrosis) in a 33-year-old woman with New York Heart Association functional class IV symptoms, currently status II listed for heart transplant (patient No. 5); **D**, Contrast-enhanced 4-chamber long-axis image in a 23-year-old man with end-stage hypertrophic cardiomyopathy: ejection fraction of 30%, LV end-diastolic cavity dimension of 53 mm, and extensive transmural LGE (arrow) occupying 21% of LV myocardial mass. Ao indicates aorta; LA, left atrium; LV, left ventricle; RA, right atrium; and RV, right ventricle.

Clinical Determinants of Heart Transplant Listing

In each of the 20 patients, the primary indication for transplant listing was a clinical history of disabling heart failure symptoms of exertional dyspnea (with or without chest pain), consistent with NYHA III/IV and refractory to optimal medical therapy. At least 1 additional clinical criteria supporting the need for transplantation was present in 18 patients, including (1) peak Vo_2 ≤14 mL/min/kg or <50% predicted for age in 12 patients (Nos. 1–4, 7, 8, 12–14, and 16–18 in Tables 2 and 3); (2) unfavorable resting hemodynamic profile, including elevated LV filling pressures or impaired cardiac index, in 14 patients (Nos. 2–4, 6–9, 11, 12, 14, 16–18, and 20); and (3) acute hemodynamic deterioration requiring inotropic therapy or mechanical support in 10 patients (Nos. 1–3, 9, 11, 12, 15, and 17–19). Therefore, 5 patients had 1 additional supporting criteria for transplant, 8 patients had 2 criteria, and 5 had 3 supporting criteria.

In the remaining 2 patients, inotropic therapy or mechanical support was not required and other traditional criteria for transplant listing were absent, including peak Vo_2 >14 mL/min/kg or ≥50% predicted for age and normal resting hemodynamic profile (patient Nos. 5 and 10). These patients were listed for transplant solely because of refractory disabling symptoms by history, judged secondary to HCM. In addition, 3 patients (No. 4, 13, and 14) were allowed exceptions by the regional transplant committee to obtain an advanced transplant status (ie., 1Ae or 1Be) than would otherwise be granted, given that traditional therapies that allow 1A or 1B listing criteria are generally not indicated in patients with HCM and preserved LV systolic function.[2]

Outcome

Twelve patients received a heart transplant and each is currently alive, without cardiovascular symptoms (NYHA functional class I), after 0.5 to 6.3 years (mean 2.3±1.7; Table I in the Data Supplement). In addition, after transplant, invasive hemodynamics parameters were significantly improved, including pulmonary capillary wedge pressure and cardiac index (P<0.001), without a significant change in EF (63±6% versus 62±4%; P=0.82; Table I in the Data Supplement). Six patients remain active on the transplant list as status 1B (n=1) or status 2 (n=5). Two patients died of unrelenting heart failure awaiting transplant.

Comparison of Patients With Preserved LV Systolic Function and End Stage

Compared with the study patients with preserved systolic function, those with EF <50% (end-stage) demonstrated evidence of adverse LV remodeling with increased cavity size (50±9 versus 39±7 mm; P<0.001), lesser degree of hypertrophy (wall thickness, 18±4 versus 22±4 mm; P=0.006), and a trend toward more extensive myocardial fibrosis on contrast-enhanced CMR (% LGE of LV myocardium, 18±10 versus 9±8; P=0.07; Table 1 and Figure 3). Particularly extensive fibrosis (LGE ≥15%) was present in 4 of 6 (67%) end-stage HCM patients compared with only 3 of 15 (20%) with preserved systolic function. Several relevant clinical variables were similar between the 2 subgroups, including peak Vo_2, LV filling pressures, age at heart failure symptom onset, and time from onset of symptoms to transplant listing (Table 1).

Discussion

Advanced heart failure has become increasingly important among patients with HCM, given the capability of sudden death prevention afforded by the implantable cardioverter defibrillator.[4–8] This evolving recognition underscores the importance of reliably identifying those HCM patients who may be candidates for major life prolonging heart failure therapies. Heart transplantation has traditionally been reserved largely for patients in the end stage of HCM, arbitrarily defined by EF <50%.[2,9,15] In this regard, we have recently recognized a subset of nonobstructive HCM patients eligible for heart transplant because of severe, unrelenting heart failure symptoms refractory to pharmacological treatment, despite evidence of preserved LV systolic function. Therefore, we describe here the clinical profile and natural history of this under-recognized patient subset within the broad disease spectrum of HCM.

By interrogating the databases of 2 major HCM referral cohorts, we found that 2% of patients were listed for heart transplantation, and among these, more than 40% demonstrated a disease phenotype distinctly different from those nonobstructive patients eligible for heart transplant in the end-stage phase, characterized by impaired systolic function and often associated with LV remodeling with regression of hypertrophy and ventricular chamber enlargement.[15,16] In contrast, the novel subgroup reported here experienced progressive and advanced heart failure refractory to maximal medical management, despite demonstrating little or no evidence of LV chamber remodeling. For example, average LV wall thickness was 22 mm (up to 34 mm), and LV cavity dimensions were normal or small, typical of that encountered in the overall HCM disease spectrum.[2] In addition, HCM transplant candidates with systolic dysfunction characteristically show diffuse (and often transmural) LV myocardial scarring grossly visible by examination of the explanted heart and also identifiable by contrast-enhanced CMR (ie, occupying on average almost 20% of total LV mass).[9,15,22] However, in contrast, most of our patients with advanced heart failure and preserved systolic function showed no or minimal myocardial fibrosis.

However, despite these substantial differences in phenotypic expression, our study patients with normal systolic function became transplant candidates in the absence of any other available therapeutic option capable of restoring reasonable expectation for an improved and acceptable quality of life with increased functional capacity. Indeed, each transplanted patient has survived without significant transplant-related complications over a 6-year period and without residual cardiovascular symptoms. Indeed, survival after heart transplant for HCM patients has been shown to be similar (if not better)[23–26] than that for patients with other cardiac diseases, with 75% and 61% survival 5- and 10-years post-transplant.[25] This experience underscores the principle that nonobstructive HCM patients with advanced heart failure symptoms, refractory to medical therapies, can (and should be) considered for cardiac transplantation as a final therapeutic option, even in the presence of normal or hyperdynamic LV systolic function and substantial increase in LV mass.

We found no relevant clinical or imaging marker that adequately predicted risk for advanced heart failure in this subset of HCM patients. Nevertheless, a disproportionate number of probands (ie, 25%) reported here with preserved systolic function had a family history of end-stage HCM with reduced EF and LV remodeling, including 2 relatives who required heart transplant. That relatives within the same HCM family (and presumably with the same disease-causing mutation) progressed to transplant with distinctly different phenotypic expressions[15,27,28] supports the principle that no definitive relationship has been established in HCM between individual sarcomere mutations and cardiac phenotype.[29–31]

The predominant mechanism responsible for the progressive symptoms of heart failure experienced by the HCM patients reported here seems to be LV diastolic dysfunction. This view is supported by evidence of abnormal LV filling at rest (or with exercise) at cardiac catheterization and with echocardiography in each patient, and in the absence of other mechanisms known to produce heart failure in HCM, for example, LV outflow tract obstruction,[10] marked mitral regurgitation,[32] and associated atherosclerotic coronary artery disease.[33] Notably, almost one half of our patients demonstrated a restrictive filling by echocardiography, previously shown to identify HCM patients at increased risk for progressive heart failure and transplant, independent of LV systolic function.[34]

Nevertheless, we recognize that the decision to pursue transplant in this subset of HCM patients is complex and challenging and ultimately requires taking into account the individual clinical profile of the patient, with the greatest weight given to the clinical history and symptom profile. Indeed, 10% of our patients with preserved systolic function were considered for transplant even in the absence of traditional parameters, such as peak Vo_2 consumption ≤14 mL/kg/min,[18] after recognition that transplant was the only therapeutic option with the capacity to restore an acceptable quality of life.

Our observations also have implications for current transplant listing criteria, which are based largely on an experience in patients with systolic heart failure and diseases other than HCM, principally ischemic and dilated cardiomyopathies.[18] This underscores the need for clinicians familiar with HCM to participate closely with multidisciplinary heart failure/transplant team to ensure optimal treatment strategies are implemented for this unique subset of HCM patients, including appropriate candidacy for heart transplant.[35]

Notably, the clinical course of HCM patients with advanced heart failure and preserved systolic function proved to be variable, and becoming transplant candidates at a broad range of ages (16–63 years), and at an average age of only 41 years. Furthermore, there were relatively modest time periods between onset of symptoms and listing for transplant (average, 8 years) and particularly between listing and the transplant itself (average, only 0.6 years). Therefore, these data underscore the importance of close longitudinal follow-up for nonobstructive HCM patients with limiting heart failure symptoms and a relatively high index of suspicion and low threshold to pursue cardiovascular evaluation for heart transplantation.[2,13,14]

Several clinical studies and expert consensus guidelines in HCM have, by convention, arbitrarily considered an EF ≥50% to represent preserved systolic function,[1,2,9,14,15,17] which served as the justification for choosing this specific EF cut point to identify our study cohort. However, most importantly, we recognize that HCM encompasses a broad range in EF (ie, from hyperdynamic to systolic dysfunction)[22] expressing a continuum of cardiac systolic function and advanced heart failure because (1) some patients with preserved LV systolic function have relatives with HCM and systolic dysfunction, including transplant candidates;[27,28] (2) several objective measures of advanced heart failure were similar between the 2 groups, including invasive measures of elevated LV filling pressures and level of functional limitation by cardiopulmonary exercise testing; and (3) a variability in the extent of myocardial fibrosis (LGE) evident by some patients with preserved LV systolic function showing substantial LGE and others with systolic dysfunction having minimal or no LGE.[15]

The number of HCM patients considered for transplant with preserved LV systolic function in this study is small (n=20). This limitation is unavoidable given the infrequency in which this subset of patient occurs in this disease. Therefore, it is unlikely that prospective studies with substantially greater numbers of these particular patients will emerge in the near future.

In conclusion, we report a novel subgroup of patients with nonobstructive HCM, who developed advanced progressive heart failure and become transplant candidates, despite preserved systolic function and in the absence of significant LV remodeling. This emerging subgroup expands the spectrum of heart failure requiring transplant in HCM and includes patients with normal LV systolic function. The pathophysiologic determinant of this novel clinical course seems to be LV diastolic dysfunction. However, the severity of symptoms was not always supported by traditional heart transplant testing criteria, and the decision to offer transplant as a final therapeutic option should be made on an individual patient basis in the presence of advanced and refractory heart failure.

Disclosures

None.

References

1. Maron BJ, Maron MS. Hypertrophic cardiomyopathy. *Lancet*. 2013;381:242–255.
2. Gersh BJ, Maron BJ, Bonow RO, Dearani JA, Fifer MA, Link MS, Naidu SS, Nishimura RA, Ommen SR, Rakowski H, Seidman CE, Towbin JA, Udelson JE, Yancy CW; American College of Cardiology Foundation/American Heart Association Task Force on Practice Guidelines; American Association for Thoracic Surgery; American Society of Echocardiography; American Society of Nuclear Cardiology; Heart Failure Society of America; Heart Rhythm Society; Society for Cardiovascular Angiography and Interventions; Society of Thoracic Surgeons. 2011 ACCF/AHA guideline for the diagnosis and treatment of hypertrophic cardiomyopathy: a report of the American College of Cardiology Foundation/American Heart Association Task Force on Practice Guidelines. *Circulation*. 2011;124:e783–e831.
3. Elliott PM, Poloniecki J, Dickie S, Sharma S, Monserrat L, Varnava A, Mahon NG, McKenna WJ. Sudden death in hypertrophic cardiomyopathy: identification of high risk patients. *J Am Coll Cardiol*. 2000;36:2212–2218.
4. O'Mahony C, Jichi F, Pavlou M, Monserrat L, Anastasakis A, Rapezzi C, Biagini E, Gimeno JR, Limongelli G, McKenna WJ, Omar RZ, Elliott PM; Hypertrophic Cardiomyopathy Outcomes Investigators. A novel clinical risk prediction model for sudden cardiac death in hypertrophic cardiomyopathy (HCM Risk-SCD). *Eur Heart J*. 2014;35:2010–2020.
5. Maron BJ, Spirito P, Shen WK, Haas TS, Formisano F, Link MS, Epstein AE, Almquist AK, Daubert JP, Lawrenz T, Boriani G, Estes NA III, Favale S, Piccininno M, Winters SL, Santini M, Betocchi S, Arribas F, Sherrid MV, Buja G, Semsarian C, Bruzzi P. Implantable cardioverter-defibrillators and prevention of sudden cardiac death in hypertrophic cardiomyopathy. *JAMA*. 2007;298:405–412.
6. Maron BJ, Spirito P, Ackerman MJ, Casey SA, Semsarian C, Estes NA III, Shannon KM, Ashley EA, Day SM, Pacileo G, Formisano F, Devoto E, Anastasakis A, Bos JM, Woo A, Autore C, Pass RH, Boriani G, Garberich RF, Almquist AK, Russell MW, Boni L, Berger S, Maron MS, Link MS. Prevention of sudden cardiac death with implantable cardioverter-defibrillators in children and adolescents with hypertrophic cardiomyopathy. *J Am Coll Cardiol*. 2013;61:1527–1535.
7. Vriesendorp PA, Schinkel AF, Van Cleemput J, Willems R, Jordaens LJ, Theuns DA, van Slegtenhorst MA, de Ravel TJ, ten Cate FJ, Michels M. Implantable cardioverter-defibrillators in hypertrophic cardiomyopathy: patient outcomes, rate of appropriate and inappropriate interventions, and complications. *Am Heart J*. 2013;166:496–502.
8. Olde Nordkamp LR, Wilde AA, Tijssen JG, Knops RE, van Dessel PF, de Groot JR. The ICD for primary prevention in patients with inherited cardiac diseases: indications, use, and outcome: a comparison with secondary prevention. *Circ Arrhythm Electrophysiol*. 2013;6:91–100.
9. Melacini P, Basso C, Angelini A, Calore C, Bobbo F, Tokajuk B, Bellini N, Smaniotto G, Zucchetto M, Iliceto S, Thiene G, Maron BJ. Clinicopathological profiles of progressive heart failure in hypertrophic cardiomyopathy. *Eur Heart J*. 2010;31:2111–2123.
10. Maron MS, Olivotto I, Betocchi S, Casey SA, Lesser JR, Losi MA, Cecchi F, Maron BJ. Effect of left ventricular outflow tract obstruction on clinical outcome in hypertrophic cardiomyopathy. *N Engl J Med*. 2003;348:295–303.
11. Ommen SR, Maron BJ, Olivotto I, Maron MS, Cecchi F, Betocchi S, Gersh BJ, Ackerman MJ, McCully RB, Dearani JA, Schaff HV, Danielson GK, Tajik AJ, Nishimura RA. Long-term effects of surgical septal myectomy on survival in patients with obstructive hypertrophic cardiomyopathy. *J Am Coll Cardiol*. 2005;46:470–476.
12. Sorajja P, Ommen SR, Holmes DR Jr, Dearani JA, Rihal CS, Gersh BJ, Lennon RJ, Nishimura RA. Survival after alcohol septal ablation for obstructive hypertrophic cardiomyopathy. *Circulation*. 2012;126:2374–2380.
13. Kato TS, Takayama H, Yoshizawa S, Marboe C, Schulze PC, Farr M, Naka Y, Mancini D, Maurer MS. Cardiac transplantation in patients with hypertrophic cardiomyopathy. *Am J Cardiol*. 2012;110:568–574.
14. Biagini E, Spirito P, Leone O, Picchio FM, Coccolo F, Ragni L, Lofiego C, Grigioni F, Potena L, Rocchi G, Bacchi-Reggiani L, Boriani G, Prandstraller D, Arbustini E, Branzi A, Rapezzi C. Heart transplantation in hypertrophic cardiomyopathy. *Am J Cardiol*. 2008;101:387–392.
15. Harris KM, Spirito P, Maron MS, Zenovich AG, Formisano F, Lesser JR, Mackey-Bojack S, Manning WJ, Udelson JE, Maron BJ. Prevalence, clinical profile, and significance of left ventricular remodeling in the end-stage phase of hypertrophic cardiomyopathy. *Circulation*. 2006;114:216–225.
16. Fernández A, Vigliano CA, Casabé JH, Diez M, Favaloro LE, Guevara E, Favaloro RR, Laguens RP. Comparison of prevalence, clinical course, and pathological findings of left ventricular systolic impairment versus normal systolic function in patients with hypertrophic cardiomyopathy. *Am J Cardiol*. 2011;108:548–555.
17. Maron BJ, McKenna WJ, Danielson GK, Kappenberger LJ, Kuhn HJ, Seidman CE, Shah PM, Spencer WH III, Spirito P, Ten Cate FJ, Wigle ED; Task Force on Clinical Expert Consensus Documents. American College of Cardiology; Committee for Practice Guidelines. European Society of Cardiology. American College of Cardiology/European Society of Cardiology clinical expert consensus document on hypertrophic cardiomyopathy. A report of the American College of Cardiology Foundation Task Force on Clinical Expert Consensus Documents and the European Society of Cardiology Committee for Practice Guidelines. *J Am Coll Cardiol*. 2003;42:1687–1713.
18. Mehra MR, Kobashigawa J, Starling R, Russell S, Uber PA, Parameshwar J, Mohacsi P, Augustine S, Aaronson K, Barr M. Listing criteria for heart transplantation: International Society for Heart and Lung Transplantation guidelines for the care of cardiac transplant candidates–2006. *J Heart Lung Transplant*. 2006;25:1024–1042.
19. Maron MS, Olivotto I, Zenovich AG, Link MS, Pandian NG, Kuvin JT, Nistri S, Cecchi F, Udelson JE, Maron BJ. Hypertrophic cardiomyopathy is predominantly a disease of left ventricular outflow tract obstruction. *Circulation*. 2006;114:2232–2239.
20. Nagueh SF, Appleton CP, Gillebert TC, Marino PN, Oh JK, Smiseth OA, Waggoner AD, Flachskampf FA, Pellikka PA, Evangelista A. Recommendations for the evaluation of left ventricular diastolic function by echocardiography. *J Am Soc Echocardiogr*. 2009;22:107–133.
21. Muthiah K, Phan J, Robson D, Macdonald PS, Keogh AM, Kotlyar E, Granger E, Dhital K, Spratt P, Jansz P, Hayward CS. Centrifugal continuous-flow left ventricular assist device in patients with hypertrophic cardiomyopathy: a case series. *ASAIO J*. 2013;59:183–187.
22. Olivotto I, Maron BJ, Appelbaum E, Harrigan CJ, Salton C, Gibson CM, Udelson JE, O'Donnell C, Lesser JR, Manning WJ, Maron MS. Spectrum and clinical significance of systolic function and myocardial fibrosis assessed by cardiovascular magnetic resonance in hypertrophic cardiomyopathy. *Am J Cardiol*. 2010;106:261–267.
23. Coutu M, Perrault LP, White M, Pelletier GB, Racine N, Poirier NC, Carrier M. Cardiac transplantation for hypertrophic cardiomyopathy: a valid therapeutic option. *J Heart Lung Transplant*. 2004;23:413–417.
24. Gajarski R, Naftel DC, Pahl E, Alejos J, Pearce FB, Kirklin JK, Zamberlan M, Dipchand AI; Pediatric Heart Transplant Study Investigators. Outcomes of pediatric patients with hypertrophic cardiomyopathy listed for transplant. *J Heart Lung Transplant*. 2009;28:1329–1334.
25. Maron MS, Kalsmith BM, Udelson JE, Li W, DeNofrio D. Survival after cardiac transplantation in patients with hypertrophic cardiomyopathy. *Circ Heart Fail*. 2010;3:574–579.
26. Warren SE, Cohn LH, Schoen FJ, Mudge GH, Lorell BH. Advanced diatolic heart failure in familial hypertrophic cardiomyopathy managed with cardiac transplant. *J Appl Cardiol* 1988;3:415–422.
27. Roberts WC, Roberts CC, Ko JM, Grayburn PA, Tandon A, Kuiper JJ, Capehart JE, Hall SA. Dramatically different phenotypic expressions of hypertrophic cardiomyopathy in male cousins undergoing cardiac transplantation with identical disease-causing gene mutation. *Am J Cardiol*. 2013;111:1818–1822.
28. Rowin EJ, Maron MS. The ever expanding spectrum of phenotypic diversity in hypertrophic cardiomyopathy. *Am J Cardiol*. 2013;112:463–464.
29. Landstrom AP, Ackerman MJ. Mutation type is not clinically useful in predicting prognosis in hypertrophic cardiomyopathy. *Circulation*. 2010;122:2441–2449; discussion 2450.

30. Maron BJ, Maron MS, Semsarian C. Genetics of hypertrophic cardiomyopathy after 20 years: clinical perspectives. *J Am Coll Cardiol.* 2012;60:705–715.
31. Garcia-Pavia P, Vázquez ME, Segovia J, Salas C, Avellana P, Gómez-Bueno M, Vilches C, Gallardo ME, Garesse R, Molano J, Bornstein B, Alonso-Pulpon L. Genetic basis of end-stage hypertrophic cardiomyopathy. *Eur J Heart Fail.* 2011;13:1193–1201.
32. Yu EH, Omran AS, Wigle ED, Williams WG, Siu SC, Rakowski H. Mitral regurgitation in hypertrophic obstructive cardiomyopathy: relationship to obstruction and relief with myectomy. *J Am Coll Cardiol.* 2000;36:2219–2225.
33. Sorajja P, Ommen SR, Nishimura RA, Gersh BJ, Berger PB, Tajik AJ. Adverse prognosis of patients with hypertrophic cardiomyopathy who have epicardial coronary artery disease. *Circulation.* 2003;108:2342–2348.
34. Biagini E, Spirito P, Rocchi G, Ferlito M, Rosmini S, Lai F, Lorenzini M, Terzi F, Bacchi-Reggiani L, Boriani G, Branzi A, Boni L, Rapezzi C. Prognostic implications of the Doppler restrictive filling pattern in hypertrophic cardiomyopathy. *Am J Cardiol.* 2009;104:1727–1731.
35. Maron BJ, Rastegar H, Udelson JE, Dearani JA, Maron MS. Contemporary surgical management of hypertrophic cardiomyopathy, the need for more myectomy surgeons and disease-specific centers, and the Tufts initiative. *Am J Cardiol.* 2013;112:1512–1515.

CLINICAL PERSPECTIVE

Heart transplantation in hypertrophic cardiomyopathy (HCM) has traditionally been reserved for patients in the end-stage phase of this disease, arbitrarily defined by ejection fraction <50%. However, a novel subset of nonobstructive HCM patients become candidates for heart transplantation with severe, unrelenting heart failure symptoms refractory to pharmacological treatment, despite evidence of preserved left ventricular systolic function (ejection fraction ≥50%). We describe the clinical profile and natural history of this under-recognized patient subset within the broad disease spectrum of HCM, by assembling 20 such patients (1% of the general HCM cohort). We found no relevant clinical or imaging marker that adequately predicted risk for advanced heart failure with unrelenting symptoms in these patients, given their typical features indistinguishable from the general HCM population: left ventricular wall thickness 22±4 mm, left ventricular cavity nondilated (39±7 mm), and no or minimal fibrosis (≤5% of left ventricular mass by cardiovascular magnetic resonance) in the majority of patients. Additionally, 10% of patients were considered for transplant even in the absence of other traditional transplant parameters, including peak Vo_2>14 mL/kg/min, because transplant was the only therapeutic option with the capacity to restore an acceptable quality of life. These findings underscore the need for clinicians familiar with HCM to participate closely with multidisciplinary heart failure teams to ensure that optimal treatment strategies are implemented in this unique subset of HCM patients, including, when appropriate, heart transplantation.

Surviving Malignant Hypertrophic Cardiomyopathy With all Major Complications in a Single Patient

Barry J. Maron, MD[a,*], Henry L. Weiner, MD[b], Martin S. Maron, MD[c], and William C. Roberts, MD[d]

The natural history and clinical course of hypertrophic cardiomyopathy (HC) is diverse, ranging from benign forms compatible with normal or extended longevity to adverse consequences requiring major interventions: surgical myectomy (or selectively alcohol septal ablation) for left ventricular (LV) outflow obstruction producing progressive heart failure; defibrillation and therapeutic hypothermia for cardiac arrest; implantable cardioverter-defibrillators (ICD) for prevention of sudden death; and heart transplant for refractory progressive heart failure in the absence of obstruction.[1,2] Patients with HC may have their clinical course importantly influenced by either of these 3 major disease complications,[1,2] but the occurrence of all 3 sequentially in a single patient over a 38 year period represents a notable and unusually aggressive form of HC. We present such a patient, prospectively followed and evaluated, who not only has incurred all major adverse consequences of HC but most importantly has survived due to effective treatment modalities available to patients with this disease.

Case Description

This patient was initially diagnosed with obstructive HC after a precordial murmur was detected at age 3 (Figure 1). Her father had experienced a resuscitated cardiac arrest from HC and one brother (age 40) has HC with an uneventful course. Surgical myectomy was performed at age 11 years to relieve outflow tract obstruction (gradient, 100 mm Hg) and heart failure symptoms, associated with massive ventricular septal hypertrophy (wall thickness, 35 mm). Symptomatic improvement ensued briefly, but at age 19, the patient was successfully resuscitated from an out-of-hospital cardiac arrest, and a secondary prevention implantable cardioverter-defibrillator (ICD) was placed and subsequently replaced at ages 24, 27 (with biventricular pacing), and 33 years. A lead extraction at age 26 was complicated by a tear in the superior vena cavae which was repaired surgically.

Appropriate ICD interventions for sustained ventricular tachycardia (VT) or ventricular fibrillation (VF) occurred at ages 25 (during tennis), 26, and 32 (sitting at beach) and 34 years. In addition, 25 episodes of monomorphic VT terminated by anti-tachycardia pacing were tabulated, as well as hundreds of spontaneously aborted runs of nonsustained VT evident on ICD interrogation.

At age 26, the patient developed progressive heart failure in NYHA class III associated with adverse LV remodeling: maximum LV wall thickness = 11 mm; LV end-diastolic cavity dimension = 56 mm, and ejection fraction = 20%. Advanced heart failure symptoms persisted for the next 12 years refractory to a variety of pharmacologic agents, including beta-blockers, verapamil, angiotensin-converting enzyme inhibitors, sotalol, mexiletine, digoxin and spironolactone. Despite her significant functional limitation, the patient held sedentary jobs and performed treadmill exercise and yoga.

During this time period, LV remodeling progressed with cavity dimension increasing to 68 mm, and ejection fraction decreasing to only 15%. Peak oxygen consumption ranged from 19 to 21 ml/kg/min; cardiac index was 2.1 L/min/m^2; pulmonary capillary wedge pressure was 18 mm Hg, and brain natriuretic peptide was 3500 pg/ml. At age 38, the patient consented to heart transplant listing, and the operation was performed at Hospital of University of Pennsylvania. Postoperative recovery has been uneventful. Genetic testing documented a pathogenic mutation in the MYBPC3 gene (c. 2441_2443 delAGA).

The explanted heart weighed 440 g. Ventricular septum was 14 mm in thickness, and the LV free wall was 16 mm (Figure 2). The LV cavity was markedly dilated, but the right ventricle was normal-sized. Extensive areas of grossly visible scarring were present involving the ventricular septum and LV free wall. The mural endocardium of ventricular septum in apposition to the anterior mitral leaflet was severely thickened by fibrous tissue, extending distally and resulting (at least in part) from the myectomy performed 27 years earlier. The LV wall at the apex was thinned, aneurysmal, and fibrotic. The epicardial coronary arteries were free of atherosclerotic plaque, and the right and left main coronary arteries arose from the aorta in normal position.

Extensive scarring of the LV wall was confirmed histologically. In addition, many myocytes in the subendocardial regions were vacuolated and enlarged. Disorganized patterns of myocyte arrangement were present in ventricular septum, associated with numerous intramural coronary arteries, increased in size with thickened walls and luminal narrowing (Figure 3), both histopathologic hallmarks of HC.

Comments

The patient presented here illustrates the most extreme example of HC and its deleterious consequences through the first 38 years of life, but nevertheless represents an important principle for this complex genetic disease. Once regarded as a disease with uniformly grim prognosis largely without effective management strategies,[2] this patient underscores the new paradigm in which HC has become

[a]Hypertrophic Cardiomyopathy Center, Minneapolis Heart Institute Foundation, Minneapolis, Minnesota; [b]Care Cardiology Consultants, Newark, New Jersey; [c]Hypertrophic Cardiomyopathy Center, Tufts Medical Center, Boston, Massachusetts; and [d]Baylor University Medical Center, Dallas, Texas. Manuscript received October 29, 2014; revised manuscript received and accepted November 3, 2014.

See page 404 for disclosure information.

*Corresponding author: Tel: +612-863-3996; fax: +612-863-3875.
E-mail address: hcm.maron@mhif.org (B.J. Maron).

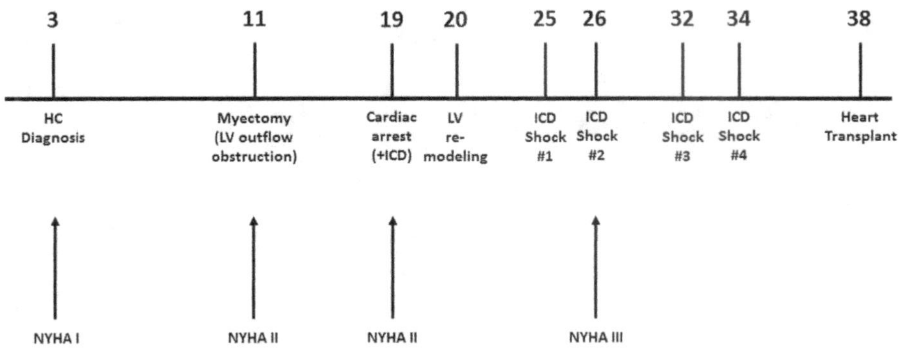

Figure 1. Time-line of cardiac events in our 38-year-old patient. The numbers at the top represent the ages when the events occurred. HC = hypertrophic cardiomyopathy; ICD = intracardiac defibrillator; LV = left ventricular; NYHA = New York Heart Association.

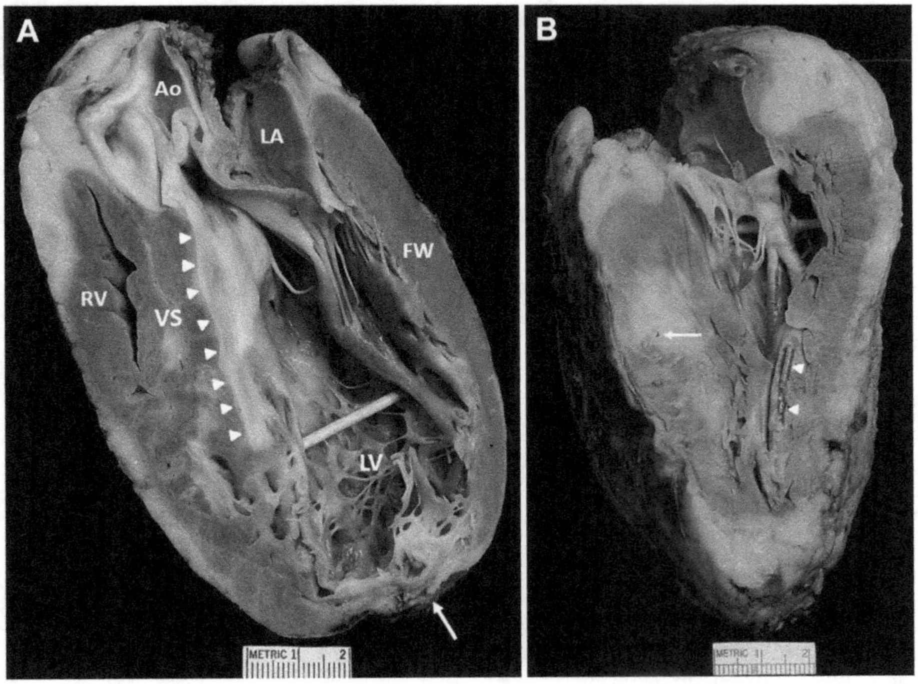

Figure 2. Parasagittal views of the heart from the left side *(A)* and from the right side *(B)*. *(A)* The left ventricle (LV) is greatly dilated, ventricular septum (VS) is focally scarred, and the apex (*white arrow*) is severely scarred, and with pressure would bulge externally (i.e., aneurysmal). The *white arrowheads* point to the mural endocardium of the septum, which is quite thickened by fibrous tissue and represents the extent of the ventricular septal myectomy performed during childhood (at age 11). The left atrium (LA) does not appear to be dilated. *(B)* View from the right side. The wall to the left represents ventricular septum which contains a large scar within which there is a large intramural coronary artery (*arrow*). Defibrillator lead is embedded in white fibrous tissue, extending from the apex into the tricuspid valve orifice (*arrowheads*). Ao = aorta; FW = free wall of left ventricle; RV = right ventricle.

a treatable cardiac disease,[3] with management options now available to target each adverse complication and prolong life, that is, surgical septal myectomy (or alcohol ablation) for limiting symptoms caused by LV outflow obstruction;[1,4,5] external defibrillation for cardiac arrest, often with therapeutic hypothermia;[6] ICD therapy to terminate potentially lethal ventricular tachyarrhythmias (VT/VF) and prevent sudden death;[7] and ultimately heart transplant only in the event that progressive end-stage heart failure intervenes associated with extreme LV remodeling (and in the absence of outflow obstruction).[8,9]

Implementation of these interventions permits most HC patients to achieve extended longevity with good quality of life, and for the present patient the prolongation of life.[1] Notably, this patient endured NYHA class III heart failure symptoms and limitations for at least 12 years before consenting to heart transplantation. Finally, despite the fact that atrial fibrillation is common in HC (in about 20% of patients), and is also linked to end-stage heart failure, our patient showed no evidence of left atrial dilatation (or atrial fibrillation).[1]

Typical of the HC end-stage there was substantial LV remodeling with striking regression from massive hypertrophy (in childhood) to virtually normal wall thickness, associated with LV chamber dilatation. The basis for the LV wall thinning was the development of extensive, diffuse and transmural myocardial scarring, presumably resulting from microvascular ischemia, and also involving the most distal LV segment where early aneurysm formation is evident.[10]

Two additional issues related to the natural history of HC are underscored by the findings in this informative patient.

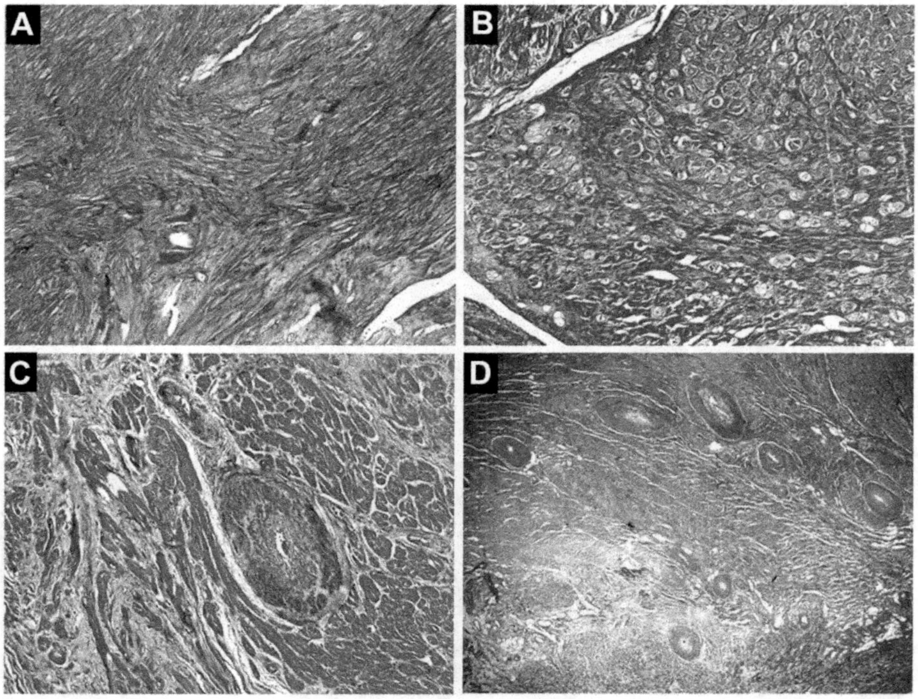

Figure 3. Histologic sections of portions of the ventricular septum *(A, C, D)* and left ventricular papillary muscle *(B)*, all stained with Masson's trichrome. *(A)* Disordered arrangement of myocytes interwoven with scar tissue (*blue*) (x20). *(B)* Large scar in the anterolateral papillary muscle; myofibers are enlarged (x20). *(C)* High power view of a single large and narrowed intramural coronary artery (x40). *(D)* Multiple large and narrowed intramural coronary arteries (*arrows*) embedded within a large scar in ventricular septum (x20).

First, the characteristic heterogeneity of disease expression and clinical course is evident in the diverse disease pathways taken by our patient's malignant course in comparison to that of her asymptomatic 40-year-old brother, with HC and the same pathogenic mutation and genetic substrate. Second, the mutation in the sarcomere MYBPC3 gene responsible for HC in our patient with highly aggressive HC has been previously regarded as benign.[11] Therefore, this patient's clinical profile is consistent with the principle that specific mutations cannot predict future outcome in individual HC patients.[11]

Disclosures

The authors have no conflicts of interest to disclose.

1. Maron BJ, Ommen SR, Semsarian C, Spirito P, Olivotto I, Maron MS. Hypertrophic cardiomyopathy: present and future, with translation into contemporary cardiovascular medicine. *J Am Coll Cardiol* 2014;64: 83–99.
2. Maron BJ, Braunwald E. Evolution of hypertrophic cardiomyopathy to a contemporary treatable disease. *Circulation* 2012;126:1640–1644.
3. Maron BJ. Recognition of hypertrophic cardiomyopathy as a contemporary, relatively common and treatable disease: International Summit V. *Am J Cardiol* 2014;113:739–744.
4. Ommen SR, Maron BJ, Olivotto I, Maron MS, Cecchi F, Betocchi S, Gersh BJ, Ackerman MJ, McCully RB, Dearani JA, Schaff HV, Danielson GK, Tajik AJ, Nishimura RA. Long-term effects of surgical septal myectomy on survival in patients with obstructive hypertrophic cardiomyopathy. *J Am Coll Cardiol* 2005;46:470–476.
5. Maron MS, Olivotto I, Betocchi S, Casey SA, Lesser JR, Losi MA, Cecchi F, Maron BJ. Effect of left ventricular outflow tract obstruction on clinical outcome in hypertrophic cardiomyopathy. *N Engl J Med* 2003;348:295–303.
6. Maron BJ, Maron MS, Maron BA, Haas TS, Altman RK, Smalley SJ, Doerer JJ, Link MS, Mooney MR. Successful therapeutic hypothermia in patients with hypertrophic cardiomyopathy. *J Am Coll Cardiol* 2011;57:2454–2456.
7. Maron BJ, Spirito P, Shen WK, Haas TS, Formisano F, Link MS, Epstein AE, Almquist AK, Daubert JP, Lawrenz T, Boriani G, Estes NA 3rd, Favale S, Piccininno M, Winters SL, Santini M, Betocchi S, Arribas F, Sherrid MV, Buja G, Semsarian C, Bruzzi P. Implantable cardioverter-defibrillators and prevention of sudden cardiac death in hypertrophic cardiomyopathy. *JAMA* 2007;298:405–412.
8. Harris KM, Spirito P, Maron MS, Zenovich AG, Formisano F, Lesser JR, Mackey-Bojack S, Manning WJ, Udelson JE, Maron BJ. Prevalence, clinical profile and significance of left ventricular remodeling in the end-stage phase of hypertrophic cardiomyopathy. *Circulation* 2006;114:216–225.
9. Rowin EJ, Maron BJ, Kiernan MS, Casey SA, Feldman DS, Hryniewicz KM, Chan RHM, Harris KM, Udelson JE, DeNofrio D, Roberts WC, Maron MS. Advanced heart failure with preserved systolic function in nonobstructive hypertrophic cardiomyopathy: under-recognized subset of candidates for heart transplant. *Circ Heart Fail* 2014;7:967–975.
10. Maron MS, Finley JJ, Bos JM, Hauser TH, Manning WJ, Haas TS, Lesser JR, Udelson JE, Ackerman MJ, Maron BJ. Prevalence, clinical significance, and natural history of left ventricular apical aneurysms in hypertrophic cardiomyopathy. *Circulation* 2008;118:1541–1549.
11. Maron BJ, Maron MS, Semsarian C. Genetics of hypertrophic cardiomyopathy after 20 years: Clinical perspectives. (State-of-the-art). *J Am Coll Cardiol* 2012;60:705–715.

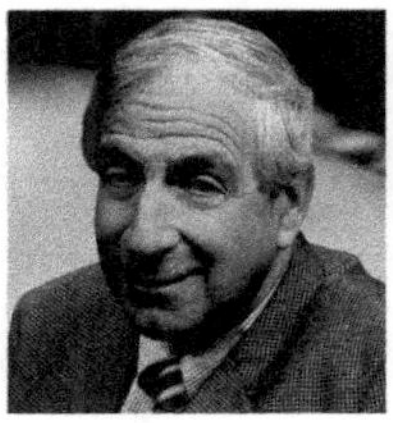
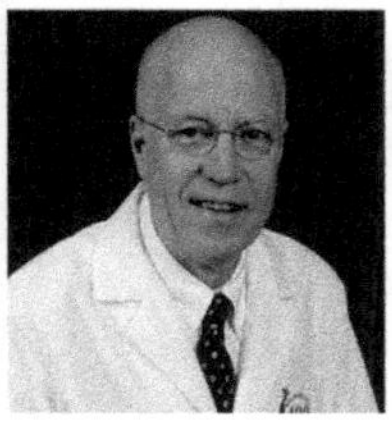

The Father of Septal Myectomy for Obstructive HCM, Who Also Had HCM

The Unbelievable Story

Barry J. Maron, MD,[a] William C. Roberts, MD[b]

Andrew Glenn Morrow, MD, was Chief of the Clinic of Surgery at the National Institutes of Health (NIH), Bethesda, Maryland, from 1953 until his death in 1982 (**Figure 1**). During that time, he established an international training program for future cardiac surgeons, and among many other accomplishments, the ventricular septal myectomy operation for obstructive hypertrophic cardiomyopathy (HCM) (1,2).

He was the first surgeon to perform the myectomy operation to relieve left ventricular (LV) outflow obstruction in patients experiencing inadequate symptom response to medical treatment, a procedure which he designed, which he performed on 299 patients, and which bears his name (1,2). A small amount of muscle is resected from the basal septum to widen the LV outflow tract (3) and abolish systolic anterior motion of the mitral valve, the mechanism responsible for subaortic obstruction. Dr. Morrow also was first to report obstruction as due to muscular hypertrophy sufficient to impede LV outflow (4).

The Morrow operation (now modified by extended muscular resection) was introduced in the early 1960s at the NIH and quickly spread to major institutions in the United States, including Mayo Clinic, and internationally (5-7). Now, >50 years later, surgical myectomy continues to benefit thousands of patients with HCM, resulting in reversal of heart failure symptoms and restoration of normal daily activity in almost 90% (5,8-12), as well as enhanced survival consistent with the general population (5). In guidelines (10) and consensus recommendations (11), myectomy remains the primary treatment option for most patients with severe drug-refractory heart failure symptoms, becoming the safest open heart procedure when performed in experienced centers (mortality, 0.3%) (6).

FIGURE 1 **Andrew Glenn Morrow, 1963**

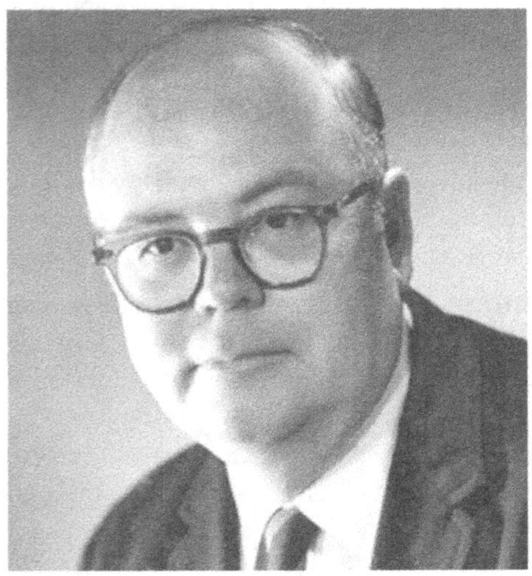

From the [a]Hypertrophic Cardiomyopathy Institute, Division of Cardiology, Tufts Medical Center, Boston, Massachusetts (formerly at Minneapolis Heart Institute Foundation, Hypertrophic Cardiomyopathy Center, Minneapolis, Minnesota); and the [b]Baylor Heart and Vascular Institute, Dallas, Texas. Both authors have reported that they have no relationships relevant to the contents of this paper to disclose.

HCM AND GLENN MORROW'S ILLNESS

It is not widely known that Dr. Morrow himself had HCM, with this diagnosis substantiated by an aggressive form of the disease identified in 2 of his children (**Figure 2**). Dr. Eugene Braunwald, Chief of Cardiology, was a close friend and colleague of Dr. Morrow. While collaborating at the NIH on the first major clinical description of HCM (13), Dr. Morrow asked Dr. Braunwald: "Gene, would you examine my heart?" (14). Solely by precordial auscultation, and recognizing the classic finding of a systolic ejection murmur due to LV outflow obstruction, Dr. Braunwald made the diagnosis of obstructive HCM at age 40 years (called "IHSS" at that time) (13,14). This diagnosis was impressive for several reasons: 1) it occurred in 1961, in the pre-echocardiographic era; and 2) it was made with auscultation when diagnostic criteria for this complex disease were just being formulated. Dr. Morrow was probably the 25th clinically identified HCM patient (13,14).

Dr. Morrow experienced exertional dyspnea and near-syncope almost daily in the morning, multiple episodes of syncope, atrial fibrillation, and ultimately, embolic stroke. He refused beta-blocker therapy, cardiac catheterization, and consideration for septal myectomy. Dr. Morrow died suddenly at only 60 years of age in his home. His heart was recovered by Dr. William Roberts with the permission of Dr. Morrow's wife. At autopsy, cardiac morphologic findings were typical of HCM with asymmetric septal hypertrophy, myocyte disarray, myocardial scarring, and structural microvascular abnormalities (**Figure 3**).

FIGURE 2 Morrow Family Pedigree

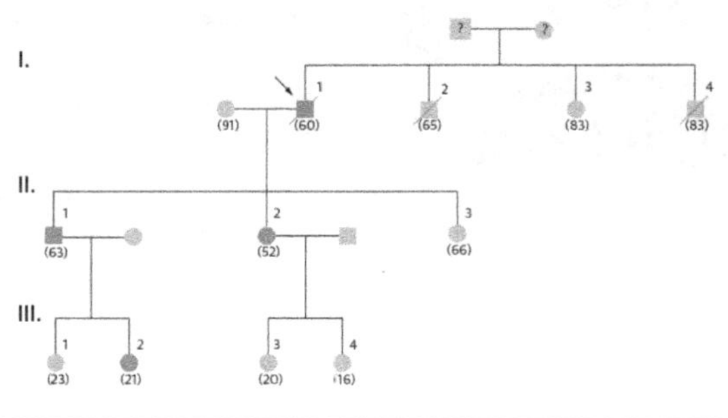

Squares indicate men; **circles** indicate women; **arrow** indicates proband (Dr. Morrow, I.1.); **solid symbols** indicate hypertrophic cardiomyopathy; and **slash** indicates deceased.

THE MORROW FAMILY DISEASE

The Morrows were married for 37 years and had 3 children, including 2 with an unusually aggressive form of HCM.

DAUGHTER. One child is a 52-year-old woman who was diagnosed with HCM at age 21 with a heart murmur due to mitral valve systolic anterior motion and ventricular septal hypertrophy (**Figures 2 and 4**). For many years, she experienced symptoms of heart failure and limited physical activity, refractory to pharmacological agents, chronic dual-chamber pacing (15), and also radiofrequency ablations that were unsuccessful in reducing symptomatic episodes of atrial fibrillation.

Although initially with a subaortic gradient of 70 mm Hg, she evolved to a nonobstructive state with end-stage heart failure (New York Heart Association functional class III to IV), associated with both preserved LV hypertrophy and systolic function (ejection fraction, 67%) (15), nondilated LV, and biatrial enlargement, characteristic of a novel subgroup of transplant candidates (16). She underwent successful heart transplant at age 51 years, and has been genotyped to a pathogenic beta-myosin heavy chain mutation (MYH7) (DNA coding c.485A>G; variant pTyr162Cys [y162c]).

SON. Another of Dr. Morrow's children is a 63-year-old man who has obstructive HCM (septal thickness, 21 mm) (**Figure 2**). For many years, he has been encumbered by recurrent episodes of syncope, symptomatic atrial fibrillation (left atrium, 48 mm)

FIGURE 3 The Heart of Dr. Morrow

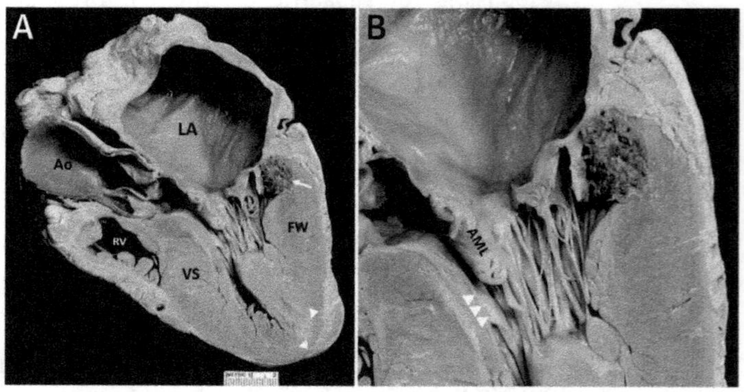

Weight, 645 g. **(A)** The ascending aorta (Ao) is free of atherosclerotic plaque, with a structurally normal aortic valve, nondilated left ventricular (LV) cavity, and greatly dilated left atrium (LA). Ventricular septal (VS) thickness is 20 mm, asymmetrically hypertrophied with respect to LV free wall (FW). Behind posterior mitral leaflet is a large calcific deposit **(arrow)**, frequent in older patients. Several small scars are evident in the VS and at the apex **(arrowheads)**. **(B)** In the subaortic region of the hypertrophied septum is a fibrous plaque **(arrowheads)** in apposition to the thickened anterior mitral leaflet (AML), evidence of prior outflow obstruction. RV = right ventricle.

FIGURE 4 The Explanted Heart of Daughter

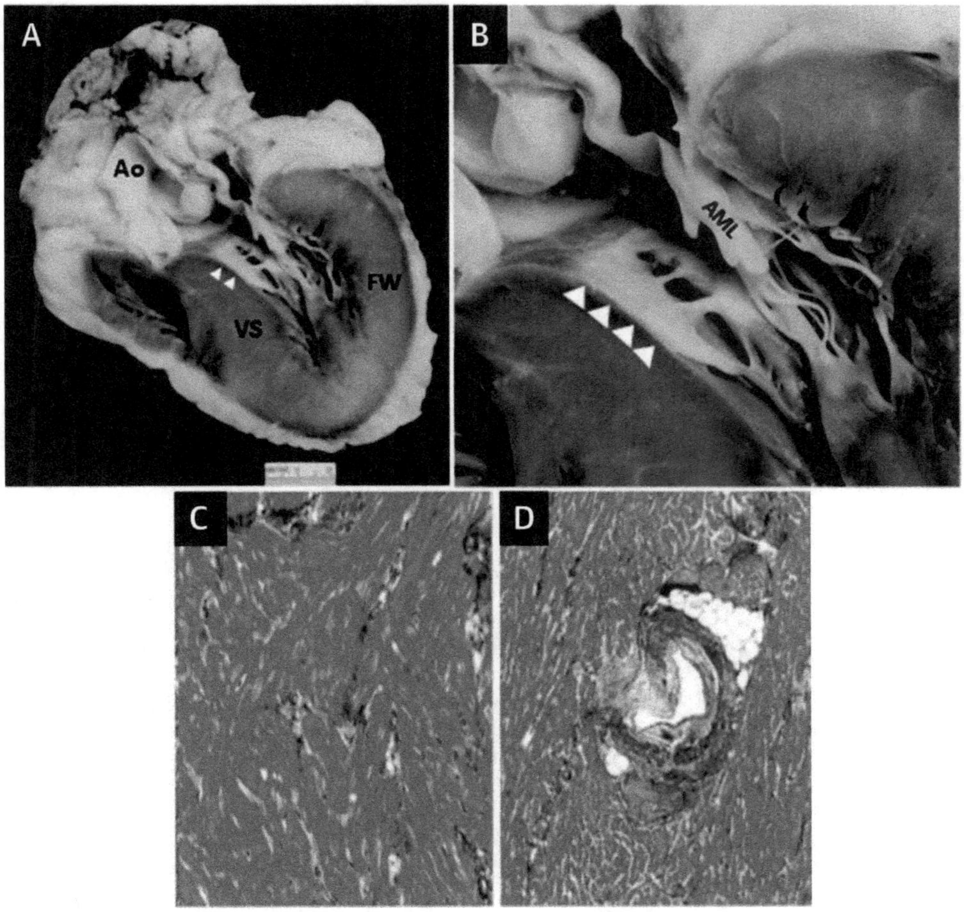

Weight 510 g. **(A)** The VS thickness is 23 mm, asymmetrically hypertrophied with respect to LV FW, and with a nondilated LV cavity. **(B)** Septal endocardial fibrous plaque **(white arrowheads)** adjacent to the thickened AML, and prior evidence of mitral valve systolic anterior motion and obstruction. **(C)** Typical disorganized myocyte arrangement in septum, and areas of interstitial fibrosis **(blue)**; myocardial scarring was absent (×400). **(D)** Intramural coronary artery with disrupted media and intimal fibrous thickening (×100). Masson trichrome stain. Abbreviations as in Figure 3.

requiring cardioversion, and 1 transient ischemic attack. At age 57 years, he developed severe progressive heart failure due to LV outflow obstruction (gradient, 55 mm Hg). He underwent successful surgical septal myectomy with symptomatic relief, remarkably with the same operation his father had developed and promoted 5 decades earlier (1,2). His 21-year-old daughter has HCM, completing a 3-generation disease transmission.

PERSPECTIVES

The saga of Dr. Glenn Morrow, HCM, and the Morrow family is of unique interest to cardiovascular medicine, and also one which has been largely unknown. It is reported here to complete the historical record. As Dr. Braunwald reflected (14), should this scenario have been encountered on television or in the movies, it would be considered impossible or ridiculous, that is, one colleague diagnosing the other while they are both collaborating on the description of the same new disease, which was then considered extraordinarily rare.

In addition, several important facets of HCM are underscored here, that is, an autosomal dominant disease with great heterogeneity in expression, the importance of atrial fibrillation, and contemporary management considerations (17). The particularly aggressive clinical variants reported here in Dr. Morrow and his offspring are considered somewhat unusual within the broad HCM disease spectrum, most often associated with normal life expectancy without major disability (12,17). Indeed, all 3 individuals were affected by a progressive disease course involving repetitive atrial fibrillation (with thromboembolism in the father), recurrent syncope (both males), heart transplant (the daughter), and subaortic obstruction causing severe heart failure symptoms in the son and reversed by the very operation designed by and named for his father.

REPRINT REQUESTS AND CORRESPONDENCE: Dr. Barry J. Maron, HCM Institute, Division of Cardiology, Tufts Medical Center, 800 Washington Street #70, Boston, Massachusetts 02111. E-mail: barrymaron1@gmail.com.

REFERENCES

1. Morrow AG, Lambrew CT, Braunwald E. Idiopathic hypertrophic subaortic stenosis. II. Operative treatment and the results of pre- and postoperative hemodynamic evaluations. Circulation 1964;30 Suppl 4:120-51.

2. Morrow AG, Reitz BA, Epstein SE, et al. Operative treatment in hypertrophic subaortic stenosis. Techniques, and the results of pre and postoperative assessments in 83 patients. Circulation 1975;52:88-102.

3. Spirito P, Maron BJ, Rosing DR. Morphologic determinants of hemodynamic state after ventricular septal myotomy-myectomy in patients with obstructive hypertrophic cardiomyopathy: M mode and two-dimensional echocardiographic assessment. Circulation 1984;70:984-5.

4. Morrow AG, Braunwald E. Functional aortic stenosis; a malformation characterized by resistance to left ventricular outflow without anatomic obstruction. Circulation 1959;20:181-9.

5. Ommen SR, Maron BJ, Olivotto I, et al. Long-term effects of surgical septal myectomy on survival in patients with obstructive hypertrophic cardiomyopathy. J Am Coll Cardiol 2005;46:470-6.

6. Maron BJ, Dearani JA, Ommen SR, et al. Low operative mortality achieved with surgical septal myectomy: role of dedicated hypertrophic cardiomyopathy centers in the management of dynamic subaortic obstruction. J Am Coll Cardiol 2015;66:1307-8.

7. Dearani JA. Septal myectomy remains the gold standard. Eur Heart J 2012;33:1999-2000.

8. Woo A, Williams WG, Choi R, et al. Clinical and echocardiographic determinants of long-term survival after surgical myectomy in obstructive hypertrophic cardiomyopathy. Circulation 2005;111:2033-41.

9. Smedira NG, Lytle BW, Lever HM, et al. Current effectiveness and risks of isolated septal myectomy for hypertrophic obstructive cardiomyopathy. Ann Thorac Surg 2008;85:127-33.

10. Gersh BJ, Maron BJ, Bonow RO, et al. 2011 ACC/AHA guideline for the diagnosis and treatment of hypertrophic cardiomyopathy: American College of Cardiology Foundation/American Heart Association task force on practice guidelines. J Am Coll Cardiol 2016;58:2703-38.

11. Maron BJ, McKenna WJ, Danielson GK, et al. American College of Cardiology/European Society of Cardiology clinical expert consensus document on hypertrophic cardiomyopathy. J Am Coll Cardiol 2003;42:1687-713.

12. Maron BJ, Ommen SR, Semsarian C, et al. Hypertrophic cardiomyopathy: present and future, with translation into contemporary cardiovascular medicine. J Am Coll Cardiol 2014;64:83-99.

13. Braunwald E, Lambrew CT, Rockoff SD, et al. Idiopathic hypertrophic subaortic stenosis. 1. A description of the disease based upon an analysis of 64 patients. Circulation 1964;30 Suppl 4:3-119.

14. Maron BJ, Braunwald E. Eugene Braunwald, MD and the early years of hypertrophic cardiomyopathy: a conversation with Dr. Barry J. Maron. Am J Cardiol 2012;109:1539-47.

15. Maron BJ, Josephson ME. Long-term consequences of the right ventricular pacing mania of the 1990s for obstructive hypertrophic cardiomyopathy. Am J Cardiol 2014;113:191-2.

16. Rowin EJ, Maron BJ, Kiernan MS, et al. Advanced heart failure with preserved systolic function in nonobstructive hypertrophic cardiomyopathy: under-recognized subset of candidates for heart transplant. Circ Heart Fail 2014;7:967-75.

17. Maron BJ, Rowin EJ, Casey SA, Maron MS. How hypertrophic cardiomyopathy became a contemporary treatable genetic disease with low mortality: shaped by 50 years of clinical research and practice. JAMA Cardiol 2016 Mar 2 [E-pub ahead of print].

www.ingramcontent.com/pod-product-compliance
Lightning Source LLC
LaVergne TN
LVHW062135200926
848484LV00007B/1816